# Dictionary of

# Medical Terms

*Specialist dictionaries*:

| | |
|---|---|
| Dictionary of Accounting | 0 7475 6991 6 |
| Dictionary of Aviation | 0 7475 7219 4 |
| Dictionary of Banking and Finance | 0 7475 6685 2 |
| Dictionary of Business | 0 7475 6980 0 |
| Dictionary of Computing | 0 7475 6622 4 |
| Dictionary of Economics | 0 7475 6632 1 |
| Dictionary of Environment and Ecology | 0 7475 7201 1 |
| Dictionary of Human Resources and Personnel Management | 0 7475 6623 2 |
| Dictionary of ICT | 0 7475 6990 8 |
| Dictionary of Law | 0 7475 6636 4 |
| Dictionary of Leisure, Travel and Tourism | 0 7475 7222 4 |
| Dictionary of Marketing | 0 7475 6621 6 |
| Dictionary of Military Terms | 0 7475 7477 4 |
| Dictionary of Nursing | 0 7475 6634 8 |
| Dictionary of Politics and Government | 0 7475 7220 8 |
| Dictionary of Science and Technology | 0 7475 6620 8 |

*Easier English™ titles*:

| | |
|---|---|
| Easier English Basic Dictionary | 0 7475 6644 5 |
| Easier English Basic Synonyms | 0 7475 6979 7 |
| Easier English Dictionary: Handy Pocket Edition | 0 7475 6625 9 |
| Easier English Intermediate Dictionary | 0 7475 6989 4 |
| Easier English Student Dictionary | 0 7475 6624 0 |
| English Thesaurus for Students | 1 9016 5931 3 |

*Check Your English Vocabulary workbooks*:

| | |
|---|---|
| Academic English | 0 7475 6691 7 |
| Business | 0 7475 6626 7 |
| Computing | 1 9016 5928 3 |
| Human Resources | 0 7475 6997 5 |
| Law | 1 9016 5921 6 |
| Leisure, Travel and Tourism | 0 7475 6996 7 |
| FCE + | 0 7475 6981 9 |
| IELTS | 0 7136 7604 3 |
| PET | 0 7475 6627 5 |
| TOEFL® | 0 7475 6984 3 |

Visit our website for full details of all our books: **www.acblack.com**

# Dictionary of
# Medical Terms

fourth edition

A & C Black • London

**www.acblack.com**

While every effort has been made to be as accurate as possible, the author, advisers, editors and publishers of this book cannot be held liable for any errors and omissions, or actions that may be taken as a consequence of using it.

First published in Great Britain in1987
as *English Medical Dictionary*

Second edition published 1993
Third edition published 2000
Fourth edition published 2004
Reprinted 2005

A & C Black Publishers Ltd
37 Soho Square, London W1D 3QZ

© P. H. Collin 1987, 1993, 2000
© Bloomsbury Publishing Plc 2004
© A & C Black Publishers Ltd 2005

A CIP record for this book is available from the British Library

ISBN 0 7136 7603 5

*Text Production and Proofreading*
Ruth Hillmore, Daisy Jackson, Sarah Lusznat, Katy McAdam, Charlotte Regan

A & C Black uses paper produced with elemental chlorine-free pulp, harvested from managed sustainable forests.

Text computer typeset by A & C Black
Printed in Italy by Legoprint

# Preface

This dictionary provides the user with the basic vocabulary currently being used in a wide range of healthcare situations. The areas covered include the technical language used in diagnosis, patient care, surgery, pathology, general practice, pharmacy, dentistry and other specialisations, as well as anatomical and physiological terms. Informal, everyday and sometimes euphemistic terms commonly used by people in discussing their condition with healthcare professionals are also included, as are common words used in reading or writing reports, articles or guidelines.

The dictionary is designed for anyone who needs to check the meaning or pronunciation of medical terms, but especially for those working in health-related areas who may not be healthcare professionals or for whom English is an additional language. Each headword is explained in clear, straightforward English. Pronunciations, uncommon plurals and uncommon verb forms are provided. Illustrations of some basic anatomical terms are also included.

Very many people have helped or advised on the compilation and checking of the dictionary in its various editions. In particular, thanks are due to Dr Judith Harvey for her helpful comments and advice on this fourth edition and to Dr Marie Condon for some revisions and clarification. Also to Lesley Bennun, Lesley Brown and Margaret Baker who copy-edited the text and Dinah Jackson who revised the pronunciations.

# Pronunciation Guide

The following symbols have been used to show the pronunciation of the main words in the dictionary.

Stress is indicated by a main stress mark ( ' ) and a secondary stress mark ( , ). Note that these are only guides, as the stress of the word changes according to its position in the sentence.

| *Vowels* | | *Consonants* | |
|---|---|---|---|
| æ | back | b | buck |
| ɑː | harm | d | dead |
| ɒ | stop | ð | other |
| aɪ | type | dʒ | jump |
| aʊ | how | f | fare |
| aɪə | hire | g | gold |
| aʊə | hour | h | head |
| ɔː | course | j | yellow |
| ɔɪ | annoy | k | cab |
| e | head | l | leave |
| eə | fair | m | mix |
| eɪ | make | n | nil |
| eʊ | go | ŋ | sing |
| ɜː | word | p | print |
| iː | keep | r | rest |
| i | happy | s | save |
| ə | about | ʃ | shop |
| ɪ | fit | t | take |
| ɪə | near | tʃ | change |
| u | annual | θ | theft |
| uː | pool | v | value |
| ʊ | book | w | work |
| ʊə | tour | x | loch |
| ʌ | shut | ʒ | measure |
| | | z | zone |

# A

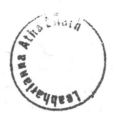

**A** /eɪ/ *noun* a human blood type of the ABO system, containing the A antigen (NOTE: Someone with type A can donate to people of the same group or of the AB group, and can receive blood from people with type A or type O.)

**AA** *abbr* Alcoholics Anonymous

**A & E** /ˌeɪ ənd ˈiː/, **A & E department** /ˌeɪ ənd ˈiː dɪˌpɑːtmənt/ *noun* same as **accident and emergency department**

**A & E medicine** /ˌeɪ ənd ˈiː ˌmed(ə)sɪn/ *noun* the medical procedures used in A & E departments

**AB** /ˌeɪ ˈbiː/ *noun* a human blood type of the ABO system, containing the A and B antigens (NOTE: Someone with type AB can donate to people of the same group and receive blood from people with type O, A, AB or B.)

**ab-** /æb/ *prefix* away from

**ABC** /ˌeɪ biː ˈsiː/ *noun* the basic initial checks of a casualty's condition. Full form **airway, breathing and circulation**

**abdomen** /ˈæbdəmən/ *noun* a space inside the body below the diaphragm, above the pelvis and in front of the spine, containing the stomach, intestines, liver and other vital organs ○ *pain in the abdomen* (NOTE: For other terms referring to the abdomen, see words beginning with **coeli-, coelio-**.)

COMMENT: The abdomen is divided for medical purposes into nine regions: at the top, the right and left hypochondriac regions with the epigastrium between them; in the centre, the right and left lumbar regions with the umbilical between them; and at the bottom, the right and left iliac regions with the hypogastrium between them.

**abdomin-** /æbdɒmɪn/ *prefix* same as **abdomino-** (*used before vowels*)

**abdominal** /æbˈdɒmɪn(ə)l/ *adjective* located in the abdomen, or relating to the abdomen

**abdominal aorta** /æbˌdɒmɪn(ə)l eɪˈɔːtə/ *noun* the part of the aorta which lies between the diaphragm and the point where the aorta divides into the iliac arteries. See illustration at KIDNEY in Supplement

**abdominal cavity** /æbˌdɒmɪn(ə)l ˈkævɪti/ *noun* the space in the body below the chest

**abdominal distension** /æbˌdɒmɪn(ə)l dɪsˈtenʃ(ə)n/ *noun* a condition in which the abdomen is stretched because of gas or fluid

**abdominal pain** /æbˈdɒmɪn(ə)l peɪn/ *noun* pain in the abdomen caused by indigestion or more serious disorders

**abdominal viscera** /æbˌdɒmɪn(ə)l ˈvɪsərə/ *plural noun* the organs which are contained in the abdomen, e.g. the stomach, liver and intestines

**abdominal wall** /æbˈdɒmɪn(ə)l wɔːl/ *noun* muscular tissue which surrounds the abdomen

**abdomino-** /æbdɒmɪnəʊ/ *prefix* referring to the abdomen

**abdominopelvic** /æbˌdɒmɪnəʊˈpelvɪk/ *adjective* referring to the abdomen and pelvis

**abdominoperineal** /æbˌdɒmɪnəʊperɪˈniːəl/ *adjective* referring to the abdomen and perineum

**abdominoperineal excision** /æbˌdɒmɪnəʊperɪˌniːəl ɪkˈsɪʒ(ə)n/ *noun* a surgical operation that involves cutting out tissue in both the abdomen and the perineum

**abdominoposterior** /æbˌdɒmɪnəʊpɒˈstɪəriə/ *adjective* referring to a position of a fetus in the uterus, where the fetus's abdomen is facing the mother's back

**abdominoscopy** /æbˌdɒmɪˈnɒskəpi/ *noun* an internal examination of the abdomen, usually with an endoscope

**abdominothoracic** /æbˌdɒmɪnəʊθɔːˈræsɪk/ *adjective* referring to the abdomen and thorax

**abduce** /æbˈdjuːs/ *verb* same as **abduct**

**abducens nerve** /æbˈdjuːs(ə)nz ˌnɜːv/ *noun* the sixth cranial nerve, which controls the muscle which makes the eyeball turn outwards

**abducent** /æbˈdjuːs(ə)nt/ *adjective* referring to a muscle which brings parts of the body away from each other or moves them away from the central line of the body or a limb. Compare **adducent**

**abducent nerve** /æbˈdjuːsənt ˌnɜːv/ *noun* same as **abducens nerve**

**abduct** /æbˈdʌkt/ *verb* (*of a muscle*) to pull a leg or arm in a direction which is away from the centre line of the body, or to pull a toe or finger away from the central line of a leg or arm. Compare **adduct**

**abduction** /æb'dʌkʃən/ *noun* the movement of a part of the body away from the centre line of the body or away from a neighbouring part. Opposite **adduction**. See illustration at **ANATOMICAL TERMS** in Supplement

'Mary was nursed in a position of not more than 90° upright with her legs in abduction.' [*British Journal of Nursing*]

**abductor** /æb'dʌktə/, **abductor muscle** /æb 'dʌktə ˌmʌs(ə)l/ *noun* a muscle which pulls a part of the body away from the centre line of the body or away from a neighbouring part. Opposite **adductor**

**aberrant** /æ'berənt/ *adjective* not usual or expected

**aberration** /ˌæbə'reɪʃ(ə)n/ *noun* an action or growth which is not usual or expected

**ablation** /æ'bleɪʃ(ə)n/ *noun* the removal of an organ or of a part of the body by surgery

**abnormal** /æb'nɔːm(ə)l/ *adjective* not usual ○ *abnormal behaviour* ○ *an abnormal movement*

'…the synovium produces an excess of synovial fluid, which is abnormal and becomes thickened. This causes pain, swelling and immobility of the affected joint.' [*Nursing Times*]

**abnormality** /ˌæbnɔː'mælɪti/ *noun* a form or condition which is not usual (NOTE: For other terms referring to abnormality, see words beginning with **terat-, terato-**.)

'Even children with the milder forms of sickle-cell disease have an increased frequency of pneumococcal infection. The reason for this susceptibility is a profound abnormality of the immune system in children with SCD.' [*Lancet*]

**abocclusion** /ˌæbɒ'kluːʒ(ə)n/ *noun* a condition in which the teeth in the top and bottom jaws do not touch

**aboral** /æb'ɔːrəl/ *adjective* situated away from or opposite the mouth

**abort** /ə'bɔːt/ *verb* to eject an embryo or fetus, or to cause an embryo or fetus to be ejected, and so end a pregnancy before the fetus is fully developed

**abortifacient** /ə,bɔːtɪ'feɪʃ(ə)nt/ *noun* a drug or instrument which provokes an abortion

**abortion** /ə'bɔːʃ(ə)n/ *noun* a situation where a fetus leaves the uterus before it is fully developed, especially during the first 28 weeks of pregnancy, or a procedure which causes this to happen □ **to have an abortion** to have an operation to make a fetus leave the uterus during the first period of pregnancy

COMMENT: In the UK, an abortion can be carried out legally if two doctors agree that the mother's life is in danger, that she risks grave permanent injury to the physical or mental health of herself or her children, or that the fetus is likely to be born with severe disabilities.

**abortionist** /ə'bɔːʃ(ə)nɪst/ *noun* a person who helps a woman abort, usually a person who performs an illegal abortion

**abortion pill** /ə'bɔːʃ(ə)n pɪl/ *noun* a drug that causes an abortion to occur very early in pregnancy

**abortion trauma syndrome** /ə,bɔːʃ(ə)n 'trɔːmə ˌsɪndrəʊm/ *noun* a set of symptoms sometimes experienced in the period after an abortion including guilt, anxiety, depression, low self-esteem, eating and sleeping disorders and suicidal thoughts

**abortive** /ə'bɔːtɪv/ *adjective* not successful ○ *an abortive attempt*

**abortive poliomyelitis** /ə,bɔːtɪv ˌpəʊliəʊ maɪə'laɪtɪs/ *noun* a mild form of polio which only affects the throat and intestines

**abortus** /ə'bɔːtəs/ *noun* a fetus which is expelled during an abortion or miscarriage

**abortus fever** /ə'bɔːtəs ˌfiːvə/ *noun* same as **brucellosis**

**ABO system** /ˌeɪ biː 'əʊ ˌsɪstəm/ *noun* a system of classifying blood groups. ◊ **blood group**

**abrasion** /ə'breɪʒ(ə)n/ *noun* a condition in which the surface of the skin has been rubbed off by a rough surface and bleeds

COMMENT: As the intact skin is an efficient barrier to bacteria, even minor abrasions can allow infection to enter the body and thus should be cleaned and treated with an antiseptic.

**abreact** /ˌæbri'ækt/ *verb* to release unconscious psychological tension by talking about or regularly remembering the events that caused it

**abreaction** /ˌæbri'ækʃən/ *noun* the treatment of a person with a neurosis by making him or her think again about past bad experiences

**abruptio placentae** /ə,brʌptiəʊ plə'sentiː/ *noun* an occasion when the placenta suddenly comes away from the uterus earlier than it should, often causing shock and bleeding

**abscess** /'æbses/ *noun* a painful swollen area where pus forms ○ *She had an abscess under a tooth.* ○ *The doctor decided to lance the abscess.* (NOTE: The formation of an abscess is often accompanied by a high temperature. The plural is **abscesses**.)

COMMENT: An acute abscess can be dealt with by opening and draining when it has reached the stage where sufficient pus has been formed. A chronic abscess is usually treated with drugs.

**absolute alcohol** /ˌæbsəluːt 'ælkəhɒl/ *noun* alcohol which contains no water

**absorb** /əb'zɔːb/ *verb* to take up or soak up something, especially a liquid, into a solid ○ *Cotton wads are used to absorb the discharge from the wound.*

**absorbable suture** /əb,zɔː'bəb(ə)l 'suːtʃə/ *noun* a suture which will eventually be absorbed into the body, and does not need to be removed

**absorbent cotton** /əb,zɔːbənt 'kɒt(ə)n/ noun a soft white material used as a dressing to put on wounds

**absorption** /əb'zɔːpʃən/ noun **1.** the process by which a liquid is taken into a solid **2.** the process of taking into the body substances such as proteins or fats which have been digested from food and enter the bloodstream from the stomach and intestines □ **absorption rate** the rate at which a liquid is absorbed by a solid

**abstainer** /əb'steɪnə/ noun a person who does not drink alcohol

**abstinence** /'æbstɪnəns/ noun a deliberate act of not doing something over a period of time, especially not eating or drinking ○ *abstinence from alcohol*

**abulia** /ə'buːliə/ noun a lack of willpower

**abuse** noun /ə'bjuːs/ **1.** the act of using something wrongly ○ *the abuse of a privilege* **2.** the illegal use of a drug or overuse of alcohol ○ *substance abuse* **3.** same as **child abuse 4.** bad treatment of a person ○ *physical abuse* ○ *sexual abuse* ■ verb /ə'bjuːz/ **1.** to use something wrongly ○ *Heroin and cocaine are drugs which are commonly abused.* □ **to abuse one's authority** to use one's powers in an illegal or harmful way **2.** to treat someone badly ○ *sexually abused children* ○ *He had physically abused his wife and child.*

**a.c.** adverb (used on prescriptions) before food. Full form **ante cibum**

**acanthosis** /ə,kæn'θəʊsɪs/ noun a disease of the prickle cell layer of the skin, where warts appear on the skin or inside the mouth

**acapnia** /eɪ'kæpniə/ noun the condition of not having enough carbon dioxide in the blood and tissues

**acariasis** /,ækə'raɪəsɪs/ noun the presence of mites or ticks on the skin

**acaricide** /ə'kærɪsaɪd/ noun a substance which kills mites or ticks

**acarophobia** /,ækərə'fəʊbiə/ noun an unusual fear of mites or ticks

**acatalasia** /eɪ,kætə'leɪziə/ noun an inherited condition which results in a lack of catalase in all tissue

**accessory** /ək'sesəri/ noun something which helps something else to happen or operate, but may not be very important in itself ■ adjective helping something else to happen or operate

**accessory nerve** /ək'sesəri ,nɜːv/ noun the eleventh cranial nerve which supplies the muscles in the neck and shoulders

**accessory organ** /ək,sesəri 'ɔːgən/ noun an organ which has a function which is controlled by another organ

**accident** /'æksɪd(ə)nt/ noun **1.** an unpleasant event which happens suddenly and harms someone's health ○ *She had an accident in the kitchen and had to go to hospital.* ○ *Three people were killed in the accident on the motorway.* **2.** chance, or something which happens by chance ○ *I met her by accident at the bus stop.*

**accidental injury** /,æksɪdent(ə)l 'ɪndʒəri/ noun an injury that happens to someone in an accident

**accident and emergency department** /,æksɪd(ə)nt ənd ɪ'mɜːdʒənsi dɪ,pɑːtmənt/ noun the part of a hospital which deals with people who need urgent treatment because they have had accidents or are in sudden serious pain. Abbr **A & E**

**accident form** /'æksɪd(ə)nt fɔːm/, **accident report form** /,æksɪd(ə)nt rɪ'pɔːt fɔːm/ noun a form to be filled in with details of an accident

**accident prevention** /,æksɪd(ə)nt prɪ'venʃən/ noun the work of taking action or changing procedures to prevent accidents from happening

**accident ward** /'æksɪd(ə)nt wɔːd/ noun a ward for urgent accident victims. Also called **casualty ward**

**accommodation** /ə,kɒmə'deɪʃ(ə)n/, **accommodation reflex** /ə,kɒmə'deɪʃ(ə)n ,riːfleks/ noun (of the lens of the eye) the ability to focus on objects at different distances, using the ciliary muscle

**accommodative squint** /ə,kɒmədeɪtɪv 'skwɪnt/ noun a squint when the eye is trying to focus on an object which is very close

**accouchement** /ə'kuːʃmɒŋ/ noun the time when a woman is being looked after because her baby is being born, or has just been born

**accretion** /ə'kriːʃ(ə)n/ noun a gradual increase in size, as through growth or external addition ○ *an accretion of calcium around the joint*

**ACE** /eɪs/ noun an enzyme that increases blood pressure

**acebutolol** /,æsɪ'bjuːtəlɒl/ noun a drug which reduces both the heart rate and how strongly the heart muscles contract, used in the treatment of high blood pressure and irregular heart rhythms

**ACE inhibitor** /'eɪs ɪn,hɪbɪtə/ noun same as **angiotensin-converting enzyme inhibitor**

**acephalus** /eɪ'sefələs/ noun a fetus born without a head

**acetabuloplasty** /,æsɪ'tæbjʊləʊ,plæsti/ noun a surgical operation to repair or rebuild the acetabulum

**acetabulum** /,æsɪ'tæbjʊləm/ noun the part of the pelvic bone, shaped like a cup, into which the head of the femur fits to form the hip joint. Also called **cotyloid cavity** (NOTE: The plural is **acetabula**.)

**acetaminophen** /əˌsiːtəˈmɪnəfən/ *noun US* same as **paracetamol**

**acetazolamide** /əˌsiːtəˈzɒləmaɪd/ *noun* a drug which helps a person to produce more urine, used in the treatment of oedema, glaucoma and epilepsy

**acetonaemia** /əˌsiːtəʊˈniːmiə/ same as **ketonaemia**

**acetone** /ˈæsɪtəʊn/ *noun* a colourless volatile substance formed in the body after vomiting or during diabetes. ◊ **ketone**

**acetonuria** /əˌsiːtəʊˈnjuːriə/ *noun* the presence of acetone in the urine, shown by the fact that the urine gives off a sweet smell

**acetylcholine** /ˌæsɪtaɪlˈkəʊliːn/ *noun* a substance released from nerve endings, which allows nerve impulses to move from one nerve to another or from a nerve to the organ it controls

COMMENT: Acetylcholine receptors are of two types, muscarinic, found in parasympathetic post-ganglionic nerve junctions, and nicotinic, found at neuromuscular junctions and in autonomic ganglia. Acetylcholine acts on both types of receptors, but other drugs act on one or the other.

**acetylcoenzyme A** /ˌæsɪtaɪlkəʊˌenzaɪm ˈeɪ/ *noun* a compound produced in the metabolism of carbohydrates, fatty acids and amino acids

**acetylsalicylic acid** /ˌæsɪtaɪlˌsæləsɪlɪk ˈæsɪd/ *noun* ♦ **aspirin**

**achalasia** /ˌækəˈleɪziə/ *noun* the condition of being unable to relax the muscles

**ache** /eɪk/ *noun* a pain which goes on for a time, but is not very severe ○ *He complained of various aches and pains.* ■ *verb* to have a pain in part of the body ○ *His tooth ached so much he went to the dentist.*

**Achilles tendon** /əˌkɪliːz ˈtendən/ *noun* a tendon at the back of the ankle which connects the calf muscles to the heel and which acts to pull up the heel when the calf muscle is contracted

**achillorrhaphy** /ˌækɪˈlɔːrəfi/ *noun* a surgical operation to stitch a torn Achilles tendon

**achillotomy** /ˌækɪˈlɒtəmi/ *noun* a surgical operation to divide the Achilles tendon

**aching** /ˈeɪkɪŋ/ *adjective* causing someone a continuous mild pain ○ *aching legs*

**achlorhydria** /ˌeɪklɔːˈhaɪdriə/ *noun* a condition in which the gastric juices do not contain hydrochloric acid, a symptom of stomach cancer or pernicious anaemia

**acholia** /eɪˈkəʊliə/ *noun* the absence or failure of the secretion of bile

**acholuria** /ˌeɪkɒˈluːriə/ *noun* the absence of bile colouring in the urine

**acholuric jaundice** /ˌeɪkəluːrɪk ˈdʒɔːndɪs/ *noun* a disease where unusually round red blood cells form, leading to anaemia, an enlarged spleen and the formation of gallstones. Also called **hereditary spherocytosis**

**achondroplasia** /ˌeɪkɒndrəˈpleɪziə/ *noun* an inherited condition in which the long bones in the arms and legs do not grow fully while the rest of the bones in the body grow as usual, resulting in dwarfism

**achromatopsia** /ˌeɪkrəʊməˈtɒpsiə/ *noun* a rare condition in which a person cannot see any colours, but only black, white and shades of grey

**achy** /ˈeɪki/ *adjective* feeling aches all over the body (*informal*)

**aciclovir** /eɪˈsaɪkləʊvɪə/ *noun* a drug that is effective against herpesviruses. Also called **acyclovir**

**acid** /ˈæsɪd/ *noun* a chemical compound containing hydrogen, which reacts with an alkali to form a salt and water

**acidaemia** /ˌæsɪˈdiːmiə/ *noun* a state in which the blood has too much acid in it. It is a feature of untreated severe diabetes.

**acid–base balance** /ˌæsɪd ˈbeɪs ˌbæləns/ *noun* the balance between acid and base, i.e. the pH level, in plasma

**acidity** /əˈsɪdɪti/ *noun* **1.** the level of acid in a liquid ○ *The alkaline solution may help to reduce acidity.* **2.** same as **hyperacidity**

**acidosis** /ˌæsɪˈdəʊsɪs/ *noun* **1.** a condition when there are more acid waste products such as urea than usual in the blood because of a lack of alkali **2.** same as **acidity**

**acidotic** /ˌæsɪˈdɒtɪk/ *adjective* relating to acidosis

**acid reflux** /ˌæsɪd ˈriːflʌks/ *noun* a condition caused by a faulty muscle in the oesophagus allowing the acid in the stomach to pass into the oesophagus

**acid stomach** /ˌæsɪd ˈstʌmək/ *noun* same as **hyperacidity**

**aciduria** /ˌæsɪˈdjʊəriə/ *noun* a condition in which there is a higher level of acidity of the urine than is desirable

**acinus** /ˈæsɪnəs/ *noun* **1.** a tiny sac which forms part of a gland **2.** part of a lobule in the lung (NOTE: The plural is **acini**.)

**acne** /ˈækni/ *noun* an inflammation of the sebaceous glands during puberty which makes blackheads appear on the skin, usually on the face, neck and shoulders. These blackheads often then become infected. ○ *She is using a cream to clear up her acne.*

**acne rosacea** /ˌækni rəʊˈzeɪʃə/ *noun* same as **rosacea**

**acne vulgaris** /ˌækni vʊlˈgɑːrɪs/ *noun* same as **acne**

**acoustic** /əˈkuːstɪk/ *adjective* relating to sound or hearing

**acoustic nerve** /əˈkuːstɪk nɜːv/ *noun* the eighth cranial nerve which governs hearing and balance

**acoustic neurofibroma** /əˌkuːstɪk ˌnjʊərəʊfaɪˈbrəʊmə/, **acoustic neuroma** /ə ˌkuːstɪk njʊəˈrəʊmə/ *noun* a tumour in the sheath of the auditory nerve, causing deafness

**acoustic trauma** /əˌkuːstɪk ˈtrɔːmə/ *noun* physical damage caused by sound waves, e.g. hearing loss, disorientation, motion sickness or dizziness

**acquired** /əˈkwaɪəd/ *adjective* referring to a condition which is neither congenital nor hereditary and which a person develops after birth in reaction to his or her environment

**acquired immunity** /əˌkwaɪəd ɪˈmjuːnɪti/ *noun* an immunity which a body acquires from having caught a disease or from immunisation, not one which is congenital

**acquired immunodeficiency syndrome** /əˌkwaɪəd ˌɪmjʊnəʊdɪˈfɪʃ(ə)nsi ˌsɪndrəʊm/, **acquired immune deficiency syndrome** /ə ˌkwaɪəd ɪmˌjuːn dɪˈfɪʃ(ə)nsi ˌsɪndrəʊm/ *noun* a viral infection which breaks down the body's immune system. Abbr **AIDS**

**acrivastine** /əˈkrɪvə stiːn/ *noun* a drug which reduces the amount of histamine produced by the body. It is used in the treatment of rhinitis, urticaria and eczema.

**acro-** /ækrəʊ/ *prefix* referring to a point or tip

**acrocephalia** /ˌækrəʊsəˈfeɪliə/ *noun* same as **oxycephaly**

**acrocephaly** /ˌækrəʊˈsefəli/ *noun* same as **oxycephaly**

**acrocyanosis** /ˌækrəʊsaɪəˈnəʊsɪs/ *noun* a blue coloration of the extremities, i.e. the fingers, toes, ears and nose, which is due to poor circulation

**acrodynia** /ˌækrəʊˈdɪniə/ *noun* a children's disease, caused by an allergy to mercury, where the child's hands, feet and face swell and become pink, and the child is also affected with fever and loss of appetite. Also called **erythroedema, pink disease**

**acromegaly** /ˌækrəʊˈmegəli/ *noun* a disease caused by excessive quantities of growth hormone produced by the pituitary gland, causing a slow enlargement of the hands and jaws in adults

**acromial** /əˈkrəʊmiəl/ *adjective* referring to the acromion

**acromioclavicular** /ˌækrəʊmaɪəʊklə ˈvɪkjʊlə/ *adjective* relating to the acromion and the clavicle

**acromion** /əˈkrəʊmiən/ *noun* the pointed top of the scapula, which forms the tip of the shoulder

**acronyx** /ˈækrɒnɪks, ˈeɪkrɒnɪks/ *noun* a condition in which a nail grows into the flesh

**acroparaesthesia** /ˌækrəʊpærɪsˈθiːziə/ *noun* a condition in which the patient experiences sharp pains in the arms and numbness in the fingers after sleep

**acrophobia** /ˌækrəˈfəʊbiə/ *noun* a fear of heights

**acrosclerosis** /ˌækrəʊskləˈrəʊsɪs/ *noun* sclerosis which affects the extremities

**ACTH** *abbr* adrenocorticotrophic hormone

**actinomycin** /ˌæktɪnəʊˈmaɪsɪn/ *noun* an antibiotic used in the treatment of children with cancer

**actinomycosis** /ˌæktɪnəʊmaɪˈkəʊsɪs/ *noun* a fungal disease transmitted to humans from cattle, causing abscesses in the mouth and lungs (pulmonary actinomycosis) or in the ileum (intestinal actinomycosis)

**action potential** /ˈækʃən pəˌtenʃəl/ *noun* a temporary change in electrical potential which occurs between the inside and the outside of a nerve or muscle fibre when a nerve impulse is sent

**active** /ˈæktɪv/ *adjective* **1.** (*of a person*) lively and energetic ○ *Although she is over eighty she is still very active.* Opposite **passive 2.** (*of a disease*) having an effect on a patient ○ *experienced two years of active rheumatoid disease* Compare **dormant 3.** (*of a drug*) having medicinal effect

**active immunity** /ˌæktɪv ɪˈmjuːnɪti/ *noun* immunity which is acquired by catching and surviving an infectious disease or by vaccination with a weakened form of the disease, which makes the body form antibodies

**active ingredient** /ˌæktɪv ɪnˈgriːdiənt/ *noun* the main medicinal ingredient of an ointment or lotion, as opposed to the base

**active movement** /ˌæktɪv ˈmuːvmənt/ *noun* movement made by a person using his or her own willpower and muscles

**active principle** /ˌæktɪv ˈprɪnsɪp(ə)l/ *noun* the main medicinal ingredient of a drug which makes it have the required effect on a person

**activities of daily living** /ækˌtɪvɪtiz əv ˌdeɪli ˈlɪvɪŋ/ *noun* a scale used by geriatricians and occupational therapists to assess the capacity of elderly or disabled people to live independently. Abbr **ADLs**

**activity** /ækˈtɪvɪti/ *noun* **1.** what someone does ○ *difficulty with activities such as walking and dressing* **2.** the characteristic behaviour of a chemical ○ *The drug's activity only lasts a few hours.* □ **antibacterial activity** effective action against bacteria

**act on** /ˈækt ɒn/, **act upon** /ˈækt əˌpɒn/ *verb* **1.** to do something as the result of something which has been said ○ *He acted on his doctor's advice and gave up smoking.* **2.** to have an effect on someone or something ○ *The antibiotic acted quickly on the infection.*

**act out** /ˌækt ˈaʊt/ *verb* to express negative feelings by behaving in a socially unacceptable way

**acuity** /əˈkjuːɪti/ *noun* keenness of sight, hearing or intellect

**acupressure** /'ækjʊpreʃə/ *noun* a treatment which is based on the same principle as acupuncture in which, instead of needles, fingers are used on specific points on the body, called pressure points

**acupuncture** /'ækjʊpʌŋktʃə/ *noun* a treatment based on needles being inserted through the skin into nerve centres in order to relieve pain or treat a disorder

**acupuncturist** /'ækjʊˌpʌŋktʃərɪst/ *noun* a person who practises acupuncture

**acute** /ə'kjuːt/ *adjective* **1.** referring to a disease or condition which develops rapidly and can be dangerous ○ *an acute abscess* Opposite **chronic 2.** referring to pain which is sharp and intense (*informal*) ○ *He felt acute chest pains.*

**acute abdomen** /əˌkjuːt 'æbdəmən/ *noun* any serious condition of the abdomen which requires surgery

**acute bed** /ə'kjuːt bed/ *noun* a hospital bed reserved for people requiring immediate treatment

'…the survey shows a reduction in acute beds in the last six years. The bed losses forced one hospital to send acutely ill patients to hospitals up to sixteen miles away.' [*Nursing Times*]

**acute care** /ə'kjuːt keə/ *noun* medical or surgical treatment in a hospital, usually for a short period, for a patient with a sudden severe illness or injury

**acute disseminated encephalomyelitis** /əˌkjuːt dɪˌsemɪneɪtɪd enˌkefələʊmaɪə'laɪtɪs/ *noun* an encephalomyelitis or myelitis believed to result from an autoimmune attack on the myelin of the central nervous system

**acute glaucoma** /əˌkjuːt glɔː'kəʊmə/ *noun* same as **angle-closure glaucoma**

**acute hospital** /ə'kjuːt ˌhɒspɪt(ə)l/ *noun* a hospital where people go for major surgery or intensive care of medical or surgical conditions

**acutely** /ə'kjuːtli/ *adverb* **1.** having or causing a suddenly developing medical condition ○ *acutely ill patients* ○ *acutely toxic chemicals* **2.** extremely (*informal*)

**acute lymphocytic leukaemia** /əˌkjuːt ˌlɪmfəsɪtɪk luː'kiːmiə/ *noun* a form of leukaemia that is the commonest cancer affecting children

**acute nonlymphocytic leukaemia** /əˌkjuːt ˌnɒnlɪmfəsɪtɪk luː'kiːmiə/ *noun* a form of leukaemia that affects adults and children and is usually treated with chemotherapy

**acute pancreatitis** /əˌkuːt ˌpæŋkriə'taɪtɪs/ *noun* inflammation after pancreatic enzymes have escaped into the pancreas, causing symptoms of acute abdominal pain

**acute respiratory distress syndrome** /əˌkjuːt rɪˌspɪrət(ə)ri dɪ'stres ˌsɪndrəʊm/ *noun* an infection of the lungs, often following injury, which prevents them functioning properly. Abbr **ARDS**

**acute rheumatism** *noun* same as **rheumatic fever**

**acute rhinitis** /əˌkjuːt raɪ'naɪtɪs/ *noun* a virus infection which causes inflammation of the mucous membrane in the nose and throat

**acute suppurative arthritis** /əˌkjuːt ˌsʌpjʊrətɪv ɑːθ'raɪtɪs/ *noun* same as **pyarthrosis**

**acute toxicity** /əˌkjuːt tɒk'sɪsɪti/ *noun* a level of concentration of a toxic substance which makes people seriously ill or can cause death

**acute yellow atrophy** /əˌkjuːt ˌjeləʊ 'ætrəfi/ ♦ **yellow atrophy**

**acyclovir** /eɪ'saɪkləʊvɪə/ *noun* same as **aciclovir**

**acystia** /eɪ'sɪstiə/ *noun* a condition in which a baby is born without a bladder

**AD** *abbr* Alzheimer's disease

**Adam's apple** /ˌædəmz 'æp(ə)l/ *noun* a part of the thyroid cartilage which projects from the neck below the chin in a man. Also called **laryngeal prominence**

**adapt** /ə'dæpt/ *verb* **1.** to change one's ideas or behaviour to fit into a new situation ○ *She has adapted very well to her new job in the children's hospital.* **2.** to change something to make it more useful ○ *The brace has to be adapted to fit the patient.*

**adaptation** /ˌædæp'teɪʃ(ə)n/ *noun* **1.** a change which has been or can be made to something **2.** the act of changing something so that it fits a new situation **3.** the process by which sensory receptors become accustomed to a sensation which is repeated

**ADD** *abbr* attention deficit disorder

**addicted** /ə'dɪktɪd/ *adjective* physically or mentally dependent on a harmful substance □ **addicted to alcohol** *or* **drugs** needing to take alcohol or a harmful drug regularly

**addictive** /ə'dɪktɪv/ *adjective* referring to a drug which is habit-forming and which people can become addicted to

**Addison's anaemia** /ˌædɪs(ə)nz ə'niːmiə/ same as **pernicious anaemia** [Described 1849. After Thomas Addison (1793–1860), from Northumberland, founder of the science of endocrinology.]

**Addison's disease** /'ædɪs(ə)nz dɪˌziːz/ *noun* a disease of the adrenal glands, causing a change in skin colour to yellow and then to dark brown and resulting in general weakness, anaemia, low blood pressure and wasting away. Treatment is with corticosteroid injections. [Described 1849. After Thomas Addison (1793–1860), from Northumberland, founder of the science of endocrinology.]

**adducent** /ə'djuːs(ə)nt/ *adjective* referring to a muscle which brings parts of the body together or moves them towards the central line of the body or a limb. Compare **abducent**

**adduct** /əˈdʌkt/ *verb* (*of a muscle*) to pull a leg or arm towards the central line of the body, or to pull a toe or finger towards the central line of a leg or arm. Opposite **abduct**

**adducted** /əˈdʌktɪd/ *adjective* referring to a body part brought towards the middle of the body

**adduction** /əˈdʌkʃən/ *noun* the movement of a part of the body towards the midline or towards a neighbouring part. Compare **abduction**. See illustration at ANATOMICAL TERMS in Supplement

**adductor** /əˈdʌktə/, **adductor muscle** /əˈdʌktə ˌmʌs(ə)l/ *noun* a muscle which pulls a part of the body towards the central line of the body. Opposite **abductor**

**aden-** /ædɪn/ *prefix* same as **adeno-** (*used before vowels*)

**adenectomy** /ˌædɪˈnektəmi/ *noun* the surgical removal of a gland

**adenine** /ˈædəniːn/ *noun* one of the four basic chemicals in DNA

**adenitis** /ˌædɪˈnaɪtɪs/ *noun* inflammation of a gland or lymph node. ◊ **lymphadenitis**

**adeno-** /ædɪnəʊ/ *prefix* referring to glands

**adenocarcinoma** /ˌædɪnəʊkɑːsɪˈnəʊmə/ *noun* a malignant tumour of a gland

**adenohypophysis** /ˌædɪnəʊhaɪˈpɒfɪsɪs/ *noun* the front lobe of the pituitary gland which secretes most of the pituitary hormones

**adenoid** /ˈædɪnɔɪd/ *adjective* like a gland

**adenoidal** /ˌædɪˈnɔɪd(ə)l/ *adjective* referring to the adenoids

**adenoidal expression** /ˌædɪnɔɪd(ə)l ɪkˈspreʃ(ə)n/ *noun* a common symptom of a child suffering from adenoids, where his or her mouth is always open, the nose is narrow and the top teeth appear to project forward

**adenoidal tissue** /ˌædɪnɔɪd(ə)l ˈtɪʃuː/ *noun* same as **adenoids**

**adenoidectomy** /ˌædɪnɔɪˈdektəmi/ *noun* the surgical removal of the adenoids

**adenoidism** /ˈædɪnɔɪdɪz(ə)m/ *noun* the condition of a person with adenoids

**adenoids** /ˈædɪnɔɪdz/ *plural noun* a mass of tissue at the back of the nose and throat that can restrict breathing if enlarged. Also called **pharyngeal tonsils**

**adenoid vegetation** /ˌædɪnɔɪd ˌvedʒəˈteɪʃ(ə)n/ *noun* a condition in children where the adenoidal tissue is covered with growths and can block the nasal passages or the Eustachian tubes

**adenolymphoma** /ˌædɪnəʊlɪmˈfəʊmə/ *noun* a benign tumour of the salivary glands

**adenoma** /ˌædɪˈnəʊmə/ *noun* a benign tumour of a gland

**adenoma sebaceum** /ˌædɪnəʊmə səˈbeɪʃəm/ *noun* a skin condition of the face shown by raised red vascular bumps appearing in late childhood or early adolescence

**adenomyoma** /ˌædɪnəʊmaɪˈəʊmə/ *noun* a benign tumour made up of glands and muscle

**adenopathy** /ˌædɪˈnɒpəθi/ *noun* a disease of a gland

**adenosclerosis** /ˌædɪnəʊskləˈrəʊsɪs/ *noun* the hardening of a gland

**adenosine** /əˈdenəʊsiːn/ *noun* a drug used to treat an irregular heartbeat

**adenosine diphosphate** /əˌdenəʊsiːn daɪˈfɒsfeɪt/ *noun* a chemical compound which provides energy for processes to take place within living cells, formed when adenosine triphosphate reacts with water. Abbr **ADP**

**adenosine triphosphate** /əˌdenəʊsiːn traɪˈfɒsfeɪt/ *noun* a chemical which occurs in all cells, but mainly in muscle, where it forms the energy reserve. Abbr **ATP**

**adenosis** /ˌædɪˈnəʊsɪs/ *noun* any disease or disorder of the glands

**adenovirus** /ˈædɪnəʊˌvaɪrəs/ *noun* a virus which produces upper respiratory infections and sore throats and can cause fatal pneumonia in infants

**ADH** *abbr* antidiuretic hormone

**ADHD** *noun* full form **attention deficit hyperactivity disorder.** ♦ **hyperactivity**

**adhesion** /ədˈhiːʒ(ə)n/ *noun* a stable connection between two parts in the body, either in a healing process or between parts which are not usually connected

**adhesive dressing** /ədˌhiːsɪv ˈdresɪŋ/ *noun* a dressing with a sticky substance on the back so that it can stick to the skin

**adhesive strapping** /ədˌhiːsɪv ˈstræpɪŋ/ *noun* overlapping strips of adhesive plaster used to protect a lesion

**adipo-** /ædɪpəʊ/ *prefix* referring to fat

**adipose** /ˈædɪpəʊs/ *adjective* containing fat, or made of fat

COMMENT: Fibrous tissue is replaced by adipose tissue when more food is eaten than is necessary.

**adipose degeneration** /ˌædɪpəʊs dɪˌdʒenəˈreɪʃ(ə)n/ *noun* an accumulation of fat in the cells of an organ such as the heart or liver, which makes the organ less able to perform its proper function. Also called **fatty degeneration**

**adipose tissue** /ˌædɪpəʊs ˈtɪʃuː/ *noun* a tissue where the cells contain fat

**adiposis** /ˌædɪˈpəʊsɪs/ *noun* a state where too much fat is accumulated in the body

**adiposis dolorosa** /ˌædɪˌpəʊsɪs ˌdɒləˈrəʊsə/ *noun* a disease of middle-aged women in which painful lumps of fatty substance form in the body. Also called **Dercum's disease**

**adiposogenitalis** /ˌædɪˌpəʊsəʊˌdʒenɪˈteɪlɪs/ *noun* same as **Fröhlich's syndrome**

**adiposuria** /ˌædɪpsəʊˈjuːriə/ *noun* the presence of fat in the urine

**adiposus** /ˌædɪˈpəʊsəs/ ♦ **panniculus adiposus**

**aditus** /ˈædɪtəs/ *noun* an opening or entrance to a passage

**adjustment** /əˈdʒʌstmənt/ *noun* a specific directional high-speed movement of a joint performed by a chiropractor

**adjuvant** /ˈædʒʊvənt/ *adjective* referring to treatment by drugs or radiation therapy after surgery for cancer ■ *noun* a substance added to a drug to enhance the effect of the main ingredient

**adjuvant therapy** /ˈædʒʊvənt ˌθerəpi/ *noun* therapy using drugs or radiation after cancer surgery

**ADLs** *abbr* activities of daily living

**administer** /ədˈmɪnɪstə/ *verb* to give someone medicine or a treatment □ **to administer orally** to give a medicine by mouth

**admission** /ədˈmɪʃ(ə)n/ *noun* the act of being registered as a hospital patient

**admit** /ədˈmɪt/ *verb* to register a patient in a hospital. ○ *He was admitted to hospital this morning.*

'80% of elderly patients admitted to geriatric units are on medication' [*Nursing Times*]

'…ten patients were admitted to the ICU before operation, the main indications being the need for evaluation of patients with a history of severe heart disease' [*Southern Medical Journal*]

**adnexa** /ædˈneksə/ *plural noun* structures attached to an organ

**adolescence** /ˌædəˈles(ə)ns/ *noun* the period of life when a child is developing into an adult

**adolescent** /ˌædəˈles(ə)nt/ *noun* a person who is at the stage of life when he or she is developing into an adult ■ *adjective* developing into an adult, or occurring at that stage of life ○ *adolescent boys and girls* ○ *adolescent fantasies*

**adopt** /əˈdɒpt/ *verb* **1.** to decide to use a particular plan or idea or way of doing something ○ *The hospital has adopted a new policy on visiting.* **2.** to become the legal parent of a child who was born to other parents

**adoptive** /əˈdɒptɪv/ *adjective* **1.** taking over the role of something else **2.** referring to people who have adopted a child or a child that has been adopted ○ *adoptive parents*

**adoptive immunotherapy** /əˌdɒptɪv ɪm jʊnəˈθerəpi/ *noun* a treatment for cancer in which the patient's own white blood cells are used to attack cancer cells

COMMENT: This technique can halt the growth of cancer cells in the body but it can have distressing toxic side-effects.

**ADP** *abbr* adenosine diphosphate

**adrenal** /əˈdriːn(ə)l/ *adjective* situated near the kidney ■ *noun* same as **adrenal gland**

**adrenal body** /əˈdriːn(ə)l ˌbɒdi/ *noun* same as **adrenal gland**

**adrenal cortex** /əˌdriːn(ə)l ˈkɔːteks/ *noun* the firm outside layer of an adrenal gland, which secretes a series of hormones affecting the metabolism of carbohydrates and water

**adrenalectomy** /əˌdriːnəˈlektəmi/ *noun* the surgical removal of one of the adrenal glands

**adrenal gland** /əˈdriːn(ə)l ɡlænd/ *noun* one of two endocrine glands at the top of the kidneys which secrete cortisone, adrenaline and other hormones. Also called **adrenal body, adrenal**. See illustration at KIDNEY in Supplement

**adrenaline** /əˈdrenəlɪn/ *noun* a hormone secreted by the medulla of the adrenal glands which has an effect similar to stimulation of the sympathetic nervous system (NOTE: The US term is **epinephrine**.)

COMMENT: Adrenaline is produced when a person experiences surprise, shock, fear or excitement and it speeds up the heartbeat and raises blood pressure. It is administered as an emergency treatment of acute anaphylaxis and in cardiopulmonary resuscitation.

**adrenal medulla** /əˌdriːn(ə)l meˈdʌlə/ *noun* the inner part of the adrenal gland which secretes adrenaline and noradrenaline. Also called **suprarenal medulla**

**adrenergic** /ˌædrəˈnɜːdʒɪk/ *adjective* referring to a neurone or receptor which is stimulated by adrenaline. ◊ **beta blocker**

**adrenergic receptor** /ˌædrənɜːdʒɪk rɪ ˈseptə/ *noun* same as **adrenoceptor**

COMMENT: Three types of adrenergic receptor act in different ways when stimulated by adrenaline. Alpha receptors constrict the bronchi, beta 1 receptors speed up the heartbeat and beta 2 receptors dilate the bronchi.

**adrenoceptor** /əˌdrenəʊˈseptə/ *noun* a cell or neurone which is stimulated by adrenaline. Also called **adrenoreceptor, adrenergic receptor**

**adrenocortical** /əˌdriːnəʊˈkɔːtɪk(ə)l/ *adjective* relating to the cortex of the adrenal glands

**adrenocorticotrophic hormone** /ə ˌdriːnəʊˌkɔːtəkəʊtrɒfɪk ˈhɔːməʊn/ *noun* a hormone secreted by the pituitary gland, which makes the cortex of the adrenal glands produce corticosteroids. Abbr **ACTH**. Also called **corticotrophin**

**adrenogenital syndrome** /əˌdriːnəʊ ˈdʒenɪt(ə)l ˌsɪndrəʊm/ *noun* a condition caused by overproduction of male sex hormones, where boys show rapid sexual development and females develop male characteristics

**adrenoleukodystrophy** /əˌdriːnəʊˌluːkəʊ ˈdɪstrəfi/ *noun* an inherited disorder of the adrenal glands in boys

**adrenolytic** /ədriːnəʊˈlɪtɪk/ *adjective* acting against the secretion of adrenaline

**adrenoreceptor** /əˌdrenəʊrɪˈseptə/ *noun* same as **adrenoceptor**

**adsorbent** /æd'sɔːbənt/ *adjective* being capable of adsorption

**adsorption** /æd'sɔːpʃ(ə)n/ *noun* the attachment of one substance to another, often the bonding of a liquid with a gas or vapour which touches its surface

**adult** /'ædʌlt, ə'dʌlt/ *adjective* grown-up ○ *Adolescents reach the adult stage about the age of eighteen or twenty.* ■ *noun* someone who is no longer a child

**adult coeliac disease** /ˌædʌlt 'siːliæk dɪ ˌziːz/ *noun* a condition in adults where the villi in the intestine become smaller and so reduce the surface which can absorb nutrients

**adult dentition** /ˌædʌlt den'tɪʃ(ə)n/ *noun* the 32 teeth which an adult has

**adulteration** /əˌdʌltə'reɪʃ(ə)n/ *noun* the act of making something less pure by adding another substance

**adult-onset diabetes** /ˌædʌlt ˌɒnset ˌdaɪə 'biːtiːz/ *noun* a form of diabetes mellitus that develops slowly in older people as the body becomes less able to use insulin effectively

**adult respiratory distress syndrome** / ˌædʌlt rɪˌspɪrət(ə)ri dɪ'stres ˌsɪndrəʊm/ *noun* a description of various lung infections which reduce the lungs' efficiency. Abbr **ARDS**

**advanced trauma life support** /əd,vɑːnst ˌtrɔːmə 'laɪf sə,pɔːt/ *noun* the management of a trauma patient during the critical first hour after injury. Abbr **ATLS**

**adventitia** /ˌædven'tɪʃə/ *noun* same as **tunica adventitia**

**adventitious** /ˌædvən'tɪʃəs/ *adjective* on the outside or in an unusual place

**adventitious bursa** /ˌædvəntɪʃəs 'bɜːsə/ *noun* a bursa which develops as a result of continued pressure or rubbing

**adverse** /'ædvɜːs/ *adjective* harmful or unfavourable □ **the treatment had an adverse effect on his dermatitis** the treatment made the dermatitis worse

**adverse occurrence** /ˌædvɜːs ə'kʌrəns/ *noun* a harmful event which occurs during treatment

**adverse reaction** /ˌædvɜːs ri'ækʃən/ *noun* a situation where someone experiences harmful effects from the application of a drug

**advocacy** /'ædvəkəsi/ *noun* active support for something, especially in order to help people who would have difficulty in gaining attention without your help

**adynamic ileus** /eɪˌdaɪnæmɪk 'ɪliəs/ *noun* same as **paralytic ileus**

**aegophony** /iː'gɒfəni/ *noun* a high sound of the voice heard through a stethoscope, where there is fluid in the pleural cavity

**aer-** /eə/ *prefix* same as **aero-** (*used before vowels*)

**aeration** /eə'reɪʃ(ə)n/ *noun* the adding of air or oxygen to a liquid

**aero-** /eərəʊ/ *prefix* referring to air

**aeroba** /eə'rəʊbə/, **aerobe** /'eərəʊb/ *noun* a tiny organism which needs oxygen to survive

**aerobic** /eə'rəʊbɪk/ *adjective* needing oxygen to live, or taking place in the presence of oxygen

**aerobic respiration** /eəˌrəʊbɪk ˌrespə'reɪʃ(ə)n/ *noun* the process where the oxygen which is breathed in is used to conserve energy as ATP

**aeroembolism** /ˌeərəʊ'embəlɪz(ə)m/ *noun* same as **air embolism**

**aerogenous** /eə'rɒdʒənəs/ *adjective* referring to a bacterium which produces gas

**aerophagia** /ˌeərə'feɪdʒə/, **aerophagy** /eə 'rɒfədʒi/ *noun* the habit of swallowing air when suffering from indigestion, so making the stomach pains worse

**aerosol** /'eərəsɒl/ *noun* tiny particles of a liquid such as a drug or disinfectant suspended in a gas under pressure in a container and used as a spray

**aetiological agent** /ˌiːtiəlɒdʒik(ə)l 'eɪdʒ(ə)nt/ *noun* an agent which causes a disease

**aetiology** /ˌiːti'ɒlədʒi/ *noun* **1.** the cause or origin of a disease **2.** the study of the causes and origins of diseases (NOTE: [all senses] The US spelling is **etiology**.)

'…a wide variety of organs or tissues may be infected by the Salmonella group of organisms, presenting symptoms which are not immediately recognised as being of Salmonella aetiology' [*Indian Journal of Medical Sciences*]

**afebrile** /eɪ'fiːbraɪl/ *adjective* with no fever

**affect** /ə'fekt/ *verb* to make something or someone change, especially to have a bad effect on something or someone ○ *Some organs are rapidly affected if the patient lacks oxygen for even a short time.* ■ *noun* same as **affection**

**affection** /ə'fekʃən/, **affect** /ə'fekt/ *noun* the general state of a person's emotions

'Depression has degrees of severity, ranging from sadness, through flatness of affection or feeling, to suicide and psychosis' [*British Journal of Nursing*]

**affective** /ə'fektɪv/ *adjective* relating to a person's moods or feelings

**affective disorder** /ə'fektɪv dɪsˌɔːdə/ *noun* a condition which changes someone's mood, making him or her depressed or excited

**afferent** /'æf(ə)rənt/ *adjective* conducting liquid or electrical impulses towards the inside. Opposite **efferent**

**afferent nerve** *noun* same as **sensory nerve**

**afferent vessel** /'æf(ə)rənt ˌves(ə)l/ *noun* a tube which brings lymph to a gland

**affinity** /ə'fɪnɪti/ *noun* an attraction between two substances

**aflatoxin** /ˌæflə'tɒksɪn/ *noun* a poison produced by some moulds in some crops such as peanuts

**African trypanosomiasis** /ˌæfrɪkən ˌtrɪpənəʊsəʊˈmaɪəsɪs/ *noun* same as **sleeping sickness**

**afterbirth** /ˈɑːtəbɜːθ/ *noun* the tissues, including the placenta and umbilical cord, which are present in the uterus during pregnancy and are expelled after the birth of a baby

**aftercare** /ˈɑːftəkeə/ *noun* **1.** the care of a person who has had an operation. Aftercare treatment involves changing dressings and helping people to look after themselves again. **2.** the care of a mother who has just given birth

**after-effect** /ˈɑːftər ɪˌfekt/ *noun* a change which appears only some time after the cause ○ *The operation had some unpleasant after-effects.*

**after-image** /ˈɑːftər ˌɪmɪdʒ/ *noun* an image of an object which remains in a person's sight after the object itself has gone

**afterpains** /ˈɑːftəpeɪnz/ *plural noun* regular pains in the uterus which are sometimes experienced after childbirth

**afunctional** /eɪ ˈfʌŋkʃən(ə)l/ *adjective* which does not function properly

**agalactia** /ˌeɪɡəˈlækʃə/ *noun* a condition in which a mother is unable to produce milk after childbirth

**agammaglobulinaemia** /eɪˌɡæməɡlɒbjʊlɪ ˈniːmiə/ *noun* a deficiency or absence of immunoglobulins in the blood, which results in a reduced ability to provide immune responses

**agar** /ˈeɪɡɑː/, **agar agar** /ˌeɪɡɑː ˈeɪɡɑː/ *noun* a culture medium based on an extract of seaweed used for growing microorganisms in laboratories

**age** /eɪdʒ/ *noun* the number of years which a person has lived ○ *What's your age on your next birthday?* ○ *He was sixty years of age.* ○ *The size varies according to age.* ■ *verb* to grow old

**age group** /ˈeɪdʒ ɡruːp/ *noun* all the people of a particular age or within a particular set of ages ○ *the age group 20–25*

**ageing** /ˈeɪdʒɪŋ/, **aging** *noun* the fact of growing old

COMMENT: Changes take place in almost every part of the body as the person ages. Bones become more brittle and skin becomes less elastic. The most important changes affect the blood vessels which are less elastic, making thrombosis more likely. This also reduces the supply of blood to the brain, which in turn reduces the mental faculties.

**ageing process** /ˈeɪdʒɪŋ ˌprəʊsəs/ *noun* the physical changes which take place in a person as he or she grows older

**agency** /ˈeɪdʒənsi/ *noun* **1.** an organisation which carries out work on behalf of another organisation, e.g. one which recruits and employs nurses and supplies them to hospitals temporarily when full-time nursing staff are unavailable **2.** the act of causing something to happen ○ *The disease develops through the agency of bacteria present in the bloodstream.*

'The cost of employing agency nurses should be no higher than the equivalent full-time staff.' [*Nursing Times*]

'Growing numbers of nurses are choosing agency careers, which pay more and provide more flexible schedules than hospitals.' [*American Journal of Nursing*]

**agenesis** /eɪˈdʒenəsɪs/ *noun* the absence of an organ, resulting from a failure in embryonic development

**agent** /ˈeɪdʒənt/ *noun* **1.** a chemical substance which makes another substance react **2.** a substance or organism which causes a disease or condition **3.** a person who acts as a representative of another person or carries out some kinds of work on his or her behalf

**agglutinate** /əˈɡluːtɪneɪt/ *verb* to form into groups or clusters, or to cause things to form into groups or clusters

**agglutination** /əˌɡluːtɪˈneɪʃ(ə)n/ *noun* the act of coming together or sticking to one another to form a clump, as of bacteria cells in the presence of serum, or blood cells when blood of different types is mixed ◇ **agglutination test 1.** a test to identify bacteria **2.** a test to identify if a woman is pregnant

**agglutinin** /əˈɡluːtɪnɪn/ *noun* a factor in a serum which makes cells stick together in clumps

**agglutinogen** /ˌæɡluːˈtɪnədʒən/ *noun* a factor in red blood cells which reacts with a specific agglutinin in serum

**aggravate** /ˈæɡrəveɪt/ *verb* to make something worse ○ *Playing football only aggravates his knee injury.* ○ *The treatment seems to aggravate the disease.*

**aggression** /əˈɡreʃ(ə)n/ *noun* the state of feeling violently angry towards someone or something

**aggressive** /əˈɡresɪv/ *adjective* referring to treatment which involves frequent high doses of medication

**aging** /ˈeɪdʒɪŋ/ *noun* another spelling of **ageing**

**agitated** /ˈædʒɪteɪtɪd/ *adjective* moving about or twitching nervously because of worry or another psychological state ○ *The person became agitated and had to be given a sedative.*

**agitation** /ˌædʒɪˈteɪʃ(ə)n/ *noun* a state of being very nervous and anxious

**aglossia** /eɪˈɡlɒsiə/ *noun* the condition of not having a tongue from birth

**agnosia** /æɡˈnəʊziə/ *noun* a brain disorder in which a person fails to recognise places, people, tastes or smells which they used to know well

**agonist** /ˈæɡənɪst/ *noun* **1.** a muscle which causes part of the body to move and another muscle to relax when it contracts. Also called

**prime mover 2.** a substance which produces an observable physiological effect by acting through specific receptors. ◊ **antagonist**

**agony** /'ægəni/ *noun* a very severe physical or emotional pain ○ *He lay in agony on the floor.* ○ *She suffered the agony of waiting for weeks until her condition was diagnosed.*

**agoraphobia** /ˌæg(ə)rə'fəubiə/ *noun* a fear of being in open spaces. Compare **claustrophobia**

**agoraphobic** /ˌæg(ə)rə'fəubik/ *adjective* afraid of being in open spaces. Compare **claustrophobic**

**agranulocytosis** /əˌgrænjuləusai'təusis/ *noun* a usually fatal disease where the number of granulocytes, a type of white blood cell, falls sharply because of a bone marrow condition

**agraphia** /ei'græfiə/ *noun* the condition of being unable to put ideas into writing

**AHF** *abbr* antihaemophilic factor

**aid** /eid/ *noun* **1.** help **2.** a machine, tool or drug which helps someone do something ○ *He uses a walking frame as an aid to exercising his legs.* ■ *verb* to help someone or something ○ *The procedure is designed to aid the repair of tissues after surgery.*

**AID** /ˌei ai 'diː/ *noun* full form **artificial insemination by donor**. Now called **DI**

**AIDS** /eidz/, **Aids** *noun* a viral infection which breaks down the body's immune system. Full form **acquired immunodeficiency syndrome**, **acquired immune deficiency syndrome**

COMMENT: AIDS is a disease caused by the human immunodeficiency virus (HIV). It is spread mostly by sexual intercourse and can affect anyone. It is also transmitted through infected blood and plasma transfusions, through using unsterilised needles for injections, and can be passed from a mother to a fetus. The disease takes a long time, usually years, to show symptoms, and many people with HIV are unaware that they are infected. It causes a breakdown of the body's immune system, making the patient susceptible to any infection and often results in the development of rare skin cancers. It is not curable.

**AIDS dementia** /ˌeidz di'menʃə/ *noun* a form of mental degeneration resulting from infection with HIV

**AIDS-related complex** /ˌeidz riˌleitid 'kɒmpleks/, **AIDS-related condition** /ˌeidz ri ˌleitid kən'diʃ(ə)n/ *noun* early symptoms shown by someone infected with the HIV virus, e.g. weight loss, fever and herpes zoster. Abbr **ARC**

**AIH** *abbr* artificial insemination by husband

**ailment** /'eilmənt/ *noun* an illness, though not generally a very serious one ○ *Chickenpox is one of the common childhood ailments.*

**ailurophobia** /ˌailuərə'fəubiə/ *noun* a fear of cats

**air** /eə/ *noun* a mixture of gases, mainly oxygen and nitrogen, which cannot be seen, but which exists all around us and which is breathed ○ *Open the window and let some fresh air into the room.* ○ *He breathed the polluted air into his lungs.*

**air bed** /'eə bed/ *noun* a mattress which is filled with air, used to prevent the formation of bedsores. ◊ **conduction**

**airborne infection** /ˌeəbɔːn in'fekʃən/ *noun* an infection which is carried in the air

**air conduction** /'eə kənˌdʌkʃən/ *noun* the process by which sounds pass from the outside to the inner ear through the auditory meatus

**air embolism** /eər 'embəliz(ə)m/ *noun* a blockage caused by bubbles of air, that stops the flow of blood in vessels

**air hunger** /'eə ˌhʌŋgə/ *noun* a condition in which the patient needs air because of lack of oxygen in the tissues

**air passage** /'eə ˌpæsidʒ/ *noun* any tube which takes air to the lungs, e.g. the nostrils, pharynx, larynx, trachea and bronchi

**air sac** /'eə sæk/ *noun* a small sac in the lungs which contains air. ◊ **alveolus**

**airsick** /'eəsik/ *adjective* feeling sick because of the movement of an aircraft

**airsickness** /'eəsiknəs/ *noun* a queasy feeling, usually leading to vomiting, caused by the movement of an aircraft

**airway** /'eəwei/ *noun* a passage through which air passes, especially the trachea

**airway clearing** /'eəwei ˌkliəriŋ/ *noun* making sure that the airways in a newborn baby or an unconscious person are free of any obstruction

**airway obstruction** /ˌeəwei əb'strʌkʃ(ə)n/ *noun* something which blocks the air passages

**akathisia** /ˌeikə'θisiə/ *noun* restlessness

**akinesia** /ˌeiki'niːziə/ *noun* a lack of voluntary movement, as in Parkinson's disease

**akinetic** /ˌeiki'netik/ *adjective* without movement

**alacrima** /ei'lækrimə/ *noun* same as **xerosis**

**alactasia** /ˌeilæk'teiziə/ *noun* a condition in which there is a deficiency of lactase in the intestine, making the patient incapable of digesting lactose, the sugar in milk

**alalia** /ei'leiliə/ *noun* a condition in which a person completely loses the ability to speak

**alanine** /'æləniːn/ *noun* an amino acid

**alanine aminotransferase** /ˌæləniːn ə ˌmiːnəu'trænsfəreiz/ *noun* an enzyme which is found in the liver and can be monitored as an indicator of liver damage. Abbr **ALT**

**alar cartilage** /ˌeilə 'kɑːtilidʒ/ *noun* cartilage in the nose

**alba** /'ælbə/ ♦ **linea alba**

**Albee's operation** /'ɔːlbiːz ɒpəˌreiʃ(ə)n/ *noun* **1.** a surgical operation to fuse two or more vertebrae **2.** a surgical operation to fuse the femur to the pelvis [After Frederick Houdlett Albee (1876–1945), US surgeon]

**albicans** /'ælbɪkænz/ ♦ **corpus albicans**

**albinism** /'ælbɪnɪz(ə)m/ *noun* a condition in which a person lacks the pigment melanin and so has pink skin and eyes and white hair. It is hereditary and cannot be treated. ◊ **vitiligo**

**albino** /æl'biːnəʊ/ *noun* a person who is deficient in melanin and has little or no pigmentation in the skin, hair or eyes

**albuginea** /,ælbjʊ'dʒɪnɪə/ *noun* a layer of white tissue covering a part of the body

**albuginea oculi** /,ælbjʊdʒɪnɪə 'ɒkjʊlaɪ/ *noun* same as **sclera**

**albuminometer** /,ælbjʊmɪ'nɒmɪtə/ *noun* an instrument for measuring the level of albumin in the urine

**albuminuria** /,ælbjʊmɪ'njʊərɪə/ *noun* a condition in which albumin is found in the urine, usually a sign of kidney disease, but also sometimes of heart failure

**albumose** /'ælbjʊməʊz/ *noun* an intermediate product in the digestion of protein

**alcohol** /'ælkəhɒl/ *noun* a pure colourless liquid which is formed by the action of yeast on sugar solutions and forms part of drinks such as wine and whisky

COMMENT: Alcohol is used medicinally to dry wounds or harden the skin. When drunk, alcohol is rapidly absorbed into the bloodstream. It is a source of energy, so any carbohydrates taken at the same time are not used by the body and are stored as fat. Alcohol is a depressant, not a stimulant, and affects the way the brain works.

**alcohol abuse** /'ælkəhɒl ə,bjuːs/ *noun* the excessive use of alcohol adversely affecting a person's health

**alcohol addiction** /'ælkəhɒl ə,dɪkʃən/ *noun* a condition in which a person is dependent on the use of alcohol

**alcohol-fast** /'ælkəhɒl fɑːst/ *adjective* referring to an organ stained for testing which is not discoloured by alcohol

**alcoholic** /,ælkə'hɒlɪk/ *adjective* **1.** containing alcohol **2.** caused by alcoholism ○ *alcoholic poisoning* ■ *noun* a person who is addicted to drinking alcohol and shows changes in behaviour and personality

**alcoholic cardiomyopathy** /,ælkəhɒlɪk ,kɑːdiəʊmaɪ'ɒpəθi/ *noun* a disease of the heart muscle arising as a result of long-term heavy alcohol consumption

**alcoholic cirrhosis** /,ælkəhɒlɪk sɪ'rəʊsɪs/ *noun* cirrhosis of the liver caused by alcoholism

**alcoholic hepatitis** /,ælkəhɒlɪk ,hepə'taɪtɪs/ *noun* inflammation of the liver as a result of long-term heavy alcohol consumption, often leading to cirrhosis

**Alcoholics Anonymous** /,ælkəhɒlɪks ə'nɒnɪməs/ *noun* an organisation of former al-

coholics which helps people to overcome their dependence on alcohol by encouraging them to talk about their problems in group therapy. Abbr **AA**

**alcoholicum** /,ælkə'hɒlɪkəm/ ♦ **delirium alcoholicum**

**alcoholism** /'ælkəhɒlɪz(ə)m/ *noun* excessive drinking of alcohol which becomes addictive

**alcohol poisoning** /'ælkəhɒl ,pɔɪz(ə)nɪŋ/ *noun* poisoning and disease caused by excessive drinking of alcohol

**alcohol rub** /'ælkəhɒl rʌb/ *noun* the act of rubbing a bedridden person with alcohol to help protect against bedsores and as a tonic

**alcoholuria** /,ælkəhɒ'ljʊərɪə/ *noun* a condition in which alcohol is present in the urine (NOTE: The level of alcohol in the urine is used as a test for drivers who are suspected of driving while drunk.)

**aldosterone** /æl'dɒstərəʊn/ *noun* a hormone secreted by the cortex of the adrenal gland, which regulates the balance of sodium and potassium in the body and the amount of body fluid

**aldosteronism** /æl'dɒst(ə)rənɪz(ə)m/ *noun* a condition in which a person produces too much aldosterone, so that there is too much salt in the blood. This causes high blood pressure and the need to drink a lot of liquids.

**alert** /ə'lɜːt/ *adjective* referring to someone who takes an intelligent interest in his or her surroundings ○ *The patient is still alert, though in great pain.*

**aleukaemic** /,eɪluː'kiːmɪk/ *adjective* **1.** referring to a state where leukaemia is not present **2.** referring to a state where leucocytes are not normal

**Alexander technique** /,ælɪg'zɑːndə tek,niːk/ *noun* a method of improving the way a person stands and moves, by making them much more aware of how muscles behave

**alexia** /eɪ'leksɪə/ *noun* a condition in which the patient cannot understand printed words. Also called **word blindness**

**alfacalcidol** /,ælfə'kælsɪdɒl/ *noun* a substance related to vitamin D, used by the body to maintain the right levels of calcium and phosphate, and also as a drug to help people who do not have enough vitamin D

**algesimeter** /,æld͡ʒɪ'sɪmɪtə/ *noun* an instrument to measure the sensitivity of the skin to pain

**-algia** /æld͡ʒɪə/ *suffix* a word ending that indicates a painful condition

**algid** /'æld͡ʒɪd/ *adjective* referring to a stage in a disease that causes fever during which the body becomes cold

**algophobia** /,ælgəʊ'fəʊbɪə/ *noun* an unusually intense fear of pain

**alienation** /ˌeɪliə'neɪʃ(ə)n/ *noun* a psychological condition in which a person develops the feeling of not being part of the everyday world, and as a result often becomes hostile to other people

**alignment** /ə'laɪnmənt/ *noun* the arrangement of something in a straight line, or in the correct position in relation to something else

**alimentary** /ˌælɪ'ment(ə)ri/ *adjective* providing food, or relating to food or nutrition

**alimentary canal** /ælɪˌment(ə)ri kə'næl/ *noun* a tube in the body going from the mouth to the anus and including the throat, stomach and intestine, through which food passes and is digested

**alimentary system** /ælɪ'ment(ə)ri ˌsɪstəm/ *noun* same as **digestive system**

**alimentation** /ˌælɪmen'teɪʃ(ə)n/ *noun* the act of providing food or nourishment

**aliquot** /'ælɪkwɒt/ *noun* a part of a larger thing, especially a sample of something which is taken to be examined

**alive** /ə'laɪv/ *adjective* living, not dead ○ *The man was still alive, even though he had been in the sea for two days.* (NOTE: **Alive** cannot be used in front of a noun: *The person is alive* but *a living person*. Note also that **live** can be used in front of a noun: *The person was injected with live vaccine*.)

**alkalaemia** /ˌælkə'liːmiə/ *noun* an excess of alkali in the blood

**alkali** /'ælkəlaɪ/ *noun* one of many substances which neutralise acids and form salts (NOTE: The UK plural is **alkalis**, but the US plural is **alkalies**.)

**alkaline** /'ælkəlaɪn/ *adjective* containing more alkali than acid

**alkalinity** /ˌælkə'lɪnɪti/ *noun* the level of alkali in a body ○ *Hyperventilation causes fluctuating carbon dioxide levels in the blood, resulting in an increase of blood alkalinity.*

COMMENT: Alkalinity and acidity are measured according to the pH scale. pH7 is neutral, and pH8 and upwards are alkaline. Alkaline solutions are used to counteract the effects of acid poisoning and also of bee stings. If strong alkali, such as ammonia, is swallowed, the patient should drink water and an acid such as orange juice.

**alkaloid** /'ælkələɪd/ *noun* one of many poisonous substances found in plants and used as medicines, e.g. atropine, morphine or quinine

**alkalosis** /ˌælkə'ləʊsɪs/ *noun* a condition in which the alkali level in the body tissue is high, producing cramps

**alkaptonuria** /ˌælkæptə'njʊəriə/ *noun* a hereditary condition where dark pigment is present in the urine

**allantoin** /ə'læntəʊɪn/ *noun* powder from the herb comfrey, used to treat skin disorders

**allantois** /ə'læntəʊɪs/ *noun* one of the membranes in the embryo, shaped like a sac, which grows out of the embryonic hindgut

**allele** /ə'liːl/ *noun* one of two or more alternative forms of a gene, situated in the same area on each of a pair of chromosomes and each producing a different effect

**allergen** /'ælədʒən/ *noun* a substance which produces hypersensitivity

COMMENT: Allergens are usually proteins and include foods, dust, hair of animals, as well as pollen from flowers. Allergic reaction to serum is known as **anaphylaxis**. Treatment of allergies depends on correctly identifying the allergen to which the patient is sensitive. This is done by patch tests in which drops of different allergens are placed on scratches in the skin. Food allergens discovered in this way can be avoided, but other allergens such as dust and pollen can hardly be avoided and have to be treated by a course of desensitising injections.

**allergenic** /ˌælə'dʒenɪk/ *adjective* producing an allergic reaction ○ *the allergenic properties of fungal spores*

**allergenic agent** /ˌælədʒenɪk 'eɪdʒənt/ *noun* a substance which produces an allergy

**allergic** /ə'lɜːdʒɪk/ *adjective* having an allergy to something ○ *She is allergic to cats.* ○ *I'm allergic to penicillin.*

**allergic agent** /ə'lɜːdʒɪk ˌeɪdʒənt/ *noun* a substance which produces an allergic reaction

**allergic purpura** /ə,lɜːdʒɪk 'pɜːpjʊrə/ *noun* a form of the skin condition purpura, found most often in children

**allergic reaction** /ə,lɜːdʒɪk ri'ækʃən/ *noun* an effect produced by a substance to which a person has an allergy, such as sneezing or a skin rash

**allergic rhinitis** /ə,lɜːdʒɪk raɪ'naɪtɪs/ *noun* inflammation in the nose and eyes caused by an allergic reaction to plant pollen, mould spores, dust mites or animal hair. ◊ **hayfever**

**allergist** /'ælədʒɪst/ *noun* a doctor who specialises in the treatment of allergies

**allergy** /'ælədʒi/ *noun* an unusual sensitivity to some substances such as pollen or dust, which cause a physical reaction such as sneezing or a rash in someone who comes into contact with them ○ *She has an allergy to household dust.* ○ *He has a penicillin allergy.* (NOTE: You **have an allergy** or you **are allergic to** something.)

**allergy bracelet** /'ælədʒi ˌbreɪslət/ *noun* ♦ **medical alert bracelet**

**alleviate** /ə'liːvieɪt/ *verb* to make pain or discomfort less severe ○ *The drug is effective in alleviating migraine headaches.*

**allied health professional** /ˌælaɪd 'helθ prə,feʃ(ə)n(ə)l/ *noun* a professional working in medicine who is not a doctor or nurse, e.g. a physiotherapist or paramedic

**allo-** /ˈæləʊ/ *prefix* different

**allodynia** /ˌæləˈdɪniə/ *noun* pain of the skin caused by something such as clothing which usually does not cause pain

**allogeneic** /ˌælədʒəˈneɪɪk/ *adjective* ((of body tissues)) genetically different and therefore incompatible when transplanted

**allograft** /ˈæləʊgrɑːft/ *noun* same as **homograft**

**allopathy** /əˈlɒpəθi/ *noun* the treatment of a condition using drugs which produce opposite symptoms to those of the condition. Compare **homeopathy**

**allopurinol** /ˌæləʊˈpjʊərɪnɒl/ *noun* a drug which helps to stop the body producing uric acid, used in the treatment of gout

**all or none law** /ˌɔːl ɔː ˈnʌn lɔː/ *noun* the rule that the heart muscle either contracts fully or does not contract at all

**allylestrenol** /ˌælaɪlˈestrənɒl/ *noun* a steroid used to encourage pregnancy

**alopecia** /ˌæləʊˈpiːʃə/ *noun* a condition in which hair is lost. Compare **hypotrichosis**

**alopecia areata** /æləʊˌpiːʃə ˌæriˈeɪtə/ *noun* a condition in which the hair falls out in patches

**alpha** /ˈælfə/ *noun* the first letter of the Greek alphabet

**alpha-adrenoceptor antagonist** /ˌælfə ə ˌdriːnəʊˈseptə ænˌtægənɪst/, **alpha-adrenoceptor blocker** /ˈælfə əˌdriːnəʊˈseptə ˌblɒkə/ *noun* a drug which can relax smooth muscle, used to treat urinary retention and hypertension. Also called **alpha blocker**

**alpha cell** /ˈælfə sel/ *noun* a type of cell found in the islets of Langerhans, in the pancreas, which produces glucagon, a hormone that raises the level of glucose in the blood. ◊ **beta cell**

**alpha-fetoprotein** /ˌælfə ˌfiːtəʊˈprəʊtiːn/ *noun* a protein produced by the liver of the human fetus, which accumulates in the amniotic fluid. A high or low concentration is tested for by amniocentesis in the antenatal diagnosis of spina bifida or Down's syndrome, respectively.

**alpha rhythm** /ˈælfə ˌrɪðəm/ *noun* the pattern of electrical activity in the brain of someone who is awake but relaxed or sleepy, registering on an electroencephalograph at 8–13 hertz

**Alport's syndrome** /ˈɔːlpɔːts ˌsɪndrəʊm/ *noun* a genetic disease of the kidneys which sometimes causes a person to lose his or her hearing and sight

**alprostadil** /ælˈprɒstədɪl/ *noun* a drug which makes blood vessels wider, used to treat impotence, prevent coagulation, and maintain babies with congenital heart conditions

**ALS** *abbr* **1.** amyotrophic lateral sclerosis **2.** antilymphocytic serum

**ALT** *abbr* alanine aminotransferase

**alternative medicine** /ɔːlˌtɜːnətɪv ˈmed(ə)sɪn/ *noun* the treatment of illness using therapies such as homoeopathy or naturopathy which are not considered part of conventional Western medicine. ◊ **complementary medicine**

**altitude sickness** /ˈæltɪtjuːd ˌsɪknəs/ *noun* a condition caused by reduced oxygen in the air above altitudes of 7000 to 8000 feet (3600 metres). Symptoms include headaches, breathlessness, fatigue, nausea and swelling of the face, hands and feet. Also called **high-altitude sickness, mountain sickness**

**aluminium** /ˌæləˈmɪniəm/ *noun* a metallic element extracted from the ore bauxite (NOTE: The US spelling is **aluminum**. The chemical symbol is **Al**.)

**aluminium hydroxide** /æləˌmɪniəm haɪ ˈdrɒksaɪd/ *noun* a chemical substance used as an antacid to treat indigestion. Formula: $Al(OH)_3$ or $Al_2O_3.3H_2O$.

**alveolar** /ˌælvɪˈəʊlə, ælˈviːələ/ *adjective* referring to the alveoli

**alveolar bone** /ˌælvɪˈəʊlə bəʊn/ *noun* part of the jawbone to which the teeth are attached

**alveolar duct** /ˌælvɪˈəʊlə dʌkt/ *noun* a duct in the lung which leads from the respiratory bronchioles to the alveoli. See illustration at LUNGS in Supplement

**alveolar wall** /ˌælvɪˈəʊlə wɔːl/ *noun* one of the walls which separate the alveoli in the lungs

**alveolitis** /ˌælviəˈlaɪtɪs/ *noun* inflammation of an alveolus in the lungs or the socket of a tooth

**alveolus** /ˌælvɪˈəʊləs, ælˈviːələs/ *noun* a small cavity, e.g. an air sac in the lungs or the socket into which a tooth fits. See illustration at LUNGS in Supplement (NOTE: The plural is **alveoli**.)

**Alzheimer plaque** /ˈæltshaɪmə plæk/ *noun* a disc-shaped plaque of amyloid found in the brain in people who have Alzheimer's disease

**Alzheimer's disease** /ˈæltshaɪməz dɪˌziːz/ *noun* a disease where a person experiences progressive dementia due to nerve cell loss in specific brain areas, resulting in loss of mental faculties including memory [Described 1906. After Alois Alzheimer (1864–1915), Bavarian physician.]

COMMENT: No single cause of Alzheimer's disease has been identified, although an early onset type occurs more frequently in some families, due to a mutation in a gene on chromosome 21. Risk factors include age, genes, head injury, lifestyle and environment.

**amalgam** /əˈmælgəm/ *noun* a mixture of metals, based on mercury and tin, used by dentists to fill holes in teeth

**amaurosis** /ˌæmɔːˈrəʊsɪs/ *noun* blindness caused by disease of the optic nerve

**amaurosis fugax** /ˌæmɔːˈrəʊsɪs ˈfjuːɡæks/ *noun* temporary blindness in one eye, caused by problems of circulation

**amaurotic familial idiocy** /ˌæmɔːˈrɒtɪk fə ˌmɪliəl ˈɪdiəsi/, **amaurotic family idiocy** /ˌæmɔːˈrɒtɪk ˌfæm(ə)li ˈɪdiəsi/ *noun* same as **Tay-Sachs disease**

**amb-** /æmb/ *prefix* same as **ambi-** (*used before vowels*)

**ambi-** /æmbi/ *prefix* both

**ambidextrous** /ˌæmbɪˈdekstrəs/ *adjective* referring to a person who can use both hands equally well and who is not right- or left-handed

**ambiguous genitalia** /æmˌbɪɡjuəs ˌdʒenɪ ˈteɪliə/ *noun* a congenital condition in which the outer genitals do not look typical of those of either sex

**ambisexual** /ˌæmbɪˈsekʃuəl/ *adjective, noun* same as **bisexual**

**amblyopia** /ˌæmbliˈəʊpiə/ *noun* a lack of normal vision without a structural cause. A common example is squint and other forms may be caused by the cyanide in tobacco smoke or by drinking methylated spirits.

**amblyopic** /ˌæmbliˈɒpɪk/ *adjective* affected by amblyopia

**amblyoscope** /ˈæmbliəʊskəʊp/ *noun* an instrument for measuring the angle of a squint and how effectively someone uses both their eyes together. Also called **orthoptoscope**

**ambulance** /ˈæmbjʊləns/ *noun* a van for taking sick or injured people to hospital ○ *The injured man was taken away in an ambulance.* ○ *The telephone number of the local ambulance service is in the phone book.* ◊ **St John Ambulance Association and Brigade**

**ambulant** /ˈæmbjələnt/ *adjective* able to walk

**ambulation** /ˌæmbjuˈleɪʃ(ə)n/ *noun* walking □ **early ambulation is recommended** patients should try to get out of bed and walk about as soon as possible after the operation

**ambulatory** /ˌæmbjuˈleɪt(ə)ri/ *adjective* referring to a patient who is not confined to bed but is able to walk

'…ambulatory patients with essential hypertension were evaluated and followed up at the hypertension clinic' [*British Medical Journal*]

**ambulatory care** /ˌæmbjuˌleɪt(ə)ri ˈkeə/ *noun* treatment of a patient which does not involve staying in hospital during the night

**ambulatory fever** /ˌæmbjuˈleɪt(ə)ri ˌfiːvə/ *noun* a mild fever where the patient can walk about and can therefore act as a carrier, e.g. during the early stages of typhoid fever

**ameba** /əˈmiːbə/ *noun US* same as **amoeba**

**amelia** /əˈmiːliə/ *noun* the absence of a limb from birth, or a condition in which a limb is short from birth

**amelioration** /əˌmiːliəˈreɪʃ(ə)n/ *noun* the process of getting better

**ameloblastoma** /ˌæmɪləʊblæˈstəʊmə/ *noun* a tumour in the jaw, usually in the lower jaw

**amenorrhoea** /eɪˌmenəˈriːə/ *noun* the absence of one or more menstrual periods, usual during pregnancy and after the menopause

**ametropia** /ˌæmɪˈtrəʊpiə/ *noun* a condition in which the eye cannot focus light correctly onto the retina, as in astigmatism, hypermetropia and myopia. Compare **emmetropia**

**amfetamine** /æmˈfetəmiːn/ *noun* an addictive drug, similar to adrenaline, used to give a feeling of wellbeing and wakefulness. Also called **amphetamine**

**amikacin** /ˌæmɪˈkeɪsɪn/ *noun* a type of antibiotic used to treat infections caused by aerobic bacteria

**amiloride** /əˈmɪləraɪd/ *noun* a drug which helps to increase the production of urine and preserve the body's supply of potassium

**amino acid** /əˌmiːnəʊ ˈæsɪd/ *noun* a chemical compound which is broken down from proteins in the digestive system and then used by the body to form its own protein

COMMENT: Amino acids all contain carbon, hydrogen, nitrogen and oxygen, as well as other elements. Some amino acids are produced in the body itself, but others have to be absorbed from food. The eight essential amino acids are: isoleucine, leucine, lysine, methionine, phenylalanine, threonine, tryptophan and valine.

**aminobutyric acid** /əˌmiːnəʊbjʊtɪrɪk ˈæsɪd/ *noun* ♦ **gamma aminobutyric acid**

**aminoglycoside** /əˌmiːnəʊˈɡlaɪkəsaɪd/ *noun* a drug used to treat many Gram-negative and some Gram-positive bacterial infections (NOTE: Aminoglycosides include drugs with names ending in **-cin**: **gentamicin**.)

**aminophylline** /ˌæmɪˈnɒfɪliːn/ *noun* a drug that makes the bronchial tubes wider, used in the treatment of asthma

**amiodarone** /ˌæmiˈɒdərəʊn/ *noun* a drug that makes the blood vessels wider, used in the treatment of irregular heartbeat

**amitosis** /ˌæmɪˈtəʊsɪs/ *noun* the multiplication of a cell by splitting of the nucleus

**amitriptyline** /ˌæmɪˈtrɪptɪliːn/ *noun* a sedative drug used to treat depression and persistent pain

**amlodipine** /æmˈlɒdɪpiːn/ *noun* a drug that helps to control the movement of calcium ions through cell membranes. It is used to treat hypertension and angina.

**ammonia** /əˈməʊniə/ *noun* a gas with a strong smell, a compound of nitrogen and hydrogen, which is a usual product of human metabolism

**ammonium** /əˈməʊniəm/ *noun* an ion formed from ammonia

**amnesia** /æmˈniːziə/ *noun* loss of memory

**amnia** /ˈæmniə/ plural of **amnion**

**amnihook** /'æmnihʊk/ *noun* a hooked instrument used to induce labour by pulling on the amniotic sac

**amnio** /'æmniəʊ/ *noun* same as **amniocentesis** (*informal*)

**amniocentesis** /ˌæmniəʊsen'tiːsɪs/ *noun* a procedure which involves taking a test sample of the amniotic fluid during pregnancy using a hollow needle and syringe

COMMENT: Amniocentesis and amnioscopy, the examination and testing of the amniotic fluid, give information about possible congenital disorders in the fetus as well as the sex of the unborn baby.

**amniography** /ˌæmni'ɒɡrəfi/ *noun* an X-ray of the womb

**amnion** /'æmniən/ *noun* the thin sac containing the amniotic fluid which covers an unborn baby in the uterus. Also called **amniotic sac**

**amnioscope** /'æmniəskəʊp/ *noun* an instrument used to examine a fetus through the cervical channel, before the amniotic sac is broken

**amnioscopy** /ˌæmni'ɒskəpi/ *noun* an examination of the amniotic fluid during pregnancy

**amniotic** /ˌæmni'ɒtɪk/ *adjective* relating to the amnion

**amniotic cavity** /ˌæmniɒtɪk 'kævɪti/ *noun* a space formed by the amnion, full of amniotic fluid

**amniotic fluid** /ˌæmniɒtɪk 'fluːɪd/ *noun* the fluid contained in the amnion which surrounds an unborn baby

**amniotic sac** /ˌæmniɒtɪk 'sæk/ *noun* same as **amnion**

**amniotomy** /ˌæmni'ɒtəmi/ *noun* a puncture of the amnion to help induce labour

**amoeba** /ə'miːbə/ *noun* a form of animal life, made up of a single cell (NOTE: The plural is **amoebae**.)

**amoebiasis** /ˌæmɪ'baɪəsɪs/ *noun* an infection caused by amoebae which can result in amoebic dysentery in the large intestine (intestinal amoebiasis) and sometimes affects the lungs (pulmonary amoebiasis)

**amoebic** /ə'miːbɪk/ *adjective* relating to or caused by amoebae

**amoebic dysentery** /əˌmiːbɪk 'dɪs(ə)ntri/ *noun* a form of dysentery mainly found in tropical areas that is caused by *Entamoeba histolytica* which enters the body through contaminated water or unwashed food

**amoebicide** /ə'miːbɪsaɪd/ *noun* a substance which kills amoebae

**amorphous** /ə'mɔːfəs/ *adjective* with no regular shape

**amoxicillin** /əˈmɒksɪsɪlɪn/ *noun* an antibiotic

**Amoxil** /ə'mɒksɪl/ a trade name for amoxicillin

**amphetamine** /æm'fetəmiːn/ *noun* same as **amfetamine**

**amphetamine abuse** /æm'fetəmiːn əˌbjuːs/ *noun* the repeated addictive use of amphetamines which in the end affects the mental faculties

**amphiarthrosis** /ˌæmfiɑː'θrəʊsɪs/ *noun* a joint which only has limited movement, e.g. one of the joints in the spine

**amphotericin** /ˌæmfəʊ'terɪsɪn/ *noun* an antifungal agent, used against *Candida*

**ampicillin** /ˌæmpɪ'sɪlɪn/ *noun* a type of penicillin, used as an antibiotic

**ampoule** /'æmpuːl/, **ampule** /'æmpjuːl/ *noun* a small glass container, closed at the neck, used to contain sterile drugs for use in injections

**ampulla** /æm'pʊlə/ *noun* a swelling of a canal or duct, shaped like a bottle (NOTE: The plural is **ampullae**.)

**amputate** /'æmpjʊteɪt/ *verb* to remove a limb or part of a limb in a surgical operation ○ *The patient's leg needs to be amputated below the knee.* ○ *After gangrene set in, surgeons had to amputate her toes.*

**amputation** /ˌæmpjʊ'teɪʃ(ə)n/ *noun* the surgical removal of a limb or part of a limb

**amputee** /ˌæmpjʊ'tiː/ *noun* someone who has had a limb or part of a limb removed in a surgical operation

**amygdala** /ə'mɪɡdələ/ *noun* an almond-shaped body in the brain, at the end of the caudate nucleus of the thalamus. Also called **amygdaloid body**

**amygdaloid body** /ə'mɪɡdəlɔɪd ˌbɒdi/ *noun* same as **amygdala**

**amyl-** /æm(ə)l/ *prefix* referring to starch

**amylase** /'æmɪleɪz/ *noun* an enzyme which converts starch into maltose

**amyl nitrate** /ˌæm(ə)l 'naɪtreɪt/ *noun* a drug used to reduce blood pressure (NOTE: Amyl nitrate is also used as a recreational drug.)

**amyloid** /'æmɪlɔɪd/ *noun* a waxy protein that forms in some tissues during the development of various diseases, e.g. forming disc-shaped plaques in the brain in Alzheimer's disease

**amyloid disease** /'æmɪlɔɪd dɪˌziːz/ *noun* same as **amyloidosis**

**amyloidosis** /ˌæmɪlɔɪ'dəʊsɪs/ *noun* a disease of the kidneys and liver, where amyloid develops in the tissues. Also called **amyloid disease**

**amyloid precursor protein** /ˌæmɪlɔɪd priˈkɜːsə ˌprəʊtiːn/ *noun* a compound found in cell membranes from which beta amyloid is derived. A mutation of the gene causes early-onset Alzheimer's disease in a few families.

**amylopsin** /ˌæmɪ'lɒpsɪn/ *noun* an enzyme which converts starch into maltose

**amylose** /'æmɪləʊz/ *noun* a carbohydrate of starch

**amyotonia** /ˌeɪmaɪə'təʊniə/ *noun* a lack of muscle tone

**amyotonia congenita** /ˌeɪmaɪətəʊniə kən'dʒenɪtə/ *noun* a congenital disease of children in which the muscles lack tone. Also called **floppy baby syndrome**

**amyotrophia** /eɪˌmaɪə'trəʊfiə/ *noun* a condition in which a muscle wastes away

**amyotrophic lateral sclerosis** /eɪˌmaɪətrɒfɪk ˌlætər(ə)l sklə'rəʊsɪs/ *noun* a motor neurone disease in which the limbs twitch and the muscles gradually waste away. Also called **Gehrig's disease**. Abbr **ALS**

**amyotrophy** /eɪˌmaɪ'ɒtrəfi/ same as **amyotrophia**

**an-** /æn/ *prefix* same as **ana-** (*used before vowels*)

**ana-** /ænə/ *prefix* without or lacking

**anabolic** /ˌænə'bɒlɪk/ *adjective* referring to a substance which synthesises protein

'...insulin, secreted by the islets of Langerhans, is the body's major anabolic hormone, regulating the metabolism of all body fuels and substrates' [*Nursing Times*]

**anabolic steroid** /ænəˌbɒlɪk 'stɪərɔɪd/ *noun* a drug which encourages the synthesis of new living tissue, especially muscle, from nutrients

**anabolism** /æ'næbəlɪz(ə)m/ *noun* the process of building up complex chemical substances on the basis of simpler ones

**anacrotism** /ə'nækrətɪz(ə)m/ *noun* a second stroke in the pulse

**anaemia** /ə'niːmiə/ *noun* a condition in which the level of red blood cells is less than usual or where the haemoglobin is less, making it more difficult for the blood to carry oxygen. The symptoms are tiredness and pale colour, especially pale lips, nails and the inside of the eyelids. The condition can be fatal if not treated. (NOTE: The US spelling is **anemia**.)

**anaemic** /ə'niːmɪk/ *adjective* having anaemia (NOTE: The US spelling is **anemic**.)

**anaerobe** /'ænərəʊb, æn'eərəʊb/ *noun* a microorganism which lives without oxygen, e.g. the tetanus bacillus

**anaerobic** /ˌænə'rəʊbɪk/ *adjective* **1.** not needing oxygen for metabolism ○ *anaerobic bacteria* **2.** without oxygen ○ *anaerobic conditions*

**anaesthesia** /ˌænəs'θiːziə/ *noun* **1.** a state, deliberately produced in a patient by a medical procedure, in which he or she can feel no pain, either in a part or in the whole of the body **2.** a loss of feeling caused by damage to nerves (NOTE: The US spelling is **anesthesia**.)

**anaesthesiologist** /ˌænəsθiːzi'ɒlədʒɪst/ *noun* US a specialist in the study of anaesthetics

**anaesthetic** /ˌænəs'θetɪk/ *adjective* inducing loss of feeling ■ *noun* a substance given to someone to remove feeling, so that he or she can undergo an operation without pain

'Spinal and epidural anaesthetics can also cause gross vasodilation, leading to heat loss' [*British Journal of Nursing*]

**anaesthetic induction** /ˌænəsθetɪk ɪn'dʌkʃən/ *noun* a method of inducing anaesthesia in a patient

**anaesthetic risk** /ˌænəsθetɪk 'rɪsk/ *noun* the risk that an anaesthetic may cause serious unwanted side effects

**anaesthetise** /ə'niːsθətaɪz/, **anaesthetize** *verb* to produce a loss of feeling in a person or in part of the person's body

**anaesthetist** /ə'niːsθətɪst/ *noun* a specialist who administers anaesthetics

**anal** /'eɪn(ə)l/ *adjective* relating to the anus

**anal canal** /ˌeɪn(ə)l kə'næl/ *noun* a passage leading from the rectum to the anus

**analeptic** /ˌænə'leptɪk/ *noun* a drug used to make someone regain consciousness or to stimulate a patient

**anal fissure** /ˌeɪn(ə)l 'fɪʃə/ *noun* a crack in the mucous membrane of the wall of the anal canal

**anal fistula** /ˌeɪn(ə)l 'fɪstjʊlə/ *noun* a fistula which develops between the rectum and the outside of the body after an abscess near the anus. Also called **fistula in ano**

**analgesia** /ˌæn(ə)l'dʒiːziə/ *noun* a reduction of the feeling of pain without loss of consciousness

**analgesic** /ˌæn(ə)l'dʒiːzɪk/ *adjective* relating to analgesia ■ *noun* a painkilling drug which produces analgesia and reduces pyrexia

COMMENT: There are two types of analgesic: non-opioid such as paracetamol and aspirin (acetylsalicylic acid), and opioid such as codeine phosphate. Opioid analgesics are used for severe pain relief such as in terminal care, as cough suppressants and to reduce gut motility in cases of diarrhoea. Analgesics are commonly used as local anaesthetics, for example in dentistry.

**anally** /'eɪn(ə)li/ *adverb* through the anus ○ *The patient is not able to pass faeces anally.*

**anal passage** /ˌeɪn(ə)l 'pæsɪdʒ/ *noun* same as **anus**

**anal sphincter** /ˌeɪn(ə)l 'sfɪŋktə/ *noun* a strong ring of muscle which closes the anus

**anal triangle** /ˌeɪn(ə)l 'traɪæŋg(ə)l/ *noun* the posterior part of the perineum. Also called **rectal triangle**

**analyse** /'ænəlaɪz/ *verb* to examine something in detail ○ *The laboratory is analysing the blood samples.* ○ *When the food was analysed it was found to contain traces of bacteria.* (NOTE: The US spelling is **analyze**.)

**analyser** /'ænəlaɪzə/ *noun* a machine which analyses blood or tissue samples automatically (NOTE: The US spelling is **analyzer**.)

**analysis** /ə'næləsɪs/ *noun* an examination of a substance to find out what it is made of (NOTE: The plural is **analyses**.)

**analyst** /'ænəlɪst/ *noun* **1.** a person who examines samples of substances or tissue, to find out what they are made of **2.** same as **psychoanalyst**

**anamnesis** /ˌænæm'niːsɪs/ *noun* someone's medical history, especially given in their own words

**anamnestic** /ˌænæm'nestɪk/ *adjective* showing a secondary immunological response to an antigen some time after immunisation

**anaphase** /'ænəfeɪz/ *noun* a stage in cell division, after the metaphase and before the telophase

**anaphylactic** /ˌænəfɪ'læktɪk/ *adjective* relating to or caused by extreme sensitivity to a substance

**anaphylactic shock** /ˌænəfɪlæktɪk 'ʃɒk/ *noun* a sudden severe reaction, which can be fatal, to something such as an injected substance or a bee sting

**anaphylaxis** /ˌænəfɪ'læksɪs/ *noun* **1.** extreme sensitivity to a substance introduced into the body **2.** same as **anaphylactic shock**

**anaplasia** /ˌænə'pleɪsiə/ *noun* the loss of a cell's typical characteristics, caused by cancer

**anaplastic** /ˌænə'plæstɪk/ *adjective* referring to anaplasia

**anaplastic neoplasm** /ˌænəplæstɪk 'niːəʊplæz(ə)m/ *noun* a cancer where the cells are not similar to those of the tissue from which they come

**anarthria** /æn'ɑːθriə/ *noun* the loss of the ability to speak words properly

**anasarca** /ˌænə'sɑːkə/ *noun* the presence of fluid in the body tissues. ◊ **oedema**

**anastomose** /ə'næstəməʊz/ *verb* to join two blood vessels or tubular structures together

**anastomosis** /əˌnæstə'məʊsɪs/ *noun* a connection made between two blood vessels or tubular structures, either naturally or by surgery

**anat.** *abbr* **1.** anatomical **2.** anatomy

**anatomical** /ˌænə'tɒmɪk(ə)l/ *adjective* relating to the anatomy ○ *the anatomical features of a fetus*

**anatomical position** /ˌænətɒmɪk(ə)l pə'zɪʃ(ə)n/ *noun* in anatomy, the standard position of the body from which all directions and positions are derived. The body is assumed to be standing, with the feet together, the arms to the side, and the head, eyes and palms facing forward.

**anatomy** /ə'nætəmi/ *noun* **1.** the structure, especially the internal structure, of the body **2.** the branch of science that studies the structure of the bodies of humans, animals and plants ○ *They are studying anatomy.* □ **the anatomy of a bone** a description of the structure and shape of a bone

**ancillary staff** /æn'sɪləri stɑːf/ *noun* the staff in a hospital who are not administrators, doctors or nurses, e.g. cleaners, porters, kitchen staff

**ancillary worker** /æn'sɪləri ˌwɜːkə/ *noun* someone who does a job for patients such cooking or cleaning which is supplementary to medical care

**anconeus** /æŋ'kəʊniəs/ *noun* a small triangular muscle at the back of the elbow

**Ancylostoma** /ˌænsɪlə'stəʊmə/ *noun* a parasitic worm in the intestine which holds onto the wall of the intestine with its teeth and lives on the blood and protein of the carrier

**ancylostomiasis** /ˌænsɪləʊstə'maɪəsɪs/ *noun* a disease of which the symptoms are weakness and anaemia, caused by a hookworm which lives on the blood of the carrier. In severe cases the person may die.

**androgen** /'ændrədʒən/ *noun* a male sex hormone, testosterone or androsterone, which increases the characteristics of the body

**androgenic** /ˌændrə'dʒenɪk/ *adjective* producing male characteristics

**androgynous** /ˌæn'drɒdʒənəs/ *adjective* same as **hermaphrodite**

**andrology** /æn'drɒlədʒi/ *noun* the study of male sexual characteristics and subjects such as impotence, infertility and the male menopause

**androsterone** /æn'drɒstərəʊn/ *noun* one of the male sex hormones

**anemia** /ə'niːmiə/ *noun* US same as **anaemia**

**anencephalous** /ˌænen'kefələs/ *adjective* having no brain

**anencephaly** /ˌænen'kefəli/ *noun* the absence of a brain, which causes a fetus to die a few hours after birth

**anergy** /'ænədʒi/ *noun* **1.** a state of severe weakness and lack of energy **2.** lack of immunity

**anesthesia, etc** /ˌænəs'θiːʒə/ US same as **anaesthesia, etc**

**aneurine** /ə'njʊərɪn/ *noun* same as **Vitamin B₁**

**aneurysm** /'ænjərɪz(ə)m/ *noun* a swelling caused by the weakening of the wall of a blood vessel

COMMENT: Aneurysm usually occurs in the wall of the aorta, 'aortic aneurysm', and is often due to atherosclerosis, and sometimes to syphilis.

**angi-** /ændʒi/ *prefix* same as **angio-** (*used before vowels*)

**angiectasis** /ˌændʒi'ektəsɪs/ *noun* a swelling of the blood vessels

**angiitis** /ˌændʒi'aɪtɪs/ *noun* an inflammation of a blood vessel

**angina** /æn'dʒaɪnə/ *noun* a pain in the chest following exercise or eating, which is caused by an inadequate supply of blood to the heart muscles because of narrowing of the arteries.

It is commonly treated with nitrates or calcium channel blocker drugs.

**anginal** /æn'dʒaɪnəl/ *adjective* referring to angina ○ *He suffered anginal pains.*

**angina pectoris** /æn,dʒaɪnə 'pektərɪs/ *noun* same as **angina**

**angio-** /ændʒiəʊ/ *prefix* referring to a blood vessel

**angiocardiogram** /,ændʒiəʊ'kɑːdiəgræm/ *noun* a series of pictures resulting from angiocardiography

**angiocardiography** /,ændʒiəʊkɑːdi'ɒgrəfi/ *noun* an X-ray examination of the cardiac system after injection with an opaque dye so that the organs show up clearly on the film

**angiodysplasia** /,ændʒiəʊdɪs'pleɪziə/ *noun* a condition where the blood vessels in the colon dilate, resulting in loss of blood

**angiogenesis** /,ændʒiəʊ'dʒenəsɪs/ *noun* the formation of new blood vessels, e.g. in an embryo or as a result of a tumour

**angiogram** /'ændʒiəʊgræm/ *noun* an X-ray picture of blood vessels

**angiography** /,ændʒi'ɒgrəfi/ *noun* an X-ray examination of blood vessels after injection with an opaque dye so that they show up clearly on the film

**angiology** /,ændʒi'ɒlədʒi/ *noun* the branch of medicine which deals with blood vessels and the lymphatic system

**angioma** /,ændʒi'əʊmə/ *noun* a benign tumour formed of blood vessels, e.g. a naevus

**angioneurotic oedema** /,ændʒiəʊnjʊˌrɒtɪk ɪ'diːmə/ *noun* a sudden accumulation of liquid under the skin, similar to nettle rash

**angiopathy** /,ændʒi'ɒpəθi/ *noun* a disease of vessels such as blood and lymphatic vessels

**angioplasty** /'ændʒiəʊˌplæsti/ *noun* plastic surgery to repair a blood vessel, e.g. a narrowed coronary artery

**angiosarcoma** /,ændʒiəʊsɑː'kəʊmə/ *noun* a malignant tumour in a blood vessel

**angioscope** /'ændʒiəʊskəʊp/ *noun* a long thin surgical instrument threaded into a patient's blood vessels to allow surgeons to observe and perform operations without making large incisions

**angiospasm** /'ændʒiəʊspæz(ə)m/ *noun* a spasm which constricts blood vessels

**angiotensin** /'ændʒiəʊtensɪn/ *noun* a polypeptide which affects blood pressure by causing vasoconstriction and increasing extracellular volume

COMMENT: The precursor protein, alpha-2-globulin is converted to angiotensin I, which is inactive. A converting enzyme changes angiotensin I into the active form, angiotensin II . Drugs which block the conversion to the active form, ACE inhibitors, are used in the treatment of hypertension and heart failure.

**angiotensin-converting enzyme inhibitor** /,ændʒiəʊtensɪn kən,vɜːtɪŋ 'enzaɪm ɪn,hɪbɪtə/ *noun* a drug which inhibits the conversion of angiotensin I to angiotensin II, which constricts arteries, used in the treatment of hypertension and heart failure. Also called **ACE inhibitor** (NOTE: ACE inhibitors have names ending in **-pril: captopril**.)

COMMENT: Contraindications include use with diuretics, when hypotension can occur and should be avoided in patients with renovascular disease.

**angle-closure glaucoma** /,æŋgəl ,kləʊʒə glɔː'kəʊmə/ *noun* an unusually high pressure of fluid inside the eyeball caused by pressure of the iris against the lens, trapping the aqueous humour. Also called **acute glaucoma**

**angular stomatitis** /,æŋgjʊlə ,stəʊmə'taɪtɪs/ *noun* a condition of the lips, mouth and cheeks characterised by cracks and fissures and caused by a bacterial infection

**angular vein** /'æŋgjʊlə veɪn/ *noun* a vein which continues the facial vein at the side of the nose

**anhedonia** /,ænhɪ'dəʊniə/ *noun* a psychological condition in which a person is unable to enjoy all the experiences that most people enjoy

**anhidrosis** /,ænhɪ'drəʊsɪs/ *noun* a condition in which sweating by the body is reduced or stops completely

**anhidrotic** /,ænhɪ'drɒtɪk/ *adjective* referring to a drug which reduces sweating

**anhydraemia** /,ænhaɪ'driːmiə/ *noun* a lack of sufficient fluid in the blood

**anhydrous** /æn'haɪdrəs/ *adjective* referring to compounds or crystals that contain no water

**anhydrous alcohol** /,ænhaɪdrəs 'ælkəhɒl/ *noun* same as **absolute alcohol**

**anidrosis** /,ænɪ'drəʊsɪs/ *noun* same as **anhidrosis**

**aniridia** /,ænɪ'rɪdiə/ *noun* a congenital absence of the iris

**anisocytosis** /,ænaɪsəʊsaɪ'təʊsɪs/ *noun* a variation in size of red blood cells

**anisomelia** /,ænaɪsəʊ'miːliə/ *noun* a difference in length of the legs

**anisometropia** /,ænaɪsəʊmə'trəʊpiə/ *noun* a state where the refraction in the two eyes is different

**ankle** /'æŋkəl/ *noun* the part of the body where the foot is connected to the leg □ **he twisted his ankle, he sprained his ankle** he hurt it by stretching it or bending it

**anklebone** /'æŋkəlˌbəʊn/ *noun* same as **talus**

**ankle jerk** /'æŋkəl dʒɜːk/ *noun* a sudden jerk as a reflex action of the foot when the back of the ankle is tapped

**ankle joint** /'æŋkəl dʒɔɪnt/ *noun* a joint which connects the bones of the lower leg (the tibia and fibula) to the talus

**ankyloblepharon** /ˌæŋkɪləʊˈblefərɒn/ noun a state where the edges of the eyelids are stuck together

**ankylose** /ˈæŋkɪləʊz/ verb to fuse together, or to cause bones to fuse together

**ankylosing spondylitis** /ˌæŋkɪləʊzɪŋ spɒndɪˈlaɪtɪs/ noun a condition occurring more frequently in young men, in which the vertebrae and sacroiliac joints are inflamed and become stiff

**ankylosis** /ˌæŋkɪˈləʊsɪs/ noun a condition in which the bones of a joint fuse together

**Ankylostoma** /ˌæŋkɪlˈstəʊmə/ noun same as **Ancylostoma**

**ankylostomiasis** /ˌæŋkɪləʊstəˈmaɪəsɪs/ noun same as **ancylostomiasis**

**ANLL** abbr acute nonlymphocytic leukaemia

**annular** /ˈænjʊlə/ adjective shaped like a ring

**annulus** /ˈænjʊləs/ noun a structure shaped like a ring

**ano-** /ænəʊ/ prefix referring to the anus

**anococcygeal** /ˌænəkɒksɪˈdʒiːəl/ adjective referring to both the anus and coccyx

**anodyne** /ˈænədaɪn/ noun a drug which reduces pain, e.g. aspirin or codeine ■ adjective referring to drugs that bring relief from pain or discomfort

**anomalous** /əˈnɒmələs/ adjective different from what is usual

**anomalous pulmonary venous drainage** /əˌnɒmələs ˌpʌlmən(ə)ri ˈviːnəs ˌdreɪ↓ nɪdʒ/ noun a condition in which oxygenated blood from the lungs drains into the right atrium instead of the left

**anomaly** /əˈnɒməli/ noun something which is different from the usual

**anomie** /ˈænəmi/ noun a psychological condition in which a person develops the feeling of not being part of the everyday world, and behaves as though they do not have any supporting social or moral framework

**anonychia** /ˌænəˈnɪkiə/ noun a congenital absence of one or more nails

**anopheles** /əˈnɒfəliːz/ noun a mosquito which carries the malaria parasite

**anoplasty** /ˈeɪnəʊplæsti/ noun surgery to repair the anus, as in treating haemorrhoids

**anorchism** /ænˈɔːkɪz(ə)m/ noun a congenital absence of testicles

**anorectal** /ˌeɪnəʊˈrekt(ə)l/ adjective referring to both the anus and rectum

**anorectic** /ˌænəˈrektɪk/ noun a medicine that suppresses the appetite ■ adjective relating to life-threatening loss of appetite

**anorexia** /ˌænəˈreksiə/ noun loss of appetite

**anorexia nervosa** /ænəˌreksiə nɜːˈvəʊsə/ noun a psychological condition, usually found in girls and young women, in which a person refuses to eat because of a fear of becoming fat

**anorexic** /ˌænəˈreksɪk/ adjective 1. referring to anorexia 2. having anorexia ○ The school has developed a programme of counselling for anorexic students.

**anosmia** /ænˈɒzmiə/ noun the lack of the sense of smell

**anovulant** /ænˈɒvjələnt/ noun a drug that prevents ovulation, e.g. a birth-control pill

**anovular** /ænˈɒvjʊlə/ adjective without an ovum

**anovular bleeding** /ænˌɒvjʊlə ˈbliːdɪŋ/ noun bleeding from the uterus when ovulation has not taken place

**anovulation** /ænˌɒvjʊˈleɪʃ(ə)n/ noun a condition in which a women does not ovulate and is therefore infertile

**anoxaemia** /ˌænɒkˈsiːmiə/ noun a reduction of the amount of oxygen in the blood

**anoxia** /ænˈɒksiə/ noun a lack of oxygen in body tissue

**anoxic** /ænˈɒksɪk/ adjective referring to anoxia or lacking oxygen

**anserina** /ˌænsəˈraɪnə/ ♦ **cutis anserina**

**antacid** /æntˈæsɪd/ adjective preventing too much acid forming in the stomach or altering the amount of acid in the stomach ■ noun a substance that stops too much acid forming in the stomach, used in the treatment of gastrointestinal conditions such as ulcers, e.g. calcium carbonate or magnesium trisilicate

**antagonism** /ænˈtæɡənɪz(ə)m/ noun 1. the opposing force that usually exists between pairs of muscles 2. the interaction between two or more chemical substances in the body that reduces the effect that each substance has individually

**antagonist** /ænˈtæɡənɪst/ adjective 1. referring to a muscle which opposes another muscle in a movement 2. referring to a substance which opposes another substance ■ noun a substance which acts through specific receptors to block the action of another substance, but which has no observable physiological effect itself ○ Atropine is a cholinergic antagonist and blocks the effects of acetylcholine.

**ante-** /ænti/ prefix before

**ante cibum** /ˌænti ˈtʃɪbəm, ˌænti ˈsiːbəm/ adverb full form of **a.c.**

**anteflexion** /ˌæntiˈflekʃən/ noun the curving forward of an organ, e.g. the usual curvature of the uterus

**antegrade amnesia** /ˌæntiɡreɪd æm ˈniːziə/ noun a form of memory loss relating to the things that happen after a traumatic event

**antemortem** /ˌæntiˈmɔːtəm/ noun the period before death

**antenatal** /ˌæntiˈneɪt(ə)l/ adjective during the period between conception and childbirth

**antenatal clinic** /ˌæntiˈneɪt(ə)l ˌklɪnɪk/ noun a clinic where expectant mothers are taught how to look after babies, do exercises and have medical checkups. Also called **maternity clinic**

**antenatal diagnosis** /ˌænti ˌneɪt(ə)l ˌdaɪəg
'nəʊsɪs/ *noun* a medical examination of a
pregnant woman to see if the fetus is developing in the usual way. Also called **prenatal diagnosis**

**antepartum** /ˌænti'pɑːtəm/ *noun* the period
of three months before childbirth ■ *adjective*
referring to the three months before childbirth

**antepartum haemorrhage** /ˌæntipɑːtəm
'hemərɪdʒ/ *noun* bleeding from the vagina before labour. Abbr **APH**

**anterior** /æn'tɪəriə/ *adjective* in front. Opposite **posterior**

**anterior aspect** /æn,tɪəriə 'æspekt/ *noun* a
view of the front of the body, or of the front of
part of the body. See illustration at **ANATOMICAL
TERMS** in Supplement

**anterior chamber** /æn,tɪəriə 'tʃeɪmbə/
*noun* part of the aqueous chamber of the eye
which is in front of the iris

**anterior fontanelle** /æn,tɪəriə fɒntə'nel/
*noun* the cartilage at the top of the head where
the frontal bone joins the two parietals

**anterior jugular** /æn,tɪəriə 'dʒʌgjʊlə/ *noun*
a small jugular vein in the neck

**anterior nares** /æn,tɪəriə 'neəriːz/ *plural
noun* the two nostrils. Also called **external
nares**

**anterior superior iliac spine** /æn,tɪəriə
sʊ,pɪəriə 'ɪliæk spaɪn/ *noun* a projection at
the front end of the iliac crest of the pelvis

**anterior synechia** /æn,tɪəriə sɪ'nekiə/
*noun* a condition of the eye, where the iris
sticks to the cornea

**anterograde amnesia** /ˌæntərəʊgreɪd æm
'niːziə/ *noun* a brain condition in which the
person cannot remember things which happened recently

**anteversion** /ˌænti'vɜːʃ(ə)n/ *noun* the tilting
forward of an organ, whether usual, as of the
uterus, or unusual

**anthelmintic** /ˌænθel'mɪntɪk/ *noun* a substance which removes worms from the intestine ■ *adjective* removing worms from the intestine

**anthracosis** /ˌænθrə'kəʊsɪs/ *noun* a lung
disease caused by breathing coal dust

**anthrax** /'ænθræks/ *noun* a disease of cattle
and sheep which can be transmitted to humans

COMMENT: Caused by *Bacillus anthracis*, anthrax can be transmitted by touching infected
skin, meat or other parts of an animal, including bone meal used as a fertiliser. It causes
pustules on the skin or in the lungs, 'woolsorter's disease'.

**anthrop-** /ænθrəp/ *prefix* referring to human
beings

**anthropometry** /ˌænθrə'pɒmətri/ *noun* the
study of human body measurements (NOTE:
The uses of anthropometry include the design of
ergonomic furniture and the examination and
comparison of populations.)

**anti-** /ænti/ *prefix* against

**antiallergenic** /ˌæntiælə'dʒenɪk/ *adjective*
referring to something such as a cosmetic
which will not aggravate an allergy

**antiarrhythmic** /ˌæntieɪ'rɪðmɪk/ *adjective*
referring to a drug which corrects an irregular
heartbeat

**antiasthmatic** /ˌæntiæs'mætɪk/ *adjective*
referring to a drug that is used to treat asthma

**antibacterial** /ˌæntibæk'tɪəriəl/ *adjective*
destroying bacteria

**antibiogram** /ˌænti'baɪəgræm/ *noun* a laboratory technique which establishes to what degree an organism is sensitive to an antibiotic

**antibiotic** /ˌæntibaɪ'ɒtɪk/ *adjective* stopping
the spread of bacteria ■ *noun* a drug which is
developed from living substances and which
stops the spread of bacteria, e.g. penicillin ○
*He was given a course of antibiotics.* ○ *Antibiotics have no effect against viral diseases.*

COMMENT: Penicillin is one of the commonest
antibiotics, together with streptomycin, tetracycline, erythromycin and many others. Although antibiotics are widely and successfully
used, new forms of bacteria have developed
which are resistant to them.

**antibody** /'æntɪbɒdi/ *noun* a protein that is
stimulated by the body to produce foreign substances such as bacteria, as part of an immune
reaction ○ *Tests showed that he had antibodies
in his blood.*

**antibody-negative** /ˌæntɪbɒdi 'negətɪv/
*adjective* showing none of a particular antibody in the blood ○ *The donor tested antibody-negative.*

**antibody-positive** /ˌæntɪbɒdi 'pɒzɪtɪv/ *adjective* showing the presence of particular antibodies in the blood ○ *The patient is HIV antibody-positive.*

**anti-cancer drug** /ˌænti 'kænsə drʌg/ *noun*
a drug which can control or destroy cancer
cells

**anticholinergic** /ˌæntikəʊlɪ'nɜːdʒɪk/ *adjective* blocking nerve impulses which are part of
the stress response ■ *noun* one of a group of
drugs which are used to control stress

**anticholinesterase** /ˌæntikəʊlɪn'estəreɪz/
*noun* a substance which blocks nerve impulses
by reducing the activity of the enzyme
cholinesterase

**anticoagulant** /ˌæntikəʊ'ægjʊlənt/ *adjective* slowing or stopping the clotting of blood ■
*noun* a drug which slows down or stops the
clotting of blood, used to prevent the formation of a thrombus (NOTE: Anticoagulants have
names ending in **-parin**: **heparin**.)

**anticonvulsant** /ˌæntikən'vʌls(ə)nt/ *adjective* acting to control convulsions ■ *noun* a
drug used to control convulsions, as in the
treatment of epilepsy, e.g. carbamazepine

**anti-D** /ˌænti 'diː/, **anti-D gamma-globulin**
/ænti ˌdiː ˌgæmə 'glɒbjʊlɪn/ *noun* Rh D im-

munoglobulin, used to treat pregnant women who develop antibodies when the mother is Rh-negative and the fetus is Rh-positive

**antidepressant** /ˌæntidɪˈpres(ə)nt/ *adjective* acting to relieve depression ■ *noun* a drug used to relieve depression by stimulating the mood of a depressed person. Examples are tricyclic antidepressants, selective serotonin reuptake inhibitors and monoamine oxidase inhibitors.

**antidiabetic** /ˌæntidaɪəˈbetɪk/ *noun* a drug used in the treatment of diabetes ■ *adjective* referring to an antidiabetic drug

**antidiarrhoeal** /ˌæntidaɪəˈriːəl/ *noun* a drug used in the treatment of diarrhoea ■ *adjective* referring to an antidiarrhoeal drug (NOTE: [all senses] The US spelling is **antidiarrheal**.)

**anti-D immunoglobulin** /ˌænti ˌdiː ɪm junəʊˈɡlɒbjʊlɪn/ *noun* immunoglobulin administered to Rh-negative mothers after the birth of an Rh-positive baby, to prevent haemolytic disease of the newborn in the next pregnancy

**antidiuretic** /ˌæntidaɪjʊˈretɪk/ *noun* a substance which stops the production of excessive amounts of urine ○ *hormones which have an antidiuretic effect on the kidneys* ■ *adjective* preventing the excessive production of urine

**antidiuretic hormone** /ˌæntidaɪjʊˌretɪk ˈhɔːməʊn/ *noun* a hormone secreted by the posterior lobe of the pituitary gland which acts on the kidneys to regulate the quantity of salt in body fluids and the amount of urine excreted by the kidneys. Also called **vasopressin**

**antidote** /ˈæntɪdəʊt/ *noun* a substance which counteracts the effect of a poison ○ *There is no satisfactory antidote to cyanide.*

**antiembolic** /ˌæntiemˈbɒlɪk/ *adjective* preventing embolism

**antiemetic** /ˌæntiɪˈmetɪk/ *noun* a drug which prevents vomiting ■ *adjective* acting to prevent vomiting

**antiepileptic drug** /ˌæntiepɪˈleptɪk drʌɡ/ *noun* a drug used in the treatment of epilepsy and convulsions, e.g. carbamazepine

**antifibrinolytic** /ˌæntifaɪbrɪnəˈlɪtɪk/ *adjective* acting to reduce fibrosis

**antifungal** /ˌæntiˈfʌŋɡəl/ *adjective* referring to a substance which kills or controls fungal and yeast infections, e.g. candida and ringworm (NOTE: Antifungal drugs have names ending in **-conazole: fluconazole**.)

**antigen** /ˈæntɪdʒən/ *noun* a substance that stimulates the body to produce antibodies, e.g. a protein on the surface of a cell or microorganism

**antigenic** /ˌæntɪˈdʒenɪk/ *adjective* referring to a substance which stimulates the formation of antibodies

**antihaemophilic factor** /ˌæntihiːməˈfɪlɪk ˌfæktə/ *noun* factor VIII, used to encourage blood-clotting in haemophiliacs. Abbr **AHF**

**antihelminthic** /ˌæntihelˈmɪnθɪk/ *noun* a drug used in the treatment of worm infections such as threadworm, hookworm or roundworm

**antihistamine** /ˌæntiˈhɪstəmiːn/ *noun* a drug used to control the effects of an allergy which releases histamine, or reduces gastric acid in the stomach for the treatment of gastric ulcers (NOTE: Antihistamines have names ending in **-tidine: loratidine** for allergies, **cimetidine** for gastric ulcers.)

**anti-HIV antibody** /ˌænti ˌeɪtʃ aɪ viː ˈænti bɒdi/ *noun* an antibody which attacks HIV

**antihypertensive** /ˌæntihaɪpəˈtensɪv/ *adjective* acting to reduce blood pressure ■ *noun* a drug used to reduce high blood pressure

**anti-inflammatory** /ˌænti ɪnˈflæmət(ə)ri/ *adjective* referring to a drug which reduces inflammation

**antilymphocytic serum** /ˌæntilɪmfəʊˈsɪtɪk ˌsɪərəm/ *noun* a serum used to produce immunosuppression in people undergoing transplant operations. Abbr **ALS**

**antimalarial** /ˌæntiməˈleəriəl/ *noun* a drug used to treat malaria and in malarial prophylaxis ■ *adjective* treating or preventing malaria

**antimetabolite** /ˌæntiməˈtæbəlaɪt/ *noun* a substance which can replace a cell metabolism, but which is not active

**antimicrobial** /ˌæntimaɪˈkrəʊbiəl/ *adjective* acting against microorganisms that cause disease

**antimigraine** /ˌæntiˈmaɪɡreɪn/ *noun* a drug used in the treatment of migraine

**antimitotic** /ˌæntimaɪˈtɒtɪk/ *adjective* preventing the division of a cell by mitosis

**antimuscarinic** /ˌæntimʌskəˈrɪnɪk/ *adjective* referring to a drug which blocks acetylcholine receptors found on smooth muscle in the gut and eye

**antimycotic** /ˌæntimaɪˈkɒtɪk/ *adjective* destroying fungi

**antinauseant** /ˌæntiˈnɔːziənt/ *adjective* referring to a drug which helps to suppress nausea

**antioxidant** /ˌæntiˈɒksɪd(ə)nt/ *noun* a substance which makes oxygen less damaging, e.g. in the body or in foods or plastics ○ *antioxidant vitamins*

**antiperistalsis** /ˌæntiperɪˈstælsɪs/ *noun* a movement in the oesophagus or intestine which causes their contents to move in the opposite direction to usual peristalsis, so leading to vomiting

**antiperspirant** /ˌæntiˈpɜːsp(ə)rənt/ *noun* a substance which prevents sweating ■ *adjective* preventing sweating

**antipruritic** /ˌæntɪprʊˈrɪtɪk/ *noun* a substance which prevents itching ■ *adjective* preventing itching

**antipsychotic** /ˌæntɪsaɪˈkɒtɪk/ *noun* a neuroleptic or major tranquilliser drug which calms disturbed people without causing sedation or confusion by blocking dopamine receptors in the brain

COMMENT: Extrapyramidal side-effects can occur from the use of antipsychotics, including Parkinsonian symptoms and restlessness.

**antipyretic** /ˌæntɪpaɪˈretɪk/ *noun* a drug which helps to reduce a fever ■ *adjective* reducing fever

**anti-Rh body** /ˌænti ɑːr ˈeɪtʃ ˌbɒdi/ *noun* an antibody formed in a mother's blood in reaction to a Rhesus antigen in the blood of the fetus

**antisepsis** /ˌæntɪˈsepsɪs/ *noun* a procedure intended to prevent sepsis

**antiseptic** /ˌæntɪˈseptɪk/ *adjective* preventing harmful microorganisms from spreading ○ *She gargled with an antiseptic mouthwash.* ■ *noun* a substance which prevents germs growing or spreading ○ *The nurse painted the wound with antiseptic.*

**antiserum** /ˌæntiˈsɪərəm/ *noun* ◈ **serum** (NOTE: The plural is **antisera**.)

**antisocial** /ˌæntiˈsəʊʃ(ə)l/ *adjective* referring to behaviour which is harmful to other people

**antispasmodic** /ˌæntispæzˈmɒdɪk/ *noun* a drug used to prevent spasms

**antitetanus serum** /ˌænti'tetənəs ˌsɪərəm/ *noun* a serum which protects a patient against tetanus. Abbr **ATS**

**antithrombin** /ˌænti'θrɒmbɪn/ *noun* a substance present in the blood which prevents clotting

**antitoxic serum** /ˌænti'tɒksɪk ˌsɪərəm/ *noun* an immunising agent, formed of serum taken from an animal which has developed antibodies to a disease, used to protect a person from that disease

**antitoxin** /ˌæntiˈtɒksɪn/ *noun* an antibody produced by the body to counteract a poison in the body

**antitragus** /ˌæntiˈtreɪgəs/ *noun* a small projection on the outer ear opposite the tragus

**antituberculous drug** /ˌæntitjʊˈbɜːkjʊləs drʌg/ *noun* a drug used to treat tuberculosis, e.g. Isoniazid or rifampicin

**antitussive** /ˌæntiˈtʌsɪv/ *noun* a drug used to reduce coughing

**antivenin** /ˌæntiˈvenɪn/, **antivenom** /ˌænti ˈvenəm/, **antivenene** /ˌæntivəˈniːn/ *noun* a substance which helps the body to fight the effects of a particular venom from a snake or insect bite

**antiviral** /ˌæntiˈvaɪrəl/ *adjective* referring to a drug or treatment which stops or reduces the damage caused by a virus ■ *noun* same as **antiviral drug**

**antiviral drug** /ˌæntiˈvaɪrəl drʌg/ *noun* a drug which is effective against a virus (NOTE: Antiviral drugs have names ending in **-ciclovir**.)

**antra** /ˈæntrə/ plural of **antrum**

**antral** /ˈæntrəl/ *adjective* referring to an antrum

**antral puncture** /ˌæntrəl ˈpʌŋktʃə/ *noun* making a hole in the wall of the maxillary sinus to remove fluid

**antrectomy** /ænˈtrektəmi/ *noun* the surgical removal of an antrum in the stomach to prevent gastrin being formed

**antroscopy** /ænˈtrɒskəpi/ *noun* an examination of an antrum

**antrostomy** /ænˈtrɒstəmi/ *noun* a surgical operation to make an opening in the maxillary sinus to drain an antrum

**antrum** /ˈæntrəm/ *noun* any cavity inside the body, especially one in bone (NOTE: The plural is **antra**.)

**anuria** /ænˈjʊəriə/ *noun* a condition in which the patient does not make urine, either because of a deficiency in the kidneys or because the urinary tract is blocked

**anus** /ˈeɪnəs/ *noun* a short passage after the rectum at the end of the alimentary canal, leading outside the body between the buttocks and through which faeces are passed. See illustration at DIGESTIVE SYSTEM in Supplement, UROGENITAL SYSTEM (MALE) in Supplement (NOTE: For other terms referring to the anus, see **anal** and words beginning with **ano-**.)

**anvil** /ˈænvɪl/ *noun* same as **incus**

**anxiety** /æŋˈzaɪəti/ *noun* the state of being very worried and afraid

**anxiety disorder** /æŋˈzaɪəti dɪsˌɔːdə/ *noun* a mental disorder where someone is very worried and afraid, e.g. a phobia

**anxiety neurosis** /æŋˈzaɪəti njʊˌrəʊsɪs/ *noun* a neurotic condition where the patient is anxious and has morbid fears

**anxiolytic** /ˌæŋksiəˈlɪtɪk/ *noun* a drug used in the treatment of anxiety ■ *adjective* treating anxiety

**anxious** /ˈæŋkʃəs/ *adjective* **1.** very worried and afraid ○ *My sister is ill – I am anxious about her.* **2.** eager ○ *She was anxious to get home.* ○ *I was anxious to see the doctor.*

**aorta** /eɪˈɔːtə/ *noun* the main artery in the body, which sends blood containing oxygen from the heart to other blood vessels around the body. See illustration at HEART in Supplement

COMMENT: The aorta is about 45 centimetres long. It leaves the left ventricle, rises where the carotid arteries branch off, then goes downwards through the abdomen and divides into the two iliac arteries. The aorta is the blood vessel which carries all arterial blood from the heart.

**aortic** /eɪˈɔːtɪk/ *adjective* relating to the aorta

**aortic aneurysm** /eɪˌɔːtɪk ˈænjə,rɪz(ə)m/ *noun* a serious aneurysm of the aorta, associated with atherosclerosis

**aortic arch** /eɪˈɔːtɪk ɑːtʃ/ *noun* a bend in the aorta which links the ascending aorta to the descending aorta

**aortic hiatus** /eɪˌɔːtɪk haɪˈeɪtəs/ *noun* an opening in the diaphragm through which the aorta passes

**aortic incompetence** /eɪˌɔːtɪk ˈɪnkɒmpɪt(ə)ns/ *noun* a condition in which the aortic valve does not close properly, causing regurgitation

**aortic regurgitation** /eɪˌɔːtɪk rɪˌɡɜːdʒɪˈteɪʃ(ə)n/ *noun* a backward flow of blood caused by a malfunctioning aortic valve

**aortic sinuses** /eɪˌɔːtɪk ˈsaɪnəsɪz/ *plural noun* swellings in the aorta from which the coronary arteries lead back into the heart itself

**aortic stenosis** /eɪˌɔːtɪk steˈnəʊsɪs/ *noun* a condition in which the aortic valve is narrow, caused by rheumatic fever

**aortic valve** /eɪˌɔːtɪk ˈvælv/ *noun* a valve with three flaps, situated at the opening into the aorta

**aortitis** /ˌeɪɔːˈtaɪtɪs/ *noun* inflammation of the aorta

**aortography** /ˌeɪɔːˈtɒɡrəfi/ *noun* an X-ray examination of the aorta after an opaque substance has been injected into it

**a.p.** *adverb* before a meal. Full form **ante prandium**

**apathetic** /ˌæpəˈθetɪk/ *adjective* referring to a person who takes no interest in anything

**apathy** /ˈæpəθi/ *noun* the condition of not being interested in anything, or of not wanting to do anything

**aperient** /əˈpɪəriənt/ *noun* a substance which causes a bowel movement, e.g. a laxative or purgative ■ *adjective* causing a bowel movement

**aperistalsis** /ˌeɪperɪˈstælsɪs/ *noun* a lack of the peristaltic movement in the bowel

**Apert's syndrome** /ˈæpɜːts ˌsɪndrəʊm/ *noun* a condition in which the skull grows tall and the lower part of the face is underdeveloped

**aperture** /ˈæpətʃə/ *noun* a hole

**apex** /ˈeɪpeks/ *noun* **1.** the top of the heart or lung **2.** the end of the root of a tooth

**apex beat** /ˈeɪpeks biːt/ *noun* a heartbeat which can be felt if the hand is placed on the heart

**Apgar score** /ˈæpɡɑː skɔː/ *noun* a method of judging the condition of a newborn baby in which the baby is given a maximum of two points on each of five criteria: colour of the skin, heartbeat, breathing, muscle tone and reaction to stimuli [Described 1952. After Virginia Apgar (1909–74), US anaesthesiologist.]

'…in this study, babies having an Apgar score of four or less had 100% mortality. The lower the Apgar score, the poorer the chance of survival' [*Indian Journal of Medical Sciences*]

**APH** *abbr* antepartum haemorrhage

**aphagia** /eɪˈfeɪdʒiə/ *noun* a condition in which a person is unable to swallow

**aphakia** /eɪˈfeɪkiə/ *noun* the absence of the crystalline lens in the eye

**aphakic** /eɪˈfeɪkɪk/ *adjective* referring to aphakia

**aphasia** /eɪˈfeɪziə/ *noun* a condition in which a person is unable to speak or write, or to understand speech or writing because of damage to the brain centres controlling speech

**apheresis** /ˌæfəˈriːsɪs/ *noun* the transfusion of blood, from which some components have been removed, back into a patient

**aphonia** /eɪˈfəʊniə/ *noun* a condition in which a person is unable to make sounds

**aphrodisiac** /ˌæfrəˈdɪziæk/ *noun* a substance which increases sexual urges ■ *adjective* increasing sexual desire

**aphtha** /ˈæfθə/ *noun* a small white ulcer which appears in groups in the mouth in people who have the fungal condition thrush (NOTE: The plural is **apthae**.)

**aphthous stomatitis** /ˌæfθəs ˌstəʊməˈtaɪtɪs/ *noun* canker sores which affect the mucous membrane in the mouth

**aphthous ulcer** /ˌæfθəs ˈʌlsə/ *noun* same as **mouth ulcer**

**apical** /ˈæpɪk(ə)l/ *adjective* situated at the top or tip of something

**apical abscess** /ˌæpɪk(ə)l ˈæbses/ *noun* an abscess in the socket around the root of a tooth

**apicectomy** /ˌæpɪˈsektəmi/ *noun* the surgical removal of the root of a tooth

**aplasia** /eɪˈpleɪziə/ *noun* a lack of growth of tissue

**aplastic** /eɪˈplæstɪk/ *adjective* unable to develop new cells or tissue

**aplastic anaemia** /eɪˌplæstɪk əˈniːmiə/ *noun* anaemia caused by the bone marrow failing to form red blood cells

**apnea** /æpˈniːə/ *noun US* same as **apnoea**

**apneusis** /æˈpnuːsɪs/ *noun* a breathing pattern caused by brain damage, in which each breath is held for a long time

**apnoea** /æpˈniːə/ *noun* the stopping of breathing (NOTE: The US spelling is **apnea**.)

**apnoeic** /æpˈniːɪk/ *adjective* where breathing has stopped (NOTE: The US spelling is **apneic**.)

**apocrine** /ˈæpəkraɪn/ *adjective* referring to apocrine glands

**apocrine gland** /ˈæpəkraɪn ɡlænd/ *noun* a gland producing body odour where parts of the gland's cells break off with the secretions, e.g. a sweat gland

**apocrinitis** /ˌæpəkrɪˈnaɪtɪs/ *noun* the formation of abscesses in the sweat glands

**apolipoprotein E** /əˌpɒlɪpəprəʊtiːn 'iː/ *noun* a compound found in three varieties which transport lipids within the cell and across cell membranes, the genes for two of which are linked with increased risk of Alzheimer's disease. Abbr **ApoE**

**apomorphine** /ˌæpəʊ'mɔːfiːn/ *noun* a substance that comes from morphine, used to make a person cough, sleep or be sick (NOTE: It is administered under the skin and is used to treat drug overdose, accidental poisoning and Parkinson's disease.)

**aponeurosis** /ˌæpəʊnjʊ'rəʊsɪs/ *noun* a band of tissue which attaches muscles to each other

**apophyseal** /æpə'fɪziəl/ *adjective* referring to apophysis

**apophysis** /ə'pɒfəsɪs/ *noun* a growth of bone, not at a joint

**apophysitis** /æpɒfɪ'saɪtɪs/ *noun* inflammation of an apophysis

**apoplexy** /'æpəpleksi/ *noun* same as **cerebrovascular accident** (*dated*)

**apoptosis** /ə'pɒptəsɪs/ *noun* a form of cell death that is necessary both to make room for new cells and to remove cells whose DNA has been damaged and which may become cancerous

**APP** *abbr* amyloid precursor protein

**apparatus** /ˌæpə'reɪtəs/ *noun* equipment used in a laboratory or hospital ○ *The hospital has installed new apparatus in the physiotherapy department.* ○ *The blood sample was tested in a special piece of apparatus.* (NOTE: No plural: use *a piece of apparatus*; *some new apparatus*.)

**appendage** /ə'pendɪdʒ/ *noun* a part of the body or piece of tissue which hangs down from another part

**appendectomy** /ˌæpən'dektəmi/ *noun US* same as **appendicectomy**

**appendiceal** /ˌæpən'dɪsiəl/ *adjective* relating to the appendix ○ *There is a risk of appendiceal infection.*

**appendiceal colic** /ˌæpəndɪsiəl 'kɒlɪk/ *noun* colic caused by an inflamed appendix

**appendicectomy** /əˌpendɪ'sektəmi/ *noun* the surgical removal of an appendix

**appendicitis** /əˌpendɪ'saɪtɪs/ *noun* inflammation of the vermiform appendix

COMMENT: Appendicitis takes several forms. In **acute appendicitis** there is a sudden attack of severe pain in the right lower part of the abdomen, accompanied by a fever. Acute appendicitis usually requires urgent surgery. In **chronic appendicitis**, the appendix is slightly inflamed, giving a dull pain or a feeling of indigestion over a period of time (a 'grumbling appendix').

**appendicular** /ˌæpən'dɪkjʊlə/ *adjective* **1.** referring to body parts which are associated with the arms and legs **2.** relating to the appendix

**appendicular skeleton** /ˌæpən'dɪkjʊlə ˌskelɪt(ə)n/ *noun* part of the skeleton, formed of the pelvic girdle, pectoral girdle and the bones of the arms and legs. Compare **axial skeleton**

**appendix** /ə'pendɪks/ *noun* **1.** a small tube attached to the caecum which serves no function but can become infected, causing appendicitis. Also called **vermiform appendix**. See illustration at DIGESTIVE SYSTEM in Supplement **2.** any small tube or sac hanging from an organ

**apperception** /ˌæpə'sepʃ(ə)n/ *noun* the conscious recognition of a stimulus

**appetite** /'æpɪtaɪt/ *noun* the feeling of wanting food □ **good appetite** interest in eating food □ **loss of appetite** becoming uninterested in eating food

**applanation tonometry** /æpləˌneɪʃ(ə)n tə 'nɒmətri/ *noun* the measuring of the thickness of the cornea

**appliance** /ə'plaɪəns/ *noun* a piece of apparatus used on the body ○ *He was wearing a surgical appliance to support his neck.*

**application** /ˌæplɪ'keɪʃ(ə)n/ *noun* **1.** the process of putting a medication or bandage on a body part ○ *Two applications of the lotion should be made each day.* **2.** the process of asking officially for something, usually in writing ○ *If you are applying for the job, you must fill in an application form.*

**applicator** /'æplɪkeɪtə/ *noun* an instrument for applying a substance

**appointment** /ə'pɔɪntmənt/ *noun* an arrangement to see someone at a particular time ○ *I have an appointment with the doctor* or *to see the doctor on Tuesday.*

**apposition** /ˌæpə'zɪʃ(ə)n/ *noun* **1.** the relative positioning of two things **2.** cell growth in which layers of new material are deposited on existing ones

**appraisal** /ə'preɪz(ə)l/ *noun* a judgment or opinion on something or somebody, especially one which decides how effective or useful they are

**apprehension** /ˌæprɪ'henʃən/ *noun* a feeling of anxiety or fear that something bad or unpleasant will happen

**approach** /ə'prəʊtʃ/ *noun* **1.** a way of dealing with a problem ○ *The authority has adopted a radical approach to the problem of patient waiting lists.* **2.** a method used by a surgeon when carrying out an operation

**approve** /ə'pruːv/ *verb* □ **to approve of something** to think that something is good ○ *I don't approve of patients staying in bed.* ○ *The Medical Council does not approve of this new treatment.*

**apraxia** /eɪ'præksiə/ *noun* a condition in which someone is unable to make proper movements

**apyrexia** /ˌeɪpaɪˈreksiə/ *noun* the absence of fever

**apyrexial** /ˌeɪpaɪˈreksiəl/ *adjective* no longer having any fever

**aqua** /ˈækwə/ *noun* water

**aqueduct** /ˈækwɪdʌkt/ *noun* a tube which carries fluid from one part of the body to another

**aqueduct of Sylvius** /ˌækwɪdʌkt əv ˈsɪlviəs/ *noun* same as **cerebral aqueduct**

**aqueous** /ˈeɪkwiəs, ˈækwiəs/ *adjective* referring to a solution made with water ■ *noun* a fluid in the eye between the lens and the cornea

**aqueous humour** /ˌeɪkwiəs ˈhjuːmə/ *noun* same as **aqueous**. see illustration at EYE in Supplement

**AR** *abbr* attributable risk

**arachidonic acid** /əˌrækɪdɒnɪk ˈæsɪd/ *noun* an essential fatty acid

**arachnidism** /əˈræknɪdɪz(ə)m/ *noun* poisoning by the bite of a spider

**arachnodactyly** /əˌræknəʊˈdæktɪli/ *noun* a congenital condition in which the fingers and toes are long and thin

**arachnoid** /əˈræknɔɪd/ *noun* the middle of the three membranes covering the brain. ◊ **dura mater**

**arachnoiditis** /əˌræknɔɪˈdaɪtɪs/ *noun* inflammation of the arachnoid

**arachnoid mater** /əˈræknɔɪd ˌmeɪtə/, **arachnoid membrane** /əˈræknɔɪd ˌmembreɪn/ *noun* same as **arachnoid**

**arachnoid villi** /əˌræknɔɪd ˈvɪlaɪ/ *plural noun* villi in the arachnoid which absorb cerebrospinal fluid

**arborisation** /ˌɑːbəraɪˈzeɪʃ(ə)n/, **arborization** *noun* the branching ends of some nerve fibres, of a motor nerve in muscle fibre or of venules, capillaries and arterioles

**arbor vitae** /ˌɑːbə ˈvaɪtiː/ *noun* the structure of the cerebellum or of the uterus which looks like a tree

**arbovirus** /ˈɑːbəʊˌvaɪrəs/ *noun* a virus transmitted by blood-sucking insects

**arc** /ɑːk/ *noun* 1. a nerve pathway 2. part of a curved structure in the body

**ARC** *abbr* AIDS-related complex *or* AIDS-related condition

**arc eye** /ˈɑːk aɪ/ *noun* temporary painful blindness caused by ultraviolet rays, especially in arc welding

**arch** /ɑːtʃ/ *noun* a curved part of the body, especially under the foot

**arch-** /ɑːtʃ/ *prefix* chief, most important

**arcuate** /ˈɑːkjuət/ *adjective* arched

**arcuate artery** /ˈɑːkjuət ˌɑːtəri/ *noun* a curved artery in the foot or kidney

**arcuate ligaments** /ˈɑːkjuət ˌɑːtəri/ *plural noun* three ligaments forming a fibrous arch to which the diaphragm is attached

**arcus** /ˈɑːkəs/ *noun* an arch

**arcus senilis** /ˌɑːkəs səˈnaɪlɪs/ *noun* an opaque circle around the cornea of the eye which can develop in old age

**ARDS** /ɑːdz/ *abbr* adult respiratory distress syndrome

**areata** /ˌæriˈeɪtə/ *noun* ♦ **alopecia areata**

**areola** /əˈriːələ/ *noun* 1. the coloured part round a nipple 2. in the eye, the part of the iris closest to the pupil

**areolar tissue** /əˈriːələ ˌtɪʃuː/ *noun* a type of connective tissue

**arginine** /ˈɑːdʒɪniːn/ *noun* an amino acid which helps the liver form urea

**argon laser** /ˈɑːgɒn ˌleɪzə/ *noun* a laser used in sealing blood vessels and destroying specific lesions

**Argyll Robertson pupil** /ɑːˌgaɪl ˈrɒbətsən ˌpjuːp(ə)l/ *noun* a condition of the eye, in which the lens is able to focus but the pupil does not react to light. It is a symptom of tertiary syphilis or of locomotor ataxia.

**ariboflavinosis** /eɪˌraɪbəʊfleɪvɪˈnəʊsɪs/ *noun* a condition caused by not having enough vitamin $B_2$. The symptoms are very oily skin and hair and small cuts in the mouth.

**arm** /ɑːm/ *noun* the part of the body from the shoulder to the hand, formed of the upper arm, the elbow and the forearm ○ *She broke her arm skiing.* ○ *Lift your arms up above your head.* (NOTE: For other terms referring to the arm see words beginning with **brachi-, brachio-**.)

**arm bones** /ˈɑːm bəʊnz/ *plural noun* the humerus, the ulna and the radius

**armpit** /ˈɑːmpɪt/ *noun* the hollow under the shoulder, between the upper arm and the body, where the upper arm joins the shoulder, containing several important blood vessels, lymph nodes and sweat glands. Also called **axilla**

**arm sling** /ˈɑːm slɪŋ/ *noun* a support for an injured arm that prevents it from moving by tying it against the chest

**Arnold-Chiari malformation** /ˌɑːnəld ki ˈeəri mælfɔːˌmeɪʃ(ə)n/ *noun* a congenital condition in which the base of the skull is malformed, allowing parts of the cerebellum into the spinal canal [Described 1894. After Julius A. Arnold (1835–1915), Professor of Pathological Anatomy at Heidelberg, Germany, and Hans von Chiari (1851–1916), Professor of Pathological Anatomy at Strasbourg and later at Prague, Czech Republic.]

**aromatherapist** /əˌrəʊməˈθerəpɪst/ *noun* a person specialising in aromatherapy

**aromatherapy** /əˌrəʊməˈθerəpi/ *noun* treatment to relieve tension and promote wellbeing in which fragrant oils and creams containing plant extracts are massaged into the skin

**arousal** /əˈraʊz(ə)l/ *noun* 1. feelings and physical signs of sexual desire 2. the act of waking up from sleep, unconsciousness or a drowsy state

**arrector pili** /əˌrektə ˈpaɪlaɪ ˌmʌs(ə)l/ *noun* a small muscle which contracts and makes the hair on the skin stand up when someone is cold or afraid

**arrest** /əˈrest/ *noun* the stopping of a bodily function. ◊ **cardiac arrest**

**arrhythmia** /əˈrɪðmiə/ *noun* a variation in the rhythm of the heartbeat

'Cardiovascular effects may include atrial arrhythmias but at 30°C there is the possibility of spontaneous ventricular fibrillation' [*British Journal of Nursing*]

**arrhythmic** /əˈrɪðmɪk/ *adjective* (*of a heartbeat or breathing*) rhythmically irregular. ◊ **antiarrhythmic**

**arsenic** /ˈɑːsnɪk/ *noun* a chemical element which forms poisonous compounds such as arsenic trioxide and which was formerly used in some medicines (NOTE: The chemical symbol is **As**.)

**ART** *abbr* assisted reproductive technology

**artefact** /ˈɑːtɪfækt/ *noun* something which is made or introduced artificially

**arter-** /ɑːtə/ *prefix* same as **arterio-** (*used before vowels*)

**arterial** /ɑːˈtɪəriəl/ *adjective* relating to arteries □ **arterial supply to the brain** the supply of blood to the brain by the internal carotid arteries and the vertebral arteries

**arterial bleeding** /ɑːˌtɪəriəl ˈbliːdɪŋ/ *noun* bleeding from an artery

**arterial block** /ɑːˈtɪəriəl blɒk/ *noun* the blocking of an artery by a blood clot

**arterial blood** /ɑːˈtɪəriəl blʌd/ *noun* same as **oxygenated blood**

**arterial haemorrhage** /ɑːˈtɪəriəl ˈhem(ə)rɪdʒ/ *noun* a haemorrhage of bright red blood from an artery

**arteriectomy** /ɑːˌtɪəriˈektəmi/ *noun* the surgical removal of an artery or part of an artery

**arterio-** /ɑːtɪəriəʊ/ *prefix* referring to arteries

**arteriogram** /ɑːˈtɪəriəʊgræm/ *noun* an X-ray photograph of an artery, taken after injection with an opaque dye

**arteriography** /ɑːˌtɪəriˈɒgrəfi/ *noun* the work of taking X-ray photographs of arteries after injection with an opaque dye

**arteriole** /ɑːˈtɪəriəʊl/ *noun* a very small artery

**arteriopathy** /ɑːˌtɪəriˈɒpəθi/ *noun* a disease of an artery

**arterioplasty** /ɑːˈtɪəriəʊplæsti/ *noun* plastic surgery to make good a damaged or blocked artery

**arteriorrhaphy** /ɑːˌtɪəriˈɔːrəfi/ *noun* the act of stitching an artery

**arteriosclerosis** /ɑːˌtɪəriəʊskləˈrəʊsɪs/ *noun* the arterial disease atherosclerosis (*dated*)

**arteriosus** /ɑːˌtɪəriˈəʊsəs/ *noun* ♦ **ductus arteriosus**

**arteriotomy** /ɑːˌtɪəriˈɒtəmi/ *noun* a puncture made in the wall of an artery

**arteriovenous** /ɑːˌtɪəriəʊˈviːnəs/ *adjective* referring to both an artery and a vein

**arteritis** /ˌɑːtəˈraɪtɪs/ *noun* inflammation of the walls of an artery

**artery** /ˈɑːtəri/ *noun* a blood vessel taking blood from the heart to the tissues of the body

COMMENT: In most arteries the blood has been oxygenated in the lungs and is bright red in colour. In the pulmonary artery, the blood is deoxygenated and so is darker. The arterial system begins with the aorta which leaves the heart and from which all the arteries branch.

**arthr-** /ɑːθr/ *prefix* same as **arthro-** (*used before vowels*)

**arthralgia** /ɑːˈθrældʒə/ *noun* pain in a joint

**arthrectomy** /ɑːˈθrektəmi/ *noun* the surgical removal of a joint

**arthritic** /ɑːˈθrɪtɪk/ *adjective* affected by or relating to arthritis ○ *She has an arthritic hip.* ■ *noun* a person suffering from arthritis

**arthritis** /ɑːˈθraɪtɪs/ *noun* a painful inflammation of a joint. ◊ **osteoarthritis, rheumatoid arthritis, reactive arthritis**

**arthro-** /ɑːθrəʊ/ *prefix* referring to a joint

**arthroclasia** /ˌɑːθrəʊˈkleɪʒə/ *noun* removal of ankylosis in a joint

**arthrodesis** /ˌɑːθrəʊˈdiːsɪs/ *noun* a surgical operation in which a joint is fused in position, so preventing pain from movement

**arthrodynia** /ˌɑːθrəʊˈdɪniə/ *noun* pain in a joint

**arthrogram** /ˈɑːθrəʊgræm/ *noun* an X-ray of the inside of a damaged joint

**arthrography** /ɑːˈθrɒgrəfi/ *noun* X-ray photography of a joint

**arthrogryposis** /ˌɑːθrəʊgrɪˈpəʊsɪs/ *noun* a group of disorders in which movement becomes progressively restricted

**arthropathy** /ɑːˈθrɒpəθi/ *noun* a disease in a joint

**arthroplasty** /ˈɑːθrəʊplæsti/ *noun* a surgical operation to repair or replace a joint

**arthroscope** /ˈɑːθrəʊskəʊp/ *noun* an instrument which is inserted into the cavity of a joint to inspect it

**arthroscopy** /ɑːˈθrɒskəpi/ *noun* a procedure to examine the inside of a joint by means of an arthroscope

**arthrosis** /ɑːˈθrəʊsɪs/ *noun* the degeneration of a joint

**arthrotomy** /ɑːˈθrɒtəmi/ *noun* a procedure that involves cutting into a joint to drain pus

**articular** /ɑːˈtɪkjʊlə/ *adjective* referring to joints

**articular cartilage** /ɑːˌtɪkjʊlə ˈkɑːtəlɪdʒ/ *noun* a layer of cartilage at the end of a bone where it forms a joint with another bone. See illustration at **BONE STRUCTURE** in Supplement, **SYNOVIAL JOINT** in Supplement

**articular facet** /ɑːˌtɪkjʊlə ˈfæsɪt/ *noun* the point at which a rib articulates with the spine

**articular process** /ɑːˌtɪkjʊlə ˈprəʊses/ *noun* a piece of bone which sticks out of the neural arch in a vertebra and links with the next vertebra

**articulate** /ɑːˈtɪkjʊleɪt/ *verb* to be linked with another bone in a joint

**articulating bone** /ɑːˈtɪkjʊleɪtɪŋ bəʊn/ *noun* a bone which forms a joint

**articulating process** /ɑːˈtɪkjʊleɪtɪŋ ˌprəʊses/ *noun* same as **articular process**

**articulation** /ɑːˌtɪkjʊˈleɪʃ(ə)n/ *noun* a joint or series of joints

**artificial** /ˌɑːtɪˈfɪʃ(ə)l/ *adjective* **1.** made by humans and not a natural part of the body ○ *artificial cartilage* ○ *artificial kidney* ○ *artificial leg* **2.** happening not as a natural process but through action by a doctor or another person or a machine ○ *artificial feeding*

**artificial insemination** /ˌɑːtɪfɪʃ(ə)l ɪnˌsemɪˈneɪʃ(ə)n/ *noun* the introduction of semen into a woman's uterus by artificial means

**artificial insemination by donor** /ˌɑːtɪ↓fɪʃ(ə)l ɪnsemɪˌneɪʃ(ə)n baɪ ˈdəʊnə/ *noun* same as **donor insemination**. Abbr **AID**

**artificial insemination by husband** /ˌɑːtɪfɪʃ(ə)l ɪnsemɪˌneɪʃ(ə)n baɪ ˈhʌzbənd/ *noun* artificial insemination using the semen of the husband. Abbr **AIH**

**artificial lung** /ˌɑːtɪfɪʃ(ə)l ˈlʌŋ/ *noun* a machine through which a person's deoxygenated blood is passed to absorb oxygen to take back to the bloodstream

**artificial pneumothorax** /ˌɑːtɪfɪʃ(ə)l ˌnjuːməʊˈθɔːræks/ *noun* a former method of treating tuberculosis, in which air was introduced between the layers of the pleura to make the lung collapse

**artificial respiration** /ˌɑːtɪfɪʃ(ə)l ˌrespɪˈreɪ↓ɪʃ(ə)n/ *noun* a way of reviving someone who has stopped breathing, e.g. mouth-to-mouth resuscitation

**artificial rupture of membranes** /ˌɑːtɪfɪʃ(ə)l ˌrʌptʃər əv ˈmembreɪnz/ *noun* the breaking of the amniotic sac with an amnihook, so releasing the amniotic fluid

**artificial ventilation** /ˌɑːtɪfɪʃ(ə)l ˌventɪˈleɪʃ(ə)n/ *noun* breathing which is assisted or controlled by a machine

**arytenoid** /ˌærɪˈtiːnɔɪd/ *adjective* located at the back of the larynx

**arytenoid cartilage** /ærɪˈtiːnɔɪd ˌkɑːtɪlɪdʒ/ *noun* a small cartilage at the back of the larynx

**arytenoidectomy** /ˌærɪˌtiːnɔɪdˈektəmi/ *noun* an operation to remove the arytenoid cartilage

**asbestosis** /ˌæsbeˈstəʊsɪs/ *noun* a disease of the lungs caused by inhaling asbestos dust

COMMENT: Asbestos was formerly widely used in cement and cladding and other types of fireproof construction materials. It is now recognised that asbestos dust can cause many lung diseases, leading in some cases to forms of cancer.

**ascariasis** /ˌæskəˈraɪəsɪs/ *noun* a disease of the intestine and sometimes the lungs, caused by infestation with *Ascaris lumbricoides*

**Ascaris lumbricoides** /ˌæskərɪs lʌmbriˈkɔɪdiːz/ *noun* a type of large roundworm which is a parasite in the human intestine

**ascending** /əˈsendɪŋ/ *adjective* going upwards

**ascending aorta** /əˌsendɪŋ eɪˈɔːtə/ *noun* the first section of the aorta as it leaves the heart and turns upwards. Compare **descending aorta**

**ascending colon** /əˌsendɪŋ ˈkəʊlɒn/ *noun* the first part of the colon which goes up the right side of the body from the caecum. Compare **descending colon**. See illustration at **DIGESTIVE SYSTEM** in Supplement

**Aschoff nodules** /ˈæʃɒf ˌnɒdjuːlz/, **Aschoff's nodules** /ˈæʃɒfs ˌnɒdjuːlz/ *plural noun* nodules which are formed mainly in or near the heart in rheumatic fever

**ascites** /əˈsaɪtiːz/ *noun* an unusual accumulation of fluid from the blood in the peritoneal cavity, occurring in heart and kidney failure or as a result of malignancy

**ascorbic acid** /əˌskɔːbɪk ˈæsɪd/ *noun* same as **Vitamin C**

COMMENT: Ascorbic acid is found in fresh fruit, especially oranges and lemons and in vegetables. Lack of Vitamin C can cause anaemia and scurvy.

**ASD** *abbr* autistic spectrum disorders

**-ase** /eɪz, eɪs/ *suffix* enzyme

**asepsis** /eɪˈsepsɪs/ *noun* the absence of microorganisms which cause infection, usually achieved by sterilisation

**aseptic** /eɪˈseptɪk/ *adjective* sterilised, or involving sterilisation, and therefore without infection

**aseptic surgery** /eɪˌseptɪk ˈsɜːdʒəri/ *noun* surgery using sterilised equipment, rather than relying on antiseptic drugs to kill harmful microorganisms. Compare **antiseptic**

**aseptic technique** /eɪˌseptɪk tekˈniːks/ *noun* a method of doing something using sterilised equipment

**asexual** /eɪˈsekʃuəl/ *adjective* not sexual, not involving sexual intercourse

**asexual reproduction** /eɪˌsekʃuəl ˌriːprəˈdʌkʃ(ə)n/ *noun* reproduction of a cell by cloning

**Asian flu** /ˌeɪʒ(ə)n ˈfluː/ *noun* ♦ flu

**-asis** /əsɪs/ ♦ **-iasis**

**asleep** /əˈsliːp/ *adjective* sleeping ○ *The patient is asleep and must not be disturbed.* (NOTE: **Asleep** cannot be used in front of a noun:

the patient is asleep but a sleeping patient.) □ she fell asleep she began to sleep □ fast asleep sleeping deeply

**asparagine** /ə'spærədʒiːn/ *noun* an amino acid

**aspartame** /ə'spɑːteɪm/ *noun* a protein produced from aspartic acid, used to make substances sweeter

**aspartate aminotransferase** /ə,spɑːteɪt ə ,miːnəʊ'trænsfəreɪz/ *noun* an enzyme found in heart muscle, liver cells, skeletal muscle cells and some other tissues. It is used in the diagnosis of liver disease and heart attacks.

**aspartic acid** /ə,spɑːtɪk 'æsɪd/ *noun* an amino acid

**aspect** /'æspekt/ *noun* a direction from which the body is viewed, e.g. the view from above is the 'superior aspect'

**Asperger's syndrome** /'æspɜːdʒəz ,sɪn drəʊm/ *noun* a developmental disorder characterised by difficulty in social interaction and a restricted range of interests, more common in boys than girls [Described 1944. After Hans Asperger (1906–80), Austrian psychiatrist.]

**aspergillosis** /,æspɜːdʒɪ'ləʊsɪs/ *noun* infection of the lungs with the fungus *Aspergillus*

**aspermia** /eɪ'spɜːmiə/ *noun* the absence of sperm in semen

**asphyxia** /æs'fɪksiə/ *noun* a condition in which someone is prevented from breathing, e.g. by strangulation or breathing poisonous gas, and therefore cannot take oxygen into the bloodstream

**asphyxia neonatorum** /æs,fɪksiə ,niːəʊn↓ eɪ'tɔːrəm/ *noun* failure to breathe in a newborn baby

**asphyxiate** /æs'fɪksieɪt/ *verb* to prevent someone from breathing, or be prevented from breathing ○ *An unconscious patient may become asphyxiated* or *may asphyxiate if left lying on his back.* ◊ **suffocate**

**asphyxiation** /əs,fɪksi'eɪʃ(ə)n/ *noun* the state of being prevented from breathing, or the act of preventing someone from breathing. ◊ **suffocation**

**aspirate** /'æspɪreɪt/ *verb* **1.** to remove liquid or gas by suction from a body cavity **2.** to inhale something, especially a liquid, into the lungs

**aspiration** /,æspɪ'reɪʃ(ə)n/ *noun* **1.** the act of removing fluid from a cavity in the body, often using a hollow needle **2.** same as **vacuum suction**

**aspiration pneumonia** /,æspɪreɪʃ(ə)n njuː'məʊniə/ *noun* a form of pneumonia in which infected matter is inhaled from the bronchi or oesophagus

**aspirator** /'æspɪreɪtə/ *noun* an instrument used to suck fluid out of a cavity such as the mouth or the site of an operation

**aspirin** /'æsprɪn/ *noun* a common pain-killing drug, or a tablet containing this drug. Also called **acetylsalicylic acid**

**assay** /'æseɪ, ə'seɪ/ *noun* the testing of a substance. ◊ **bioassay, immunoassay**

**assimilate** /ə'sɪmɪ,leɪt/ *verb* to take into the body's tissues substances which have been absorbed into the blood from digested food

**assimilation** /ə,sɪmɪ'leɪʃ(ə)n/ *noun* the action of assimilating food substances

**assistance** /ə'sɪst(ə)ns/ *noun* help

**assistant** /ə'sɪst(ə)nt/ *noun* a person who helps someone, usually as a job

**assisted conception** /ə,sɪstɪd kən 'sepʃ(ə)n/, **assisted reproduction** /ə,sɪstɪd ,riːprə'dʌkʃ(ə)n/ *noun* the use of a technique such as in vitro fertilisation to help someone to become pregnant

**assisted respiration** /ə,sɪstɪd ,respə'reɪ↓ ɪʃ(ə)n/ *noun* the use of a machine to help breathing

**assisted suicide** /ə,sɪstɪd 'suːɪsaɪd/ *noun* the suicide of someone who is terminally ill with the help of a doctor or friend at the request of the person who is dying

**associate** /ə'səʊsieɪt/ *verb* to be related to or connected with something ○ *side effects which may be associated with the drug* ○ *The condition is often associated with diabetes.*

**associate nurse** /ə,səʊsiət 'nɜːs/ *noun* a nurse who assists a primary nurse by carrying out agreed care for someone based on a plan designed by a primary nurse

**association area** /ə,səʊsi'eɪʃ(ə)n ,eəriə/ *noun* an area of the cortex of the brain which is concerned with relating stimuli coming from different sources

**association neuron** /ə,səʊsi'eɪʃ(ə)n ,njuərɒn/ *noun* a neuron which links an association area to the main parts of the cortex

**association tract** /ə,səʊsi'eɪʃ(ə)n trækt/ *noun* one of the tracts which link areas of the cortex in the same cerebral hemisphere

**asthenia** /æs'θiːniə/ *noun* a condition in which someone is weak and does not have any strength

**asthenic** /æs'θenɪk/ *adjective* referring to a general condition in which someone has no strength and no interest in things

**asthenopia** /,æsθɪ'nəʊpiə/ *noun* same as **eyestrain**

**asthma** /'æsmə/ *noun* a lung condition characterised by narrowing of the bronchial tubes, in which the muscles go into spasm and the person has difficulty breathing. ◊ **cardiac asthma**

**asthmatic** /æs'mætɪk/ *adjective* having the lung disease asthma, or relating to asthma ○ *He has an asthmatic attack every spring.* □ **acute asthmatic attack** a sudden attack of asthma ■ *noun* a person who has asthma

**asthmatic bronchitis** /æsˌmætɪk brɒŋ
ˈkaɪtɪs/ *noun* asthma associated with bronchitis

**asthmaticus** /æsˈmætɪkəs/ *adjective* ♦ **status asthmaticus**

**astigmatic** /ˌæstɪɡˈmætɪk/ *adjective* referring to astigmatism □ **he is astigmatic** he has astigmatism

**astigmatism** /əˈstɪɡmətɪz(ə)m/ *noun* a condition in which the eye cannot focus vertical and horizontal lines simultaneously, leading to blurring of vision

**astragalus** /əˈstræɡələs/ *noun* an old name for the talus (anklebone)

**astringent** /əˈstrɪndʒənt/ *noun* a substance which makes the skin tissues contract and harden ■ *adjective* referring to an astringent

**astrocyte** /ˈæstrəsaɪt/ *noun* a star-shaped cell of the connective tissue of the nervous system

**astrocytoma** /ˌæstrəsaɪˈtəʊmə/ *noun* a type of brain tumour which develops slowly in the connective tissue of the nervous system

**asymmetric** /ˌæsɪˈmetrɪk/ *adjective* shaped or arranged so that the two sides do not match or balance each other

**asymmetry** /æˈsɪmətri/ *noun* a state in which the two sides of the body or of an organ do not resemble each other

**asymptomatic** /ˌeɪsɪmptəˈmætɪk/ *adjective* not showing any symptoms of disease

**asynclitism** /æˈsɪŋklɪtɪz(ə)m/ *noun* in childbirth, a situation in which the head of the baby enters the vagina at an angle

**asynergia** /ˌæsɪˈnɜːdʒə/, **asynergy** /æˈsɪnədʒi/ *noun* awkward movements and bad coordination, caused by a disorder of the cerebellum. Also called **dyssynergia**

**asystole** /eɪˈsɪstəli/ *noun* a state in which the heart has stopped beating

**ataractic** /ˌætəˈræktɪk/ *noun* a drug which has a calming effect ■ *adjective* calming

**ataraxia** /ˌætəˈræksiə/, **ataraxis** /ˌætəˈræksɪs/ *noun* the state of being calm and not worrying

**ataraxic** /ˌætəˈræksɪk/ *noun, adjective* same as **ataractic**

**ataxia** /əˈtæksiə/ *noun* a failure of the brain to control movements

**ataxic** /əˈtæksɪk/ *adjective* having ataxia, or relating to ataxia

**ataxic gait** /əˌtæksɪk ˈɡeɪt/ *noun* a way of walking in which the person walks unsteadily due to a disorder of the nervous system

**ataxy** /əˈtæksi/ *noun* same as **ataxia**

**atelectasis** /ˌætəˈlektəsɪs/ *noun* the failure of a lung to expand properly

**atenolol** /əˈtenəlɒl/ *noun* a drug used in controlling blood pressure and angina

**ateriovenous malformation** /ɑːˌtɪəriəʊ
ˌviːnəs mælfɔːˈmeɪʃ(ə)n/ *noun* a condition in which the arteries and veins in the brain are not properly formed, leading to strokes or epilepsy. Abbr **AVM**

**atherogenesis** /ˌæθerəʊˈdʒenɪsɪs/ *noun* the formation of fatty deposits (**atheromas**) in arteries

**atherogenic** /ˌæθərəʊˈdʒenɪk/ *adjective* referring to something which may produce atheroma

**atheroma** /ˌæθəˈrəʊmə/ *noun* thickening of the walls of an artery by deposits of a fatty substance such as cholesterol

**atheromatous** /ˌæθəˈrɒmətəs/ *adjective* referring to atheroma

**atherosclerosis** /ˌæθərəʊskləˈrəʊsɪs/ *noun* a condition in which deposits of fats and minerals form on the walls of an artery, especially the aorta or one of the coronary or cerebral arteries, and prevent blood from flowing easily

**atherosclerotic** /ˌæθərəʊskləˈrɒtɪk/ *adjective* referring to atherosclerosis

**atherosclerotic plaque** /ˌæθərəʊsklərɒtɪk
ˈplæk/ *noun* a deposit on the walls of arteries

**athetosis** /ˌæθəˈtəʊsɪs/ *noun* repeated slow movements of the limbs, caused by a brain disorder such as cerebral palsy

**athlete's foot** /ˌæθliːts ˈfʊt/ *noun* an infectious skin disorder between the toes, caused by a fungus. Also called **tinea pedis**

**atlas** /ˈætləs/ *noun* the top vertebra in the spine, which supports the skull and pivots on the axis or second vertebra

**atmospheric pressure** /ˌætməsferɪk
ˈpreʃə/ *noun* the pressure of the air on the surface of the Earth

COMMENT: Disorders due to variations in atmospheric pressure include mountain sickness and caisson diseases.

**atomic cocktail** /əˌtɒmɪk ˈkɒkteɪl/ *noun* a radioactive substance in liquid form, used to diagnose or treat cancer (*informal*)

**atomiser** /ˈætəmaɪzə/ *noun* an instrument which sprays liquid in the form of very small drops like mist. Also called **nebuliser**

**atonic** /eɪˈtɒnɪk/ *adjective* referring to lack of muscle tone or tension

**atony** /ˈætəni/ *noun* a lack of tone or tension in the muscles

**atopen** /ˈætəpen/ *noun* an allergen which causes an atopy

**atopic** /eɪˈtɒpɪk/ *adjective* referring to conditions arising from an inherited tendency to react to specific allergens, as in hay fever, some skin conditions and asthma

**atopic eczema** /eɪˌtɒpɪk ˈeksɪmə/, **atopic dermatitis** /eɪˌtɒpɪk dɜːməˈtaɪtɪs/ *noun* a type of eczema often caused by a hereditary allergy

**atopy** /ˈætəpi/ *noun* a hereditary allergic reaction

**ATP** *abbr* adenosine triphosphate

**atracurium** /ˌætrəˈkjʊəriəm/ *noun* a drug used as a relaxant

**atresia** /əˈtriːziə/ *noun* an unusual closing or absence of a tube in the body

**atretic** /əˈtretɪk/ *adjective* referring to atresia

**atretic follicle** /əˌtretɪk ˈfɒlɪk(ə)l/ *noun* the scarred remains of an ovarian follicle

**atri-** /eɪtri/ *prefix* referring to an atrium

**atria** /ˈeɪtriə/ plural of **atrium**

**atrial** /ˈeɪtriəl/ *adjective* referring to one or both of the atria of the heart

**atrial fibrillation** /ˌeɪtriəl faɪbrɪˈleɪʃ(ə)n/ *noun* a rapid uncoordinated fluttering of the atria of the heart, which causes an irregular heartbeat

**atrial septal defect** /ˌeɪtriəl ˈsept(ə)l ˌdiːfekt/ *noun* a congenital condition in which a hole in the wall between the two atria of the heart allows blood to flow through the heart and lungs. Compare **ventricular septal defect**

**atrioventricular** /ˌeɪtriəʊvenˈtrɪkjʊlə/ *adjective* referring to the atria and ventricles

**atrioventricular bundle** /ˌeɪtriəʊven ˌtrɪkjʊlə ˈbʌnd(ə)l/ *noun* a bundle of modified cardiac muscle which conducts impulses from the atrioventricular node to the septum and then divides to connect with the ventricles. Also called **AV bundle, bundle of His**

**atrioventricular groove** /ˌeɪtriəʊven ˌtrɪkjʊlə ˈgruːv/ *noun* a groove round the outside of the heart, showing the division between the atria and ventricles

**atrioventricular node** /ætriəʊvenˈtrɪkjʊlə nəʊd/ *noun* a mass of conducting tissue in the right atrium of the heart, which continues as the atrioventricular bundle, and passes impulses from the atria to the ventricles. Also called **AV node**

**at-risk** /ət ˈrɪsk/ *adjective* exposed to danger or harm of some kind ○ *at-risk children*

**atrium** /ˈeɪtriəm/ *noun* **1.** one of the two upper chambers in the heart. See illustration at HEART in Supplement **2.** a cavity in the ear behind the eardrum (NOTE: The plural is **atria.**)

COMMENT: The two atria in the heart both receive blood from veins. The right atrium receives venous blood from the superior and inferior venae cavae and the left atrium receives oxygenated blood from the pulmonary veins.

**atrophic cirrhosis** /æˌtrɒfɪk sɪˈrəʊsɪs/ *noun* advanced portal cirrhosis in which the liver has become considerably smaller and clumps of new cells are formed on the surface of the liver where fibrous tissue has replaced damaged liver cells. Also called **hobnail liver**

**atrophic gastritis** /æˌtrɒfɪk gæˈstraɪtɪs/ *noun* inflammation of the stomach caused by being unable to produce enough acid to kill bacteria

**atrophic vaginitis** /æˌtrɒfɪk ˌvædʒɪˈnaɪtɪs/ *noun* inflammation, thinning and shrinking of the tissues of the vagina caused by a lack of oestrogen

**atrophy** /ˈætrəfi/ *noun* the wasting of an organ or part of the body ■ *verb* (*of an organ or part of the body*) to waste away

**atropine** /ˈætrəpiːn/ *noun* an alkaloid substance derived from the poisonous plant belladonna and used, among other things, to enlarge the pupil of the eye, to reduce salivary and bronchial secretions during anaesthesia and as a muscarinic antagonist

**ATS** /ˌeɪ tiː ˈes/ *abbr* antitetanus serum

**attack** /əˈtæk/ *noun* a sudden occurrence of an illness ○ *He had an attack of fever.* ○ *She had two attacks of laryngitis during the winter.*

**attempted suicide** /əˌtemptɪd ˈsuːɪsaɪd/ *noun* an unsuccessful attempt to kill oneself

**attending physician** /əˌtendɪŋ fɪˈzɪʃ(ə)n/ *noun* a doctor who is looking after a particular patient ○ *He was referred to the hypertension unit by his attending physician.*

**attention deficit disorder** /əˌtenʃən ˈde fɪsɪt dɪsˌɔːdə/ *noun* a condition in which a person is unable to concentrate, does things without considering their actions properly and has little confidence. It occurs mainly in children. Abbr **ADD**

**attention deficit hyperactivity disorder** /əˌtenʃən ˌdefɪsɪt ˌhaɪpərækˈtɪvɪti dɪs ˌɔːdə/ *noun* a condition in which a child has an inability to concentrate and shows disruptive behaviour. Abbr **ADHD**

**attention deficit syndrome** /əˌtenʃən ˈde fɪsɪt ˌsɪndrəʊm/ *noun* same as **attention deficit disorder**

**attenuation** /əˌtenjuˈeɪʃ(ə)n/ *noun* a reduction in the effect or strength of something such as a virus, either because of environmental conditions or as a result of a laboratory procedure

**atticotomy** /ˌætɪˈkɒtəmi/ *noun* the removal of the wall in the inner ear. Also called **cortical mastoidectomy**

**attitude** /ˈætɪtjuːd/ *noun* **1.** an opinion or general feeling about something ○ *a positive attitude towards the operation* **2.** a way of standing or sitting

**attributable risk** /əˌtrɪbjʊtəb(ə)l ˈrɪsk/ *noun* a measure of the excess risk of disease due to exposure to a particular risk. The excess risk of bacteriuria in oral contraceptive users attributable to the use of oral contraceptives is 1,566 per 100,000. Abbr **AR**

**attrition** /əˈtrɪʃ(ə)n/ *noun* the condition of being worn away, as may be caused by friction ○ *Examination showed attrition of two extensor tendons.*

**atypical** /eɪˈtɪpɪk(ə)l/ *adjective* not usual or expected ○ *an atypical renal cyst*

**audi-** /ɔːdi/ *prefix* same as **audio-** (*used before vowels*)

**audible limits** /ˌɔːdəb(ə)l ˈlɪmɪts/ *plural noun* upper and lower limits of the sound frequencies which can be heard by humans

**audio-** /ɔːdiəʊ/ *prefix* referring to hearing or sound

**audiogram** /ˈɔːdiəʊgræm/ *noun* a graph drawn by an audiometer

**audiologist** /ˌɔːdiˈɒlədʒɪst/ *noun* a specialist who deals in the treatment of hearing disorders

**audiology** /ˌɔːdiˈɒlədʒi/ *noun* the scientific study of hearing, especially for diagnosing and treating hearing loss

**audiometer** /ˌɔːdiˈɒmɪtə/ *noun* an apparatus for testing hearing, especially for testing the range of sounds that the human ear can detect

**audiometry** /ˌɔːdiˈɒmətri/ *noun* the science of testing hearing

**audit** /ˈɔːdɪt/ *noun* a check on figures, scientific data or procedures ○ *a medical audit regarding the outpatient appointment system*

**audit cycle** /ˈɔːdɪt ˌsaɪk(ə)l/ *noun* the cycle in which medical topics are selected for review, observation and comparison with agreed standards and changes are decided on

**auditory** /ˈɔːdɪt(ə)ri/ *adjective* relating to hearing

**auditory acuity** /ˌɔːdɪt(ə)ri əˈkjuːɪti/ *noun* the ability to hear sounds clearly

**auditory canals** /ˌɔːdɪt(ə)ri kəˈnælz/ *plural noun* the external and internal passages of the ear

**auditory nerve** /ˈɔːdɪt(ə)ri nɜːv/ *noun* the eighth cranial nerve which governs hearing and balance. See illustration at EAR in Supplement. Also called **vestibulocochlear nerve**

**auditory ossicles** /ˌɔːdɪt(ə)ri ˈɒsɪk(ə)lz/ *plural noun* the three little bones, the malleus, incus and stapes, in the middle ear

**Auerbach's plexus** /ˌaʊərbɑːks ˈpleksəs/ *noun* a group of nerve fibres in the intestine wall [Described 1862. After Leopold Auerbach (1828–97), Professor of Neuropathology at Breslau, now in Poland.]

**aura** /ˈɔːrə/ *noun* a warning sensation which is experienced before an attack of epilepsy, migraine or asthma

**aural** /ˈɔːrəl/ *adjective* referring to the ear

**aural polyp** /ˌɔːrəl ˈpɒlɪp/ *noun* a polyp in the middle ear

**aural surgery** /ˌɔːrəl ˈsɜːdʒəri/ *noun* surgery on the ear

**auricle** /ˈɔːrɪk(ə)l/ *noun* the tip of each atrium in the heart

**auriculae** /ɔːˈrɪkjʊli/ ♦ **concha auriculae**

**auricular** /ɔːˈrɪkjʊlə/ *adjective* **1.** referring to the ear **2.** referring to an auricle

**auricular vein** /ɔːˈrɪkjʊlə veɪn/ *noun* a vein which leads into the posterior facial vein

**auriscope** /ˈɔːrɪskəʊp/ *noun* an instrument for examining the ear and eardrum. Also called **otoscope**

**auscultation** /ˌɔːskəlˈteɪʃ(ə)n/ *noun* the act of listening to the sounds of the body using a stethoscope

**auscultatory** /ɔːˈskʌltət(ə)ri/ *adjective* referring to auscultation

**Australia antigen** /ɔːˈstreɪliə ˌæntɪdʒən/ *noun* an antigen produced on the surface of liver cells infected with the hepatitis B virus

**autism** /ˈɔːtɪz(ə)m/ *noun* a condition developing in childhood, characterised by difficulty in social interaction, language and communication problems, learning difficulties and obsessional repetitive behaviour (NOTE: Autism is more common in boys than in girls.)

**autistic** /ɔːˈtɪstɪk/ *adjective* affected by, or relating to, autism

**autistic spectrum disorders** /ɔːˌtɪstɪk ˌspektrəm dɪsˈɔːdəz/ *plural noun* autism in all its forms and degrees of severity. Abbr **ASD**

**auto-** /ɔːtəʊ/ *prefix* self

**autoantibody** /ˌɔːtəʊˈæntɪbɒdi/ *noun* an antibody formed to attack antigens in the body's own cells

**autoclavable** /ˈɔːtəʊˌkleɪvəb(ə)l/ *adjective* able to be sterilised in an autoclave ○ *Waste should be put into autoclavable plastic bags.*

**autoclave** /ˈɔːtəʊkleɪv/ *noun* equipment for sterilising surgical instruments using heat under high pressure ■ *verb* to sterilise equipment using heat under high pressure ○ *Autoclaving is the best method of sterilisation.*

**autogenous** /ɔːˈtɒdʒənəs/, **autogenic** /ˌɔːtəʊˈdʒenɪk/ *adjective* produced either in the person's body, or using tissue from the person's own body ○ *an autogenous vein graft*

**autograft** /ˈɔːtəʊɡrɑːft/ *noun* a transplant made using parts of the person's own body

**autoimmune** /ˌɔːtəʊˈɪmjuːn/ *adjective* referring to an immune reaction in a person against antigens in their own cells

**autoimmune disease** /ˌɔːtəʊˌɪmjuːn dɪˈziːz/ *noun* a disease in which the person's own cells are attacked by autoantibodies ○ *Rheumatoid arthritis is thought to be an autoimmune disease.*

**autoimmunisation** /ˌɔːtəʊˌɪmjʊnaɪˈzeɪʃ(ə)n/, **autoimmunization** *noun* the process leading to an immune reaction in a person to antigens produced in their own body

**autoimmunity** /ˌɔːtəʊɪˈmjuːnɪti/ *noun* a condition in which a person's own cells are attacked by autoantibodies

**autoinfection** /ˌɔːtəʊɪnˈfekʃ(ə)n/ *noun* an infection by a microorganism already in the body, or infection of one part of the body by another part

**autointoxication** /ˌɔːtəʊɪntɒksɪˈkeɪʃ(ə)n/ *noun* the poisoning of the body by toxins produced in the body itself

**autologous** /ɔːˈtɒləgəs/ *adjective* referring to a graft or other material coming from the same source

**autologous transfusion** /ɔːˌtɒləgəs trænsˈfjuːʒ(ə)n/ *noun* a blood transfusion in which the blood is removed from the body for later transfusion after an operation. ◊ **transfusion**

**autolysis** /ɔːˈtɒləsɪs/ *noun* a situation in which cells destroy themselves within their own enzymes

**automatic** /ˌɔːtəˈmætɪk/ *adjective* **1.** done without conscious thought ○ *an automatic reaction* **2.** (*of a machine or process*) able to work by itself, without anyone giving instructions

**automatism** /ɔːˈtɒmətɪz(ə)m/ *noun* a state in which a person acts without consciously knowing that he or she is acting

COMMENT: Automatic acts can take place after concussion or epileptic fits. In law, automatism can be a defence to a criminal charge when the accused states that he or she acted without knowing what they were doing.

**autonomic** /ˌɔːtəˈnɒmɪk/ *adjective* governing itself independently

**autonomic nervous system** /ɔːtəˌnɒmɪk ˈnɜːvəs ˌsɪstəm/ *noun* the nervous system formed of ganglia linked to the spinal column. It regulates the automatic functioning of the main organs such as the heart and lungs and works when a person is asleep or even unconscious. ◊ **parasympathetic nervous system, sympathetic nervous system**

**autonomy** /ɔːˈtɒnəmi/ *noun* the state of being free to act as one wishes

**autoplasty** /ˈɔːtəʊplæsti/ *noun* the repair of someone's body using tissue taken from another part of their body

**autopsy** /ˈɔːtɒpsi/ *noun* the examination of a dead body by a pathologist to find out the cause of death ○ *The autopsy showed that he had been poisoned.* Also called **post mortem**

**autosomal** /ˌɔːtəʊˈsəʊm(ə)l/ *adjective* referring to an autosome

**autosome** /ˈɔːtəʊsəʊm/ *noun* a chromosome that is not a sex chromosome

**autotransfusion** /ˌɔːtəʊtrænsˈfjuːʒ(ə)n/ *noun* an infusion into a person of their own blood

**auxiliary** /ɔːgˈzɪliəri/ *adjective* providing help ○ *The hospital has an auxiliary power supply in case the electricity supply breaks down.* ■ *noun* an assistant

**avascular** /eɪˈvæskjʊlə/ *adjective* with no blood vessels, or with a deficient blood supply

**avascular necrosis** /əˌvæskjʊlə neˈkrəʊsɪs/ *noun* a condition in which tissue cells die because their supply of blood has been cut

**AV bundle** /ˌeɪ ˈviː ˈbʌnd(ə)l/ *noun* same as **atrioventricular bundle**

**average** /ˈæv(ə)rɪdʒ/ *noun* **1.** the usual amount, size, rate, etc. ○ *Her weight is above (the) average.* **2.** a value calculated by adding together several quantities and then dividing the total by the number of quantities ■ *adjective* **1.** usual ○ *Their son is of above average weight.* **2.** calculated by adding together several quantities and then dividing the total by the number of quantities ○ *The average age of the group is 25.*

**aversion therapy** /əˈvɜːʃ(ə)n ˌθerəpi/ *noun* a treatment by which someone is cured of a type of behaviour by making him or her develop a great dislike for it

**avitaminosis** /eɪˌvɪtəmɪˈnəʊsɪs/ *noun* a disorder caused by a lack of vitamins

**AVM** *abbr* arteriovenous malformation

**AV node** /ˌeɪ ˈviː ˈnəʊd/ *noun* same as **atrioventricular node**

**AVPU** *noun* a method of rating if a person is conscious: A = alert; V = verbal, responding to verbal commands; P = pain, responding to pain; U = unconscious

**avulse** /əˈvʌls/ *verb* to tear tissue or a body part away by force

**avulsion** /əˈvʌlʃən/ *noun* an act of pulling away tissue or a body part by force

**avulsion fracture** /əˌvʌlʃ(ə)n ˈfræktʃə/ *noun* a fracture in which a tendon pulls away part of the bone to which it is attached

**awake** /əˈweɪk/ *adjective* not asleep ○ *He was still awake at 2 o'clock in the morning.* □ **wide awake** very awake

**aware** /əˈweə/ *adjective* **1.** conscious enough to know what is happening ○ *She is not aware of what is happening around her.* **2.** knowing about something ○ *The surgeon became aware of a problem with the heart-lung machine.*

**awareness** /əˈweənəs/ *noun* the fact of being aware, especially of a problem

'…doctors should use the increased public awareness of whooping cough during epidemics to encourage parents to vaccinate children' [*Health Visitor*]

**axial** /ˈæksiəl/ *adjective* referring to an axis

**axial skeleton** /ˌæksiəl ˈskelɪt(ə)n/ *noun* the bones that make up the vertebral column and the skull. Compare **appendicular skeleton**

**axilla** /ækˈsɪlə/ *noun* same as **armpit** (*technical*) (NOTE: The plural is **axillae**.)

**axillary** /ækˈsɪləri/ *adjective* referring to the armpit

**axillary artery** /ækˌsɪləri ˈɑːtəri/ *noun* an artery leading from the subclavian artery in the armpit

**axillary nodes** /ækˈsɪləri nəʊdz/ *plural noun* part of the lymphatic system in the arm

**axillary temperature** /ækˌsɪləri ˌtemprɪ ˈtʃə/ *noun* the temperature in the armpit

**axis** /ˈæksɪs/ *noun* **1.** an imaginary line through the centre of the body **2.** a central vessel which divides into other vessels **3.** the second vertebra on which the atlas sits (NOTE: The plural is **axes.**)

**axodendrite** /ˌæksəʊˈdendraɪt/ *noun* an appendage like a fibril on the axon of a nerve

**axolemma** /ˌæksəˈlemə/ *noun* a membrane covering an axon

**axon** /ˈæksɒn/ *noun* a nerve fibre which sends impulses from one neurone to another, linking with the dendrites of the other neurone. See illustration at NEURONE in Supplement

**axon covering** /ˈæksɒn ˌkʌv(ə)rɪŋ/ *noun* the myelin sheath which covers a nerve

**Ayurvedic medicine** /ˌaɪəveɪdɪk ˈmed(ə)s(ə)n/ *noun* a traditional Hindu system of healing that reviews a person's state of health and lifestyle and recommends treatment based on herbal products, dietary control and spiritual practices

**azathioprine** /ˌeɪzəˈθaɪəpriːn/ *noun* a drug which suppresses the immune response, used after transplant surgery to prevent rejection

**-azepam** /æzɪpæm/ *suffix* used in names of benzodiazepines ○ *diazepam*

**azidothymidine** /ˌeɪzɪdəʊˈθaɪmɪdiːn/ *noun* a drug used in the treatment of AIDS. Abbr **AZT**. Also called **zidovudine**

**azo-** /eɪzəʊ/ *prefix* containing a nitrogen group

**azoospermia** /ˌeɪzəʊəˈspɜːmiə/ *noun* the absence of sperm

**azotaemia** /ˌeɪzəʊˈtiːmiə/ *noun* the presence of urea or other nitrogen compounds in the blood

**azoturia** /ˌeɪzəʊˈtjʊəriə/ *noun* the presence of urea or other nitrogen compounds in the urine, caused by kidney disease

**AZT** *abbr* azidothymidine

**azygous** /ˈæzɪɡəs/ *adjective* single, not one of a pair

**azygous vein** /ˈæzɪɡəs veɪn/ *noun* a vein which brings blood back into the vena cava from the abdomen

# B

**babesiosis** /bə,biːziˈəʊsɪs/ *noun* a disease caused by infection of red blood cells by a protozoan introduced by a tick bite

**Babinski reflex** /bə,bɪnski ˈriːfleks/, **Babinski's reflex** /bə,bɪnskiz ˈriːfleks/ *noun* an unusual curling upwards of the big toe when a finger is lightly run across the sole of the foot, while the others turn down and spread out, a sign of hemiplegia and pyramidal tract disease. Compare **plantar reflex** [Described 1896. After Joseph François Felix Babinski (1857–1932), French-born son of Polish refugees. A pupil of Charcot, he was head of the Neurological clinic at Hôpital de la Pitié, 1890–1927.]

**Babinski test** /bəˈbɪnski test/ *noun* a test for a Babinski reflex

**baby** /ˈbeɪbi/ *noun* a very young child who is not yet old enough to talk or walk ○ *Babies start to walk when they are about 12 months old.* (NOTE: If you do not know the sex of a baby you can refer to the child as **it**: *The baby was sucking its thumb*)

**baby blues** /ˈbeɪbi bluːz/ *plural noun* same as **postnatal depression** (*informal*)

**baby care** /ˈbeɪbi keə/ *noun* the act of looking after babies

**baby clinic** /ˈbeɪbi ˌklɪnɪk/ *noun* a special clinic which deals with babies

**bacillaemia** /ˌbæsɪˈliːmiə/ *noun* an infection of the blood by bacilli

**bacillary** /bəˈsɪləri/ *adjective* referring to bacilli

**bacillary dysentery** /bə,sɪləri ˈdɪs(ə)ntri/ *noun* dysentery caused by the bacillus *Shigella* in contaminated food

**bacille Calmette-Guérin** /bæ,siːl ˌkælmet ˈɡeræn/ *noun* full form of **BCG** [After A. Calmette (1863–1933) and C. Guérin (1872–1961), French bacteriologists.]

**bacilluria** /ˌbæsɪˈljʊəriə/ *noun* the presence of bacilli in the urine

**bacillus** /bəˈsɪləs/ *noun* a bacterium shaped like a rod (NOTE: The plural is **bacilli**.)

**back** /bæk/ *noun* **1.** the part of the body from the neck downwards to the waist, which is made up of the spine and the bones attached to it (NOTE: For other terms referring to the back,

see **dorsal** and words beginning with **dorsi-, dorso-**.) **2.** the other side from the front ○ *She has a swelling on the back of her hand.* ◊ **dorsum**

**backache** /ˈbækeɪk/ *noun* pain in the back, often without a specific cause

COMMENT: Backache can result from bad posture or muscle strain, but it can also be caused by rheumatism (lumbago), fevers such as typhoid fever and osteoarthritis. Pains in the back can also be referred pains from gallstones or kidney disease.

**backbone** /ˈbækbəʊn/ *noun* a series of bones, the vertebrae, linked together to form a flexible column running from the pelvis to the skull. Also called **rachis, spine**

**background carboxyhaemoglobin level** /ˌbækɡraʊnd kɑː,bɒksi hiːməˈɡləʊbɪn ˌlev(ə)l/ *noun* the level of carboxyhaemoglobin in the blood of a person who is not exposed to high levels of carbon monoxide

**back muscles** /ˈbæk ˌmʌs(ə)lz/ *plural noun* the strong muscles in the back which help hold the body upright

**back pain** /ˈbæk peɪn/ *noun* pain in the back, especially long-lasting or severe pain

**backside** /ˈbæksaɪd/ *noun* someone's buttocks (*informal*)

**back strain** /ˈbæk streɪn/ *noun* a condition in which the muscles or ligaments in the back have been strained

**baclofen** /ˈbækləʊfen/ *noun* a drug that relaxes skeletal muscles which are in spasm, either because of injury or as a result of multiple sclerosis

**bacteraemia** /ˌbæktəˈriːmiə/ *noun* the fact of having bacteria in the blood. Bacteraemia is not necessarily a serious condition. Compare **septicaemia**. ◊ **blood poisoning**

**bacteria** /bækˈtɪəriə/ *plural of* **bacterium**

**bacterial** /bækˈtɪəriəl/ *adjective* relating to bacteria or caused by bacteria ○ *Children with sickle-cell anaemia are susceptible to bacterial infection.*

**bacterial plaque** /bækˈtɪəriəl ˌplæk/ *noun* a hard smooth bacterial deposit on teeth

**bacterial pneumonia** /bæk,tɪəriəl njuː'məʊniə/ *noun* a form of pneumonia caused by pneumococcus. ◊ **bronchopneumonia**

**bacterial strain** /bæk,tɪəriəl 'streɪn/ *noun* a group of bacteria which are different from others of the same general type

**bactericidal** /bæktɪərɪ'saɪd(ə)l/ *adjective* referring to a substance which destroys bacteria

**bactericide** /bæk'tɪərɪsaɪd/ *noun* a substance which destroys bacteria

**bacteriological** /bæktɪərɪə'lɒdʒɪk(ə)l/ *adjective* referring to bacteriology

**bacteriologist** /bæk,tɪəri'ɒlədʒɪst/ *noun* a doctor who specialises in the study of bacteria

**bacteriology** /bæk,tɪəri'ɒlədʒi/ *noun* the scientific study of bacteria

**bacteriolysin** /bæk,tɪəri'ɒlɪsɪn/ *noun* a protein, usually an immunoglobulin, which destroys bacterial cells

**bacteriolysis** /bæk,tɪəri'ɒlɪsɪs/ *noun* the destruction of bacterial cells

**bacteriolytic** /bæk,tɪəriə'lɪtɪk/ *adjective* referring to a substance which can destroy bacteria

**bacteriophage** /bæk'tɪəriəfeɪdʒ/ *noun* a virus which affects bacteria

**bacteriostasis** /bæk,tɪəriəʊ'steɪsɪs/ *noun* the action of stopping bacteria from multiplying

**bacteriostatic** /bæk,tɪəriəʊ'stætɪk/ *adjective* referring to a substance which does not kill bacteria but stops them from multiplying

**bacterium** /bæk'tɪəriəm/ *noun* a microscopic organism. Some types are permanently present in the gut and can break down food tissue, but many can cause disease. (NOTE: The plural is **bacteria**.)

COMMENT: Bacteria can be shaped like rods (bacilli), like balls (cocci) or have a spiral form (spirochaetes). Bacteria, especially bacilli and spirochaetes, can move and reproduce very rapidly.

**bacteriuria** /bæk,tɪəri'jʊəriə/ *noun* a condition in which bacteria are present in the urine

**Bactrim** /'bæktrɪm/ a trade name for co-trimoxazole

**bad breath** /,bæd 'breθ/ *noun* same as **halitosis** (*informal*)

**Baghdad boil** /,bægdæd 'bɔɪl/, **Baghdad sore** /,bægdæd 'sɔː/ *noun* a skin disease of tropical countries caused by the parasite *Leishmania*. Also called **Oriental sore**

**bag of waters** /,bæg əv 'wɔːtəz/ *noun* part of the amnion which covers an unborn baby in the uterus and contains the amniotic fluid

**BAHA** *abbr* bone anchored hearing aid

**Baker's cyst** /,beɪkəz 'sɪst/ *noun* a swelling filled with synovial fluid, at the back of the knee, caused by weakness of the joint membrane [Described 1877. After William Morrant Baker (1838–96), member of staff at St Bartholomew's Hospital, London, UK.]

**baker's itch** /,beɪkəz 'ɪtʃ/, **baker's dermatitis** /'beɪkəz dɜːmə'taɪtɪs/ *noun* an irritation of the skin caused by handling yeast

**BAL** *abbr* British anti-lewisite

**balance** /'bæləns/ *noun* **1.** the act of staying upright, not falling □ **he stood on top of the fence and kept his balance** he did not fall off **2.** the proportions of substances in a mixture, e.g. in the diet ○ *to maintain a healthy balance of vitamins in the diet*

**balanced diet** /,bælənst 'daɪət/ *noun* a diet which provides all the nutrients needed in the correct proportions

**balance of mind** /,bæləns əv 'maɪnd/ *noun* someone's mental state □ **disturbed balance of mind** a state of mind when someone is for a time incapable of reasoned action, because of illness or depression

**balanitis** /,bælə'naɪtɪs/ *noun* inflammation of the glans of the penis

**balanoposthitis** /,bælənəʊpɒs'θaɪtɪs/ *noun* inflammation of the foreskin and the end of the penis

**balantidiasis** /,bæləntɪ'daɪəsɪs/ *noun* an infestation of the large intestine by a parasite *Balantidium coli*, which causes ulceration of the wall of the intestine, leading to diarrhoea and finally dysentery

**balanus** /'bælənəs/ *noun* the round end of the penis. ◊ **glans**

**bald** /bɔːld/ *adjective* with no hair, especially on the head □ **he is going bald** *or* **he is becoming bald** he is beginning to lose his hair

**baldness** /'bɔːldnəs/ *noun* the state of not having any hair

COMMENT: Baldness in men is hereditary; it can also occur in both men and women as a reaction to an illness or to a drug.

**Balkan frame** /,bɔːlkən 'freɪm/, **Balkan beam** /,bɔːlkən 'biːm/ *noun* a frame fitted above a bed to which a leg in plaster can be attached. ◊ **Pearson bed**

**ball** /bɔːl/ *noun* **1.** the soft part of the hand below the thumb **2.** the soft part of the foot below the big toe

**ball and cage valve** /,bɔːl ən 'keɪdʒ vælv/ *noun* an artificial heart valve, formed of a silicon ball which moves inside a metal cage to open and shut the valve

**ball and socket joint** /,bɔːl ənd 'sɒkɪt dʒɔɪnt/ *noun* a joint where the round end of a long bone is attached to a cup-shaped hollow in another bone in such a way that the long bone can move in almost any direction. Compare **ginglymus**

**balloon** /bə'luːn/ *noun* a bag of light material inflated with air or a gas, used to unblock arteries

**balloon angioplasty** /bəˌluːn ˌændʒɪə 'plæsti/ *noun* same as **percutaneous angioplasty**

**balloon catheter** /bəˈluːn ˌkæθɪtə/ *noun* a tube that can be inserted into a blood vessel or other body part and then inflated, e.g. to widen a narrow artery

**ballottement** /bəˈlɒtmənt/ *noun* a method of examining the body by tapping or moving a part, especially during pregnancy

**balneotherapy** /ˌbælnɪəʊˈθerəpi/ *noun* the treatment of diseases by bathing in hot water or water containing beneficial natural chemicals

**balsam** /ˈbɔːls(ə)m/ *noun* a mixture of resin and oil, used to rub on sore joints or to put in hot water and use as an inhalant. ◊ **friar's balsam**

**ban** /bæn/ *verb* to say that something is not permitted ○ *Smoking is banned throughout the building.* ○ *Use of this drug has been banned.*

**bandage** /ˈbændɪdʒ/ *noun* a piece of cloth which is wrapped around a wound or an injured limb ○ *His head was covered with bandages.* ■ *verb* to wrap a piece of cloth around a wound ○ *She bandaged his leg.* ○ *His arm is bandaged up.*

**Bandl's ring** /ˈbænd(ə)lz rɪŋ/ same as **retraction ring** [After Ludwig Bandl (1842–92), German obstetrician]

**bank** /bæŋk/ *noun* a place where blood or organs from donors can be stored until needed. ◊ **blood bank**

**Bankart's operation** /ˈbæŋkɑːts ɒpəˌreɪ↓ ɪʃ(ə)n/ *noun* an operation to repair a recurrent dislocation of the shoulder [First performed 1923. After Arthur Sydney Blundell Bankart (1879–1951), first orthopaedic surgeon at the Middlesex Hospital, London, UK.]

**Banti's syndrome** /ˈbæntiz ˌsɪndrəʊm/, **Banti's disease** /ˈbæntiz dɪˌziːz/ *noun* same as **splenic anaemia** [Described 1882. After Guido Banti (1852–1925), Florentine pathologist and physician.]

**Barbados leg** /bɑːˌbeɪdɒs 'leg/ *noun* a form of elephantiasis, a large swelling of the leg due to a Filaria worm

**barber's itch** /ˌbɑːbəz 'ɪtʃ/, **barber's rash** /ˌbɑːbəz 'ræʃ/ *noun* same as **sycosis barbae**

**barbital** /ˈbɑːbɪtəl/ *noun* US same as **barbitone**

**barbitone** /ˈbɑːbɪtəʊn/ *noun* a type of barbiturate

**barbiturate** /bɑːˈbɪtʃʊrət/ *noun* a sedative drug

**barbiturate abuse** /bɑːˈbɪtʃʊrət əˌbjuːs/ *noun* repeated addictive use of barbiturates which in the end affects the brain

**barbiturate dependence** /bɑːˈbɪtʃʊrət dɪˌpendəns/ *noun* being dependent on regularly taking barbiturate tablets

**barbiturate poisoning** /bɑːˈbɪtʃʊrət ˌpɔɪz(ə)nɪŋ/ *noun* poisoning caused by an overdose of barbiturates

**barbotage** /ˌbɑːbɔːˈtɑːʒ/ *noun* a method of spinal analgesia by which cerebrospinal fluid is withdrawn and then injected back

**bare** /beə/ *adjective* with no covering □ **bare area of the liver** a large triangular part of the liver not covered with peritoneum

**bariatrics** /ˌbæriˈætrɪks/ *noun* the medical treatment of obesity

**barium** /ˈbeəriəm/ *noun* a chemical element, forming poisonous compounds, used as a contrast medium when taking X-ray photographs of soft tissue (NOTE: The chemical symbol is **Ba**.)

**barium enema** /ˌbeəriəm 'enɪmə/ *noun* a liquid solution containing barium sulphate which is put into the rectum to increase the contrast of an X-ray of the lower intestine

**barium meal** /ˌbeəriəm 'miːl/, **barium solution** /ˌbeəriəm səˈluːʃ(ə)n/ *noun* a liquid solution containing barium sulphate which someone drinks to increase the contrast of an X-ray of the alimentary tract

**barium sulphate** /ˌbeəriəm 'sʌlfeɪt/ *noun* a salt of barium not soluble in water and which shows as opaque in X-ray photographs

**Barlow's disease** /ˈbɑːləʊz dɪˌziːz/ *noun* scurvy in children, caused by a lack of vitamin C [Described 1882. After Sir Thomas Barlow (1845–1945), physician at various London hospitals and to Queen Victoria, King Edward VII and King George V.]

**Barlow's sign** /ˈbɑːləʊz saɪn/ *noun* a test for congenital dislocation of the hip, in which a sudden movement is felt and sometimes a sound is heard when the joint is manipulated

**baroreceptor** /ˌbærəʊrɪˈseptə/ *noun* one of a group of nerves near the carotid artery and aortic arch, which senses changes in blood pressure

**barotitis** /ˌbærəʊˈtaɪtɪs/ *noun* pain in the ear caused by differences in air pressure, e.g. during air travel

**barotrauma** /ˌbærəʊˈtrɔːmə/ *noun* an injury caused by a sharp increase in pressure

**Barr body** /ˈbɑː ˌbɒdi/ *noun* a dense clump of chromatin found only in female cells, which can be used to identify the sex of a baby before birth [Described 1949. After Murray Llewellyn Barr (1908–95), head of the Department of Anatomy at the University of Western Ontario, Canada.]

**Barre-Guillain syndrome** /ˌbæreɪ 'giː jæn ˌsɪndrəʊm/ *noun* ♦ **Guillain-Barré syndrome**

**barrel chest** /ˌbærəl 'tʃest/ *noun* a chest formed like a barrel, caused by asthma or emphysema

**barrier cream** /ˈbæriə kriːm/ *noun* a cream put on the skin to prevent the skin coming into contact with irritating substances

**barrier method** /ˈbæriə ˌmeθəd/ *noun* a method of contraception in which the entry of sperm to the womb is blocked by a protective device such as a condom or diaphragm

**barrier nursing** /ˈbæriə ˌnɜːsɪŋ/ *noun* the nursing of someone who has an infectious disease. It involves keeping them away from other patients and making sure that faeces and soiled bedclothes do not carry the infection to other patients.

'…those affected by salmonella poisoning are being nursed in five isolation wards and about forty suspected sufferers are being barrier nursed in other wards' [*Nursing Times*]

**bartholinitis** /ˌbɑːθəlɪˈnaɪtɪs/ *noun* inflammation of the Bartholin's glands

**Bartholin's glands** /ˈbɑːθəlɪnz ɡlændz/ *plural noun* two glands at the side of the vagina and between it and the vulva, which secrete a lubricating substance. Also called **greater vestibular glands** [After Caspar Bartholin (1655–1748), Danish anatomist]

**basal** /ˈbeɪs(ə)l/ *adjective* located at the bottom of something, or forming its base

**basal cell** /ˈbeɪs(ə)l sel/ *noun* a cell from the stratum germinativum. ◊ **stratum**

**basal cell carcinoma** /ˌbeɪs(ə)l ˌsel ˌkɑːsɪˈnəʊmə/ *noun* same as **rodent ulcer**

**basale** /bəˈseɪli/ *adjective* ♦ **stratum**

**basal ganglia** /ˌbeɪs(ə)l ˈɡæŋɡliə/ *noun* masses of grey matter at the base of each cerebral hemisphere which receive impulses from the thalamus and influence the motor impulses from the frontal cortex

**basalis** /bəˈseɪlɪs/ ♦ **decidua**

**basal metabolic rate** /ˌbeɪsɪk metəˈbɒlɪk reɪt/ *noun* the amount of energy used by the body in exchanging oxygen and carbon dioxide when at rest. It was formerly used as a way of testing thyroid gland activity. Abbr **BMR**

**basal metabolism** /ˌbeɪs(ə)l məˈtæbəlɪz(ə)m/ *noun* the minimum amount of energy needed to keep the body functioning and the temperature standard when at rest

**basal narcosis** /ˌbeɪs(ə)l nɑːˈkəʊsɪs/ *noun* the administration a narcotic before a general anaesthetic

**basal nuclei** /ˌbeɪs(ə)l ˈnuːkliaɪ/ *plural noun* masses of grey matter at the bottom of each cerebral hemisphere

**base** /beɪs/ *noun* **1.** the bottom part ○ *the base of the spine* □ **base of the brain** the bottom surface of the cerebrum **2.** the main ingredient of an ointment, as opposed to the active ingredient **3.** a substance which reacts with an acid to form a salt ■ *verb* to use something as a base □ **cream based on zinc oxide** cream which uses zinc oxide as a base

**Basedow's disease** /ˈbæzɪdəʊz dɪˌziːz/ *noun* a form of hyperthyroidism [Described 1840. After Carl Adolph Basedow (1799–1854), general practitioner in Mersburg, Germany.]

**basement membrane** /ˈbeɪsmənt ˌmembreɪn/ *noun* a membrane at the base of an epithelium

**basic** /ˈbeɪsɪk/ *adjective* **1.** very simple, from which everything else comes □ **basic structure of the skin** the two layers of skin, the inner dermis and the outer epidermis **2.** referring to a chemical substance which reacts with an acid to form a salt

**basic salt** /ˌbeɪsɪk ˈsɔːlt/ *noun* a chemical compound formed when an acid reacts with a base

**basilar** /ˈbæzɪlə/ *adjective* referring to a base

**basilar artery** /ˌbæzɪlə ˈɑːtəri/ *noun* an artery which lies at the base of the brain

**basilar membrane** /ˌbæzɪlə ˈmembreɪn/ *noun* a membrane in the cochlea which transmits nerve impulses from sound vibrations to the auditory nerve

**basilic** /bəˈsɪlɪk/ *adjective* important or prominent

**basilic vein** /bəˌzɪlɪk ˈveɪn/ *noun* a large vein running along the inside of the arm

**basin** /ˈbeɪs(ə)n/ *noun* a large bowl

**basophil** /ˈbeɪsəfɪl/ *noun* a type of white blood cell which has granules in its cytoplasm and contains histamine and heparin

**basophilia** /ˌbeɪsəˈfɪliə/ *noun* an increase in the number of basophils in the blood

**basophilic granulocyte** /ˌbeɪsəfɪlɪk ˈɡrænjʊləsaɪt/ *noun* same as **basophil**

**basophilic leucocyte** /ˌbeɪsəfɪlɪk ˈluːkəsaɪt/ *noun* same as **basophil**

**Batchelor plaster** /ˈbætʃələ ˌplɑːstə/ *noun* a plaster cast which keeps both legs apart [After J.S. Bachelor (b. 1905), British orthopaedic surgeon]

**bathe** /beɪð/ *verb* to wash a wound ○ *He bathed the grazed knee with boiled water.*

**Batten's disease** /ˈbæt(ə)nz dɪˌziːz/ *noun* a hereditary disease which affects the enzymes of the brain, causing cells in the brain and eye to die

**battered baby syndrome** /ˈbætəd ˌbeɪbi ˌsɪndrəʊm/, **battered child syndrome** /ˈbætəd ˈtʃaɪld ˈsɪndrəʊm/ *noun* a condition in which a baby or small child is frequently beaten, usually by one or both of its parents, sustaining injuries such as multiple fractures

**battledore placenta** /ˈbæt(ə)ldɔː pləˌsentə/ *noun* a placenta where the umbilical cord is attached at the edge and not at the centre

**Bazin's disease** /ˈbeɪzɪnz dɪˌziːz/ *noun* same as **erythema induratum** [Described 1861. After Pierre Antoine Ernest Bazin (1807–78), dermatologist at Hôpital St Louis, Paris, France.]

He was an expert in parasitology associated with skin conditions.]

**BC** *abbr* bone conduction. ✦ **osteophony**

**BCC** *abbr* Breast Cancer Campaign

**B cell** /'biː sel/ *noun* same as **beta cell**

**BCG** /ˌbiː siː 'dʒiː/, **BCG vaccine** *noun* a vaccine which immunises against tuberculosis. Full form **bacille Calmette-Guérin**

**BCh** *abbr* Bachelor of Surgery

**BDA** *abbr* British Dental Association

**bearing down** /ˌbeərɪŋ 'daʊn/ *noun* a stage in childbirth when the woman starts to push out the baby from the uterus

**bearing-down pain** /ˌbeərɪŋ 'daʊn peɪn/ *noun* pain felt in the uterus during the second stage of labour (NOTE: Bearing-down pain is also associated with uterine prolapse.)

**beat joint** /'biːt dʒɔɪnt/ *noun* an inflammation of a joint such as the elbow (beat elbow) or knee (beat knee) caused by frequent sharp blows or other pressure

**Beck inventory of depression** /ˌbek ˌɪnvənt(ə)ri əv dɪ'preʃ(ə)n/ *noun* one of the rating scales for depression, in which a series of 21 questions refers to attitudes frequently shown by people suffering from depression

**beclomethasone** /ˌbeklə'meθəsəʊn/ *noun* a steroid drug usually used in an inhaler to treat asthma or hay fever

**becquerel** /'bekərel/ *noun* an SI unit of measurement of radiation. Abbr **Bq** (NOTE: Now used in place of the **curie**.)

**bed bath** /'bed bɑːθ/ *noun* an act of washing the whole body of someone who is unable to get up to wash. Also called **blanket bath**

**bed blocker** /'bed ˌblɒkə/ *noun* a patient who does not need medical attention but continues to stay in hospital because suitable care is not available elsewhere

**bed blocking** /'bed ˌblɒkɪŋ/ *noun* the fact of people being kept in hospital because other forms of care are not available, which means that other people cannot be treated

**bedbug** /'bedbʌg/ *noun* a small insect which lives in dirty bedclothes and sucks blood

**bed occupancy** /'bed ˌɒkjʊpənsi/ *noun* the percentage of beds in a hospital which are occupied

**bed occupancy rate** /bed 'ɒkjʊpənsi ˌreɪt/ *noun* the number of beds occupied in a hospital shown as a percentage of all the beds in the hospital

**bedpan** /'bedpæn/ *noun* a dish into which someone can urinate or defecate without getting out of bed

**bed rest** /'bed rest/ *noun* a period of time spent in bed in order to rest and recover from an illness

**bedridden** /'bed,rɪd(ə)n/ *adjective* referring to someone who has been too ill to get out of bed over a long period of time

**bedside manner** /ˌbedsaɪd 'mænə/ *noun* the way in which a doctor behaves towards a patient, especially a patient who is in bed □ **a good bedside manner** the ability to make patients feel comforted and reassured

**bedsore** /'bedsɔː/ *noun* an inflamed patch of skin on a bony part of the body, which develops into an ulcer, caused by pressure of the part on the mattress after lying for some time in one position. Special beds such as air beds, ripple beds and water beds are used to try to prevent the formation of bedsores. Also called **pressure sore, decubitus ulcer**

**bedtable** /'bedteɪb(ə)l/ *noun* a specially designed table which can be used by a person sitting up in bed

**bedwetting** /'bedwetɪŋ/ *noun* same as **nocturnal enuresis** (NOTE: This term is used mainly about children.)

**Beer's knife** /'bɪəz naɪf/ *noun* a knife with a triangular blade, used in eye operations [After George Joseph Beer (1763–1821), German ophthalmologist]

**behaviour** /bɪ'heɪvjə/ *noun* a way of acting ○ *His behaviour was very aggressive.* (NOTE: The US spelling is **behavior**.)

**behavioural** /bɪ'heɪvjərəl/ *adjective* relating to behaviour (NOTE: The US spelling is **behavioral**.)

**behavioural scientist** /bɪˌheɪvjərəl 'saɪəntɪst/ *noun* a person who specialises in the study of behaviour

**behaviourism** /bɪ'heɪvjərɪz(ə)m/ *noun* a psychological theory proposing that only someone's behaviour should be studied to discover their psychological problems

**behaviourist** /bɪ'heɪvjərɪst/ *noun* a psychologist who follows behaviourism

**behaviour therapy** /bɪˌheɪvjə 'θerəpi/ *noun* a form of psychiatric treatment in which someone learns how to improve their condition

**Behçet's syndrome** /'beɪsets ˌsɪndrəʊm/ *noun* a chronic condition of the immune system with no known cause, experienced as a series of attacks of inflammation of small blood vessels accompanied by mouth ulcers and sometimes genital ulcers, skin lesions and inflamed eyes [Described 1937. After Halushi Behçet (1889–1948), Turkish dermatologist.]

**behind** /bɪ'haɪnd/ *noun* same as **buttock** (*informal*)

**bejel** /'bedʒəl/ *noun* a non-venereal form of syphilis which is endemic among children in some areas of the Middle East and elsewhere and is caused by a spirochaete strain of bacteria

**belch** /beltʃ/ *noun* the action of allowing air in the stomach to come up through the mouth ■ *verb* to allow air in the stomach to come up through the mouth

**belching** /'beltʃɪŋ/ *noun* the action of allowing air in the stomach to come up through the mouth. Also called **eructation**

**belladonna** /ˌbelə'dɒnə/ *noun* 1. a poisonous plant with berries containing atropine. Also called **deadly nightshade** 2. a form of atropine extracted from the belladonna plant

**belle indifférence** /ˌbel æn'dɪferɑːns/ *noun* an excessively calm state in a person, in a situation which would usually produce a show of emotion

**Bellocq's cannula** /beˌlɒks 'kænjʊlə/, **Bellocq's sound** /beˌlɒks 'saʊnd/ *noun* an instrument used to control a nosebleed [After Jean Jacques Bellocq (1732–1807), French surgeon]

**Bell's mania** /ˌbelz 'meɪniə/ *noun* a form of acute mania with delirium [After Luther Vose Bell (1806–62), American physiologist]

**Bell's palsy** /ˌbelz 'pɔːlzi/ *noun* paralysis of the facial nerve on one side of the face, preventing one eye being closed. Also called **facial paralysis** [Described 1821. After Sir Charles Bell (1774–1842), Scottish surgeon. He ran anatomy schools, first in Edinburgh and then in London. Professor of Anatomy at the Royal Academy.]

**belly** /'beli/ *noun* 1. same as **abdomen** 2. the fatter central part of a muscle

**bellyache** /'belieɪk/ *noun* a pain in the abdomen or stomach

**belly button** /'beli ˌbʌt(ə)n/ *noun* the navel (*informal*)

**Bence Jones protein** /ˌbens 'dʒəʊnz ˌprəʊtiːn/ *noun* a protein found in the urine of people who have myelomatosis, lymphoma, leukaemia and some other cancers [Described 1848. After Henry Bence Jones (1814–73), physician at St George's Hospital, London, UK.]

**bends** /bendz/ *plural noun* □ **the bends ♦ caisson disease**

**Benedict's solution** /'benɪdɪkts səˌluːʃ(ə)n/ *noun* a solution used to carry out Benedict's test

**Benedict's test** /'benɪdɪkts test/ *noun* a test to see if sugar is present in the urine [Described 1915. After Stanley Rossiter Benedict (1884–1936), physiological chemist at Cornell University, New York, USA.]

**benign** /bə'naɪn/ *adjective* generally harmless

**benign growth** /bə'naɪn grəʊθ/ *noun* same as **benign tumour**

**benign pancreatic disease** /bəˌnaɪn ˌpæŋkri'ætɪk dɪˌziːz/ *noun* chronic pancreatitis

**benign prostatic hypertrophy** /bɪˌnaɪn prɒˌstætɪk haɪ'pɜːtrəfi/ *noun* a nonmalignant enlargement of the prostate. Abbr **BPH**

**benign tumour** /bəˌnaɪn 'tjuːmə/ *noun* a tumour which will not grow again or spread to other parts of the body if it is removed surgi-

cally, but which can be fatal if not treated. Also called **benign growth**. Opposite **malignant tumour**

**Bennett's fracture** /ˌbenɪts 'fræktʃə/ *noun* a fracture of the first metacarpal, the bone between the thumb and the wrist [Described 1886. After Edward Halloran Bennett (1837–1907), Irish anatomist, later Professor of Surgery at Trinity College, Dublin, Ireland.]

**bent** /bent/ *adjective* □ **bent double** bent over completely so that the face is towards the ground ○ *He was bent double with pain.*

**benzocaine** /'benzəkeɪn/ *noun* a drug with anaesthetic properties used in some throat lozenges and skin creams

**benzodiazepine** /ˌbenzəʊdaɪ'æzəpiːn/ *noun* a drug which acts on receptors in the central nervous system to relieve symptoms of anxiety and insomnia, although prolonged use is to be avoided (NOTE: Benzodiazepines have names ending in **-azepam**: **diazepam**.)

**benzoin** /'benzəʊɪn/ *noun* a resin used to make friar's balsam

**benzyl benzoate** /ˌbenzɪl 'benzəʊeɪt/ *noun* a colourless oily liquid which occurs naturally in balsams, used in medicines and perfumes

**benzylpenicillin** /ˌbenzɪl penɪ'sɪlɪn/ *noun* an antibacterial drug used against streptococcal infections, meningococcal meningitis and other serious infections

**bereavement** /bɪ'riːvmənt/ *noun* the loss of someone, especially a close relative or friend, through death

**beriberi** /ˌberi'beri/ *noun* a disease of the nervous system caused by lack of vitamin $B_1$
  COMMENT: Beriberi is prevalent in tropical countries where the diet is mainly formed of white rice, which is deficient in thiamine.

**berylliosis** /bəˌrɪli'əʊsɪs/ *noun* poisoning caused by breathing in particles of the poisonous chemical compound beryllium oxide

**Besnier's prurigo** /ˌbenieɪz prʊ'raɪgəʊ/ *noun* an itchy skin rash on the backs of the knees and the insides of the elbows [After Ernest Besnier (1831–1909), French dermatologist]

**beta** /'biːtə/ *noun* the second letter of the Greek alphabet

**beta-adrenergic receptor** /ˌbiːtə ˌædrə'nɜːdʒɪk/ *noun* one of two types of nerve endings that respond to adrenaline by speeding up the heart rate or dilating the bronchi

**beta amyloid** /ˌbiːtə 'æmɪlɔɪd/ *noun* a wax-like protein formed from amyloid precursor protein in nerve cells which aggregates in Alzheimer's disease to form plaques

**beta blocker** /'biːtə ˌblɒkə/ *noun* a drug which reduces the activity of the heart (NOTE: Beta blockers have names ending in **-olol**: **atenolol, propranolol hydrochloride**.)

**beta cell** /'biːtə sel/ *noun* a type of cell found in the islets of Langerhans, in the pancreas, which produces insulin. Also called **B cell.** ◊ **alpha cell**

**Betadine** /'biːtədiːn/ *noun* a trade name for a form of iodine

**betamethasone** /ˌbiːtə'meθəsəʊn/ *noun* a very strong corticosteroid drug

**beta rhythm** /'biːtə ˌrɪθəm/ *noun* a pattern of electrical waves in the brain of someone who is awake and active, registering on an electro-encephalograph at 18–30 hertz

**betaxolol** /bɪ'tæksəlɒl/ *noun* a beta blocker drug used in the treatment of high blood pressure and glaucoma

**bethanechol** /be'θænɪkɒl/ *noun* an agonist drug used to increase muscle tone after surgery

**Betnovate** /'betnəveɪt/ *noun* a trade name for an ointment containing betamethasone

**bi-** /baɪ/ *prefix* two or twice

**bias** /'baɪəs/ *noun* a systematic error in the design or conduct of a study which could explain the results

**bicarbonate of soda** /baɪ'kɑːbənət əv 'səʊdə/ *noun* same as **sodium bicarbonate**

**bicellular** /baɪ'seljʊlə/ *adjective* having two cells

**biceps** /'baɪseps/ *noun* any muscle formed of two parts joined to form one tendon, especially the muscles in the front of the upper arm (biceps brachii) and the back of the thigh (biceps femoris). ◊ **triceps** (NOTE: The plural is **biceps.**)

**bicipital** /baɪ'sɪpɪt(ə)l/ *adjective* **1.** referring to a biceps muscle **2.** with two parts

**biconcave** /baɪ'kɒnkeɪv/ *adjective* referring to a lens which is concave on both sides

**biconvex** /baɪ'kɒnveks/ *adjective* referring to a lens which is convex on both sides

**bicornuate** /baɪ'kɔːnjuət/ *adjective* divided into two parts (NOTE: The word is sometimes applied to a malformation of the uterus.)

**bicuspid** /baɪ'kʌspɪd/ *adjective* with two points ■ *noun* a premolar tooth

**bicuspid valve** /ˌbaɪ'kʌspɪd ˌvælv/ *noun* same as **mitral valve.** see illustration at HEART in Supplement

**b.i.d.** *adverb* (*used on prescriptions*) twice daily. Full form **bis in die**

**bifid** /'baɪfɪd/ *adjective* in two parts

**bifida** /'bɪfɪdə/ ◆ **spina bifida**

**bifocal** /baɪ'fəʊk(ə)l/ *adjective* referring to lenses made with two sections which have different focal lengths, one for looking at things which are near, the other for looking at things which are far away

**bifocal glasses** /baɪˌfəʊk(ə)l 'glɑːsɪz/, **bifocal lenses** /baɪ'fəʊk(ə)l 'lenzɪz/, **bifocals** /baɪ'fəʊk(ə)lz/ *plural noun* spectacles with lenses which have two types of lens combined in the same piece of glass, the top part being used for seeing at a distance and the lower part for reading

**bifurcate** /'baɪfəkeɪt/ *adjective* separating or branching off into two parts ■ *verb* to split or branch off into two parts

**bifurcation** /ˌbaɪfə'keɪʃ(ə)n/ *noun* a place where something divides into two parts

**bigeminy** /baɪ'dʒemɪni/ *noun* same as **pulsus bigeminus**

**big toe** /bɪg 'təʊ/ *noun* the largest of the five toes, on the inside of the foot. Also called **great toe**

**biguanide** /baɪ'gwɑːnaɪd/ *noun* a drug which lowers blood sugar, used in the treatment of Type II diabetes

**bilateral** /baɪ'læt(ə)rəl/ *adjective* affecting both sides

**bilateral adrenalectomy** /baɪˌlæt(ə)rəl əˌdriːnə'lektəmi/ *noun* the surgical removal of both adrenal glands

**bilateral pneumonia** /baɪˌlæt(ə)rəl njuː'məʊniə/ *noun* pneumonia affecting both lungs

**bilateral vasectomy** /baɪˌlæt(ə)rəl və'sektəmi/ *noun* a surgical operation to cut both vasa deferentia and so make a man sterile

**bile** /baɪl/ *noun* a thick bitter brownish yellow fluid produced by the liver, stored in the gall bladder and used to digest fatty substances and neutralise acids (NOTE: For other terms referring to bile, see words beginning with **chol-**.)

COMMENT: In jaundice, excess bile pigments flow into the blood and cause the skin to turn yellow.

**bile acid** /'baɪl ˌæsɪd/ *noun* an acid found in the bile, e.g. cholic acid

**bile canal** /'baɪl kəˌnæl/ *noun* a very small vessel leading from a hepatic cell to the bile duct

**bile duct** /'baɪl dʌkt/ *noun* a tube which links the cystic duct and the hepatic duct to the duodenum

**bile pigment** /'baɪl ˌpɪgmənt/ *noun* colouring matter in bile

**bile salts** /'baɪl sɔːltz/ *plural noun* sodium salts of bile acids

**bilharzia** /bɪl'hɑːtsiə/ *noun* **1.** a fluke which enters the bloodstream and causes bilharziasis. Also called **Schistosoma 2.** same as **bilharziasis** (NOTE: Although strictly speaking, **bilharzia** is the name of the fluke, it is also generally used for the name of the disease: *bilharzia patients*; *six cases of bilharzia*.)

**bilharziasis** /ˌbɪlhɑː'tsaɪəsɪs/ *noun* a tropical disease caused by flukes in the intestine or bladder. Also called **bilharzia, schistosomiasis**

COMMENT: The larvae of the fluke enter the skin through the feet and lodge in the walls of the intestine or bladder. They are passed out of the body in stools or urine and return to water, where they lodge and develop in the water snail, the secondary host, before going back into humans. Patients experience fever and anaemia.

**bili-** /ˈbɪli/ *prefix* referring to bile (NOTE: For other terms referring to bile, see words beginning with **chol-, chole-**.)

**biliary** /ˈbɪliəri/ *adjective* referring to bile

**biliary colic** /ˌbɪliəri ˈkɒlɪk/ *noun* pain in the abdomen caused by gallstones in the bile duct or by inflammation of the gall bladder

**biliary fistula** /ˌbɪliəri ˈfɪstjʊlə/ *noun* an opening which discharges bile on to the surface of the skin from the gall bladder, bile duct or liver

**bilious** /ˈbɪliəs/ *adjective* **1.** referring to bile **2.** referring to nausea (*informal*)

**biliousness** /ˈbɪliəsnəs/ *noun* a feeling of indigestion and nausea (*informal*)

**bilirubin** /ˌbɪliˈruːbɪn/ *noun* a red pigment in bile

**bilirubinaemia** /ˌbɪliruːbɪˈniːmiə/ *noun* an excess of bilirubin in the blood

**biliuria** /ˌbɪliˈjʊəriə/ *noun* the presence of bile in the urine. Also called **choluria**

**biliverdin** /ˌbɪliˈvɜːdɪn/ *noun* a green pigment in bile, produced by oxidation of bilirubin

**Billings method** /ˈbɪlɪŋz ˌmeθəd/ *noun* a method of birth control which uses the colour and consistency of the cervical mucus as guides to whether ovulation is taking place

**Billroth's operations** /ˈbɪlrɒθs ɒpəˌreɪʃ(ə)nz/ *plural noun* surgical operations in which the lower part of the stomach is removed and the part which is left is linked to the duodenum (Billroth I) or jejunum (Billroth II) [Described 1881. After Christian Albert Theodore Billroth (1829–94), Prussian surgeon.]

**bilobate** /baɪˈləʊbeɪt/ *adjective* with two lobes

**bimanual** /baɪˈmænjuəl/ *adjective* done with two hands, or needing both hands to be done

**binary** /ˈbaɪnəri/ *adjective* made of two parts

**binary fission** /ˌbaɪnəri ˈfɪʃ(ə)n/ *noun* the process of splitting into two parts in some types of cell division

**binaural** /baɪnˈɔːrəl/ *adjective* using, or relating to, both ears

**binder** /ˈbaɪndə/ *noun* a bandage which is wrapped round a limb to support it

**Binet's test** /ˈbɪneɪz test/ *noun* an intelligence test for children [Originally described 1905 but later modified at Stanford University, California, USA. After Alfred Binet (1857–1911), French psychologist and physiologist.]

**binocular** /bɪˈnɒkjʊlə/ *adjective* referring to the two eyes

**binocular vision** /bɪˌnɒkjʊlə ˈvɪʒ(ə)n/ *noun* ability to see with both eyes at the same time, which gives a stereoscopic effect and allows a person to judge distances. Compare **monocular**

**binovular** /bɪˈnɒvjʊlə/ *adjective* referring to twins who develop from two different ova

**bio-** /baɪəʊ/ *prefix* referring to living organisms

**bioactive** /ˌbaɪəʊˈæktɪv/ *adjective* producing an effect in living tissue or in a living organism

**bioassay** /ˌbaɪəʊəˈseɪ/ *noun* a test of the strength of a drug, hormone, vitamin or serum, by examining the effect it has on living animals or tissue

**bioavailability** /ˌbaɪəʊəveɪləˈbɪlɪti/ *noun* the extent to which a nutrient or medicine can be taken up by the body

**biochemical** /ˌbaɪəʊˈkemɪk(ə)l/ *adjective* referring to biochemistry

**biochemistry** /ˌbaɪəʊˈkemɪstri/ *noun* the chemistry of living tissues

**biocide** /ˈbaɪəʊsaɪd/ *noun* a substance which kills living organisms

**biocompatibility** /ˌbaɪəʊkəmpætəˈbɪlɪti/ *noun* the compatibility of a donated organ or artificial limb with the living tissue into which it has been introduced or with which it is brought into contact

**biodegradable** /ˌbaɪəʊdɪˈgreɪdəb(ə)l/ *adjective* easily decomposed by organisms such as bacteria or by the effect of sunlight, the sea, etc.

**bioengineering** /ˌbaɪəʊendʒɪˈnɪərɪŋ/ *noun* same as **biomedical engineering**

**bioethics** /ˈbaɪəʊˌeθɪks/ *noun* the study of the moral and ethical choices in medical research and treatment of patients, especially when advanced technology is available

**biofeedback** /ˌbaɪəʊˈfiːdbæk/ *noun* the control of the autonomic nervous system by someone's conscious thought, as he or she sees the results of tests or scans

**biogenesis** /ˌbaɪəʊˈdʒenəsɪs/ *noun* a theory that living organisms can only develop from other living organisms

**biohazard** /ˈbaɪəʊˌhæzəd/ *noun* a danger to human beings or their environment, especially one from a poisonous or infectious agent

**bioinstrumentation** /ˌbaɪəʊɪnstrəmenˈteɪʃ(ə)n/ *noun* instruments used to record and display information about the body's functions, or the use of such instruments

**biological** /ˌbaɪəˈlɒdʒɪk(ə)l/ *adjective* referring to biology

**biological clock** /ˌbaɪəlɒdʒɪk(ə)l ˈklɒk/ *noun* the rhythm of daily activities and bodily processes such as eating, defecating or sleeping, frequently controlled by hormones, which repeats every twenty-four hours. Also called **circadian rhythm**

**biological parent** /ˌbaɪəˌlɒdʒɪk(ə)l ˈpeərəmt/ *noun* a parent who was physically involved in producing a child

**biologist** /baɪˈɒlədʒɪst/ *noun* a scientist who specialises in biology

**biology** /baɪˈɒlədʒi/ *noun* the study of living organisms

**biomaterial** /ˌbaɪəʊmə'tɪərɪəl/ *noun* a synthetic material which can be used as an implant in living tissue

**biomedical engineering** /ˌbaɪəʊmedɪk(ə)lˌendʒɪ'nɪərɪŋ/ *noun* the application of engineering science such as robotics and hydraulics to medicine

**biomedicine** /ˈbaɪəʊˌmed(ə)s(ə)n/ *noun* **1.** the use of the principles of biology, biochemistry, physiology and other basic sciences to solve problems in clinical medicine **2.** the study of the body's ability to withstand unusual or extreme environments

**biometry** /baɪ'ɒmətri/ *noun* the science which applies statistics to the study of living things □ **biometry of the eye** measurement of the eye by ultrasound □ **biometry of a fetus** the measurement of the key parameters of growth of a fetus by ultrasound

**biomonitoring** /ˈbaɪəʊˌmɒnɪt(ə)rɪŋ/ *noun* the measurement and tracking of a chemical substance in a living organism or biological material such as blood or urine, usually to check environmental pollution or chemical exposure

**bionic ear** /baɪ'ɒnɪk ɪə/ *noun* a cochlear implant (*informal*)

**bionics** /baɪ'ɒnɪks/ *noun* the process of applying knowledge of biological systems to mechanical and electronic devices

**biopharmaceutical** /ˌbaɪəʊfɑːmə'suːtɪk(ə)l/ *noun* a drug produced by biotechnological methods

**biophysical profile** /ˌbaɪəʊfɪzɪk(ə)l 'prəʊfaɪl/ *noun* a profile of a fetus, based on such things as its breathing movement and body movement

**biopsy** /ˈbaɪɒpsi/ *noun* the process of taking a small piece of living tissue for examination and diagnosis ○ *The biopsy of the tissue from the growth showed that it was benign.*

**biorhythm** /ˈbaɪəʊrɪð(ə)m/ *noun* a regular process of change which takes place within living organisms, e.g. sleeping, waking or the reproductive cycle (NOTE: Some people believe that biorhythms affect behaviour and mood.)

**biosensor** /ˈbaɪəʊˌsensə/ *noun* a device that uses a biological agent such as an enzyme or organelle to detect, measure or analyse chemicals (NOTE: Biosensors are increasingly used in tests to diagnose medical conditions such as blood pressure.)

**biostatistics** /ˌbaɪəʊstə'tɪstɪks/ *plural noun* statistics used in medicine and the study of disease

**biosurgery** /ˈbaɪəʊˌsɜːdʒəri/ *noun* the use of living organisms in surgery and post-surgical treatment, especially the use of maggots or leeches to clean wounds

**biotechnology** /ˌbaɪəʊtek'nɒlədʒi/ *noun* **1.** the use of biological processes in industrial production, e.g. in the production of drugs **2.** same as **genetic modification**

**biotherapy** /ˈbaɪəʊˌθerəpi/ *noun* the treatment of disease with substances produced through the activity of living organisms such as sera, vaccines or antibiotics

**biotin** /ˈbaɪətɪn/ *noun* a type of vitamin B found in egg yolks, liver and yeast

**biparietal** /ˌbaɪpə'raɪət(ə)l/ *adjective* referring to the two parietal bones

**biparous** /ˈbɪpərəs/ *adjective* producing twins

**bipennate** /baɪ'peneɪt/ *adjective* referring to a muscle with fibres which rise from either side of the tendon

**bipolar** /baɪ'pəʊlə/ *adjective* with two poles. See illustration at NEURONE in Supplement

**bipolar disorder** /ˌbaɪˌpəʊlə dɪs'ɔːdə/ *noun* a psychological condition in which someone moves between mania and depression and experiences delusion. Also called **manic-depressive illness, manic depression**

**bipolar neurone** /ˌbaɪˌpəʊlə 'njʊərəʊn/ *noun* a nerve cell with two processes, a dendrite and an axon, found in the retina. See illustration at NEURONE in Supplement. Compare **multipolar neurone, unipolar neurone**

**birth** /bɜːθ/ *noun* the act of being born □ **to give birth** to have a baby ○ *She gave birth to twins.*

**birth canal** /ˈbɜːθ kəˌnæl/ *noun* the uterus, vagina and vulva

**birth control** /ˈbɜːθ kənˌtrəʊl/ *noun* same as **contraception**

**birth control pill** /ˈbɜːθ kənˌtrəʊl pɪl/ *noun* same as **oral contraceptive**

**birth defect** /ˈbɜːθ ˌdiːfekt/ *noun* same as **congenital anomaly** (NOTE: The word 'defect' is now avoided.)

**birthing** /ˈbɜːθɪŋ/ *noun* the process of giving birth using natural childbirth methods ■ *adjective* designed to help in childbirth

**birthing chair** /ˈbɜːθɪŋ tʃeə/ *noun* a special chair in which a woman sits to give birth

**birthing pool** /ˈbɜːθɪŋ puːl/ *noun* a special large bath in which pregnant women can relax before and when giving birth

**birthing room** /ˈbɜːθɪŋ ruːm/ *noun* an area set up for childbirth in a hospital or other building to provide comfortable and homely surroundings

**birth injury** /ˈbɜːθ ˌɪndʒəri/ *noun* an injury which a baby experiences during a difficult birth, e.g. brain damage

**birthmark** /ˈbɜːθmɑːk/ *noun* an unusual coloured or raised area on the skin which someone has from birth. Also called **naevus**

**birth mother** /ˈbɜːθ ˌmʌðə/ *noun* the woman who gave birth to a child

**birth parent** /ˈbɜːθ ˌpeərənt/ *noun* one of the parents that physically produced a child

**birth plan** /ˈbɜːθ plæn/ *noun* a list of a pregnant woman's wishes about how the birth of her baby should take place, e.g. whether she wants a natural birth and what pain relief she should be given

**birth rate** /ˈbɜːθ reɪt/ *noun* the number of births per year, shown per thousand of the population ○ *a birth rate of 15 per thousand* ○ *There has been a severe decline in the birth rate.*

**birth trauma** /ˈbɜːθ ˌtrɔːmə/ *noun* an injury caused to a baby during delivery

**birth weight** /ˈbɜːθ weɪt/ *noun* the weight of a baby at birth

**bisacodyl** /ˌbaɪsəˈkəʊdɪl/ *noun* a laxative drug

**bisexual** /baɪˈsekʃuəl/ *noun* someone who has both male and female sexual partners ■ *adjective* referring to a person who is sexually attracted to both males and females. Compare **heterosexual, homosexual**

**bisexuality** /ˌbaɪsekʃuˈælɪti/ *noun* the state of being sexually attracted to both males and females

**bis in die** /ˌbɪs ɪn ˈdiːeɪ/ *adverb* full form of **b.i.d.**

**bismuth** /ˈbɪzməθ/ *noun* a chemical element (NOTE: The chemical symbol is **Bi**.)

**bismuth salts** /ˈbɪzməθ sɔːlts/ *plural noun* salts used to treat acid stomach and formerly used in the treatment of syphilis

**bistoury** /ˈbɪstəri/ *noun* a sharp thin surgical knife

**bite** /baɪt/ *verb* **1.** to cut into something with the teeth ○ *He bit a piece out of the apple.* □ **to bite on something** to hold onto something with the teeth ○ *The dentist told him to bite on the bite wing.* **2.** (*of an insect*) to puncture someone's skin ■ *noun* **1.** the action of biting or of being bitten **2.** a place or mark where someone has been bitten ○ *a dog bite* ○ *an insect bite*

**bite wing** /ˈbaɪt wɪŋ/ *noun* a holder for dental X-ray film, which a person clenches between the teeth, so allowing an X-ray of both upper and lower teeth to be taken

**Bitot's spots** /ˌbiːtəʊz ˈspɒts/ *plural noun* small white spots on the conjunctiva, caused by vitamin A deficiency [Described 1863. After Pierre A. Bitot (1822–88), French physician.]

**bivalve** /ˈbaɪvælv/ *noun* an organ which has two valves ■ *adjective* referring to a bivalve organ

**black eye** /ˌblæk ˈaɪ/ *noun* bruising and swelling of the tissues round an eye, usually caused by a blow

**blackhead** /ˈblækhed/ *noun* same as **comedo** (*informal*)

**black heel** /ˈblæk ˌhiːl/ *noun* a haemorrhage inside the heel, characterised by black spots

**black out** /ˌblæk ˈaʊt/ *verb* to have sudden loss of consciousness ○ *I suddenly blacked out and I can't remember anything more*

**blackout** /ˈblækaʊt/ *noun* a sudden loss of consciousness (*informal*) ○ *She must have had a blackout while driving.* Also called **fainting fit**

**black spots** /ˌblæk ˈspɒts/ *plural noun* □ **black spots in front of the eyes** moving black dots seen when looking at something, more noticeable when a person is tired or run-down, and more common in shortsighted people

**blackwater fever** /ˈblækwɔːtə ˌfiːvə/ *noun* a form of malaria where haemoglobin from red blood cells is released into plasma and makes the urine dark

**bladder** /ˈblædə/ *noun* any sac in the body, especially the sac where the urine collects before being passed out of the body ○ *He is suffering from bladder trouble.* ○ *She is taking antibiotics for a bladder infection.*

**Blalock's operation** /ˈbleɪlɒks ɒpəˌreɪʃ(ə)n/, **Blalock-Taussig operation** /ˌbleɪlɒk ˈtɔːsɪg ɒpəˌreɪʃ(ə)n/ *noun* a surgical operation to connect the pulmonary artery to the subclavian artery, in order to increase blood flow to the lungs of someone who has tetralogy of Fallot

**bland** /blænd/ *adjective* referring to food which is not spicy, irritating or acid

**bland diet** /ˌblænd ˈdaɪət/ *noun* a diet in which someone eats mainly milk-based foods, boiled vegetables and white meat, as a treatment for peptic ulcers

**blanket bath** /ˈblæŋkɪt bɑːθ/ *noun* same as **bed bath**

**blast** /blɑːst/ *noun* **1.** a wave of air pressure from an explosion which can cause concussion **2.** an immature form of a cell before distinctive characteristics develop

**-blast** /blæst/ *suffix* referring to a very early stage in the development of a cell

**blast injury** /ˈblɑːst ˌɪndʒəri/ *noun* a severe injury to the chest following a blast

**blasto-** /blæstəʊ/ *prefix* referring to a germ cell

**blastocoele** /ˈblæstəʊsiːl/ *noun* a cavity filled with fluid in a morula (NOTE: The US spelling is **blastocele**.)

**blastocyst** /ˈblæstəʊsɪst/ *noun* an early stage in the development of an embryo

**Blastomyces** /ˌblæstəʊˈmaɪsiːz/ *noun* a type of parasitic fungus which affects the skin

**blastomycosis** /ˌblæstəʊmaɪˈkəʊsɪs/ *noun* an infection caused by *Blastomyces*

**blastula** /ˈblæstjʊlə/ *noun* the first stage of the development of an embryo in animals

**bleb** /bleb/ *noun* a blister. Compare **bulla**

**bled** /bled/ ♦ **bleed**

**bleed** /bliːd/ *verb* to lose blood ○ *His knee was bleeding.* ○ *He was bleeding from a cut on the head.* (NOTE: **bleeding – bled**)

**bleeder** /ˈbliːdə/ *noun* **1.** a blood vessel which bleeds during surgery **2.** a person who has haemophilia (*informal*)

**bleeding** /ˈbliːdɪŋ/ *noun* an unusual loss of blood from the body through the skin, through an orifice or internally

COMMENT: Blood lost through bleeding from an artery is bright red and can rush out because it is under pressure. Blood from a vein is darker red and flows more slowly.

**bleeding point** /ˈbliːdɪŋ pɔɪnt/, **bleeding site** /ˈbliːdɪŋ saɪt/ *noun* a place in the body where bleeding is taking place

**bleeding time** /ˈbliːdɪŋ taɪm/ *noun* a test of the clotting ability of someone's blood, by timing the length of time it takes for the blood to congeal

**blenno-** /blenəʊ/ *prefix* referring to mucus

**blennorrhagia** /ˌblenəʊˈreɪdʒə/ *noun* **1.** the discharge of mucus **2.** gonorrhoea

**blennorrhoea** /ˌblenəˈriːə/ *noun* **1.** the discharge of watery mucus **2.** gonorrhoea

**bleomycin** /ˌbliːəʊˈmaɪsɪn/ *noun* an antibiotic used to treat forms of cancer such as Hodgkin's disease

**blephar-** /blefər/ *prefix* same as **blepharo-** (*used before vowels*)

**blepharitis** /ˌblefəˈraɪtɪs/ *noun* inflammation of the eyelid

**blepharo-** /blefərəʊ/ *prefix* referring to eyelid

**blepharoconjunctivitis** /ˌblefərəʊkən ˌdʒʌŋktɪˈvaɪtɪs/ *noun* inflammation of the conjunctiva of the eyelids

**blepharon** /ˈblefərɒn/ *noun* an eyelid

**blepharospasm** /ˈblefərəʊspæz(ə)m/ *noun* a sudden contraction of the eyelid, as when a tiny piece of dust gets in the eye

**blepharotosis** /ˌblefərəʊˈtəʊsɪs/ *noun* a condition in which the upper eyelid is half closed because of paralysis of the muscle or nerve

**blind** /blaɪnd/ *adjective* not able to see ■ *plural noun* □ **the blind** people who are blind. ◊ **visually impaired** ■ *verb* to make someone blind ○ *He was blinded in the accident.*

**blind gut** /ˌblaɪnd ˈɡʌt/ *noun* same as **caecum**

**blind loop syndrome** /blaɪnd ˈluːp ˌsɪn drəʊm/ *noun* a condition which occurs in cases of diverticulosis or of Crohn's disease, with steatorrhoea, abdominal pain and megaloblastic anaemia

**blindness** /ˈblaɪndnəs/ *noun* the fact of not being able to see

**blind spot** /ˈblaɪnd spɒt/ *noun* the point in the retina where the optic nerve joins it, which does not register light

**blind study** /ˌblaɪnd ˈstʌdi/ *noun* an investigation to test an intervention such as giving a drug, in which a person does not know if he or she has taken the active medicine or the placebo

**blink** /blɪŋk/ *verb* to close and open the eyelids rapidly several times or once ○ *He blinked in the bright light.*

**blister** /ˈblɪstə/ *noun* a swelling on the skin containing serum from the blood, caused by rubbing, burning or a disease such as chickenpox ■ *verb* to produce blisters

**bloated** /ˈbləʊtɪd/ *adjective* experiencing the uncomfortable sensation of a very full stomach

**block** /blɒk/ *noun* **1.** the stopping of a function **2.** something which obstructs **3.** a large piece of something ○ *A block of wood fell on his foot.* **4.** a period of time ○ *The training is in two three-hour blocks.* **5.** one of the different buildings forming a section of a hospital ○ *The patient is in Block 2, Ward 7.* ○ *She is having treatment in the physiotherapy block.* ■ *verb* to fill the space in something and stop other things passing through it ○ *The artery was blocked by a clot.* ○ *He swallowed a piece of plastic which blocked his oesophagus.*

**blockage** /ˈblɒkɪdʒ/ *noun* **1.** something which obstructs ○ *There is a blockage in the rectum.* **2.** the act of being obstructed ○ *The blockage of the artery was caused by a blood clot.*

**blocker** /ˈblɒkə/ *noun* a substance which blocks an action. ♦ **beta blocker**

**blocking** /ˈblɒkɪŋ/ *noun* a psychiatric disorder, in which someone suddenly stops one train of thought and switches to another

**blood** /blʌd/ *noun* a red liquid moved around the body by the pumping action of the heart (NOTE: For other terms referring to blood, see words beginning with **haem-, haemo-, haemato-.**) ◊ **blood chemistry** or **chemistry of the blood 1.** the substances which make up blood can be analysed in blood tests, the results of which are useful in diagnosing disease **2.** the record of changes which take place in blood during disease and treatment

COMMENT: Blood is formed of red and white cells, platelets and plasma. It circulates round the body, going from the heart and lungs along arteries, and returns to the heart through the veins. As it moves round the body it takes oxygen to the tissues and removes waste material which is cleaned out through the kidneys or exhaled through the lungs. It also carries hormones produced by glands to the various organs which need them. The body of an average adult contains about six litres or ten pints of blood.

**blood bank** /ˈblʌd bæŋk/ *noun* a section of a hospital or a special centre where blood given by donors is stored for use in transfusions

**blood blister** /ˈblʌd ˌblɪstə/ noun a swelling on the skin with blood inside, caused by nipping the flesh

**blood-borne virus** /ˌblʌd bɔːn ˈvaɪrəs/ noun a virus carried by the blood

**blood-brain barrier** /ˌblʌd breɪn ˈbæriə/ noun the process by which some substances, which in other parts of the body will diffuse from capillaries, are held back by the endothelium of cerebral capillaries, preventing them from coming into contact with the fluids round the brain

**blood casts** /ˈblʌd kɑːsts/ plural noun pieces of blood cells which are secreted by the kidneys in kidney disease

**blood cell** /ˈblʌd sel/ noun a red or a white cell in the blood

**blood clot** /ˈblʌd klɒt/ noun a soft mass of coagulated blood in a vein or an artery. Also called **thrombus**

**blood clotting** /ˈblʌd ˌklɒtɪŋ/ noun the process by which blood changes from being liquid to being semi-solid and so stops flowing

**blood corpuscle** /ˈblʌd ˌkɔːpʌs(ə)l/ noun ♦ **blood cell**

**blood count** /ˈblʌd kaʊnt/ noun a test to count the number and types of different blood cells in a sample of blood, in order to give an indication of the condition of the person's blood as a whole

**blood culture** /ˈblʌd ˌkʌltʃə/ noun a method of testing a sample of blood by placing it on a culture medium to see if foreign organisms in it grow

**blood donor** /ˈblʌd ˌdəʊnə/ noun a person who gives blood which is then used in transfusions to other people

**blood dyscrasia** /ˌblʌd dɪsˈkreɪziə/ noun any unusual blood condition such as a low cell count or platelet count

**blood formation** /ˈblʌd fɔːˌmeɪʃ(ə)n/ noun same as **haemopoiesis**

**blood-glucose level** /ˌblʌd ˈɡluːkəʊz ˌlev(ə)l/ noun the amount of glucose present in the blood. The usual blood-glucose level is about 60–100 mg of glucose per 100 ml of blood.

**blood group** /ˈblʌd ɡruːp/ noun one of the different groups into which human blood is classified. Also called **blood type**

COMMENT: Blood is classified in various ways. The most common classifications are by the agglutinogens (factors A and B) in red blood cells and by the Rhesus factor. Blood can therefore have either factor (Group A and Group B) or both factors (Group AB) or neither (Group O) and each of these groups can be Rhesus negative or positive.

**blood grouping** /ˈblʌd ˌɡruːpɪŋ/ noun the process of classifying people according to their blood groups

**blood-letting** /ˈblʌd ˌletɪŋ/ noun same as **phlebotomy**

**blood loss** /ˈblʌd lɒs/ noun loss of blood from the body by bleeding

**blood picture** /ˈblʌd ˌpɪktʃə/ noun US a full blood count

**blood pigment** /ˈblʌd ˌpɪɡmənt/ noun same as **haemoglobin**

**blood plasma** /ˈblʌd ˌplæzmə/ noun a yellow watery liquid which makes up the main part of blood

**blood platelet** /ˈblʌd ˌpleɪtlət/ noun a small blood cell which releases thromboplastin and which multiplies rapidly after an injury, encouraging the coagulation of blood

**blood poisoning** /ˈblʌd ˌpɔɪz(ə)nɪŋ/ noun a condition in which bacteria are present in the blood and cause illness (informal) ♦ **septicaemia, bacteraemia, toxaemia**

**blood pressure** /ˈblʌd ˌpreʃə/ noun the pressure, measured in millimetres of mercury, at which the blood is pumped round the body by the heart □ **high blood pressure** or **raised blood pressure** a level of blood pressure which is higher than usual

'…raised blood pressure may account for as many as 70% of all strokes. The risk of stroke rises with both systolic and diastolic blood pressure in the normotensive and hypertensive ranges. Blood pressure control reduces the incidence of first stroke and aspirin appears to reduce the risk of stroke after TIAs' [British Journal of Hospital Medicine]

COMMENT: Blood pressure is measured using a sphygmomanometer. A rubber tube is wrapped round the patient's arm and inflated and two readings of blood pressure are taken: the systolic pressure, when the heart is contracting and so pumping out, and the diastolic pressure, which is always a lower figure, when the heart relaxes. Healthy adult values are considered to be 160/95, unless the patient is diabetic or has heart disease, when lower target values are set.

**blood product** /ˈblʌd ˌprɒdʌkt/ noun a substance such as plasma taken out of blood and used in the treatment of various medical conditions

**blood relationship** /ˌblʌd rɪˈleɪʃ(ə)nʃɪp/ noun a relationship between people who come from the same family and have the same parents, grandparents or ancestors, as opposed to a relationship by marriage

**blood sample** /ˈblʌd ˌsɑːmpəl/ noun a sample of blood, taken for testing

**blood serum** /ˈblʌd ˌsɪərəm/ noun ♦ **serum**

**bloodshot** /ˈblʌdʃɒt/ adjective referring to an eye with small specks of blood in it from a small damaged blood vessel

**bloodstained** /ˈblʌdsteɪnd/ adjective having blood in or on it ○ He coughed up blood-stained sputum.

**bloodstream** /ˈblʌdstriːm/ noun the blood flowing round the body ○ Hormones are secreted by the glands into the bloodstream.

**blood sugar** /ˌblʌd ˈʃʊɡə/ noun glucose present in the blood

**blood sugar level** /ˌblʌd ˈʃʊɡə ˌlev(ə)l/ noun the amount of glucose in the blood, which is higher after meals and in people with diabetes

**blood test** /ˈblʌd test/ noun a laboratory test of a blood sample to analyse its chemical composition ○ The patient will have to have a blood test.

**blood transfusion** /ˈblʌd trænsˌfjuːʒ(ə)n/ noun a procedure in which blood given by another person or taken from the patient at an earlier stage is transferred into the patient's vein

**blood type** /ˈblʌd taɪp/ noun same as **blood group**

**blood typing** /ˈblʌd ˌtaɪpɪŋ/ noun the analysis of blood for transfusion factors and blood group

**blood urea** /ˌblʌd jʊˈriːə/ noun urea present in the blood. A high level occurs following heart failure or kidney disease.

**blood vessel** /ˈblʌd ˌves(ə)l/ noun any tube which carries blood round the body, e.g. an artery, vein or capillary (NOTE: For other terms referring to blood vessels, see words beginning with **angi-, angio-**.)

**blood volume** /ˈblʌd ˌvɒljuːm/ noun the total amount of blood in the body

**blotch** /blɒtʃ/ noun a reddish patch on the skin

**blot test** /ˈblɒt test/ noun ♦ **Rorschach test**

**blue baby** /ˌbluː ˈbeɪbi/ noun a baby who has congenital cyanosis, born either with a congenital heart condition or with a collapsed lung, which prevents an adequate supply of oxygen reaching the tissues, giving the baby's skin a slight blue colour (informal)

**blue disease** /ˈbluː dɪˈziːz/, **blueness** /ˈbluːnəs/ noun ♦ **cyanosis**

**blue litmus** /ˌbluː ˈlɪtməs/ noun treated paper which indicates the presence of acid by turning red

**blurred vision** /ˌblɜːd ˈvɪʒ(ə)n/ noun a condition in which someone does not see objects clearly

**blush** /blʌʃ/ noun a rush of red colour to the skin of the face, caused by emotion ■ verb to go red in the face because of emotion

**bm** abbr bowel movement

**BM** abbr Bachelor of Medicine

**BMA** abbr British Medical Association

**BMI** abbr body mass index

**BMJ** abbr British Medical Journal

**BMR** abbr basal metabolic rate

**BMR test** /ˌbiː ˌem ˈɑː test/ noun a test of thyroid function

**BNF** abbr British National Formulary

**bodily** /ˈbɒdɪli/ adjective referring to the body ○ The main bodily functions are controlled by the sympathetic nervous system.

**body** /ˈbɒdi/ noun **1.** the physical structure of a person, as opposed to the mind **2.** the main part of a person's body, not including the head or arms and legs **3.** a dead person ■ an amount of something ■ noun **1.** the main part of something □ **body of sternum** the main central part of the breastbone □ **body of vertebra** the main part of a vertebra which supports the weight of the body □ **body of the stomach** main part of the stomach between the fundus and the pylorus. See illustration at STOMACH in Supplement **2.** ♦ **foreign body**

**body cavity** /ˈbɒdi ˌkævɪti/ noun an opening in the body, e.g. the mouth, oesophagus, vagina, rectum or ear

**body fat** /ˈbɒdi fæt/ noun tissue where the cells contain fat which replaces the fibrous tissue when too much food is eaten

**body fluid** /ˈbɒdi ˌfluːɪd/ noun a liquid in the body, e.g. water, blood or semen

**body image** /ˈbɒdi ˈɪmɪdʒ/ noun the mental image which a person has of their own body. Also called **body schema**

**body language** /ˈbɒdi ˌlæŋɡwɪdʒ/ noun the expression on your face, or the way you hold your body, interpreted by other people as unconsciously revealing your feelings

**body mass index** /ˌbɒdi ˈmæs ˌɪndeks/ noun a figure obtained by dividing someone's weight in kilos by the square of his or her height in metres. 19–25 is considered usual. Abbr **BMI**

COMMENT: If a person is 1.70m (5ft 7in.) and weighs 82kg (180 lbs), his or her BMI is 28 and so above average.

**body odour** /ˌbɒdi ˈəʊdə/ noun an unpleasant smell caused by perspiration

**body scan** /ˈbɒdi skæn/ noun an examination of the whole of the body using ultrasound or other scanning techniques

**body schema** /ˌbɒdi ˈskiːmə/ noun same as **body image**

**body substance isolation** /ˈbɒdi ˌsʌbstəns aɪsəˌleɪʃ(ə)n/ noun making sure that a trauma victim is kept isolated from the possibility of infection from moist body substances

**body temperature** /ˈbɒdi ˌtemprɪˌtʃə/ noun the internal temperature of the human body, usually about 37°C

**Boeck's disease** /ˈbeks dɪˌziːz/, **Boeck's sarcoid** /ˈbeks ˌsɑːkɔɪd/ noun same as **sarcoidosis** [Described 1899. After Caesar Peter Moeller Boeck (1845–1913), Professor of Dermatology at Oslo, Norway.]

**Bohn's nodules** /ˌbɔːnz ˈnɒdjuːlz/, **Bohn's epithelial pearls** plural noun tiny cysts found in the mouths of healthy infants

**boil** /bɔɪl/ *noun* a tender raised mass of infected tissue and skin, usually caused by infection of a hair follicle by the bacterium *Staphylococcus aureus*. Also called **furuncle**

**bolus** /'bəʊləs/ *noun* **1.** a mass of food which has been chewed and is ready to be swallowed **2.** a mass of food passing along the intestine

**bonding** /'bɒndɪŋ/ *noun* the process by which a psychological link is formed between a baby and its mother ○ *In autistic children bonding is difficult.*

**bone** /bəʊn/ *noun* **1.** calcified connective tissue **2.** one of the calcified pieces of connective tissue which make the skeleton ○ *There are several small bones in the human ear.* See illustration at **SYNOVIAL JOINT** in Supplement ◇ **bone structure 1.** the system of jointed bones forming the body **2.** the arrangement of the various components of a bone

COMMENT: Bones are formed of a hard outer layer (compact bone) which is made up of a series of layers of tissue (Haversian systems) and a softer inner part (cancellous bone *or* spongy bone) which contains bone marrow.

**bone-anchored hearing aid** /ˌbəʊn ˌæŋkəd 'hɪərɪŋ eɪd/ *noun* a hearing aid that is fitted surgically into the skull, usually behind the ear. Abbr **BAHA**

**bone conduction** /'bəʊn kənˌdʌkʃ(ə)n/ *noun* same as **osteophony**

**bone damage** /'bəʊn ˌdæmɪdʒ/ *noun* damage caused to a bone ○ *extensive bruising but no bone damage*

**bone graft** /'bəʊn grɑːft/ *noun* a piece of bone taken from one part of the body to repair a another bone

**bone marrow** /'bəʊn ˌmærəʊ/ *noun* soft tissue in cancellous bone (NOTE: For other terms referring to bone marrow, see words beginning with **myel-**, **myelo-**.)

COMMENT: Two types of bone marrow are to be found: red bone marrow or myeloid tissue, which forms red blood cells and is found in cancellous bone in the vertebrae, the sternum and other flat bones. As a person gets older, fatty yellow bone marrow develops in the central cavity of long bones.

**bone marrow transplant** /ˌbəʊn 'mærəʊ ˌtrænsplɑːnt/ *noun* the transplant of marrow from a donor to a recipient

**bone scan** *noun* a scan which tracks a radioactive substance injected into the body to find areas where a bone is breaking down or repairing itself

**Bonney's blue** /ˌbɒniz 'bluː/ *noun* a blue dye used as a disinfectant [After William Francis Victor Bonney (1872–1953), British gynaecologist]

**bony** /'bəʊni/ *adjective* **1.** relating to bones, or made of bone **2.** referring to a part of the body where the structure of the bones underneath can be seen ○ *thin bony hands*

**bony labyrinth** /ˌbəʊni 'læbərɪnθ/ *noun* a hard part of the temporal bone surrounding the membranous labyrinth in the inner ear. Also called **osseous labyrinth**

**booster** /'buːstər ɪnˌdʒekʃ(ə)n/, **booster injection** *noun* a repeat injection of vaccine given some time after the first injection to maintain the immunising effect

**boracic acid** /bəˌræsɪk 'æsɪd/ *noun* a soluble white powder used as a general disinfectant. Also called **boric acid**

**borax** /'bɔːræks/ *noun* a white powder used as a household cleaner and disinfectant

**borborygmus** /ˌbɔːbə'rɪgməs/ *noun* a rumbling noise in the abdomen, caused by gas in the intestine (NOTE: The plural is **borborygmi**.)

**borderline** /'bɔːdəlaɪn/ *adjective* **1.** not clearly belonging to either one of two categories ○ *a borderline case* **2.** referring to a medical condition likely to develop in someone unless an effort is made to prevent it **3.** characterised by emotional instability and self-destructive behaviour ○ *a borderline personality*

**Bordetella** /ˌbɔːdə'telə/ *noun* a bacterium of the family *Brucellaceae* (NOTE: *Bordetella pertussis* causes whooping cough.)

**boric acid** /ˌbɔːrɪk 'æsɪd/ *noun* same as **boracic acid**

**born** /bɔːn/ *verb* □ **to be born** to begin to live outside the mother's uterus

**Bornholm disease** /'bɔːnhəʊm dɪˌziːz/ *noun* same as **epidemic pleurodynia**

**bottle-fed** /'bɒt(ə)l fed/ *adjective* referring to a baby which is fed from a bottle. Compare **breast-fed**

**bottle feeding** /ˌbɒt(ə)l 'fiːdɪŋ/ *noun* the act of giving a baby milk from a bottle, as opposed to breast feeding. Compare **breast feeding**

**bottom** /'bɒtəm/ *noun* **1.** the part of the body on which you sit. ◊ **buttock 2.** the anus (*informal*)

**bottom shuffling** /'bɒtəm ˌʃʌf(ə)lɪŋ/ *noun* the process by which a baby who cannot yet walk moves around by moving itself along on its hands and buttocks

**botulinum toxin** /ˌbɒtjʊ'laɪnəm ˌtɒksɪn/ *noun* a poison produced by the bacterium *Clostridium botulinum* and used, in small doses, to treat muscular cramps and spasms

**botulism** /'bɒtjʊlɪz(ə)m/ *noun* a type of food poisoning, often fatal, caused by a toxin of *Clostridium botulinum* in badly canned or preserved food. Symptoms include paralysis of the muscles, vomiting and hallucinations.

**bougie** /'buːʒiː/ *noun* a thin tube which can be inserted into passages in the body such as the oesophagus or rectum, either to allow liquid to be introduced or to dilate the passage

**bout** /baʊt/ *noun* a sudden attack of a disease, especially one which recurs ○ *He is recovering from a bout of flu.* □ **bout of fever** a period when someone is feverish ○ *She has recurrent bouts of malarial fever.*

**bovine spongiform encephalopathy** /ˌbəʊvaɪn ˌspʌndʒɪfɔːm enˌkefəˈlɒpəθi/ *noun* a fatal brain disease of cattle. Abbr **BSE**. ◊ **Creutzfeldt-Jakob disease**. Also called **mad cow disease**

**bowel** /ˈbaʊəl/ *noun* the intestine, especially the large intestine (NOTE: **Bowel** is often used in the plural in everyday language.) □ **to open the bowels** to have a bowel movement

**bowel movement** /ˈbaʊəl ˌmuːvmənt/ *noun* **1.** an act of passing faeces out of the body through the anus ○ *The patient had a bowel movement this morning.* Also called **motion**. ◊ **defecation 2.** the amount of faeces passed through the anus

**bowels** /ˈbaʊəlz/ *plural noun* same as **bowel**

**Bowen's disease** /ˈbəʊɪnz dɪˌziːz/ *noun* a form of carcinoma, appearing as red plaques on the skin

**bowl** /bəʊl/ *noun* a wide shallow container used for holding liquids

**bow-legged** /ˌbəʊ ˈlegɪd/ *adjective* with bow legs

**bow legs** /bəʊ ˈlegz/ *noun* a state where the ankles touch and the knees are apart when a person is standing straight. Also called **genu varum**

**Bowman's capsule** /ˌbəʊmənz ˈkæpsjuːl/ *noun* the expanded end of a renal tubule, surrounding a glomerular tuft in the kidney, which filters plasma in order to reabsorb useful foodstuffs and eliminate waste. Also called **Malpighian glomerulus, glomerular capsule** [Described 1842. After Sir William Paget Bowman (1816–92), surgeon in Birmingham and later in London, who was a pioneer in work on the kidney and in ophthalmology.]

**BP** *abbr* **1.** blood pressure **2.** British Pharmacopoeia

**BPH** *abbr* benign prostatic hypertrophy

**Bq** *symbol* becquerel

**brace** /breɪs/ *noun* any type of splint or appliance worn for support, e.g. a metal support used on children's legs to make the bones straight or on teeth which are forming badly ○ *She wore a brace on her front teeth.*

**bracelet** /ˈbreɪslət/ *noun* ♦ **identity bracelet, medical alert bracelet**

**brachi-** /ˈbreɪki/ *prefix* same as **brachio-** (*used before vowels*)

**brachial** /ˈbreɪkiəl/ *adjective* referring to the arm, especially the upper arm

**brachial artery** /ˈbreɪkiəl ˌɑːtəri/ *noun* an artery running down the arm from the axillary artery to the elbow, where it divides into the radial and ulnar arteries

**brachialis muscle** /ˌbreɪkiˈeɪlɪs ˌmʌs(ə)l/ *noun* a muscle that causes the elbow to bend

**brachial plexus** /ˌbreɪkiəl ˈpleksəs/ *noun* a group of nerves at the armpit and base of the neck which lead to the nerves in the arms and hands. Injury to the brachial plexus at birth leads to Erb's palsy.

**brachial pressure point** /ˌbreɪkiəl ˈpreʃə pɔɪnt/ *noun* the point on the arm where pressure will stop bleeding from the brachial artery

**brachial vein** /ˈbreɪkiəl veɪn/ *noun* a vein accompanying the brachial artery, draining into the axillary vein

**brachio-** /breɪkiəʊ/ *prefix* referring to the arm

**brachiocephalic artery** /ˌbreɪkiəʊsəˌfælɪk ˈɑːtəri/ *noun* the largest branch of the arch of the aorta, which continues as the right common carotid and right subclavian arteries

**brachiocephalic vein** /ˌbreɪkiəʊsəˌfælɪk ˈveɪn/ *noun* one of a pair of large veins on opposite sides of the neck that join to form the superior vena cava. Also called **innominate vein**

**brachium** /ˈbreɪkiəm/ *noun* an arm, especially the upper arm between the elbow and the shoulder (NOTE: The plural is **brachia**.)

**brachy-** /ˈbræki/ *prefix* short

**brachycephaly** /ˌbræki'sefəli/ *noun* a condition in which the skull is shorter than usual

**brachytherapy** /ˌbræki'θerəpi/ *noun* a radioactive treatment in which the radioactive material actually touches the tissue being treated

**Bradford's frame** /ˈbrædfədz freɪm/ *noun* a frame of metal and cloth, used to support a patient [After Edward Hickling Bradford (1848–1926), US orthopaedic surgeon]

**brady-** /ˈbrædɪ/ *prefix* slow

**bradycardia** /ˌbrædɪˈkɑːdiə/ *noun* a slow rate of heart contraction, shown by a slow pulse rate of less than 70 beats per minute

**bradykinesia** /ˌbrædɪkaɪˈniːziə/ *noun* a condition in which the someone walks slowly and makes slow movements because of disease

**bradykinin** /ˌbrædɪˈkaɪnɪn/ *noun* a chemical produced in the blood when tissues are injured, that plays a role in inflammation. ◊ **kinin**

**bradypnoea** /ˌbrædɪpˈniːə/ *noun* unusually slow breathing (NOTE: The US spelling is **bradypnea**.)

**Braille** /breɪl/ *noun* a system of writing using raised dots on the paper to indicate letters which a blind person can read by passing their fingers over the page ○ *The book has been published in Braille.* [Introduced 1829–30. After Louis Braille (1809–52), blind Frenchman and teacher of the blind; he introduced the system which had originally been proposed by Charles Barbier in 1820.]

**brain** /breɪn/ *noun* the part of the central nervous system situated inside the skull. Also called **encephalon**. See illustration at **BRAIN** in Supplement

COMMENT: The main part of the brain is the cerebrum, formed of two sections or hemispheres, which relate to thought and to sensations from either side of the body. At the back of the head and beneath the cerebrum is the cerebellum which coordinates muscle reaction and balance. Also in the brain are the hypothalamus which governs body temperature, hunger, thirst and sexual urges, and the tiny pituitary gland which is the most important endocrine gland in the body.

**brain covering** /ˈbreɪn ˌkʌv(ə)rɪŋ/ *noun* ♦ **meninges**

**brain damage** /ˈbreɪn ˌdæmɪdʒ/ *noun* damage caused to the brain as a result of oxygen and sugar deprivation, e.g. after a haemorrhage, accident, or though disease

**brain-damaged** /ˈbreɪn ˌdæmɪdʒd/ *adjective* referring to someone who has experienced brain damage

**brain death** /ˈbreɪn deθ/ *noun* a condition in which the nerves in the brain stem have died, and the person can be certified as dead, although the heart may not have stopped beating

**brain haemorrhage** /breɪn ˈhem(ə)rɪdʒ/ *noun* same as **cerebral haemorrhage**

**brain scan** /ˈbreɪn skæn/ *noun* an examination of the inside of the brain, made by passing X-rays through the head, using a scanner, and reconstituting the images on a computer monitor

**brain scanner** /ˈbreɪn ˌskænə/ *noun* a machine which scans the interior of the body, used to examine the brain

**brain stem** /ˈbreɪn stem/ *noun* the lower narrow part of the brain which connects the brain to the spinal cord

**brain tumour** /ˈbreɪn tjuːmə/ *noun* a tumour which grows in the brain

COMMENT: Tumours may grow in any part of the brain. The symptoms of brain tumour are usually headaches and dizziness, and as the tumour grows it may affect the senses or mental faculties. Operations to remove brain tumours can be very successful.

**brain wave** /breɪn stem/ *noun* a rhythmic wave of voltage produced by electrical activity in the brain tissue

**bran** /bræn/ *noun* the outside covering of the wheat seed, removed when making white flour, but an important source of roughage in the diet

**branch** /brɑːntʃ/ *noun* any part which grows out of a main part ■ *verb* to split out into smaller parts ○ *The radial artery branches from the brachial artery at the elbow.*

**branchia** /ˈbræŋkiə/ *noun* a breathing organ similar to the gill of a fish found in human embryos in the early stages of development (NOTE: The plural is **branchiae**.)

**branchial** /ˈbræŋkiəl/ *adjective* referring to the branchiae

**branchial cyst** /ˌbræŋkiəl ˈsɪst/ *noun* a cyst on the side of the neck of an embryo

**branchial pouch** /ˌbræŋkiəl ˈpautʃ/ *noun* a pouch on the side of the neck of an embryo

**Braun's frame** /ˌbraʊnz ˈfreɪm/, **Braun's splint** /ˌbraʊnz ˈsplɪnt/ *noun* a metal splint and frame to which pulleys are attached, used for holding up a fractured leg while the person is lying in bed [After Heinrich Friedrich Wilhelm Braun (1862–1934), German surgeon]

**Braxton-Hicks contractions** /ˌbrækstən ˈhɪks kənˌtrækʃənz/ *plural noun* contractions of the uterus which occur throughout a pregnancy and become more frequent and stronger towards the end [After Dr Braxton-Hicks, 19th century British physician]

**break** /breɪk/ *noun* the point at which a bone has broken □ **clean break** a break in a bone which is not complicated and where the two parts will join again easily

**breakbone fever** /ˈbreɪkbəʊn ˌfiːvə/ *noun* same as **dengue**

**break down** /ˌbreɪk ˈdaʊn/ *verb* **1.** to experience a sudden physical or psychological illness (*informal*) ○ *After she lost her husband, her health broke down.* **2.** to start to cry and become upset (*informal*) ○ *She broke down as she described the symptoms to the doctor.* **3.** to split or cause to split into smaller chemical components, as in the digestion of food

**breakdown** /ˈbreɪkdaʊn/ *noun* ♦ **nervous breakdown**

**breakdown product** /ˈbreɪkdaʊn ˌprɒdʌkt/ *noun* a substance which is produced when a compound is broken down into its parts

**breast** /brest/ *noun* one of two glands in a woman which secrete milk. Also called **mamma** (NOTE: For other terms referring to breasts, see words beginning with **mamm-, mammo-, mast-, masto-**.)

**breast augmentation** /ˈbrest ˌɔːgmenteɪʃ(ə)n/ *noun* a surgical procedure to increase the size of the breast for cosmetic purposes

**breastbone** /ˈbrestbəʊn/ *noun* a bone which is in the centre of the front of the thorax and to which the ribs are connected. Also called **sternum**

**breast cancer** /ˈbrest ˌkænsə/ *noun* a malignant tumour in a breast

**breast-fed** /ˈbrest fed/ *adjective* referring to a baby which is fed from the mother's breasts ○ *She was breast-fed for the first two months.*

**breast feeding** /ˈbrest ˌfiːdɪŋ/ *noun* feeding a baby from the mother's breasts as opposed to from a bottle. Compare **bottle feeding**

**breast implant** /ˈbrest ˌɪmplɑːnt/ *noun* a sac containing silicone, implanted to improve the appearance of a breast

**breast milk** /ˈbrest mɪlk/ *noun* the milk produced by a woman who has recently had a baby

**breast palpation** /ˈbrest ˌpælˌpeɪʃ(ə)n/ noun feeling a breast to see if a lump is present which might indicate breast cancer

**breast pump** /ˈbrest pʌmp/ noun an instrument for taking milk from a breast

**breast reconstruction** noun the construction of a new breast for a woman who has had a breast removed because of cancer

**breast reduction** /ˈbrest rɪˌdʌkʃ(ə)n/ noun a reduction of the size of the breast for cosmetic purposes

**breath** /breθ/ noun air which goes in and out of the body when you breathe ○ *He ran so fast he was out of breath.* ○ *Stop for a moment to get your breath back.* ○ *She took a deep breath and dived into the water.* □ **to hold your breath** to stop breathing out, after having inhaled deeply

**breathe** /briːð/ verb to take air in and blow air out through the nose or mouth ○ *The patient has begun to breathe normally.* □ **to breathe in** to take air into your lungs □ **to breathe out** to let the air out of your lungs ○ *He breathed in the smoke from the fire and it made him cough.* ○ *The doctor told him to take a deep breath and breathe out slowly.*

COMMENT: Children breathe about 20 to 30 times per minute, men 16–18 per minute, and women slightly faster. The breathing rate increases if the person is taking exercise or has a fever. Some babies and young children hold their breath and go blue in the face, especially when crying or during a temper tantrum.

**breath-holding attack** /ˈbreθ ˌhəʊldɪŋ əˌtæk/ noun a period when a young child stops breathing, usually because he or she is angry

**breathing** /ˈbriːðɪŋ/ noun same as **respiration** ○ *If breathing is difficult or has stopped, begin artificial ventilation immediately.* (NOTE: For other terms referring to breathing see words beginning with **pneum-, pneumo-, pneumat-, pneumato-**.)

**breathing rate** /ˈbriːðɪŋ reɪt/ noun the number of times a person breathes in and out in a specific period

**breathless** /ˈbreθləs/ adjective referring to someone who finds it difficult to breathe enough air ○ *After running upstairs she became breathless and had to sit down.*

**breathlessness** /ˈbreθləsnəs/ noun difficulty in breathing enough air

'26 patients were selected from the outpatient department on grounds of disabling breathlessness present for at least five years' [*Lancet*]

**breath sounds** /ˈbreθ saʊndz/ noun hollow sounds made by the lungs and heard through a stethoscope placed on a person's chest, used in diagnosis

**breech** /briːtʃ/ noun the buttocks, especially of a baby

**breech birth** /ˈbriːtʃ ˌbɜːθ/, **breech delivery** /ˈbriːtʃ dɪˌlɪv(ə)ri/ noun a birth in which the baby's buttocks appear first rather than its head

**breech presentation** /briːtʃ ˌprez(ə)n ˈteɪʃ(ə)n/ noun a position of the baby in the uterus in which the buttocks will appear first during childbirth

**breed** /briːd/ verb to reproduce, or reproduce animals or plants ○ *The bacteria breed in dirty water.* ○ *Insanitary conditions help to breed disease.*

**bregma** /ˈbregmə/ noun the point at the top of the head where the soft gap between the bones of a baby's skull hardens

**bretylium tosylate** /brəˌtɪliəm ˈtɒsɪleɪt/ noun an agent used to block adrenergic transmitter release

**bridge** /brɪdʒ/ noun **1.** the top part of the nose where it joins the forehead **2.** an artificial tooth or set of teeth which is joined to natural teeth which hold it in place **3.** a part joining two or more other parts

**Bright's disease** /ˈbraɪts dɪˌziːz/ noun inflammation of the kidneys, characterised by albuminuria and high blood pressure. Also called **glomerulonephritis** [Described 1836. After Richard Bright (1789–1858), physician at Guy's Hospital, London, UK.]

**bring up** /ˌbrɪŋ ˈʌp/ verb **1.** to look after and educate a child **2.** to cough up material such as mucus from the lungs or throat **3.** to vomit (*informal*)

**British anti-lewisite** /ˌbrɪtɪʃ ˌænti ˈluːɪsaɪt/ noun an antidote for gases which cause blistering, also used to treat cases of poisoning such as mercury poisoning. Abbr **BAL**

**British Dental Association** /ˌbrɪtɪʃ ˈdent(ə)l əsəʊsiˌeɪʃ(ə)n/ noun in the UK, a professional association of dentists. Abbr **BDA**

**British Medical Association** /ˌbrɪtɪʃ ˈmedɪk(ə)l əsəʊsiˌeɪʃ(ə)n/ noun in the UK, a professional association of doctors. Abbr **BMA**

**British National Formulary** /ˌbrɪtɪʃ ˌnæʃ(ə)nəl ˈfɔːmjʊləri/ noun a book listing key information on the prescribing, dispensing and administration of prescription drugs used in the UK. Abbr **BNF**

**British Pharmacopoeia** /ˌbrɪtɪʃ ˌfɑːməkə ˈpiːə/ noun a book listing drugs approved in the UK and their dosages. Abbr **BP**

COMMENT: Drugs listed in the British Pharmacopoeia have the letters BP written after them on labels.

**brittle** /ˈbrɪt(ə)l/ adjective easily broken ○ *The people's bones become brittle as they get older.*

**brittle bone disease** /ˌbrɪt(ə)l ˈbəʊn dɪˌziːz/ noun **1.** same as **osteogenesis imperfecta 2.** same as **osteoporosis**

**Broadbent's sign** /ˈbrɔːdbents saɪn/ noun a movement of someone's left side near the lower ribs at each beat of the heart, indicating adhesion between the diaphragm and pericardium in cases of pericarditis [After Sir William

Henry Broadbent (1835–1907), British physician]

**broad ligament** /ˌbrɔːd ˈlɪɡəmənt/ *noun* peritoneal folds supporting the uterus on each side

**broad-spectrum antibiotic** /ˌbrɔːd ˌspektrəm ˌæntibaɪˈɒtɪk/ *noun* an antibiotic used to control many types of microorganism

**Broca's aphasia** /ˌbrəʊkəz əˈfeɪziə/ *noun* a condition in which someone is unable to speak or write, as a result of damage to Broca's area

**Broca's area** /ˈbrəʊkəz ˌeəriə/ *noun* an area on the left side of the brain which governs the motor aspects of speaking [Described 1861. After Pierre Henri Paul Broca (1824–80), French surgeon and anthropologist. A pioneer of neurosurgery, he also invented various instruments, described muscular dystrophy before Duchenne, and recognised rickets as a nutritional disorder before Virchow.]

**Brodie's abscess** /ˌbrəʊdiz ˈæbses/ *noun* an abscess of a bone, caused by staphylococcal osteomyelitis [Described 1832. After Sir Benjamin Collins Brodie (1783–1862), British surgeon.]

**bromhidrosis** /ˌbrɒmhɪˈdrəʊsɪs/ *noun* a condition in which body sweat has an unpleasant smell

**bromide** /ˈbrəʊmaɪd/ *noun* a bromine salt (NOTE: Bromides are used as sedatives.)

**bromine** /ˈbrəʊmiːn/ *noun* a chemical element (NOTE: The chemical symbol is **Br**.)

**bromism** /ˈbrəʊmɪz(ə)m/ *noun* chronic ill health caused by excessive use of bromides

**bromocriptine** /ˌbrəʊməʊˈkrɪptiːn/ *noun* a drug which functions like dopamine, used to treat excessive lactation, breast pain, some forms of infertility, growth disorder and Parkinson's disease

**bronch-** /brɒŋk/, **bronchi-** /brɒŋki/ *prefix* same as **broncho-** (*used before vowels*)

**bronchi** /ˈbrɒŋkaɪ/ *plural of* **bronchus**

**bronchial** /ˈbrɒŋkiəl/ *adjective* referring to the bronchi

**bronchial asthma** /ˌbrɒŋkiəl ˈæsmə/ *noun* a type of asthma mainly caused by an allergen or by exertion

**bronchial breath sounds** /ˌbrɒŋkiəl ˈbreθ ˌsaʊndz/ *plural noun* distinctive breath sounds from the lungs which help diagnosis

**bronchial pneumonia** /ˌbrɒŋkiəl njuːˈməʊniə/ *noun* same as **bronchopneumonia**

**bronchial tree** /ˈbrɒŋkiəl triː/ *noun* a system of tubes (bronchi and bronchioles) which take the air from the trachea into the lungs

**bronchiectasis** /ˌbrɒŋkiˈektəsɪs/ *noun* a disorder of the bronchi which become wide, infected and filled with pus (NOTE: Bronchiectasis can lead to pneumonia.)

**bronchio-** /ˈbrɒŋkiəʊ/ *prefix* referring to the bronchioles

**bronchiolar** /ˌbrɒŋkiˈəʊlə/ *adjective* referring to the bronchioles

**bronchiole** /ˈbrɒŋkiəʊl/ *noun* a very small air tube in the lungs leading from a bronchus to the alveoli. See illustration at **LUNGS** in Supplement

**bronchiolitis** /ˌbrɒŋkiəʊˈlaɪtɪs/ *noun* inflammation of the bronchioles, usually in small children

**bronchitic** /brɒŋˈkɪtɪk/ *adjective* **1.** referring to bronchitis **2.** referring to a person who has bronchitis

**bronchitis** /brɒŋˈkaɪtɪs/ *noun* inflammation of the mucous membrane of the bronchi □ **acute bronchitis** an attack of bronchitis caused by a virus or by exposure to cold and wet

**broncho-** /brɒŋkəʊ/ *prefix* referring to the windpipe

**bronchoconstrictor** /ˌbrɒŋkəʊkənˈstrɪktə/ *noun* a drug which narrows the bronchi

**bronchodilator** /ˌbrɒŋkəʊdaɪˈleɪtə/ *noun* a drug which makes the bronchi wider, used in the treatment of asthma and allergy (NOTE: Bronchodilators usually have names ending in -**terol**; however, the most common bronchodilator is **salbutamol**.)

'19 children with mild to moderately severe perennial bronchial asthma were selected. These children gave a typical history of exercise-induced asthma and their symptoms were controlled with oral or aerosol bronchodilators' [*Lancet*]

**bronchogram** /ˈbrɒŋkəʊɡræm/ *noun* an X-ray picture of the bronchial tubes obtained by bronchography

**bronchography** /brɒŋˈkɒɡrəfi/ *noun* an X-ray examination of the lungs after an opaque substance has been put into the bronchi

**bronchomediastinal trunk** /ˌbrɒŋkəʊ miːdiəˌstaɪn(ə)l ˈtrʌŋk/ *noun* the set of lymph nodes draining part of the chest

**bronchomycosis** /ˌbrɒŋkəʊmaɪˈkəʊsɪs/ *noun* an infection of the bronchi by a fungus

**bronchophony** /brɒŋˈkɒfəni/ *noun* vibrations of the voice heard over the lungs, indicating solidification in the lungs

**bronchopleural** /ˌbrɒŋkəʊˈpluərəl/ *adjective* referring to a bronchus and the pleura

**bronchopneumonia** /ˌbrɒŋkəʊnjuːˈməʊniə/ *noun* an infectious inflammation of the bronchioles, which may lead to general infection of the lungs

**bronchopulmonary** /ˌbrɒŋkəʊˈpʌlmən(ə)ri/ *adjective* referring to the bronchi and the lungs

**bronchorrhoea** /ˌbrɒŋkəʊˈriːə/ *noun* the secretion of mucus by the bronchi

**bronchoscope** /ˈbrɒŋkəʊskəʊp/ *noun* an instrument which is passed down the trachea into the lungs, which a doctor can use to inspect the inside passages of the lungs

**bronchoscopy** /brɒŋ'kɒskəpi/ *noun* an examination of a person's bronchi using a bronchoscope

**bronchospasm** /'brɒŋkəʊspæz(ə)m/ *noun* a tightening of the bronchial muscles which causes the tubes to contract, as in asthma

**bronchospirometer** /ˌbrɒŋkəʊspaɪ'rɒmɪtə/ *noun* an instrument for measuring the volume of the lungs

**bronchospirometry** /ˌbrɒŋkəʊspaɪ'rɒmɪtri/ *noun* a procedure for measuring the volume of the lungs

**bronchostenosis** /ˌbrɒŋkəʊste'nəʊsɪs/ *noun* an unusual constriction of the bronchial tubes

**bronchotracheal** /ˌbrɒŋkəʊtrə'kiːəl/ *adjective* referring to the bronchi and the trachea

**bronchus** /'brɒŋkəs/ *noun* one of the two air passages leading from the trachea into the lungs, where they split into many bronchioles. See illustration at **LUNGS** in Supplement (NOTE: The plural is **bronchi**.)

**bronze diabetes** /ˌbrɒnz daɪə'biːtiːz/ *noun* same as **haemochromatosis**

**Broviac catheter** /'brəʊviæk ˌkæθɪtə/ *noun* a type of thin catheter used to insert into a vein

**brow** /braʊ/ *noun* 1. same as **forehead** 2. same as **eyebrow**

**brown fat** /braʊn 'fæt/ *noun* dark-coloured body fat that can easily be converted to energy and helps to control body temperature

**Brown-Séquard syndrome** /ˌbraʊn 'seɪkɑː ˌsɪndrəʊm/ *noun* a condition in which the spinal cord has been partly severed or compressed, with the result that the lower half of the body is paralysed on one side and loses feeling in the other side [Described 1851. After Charles Edouard Brown-Séquard (1817–94), French physiologist.]

**Brucella** /bruː'selə/ *noun* a type of rod-shaped bacterium

**brucellosis** /ˌbruːsɪ'ləʊsɪs/ *noun* a disease which can be caught from cattle or goats or from drinking infected milk, spread by a species of the bacterium *Brucella*. The symptoms include tiredness, arthritis, headache, sweating, irritability and swelling of the spleen. Also called **abortus fever, Malta fever, mountain fever, undulant fever**

**Brufen** /'bruːfən/ a trade name for ibuprofen

**bruise** /bruːz/ *noun* a dark painful area on the skin, where blood has escaped under the skin following a blow. ◊ **black eye** ■ *verb* to cause a bruise on part of the body ○ *She bruised her knee on the corner of the table.* □ **she bruises easily** even a soft blow will give her a bruise

**bruised** /bruːzd/ *adjective* painful after a blow or showing the marks of a bruise ○ *a badly bruised leg*

**bruising** /'bruːzɪŋ/ *noun* an area of bruises ○ *The baby has bruising on the back and legs.*

**bruit** /bruːt/ *noun* an unusual noise heard through a stethoscope

**Brunner's glands** /'brʊnəz ˌglændz/ *plural noun* glands in the duodenum and jejunum [Described 1687. After Johann Konrad Brunner (1653–1727), Swiss anatomist at Heidelberg, then at Strasbourg.]

**bruxism** /'brʌksɪz(ə)m/ *noun* the action of grinding the teeth, as a habit

**BSE** *abbr* bovine spongiform encephalopathy

**bubo** /'bjuːbəʊ/ *noun* a swelling of a lymph node in the groin or armpit

**bubonic plague** /bjuːˌbɒnɪk 'pleɪg/ *noun* a usually fatal infectious disease caused by *Yersinia pestis* in the lymph system, transmitted to humans by fleas from rats

COMMENT: Bubonic plague was the Black Death of the Middle Ages. Its symptoms are fever, delirium, vomiting and swelling of the lymph nodes.

**buccal** /'bʌk(ə)l/ *adjective* referring to the cheek or mouth

**buccal cavity** /'bʌk(ə)l ˌkævɪti/ *noun* the mouth

**buccal fat** /'bʌk(ə)l fæt/ *noun* a pad of fat separating the buccinator muscle from the masseter

**buccal smear** /'bʌk(ə)l smɪə/ *noun* a gentle scraping of the inside of the cheek with a spatula to obtain cells for testing

**buccinator** /'bʌksɪneɪtə/ *noun* a cheek muscle which helps the jaw to move when chewing

**Budd–Chiari syndrome** /ˌbʌd kɪ'eəri ˌsɪndrəʊm/ *noun* a disease of the liver, where thrombosis has occurred in the hepatic veins [Described 1845. After George Budd (1808–82), Professor of Medicine at King's College Hospital, London; Hans von Chiari (1851–1916), Viennese pathologist who was Professor of Pathological Anatomy at Strasbourg and later at Prague.]

**budesonide** /bjuː'desənaɪd/ *noun* a corticosteroid drug taken by inhalation or in tablets, used in the treatment of hay fever and nasal polyps

**Buerger's disease** /'bɜːgəz dɪˌziːz/ *noun* same as **thromboangiitis obliterans** [Described 1908. After Leo Buerger (1879–1943), New York physician of Viennese origin.]

**buffer** /'bʌfə/ *noun* 1. a substance that keeps a constant balance between acid and alkali 2. a solution where the pH is not changed by adding acid or alkali ■ *verb* to prevent a solution from becoming acid

**buffer action** /'bʌfə ˌækʃən/ *noun* the balancing process between acid and alkali

**buffered** /'bʌfəd/ *adjective* prevented from becoming acid ○ *buffered aspirin*

**bug** /bʌg/ *noun* an infectious disease (*informal*) ○ *He caught a bug on holiday.* ○ *Half the staff have got a stomach bug.*

**build** /bɪld/ *noun* the general size and shape of a person's body ○ *He has a heavy build for his height.* ○ *The girl is of slight build.*

**build up** /ˌbɪld ˈʌp/ *verb* to form gradually by being added to, or to form something in this way (NOTE: **building – built**)

**build-up** /ˈbɪld ʌp/ *noun* a gradual process of being added to ○ *a build-up of fatty deposits on the walls of the arteries*

**built** /bɪlt/ *adjective* referring to the general size of a person's body ○ *a heavily built man* ○ *She's slightly built.*

**bulb** /bʌlb/ *noun* a round part at the end of an organ or bone □ **bulb of the penis** the round end of the penis. Also called **glans penis**

**bulbar** /ˈbʌlbə/ *adjective* **1.** referring to a bulb **2.** referring to the medulla oblongata

**bulbar paralysis** /ˌbʌlbə pəˈræləsɪs/, **bulbar palsy** /ˌbʌlbə ˈpɔːlzi/ *noun* a form of motor neurone disease which affects the muscles of the mouth, jaw and throat

**bulbar poliomyelitis** /ˌbʌlbə ˌpəʊliəʊmaɪəˈlaɪtɪs/ *noun* a type of polio affecting the brain stem, which makes it difficult for a person to swallow or breathe

**bulbospongiosus muscle** /ˌbʌlbəʊspʌndʒiˈəʊsəs ˌmʌsəl/ *noun* a muscle in the perineum behind the penis

**bulbourethral gland** /ˌbʌlbəʊjuˈriːθrəl ˌglænd/ *noun* one of two glands at the base of the penis which secrete into the urethra. ♦ **gland**

**bulge** /bʌldʒ/ *verb* to push out ○ *The wall of the abdomen becomes weak and part of the intestine bulges through.*

**bulging** /ˈbʌldʒɪŋ/ *adjective* sticking out ○ *bulging eyes*

**bulimia** /buˈlɪmiə/, **bulimia nervosa** /buˌlɪmiə nəˈvəʊsə/ *noun* a psychological condition in which a person eats too much and is incapable of controlling his or her eating. The eating is followed by behaviour designed to prevent weight gain, e.g. vomiting, use of laxatives or excessive exercise.

**bulimic** /buˈlɪmɪk/ *adjective* **1.** referring to bulimia **2.** having bulimia ■ *noun* someone who has bulimia

**bulla** /ˈbʊlə/ *noun* a large blister (NOTE: The plural is **bullae**.)

**bumetanide** /bjuːˈmetənaɪd/ *noun* a drug which helps a patient to produce urine, used in the treatment of swelling caused by fluid accumulating in the tissues

**bump** /bʌmp/ *noun* a slightly swollen part on the skin, caused by something such as a blow or sting

**bumper fracture** /ˈbʌmpə ˌfræktʃə/ *noun* a fracture in the upper part of the tibia (NOTE: It has this name because it can be caused by a blow from the bumper of a car.)

**bundle** /ˈbʌnd(ə)l/ *noun* a group of nerves running in the same direction

**bundle branch block** /ˈbʌnd(ə)l brɑːntʃ ˌblɒk/ *noun* an unusual condition of the heart's conduction tissue

**bundle of His** /ˌbʌnd(ə)l əv ˈhɪs/ *noun* same as **atrioventricular bundle** [Described 1893. After Ludwig His (1863–1934), Professor of Anatomy successively at Leipzig, Basle, Göttingen and Berlin.]

**bunion** /ˈbʌnjən/ *noun* an inflammation and swelling of the big toe, caused by tight shoes which force the toe sideways so that a callus develops over the joint between the toe and the metatarsal

**buphthalmos** /bʌfˈθælməs/ *noun* a type of congenital glaucoma occurring in infants

**bupivacaine** /bjuːˈpɪvəkeɪn/ *noun* a powerful local anaesthetic, used in epidural anaesthesia

**buprenorphine** /bjuːˈprenəfiːn/ *noun* an opiate drug used in the relief of moderate to severe pain, and as an opioid substitute in treating drug addiction

**Burkitt's tumour** /ˌbɜːkɪts ˈtjuːmə/, **Burkitt's lymphoma** /ˌbɜːkɪts lɪmˈfəʊmə/ *noun* a malignant tumour, usually on the maxilla, found especially in children in Africa [Described 1957. After Denis Parsons Burkitt (1911–93), formerly Senior Surgeon, Kampala, Uganda; later a member of the Medical Research Council (UK).]

**burn** /bɜːn/ *noun* an injury to skin and tissue caused by light, heat, radiation, electricity or chemicals ■ *verb* to harm or destroy something by fire ○ *She burnt her hand on the hot frying pan.* ○ *Most of his hair or his skin was burnt off.* (NOTE: **burning – burnt** *or* **burned**)

COMMENT: The modern classification of burns is into two categories: deep and superficial. Burns were formerly classified as first, second or third degree and are still sometimes referred to in this way.

**burning** /ˈbɜːnɪŋ/ *adjective* referring to a feeling similar to that of being hurt by fire ○ *She had a burning pain or in her chest.*

**burnout** /ˈbɜːnaʊt/ *noun* a feeling of depression, fatigue and lack of energy caused by stress and being overworked ○ *He suffered a burnout and had to go on leave.*

**burns unit** /ˈbɜːnz ˌjuːnɪt/ *noun* a special department in a hospital which deals with burns

**burp** /bɜːp/ (*informal*) *noun* an act of allowing air in the stomach to come up through the mouth ■ *verb* to allow air in the stomach to come up through the mouth □ **to burp a baby** to pat a baby on the back until it burps

**burr** /bɜː/ *noun* a bit used with a drill to make holes in a bone such as the cranium or in a tooth

**bursa** /ˈbɜːsə/ *noun* a sac containing fluid, forming part of the usual structure of a joint such as the knee and elbow, where it protects against frequent pressure and rubbing (NOTE: The plural is **bursae**.)

**bursitis** /bɜːˈsaɪtɪs/ *noun* the inflammation of a bursa, especially in the shoulder

**Buscopan** /ˈbʌskəpæn/ a trade name for a form of hyoscine

**butobarbitone** /ˌbjuːtəʊˈbɑːbɪtəʊn/ *noun* a barbiturate drug used as a sedative and hypnotic

**buttock** /ˈbʌtək/ *noun* one of the two fleshy parts below the back, on which a person sits, made up mainly of the gluteal muscles. Also called **nates**

**buttonhole surgery** /ˈbʌt(ə)nhəʊl ˌsɜːdʒəri/ *noun* a surgical operation through a small hole in the body, using an endoscope

**bypass** /ˈbaɪpɑːs/ *noun* **1.** a surgical operation to redirect the blood, usually using a grafted blood vessel and usually performed when one of the person's own blood vessels is blocked **2.** a new route for the blood created by a bypass operation

**byssinosis** /ˌbɪsɪˈnəʊsɪs/ *noun* a lung disease which is a form of pneumoconiosis caused by inhaling cotton dust

# C

**c** *symbol* centi-

**C** *symbol* Celsius

**CABG** *abbr* coronary artery bypass graft

**cachet** /ˈkæʃeɪ/ *noun* a quantity of a drug wrapped in paper, to be swallowed

**cachexia** /kæˈkeksiə/ *noun* a state of ill health characterised by wasting and general weakness

**cadaver** /kəˈdævə/ *noun* a dead body, especially one used for dissection

**cadaveric** /kəˈdævərɪk/, **cadaverous** /kəˈdæv(ə)rəs/ *adjective* referring to a person who is thin or wasting away

**caeca** /ˈsiːkə/ plural of **caecum**

**caecal** /ˈsiːk(ə)l/ *adjective* referring to the caecum

**caecosigmoidostomy** /ˌsiːkəʊˌsɪɡmɔɪˈdɒstəmi/ *noun* an operation to open up a connection between the caecum and the sigmoid colon

**caecostomy** /siːˈkɒstəmi/ *noun* a surgical operation to make an opening between the caecum and the abdominal wall to allow faeces to be passed without going through the rectum and anus

**caecum** /ˈsiːkəm/ *noun* the wider part of the large intestine in the lower right-hand side of the abdomen at the point where the small intestine joins it and which has the appendix attached to it. See illustration at **DIGESTIVE SYSTEM** in Supplement. Also called **cecum** (NOTE: The plural is **caeca**.)

**caesarean** /sɪˈzeəriən/, **caesarean section** /sɪˈzeəriən ˌsekʃən/ *noun* a surgical operation to deliver a baby by cutting through the abdominal wall into the uterus. Compare **vaginal delivery** (NOTE: The US spelling is **cesarean**.)

COMMENT: A caesarean section is performed only when it appears that natural childbirth is impossible or might endanger mother or child, and only after the 28th week of gestation.

**caesium** /ˈsiːziəm/ *noun* a radioactive element, used in treatment by radiation (NOTE: The chemical symbol is **Cs**.)

**caesium-137** /ˌsiːziəm wʌn θriː ˈsev(ə)n/ *noun* a radioactive substance used in radiology

**café au lait spots** /ˌkæfeɪ əʊ ˈleɪ spɒts/ *plural noun* brown spots on the skin, which are an indication of von Recklinghausen's disease

**caffeine** /ˈkæfiːn/ *noun* an alkaloid found in coffee, tea and chocolate, which acts as a stimulant

COMMENT: Apart from acting as a stimulant, caffeine also helps in the production of urine. It can be addictive, and exists in both tea and coffee in about the same percentages as well as in chocolate and other drinks.

**caisson disease** /ˈkeɪs(ə)n dɪˌziːz/ *noun* a condition in which a person experiences pains in the joints and stomach, and dizziness caused by nitrogen in the blood. Also called **the bends, compressed air sickness, decompression sickness**

COMMENT: The disease occurs in a person who has moved rapidly from high atmospheric pressure to a lower pressure area, such as a diver who has come back to the surface too quickly after a deep dive. The first symptoms, pains in the joints, are known as 'the bends'. The disease can be fatal.

**calamine** /ˈkæləmaɪn/, **calamine lotion** /ˈkæləmaɪn ˌləʊʃ(ə)n/ *noun* a lotion, based on zinc oxide, which helps relieve skin irritation, caused e.g. by sunburn or chickenpox

**calc-** /kælk/ *prefix* same as **calci-** (*used before vowels*)

**calcaemia** /kælˈsiːmiə/ *noun* a condition in which the blood contains an unusually large amount of calcium

**calcaneal** /kælˈkeɪniəl/ *adjective* referring to the calcaneus

**calcaneal tendon** /kælˌkeɪniəl ˈtendən/ *noun* the Achilles tendon, the tendon at the back of the ankle which connects the calf muscles to the heel and which acts to pull up the heel when the calf muscle is contracted

**calcaneus** /kælˈkeɪniəs/, **calcaneum** /kælˈkeɪniəm/ *noun* the heel bone, situated underneath the talus. See illustration at **FOOT** in Supplement

**calcareous degeneration** /kælˌkeəriəs dɪˌdʒenəˈreɪʃ(ə)n/ *noun* the formation of calcium on bones or at joints in old age

**calci-** /kælsɪ/ *prefix* referring to calcium

**calcification** /ˌkælsɪfɪ'keɪʃ(ə)n/ noun a process of hardening caused by the formation of deposits of calcium salts

COMMENT: Calcification can be expected in the formation of bones, but can occur unusually in joints, muscles and organs, where it is known as calcinosis.

**calcified** /'kælsɪfaɪd/ adjective made hard ○ *Bone is calcified connective tissue.*

**calcinosis** /ˌkælsɪ'nəʊsɪs/ noun a medical condition where deposits of calcium salts form in joints, muscles and organs

**calcitonin** /ˌkælsɪ'təʊnɪn/ noun a hormone produced by the thyroid gland, which is believed to regulate the level of calcium in the blood. Also called **thyrocalcitonin**

**calcium** /'kælsiəm/ noun a metallic chemical element which is a major component of bones and teeth and which is essential for various bodily processes such as blood clotting (NOTE: The chemical symbol is **Ca**.)

COMMENT: Calcium is an important element in a balanced diet. Milk, cheese, eggs and certain vegetables are its main sources. Calcium deficiency can be treated by injections of calcium salts.

**calcium antagonist** /'kælsiəm æn ˌtægənɪst/ noun a drug which makes the arteries wider and slows the heart rate. It is used in the treatment of angina.

**calcium channel blocker** /'kælsiəm ˌtʃæn(ə)l ˌblɒkə/, **calcium blocker** /'kælsiəm ˌblɒkə/ noun a drug which affects the smooth muscle of the cardiovascular system, used in the treatment of angina and hypertension (NOTE: Calcium channel blockers have names ending in **-dipine: nifedipine**. Not to be used in heart failure as they reduce cardiac function further.)

**calcium deficiency** /'kælsiəm dɪˌfɪʃ(ə)nsi/ noun a lack of calcium in the bloodstream

**calcium phosphate** /ˌkælsiəm 'fɒsfeɪt/ noun the main constituent of bones

**calcium supplement** /'kælsiəm ˌsʌplɪmənt/ noun the addition of calcium to the diet, or as injections, to improve the level of calcium in the bloodstream

**calculosis** /ˌkælkjʊ'ləʊsɪs/ noun a condition in which calculi exist in an organ

**calculus** /'kælkjʊləs/ noun a hard mass like a little piece of stone, which forms inside the body. Also called **stone** (NOTE: The plural is **calculi**.)

COMMENT: Calculi are formed of cholesterol and various inorganic substances, and are commonly found in the bladder, the gall bladder (gallstones) and various parts of the kidney.

**Caldwell–Luc operation** /ˌkɔːldwel 'luːk ɒpəˌreɪʃ(ə)n/ noun a surgical operation to drain the maxillary sinus by making an incision above the canine tooth [Described 1893. After George Walter Caldwell (1834–1918), US

physician; Henri Luc (1855–1925), French laryngologist.]

**calf** /kɑːf/ noun a muscular fleshy part at the back of the lower leg, formed by the gastrocnemius muscles (NOTE: The plural is **calves**.)

**caliber** /'kælɪbə/ noun US same as **calibre**

**calibrate** /'kælɪbreɪt/ verb 1. to measure the inside diameter of a tube or passage 2. to measure the sizes of two parts of the body to be joined together in surgery 3. to adjust an instrument or piece of equipment against a known standard

**calibrator** /'kælɪbreɪtə/ noun 1. an instrument used to enlarge a tube or passage 2. an instrument for measuring the diameter of a tube or passage

**calibre** /'kælɪbə/ noun the interior diameter of a tube or of a blood vessel

**caliectasis** /ˌkeɪli'ektəsɪs/ noun swelling of the calyces

**caliper** /'kælɪpə/ noun 1. an instrument with two legs, used for measuring the width of the pelvic cavity 2. an instrument with two sharp points which are put into a fractured bone and weights attached to cause traction 3. a leg splint made of rods and straps and usually fastened to the lower leg to enable the hip bone rather than the foot to support the person's weight when walking

**calliper** /'kælɪpə/ noun same as **caliper 3**

**callisthenic** /ˌkælɪs'θenɪk/ adjective relating to callisthenics

**callisthenics** /ˌkælɪs'θenɪks/ plural noun energetic physical exercises for improving fitness and muscle tone, including push-ups, sit-ups and star jumps

**callosity** /kə'lɒsɪti/ noun a hard patch on the skin, e.g. a corn, resulting from frequent pressure or rubbing. Also called **callus**

**callosum** /kə'ləʊs(ə)m/ ♦ **corpus callosum**

**callus** /'kæləs/ noun 1. same as **callosity 2**. tissue which forms round a broken bone as it starts to mend, leading to consolidation ○ *Callus formation is more rapid in children and young adults than in elderly people.*

**calm** /kɑːm/ adjective quiet, not upset ○ *The patient was delirious but became calm after the injection.*

**calomel** /'kæləmel/ noun mercurous chloride, a poisonous substance used to treat pinworms in the intestine. Formula: $Hg_2Cl_2$.

**calor** /'kælə/ noun heat

**caloric** /kə'lɒrɪk/ adjective referring to calories or to heat

**caloric energy** /kəˌlɒrɪk 'enədʒi/ noun the amount of energy shown as a number of calories

**caloric requirement** /kəˌlɒrɪk rɪ'kwaɪəmənt/ noun the amount of energy shown in calories which a person needs each day

**calorie** /ˈkæləri/ *noun* **1.** a unit of measurement of heat or energy, equivalent to the amount of heat needed to raise the temperature of 1g of water by 1°C. Now called **joule 2.** also **Calorie** a unit of measurement of energy in food (*informal*) ○ *a low-calorie diet* Now called **joule** □ **to count calories** to be careful about how much you eat

**calvaria** /kælˈveəriə/, **calvarium** /kælˈveəriəm/ *noun* the top part of the skull

**calyx** /ˈkeɪlɪks/ *noun* a part of the body shaped like a cup especially the tube leading to a renal pyramid. See illustration at KIDNEY in Supplement (NOTE: The plural is **calyces**.)

COMMENT: The renal pelvis is formed of three major calyces, which themselves are formed of several smaller minor calyces.

**CAM** *abbr* complementary and alternative medicine

**camphor** /ˈkæmfə/ *noun* white crystals with a strong smell, made from a tropical tree, used to keep insects away or as a liniment

**camphor oil** /ˈkæmfə ɔɪl/, **camphorated oil** /ˈkæmfəreɪtɪd ɔɪl/ *noun* a mixture of 20% camphor and oil, used as a rub

**Campylobacter** /ˈkæmpɪləʊˌbæktə/ *noun* a bacterium which is a common cause of food poisoning in humans and of spontaneous abortion in farm animals

**canal** /kəˈnæl/ *noun* a tube along which something flows

**canaliculitis** /ˌkænəlɪkjʊˈlaɪtɪs/ *noun* inflammation of the tear duct canal

**canaliculotomy** /ˌkænəlɪkjʊˈlɒtəmi/ *noun* a surgical operation to open up a little canal

**canaliculus** /ˌkænəˈlɪkjʊləs/ *noun* a little canal, e.g. a canal leading to the Haversian systems in compact bone, or a canal leading to the lacrimal duct (NOTE: The plural is **canaliculi**.)

**cancellous bone** /ˈkænsələs ˈbəʊn/ *noun* a light spongy bone tissue which forms the inner core of a bone and also the ends of long bones. See illustration at BONE STRUCTURE in Supplement

**cancer** /ˈkænsə/ *noun* a malignant growth or tumour which develops in tissue and destroys it, which can spread by metastasis to other parts of the body and which cannot be controlled by the body itself ○ *Cancer cells developed in the lymph.* ○ *She has been diagnosed as having lung cancer* or *as having cancer of the lung.* (NOTE: For other terms referring to cancer, see words beginning with **carcin-**.)

COMMENT: Cancers can be divided into cancers of the skin (**carcinomas**) or cancers of connective tissue such as bone or muscle (**sarcomas**). They have many causes. Many are curable by surgery, by chemotherapy or by radiation, especially if they are detected early.

**cancerophobia** /ˌkænsərəʊˈfəʊbiə/ *noun* a fear of cancer

**cancerous** /ˈkænsərəs/ *adjective* referring to cancer ○ *The X-ray revealed a cancerous growth in the breast.*

**cancer phobia** /ˈkænsə ˌfəʊbiə/ *noun* same as **cancerophobia**

**cancrum oris** /ˌkæŋkrəm ˈɔːrɪs/ *noun* severe ulcers in the mouth, leading to gangrene. Also called **noma**

**Candida** /ˈkændɪdə/ *noun* a type of fungus which causes mycosis. Also called **Monilia**

'It is incorrect to say that oral candida is an infection. Candida is easily isolated from the mouths of up to 50% of healthy adults and is a normal commensal.' [*Nursing Times*]

**Candida albicans** /ˌkændɪdə ˈælbɪkænz/ *noun* one type of Candida which is usually present in the mouth and throat without causing any illness, but which can cause thrush

**candidate** /ˈkændɪdeɪt/ *noun* someone who could have an operation ○ *These types of patients may be candidates for embolisation.*

**candidate vaccine** /ˈkændɪdeɪt ˌvæksiːn/ *noun* a vaccine which is being tested for use in immunisation

**candidiasis** /ˌkændɪˈdaɪəsɪs/, **candidosis** /ˌkændɪˈdəʊsɪs/ *noun* infection with a species of the fungus Candida

COMMENT: When the infection occurs in the vagina or mouth it is known as 'thrush'. Thrush in the mouth usually affects small children.

**canicola fever** /kəˈnɪkələ ˌfiːvə/ *noun* a form of leptospirosis, giving high fever and jaundice

**canine** /ˈkeɪnaɪn/, **canine tooth** /ˈkeɪnaɪn ˌtuːθ/ *noun* a pointed tooth next to an incisor. See illustration at TEETH in Supplement

COMMENT: There are four canines in all, two in the upper jaw and two in the lower. Those in the upper jaw are referred to as the 'eyeteeth'.

**canities** /kəˈnɪʃiːz/ *noun* a loss of pigments, which makes the hair turn white

**canker sore** /ˈkæŋkə ˌsɔː/ *noun* same as **mouth ulcer**

**cannabis** /ˈkænəbɪs/ *noun* a drug made from the dried leaves or flowers of the Indian hemp plant. Recreational use of cannabis is illegal and its use to relieve the pain associated with conditions such as multiple sclerosis is controversial. Also called **hashish, marijuana**

COMMENT: Cannabis has analgesic properties, and the possibility that it should be legalised for therapeutic use in conditions of chronic pain is being debated.

**cannabis resin** /ˌkænəbɪs ˈrezɪn/ *noun* an addictive drug, a purified extract made from the flowers of the Indian hemp plant

**cannula** /ˈkænjʊlə/ *noun* a tube with a trocar or blunt needle inside, inserted into the body to introduce fluids

**cannulate** /ˈkænjʊleɪt/ *verb* to put a cannula into a vein or cavity to give drugs or to drain away fluid

**canthal** /'kænθəl/ *adjective* referring to the corner of the eye

**cantholysis** /kæn'θɒləsɪs/ *noun* same as **canthoplasty**

**canthoplasty** /'kænθəplæsti/ *noun* **1.** an operation to repair the canthus of the eye **2.** an operation to cut through the canthus to enlarge the groove in the eyelid

**canthus** /'kænθəs/ *noun* a corner of the eye

**canula** *noun* another spelling of **cannula**

**canulate** *verb* another spelling of **cannulate**

**cap** /kæp/ *noun* **1.** a covering which protects something **2.** an artificial hard covering for a damaged or broken tooth

**CAPD** *abbr* continuous ambulatory peritoneal dialysis

**capeline bandage** /'kæpəlaɪn ˌbændɪdʒ/ *noun* a bandage shaped like a cap, either for the head, or to cover a stump after amputation

**capillary** /kə'pɪləri/ *noun* **1.** a tiny blood vessel between the arterioles and the venules, which carries blood and nutrients into the tissues **2.** any tiny tube carrying a liquid in the body

**capillary bleeding** /kəˌpɪləri 'bliːdɪŋ/ *noun* bleeding where blood oozes out from small blood vessels

**capita** /'kæpɪtə/ plural of **caput**

**capitate** /'kæpɪteɪt/, **capitate bone** /ˈkæpɪteɪt ˌbəʊn/ *noun* the largest of the eight small carpal bones in the wrist. See illustration at HAND in Supplement

**capitellum** /ˌkæpɪ'teləm/ *noun* a rounded enlarged part at the end of a bone, especially this part of the upper arm bone, the humerus, that forms the elbow joint with one of the lower bones, the radius. Also called **capitulum of humerus** (NOTE: The plural is **capitella**.)

**capitis** /kə'paɪtɪs/ ♦ **corona capitis**

**capitular** /kə'pɪtjʊlə/ *adjective* describing the rounded end (**capitulum**) of a bone

**capitulum** /kə'pɪtjʊləm/ *noun* the rounded end of a bone which articulates with another bone, e.g. the distal end of the humerus (NOTE: The plural is **capitula**.)

**capitulum of humerus** /kəˌpɪtjʊləm əv 'hjuːmərəs/ *noun* same as **capitellum**

**caplet** /'kæplət/ *noun* a small oblong tablet with a covering that dissolves easily and which usually cannot be broken in two

**caps.** *abbr* capsule

**capsular** /'kæpsjʊlə/ *adjective* referring to a capsule

**capsule** /'kæpsjuːl/ *noun* **1.** a membrane round an organ or joint **2.** a small hollow digestible case filled with a drug that is taken by swallowing ○ *She swallowed three capsules of painkiller.* ○ *The doctor prescribed the drug in capsule form.*

**capsulectomy** /ˌkæpsjʊ'lektəmi/ *noun* the surgical removal of the capsule round a joint

**capsulitis** /ˌkæpsjʊ'laɪtɪs/ *noun* inflammation of a capsule

**capsulotomy** /ˌkæpsjʊ'lɒtəmi/ *noun* a surgical procedure involving cutting into the capsule around a body part, e.g. cutting into the lens of the eye during the removal of a cataract

**captopril** /'kæptəprɪl/ *noun* a drug which helps to prevent the arteries from being made narrower by an angiotensin. It is used to control high blood pressure.

**caput** /'kæpət/ *noun* **1.** the head **2.** the top of part of something (NOTE: [all senses] The plural is **capita**.)

**carbamazepine** /ˌkɑːbə'mæzəpiːn/ *noun* a drug which reduces pain and helps to prevent convulsions. It is used in the treatment of epilepsy, pain and bipolar disorder.

**carbenoxolone** /ˌkɑːbə'nɒksələʊn/ *noun* a liquorice agent, used to treat stomach ulcers

**carbidopa** /ˌkɑːbɪ'dəʊpə/ *noun* an inhibitor used to enable levodopa to enter the brain in larger quantities in the treatment of Parkinson's disease

**carbimazole** /kɑː'bɪməzəʊl/ *noun* a drug which helps to prevent the formation of thyroid hormones, used in the management of hyperthyroidism

**carbohydrate** /ˌkɑːbəʊ'haɪdreɪt/ *noun* **1.** a biological compound containing carbon, hydrogen and oxygen. Carbohydrates derive from sugar and are an important source of food and energy. **2.** food containing carbohydrates ○ *high carbohydrate drinks*

**carbolic acid** /kɑːˌbɒlɪk 'æsɪd/ *noun* same as **phenol**

**carbon** /'kɑːbən/ *noun* one of the common non-metallic elements, an essential component of living matter and organic chemical compounds (NOTE: The chemical symbol is **C**.)

**carbon dioxide** /ˌkɑːbən daɪ'ɒksaɪd/ *noun* a colourless gas produced by the body's metabolism as the tissues burn carbon, and breathed out by the lungs as waste (NOTE: The chemical symbol is $CO_2$.)

COMMENT: Carbon dioxide can be solidified at low temperatures and is known as 'dry ice' or 'carbon dioxide snow', being used to remove growths on the skin.

**carbon dioxide snow** /ˌkɑːbən daɪˌɒksaɪd 'snəʊ/ *noun* solid carbon dioxide, used in treating skin growths such as warts, or to preserve tissue samples

**carbonic anhydrase** /kɑːˌbɒnɪk æn'haɪdreɪz/ *noun* an enzyme which acts as a buffer and regulates the body's water balance, including gastric acid secretion and aqueous humour production

**carbon monoxide** /ˌkɑːbən mə'nɒksaɪd/ *noun* a poisonous gas found in fumes from car engines, from burning gas and cigarette smoke (NOTE: The chemical symbol is **CO**.)

COMMENT: Carbon monoxide is dangerous because it is easily absorbed into the blood and takes the place of the oxygen in the blood, combining with haemoglobin to form carboxyhaemoglobin, which has the effect of starving the tissues of oxygen. Carbon monoxide has no smell and people do not realise that they are being poisoned by it. They become unconscious, with a characteristic red colouring to the skin. Poisoning with car exhaust fumes is sometimes used as a method of suicide. The treatment for carbon monoxide poisoning is very rapid inhalation of fresh air together with carbon dioxide if this can be provided.

**carbon monoxide poisoning** /ˌkɑːbən məˈnɒksaɪd ˌpɔɪz(ə)nɪŋ/ noun poisoning caused by breathing carbon monoxide

**carboxyhaemoglobin** /kɑːˌbɒksihiːmə ˈgləʊbɪn/ noun a compound of carbon monoxide and haemoglobin formed when a person breathes in carbon monoxide from tobacco smoke or car exhaust fumes

**carboxyhaemoglobinaemia** /kɑːˌbɒksi hiːmə,gləʊbɪˈniːmiə/ noun the presence of carboxyhaemoglobin in the blood

**carbuncle** /ˈkɑːbʌŋkəl/ noun a localised staphylococcal infection, which goes deep into the tissue

**carcin-** /kɑːsɪn/ prefix same as **carcino-** (used before vowels)

**carcino-** /kɑːsɪnə/ prefix referring to carcinoma or cancer

**carcinogen** /kɑːˈsɪnədʒən/ noun a substance which produces a carcinoma or cancer

COMMENT: Carcinogens are found in pesticides such as DDT, in asbestos, tobacco, aromatic compounds such as benzene and radioactive substances.

**carcinogenesis** /ˌkɑːsɪnəˈdʒenəsɪs/ noun the process of forming a carcinoma in tissue

**carcinogenic** /ˌkɑːsɪnəˈdʒenɪk/ adjective causing a carcinoma or cancer

**carcinoid** /ˈkɑːsɪnɔɪd/ noun an intestinal tumour, especially in the appendix, which causes diarrhoea

**carcinoid syndrome** /ˈkɑːsɪnɔɪd ˌsɪndrəʊm/ noun a group of symptoms which are associated with a carcinoid tumour

**carcinoid tumour** /ˈkɑːsɪnɔɪd ˌtjuːmə/ same as **carcinoid**

**carcinoma** /ˌkɑːsɪˈnəʊmə/ noun a cancer of the epithelium or glands

**carcinoma in situ** /kɑːsɪˌnəʊmə ɪn ˈsɪtjuː/ noun the first stage in the development of a cancer, where the epithelial cells begin to change

**carcinomatosis** /ˌkɑːsɪnəʊməˈtəʊsɪs/ noun a carcinoma which has spread to many sites in the body

**carcinomatous** /ˌkɑːsɪˈnɒmətəs/ adjective referring to carcinoma

**carcinosarcoma** /ˌkɑːsɪnəʊsɑːˈkəʊmə/ noun a malignant tumour containing elements of both a carcinoma and a sarcoma

**cardi-** /kɑːdi/ prefix same as **cardio-** (used before vowels)

**cardia** /ˈkɑːdiə/ noun 1. an opening at the top of the stomach which joins it to the gullet 2. the heart

**cardiac** /ˈkɑːdiæk/ adjective 1. referring to the heart 2. referring to the cardia

**cardiac achalasia** /ˌkɑːdiæk ˌækəˈleɪziə/ noun a condition in which the patient is unable to relax the cardia, the muscle at the entrance to the stomach, with the result that food cannot enter the stomach. ◊ **cardiomyotomy**

**cardiac arrest** /ˌkɑːdiæk əˈrest/ noun a condition in which the heart muscle stops beating

**cardiac asthma** /ˌkɑːdiæk ˈæsmə/ noun difficulty in breathing caused by heart failure

**cardiac catheter** /ˌkɑːdiæk ˈkæθɪtə/ noun a catheter passed through a vein into the heart, to take blood samples, to record pressure or to examine the interior of the heart before surgery

**cardiac catheterisation** /ˌkɑːdiæk ˌkæθɪtəraɪˈzeɪʃ(ə)n/ noun a procedure which involves passing a catheter into the heart

**cardiac cirrhosis** /ˌkɑːdiæk sɪˈrəʊsɪs/ noun cirrhosis of the liver caused by heart disease

**cardiac compression** /ˌkɑːdiæk kəmˈpreʃ(ə)n/ noun the compression of the heart by fluid in the pericardium

**cardiac conducting system** /ˌkɑːdiæk kənˈdʌktɪŋ ˌsɪstəm/ noun the nerve system in the heart which links an atrium to a ventricle, so that the two beat at the same rate

**cardiac cycle** /ˌkɑːdiæk ˈsaɪk(ə)l/ noun the repeated beating of the heart, formed of the diastole and systole

**cardiac decompression** /ˌkɑːdiæk ˌdiːkəmˈpreʃ(ə)n/ noun the removal of a haematoma or constriction of the heart

**cardiac failure** /ˌkɑːdiæk ˈfeɪljə/ noun same as **heart failure**

**cardiac glycoside** /ˌkɑːdiæk ˈglaɪkəsaɪd/ noun a drug used in the treatment of tachycardia and atrial fibrillation, e.g. digoxin

**cardiac impression** /ˌkɑːdiæk ɪmˈpreʃ(ə)n/ noun 1. a concave area near the centre of the upper surface of the liver under the heart 2. a depression on the mediastinal part of the lungs where they touch the pericardium

**cardiac index** /ˌkɑːdiæk ˈɪndeks/ noun the cardiac output per square metre of body surface, usually between 3.1 and 3.8l/min/m$^2$ (litres per minute per square metre)

**cardiac infarction** /ˌkɑːdiæk ɪnˈfɑːkʃən/ noun same as **myocardial infarction**

**cardiac monitor** /ˌkɑːdiæk ˈmɒnɪtə/ noun same as **electrocardiograph**

**cardiac murmur** /ˌkɑːdiæk ˈmɜːmə/ noun same as **heart murmur**

**cardiac muscle** /ˈkɑːdiæk ˌmʌs(ə)l/ *noun* a muscle in the heart which makes the heart beat

**cardiac neurosis** /ˌkɑːdiæk njʊˈrəʊsɪs/ *noun* same as **disordered action of the heart**

**cardiac notch** /ˌkɑːdiæk ˈnɒtʃ/ *noun* **1.** a point in the left lung, where the right inside wall is bent. See illustration at LUNGS in Supplement **2.** a notch at the point where the oesophagus joins the greater curvature of the stomach

**cardiac orifice** /ˌkɑːdiæk ˈɒrɪfɪs/ *noun* an opening where the oesophagus joins the stomach

**cardiac output** /ˌkɑːdiæk ˈaʊtpʊt/ *noun* the volume of blood expelled by each ventricle in a specific time, usually between 4.8 and 5.3l/min (litres per minute)

**cardiac pacemaker** /ˌkɑːdiæk ˈpeɪsↆmeɪkə/ *noun* an electronic device implanted on a patient's heart, or which a patient wears attached to the chest, which stimulates and regulates the heartbeat

**cardiac patient** /ˈkɑːdiæk ˌpeɪʃ(ə)nt/ *noun* a patient who has a heart disorder

**cardiac reflex** /ˌkɑːdiæk ˈriːfleks/ *noun* the reflex which controls the heartbeat automatically

**cardiac surgery** /ˌkɑːdiæk ˈsɜːdʒəri/ *noun* surgery to the heart

**cardiac tamponade** /ˌkɑːdiæk ˌtæmpəˈneɪd/ *noun* pressure on the heart when the pericardial cavity fills with blood. Also called **heart tamponade**

**cardiac vein** /ˈkɑːdiæk veɪn/ *noun* one of the veins which lead from the myocardium to the right atrium

**cardinal** /ˈkɑːdɪn(ə)l/ *adjective* most important

**cardinal ligaments** /ˌkɑːdɪn(ə)l ˈlɪgəmənts/ *plural noun* ligaments forming a band of connective tissue that extends from the uterine cervix and vagina to the pelvic walls. Also called **Mackenrodt's ligaments**

**cardio-** /kɑːdiəʊ/ *prefix* referring to the heart

**cardiogenic** /ˌkɑːdiəˈdʒenɪk/ *adjective* resulting from activity or disease of the heart

**cardiogram** /ˈkɑːdiəgræm/ *noun* a graph showing the heartbeat, produced by a cardiograph

**cardiograph** /ˈkɑːdiəgrɑːf/ *noun* an instrument which records the heartbeat

**cardiographer** /ˌkɑːdiˈɒgrəfə/ *noun* a technician who operates a cardiograph

**cardiography** /ˌkɑːdiˈɒgrəfi/ *noun* the action of recording the heartbeat

**cardiologist** /ˌkɑːdiˈɒlədʒɪst/ *noun* a doctor who specialises in the study of the heart

**cardiology** /ˌkɑːdiˈɒlədʒi/ *noun* the study of the heart, its diseases and functions

**cardiomegaly** /ˌkɑːdiəʊˈmegəli/ *noun* an enlarged heart

**cardiomyopathy** /ˌkɑːdiəʊmaɪˈɒpəθi/ *noun* a disease of the heart muscle

**cardiomyoplasty** /ˌkɑːdiəʊˈmaɪəʊˌplæsti/ *noun* an operation to improve the functioning of the heart, by using the latissimus dorsi as a stimulant

**cardiomyotomy** /ˌkɑːdiəʊmaɪˈɒtəmi/ *noun* an operation to treat cardiac achalasia by splitting the ring of muscles where the oesophagus joins the stomach. Also called **Heller's operation**

**cardiopathy** /ˌkɑːdiˈɒpəθi/ *noun* any kind of heart disease

**cardiophone** /ˈkɑːdiəfəʊn/ *noun* a microphone attached to a patient to record sounds, usually used to record the heart of an unborn baby

**cardioplegia** /ˌkɑːdiəʊˈpliːdʒiə/ *noun* the stopping of a patient's heart, by chilling it or using drugs, so that heart surgery can be performed

**cardiopulmonary** /ˌkɑːdiəʊˈpʌlmən(ə)ri/ *adjective* relating to both the heart and the lungs

**cardiopulmonary bypass** /ˌkɑːdiəʊ ˌpʌlmən(ə)ri ˈbaɪpɑːs/ *noun* a machine or method for artificially circulating the patient's blood during open-heart surgery. The heart and lungs are cut off from the circulation and replaced by a pump.

**cardiopulmonary resuscitation** /ˌkɑːdiəʊˌpʌlmən(ə)ri rɪˌsʌsɪˈteɪʃ(ə)n/ *noun* an emergency technique to make a person's heart start beating again. It involves clearing the airways and then alternately pressing on the chest and breathing into the mouth. Abbr **CPR**

**cardiopulmonary system** /ˌkɑːdiəʊ ˈpʌlmən(ə)ri ˌsɪstəm/ *noun* the heart and lungs considered together as a functional unit

**cardiorespiratory** /ˌkɑːdiəʊrɪˈspɪrɪt(ə)ri/ *adjective* referring to both the heart and the respiratory system

**cardioscope** /ˈkɑːdiəskəʊp/ *noun* an instrument formed of a tube with a light at the end, used to inspect the inside of the heart

**cardiospasm** /ˈkɑːdiəʊspæz(ə)m/ *noun* same as **cardiac achalasia**

**cardiothoracic** /ˌkɑːdiəʊθɒˈræsɪk/ *adjective* referring to the heart and the chest region ○ *a cardiothoracic surgeon*

**cardiotocography** /ˌkɑːdiəʊtɒˈkɒgrəfi/ *noun* the recording of the heartbeat of a fetus

**cardiotomy** /ˌkɑːdiˈɒtəmi/ *noun* an operation that involves cutting the wall of the heart

**cardiotomy syndrome** /ˌkɑːdiˈɒtəmi ˌsɪndrəʊm/ *noun* fluid in the membranes round the heart after cardiotomy

**cardiotoxic** /ˌkɑːdiəʊˈtɒksɪk/ *adjective* which is toxic to the heart

**cardiovascular** /ˌkɑːdiəʊˈvæskjʊlə/ adjective referring to the heart and the blood circulation system

**cardiovascular disease** /ˌkɑːdiəʊ ˈvæskjʊlə dɪˌziːz/ noun any disease which affects the circulatory system, e.g. hypertension

'…cardiovascular diseases remain the leading cause of death in the United States' [*Journal of the American Medical Association*]

**cardiovascular system** /ˌkɑːdiəʊ ˈvæskjʊlə ˌsɪstəm/ noun the system of organs and blood vessels by means of which the blood circulates round the body and which includes the heart, arteries and veins

**cardioversion** /ˌkɑːdiəʊˈvɜːʃ(ə)n/ noun a procedure to correct an irregular heartbeat by applying an electrical impulse to the chest wall. ◊ **defibrillation**

**carditis** /kɑːˈdaɪtɪs/ noun inflammation of the connective tissue of the heart

**caregiver** /ˈkeəˌgɪvə/ noun same as **carer**

**care pathway** /ˈkeə ˌpɑːθweɪ/ noun the entire process of diagnosis, treatment and care that a patient goes through

**care plan** /ˈkeə plæn/ noun a plan drawn up by the nursing staff for the treatment of an individual patient

'…all relevant sections of the nurses' care plan and nursing process had been left blank' [*Nursing Times*]

**carer** /ˈkeərə/, **caregiver** /ˈkeəˌgɪvə/ noun someone who looks after a sick or dependent person

'…most research has focused on those caring for older people or for adults with disability and chronic illness. Most studied are the carers of those who might otherwise have to stay in hospital for a long time' [*British Medical Journal*]

**caries** /ˈkeərɪz/ noun decay in a tooth or bone

**carina** /kəˈriːnə/ noun a structure shaped like the bottom of a boat, e.g. the cartilage at the point where the trachea branches into the bronchi

**cariogenic** /ˌkeəriəʊˈdʒenɪk/ adjective referring to a substance which causes caries

**carminative** /ˈkɑːmɪnətɪv/ noun a substance which relieves colic or indigestion ■ adjective relieving colic or indigestion

**carneous mole** /ˌkɑːniəs ˈməʊl/ noun matter in the uterus after the death of a fetus

**carotenaemia** /ˌkærətɪˈniːmiə/ noun an excessive amount of carotene in the blood, usually as a result of eating too many carrots or tomatoes, which gives the skin a yellow colour. Also called **xanthaemia**

**carotene** /ˈkærətiːn/ noun an orange or red pigment in carrots, egg yolk and some oils, which is converted by the liver into vitamin A

**carotid** /kəˈrɒtɪd/, **carotid artery** /kəˌrɒtɪd ˈɑːtəri/ noun either of the two large arteries in the neck which supply blood to the head

COMMENT: The common carotid artery is in the lower part of the neck and branches upwards into the external and internal carotids. The ca-

rotid body is situated at the point where the carotid divides.

**carotid artery thrombosis** /kəˌrɒtɪd ˌɑːtəri θrɒmˈbəʊsɪs/ noun the formation of a blood clot in the carotid artery

**carotid body** /kæˌrɒtɪd ˈbɒdi/ noun tissue in the carotid sinus which is concerned with cardiovascular reflexes

**carotid pulse** /kəˌrɒtɪd ˈpʌls/ noun a pulse felt in the carotid artery at the side of the neck

**carotid sinus** /kæˌrɒtɪd ˈsaɪnəs/ noun an expanded part attached to the carotid artery, which monitors blood pressure in the skull

**carp-** /kɑːp/ prefix same as **carpo-** (*used before vowels*)

**carpal** /ˈkɑːp(ə)l/ adjective referring to the wrist

**carpal bones** /ˈkɑːp(ə)l bəʊnz/, **carpals** /ˈkɑːp(ə)lz/ plural noun the eight bones which make up the carpus or wrist. See illustration at HAND in Supplement

**carpal tunnel release** /ˌkɑːp(ə)l ˈtʌn(ə)l rɪˌliːs/ noun an operation to relieve the compression of the median nerve

**carpal tunnel syndrome** /ˌkɑːp(ə)l ˈtʌn(ə)l ˌsɪndrəʊm/ noun a condition, usually affecting women, in which the fingers tingle and hurt at night. It is caused by compression of the median nerve.

**carphology** /kɑːˈfɒlədʒi/ noun the action of pulling at the bedclothes, a sign of delirium in typhoid and other fevers. Also called **floccitation**

**carpi** /ˈkɑːpi/ plural of **carpus**

**carpo-** /kɑːpəʊ/ prefix referring to the wrist

**carpometacarpal joint** /ˌkɑːpəʊmetə ˈkɑːp(ə)l dʒɔɪnt/ noun one of the joints between the carpals and metacarpals. Also called **CM joint**

**carpopedal spasm** /ˌkɑːpəʊpiːd(ə)l ˈspæz(ə)m/ noun a spasm in the hands and feet caused by lack of calcium

**carpus** /ˈkɑːpəs/ noun the bones by which the lower arm is connected to the hand. Also called **wrist**. See illustration at HAND in Supplement (NOTE: The plural is **carpi**.)

COMMENT: The carpus is formed of eight small bones (the carpals): the capitate, hamate, lunate, pisiform, scaphoid, trapezium, trapezoid and triquetral.

**carrier** /ˈkæriə/ noun **1.** a person who carries bacteria of a disease in his or her body and who can transmit the disease to others without showing any signs of being infected with it ○ *Ten per cent of the population are believed to be unwitting carriers of the bacteria.* **2.** an insect which carries disease and infects humans **3.** a healthy person who carries a chromosome variation that gives rise to a hereditary disease such as haemophilia or Duchenne muscular dystrophy

**carry** /'kæri/ *verb* to have a disease and be capable of infecting others

**cartilage** /'kɑːtɪlɪdʒ/ *noun* thick connective tissue which lines and cushions the joints and which forms part of the structure of an organ. Cartilage in small children is the first stage in the formation of bones.

**cartilaginous** /ˌkɑːtɪ'lædʒɪnəs/ *adjective* made of cartilage

**cartilaginous joint** /ˌkɑːtɪ'lædʒɪnəs dʒɔɪnt/ *noun* **1. primary cartilaginous joint** same as **synchondrosis 2. secondary cartilaginous joint** same as **symphysis**

**caruncle** /kə'rʌŋkəl/ *noun* a small swelling

**cascara** /kæ'skɑːrə/, **cascara sagrada** /kæ ˌskɑːrə sə'grɑːdə/ *noun* a laxative made from the bark of a tropical tree

**case** /keɪs/ *noun* **1.** a single occurrence of a disease ○ *There were two hundred cases of cholera in the recent outbreak.* **2.** a person who has a disease or who is undergoing treatment ○ *The hospital is only admitting urgent cases.*

**caseation** /ˌkeɪsi'eɪʃ(ə)n/ *noun* the process by which dead tissue decays into a firm and dry mass. It is characteristic of tuberculosis.

**case control study** /keɪs kən'trəʊl ˌstʌdi/ *noun* an investigation in which a group of patients with a disease are compared with a group without the disease in order to study possible causes

**case history** /'keɪs ˌhɪst(ə)ri/ *noun* details of what has happened to a patient undergoing treatment

**casein** /'keɪsiːn/ *noun* one of the proteins found in milk

**caseinogen** /ˌkeɪsi'ɪnədʒən/ *noun* the main protein in milk, from which casein is formed

**Casey's model** /'keɪsiz ˌmɒd(ə)l/ *noun* a model for the care of child patients, where the parents are involved in the treatment

**cast** /kɑːst/ *noun* a mass of material formed in a hollow organ or tube and excreted in fluid

**castor oil** /ˌkɑːstər 'ɔɪl/ *noun* a plant oil which acts as a laxative

**castration** /kæ'streɪʃ(ə)n/ *noun* the surgical removal of the sexual organs, usually the testicles, in males

**casualty** /'kæʒuəlti/ *noun* **1.** a person who has had an accident or who is suddenly ill ○ *The fire caused several casualties.* ○ *The casualties were taken by ambulance to the nearest hospital.* **2.** also **casualty department** same as **accident and emergency department** ○ *The accident victim was rushed to casualty.*

**casualty ward** /'kæʒuəlti wɔːd/ *noun* same as **accident ward**

**CAT** /kæt/ *noun* same as **computerised axial tomography**

**cata-** /kætə/ *prefix* downwards

**catabolic** /ˌkætə'bɒlɪk/ *adjective* referring to catabolism

**catabolism** /kə'tæbəlɪz(ə)m/ *noun* the process of breaking down complex chemicals into simple chemicals

**catalase** /'kætəleɪz/ *noun* an enzyme present in the blood and liver which catalyses the breakdown of hydrogen peroxide into water and oxygen

**catalepsy** /'kætəlepsi/ *noun* a condition often associated with schizophrenia, where a person becomes incapable of sensation, the body is rigid and he or she does not move for long periods

**catalyse** /'kætəlaɪz/ *verb* to act as a catalyst and help make a chemical reaction take place (NOTE: The US spelling is **catalyze**.)

**catalysis** /kə'tæləsɪs/ *noun* a process where a chemical reaction is helped by a substance (the catalyst) which does not change during the process

**catalyst** /'kætəlɪst/ *noun* a substance which produces or helps a chemical reaction without itself changing ○ *an enzyme which acts as a catalyst in the digestive process*

**catalytic** /ˌkætə'lɪtɪk/ *adjective* referring to catalysis

**catalytic reaction** /ˌkætəlɪtɪk ri'ækʃən/ *noun* a chemical reaction which is caused by a catalyst which does not change during the reaction

**catamenia** /ˌkætə'miːniə/ *noun* menstruation (*technical*)

**cataplexy** /'kætəpleksi/ *noun* a condition in which a person's muscles become suddenly rigid and he or she falls without losing consciousness, possibly caused by a shock

**cataract** /'kætərækt/ *noun* a condition in which the lens of the eye gradually becomes hard and opaque

COMMENT: Cataracts form most often in people after the age of 50. They are sometimes caused by a blow or an electric shock. Cataracts can easily and safely be removed by surgery.

**cataract extraction** /'kætərækt ɪk ˌstrækʃ(ə)n/ *noun* the surgical removal of a cataract from the eye

**cataractous lens** /kætə'ræktəs lenz/ *noun* a lens on which a cataract has formed

**catarrh** /kə'tɑː/ *noun* inflammation of the mucous membranes in the nose and throat, creating an excessive amount of mucus

**catarrhal** /kə'tɑːrəl/ *adjective* referring to catarrh ○ *a catarrhal cough*

**catatonia** /ˌkætə'təʊniə/ *noun* a condition in which a psychiatric patient is either motionless or shows violent reactions to stimulation

**catatonic** /ˌkætə'tɒnɪk/ *adjective* referring to behaviour in which a person is either motionless or extremely violent

**catatonic schizophrenia** /ˌkætətɒnɪk ˌskɪtsəʊ'friːniə/ *noun* a type of schizophrenia where the patient is alternately apathetic or very active and disturbed

**catching** /'kætʃɪŋ/ *adjective* infectious (*informal*) ○ *Is the disease catching?*

**catchment area** /'kætʃmənt ˌeəriə/ *noun* an area around a hospital which is served by that hospital

**catecholamines** /ˌkætə'kɒləmiːnz/ *plural noun* the hormones adrenaline and noradrenaline which are released by the adrenal glands

**category** /'kætɪɡ(ə)ri/ *noun* a classification, the way in which things can be classified ○ *His condition is of a non-urgent category.*

**catgut** /'kætɡʌt/ *noun* a thread made from part of the intestines of sheep, now usually artificially hardened, used to sew up cuts made during surgery

> COMMENT: Catgut is slowly dissolved by fluids in the body after the wound has healed and therefore does not need to be removed. Ordinary catgut will dissolve in five to ten days; hardened catgut takes up to three or four weeks.

**catharsis** /kə'θɑːsɪs/ *noun* purgation of the bowels

**cathartic** /kə'θɑːtɪk/ *adjective* laxative or purgative

**catheter** /'kæθɪtə/ *noun* a tube passed into the body along one of the passages in the body

**catheterisation** /ˌkæθɪtəraɪ'zeɪʃ(ə)n/, **catheterization** *noun* the act of putting a catheter into a patient's body

> '…high rates of disconnection of closed urine drainage systems, lack of hand washing and incorrect positioning of urine drainage bags have been highlighted in a new report on urethral catheterisation' [*Nursing Times*]

> '…the technique used to treat aortic stenosis is similar to that for any cardiac catheterisation. A catheter introduced through the femoral vein is placed across the aortic valve and into the left ventricle.' [*Journal of the American Medical Association*]

**catheterise** /'kæθɪtəraɪz/, **catheterize** *verb* to insert a catheter into a patient

**CAT scan** /'kæt skæn/, **CT scan** /ˌsiː 'tiː skæn/ *noun* same as **CT scan**

**cat-scratch disease** /'kæt skrætʃ dɪˌziːz/, **cat-scratch fever** /'kæt skrætʃ ˌfiːvə/ *noun* an illness in which the patient has a fever and swollen lymph glands, thought to be caused by a bacterium transmitted to humans by the scratch of a cat. It may also result from scratching with other sharp points.

**cauda equina** /ˌkɔːdə ɪ'kwaɪnə/ *noun* a group of nerves which go from the spinal cord to the lumbar region and the coccyx

**caudal** /'kɔːd(ə)l/ *adjective* (*in humans*) referring to the cauda equina

**caudal anaesthetic** /ˌkɔːd(ə)l ˌænəs'θetɪk/ *noun* an anaesthetic, injected into the base of the spine to remove feeling in the lower part of the body. It is often used in childbirth.

**caudal analgesia** /ˌkɔːd(ə)l ˌæn(ə)l'dʒiːziə/ *noun* a method of pain relief that involves injecting an anaesthetic into the base of the spine to remove feeling in the lower part of the body

**caudal block** /'kɔːd(ə)l blɒk/ *noun* a local analgesia of the cauda equina nerves in the lower spine

**caudate** /'kɔːdeɪt/ *adjective* like a tail

**caudate lobe** /'kɔːdeɪt ləʊb/ *noun* a lobe at the back of the liver, behind the right and left lobes. Also called **posterior lobe**

**caul** /kɔːl/ *noun* **1.** a membrane which sometimes covers a baby's head at birth **2.** same as **omentum**

**cauliflower ear** /ˌkɒliflaʊər 'ɪə/ *noun* a permanently swollen ear, caused by blows in boxing

**causalgia** /kɔː'zældʒə/ *noun* burning pain in a limb, caused by a damaged nerve

**causal organism** /ˌkɔːz(ə)l 'ɔːɡənɪz(ə)m/ *noun* an organism that causes a particular disease

**caustic** /'kɔːstɪk/ *noun* a chemical substance that destroys tissues that it touches ■ *adjective* corrosive and destructive

**cauterisation** /ˌkɔːtəraɪ'zeɪʃ(ə)n/, **cauterization** *noun* the act of cauterising ○ *The growth was removed by cauterisation.*

**cauterise** /'kɔːtəraɪz/, **cauterize** *verb* to use burning, radiation or laser beams to remove tissue or to stop bleeding

**cautery** /'kɔːtəri/ *noun* a surgical instrument used to cauterise a wound

**cava** /'keɪvə/ ♦ vena cava

**cavernosum** /ˌkævə'nəʊsəm/ ♦ corpus cavernosum

**cavernous breathing sounds** /ˌkævənəs 'briːðɪŋ ˌsaʊndz/ *plural noun* hollow sounds made by the lungs and heard through a stethoscope placed on a patient's chest, used in diagnosis

**cavernous haemangioma** /ˌkævənəs ˌhiːmændʒɪ'əʊmə/ *noun* a tumour in connective tissue with wide spaces which contain blood

**cavernous sinus** /ˌkævənəs 'saɪnəs/ *noun* one of two cavities in the skull behind the eyes, which form part of the venous drainage system

**cavitation** /ˌkævɪ'teɪʃ(ə)n/ *noun* the forming of a cavity

**cavity** /'kævɪti/ *noun* a hole or space inside the body

**cc** *abbr* cubic centimetre

**CCU** *abbr* coronary care unit

**CD4** /ˌsiː diː 'fɔː/ *noun* a compound consisting of a protein combined with a carbohydrate which is found in some cells and helps to protect the body against infection □ **CD4 count** a test used to monitor how many CD4 cells have been destroyed in people with HIV

# 65

**centre**

**CDH** *abbr* congenital dislocation of the hip

**cecum** /'siːkəm/ *noun US* same as **caecum**

**cefaclor** /'sefəklɔː/ *noun* an antibacterial drug used to treat septicaemia

**cefotaxime** /ˌsefə'tæksiːm/ *noun* a synthetic cephalosporin used to treat bacterial infection by pseudomonads

**-cele** /siːl/ *suffix* referring to a swelling

**celiac** /'siːliæk/ *adjective US* same as **coeliac**

**cell** /sel/ *noun* a tiny unit of matter which is the base of all plant and animal tissue (NOTE: For other terms referring to cells, see words beginning with **cyt-, cyto-**.)

COMMENT: The cell is a unit which can reproduce itself. It is made up of a jelly-like substance (cytoplasm) which surrounds a nucleus and contains many other small structures which are different according to the type of cell. Cells reproduce by division (mitosis) and their process of feeding and removing waste products is metabolism. The division and reproduction of cells is the way the human body is formed.

**cell body** /'sel ˌbɒdi/ *noun* the part of a nerve cell which surrounds the nucleus and from which the axon and dendrites begin

**cell division** /'sel dɪˌvɪʒ(ə)n/ *noun* the way in which a cell reproduces itself. ♦ **mitosis, meiosis**

**cell membrane** /'sel ˌmembreɪn/ *noun* a membrane enclosing the cytoplasm of a cell. ◊ **columnar cell, target cell**

**cellular** /'seljʊlə/ *adjective* **1.** referring to cells, or formed of cells **2.** made of many similar parts connected together

**cellular tissue** /ˌseljʊlə 'tɪʃuː/ *noun* a form of connective tissue with large spaces

**cellulite** /'seljʊlaɪt/ *noun* lumpy deposits of subcutaneous fat, especially in the thighs and buttocks

**cellulitis** /ˌseljʊ'laɪtɪs/ *noun* a usually bacterial inflammation of connective tissue or of the subcutaneous tissue

**cellulose** /'seljʊləʊs/ *noun* a carbohydrate which makes up a large percentage of plant matter

COMMENT: Cellulose is not digestible and is passed through the digestive system as roughage.

**Celsius** /'selsiəs/ *noun* a metric scale of temperature on which 0° is the point at which water freezes and 100° is the point at which water boils under average atmospheric conditions. Also called **centigrade**. ◊ **Fahrenheit** (NOTE: It is usually written as a **C** after the degree sign: **52°C** (say: 'fifty-two degrees Celsius').) [Described 1742. After Anders Celsius (1701–44), Swedish astronomer and scientist.]

COMMENT: To convert Celsius temperatures to Fahrenheit, multiply by 1.8 and add 32. So 20°C is equal to 68°F. Celsius is used in many countries, though not in the US, where the Fahrenheit system is still preferred.

**Celsius temperature** /'selsiəs ˌtemprɪtʃə/ *noun* temperature as measured on the Celsius scale

**CEMACH** /'siːmæʃ/ *noun* a UK research project investigating the causes of infant deaths and stillbirths. Full form **Confidential Enquiry into Maternal and Child Health**

**cement** /sɪ'ment/ *noun* **1.** an adhesive used in dentistry to attach a crown to the base of a tooth **2.** same as **cementum**

**cementum** /sɪ'mentəm/ *noun* a layer of thick hard material which covers the roots of teeth

**census** /'sensəs/ *noun* a systematic count or survey

**center** /'sentə/ *noun US* same as **centre**

**-centesis** /sentiːsɪs/ *suffix* puncture

**centi-** /senti/ *prefix* one hundredth ($10^{-2}$). Symbol **c**

**centigrade** /'sentɪgreɪd/ *noun* same as **Celsius**

**centile chart** /'sentaɪl tʃɑːt/ *noun* a chart showing the number of babies who fall into each percentage category, as regards, e.g., birth weight

**centilitre** /'sentɪliːtə/, **centiliter** *noun* a unit of measurement of liquid equal to one hundredth of a litre. Symbol **cl**

**centimetre** /'sentɪmiːtə/, **centimeter** *noun* a unit of measurement of length equal to one hundredth of a metre. Symbol **cm**

**central** /'sentrəl/ *adjective* referring to the centre

**central canal** /ˌsentrəl kə'næl/ *noun* a thin tube in the centre of the spinal cord containing cerebrospinal fluid

**central line** /'sentrəl laɪn/ *noun* a catheter inserted through the neck, used to monitor central venous pressure in conditions such as shock where fluid balance is severely upset

**central nervous system** /ˌsentrəl 'nɜːvəs ˌsɪstəm/ *noun* the brain and spinal cord which link together all the nerves

**central sulcus** /ˌsentrəl 'sʌlkəs/ *noun* one of the grooves which divide a cerebral hemisphere into lobes

**central temperature** /ˌsentrəl 'temprɪtʃə/ *noun* the temperature of the brain, thorax and abdomen, which is constant

**central vein** /ˌsentrəl 'veɪn/ *noun* a vein in the liver

**central venous pressure** /ˌsentrəl 'viːnəs ˌpreʃə/ *noun* blood pressure in the right atrium of the heart, which can be measured by means of a catheter

**centre** /'sentə/ *noun* **1.** the middle point, or the main part of something ○ *The aim of the examination is to locate the centre of infection.* **2.** a large building **3.** the point where a group of nerves come together (NOTE: [all senses] The US spelling is **center**.)

**centrifugal** /ˌsentrɪˈfjuːg(ə)l, senˈtrɪfjʊg(ə)l/ adjective moving away from the centre

**centrifugation** /ˌsentrɪfjuːˈɡeɪʃ(ə)n/, **centrifuging** /ˈsentrɪfjuːdʒɪŋ/ noun the process of separating the components of a liquid in a centrifuge

**centrifuge** /ˈsentrɪfjuːdʒ/ noun a device to separate the components of a liquid by rapid spinning

**centriole** /ˈsentriəʊl/ noun a small structure found in the cytoplasm of a cell, which involved in forming the spindle during cell division

**centripetal** /ˌsentrɪˈpiːt(ə)l, senˈtrɪpɪt(ə)l/ adjective moving towards the centre

**centromere** /ˈsentrəmɪə/ noun a constricted part of a chromosome, seen as a cell divides

**centrosome** /ˈsentrəsəʊm/ noun the structure in the cytoplasm of a cell, near the nucleus, and containing the centrioles

**centrum** /ˈsentrəm/ noun the central part of an organ (NOTE: The plural is **centra**.)

**cephal-** /sefəl/ prefix same as **cephalo-** (used before vowels)

**cephalalgia** /ˌsefəˈlældʒə/ noun same as **headache**

**cephalexin** /ˌsefəˈleksɪn/ noun an antibiotic used to treat infections of the urinary system or respiratory tract

**cephalhaematoma** /ˌsefəlhiːməˈtəʊmə/ noun a swelling found mainly on the head of babies delivered with forceps

**cephalic** /səˈfælɪk/ adjective referring to the head

**cephalic index** /səˌfælɪk ˈɪndeks/ noun a measurement of the shape of the skull

**cephalic presentation** /səˌfælɪk ˌprez(ə)nˈteɪʃ(ə)n/ noun the usual position of a baby in the uterus, where the baby's head will appear first

**cephalic version** /səˌfælɪk ˈvɜːʃ(ə)n/ noun turning a wrongly positioned fetus round in the uterus, so that the head will appear first at birth

**cephalo-** /sefələʊ/ prefix referring to the head

**cephalocele** /ˈsefələʊsiːl/ noun a swelling caused by part of the brain passing through a weak point in the bones of the skull

**cephalogram** /ˈsefələʊɡræm/ noun an X-ray photograph of the bones of the skull

**cephalometry** /ˌsefəˈlɒmɪtri/ noun measurement of the head

**cephalopelvic** /ˌsefələʊˈpelvɪk/ adjective referring to the head of the fetus and the pelvis of the mother

**cephalopelvic disproportion** /ˌsefələʊ ˌpelvɪk ˌdɪsprəˈpɔːʃ(ə)n/ noun a condition in which the pelvic opening of the mother is not large enough for the head of the fetus

**cephalosporin** /ˌsefələʊˈspɔːrɪn/ noun a drug used in the treatment of bacterial infection

**cephradine** /ˈsefrədiːn/ noun an antibacterial drug used to treat sinusitis and urinary tract infections

**cerclage** /sɜːˈklɑːʒ/ noun the act of tying things together with a ring

**cerea** /ˈsɪəriə/ ♦ **flexibilitas cerea**

**cerebellar** /ˌserəˈbelə/ adjective referring to the cerebellum

**cerebellar ataxia** /ˌserəbelər əˈtæksiə/ noun a disorder where a person staggers and cannot speak clearly, due to a disease of the cerebellum

**cerebellar cortex** /ˌserəbelə ˈkɔːteks/ noun the outer covering of grey matter which covers the cerebellum

**cerebellar gait** /ˌserəbelə ˈɡeɪt/ noun a way of walking where a person staggers along, caused by a disease of the cerebellum

**cerebellar peduncle** /ˌserəbelə pɪˈdʌŋk(ə)l/ noun a band of nerve tissue connecting parts of the cerebellum

**cerebellar syndrome** /ˌserəbelə ˈsɪndrəʊm/ noun a disease affecting the cerebellum, the symptoms of which are lack of muscle coordination, spasms in the eyeball and impaired speech

**cerebellum** /ˌserəˈbeləm/ noun a section of the hindbrain, located at the back of the head beneath the back part of the cerebrum. See illustration at BRAIN in Supplement

COMMENT: The cerebellum is formed of two hemispheres with the vermis in the centre. Fibres go into or out of the cerebellum through the peduncles. The cerebellum is the part of the brain where voluntary movements are coordinated and is associated with the sense of balance.

**cerebr-** /serəbr/ prefix same as **cerebro-** (used before vowels)

**cerebra** /səˈriːbrə/ plural of **cerebrum**

**cerebral** /ˈserəbrəl/ adjective referring to the cerebrum or to the brain in general

**cerebral aqueduct** /ˌserəbrəl ˈækwɪdʌkt/ noun a canal connecting the third and fourth ventricles in the brain. Also called **aqueduct of Sylvius**

**cerebral artery** /ˌserəbrəl ˈɑːtəri/ noun one of the main arteries which take blood into the brain

**cerebral cavity** /ˌserəbrəl ˈkævɪti/ noun one of the four connected fluid-filled spaces in the brain

**cerebral cortex** /ˌserəbrəl ˈkɔːteks/ noun the outer layer of grey matter which covers the cerebrum

**cerebral decompression** /ˌserəbrəl ˌdiːkəmˈpreʃ(ə)n/ noun the removal of part of the skull to relieve pressure on the brain

**cerebral dominance** /ˌserəbrəl ˈdɒmɪnəns/ noun the usual condition where the centres for various functions are located in one cerebral hemisphere

**cerebral haemorrhage** /ˌserəbrəl ˈhem(ə)rɪdʒ/ *noun* bleeding inside the brain from a cerebral artery. Also called **brain haemorrhage**

**cerebral hemisphere** /ˌserəbrəl ˈhemɪsfɪə/ *noun* one of the two halves of the cerebrum

**cerebral infarction** /ˌserəbrəl ɪnˈfɑːkʃən/ *noun* the death of brain tissue as a result of reduction in the blood supply to the brain

**cerebral ischaemia** /ˌserəbrəl ɪˈskiːmiə/ *noun* failure in the blood supply to the brain

**cerebral palsy** /ˌserəbrəl ˈpɔːlzi/ *noun* a disorder mainly due to brain damage occurring before birth, or due to lack of oxygen during birth, associated with poor coordination of muscular movements, impaired speech, hearing and sight, and sometimes mental impairment (NOTE: Premature babies are at higher risk.)

**cerebral peduncle** /ˌserəbrəl pɪˈdʌŋk(ə)l/ *noun* a mass of nerve fibres connecting the cerebral hemispheres to the midbrain. See illustration at BRAIN in Supplement

**cerebral thrombosis** /ˌserəbrəl θrɒmˈbəʊsɪs/ *noun* same as **cerebrovascular accident**

**cerebral vascular accident** /ˌserəbrəl ˌvæskjʊlər ˈæksɪd(ə)nt/ *noun* same as **cerebrovascular accident**

**cerebration** /ˌserəˈbreɪʃ(ə)n/ *noun* brain activity

**cerebro-** /ˈserəbrəʊ/ *prefix* referring to the cerebrum

**cerebrospinal** /ˌserəbrəʊˈspaɪn(ə)l/ *adjective* referring to the brain and the spinal cord

**cerebrospinal fever** /ˌserəbrəʊspaɪn(ə)l ˈfiːvə/ *noun* same as **meningococcal meningitis**

**cerebrospinal fluid** /ˌserəbrəʊspaɪn(ə)l ˈfluːɪd/ *noun* fluid which surrounds the brain and the spinal cord. Abbr **CSF**

COMMENT: CSF is found in the space between the arachnoid mater and pia mater of the brain, within the ventricles of the brain and in the central canal of the spinal cord. It consists mainly of water, with some sugar and sodium chloride. Its function is to cushion the brain and spinal cord and it is continually formed and absorbed to maintain the correct pressure.

**cerebrospinal meningitis** /ˌserəbrəʊ spaɪn(ə)l ˌmenɪnˈdʒaɪtɪs/ *noun* same as **meningococcal meningitis**

**cerebrospinal tract** /ˌserəbrəʊspaɪn(ə)l ˈtrækt/ *noun* one of the main motor pathways in the anterior and lateral white columns of the spinal cord

**cerebrovascular** /ˌserəbrəʊˈvæskjʊlə/ *adjective* referring to the blood vessels in the brain

**cerebrovascular accident** /ˌserəbrəʊ ˌvæskjʊlər ˈæksɪd(ə)nt/ *noun* a sudden

blocking of or bleeding from a blood vessel in the brain resulting in temporary or permanent paralysis or death. Also called **stroke**

**cerebrovascular disease** /ˌserəbrəʊ ˌvæskjʊlə dɪˈziːz/ *noun* a disease of the blood vessels in the brain

**cerebrum** /səˈriːbrəm/ *noun* the largest part of the brain, formed of two sections, the cerebral hemispheres, which run along the length of the head. The cerebrum controls the main mental processes, including the memory. Also called **telencephalon**

**certificate** /səˈtɪfɪkət/ *noun* an official paper which states something

**certify** /ˈsɜːtɪfaɪ/ *verb* to make an official statement in writing about something ○ *He was certified dead on arrival at hospital.*

**cerumen** /səˈruːmen/ *noun* wax which forms inside the ear. Also called **earwax**

**ceruminous gland** /səˈruːmɪnəs ˌglænd/ *noun* a gland which secretes earwax. See illustration at EAR in Supplement

**cervic-** /ˈsɜːvɪk/ *prefix* same as **cervico-** (*used before vowels*)

**cervical** /ˈsɜːvɪk(ə)l, səˈvaɪk(ə)l/ *adjective* **1.** referring to the neck **2.** referring to any part of the body which is shaped like a neck, especially the cervix of the uterus

**cervical canal** /ˌsɜːvɪk(ə)l kəˈnæl/ *noun* a tube running through the cervix, from the point where the uterus joins the vagina to the entrance of the uterine cavity. Also called **cervicouterine canal**

**cervical cancer** /ˌsɜːvɪk(ə)l ˈkænsə/ *noun* a cancer of the cervix of the uterus

**cervical collar** /ˌsɜːvɪk(ə)l ˈkɒlə/ *noun* a special strong orthopaedic collar to support the head of a person with neck injuries or a condition such as cervical spondylosis

**cervical erosion** /ˌsɜːvɪk(ə)l ɪˈrəʊʒ(ə)n/ *noun* a condition in which the epithelium of the mucous membrane lining the cervix uteri extends outside the cervix

**cervical ganglion** /ˌsɜːvɪk(ə)l ˈgæŋɡliən/ *noun* one of the bundles of nerves in the neck

**cervical incompetence** /ˌsɜːvɪk(ə)l ˈɪnkɒmpɪt(ə)ns/ *noun* a dysfunction of the cervix of the uterus which is often the cause of spontaneous abortions and premature births and can be remedied by Shirodkar's operation

**cervical intraepithelial neoplasia** /ˌsɜːvɪk(ə)l ˌɪntrəepɪˌθiːliəl niːəʊˈpleɪʒə/ *noun* changes in the cells of the cervix which may lead to cervical cancer. Abbr **CIN**

**cervical nerve** /ˌsɜːvɪk(ə)l ˈnɜːv/ *noun* spinal nerve in the neck

**cervical node** /ˌsɜːvɪk(ə)l ˈnəʊd/ *noun* lymph node in the neck

**cervical plexus** /ˌsɜːvɪk(ə)l ˈpleksəs/ *noun* a group of nerves in front of the vertebrae in the neck, which lead to nerves supplying the skin and muscles of the neck, and also the phrenic nerve which controls the diaphragm

**cervical rib** /ˌsɜːvɪk(ə)l ˈrɪb/ *noun* an extra rib sometimes found attached to the vertebrae above the other ribs and which may cause thoracic inlet syndrome

**cervical smear** /ˌsɜːvɪk(ə)l ˈsmɪə/ *noun* a test for cervical cancer, where cells taken from the mucus in the cervix of the uterus are examined

**cervical spondylosis** /ˌsɜːvɪk(ə)l spɒndɪˈləʊsɪs/ *noun* a degenerative change in the neck bones. ◊ **spondylosis**

**cervical vertebrae** /ˌsɜːvɪk(ə)l ˈvɜːtɪbriː/ *plural noun* the seven bones which form the neck

**cervicectomy** /ˌsɜːvɪˈsektəmi/ *noun* the surgical removal of the cervix uteri

**cervices** /ˈsɜːvɪsiːz/ *plural of* **cervix**

**cervicitis** /ˌsɜːvɪˈsaɪtɪs/ *noun* inflammation of the cervix uteri

**cervico-** /sɜːvɪkəʊ/ *prefix* **1.** referring to the neck **2.** referring to the cervix of the uterus

**cervicography** /ˌsɜːvɪˈkɒɡrəfi/ *noun* the act of photographing the cervix uteri, used as a method of screening for cervical cancer

**cervicouterine canal** /ˌsɜːvɪkəʊˌjuːtəraɪn kəˈnæl/ *noun* same as **cervical canal**

**cervix** /ˈsɜːvɪks/ *noun* **1.** any narrow neck of an organ **2.** the neck of the uterus, the narrow lower part of the uterus leading into the vagina. Also called **cervix uteri**

**CESDI** *noun* full form **Confidential Enquiry into Stillbirths and Deaths in Infancy.** ✦ **CEMACH**

**cesium** /ˈsiːziəm/ *noun US* same as **caesium**

**cestode** /ˈsestəʊd/ *noun* a type of tapeworm

**cetrimide** /ˈsetrɪmaɪd/ *noun* a mixture of ammonium compounds, used in disinfectants and antiseptics

**CF** *abbr* cystic fibrosis

**CFT** *abbr* complement fixation test

**chafe** /tʃeɪf/ *verb* to rub something, especially to rub against the skin ○ *The rough cloth of the collar chafed the girl's neck.*

**chafing** /ˈtʃeɪfɪŋ/ *noun* irritation of the skin due to rubbing ○ *She was experiencing chafing of the thighs.*

**Chagas' disease** /ˈʃɑːɡəs dɪˌziːz/ *noun* a type of sleeping sickness found in South America, transmitted by insect bites which pass trypanosomes into the bloodstream. Children are mainly affected and if untreated the disease can cause fatal heart block in early adult life. [Described 1909. After Carlos Chagas (1879–1934), Brazilian scientist and physician.]

**CHAI** *abbr* Commission for Healthcare Audit and Improvement

**chalasia** /tʃəˈleɪziə/ *noun* an excessive relaxation of the oesophageal muscles, which causes regurgitation

**chalazion** /kəˈleɪziən/ *noun* same as **meibomian cyst**

**challenge** /ˈtʃælɪndʒ/ *verb* to expose someone to a substance to determine whether an allergy or other adverse reaction will occur ■ *noun* exposure of someone to a substance to determine whether an allergy or other adverse reaction will occur

**chalone** /ˈkeɪləʊn, ˈkæləʊn/ *noun* a hormone which stops a secretion, as opposed to those hormones which stimulate secretion

**chamber** /ˈtʃeɪmbə/ *noun* a hollow space (atrium or ventricle) in the heart where blood is collected

**chancre** /ˈʃæŋkə/ *noun* a sore on the lip, penis or eyelid which is the first symptom of syphilis

**chancroid** /ˈʃæŋkrɔɪd/ *noun* a venereal sore with a soft base, situated in the groin or on the genitals and caused by the bacterium *Haemophilus ducreyi.* Also called **soft chancre**

**change of life** /ˌtʃeɪndʒ əv ˈlaɪf/ *noun* same as **menopause** (*dated informal*)

**chapped** /tʃæpt/ *adjective* referring to skin which is cracked due to cold

**characterise** /ˈkærɪktəraɪz/, **characterize** *verb* to be a typical or special quality or feature of something or someone ○ *The disease is characterised by the development of lesions throughout the body.*

**characteristic** /ˌkærɪktəˈrɪstɪk/ *noun* a quality which allows something to be recognised as different ○ *Cancer destroys the cell's characteristics.* ■ *adjective* being a typical or distinguishing quality ○ *symptoms characteristic of anaemia* ○ *The inflammation is characteristic of shingles.*

**charcoal** /ˈtʃɑːkəʊl/ *noun* a highly absorbent substance, formed when wood is burnt in the absence of oxygen, used to relieve diarrhoea or intestinal gas and in cases of poisoning

COMMENT: Charcoal tablets can be used to relieve diarrhoea or flatulence.

**Charcot's joint** /ˌʃɑːkəʊz ˈdʒɔɪnt/ *noun* a joint which becomes deformed because the patient cannot feel pain in it when the nerves have been damaged by syphilis, diabetes or leprosy [Described 1868. After Jean-Martin Charcot (1825–93), French neurologist.]

**Charcot's triad** /ˌʃɑːkəʊz ˈtraɪæd/ *noun* three symptoms of multiple sclerosis: rapid eye movement, tremor and scanning speech

**charleyhorse** /ˈtʃɑːlihɔːs/ *noun US* a painful cramp in a leg or thigh (*informal*)

**Charnley clamps** /ˌtʃɑːnli ˈklæmps/ *plural noun* metal clamps fixed to a rod through a bone to hold it tight

**chart** /tʃɑːt/ *noun* a record of information shown as a series of lines or points on graph paper ○ *a temperature chart*

**charting** /'tʃɑːtɪŋ/ *noun* the preparation and updating of a hospital patient's chart by nurses and doctors

**ChB** *abbr* bachelor of surgery

**CHC** *abbr* **1.** child health clinic **2.** community health council

**CHD** *abbr* coronary heart disease

**check-up** /'tʃek ʌp/ *noun* a general examination by a doctor or dentist ○ *She went for a check-up.* ○ *He had a heart check-up last week.*

**cheek** /tʃiːk/ *noun* **1.** one of two fleshy parts of the face on each side of the nose **2.** either side of the buttocks (*informal*)

**cheekbone** /'tʃiːkbəʊn/ *noun* an arch of bone in the face beneath the cheek which also forms the lower part of the eye socket

**cheil-** /kaɪl/ *prefix* same as **cheilo-** (*used before vowels*)

**cheilitis** /kaɪ'laɪtɪs/ *noun* inflammation of the lips

**cheilo-** /kaɪləʊ/ *prefix* referring to the lips

**cheiloschisis** /ˌkaɪləʊ'ʃaɪsɪs/ *noun* a double cleft upper lip

**cheilosis** /kaɪ'ləʊsɪs/ *noun* swelling and cracks on the lips and corners of the mouth caused by lack of vitamin B

**cheiro-** /keɪrəʊ/ *prefix* referring to the hand

**cheiropompholyx** /ˌkeɪrəʊ'pɒmfəlɪks/ *noun* a disorder of the skin in which tiny blisters appear on the palms of the hand

**chelate** /'kiːleɪt/ *verb* to treat someone with a chelating agent in order to remove a heavy metal such as lead from the bloodstream

**chelating agent** /'kiːleɪtɪŋ ˌeɪdʒənt/ *noun* a chemical compound which can combine with some metals, used as a treatment for metal poisoning

**cheloid** /'kiːlɔɪd/ *noun* same as **keloid**

**chemical** /'kemɪk(ə)l/ *adjective* referring to chemistry ■ *noun* a substance produced by a chemical process or formed of chemical elements

> 'The MRI body scanner is able to provide a chemical analysis of tissues without investigative surgery' [*Health Services Journal*]

**chemical composition** /ˌkemɪk(ə)l ˌkɒmpə'zɪʃ(ə)n/ *noun* the chemicals which make up a substance ○ *They analysed the blood samples to find out their chemical composition.*

**chemical symbol** /ˌkemɪk(ə)l 'sɪmbəl/ *noun* letters which represent a chemical substance ○ *Na is the symbol for sodium.*

**chemist** /'kemɪst/ *noun* a shop where you can buy medicine, toothpaste, soap and similar items ○ *Go to the chemist to get some cough medicine.* ○ *The tablets are sold at all chemists.* ○ *There's a chemist on the corner.*

**chemistry** /'kemɪstri/ *noun* the study of substances, elements and compounds and their reactions with each other ◇ **blood chemistry** or **chemistry of the blood 1.** substances which make up blood, which can be analysed in blood tests, the results of which are useful in diagnosing disease **2.** a record of changes which take place in blood during disease and treatment

**chemo** /'kiːməʊ/ *noun* chemotherapy (*informal*)

**chemo-** /kiːməʊ/ *prefix* referring to chemistry

**chemoreceptor** /ˌkiːməʊrɪ'septə/ *noun* a cell which responds to the presence of a chemical compound by activating a nerve, e.g. a taste bud reacting to food or cells in the carotid body reacting to lowered oxygen and raised carbon dioxide in the blood

**chemosis** /kiː'məʊsɪs/ *noun* swelling of the conjunctiva

**chemotaxis** /ˌkiːməʊ'tæksɪs/ *noun* the movement of a cell when it is attracted to or repelled by a chemical substance

**chemotherapeutic agent** /ˌkiːməʊθerə'pjuːtɪk ˌeɪdʒənt/ *noun* a chemical substance used to treat a disease

**chemotherapy** /ˌkiːməʊ'θerəpi/ *noun* the use of drugs such as antibiotics, painkillers or antiseptic lotions to fight a disease, especially using toxic chemicals to destroy rapidly developing cancer cells

**chest** /tʃest/ *noun* **1.** the upper front part of the body between the neck and stomach. Also called **thorax 2.** same as **thorax** (NOTE: For other terms referring to the chest, see **pectoral** and words beginning with **steth-, thorac-, thoraco-**.)

**chest cavity** /'tʃest ˌkævɪti/ *noun* a space in the body containing the diaphragm, heart and lungs

**chest examination** /'tʃest ɪgˌzæmɪneɪʃ(ə)n/ *noun* an examination of someone's chest by percussion, stethoscope or X-ray

**chest muscle** /'tʃest ˌmʌs(ə)l/ *noun* same as **pectoral muscle**

**chest pain** /'tʃest peɪn/ *noun* pain in the chest which may be caused by heart disease

**chesty** /'tʃesti/ *adjective* having phlegm in the lungs, or having a tendency to chest complaints

**Cheyne–Stokes respiration** /ˌtʃeɪn 'stəʊks respɪˌreɪʃ(ə)n/, **Cheyne–Stokes breathing** /'briːðɪŋ/ *noun* irregular breathing, usually found in people who are unconscious, with short breaths gradually increasing to deep breaths, then reducing again, until breathing appears to stop

**CHI** *abbr* Commission for Health Improvement

**chiasm** /'kaɪæz(ə)m/, **chiasma** /kaɪ'æzmə/ noun ♦ optic chiasma

**chickenpox** /'tʃɪkɪnˌpɒks/ noun an infectious disease of children, with fever and red spots which turn into itchy blisters. Also called **varicella**

COMMENT: Chickenpox is caused by a herpesvirus. In later life, shingles is usually a re-emergence of a dormant chickenpox virus and an adult with shingles can infect a child with chickenpox.

**Chief Medical Officer** /tʃiːf 'medɪk(ə)l ˌɒfɪsə/ noun in the UK, a government official responsible for all aspects of public health. Abbr **CMO**

**Chief Nursing Officer** /tʃiːf 'nɜːsɪŋ ˌɒfɪsə/ noun in the UK, an official appointed by the Department of Health to advise Government Ministers and provide leadership to nurses and midwives. Abbr **CNO**

**chilblain** /'tʃɪlbleɪn/ noun a condition in which the skin of the fingers, toes, nose or ears becomes red, swollen and itchy because of exposure to cold. Also called **erythema pernio**

**child** /tʃaɪld/ noun a young boy or girl. Child is the legal term for a person under 14 years of age. (NOTE: The plural is **children**. For other terms referring to children, see words beginning with **paed-, paedo-** or **ped-, pedo-**.)

**child abuse** /'tʃaɪld əˌbjuːs/ noun cruel treatment of a child by an adult, including physical and sexual harm

**childbearing** /'tʃaɪldbeərɪŋ/ noun the act of carrying and giving birth to a child

**childbirth** /'tʃaɪldbɜːθ/ noun the act of giving birth. Also called **parturition**

**child care** /'tʃaɪld keə/ noun the care of young children and study of their special needs

**child health clinic** /tʃaɪld 'helθ ˌklɪnɪk/ noun a special clinic for checking the health and development of small children under school age. Abbr **CHC**

**childhood illness** /ˌtʃaɪldhʊd 'ɪlnəs/ noun an illness which mainly affects children and not adults

**child-proof** /'tʃaɪld pruːf/ adjective designed so that a child cannot use it ○ child-proof containers ○ The pills are sold in bottles with child-proof lids or caps.

**child protection** /ˌtʃaɪld prə'tekʃən/ noun the measures taken to avoid abuse, neglect or exploitation of any kind towards children

**children** /'tʃɪldrən/ plural of **child**

**children's hospital** /'tʃɪldrənz ˌhɒspɪt(ə)l/ noun a hospital which specialises in treating children

**chill** /tʃɪl/ noun a short illness causing a feeling of being cold and shivering, usually the sign of the beginning of a fever, of flu or a cold

**chin** /tʃɪn/ noun the bottom part of the face, beneath the mouth

**Chinese medicine** /ˌtʃaɪniːz 'med(ə)sɪn/ noun a system of diagnosis, treatment and prevention of illness developed in China over many centuries. It uses herbs, minerals and animal products, exercise, massage and acupuncture.

**Chinese restaurant syndrome** /ˌtʃaɪniːz 'rest(ə)rɒnt ˌsɪndrəʊm/ noun an allergic condition which gives people severe headaches after eating food flavoured with monosodium glutamate (informal)

**chiro-** /kaɪrəʊ/ prefix referring to the hand

**chiropodist** /kɪ'rɒpədɪst/ noun a person who specialises in treatment of minor disorders of the feet

**chiropody** /kɪ'rɒpədi/ noun the study and treatment of minor diseases and disorders of the feet

**chiropractic** /ˌkaɪrəʊ'præktɪk/ noun the treatment and prevention of disorders of the neuromusculoskeletal system by making adjustments primarily to the bones of the spine

**chiropractor** /'kaɪrəʊˌpræktə/ noun a person who treats musculoskeletal disorders by making adjustments primarily to the bones of the spine

**chiropracty** /'kaɪrəʊˌprækti/ noun same as **chiropractic** (informal)

**Chlamydia** /klə'mɪdiə/ noun a bacterium that causes trachoma and urogenital diseases in humans and psittacosis in birds, which can be transmitted to humans. It is currently a major cause of sexually transmitted disease.

**chlamydial** /klə'mɪdiəl/ adjective referring to infections caused by Chlamydia

**chloasma** /kləʊ'æzmə/ noun the presence of brown spots on the skin from various causes

**chlor-** /klɔːr/ prefix same as **chloro-** (used before vowels)

**chlorambucil** /klɔːr'æmbjʊsɪl/ noun a drug which is toxic to cells, used in cancer treatment

**chloramphenicol** /ˌklɔːræm'fenɪkɒl/ noun a powerful antibiotic which sometimes causes the collapse of blood cell production, so is used only for treating life-threatening diseases such as meningitis

**chlordiazepoxide** /ˌklɔːdaɪˌæzɪ'pɒksaɪd/ noun a yellow crystalline powder, used as a tranquilliser and treatment for alcoholism

**chlorhexidine** /klɔː'heksɪdiːn/ noun a disinfectant mouthwash

**chloride** /'klɔːraɪd/ noun a salt of hydrochloric acid

**chlorination** /ˌklɔːrɪ'neɪʃ(ə)n/ noun sterilisation by adding chlorine

COMMENT: Chlorination is used to kill bacteria in drinking water, in swimming pools and sewage farms, and has many industrial applications such as sterilisation in food processing.

**chlorinator** /'klɔːrɪneɪtə/ noun apparatus for adding chlorine to water

**chlorine** /ˈklɔːriːn/ noun a powerful greenish gas, used to sterilise water (NOTE: The chemical symbol is **Cl**.)

**chlormethiazole** /ˌklɔːmeˈθaɪəzəʊl/ noun a sedative used in the treatment of people with alcoholism

**chloro-** /klɔːrəʊ/ prefix referring to chlorine

**chloroform** /ˈklɒrəfɔːm/ noun a powerful drug formerly used as an anaesthetic

**chloroma** /klɔːˈrəʊmə/ noun a bone tumour associated with acute leukaemia

**chloroquine** /ˈklɔːrəkwɪn/ noun a drug used to prevent and treat malaria, but to which resistance has developed in some parts of the world

**chlorosis** /klɔːˈrəʊsɪs/ noun a type of severe anaemia due to iron deficiency, affecting mainly young girls

**chlorothiazide** /ˌklɔːrəʊˈθaɪəzaɪd/ noun a drug which helps the body to produce more urine, used in the treatment of high blood pressure, swelling and heart failure

**chloroxylenol** /ˌklɔːrəʊˈzaɪlənɒl/ noun a chemical used as an antimicrobial agent in skin creams and in disinfectants

**chlorpheniramine** /ˌklɔːfenˈaɪrəmiːn/, **chlorpheniramine maleate** /ˌklɔːfenaɪrəmiːn ˈmæliːeɪt/ noun an antihistamine drug

**chlorpromazine hydrochloride** /klɔːˌprəʊməziːn ˌhaɪdrəʊˈklɔːraɪd/ noun a drug used to treat schizophrenia and other psychoses

**chlorpropamide** /klɔːˈprəʊpəmaɪd/ noun a drug which lowers blood sugar, used in the treatment of diabetes

**chlorthalidone** /klɔːˈθælɪdəʊn/ noun a diuretic

**ChM** abbr Master of Surgery

**choana** /ˈkəʊənə/ noun any opening shaped like a funnel, especially the one leading from the nasal cavity to the pharynx (NOTE: The plural is **choanae**.)

**chocolate cyst** /ˌtʃɒklət ˈsɪst/ noun an ovarian cyst containing old brown blood

**choke** /tʃəʊk/ verb to stop breathing because the windpipe becomes blocked by a foreign body or by inhalation of water, or to stop someone breathing by blocking the windpipe □ **to choke on (something)** to take something into the windpipe instead of the gullet, so that the breathing is interrupted ○ *A piece of bread made him choke* or *He choked on a piece of bread.*

**choking** /ˈtʃəʊkɪŋ/ noun a condition in which someone is prevented from breathing. ◊ **asphyxia**

**chol-** /kɒl/ prefix same as **chole-** (*used before vowels*)

**cholaemia** /kəˈliːmiə/ noun the presence of an unusual amount of bile in the blood

**cholagogue** /ˈkɒləgɒg/ noun a drug which encourages the production of bile

**cholangiocarcinoma** /kəˌlændʒiəʊˌkɑːsɪˈnəʊmə/ noun a rare cancer of the cells of the bile ducts

**cholangiography** /kəˌlændʒiˈɒgrəfi/ noun an X-ray examination of the bile ducts and gall bladder

**cholangiolitis** /kəˌlændʒiəʊˈlaɪtɪs/ noun inflammation of the small bile ducts

**cholangiopancreatography** /kəˌlændʒiəʊˌpæŋkriəˈtɒgrəfi/ noun an X-ray examination of the bile ducts and pancreas

**cholangitis** /ˌkəʊlænˈdʒaɪtɪs/ noun inflammation of the bile ducts

**chole-** /kɒli/ prefix referring to bile

**cholecalciferol** /ˌkɒlikælˈsɪfərɒl/ noun a form of vitamin D found naturally in fish-liver oils and egg yolks

**cholecystectomy** /ˌkɒlɪsɪˈstektəmi/ noun the surgical removal of the gall bladder

**cholecystitis** /ˌkɒlɪsɪˈstaɪtɪs/ noun inflammation of the gall bladder

**cholecystoduodenostomy** /ˌkɒlɪsɪstəˌdjuːədɪˈnɒstəmi/ noun a surgical operation to join the gall bladder to the duodenum to allow bile to pass into the intestine when the main bile duct is blocked

**cholecystogram** /ˌkɒlɪˈsɪstəgræm/ noun an X-ray photograph of the gall bladder

**cholecystography** /ˌkɒlɪsɪˈstɒgrəfi/ noun an X-ray examination of the gall bladder

**cholecystokinin** /ˌkɒlɪsɪstəʊˈkaɪnɪn/ noun a hormone released by cells at the top of the small intestine. It stimulates the gall bladder, making it contract and release bile.

**cholecystotomy** /ˌkɒlɪsɪˈstɒtəmi/ noun a surgical operation to make a cut in the gall bladder, usually to remove gallstones

**choledoch-** /kəˈledək/ prefix referring to the common bile duct

**choledocholithiasis** /kəˌledəkəlɪˈθaɪəsɪs/ noun same as **cholelithiasis**

**choledocholithotomy** /kəˌledɪkəʊlɪˈθɒtəmi/ noun a surgical operation to remove a gallstone by cutting into the bile duct

**choledochostomy** /kəˌledəˈkɒstəmi/ noun a surgical operation to make an opening in a bile duct

**choledochotomy** /kəledəˈkɒtəmi/ noun a surgical operation to make a cut in the common bile duct to remove gallstones

**cholelithiasis** /ˌkɒlɪlɪˈθaɪəsɪs/ noun a condition in which gallstones form in the gall bladder or bile ducts. Also called **choledocholithiasis**

**cholelithotomy** /ˌkɒlɪlɪˈθɒtəmi/ noun the surgical removal of gallstones by cutting into the bile duct

**cholera** /ˈkɒlərə/ noun a serious bacterial disease spread through food or water which has been infected by *Vibrio cholerae* ○ *A cholera epidemic broke out after the flood.*

COMMENT: The infected person experiences diarrhoea, cramp in the intestines and dehydration. The disease is often fatal and vaccination is only effective for a relatively short period.

**choleresis** /kəˈlɪərəsɪs/ *noun* the production of bile by the liver

**choleretic** /ˌkɒlɪˈretɪk/ *adjective* referring to a substance which increases the production and flow of bile

**cholestasis** /ˌkɒlɪˈsteɪsɪs/ *noun* a condition in which all bile does not pass into the intestine but some remains in the liver and causes jaundice

**cholesteatoma** /kəˌlestɪəˈtəʊmə/ *noun* a cyst containing some cholesterol found in the middle ear and also in the brain

**cholesterol** /kəˈlestərɒl/ *noun* a fatty substance found in fats and oils, also produced by the liver and forming an essential part of all cells

COMMENT: Cholesterol is found in brain cells, the adrenal glands, liver and bile acids. High levels of cholesterol in the blood are found in diabetes. Cholesterol is formed by the body, and high blood cholesterol levels are associated with diets rich in animal fat, such as butter and fat meat. Excess cholesterol can be deposited in the walls of arteries, causing atherosclerosis.

**cholesterolaemia** /kəˌlestərəˈliːmiə/ *noun* a high level of cholesterol in the blood

**cholesterosis** /kəˌlestəˈrəʊsɪs/ *noun* inflammation of the gall bladder with deposits of cholesterol

**cholic acid** /ˌkəʊlɪk ˈæsɪd/ *noun* one of the bile acids

**choline** /ˈkəʊliːn/ *noun* a compound involved in fat metabolism and the precursor for acetylcholine

**cholinergic** /ˌkəʊlɪˈnɜːdʒɪk/ *adjective* referring to a neurone or receptor which responds to acetylcholine

**cholinesterase** /ˌkəʊlɪˈnestəreɪz/ *noun* an enzyme which breaks down a choline ester

**choluria** /kəʊˈljʊəriə/ *noun* same as **biliuria**

**chondr-** /kɒndr/ *prefix* referring to cartilage

**chondritis** /kɒnˈdraɪtɪs/ *noun* inflammation of a cartilage

**chondroblast** /ˈkɒndrəʊblæst/ *noun* a cell from which cartilage develops in an embryo

**chondrocalcinosis** /ˌkɒndrəʊˌkælsɪˈnəʊsɪs/ *noun* a condition in which deposits of calcium phosphate are found in articular cartilage

**chondrocyte** /ˈkɒndrəʊsaɪt/ *noun* a mature cartilage cell

**chondrodysplasia** /ˌkɒndrəʊdɪsˈpleɪziə/ *noun* a hereditary disorder of cartilage which is linked to dwarfism

**chondrodystrophy** /ˌkɒndrəʊˈdɪstrəfi/ *noun* any disorder of cartilage

**chondroma** /kɒnˈdrəʊmə/ *noun* a tumour formed of cartilaginous tissue

**chondromalacia** /ˌkɒndrəʊməˈleɪʃə/ *noun* degeneration of the cartilage of a joint

**chondrosarcoma** /ˌkɒndrəʊsɑːˈkəʊmə/ *noun* a malignant, rapidly growing tumour involving cartilage cells

**chorda** /ˈkɔːdə/ *noun* a cord or tendon (NOTE: The plural is **chordae**.)

**chordae tendineae** /ˌkɔːdaɪ tenˈdɪniaɪ/ *plural noun* tiny fibrous ligaments in the heart which attach the edges of some of the valves to the walls of the ventricles

**chordee** /ˈkɔːdiː/ *noun* a painful condition where the erect penis is curved, a complication of gonorrhoea

**chorditis** /kɔːˈdaɪtɪs/ *noun* inflammation of the vocal cords

**chordotomy** /kɔːˈdɒtəmi/ *noun* a surgical operation to cut a cord such as a nerve pathway in the spinal cord in order to relieve intractable pain

**chorea** /kɔːˈriːə/ *noun* a sudden severe twitching, usually of the face and shoulders, which is a symptom of disease of the nervous system

**chorion** /ˈkɔːriən/ *noun* a membrane covering the fertilised ovum

**chorionic** /ˌkɔːriˈɒnɪk/ *adjective* referring to the chorion

**chorionic gonadotrophin** /kɔːriˌɒnɪk gəʊnədəʊˈtrəʊfɪn/ *noun* ♦ **human chorionic gonadotrophin**

**chorionic villi** /kɔːriˌɒnɪk ˈvɪlaɪ/ *plural noun* tiny finger-like folds in the chorion

**chorionic villus sampling** /kɔːriˌɒnɪk ˈvɪləs ˌsɑːmplɪŋ/ *noun* an antenatal screening test carried out by examining cells from the chorionic villi of the outer membrane surrounding an embryo, which have the same DNA as the fetus

**choroid** /ˈkɔːrɔɪd/ *noun* the middle layer of tissue which forms the eyeball, between the sclera and the retina. See illustration at EYE in Supplement

**choroiditis** /ˌkɔːrɔɪˈdaɪtɪs/ *noun* inflammation of the choroid in the eyeball

**choroidocyclitis** /ˌkɔːˌrɔɪdəʊsaɪˈklaɪtɪs/ *noun* inflammation of the choroids and ciliary body

**choroid plexus** /ˌkɔːrɔɪd ˈpleksəs/ *noun* part of the pia mater, a network of small blood vessels in the ventricles of the brain which produce cerebrospinal fluid. See illustration at EYE in Supplement

**Christmas disease** /ˈkrɪsməs dɪˌziːz/ *noun* same as **haemophilia B** [After Mr Christmas, the person in whom the disease was first studied in detail]

**Christmas factor** /ˈkrɪsməs ˌfæktə/ *noun* same as **Factor IX**

**chrom-** /krəʊm/ *prefix* same as **chromo-** (*used before vowels*)

**-chromasia** /krəmeɪziə/ *suffix* referring to colour

**chromatid** /ˈkrəʊmətɪd/ *noun* one of two parallel filaments making up a chromosome

**chromatin** /ˈkrəʊmətɪn/ *noun* a network which forms the nucleus of a cell and can be stained with basic dyes

**chromatography** /ˌkrəʊməˈtɒɡrəfi/ *noun* a method of separating chemicals through a porous medium, used in analysing compounds and mixtures

**chromatophore** /krəʊˈmætəfɔː/ *noun* any pigment-bearing cell in the eyes, hair and skin

**chromic acid** /ˌkrəʊmɪk ˈæsɪd/ *noun* an unstable acid existing only in solution or in the form of a salt, sometimes used in the removal of warts

**chromicised catgut** /ˌkrəʊmɪsaɪzd ˈkætɡʌt/ *noun* catgut which is hardened with chromium to make it slower to dissolve in the body

**chromium** /ˈkrəʊmiəm/ *noun* a metallic trace element (NOTE: The chemical symbol is **Cr.**)

**chromo-** /krəʊməʊ/ *prefix* referring to colour

**chromosomal** /ˌkrəʊməˈsəʊm(ə)l/ *adjective* referring to chromosomes

**chromosomal aberration** /ˌkrəʊmə ˈsəʊm(ə)l ˌæbəˈreɪʃ(ə)n/ *noun* same as **chromosome aberration**

**chromosome** /ˈkrəʊməsəʊm/ *noun* a rod-shaped structure in the nucleus of a cell, formed of DNA, which carries the genes

COMMENT: Each human cell has 46 chromosomes, 23 inherited from each parent. The female has one pair of X chromosomes, and the male one pair of XY chromosomes, which are responsible for the sexual difference. Sperm from a male have either an X or a Y chromosome. If a Y chromosome sperm fertilises the female's ovum the child will be male.

**chromosome aberration** /ˈkrəʊməsəʊm ˌæbəreɪʃ(ə)n/ *noun* a change from the usual number or arrangement of chromosomes

**chromosome mapping** /ˈkrəʊməsəʊm ˌmæpɪŋ/ *noun* a procedure by which the position of genes on a chromosome is established

**chronic** /ˈkrɒnɪk/ *adjective* **1.** referring to a disease or condition which lasts for a long time ○ *He has a chronic chest complaint.* Opposite **acute 2.** referring to serious pain (*informal*)

**chronic abscess** /ˌkrɒnɪk ˈæbses/ *noun* an abscess which develops slowly over a period of time

**chronic appendicitis** /ˌkrɒnɪk əˌpendɪ ˈsaɪtɪs/ *noun* a condition in which the vermiform appendix is always slightly inflamed. ◊ **grumbling appendix**

**chronic catarrhal rhinitis** /ˌkrɒnɪk kə ˌtɑːrəl raɪˈnaɪtɪs/ *noun* a persistent form of inflammation of the nose where excess mucus is secreted by the mucous membrane

**chronic fatigue syndrome** /ˌkrɒnɪk fə ˈtiːɡ ˌsɪndrəʊm/ *noun* same as **myalgic encephalomyelitis**

**chronic glaucoma** /ˌkrɒnɪk ɡlɔːˈkəʊmə/ *noun* same as **open-angle glaucoma**

**chronic granulomatous disease** /ˌkrɒnɪk ˌɡrænjʊˈləʊmətəs dɪˌziːz/ *noun* a type of inflammation where macrophages are converted into epithelial-like cells as a result of infection, as in tuberculosis or sarcoidosis

**chronic obstructive airways disease** /ˌkrɒnɪk əbˌstrʌktɪv ˈeəweɪz dɪˌziːz/ *noun* Abbr **COAD**. Now called **chronic obstructive pulmonary disease**

**chronic obstructive pulmonary disease** /ˌkrɒnɪk əbˌstrʌktɪv ˈpʌlmən(ə)ri dɪˌziːz/ *noun* any of a group of progressive respiratory disorders where someone experiences loss of lung function and shows little or no response to steroid or bronchodilator drug treatments, e.g. emphysema and chronic bronchitis. Abbr **COPD**

**chronic pancreatitis** /ˌkrɒnɪk pæŋkriə ˈtaɪtɪs/ *noun* a persistent inflammation occurring after repeated attacks of acute pancreatitis, where the gland becomes calcified

**chronic periarthritis** /ˌkrɒnɪk periɑː ˈθraɪtɪs/ *noun* inflammation of tissues round the shoulder joint. Also called **scapulohumeral arthritis**

**chronic pericarditis** /ˌkrɒnɪk perikɑː ˈdaɪtɪs/ *noun* a condition in which the pericardium becomes thickened and prevents the heart from functioning normally. Also called **constrictive pericarditis**

**Chronic Sick and Disabled Persons Act 1970** /ˌkrɒnɪk ˌsɪk ən dɪsˌeɪb(ə)ld ˈpɜːs(ə)nz ækt/ *noun* an Act of Parliament in the UK which provides benefits such as alterations to their homes for people with long-term conditions

**chronic toxicity** /ˌkrɒnɪk tɒkˈsɪsɪti/ *noun* exposure to harmful levels of a toxic substance over a period of time

**chrysotherapy** /ˌkraɪsəʊˈθerəpi/ *noun* treatment which involves gold injections

**Chvostek's sign** /tʃəˈvɒsteks saɪn/ *noun* an indication of tetany, where a spasm is produced if the facial muscles are tapped

**chyle** /kaɪl/ *noun* a fluid in the lymph vessels in the intestine, which contains fat, especially after a meal

**chylomicron** /ˌkaɪləʊˈmaɪkrɒn/ *noun* a particle of chyle present in the blood

**chyluria** /kaɪˈljʊəriə/ *noun* the presence of chyle in the urine

**chyme** /kaɪm/ *noun* a semi-liquid mass of food and gastric juices, which passes from the stomach to the intestine

**chymotrypsin** /ˌkaɪməʊˈtrɪpsɪn/ *noun* an enzyme which digests protein

**Ci** *abbr* curie

**cicatrise** /ˈsɪkətraɪz/, **cicatrize** *verb* to heal and form a scar, or to cause a wound to heal and form a scar

**cicatrix** /ˈsɪkətrɪks/ *noun* same as **scar**

**-ciclovir** /sɪkləvɪə/ *suffix* used in the names of antiviral drugs

**-cide** /saɪd/ *suffix* referring to killing

**cilia** /ˈsɪliə/ plural of **cilium**

**ciliary** /ˈsɪliəri/ *adjective* 1. referring to the eyelid or eyelashes 2. referring to cilia

**ciliary body** /ˈsɪliəri ˌbɒdi/ *noun* the part of the eye which connects the iris to the choroid. See illustration at EYE in Supplement

**ciliary ganglion** /ˌsɪliəri ˈgæŋgliən/ *noun* a parasympathetic ganglion in the orbit of the eye, supplying the intrinsic eye muscles

**ciliary muscle** /ˈsɪliəri ˌmʌs(ə)l/ *noun* a muscle which makes the lens of the eye change its shape to focus on objects at different distances. See illustration at EYE in Supplement

**ciliary processes** /ˌsɪliəri ˈprəʊsesiz/ *plural noun* the ridges behind the iris to which the lens of the eye is attached

**ciliated epithelium** /ˌsɪlieɪtɪd epɪˈθiːliəm/ *noun* simple epithelium where the cells have tiny hairs or cilia

**cilium** /ˈsɪliəm/ *noun* 1. an eyelash 2. one of many tiny hair-like processes which line cells in passages in the body and by moving backwards and forwards drive particles or fluid along the passage (NOTE: The plural is **cilia**.)

**-cillin** /sɪlɪn/ *suffix* used in the names of penicillin drugs ○ *amoxycillin*

**cimetidine** /sɪˈmetɪdiːn/ *noun* a drug which reduces the production of stomach acid, used in peptic ulcer treatment

**cimex** /ˈsaɪmeks/ *noun* a bedbug or related insect which feeds on birds, humans and other mammals (NOTE: The plural is **cimices**.)

**CIN** *abbr* cervical intraepithelial neoplasia

**-cin** /sɪn/ *suffix* referring to aminoglycosides ○ *gentamicin*

**cinematics** /ˌsɪnɪˈmætɪks/ *noun* the science of movement, especially of body movements

**cineplasty** /ˈsɪnɪplæsti/ *noun* an amputation where the muscles of the stump of the amputated limb are used to operate an artificial limb

**cineradiography** /ˌsɪnireɪdiˈɒgrəfi/ *noun* the practice of taking a series of X-ray photographs for diagnosis, or to show how something moves or develops in the body

**cinesiology** /sɪˌniːsiˈɒlədʒi/ *noun* the study of muscle movements, particularly in relation to treatment

**cingulectomy** /ˌsɪŋgjʊˈlektəmi/ *noun* a surgical operation to remove the cingulum

**cingulum** /ˈsɪŋgjʊləm/ *noun* a long curved bundle of nerve fibres in the cerebrum (NOTE: The plural is **cingula**.)

**cinnarizine** /ˈsɪnərəziːn/ *noun* an antihistaminic used to treat Ménière's disease

**ciprofloxacin** /ˌsaɪprəʊˈflɒksəsɪn/ *noun* a powerful antibiotic used in eye drops to treat corneal ulcers and surface infections of the eye, and in the treatment of anthrax in humans

**circadian** /sɜːˈkeɪdiən/ *adjective* referring to a pattern which is repeated approximately every 24 hours

**circadian rhythm** /sɜːˌkeɪdiən ˈrɪð(ə)m/ *noun* same as **biological clock**

**circle of Willis** /ˌsɜːk(ə)l əv ˈwɪlɪs/ *noun* a circle of branching arteries at the base of the brain formed by the basilar artery, the anterior and posterior cerebral arteries, the anterior and posterior communicating arteries and the internal carotid arteries [Described 1664. After Thomas Willis (1621–75), English physician and anatomist.]

**circular fold** /ˈsɜːkjʊlə fəʊld/ *noun* a large transverse fold of mucous membrane in the small intestine

**circulation** /ˌsɜːkjʊˈleɪʃ(ə)n/ *noun* □ **circulation (of the blood)** movement of blood around the body from the heart through the arteries to the capillaries and back to the heart through the veins ○ *She has poor circulation in her legs.* ○ *Rub your hands to get the circulation going.*

COMMENT: Blood circulates around the body, carrying oxygen from the lungs and nutrients from the liver through the arteries and capillaries to the tissues. The capillaries exchange the oxygen for waste matter such as carbon dioxide which is taken back to the lungs to be expelled. At the same time the blood obtains more oxygen in the lungs to be taken to the tissues. The circulation pattern is as follows: blood returns through the veins to the right atrium of the heart. From there it is pumped through the right ventricle into the pulmonary artery, and then into the lungs. From the lungs it returns through the pulmonary veins to the left atrium of the heart and is pumped from there through the left ventricle into the aorta and from the aorta into the other arteries.

**circulatory** /ˌsɜːkjʊˈleɪt(ə)ri/ *adjective* referring to the circulation of the blood

**circulatory system** /ˌsɜːkjʊˈleɪt(ə)ri ˌsɪstəm/ *noun* a system of arteries and veins, together with the heart, which makes the blood circulate around the body

**circum-** /sɜːkəm/ *prefix* around

**circumcise** /ˈsɜːkəmsaɪz/ *verb* to remove the foreskin of the penis

**circumcision** /ˌsɜːkəmˈsɪʒ(ə)n/ *noun* the surgical removal of the foreskin of the penis

**circumduction** /ˌsɜːkəmˈdʌkʃən/ noun the action of moving a limb so that the end of it makes a circular motion

**circumflex** /ˈsɜːkəmfleks/ adjective bent or curved

**circumflex artery** /ˈsɜːkəmfleks ˌɑːtəri/ noun a branch of the femoral artery in the upper thigh

**circumflex nerve** /ˈsɜːkəmfleks nɜːv/ noun a sensory and motor nerve in the upper arm

**circumoral** /ˌsɜːkəmˈɔːrəl/ adjective referring to rashes surrounding the lips

**circumvallate papillae** /sɜːkəmˌvæleɪt pəˈpɪliː/ plural noun large papillae at the base of the tongue, which have taste buds

**cirrhosis** /səˈrəʊsɪs/ noun a progressive disease of the liver, often associated with alcoholism, in which healthy cells are replaced by scar tissue □ **cirrhosis of the liver** hepatocirrhosis, a condition where some cells of the liver die and are replaced by hard fibrous tissue

COMMENT: Cirrhosis can have many causes: the commonest cause is alcoholism (alcoholic cirrhosis or Laennec's cirrhosis). It can also be caused by heart disease (cardiac cirrhosis), by viral hepatitis (postnecrotic cirrhosis), by autoimmune disease (primary biliary cirrhosis) or by obstruction or infection of the bile ducts (biliary cirrhosis).

**cirrhotic** /sɪˈrɒtɪk/ adjective referring to cirrhosis ○ The patient had a cirrhotic liver.

**cirs-** /sɜːs/ prefix referring to dilation

**cirsoid** /ˈsɜːsɔɪd/ adjective referring to a varicose vein which is dilated

**cirsoid aneurysm** /ˌsɜːsɔɪd ˈænjərɪz(ə)m/ noun a condition in which arteries become swollen and twisted

**cisplatin** /sɪsˈpleɪtɪn/ noun a chemical substance which may help fight cancer by binding to DNA. It is used in the treatment of ovarian and testicular cancer.

**cistern** /ˈsɪstən/, **cisterna** /sɪˈstɜːnə/ noun a space containing fluid

**cisterna magna** /sɪˌstɜːnə ˈmæɡnə/ noun a large space containing cerebrospinal fluid, situated underneath the cerebellum and behind the medulla oblongata

**citric acid** /ˌsɪtrɪk ˈæsɪd/ noun an acid found in fruit such as oranges, lemons and grapefruit

**citric acid cycle** /ˌsɪtrɪk ˈæsɪd ˌsaɪk(ə)l/ noun an important series of events concerning amino acid metabolism, which takes place in the mitochondria in the cell. Also called **Krebs cycle**

**citrullinaemia** /ˌsɪtrʊlɪˈniːmiə/ noun a deficiency of an enzyme which helps break down proteins

**citrulline** /ˈsɪtrʊliːn, ˈsɪtrʊlaɪn/ noun an amino acid

**CJD** abbr Creutzfeldt-Jakob disease

**cl** abbr centilitre

**clamp** /klæmp/ noun a surgical instrument to hold something tightly, e.g. a blood vessel during an operation ■ verb to hold something tightly

**clap** /klæp/ noun same as **gonorrhoea** (slang)

**classic** /ˈklæsɪk/ adjective referring to a typically well-known symptom ○ She showed classic heroin withdrawal symptoms: sweating, fever, sleeplessness and anxiety.

**classification** /ˌklæsɪfɪˈkeɪʃ(ə)n/ noun the work of putting references or components into order so as to be able to refer to them again and identify them easily ○ the ABO classification of blood

**classify** /ˈklæsɪfaɪ/ verb to put references or components into order so as to be able to refer to them again and identify them easily ○ The medical records are classified under the surname of the patient. ○ Blood groups are classified according to the ABO system.

**claudication** /ˌklɔːdɪˈkeɪʃ(ə)n/ noun the fact of limping or being lame

COMMENT: At first, the person limps after having walked a short distance, then finds walking progressively more difficult and finally impossible. The condition improves after rest.

**claustrophobia** /ˌklɔːstrəˈfəʊbiə/ noun a fear of enclosed spaces or crowded rooms. Compare **agoraphobia**

**claustrophobic** /ˌklɔːstrəˈfəʊbɪk/ adjective afraid of being in enclosed spaces or crowded rooms. Compare **agoraphobic**

**clavicle** /ˈklævɪk(ə)l/ noun same as **collarbone**

**clavicular** /kləˈvɪkjʊlə/ adjective referring to the clavicle

**clavus** /ˈkleɪvəs/ noun 1. a corn on the foot 2. severe pain in the head, like a nail being driven in

**claw foot** /ˌklɔː ˈfʊt/ noun a deformed foot with the toes curved towards the instep and with a very high arch. Also called **pes cavus**

**claw hand** /ˌklɔː ˈhænd/ noun a deformed hand with the fingers, especially the ring finger and little finger, bent towards the palm, caused by paralysis of the muscles

**clean** /kliːn/ adjective 1. free from dirt, waste products or unwanted substances 2. sterile or free from infection ○ a clean dressing ○ a clean wound 3. not using recreational drugs

**cleanliness** /ˈklenlinəs/ noun the state of being clean ○ The report praised the cleanliness of the hospital kitchen.

**clear** /klɪə/ adjective 1. easily understood ○ The doctor made it clear that he wanted the patient to have a home help. ○ The words on the medicine bottle are not very clear. 2. not cloudy and easy to see through ○ a clear glass bottle ○ The urine sample was clear. 3. □ **clear of** free from ○ The area is now clear of infection. ■ verb to take away a blockage ○ The inhalant will clear your blocked nose. ○ He is on *antibiotics to try to clear the congestion in his lungs.*

**clear up** /ˌklɪər ˈʌp/ *verb* to get better ○ *His infection should clear up within a few days.* ○ *I hope your cold clears up before the holiday.*

**cleavage** /ˈkliːvɪdʒ/ *noun* the repeated division of cells in an embryo

**cleavage lines** *plural noun* same as **Langer's lines**

**cleft** /kleft/ *noun* a small opening or hollow place in a surface or body part ■ *adjective* referring to a surface or body part which has separated into two or more sections

**cleft foot** /ˌkleft ˈfʊt/ *noun* same as **talipes**

**cleft lip** /ˌkleft ˈlɪp/ *noun* a congenital condition in which the upper lip fails to form in the usual way during fetal development. Also called **harelip**

**cleft palate** /ˌkleft ˈpælət/ *noun* a congenital condition in which the palate does not fuse during fetal development, causing a gap between the mouth and nasal cavity in severe cases

COMMENT: A cleft palate is usually associated with a cleft lip. Both can be successfully corrected by surgery.

**cleido-** /klaɪdəʊ/ *prefix* referring to the clavicle

**cleidocranial dysostosis** /ˌklaɪdəʊkreɪniəl ˌdɪsɒsˈtəʊsɪs/ *noun* a hereditary bone malformation, with protruding jaw, lack of collarbone and malformed teeth

**clerking** /ˈklɑːkɪŋ/ *noun* the practice of writing down the details of a person on admission to a hospital (*informal*)

**client** /ˈklaɪənt/ *noun* a person visited by a health visitor or social worker

**climacteric** /klaɪˈmæktərɪk/ *noun* 1. same as **menopause** 2. a period of diminished sexual activity in a man who reaches middle age

**climax** /ˈklaɪmæks/ *noun* 1. an orgasm 2. the point where a disease is at its worst ■ *verb* to have an orgasm

**clindamycin** /ˌklɪndəˈmaɪsɪn/ *noun* a powerful antibiotic used to treat severe infections and acne

**clinic** /ˈklɪnɪk/ *noun* 1. a small hospital or a department in a large hospital which deals only with out-patients or which specialises in the treatment of particular medical conditions ○ *He is being treated in a private clinic.* ○ *She was referred to an antenatal clinic.* 2. a group of students under a doctor or surgeon who examine patients and discuss their treatment

**clinical** /ˈklɪnɪk(ə)l/ *adjective* 1. referring to the physical assessment and treatment of patients by doctors, as opposed to a surgical operation, a laboratory test or experiment 2. referring to instruction given to students at the bedside of patients as opposed to class instruction with no patient present 3. referring to a clinic

'…we studied 69 patients who met the clinical and laboratory criteria of definite MS' [*Lancet*]

'…the allocation of students to clinical areas is for their educational needs and not for service requirements' [*Nursing Times*]

**clinical audit** /ˌklɪnɪk(ə)l ˈɔːdɪt/ *noun* an evaluation of the standard of clinical care

**clinical care** /ˌklɪnɪk(ə)l ˈkeə/ *noun* the care and treatment of patients in hospital wards or in doctors' surgeries

**clinical effectiveness** /ˌklɪnɪk(ə)l ɪˈfektɪvnəs/ *noun* the ability of a procedure or treatment to achieve the desired result

**clinical governance** /ˌklɪnɪk(ə)l ˈgʌv(ə)nəns/ *noun* the responsibility given to doctors to coordinate audit, research, education, use of guidelines and risk management to develop a strategy to raise the quality of medical care

**clinically** /ˈklɪnɪkli/ *adverb* using information gathered from the treatment of patients in a hospital ward or in the doctor's surgery ○ *Smallpox is now clinically extinct.*

**clinical medicine** /ˌklɪnɪk(ə)l ˈmed(ə)s(ə)n/ *noun* the study and treatment of patients in a hospital ward or in the doctor's surgery, as opposed to in the operating theatre or laboratory

**clinical nurse manager** /ˌklɪnɪk(ə)l ˈnɜːs ˌmænɪdʒə/ *noun* the administrative manager of the clinical nursing staff of a hospital

**clinical nurse specialist** /ˌklɪnɪk(ə)l nɜːs ˈspeʃ(ə)lɪst/ *noun* a nurse who specialises in a particular branch of clinical care

**clinical pathology** /ˌklɪnɪk(ə)l pəˈθɒlədʒi/ *noun* the study of disease as applied to the treatment of patients

**clinical psychologist** /ˌklɪnɪk(ə)l saɪˈkɒlədʒɪst/ *noun* a psychologist who studies and treats sick patients in hospital

**clinical thermometer** /ˌklɪnɪk(ə)l θəˈmɒmɪtə/ *noun* a thermometer used in a hospital or by a doctor for measuring a person's body temperature

**clinical trial** /ˌklɪnɪk(ə)l ˈtraɪəl/ *noun* a trial carried out in a medical laboratory on a person or on tissue from a person

**clinician** /klɪˈnɪʃ(ə)n/ *noun* a doctor, usually not a surgeon, who has considerable experience in treating patients

**clinodactyly** /ˌklaɪnəʊˈdæktɪli/ *noun* the permanent bending of a finger to one side

**clip** /klɪp/ *noun* a piece of metal with a spring, used to attach things together

**clitoris** /ˈklɪtərɪs/ *noun* a small erectile female sex organ, situated at the anterior angle of the vulva, which can be excited by sexual activity. See illustration at UROGENITAL SYSTEM (FEMALE) in Supplement

**cloaca** /kləʊˈeɪkə/ *noun* the end part of the hindgut in an embryo

**clomipramine** /kləʊˈmɪprəmiːn/ *noun* a drug used to treat depression, phobias and obsessive-compulsive disorder

**clonazepam** /kləʊˈnæzɪpæm/ *noun* a drug used to treat epilepsy

**clone** /kləʊn/ *noun* a group of cells derived from a single cell by asexual reproduction and so identical to the first cell ■ *verb* to reproduce an individual organism by asexual means

**clonic** /ˈklɒnɪk/ *adjective* 1. referring to clonus 2. having spasmodic contractions

**clonic spasms** /ˌklɒnɪk ˈspæz(ə)mz/ *plural noun* spasms which recur regularly

**clonidine** /ˈklɒnɪdiːn/ *noun* a drug which relaxes and widens the arteries, used in the treatment of hypertension, migraine headaches and heart failure

**cloning** /ˈkləʊnɪŋ/ *noun* the reproduction of an individual organism by asexual means

**clonorchiasis** /ˌkləʊnəˈkaɪəsɪs/ *noun* a liver condition, common in the Far East, caused by the fluke *Clonorchis sinensis*

**clonus** /ˈkləʊnəs/ *noun* the rhythmic contraction and relaxation of a muscle, usually a sign of upper motor neurone lesions

**close** /kləʊz/ *verb* 1. to become covered with new tissue as part of the healing process 2. to fix together the sides of a wound after surgery to allow healing to take place

**closed fracture** /ˌkləʊzd ˈfræktʃə/ *noun* same as **simple fracture**

**Clostridium** /klɒˈstrɪdiəm/ *noun* a type of bacteria

COMMENT: Species of Clostridium cause botulism, tetanus and gas gangrene.

**clot** /klɒt/ *noun* a soft mass of coagulated blood in a vein or an artery ○ *The doctor diagnosed a blood clot in the brain.* ○ *Blood clots occur in thrombosis.* ■ *verb* to change from a liquid to a semi-solid state, or to cause a liquid to do this ○ *His blood does not clot easily.* (NOTE: **clotting – clotted**)

**clotrimazole** /klɒˈtrɪməzəʊl/ *noun* a drug used to treat yeast and fungal infections

**clotting** /ˈklɒtɪŋ/ *noun* the action of coagulating

**clotting factors** /ˌklɒtɪŋ ˈfæktəz/ *plural noun* substances in plasma, called Factor I, Factor II, and so on, which act one after the other to make the blood coagulate when a blood vessel is damaged

COMMENT: Deficiency in one or more of the clotting factors results in haemophilia.

**clotting time** /ˈklɒtɪŋ taɪm/ *noun* the time taken for blood to coagulate under usual conditions. Also called **coagulation time**

**cloud** /klaʊd/ *noun* the disturbed sediment in a liquid

**cloudy** /ˈklaʊdi/ *adjective* referring to liquid which is not transparent but which has an opaque substance in it

**clubbing** /ˈklʌbɪŋ/ *noun* a thickening of the ends of the fingers and toes, a sign of many different diseases

**club foot** /ˌklʌb ˈfʊt/ *noun* same as **talipes**

**cluster** /ˈklʌstə/ *noun* 1. a group of small items which cling together 2. a significant subset in a statistical sample, e.g. of numbers of people affected by a particular disease or condition

**cluster headache** /ˈklʌstə ˌhedeɪk/ *noun* a headache which occurs behind one eye for a short period

**Clutton's joint** /ˈklʌt(ə)nz ˌdʒɔɪnt/ *noun* a swollen knee joint occurring in congenital syphilis [Described 1886. After Henry Hugh Clutton (1850–1909), surgeon at St Thomas's Hospital, London, UK.]

**cm** *abbr* centimetre

**CMHN** *abbr* community mental health nurse

**CM joint** /ˌsiː ˈem dʒɔɪnt/ *plural noun* same as **carpometacarpal joint**

**CMO** *abbr* Chief Medical Officer

**CMV** *abbr* cytomegalovirus

**C/N** *abbr* charge nurse

**CNS** *abbr* central nervous system

**COAD** *abbr* chronic obstructive airways disease

**coagulant** /kəʊˈægjʊlənt/ *noun* a substance which can make blood clot

**coagulase** /kəʊˈægjʊleɪz/ *noun* an enzyme produced by a staphylococcal bacteria which makes blood plasma clot

**coagulate** /kəʊˈægjʊleɪt/ *verb* to change from liquid to semi-solid, or cause a liquid to do this ○ *His blood does not coagulate easily.* ◊ **clot**

COMMENT: Blood coagulates when fibrinogen, a protein in the blood, converts into fibrin under the influence of the enzyme thrombokinase.

**coagulation** /kəʊˌægjʊˈleɪʃ(ə)n/ *noun* the action of clotting

**coagulation time** /kəʊægjuˈleɪʃ(ə)n taɪm/ *noun* same as **clotting time**

**coagulum** /kəʊˈægjʊləm/ *noun* same as **blood clot** (NOTE: The plural is **coagula**.)

**coalesce** /ˌkəʊəˈles/ *verb* to combine, or to cause things to combine, into a single body or group

**coalescence** /ˌkəʊəˈles(ə)ns/ *noun* the process by which wound edges come together when healing

**coarctation** /ˌkəʊɑːkˈteɪʃ(ə)n/ *noun* the process of narrowing □ **coarctation of the aorta** congenital narrowing of the aorta, which results in high blood pressure in the upper part of the body and low blood pressure in the lower part

**coarse tremor** /ˌkɔːs ˈtremə/ *noun* severe trembling

**coat** /kəʊt/ *noun* a layer of material covering an organ or a cavity ■ *verb* to cover something with something else

**coated tongue** /ˌkəʊtɪd ˈtʌŋ/ *noun* same as **furred tongue**

**coating** /ˈkəʊtɪŋ/ *noun* a thin covering ○ *a pill with a sugar coating*

**cobalt** /ˈkəʊbɔːlt/ *noun* a metallic element (NOTE: The chemical symbol is **Co**.)

**cobalt 60** /ˌkəʊbɔːlt ˈsɪksti/ *noun* a radioactive isotope which is used in radiotherapy to treat cancer

**cocaine** /kəʊˈkeɪn/ *noun* a narcotic drug not generally used in medicine because its use leads to addiction, but sometimes used as a surface anaesthetic

**cocci** /ˈkɒki/ *plural of* **coccus**

**coccidioidomycosis** /kɒkˌsɪdiɔɪˌdəʊmaɪˈkəʊsɪs/ *noun* a lung disease, caused by inhaling spores of the fungus *Coccidioides immitis*

**coccus** /ˈkɒkəs/ *noun* a bacterium shaped like a ball (NOTE: The plural is **cocci**.)

COMMENT: Cocci grow together in groups: either in clusters (staphylococci) or in long chains (streptococci).

**coccy-** /kɒksi/ *prefix* referring to the coccyx

**coccydynia** /ˌkɒksiˈdɪniə/ *noun* a sharp pain in the coccyx, usually caused by a blow. Also called **coccygodynia**

**coccygeal vertebrae** /kɒkˌsɪdʒiəl ˈvɜːtɪˌbreɪ/ *plural noun* the fused bones in the coccyx

**coccyges** /kɒkˈsaɪdʒiːz/ *plural of* **coccyx**

**coccygodynia** /ˌkɒksɪgəʊˈdɪniə/ *noun* same as **coccydynia**

**coccyx** /ˈkɒksɪks/ *noun* the lowest bone in the backbone (NOTE: The plural is **coccyges**.)

COMMENT: The coccyx is a rudimentary tail made of four bones which have fused together into a bone in the shape of a triangle.

**cochlea** /ˈkɒkliə/ *noun* a spiral tube inside the inner ear, which is the essential organ of hearing. See illustration at EAR in Supplement (NOTE: The plural is **cochleae**.)

COMMENT: Sounds are transmitted as vibrations to the cochlea from the ossicles through the oval window. The lymph fluid in the cochlea passes the vibrations to the organ of Corti which in turn is connected to the auditory nerve.

**cochlear** /ˈkɒkliə/ *adjective* referring to the cochlea

**cochlear duct** /ˈkɒkliə dʌkt/ *noun* a spiral channel in the cochlea

**cochlear implant** /ˌkɒkliə ˈɪmplɑːnt/ *noun* a type of hearing aid for profound hearing loss

**cochlear nerve** /ˈkɒkliə nɜːv/ *noun* a division of the auditory nerve

**Cochrane database** /ˌkɒkrən ˈdeɪtəbeɪs/ *noun* a database of regular reviews carried out on research

**code** /kəʊd/ *noun* **1.** a system of numbers, letters or symbols used to represent language or information **2.** same as **genetic code** ■ *verb* **1.** to convert instructions or data into another form **2.** (*of a codon or gene*) to provide the genetic information which causes a specific amino acid to be produced ○ *Genes are sections of DNA that code for a specific protein sequence.*

**codeine** /ˈkəʊdiːn/, **codeine phosphate** /ˌkəʊdiːn ˈfɒsfeɪt/ *noun* a common painkilling drug that can also be used to suppress coughing and in the treatment of diarrhoea

**code of conduct** /ˌkəʊd əv ˈkɒndʌkt/ *noun* a set of general rules showing how a group of people such as doctors or nurses should work

**cod liver oil** /ˌkɒd lɪvər ˈɔɪl/ *noun* a fish oil which is rich in calories and vitamins A and D

**-coele** /siːl/ *suffix* referring to a hollow (NOTE: The US spelling is usually **-cele**.)

**coeli-** /siːli/ *prefix* same as **coelio-** (*used before vowels*) (NOTE: The US spelling is usually **celi-**.)

**coeliac** /ˈsiːliæk/ *adjective* referring to the abdomen

**coeliac artery** /ˌsiːliæk ˈɑːtəri/, **coeliac axis** /ˌsiːliæk ˈæksɪs/ *noun* the main artery in the abdomen leading from the abdominal aorta and dividing into the left gastric, hepatic and splenic arteries. Also called **coeliac trunk**

**coeliac disease** /ˌsiːliæk dɪˈziːz/ *noun* same as **gluten-induced enteropathy**

**coeliac ganglion** /ˌsiːliæk ˈɡæŋgliən/ *noun* a ganglion on each side of the origins of the diaphragm, connected with the coeliac plexus

**coeliac plexus** /ˌsiːliæk ˈpleksəs/ *noun* a network of nerves in the abdomen, behind the stomach

**coeliac trunk** /ˌsiːliæk ˈtrʌŋk/ *noun* same as **coeliac artery**

**coelio-** /siːliəʊ/ *prefix* referring to a hollow, usually the abdomen (NOTE: The US spelling is usually **celio-**.)

**coelioscopy** /ˌsiːliˈɒskəpi/ *noun* an examination of the peritoneal cavity by inflating the abdomen with sterile air and passing an endoscope through the abdominal wall (NOTE: The plural is **coelioscopies**.)

**coelom** /ˈsiːləm/ *noun* a body cavity in an embryo, which divides to form the thorax and abdomen (NOTE: The plural is **coeloms** or **coelomata**.)

**coffee ground vomit** /ˈkɒfi ɡraʊnd ˌvɒmɪt/ *noun* vomit containing dark pieces of blood, indicating that the person is bleeding from the stomach or upper intestine

**cognition** /kɒɡˈnɪʃ(ə)n/ *noun* the mental action or process of gaining knowledge by using your mind or your senses, or knowledge gained in this way

**cognitive** /ˈkɒɡnɪtɪv/ *adjective* referring to the mental processes of perception, memory, judgment and reasoning ○ *a cognitive impairment*

**cognitive disorder** /ˌkɒgnɪtɪv dɪsˈɔːdə/ *noun* impairment of any of the mental processes of perception, memory, judgment and reasoning

**cognitive therapy** /ˌkɒgnɪtɪv ˈθerəpi/ *noun* a treatment of psychiatric disorders such as anxiety or depression which encourages people to deal with their negative ways of thinking

**cohort** /ˈkəʊhɔːt/ *noun* a group of people sharing a particular characteristic such as age or gender who are studied in a scientific or medical investigation

**cohort study** /ˈkəʊhɔːt ˌstʌdi/ *noun* an investigation in which a group of people are classified according to their exposure to various risks and studied over a period of time to see if they develop a specific disease, in order to evaluate the links between risk and disease

**coil** /kɔɪl/ *noun* a former name for an intrauterine contraceptive device

**coinfection** /ˌkəʊɪnˈfekʃ(ə)n/ *noun* infection with two or more diseases or viruses at the same time

**coital** /ˈkəʊɪt(ə)l/ *adjective* referring to sexual intercourse

**coitus** /ˈkəʊɪtəs/, **coition** /kəʊˈɪʃ(ə)n/ *noun* same as **sexual intercourse**

**coitus interruptus** /ˌkəʊɪtəs ɪntəˈrʌptəs/ *noun* removal of the penis from the vagina before ejaculation, sometimes used as a method of contraception although it is not very efficient

**cold** /kəʊld/ *adjective* not warm or hot ■ *noun* an illness, with inflammation of the nasal passages, in which someone sneezes and coughs and has a blocked and running nose ○ *She had a heavy cold.* Also called **common cold, coryza**

COMMENT: A cold usually starts with a virus infection which causes inflammation of the mucous membrane in the nose and throat. Symptoms include running nose, cough and loss of taste and smell. Coronaviruses have been identified in people with colds, but there is no cure for a cold at present.

**cold burn** /ˈkəʊld bɜːn/ *noun* an injury to the skin caused by exposure to extreme cold or by touching a very cold surface

**cold cautery** /kəʊld ˈkɔːtəri/ *noun* the removal of a skin growth using carbon dioxide snow

**cold compress** /kəʊld ˈkɒmpres/ *noun* a wad of cloth soaked in cold water, used to relieve a headache or bruise

**cold pack** /ˈkəʊld pæk/ *noun* a cloth or a pad filled with gel or clay which is chilled and put on the body to reduce or increase the temperature

**cold sore** /ˈkəʊld sɔː/ *noun* a painful blister, usually on the lips or nose, caused by herpes simplex Type I

**colectomy** /kəˈlektəmi/ *noun* a surgical operation to remove the whole or part of the colon (NOTE: The plural is **colectomies**.)

**colic** /ˈkɒlɪk/ *noun* **1.** pain in any part of the intestinal tract. Also called **enteralgia, tormina 2.** crying and irritability in babies, especially from stomach pains

COMMENT: Although colic can refer to pain caused by indigestion, it can also be caused by stones in the gall bladder or kidney.

**colicky** /ˈkɒlɪki/ *adjective* referring to colic ○ *She had colicky pains in her abdomen.*

**coliform bacterium** /ˌkəʊlifɔːm bækˈtɪəriəm/ *plural noun* any bacterium which is similar to *Escherichia coli*

**colistin** /kɒˈlɪstɪn/ *noun* an antibiotic which is effective against a wide range of organisms and is used to treat gastrointestinal infections

**colitis** /kəˈlaɪtɪs/ *noun* inflammation of the colon. Also called **colonitis**

**collagen** /ˈkɒlədʒən/ *noun* a thick protein fibre forming bundles, which make up the connective tissue, bone and cartilage

**collagen disease** /ˈkɒlədʒən dɪˌziːz/ *noun* any disease of the connective tissue

COMMENT: Collagen diseases include rheumatic fever, rheumatoid arthritis, periarteritis nodosa, scleroderma and dermatomyositis.

**collagenous** /kəˈlædʒɪnəs/ *adjective* **1.** containing collagen **2.** referring to collagen disease

**collapse** /kəˈlæps/ *noun* **1.** a condition in which someone is extremely exhausted or semi-conscious ○ *She was found in a state of collapse.* **2.** a condition in which an organ becomes flat or loses air ○ *lung collapse* ■ *verb* **1.** to fall down in a semi-conscious state ○ *After running to catch his train he collapsed.* **2.** to become flat, or lose air

**collapsed lung** /kəˈlæpsd lʌŋ/ *noun* same as **pneumothorax**

**collarbone** /ˈkɒləbəʊn/ *noun* one of two long thin bones which join the shoulder blades to the breastbone. Also called **clavicle** (NOTE: Collarbone fracture is one of the most frequent fractures in the body.)

**collateral** /kəˈlæt(ə)rəl/ *adjective* secondary or less important

'...embolisation of the coeliac axis is an effective treatment for severe bleeding in the stomach or duodenum, localized by endoscopic examination. A good collateral blood supply makes occlusion of a single branch of the coeliac axis safe.' [*British Medical Journal*]

**collateral circulation** /kəˌlæt(ə)rəl ˌsɜːkjʊ ˈleɪʃ(ə)n/ *noun* an enlargement of some secondary blood vessels as a response when the main vessels become slowly blocked

**collection chamber** /kəˈlekʃən ˌtʃeɪmbə/ *noun* a section of the heart where blood collects before being pumped out

**Colles' fracture** /ˈkɒlɪs(ɪz) ˌfræktʃə/ *noun* a fracture of the lower end of the radius with displacement of the wrist backwards, usually when someone has stretched out a hand to try to break a fall [After Abraham Colles (1773–1843), Irish surgeon]

**colliculus** /kə'lıkjʊləs/ noun one of four small projections (**superior colliculi** and **inferior colliculi**) in the midbrain. See illustration at BRAIN in Supplement (NOTE: The plural is **colliculi**.)

**collodion** /kə'ləʊdiən/ noun a liquid used for painting on a clean wound, where it dries to form a flexible covering

**colloid** /'kɒlɔɪd/ noun **1.** a mass of tiny particles of one substance dispersed in another substance **2.** the particles which are suspended in a colloid **3.** a thick jelly-like substance which stores hormones, produced in the thyroid gland ■ adjective relating to or resembling a colloid ○ colloid acne

**collyrium** /kə'lıriəm/ noun a solution used to bathe the eyes (NOTE: The plural is **collyria**.)

**colo-** /kɒləʊ/ prefix referring to the colon

**coloboma** /,kɒləʊ'bəʊmə/ noun a condition in which part of the eye, especially part of the iris, is missing

**colon** /'kəʊlɒn/ noun the main part of the large intestine, running from the caecum at the end of the small intestine to the rectum

COMMENT: The colon is about 1.35 metres in length, and rises from the end of the small intestine up the right side of the body, then crosses beneath the stomach and drops down the left side of the body to end as the rectum. In the colon, water is extracted from the waste material which has passed through the small intestine, leaving only the faeces which are pushed forward by peristaltic movements and passed out of the body through the rectum.

**colonic** /kə'lɒnık/ adjective referring to the colon

**colonic irrigation** /kə,lɒnık ırı'geıʃ(ə)n/ noun the washing out of the contents of the large intestine using a tube inserted in the anus

**colonitis** /,kɒlə'naıtıs/ noun same as **colitis**

**colonoscope** /kə'lɒnəskəʊp/ noun a surgical instrument for examining the interior of the colon

**colonoscopy** /,kɒlə'nɒskəpi/ noun an examination of the inside of the colon, using a colonoscope passed through the rectum (NOTE: The plural is **colonoscopies**.)

**colony** /'kɒləni/ noun a group or culture of microorganisms

**colorectal** /,kəʊləʊ'rekt(ə)l/ adjective referring to both the colon and rectum

**colostomy** /kə'lɒstəmi/ noun a surgical operation to make an opening between the colon and the abdominal wall to allow faeces to be passed out without going through the rectum (NOTE: The plural is **colostomies**.)

COMMENT: A colostomy is carried out when the colon or rectum is blocked, or where part of the colon or rectum has had to be removed.

**colostomy bag** /kə'lɒstəmi bæg/ noun a bag attached to the opening made by a colostomy, to collect faeces as they are passed out of the body

**colostrum** /kə'lɒstrəm/ noun a fluid rich in antibodies and low in fat, secreted by the mother's breasts at the birth of a baby, before the true milk starts to flow

**colour blindness** /'kʌlə ,blaındnəs/ noun a condition of being unable to tell the difference between specific colours

COMMENT: Colour blindness is a condition which almost never occurs in women. The commonest form is the inability to tell the difference between red and green. The Ishihara test is used to test for colour blindness.

**colour index** /'kʌlər ,ındeks/ noun the ratio between the amount of haemoglobin and the number of red blood cells in a specific amount of blood

**colouring** /'kʌlərıŋ ,mætə/, **colouring matter** noun a substance which colours an organ

**colp-** /kɒlp/ prefix same as **colpo-** (used before vowels)

**colpitis** /kɒl'paıtıs/ noun same as **vaginitis**

**colpo-** /kɒlpəʊ/ prefix referring to the vagina

**colpocele** /'kɒlpəsiːl/ noun same as **colpoptosis**

**colpocystitis** /,kɒlpəʊsı'staıtıs/ noun inflammation of both the vagina and the urinary bladder

**colpocystopexy** /,kɒlpə'sıstəpeksi/ noun a surgical operation to lift and stitch the vagina and bladder to the abdominal wall (NOTE: The plural is **colpocystopexies**.)

**colpohysterectomy** /,kɒlpəʊhıstə'rektəmi/ noun a surgical operation in which the womb is removed through the vagina (NOTE: The plural is **colpohysterectomies**.)

**colpopexy** /'kɒlpəpeksi/ noun a surgical operation to fix a prolapsed vagina to the abdominal wall (NOTE: The plural is **colpopexies**.)

**colpoplasty** /'kɒlpəplæsti/ noun a surgical operation to repair a damaged vagina (NOTE: The plural is **colpoplasties**.)

**colpoptosis** /,kɒlpə'təʊsıs/ noun a prolapse of the walls of the vagina. Also called **colpocele** (NOTE: The plural is **colpoptoses**.)

**colporrhaphy** /kɒl'pɒrəfi/ noun a surgical operation to stitch a prolapsed vagina (NOTE: The plural is **colporrhaphies**.)

**colposcope** /'kɒlpəskəʊp/ noun a surgical instrument used to examine the inside of the vagina. Also called **vaginoscope**

**colposcopy** /kɒl'pɒskəpi/ noun an examination of the inside of the vagina (NOTE: The plural is **colposcopies**.)

**colposuspension** /,kɒlpəʊsə'spenʃən/ noun a surgical operation to strengthen the pelvic floor muscles to prevent incontinence

**colpotomy** /kɒlˈpɒtəmi/ *noun* a surgical operation to make a cut in the vagina (NOTE: The plural is **colpotomies**.)

**column** /ˈkɒləm/ *noun* ♦ **vertebral column**

**columnar** /kəˈlʌmnə/ *adjective* shaped like a column

**columnar cell** /kəˈlʌmnə sel/ *noun* a type of epithelial cell shaped like a column

**coma** /ˈkəʊmə/ *noun* a state of unconsciousness from which a person cannot be awakened by external stimuli

COMMENT: A coma can have many causes: head injuries, diabetes, stroke or drug overdose. A coma is often fatal, but a patient may continue to live in a coma for a long time, even several months, before dying or regaining consciousness.

**comatose** /ˈkəʊmətəʊs/ *adjective* **1.** unconscious or in a coma **2.** like a coma

**combined therapy** /kəmˌbaɪnd ˈθerəpi/ *noun* the use of two or more treatments at the same time

**comedo** /ˈkɒmɪdəʊ/ *noun* a small point of dark, hard matter in a sebaceous follicle, often found associated with acne on the skin of adolescents (NOTE: The plural is **comedones**.)

**come down with** /ˌkʌm ˈdaʊn wɪθ/ *verb* to catch a cold, flu or other minor illness (*informal*)

**come out in** /ˌkʌm ˈaʊt ɪn/ *verb* to have something such as spots or a rash appear on the skin (*informal*)

**come round** /ˌkʌm ˈraʊnd/ *verb* to regain consciousness, e.g. after being knocked out

**comfort** /ˈkʌmfət/ *verb* to help make someone less anxious or unhappy, especially when something bad has just happened

**comfortable** /ˈkʌmf(ə)təb(ə)l/ *adjective* in a stable physical condition

**comforter** /ˈkʌmfətə/ *noun* **1.** someone who helps to make another person less anxious or unhappy **2.** a baby's dummy

**commando operation** /kəˈmɑːndəʊ ˌɒpəreɪʃ(ə)n/, **commando procedure** /kəˈmɑːndəʊ prəˌsiːdʒə/ *noun* a major operation to combat cancer of the face and neck. It involves the removal of facial features, which are later rebuilt.

**commensal** /kəˈmens(ə)l/ *noun* an animal or plant which lives on another animal or plant but does not harm it in any way. Both may benefit from the association. ○ *Candida is a commensal in the mouths of 50% of healthy adults.* (NOTE: If a commensal causes harm, it is a **parasite**.) ■ *adjective* living on another animal or plant

**comminuted fracture** /ˌkɒmɪnjuːtɪd ˈfræktʃə/ *noun* a fracture where the bone is broken in several places

**Commission for Health Improvement** in the UK, the independent inspection body for the National Health Service, with the role of helping to raise standards of patient care. It aims to identify where improvement is required and share good practice. Abbr **CHI**

**commissure** /ˈkɒmɪsjʊə/ *noun* a structure which joins two similar tissues, e.g. a group of nerves which crosses from one part of the central nervous system to another. ◊ **corpus callosum, grey commissure, white commissure**

**commit** /kəˈmɪt/ *verb* to arrange legally for someone to enter a mental health facility, perhaps without the person's consent

**commitment** /kəˈmɪtmənt/ *noun* an act of legally making someone enter a mental health facility

**Committee on Safety of Medicines** /kə ˌmɪti ɒn ˌseɪfti əv ˈmed(ə)sɪnz/ *noun* the official body which advises the British Government on the safety and quality of medicines

**commode** /kəˈməʊd/ *noun* a special chair with a removable basin used as a toilet by people with limited mobility

**common** /ˈkɒmən/ *adjective* **1.** frequently occurring **2.** shared □ **(in) common** belonging to more than one thing or person ○ *These viral diseases have several symptoms in common.*

**common bile duct** /ˌkɒmən ˈbaɪl dʌkt/ *noun* a duct leading to the duodenum, formed of the hepatic and cystic ducts

**common carotid artery** /ˌkɒmən kəˈrɒtɪd ˌɑːtəri/ *noun* the main artery running up each side of the lower part of the neck. Also called **carotid**

**common cold** /ˌkɒmən ˈkəʊld/ *noun* same as **cold**

**common hepatic duct** /ˌkɒmən hɪˈpætɪk dʌkt/ *noun* a duct from the liver formed when the right and left hepatic ducts join

**common iliac artery** /ˌkɒmən ˈɪliæk ˌɑːtəri/ *noun* one of two arteries which branch from the aorta in the abdomen and in turn divide into the internal iliac artery, leading to the pelvis, and the external iliac artery, leading to the leg

**common iliac vein** /ˌkɒmən ˈɪliæk veɪn/ *noun* one of the veins draining the legs, pelvis and abdomen, which unite to form the inferior vena cava

**common salt** /ˌkɒmən ˈsɔːlt/ *noun* a white powder used to make food, especially meat, fish and vegetables, taste better. Also called **sodium chloride**

COMMENT: Too much salt in the diet is to be avoided, as it is implicated in hypertension. Persistent diarrhoea or vomiting can lead to a dangerous loss of salt from the body.

**common wart** /ˌkɒmən ˈwɔːt/ *noun* a wart which appears mainly on the hands

**communicable disease** /kə ˌmjuːnɪkəb(ə)l dɪˈziːz/ *noun* a disease which can be passed from one person to another or from an animal to a person. ◊ **contagious disease, infectious disease**

**communicating artery** /kə'mjuːnɪkeɪtɪŋ ˌɑːtəri/ *noun* one of the arteries which connect the blood supply from each side of the brain, forming part of the circle of Willis

**community** /kə'mjuːnɪti/ *noun* a group of people who live and work in a district ○ *The health services serve the local community.*

**community care** /kəˌmjuːnɪti 'keə/ *noun* the providing of help to people such as those who are elderly or mentally ill in order to allow them to stay in their own homes, rather than requiring them to be cared for in hospitals or care homes

**community health** /kəˌmjuːnɪti 'helθ/ *noun* the health of a local community, or provision of services for a local community

**community health council** /kəˌmjuːnɪti 'helθ ˌkaʊnsəl/ *noun* a statutory body of interested people from outside the medical professions charged with putting forward the patients' point of view on local health issues. Abbr **CHC**

**community hospital** /kə'mjuːnɪti ˌhɒspɪt(ə)l/ *noun* a hospital serving a local community

**community medicine** /kə'mjuːnɪti 'med(ə)s(ə)n/ *noun* the study of medical practice which examines groups of people and the health of the community, including housing, pollution and other environmental factors

**community mental health nurse** /kəˌmjuːnɪti ˌment(ə)l 'helθ ˌnɜːs/ *noun* a specialist nurse who works in a particular district visiting people in the area with mental health problems. Abbr **CMHN**

**community midwife** /kəˌmjuːnɪti 'mɪdwaɪf/ *noun* a midwife who works in a community as part of a primary health care team

**community nurse** /kəˌmjuːnɪti 'nɜːs/ *noun* a nurse who treats people in a local community

**community psychiatric nurse** /kəˌmjuːnɪti ˌsaɪki'ætrɪk/ *noun* . Also called **community mental health nurse**. Abbr **CPN**

**community services** /kəˌmjuːnɪti 'sɜːvɪsɪz/ *plural noun* nursing services which are available to the community

**community trust** /kəˌmjuːnɪti 'trʌst/ *noun* an independent non-profit-making body set up to represent an area of public concern

**compact bone** /ˌkɒmpækt 'bəʊn/ *noun* a type of bone tissue which forms the hard outer layer of a bone. See illustration at **BONE STRUCTURE** in Supplement

**compatibility** /kəmˌpætɪ'bɪlɪti/ *noun* **1.** the ability of two drugs not to interfere with each other when administered together **2.** the ability of a body to accept organs, tissue or blood from another person and not to reject them

**compatible** /kəm'pætɪb(ə)l/ *adjective* able to function together without being rejected ○ *The surgeons are trying to find a compatible*

donor or *a donor with a compatible blood group.*

**compensate** /'kɒmpənseɪt/ *verb* **1.** to give someone an amount of money or something else to pay for loss or damage **2.** (*of an organ*) to make good the failure of an organ by making another organ, or the undamaged parts of the same organ, function at a higher level ○ *The heart has to beat more strongly to compensate for the narrowing of the arteries.* **3.** to emphasise a particular ability or personality characteristic in order to make the lack of another one seem less bad

**compensation** /ˌkɒmpən'seɪʃ(ə)n/ *noun* **1.** something which makes something else seem less bad or less serious **2.** an amount of money or something else given to pay for loss or damage ○ *The drugs caused him to develop breathing problems, so he thinks he's entitled to medical compensation.* **3.** the act of giving money to pay for loss or damage ○ *compensation for loss of a limb* **4.** a situation where the body helps to correct a problem in a particular organ by making another organ, or the undamaged parts of the same organ, function at a higher level **5.** behaviour that emphasises a particular ability or personality characteristic in order to make the lack of another one seem less bad

**competence** /'kɒmpɪt(ə)ns/ *noun* the ability to do something well, measured against a standard, especially ability which you get through experience or training ○ *encouraging the development of professional competence in the delivery of care to patients*

**complaint** /kəm'pleɪnt/ *noun* **1.** an expression of dissatisfaction about something or someone ○ *The hospital administrator wouldn't listen to the complaints of the consultants.* **2.** an illness ○ *a chest complaint* ○ *a nervous complaint*

**complement** *noun* /'kɒmplɪmənt/ a substance which forms part of blood plasma and is essential to the work of antibodies and antigens ■ *verb* /'kɒmplɪment/ to complete something by providing useful or pleasing qualities which it does not itself have

**complementary** /ˌkɒmplɪ'ment(ə)ri/ *adjective* **1.** combining with or adding to something else ○ *Ultrasound and CT provide complementary information.* **2.** used in or using complementary medicine ○ *complementary therapies* **3.** referring to genes which are necessary to each other and produce their effect only when they are present together

**complementary medicine** /ˌkɒmplɪment(ə)ri 'med(ə)sɪn/ *noun* alternative medicine in the forms which are now accepted by practitioners of conventional Western medicine, e.g. acupuncture and osteopathy

**complement fixation test** /ˌkɒmplɪˌment fɪk'seɪʃ(ə)n test/ *noun* a test to measure the amount of complement in antibodies and antigens. Abbr **CFT**

**complete abortion** /kəm,pliːt ə'bɔːʃ(ə)n/ *noun* an abortion where the whole contents of the uterus are expelled

**complete blood count** /kəm,pliːt 'blʌd kaʊnt/ *noun* a test to find the exact numbers of each type of blood cell in a sample of blood. Abbr **CBC**

**complex** /'kɒmpleks/ *noun* **1.** (*in psychiatry*) a group of ideas which are based on the experience a person has had in the past and which influence the way he or she behaves **2.** a group of items, buildings or organs ○ *He works in the new laboratory complex.* **3.** a group of signs and symptoms due to a particular cause. ◊ **syndrome ■** *adjective* complicated ○ *A gastrointestinal fistula can cause many complex problems, including fluid depletion.*

**complexion** /kəm'plekʃən/ *noun* the general colour of the skin on the face ○ *People with fair complexions burn easily in the sun.*

**compliance** /kəm'plaɪəns/ *noun* the agreement of a patient to co-operate with a treatment

**complicated fracture** /,kɒmplɪkeɪtɪd 'fræktʃə/ *noun* a fracture with an associated injury of tissue, as when a bone has punctured an artery

**complication** /,kɒmplɪ'keɪʃ(ə)n/ *noun* **1.** a condition in which two or more conditions exist in someone, whether or not they are connected ○ *He was admitted to hospital suffering from pneumonia with complications.* **2.** a situation in which someone develops a second condition which changes the course of treatment for the first ○ *She appeared to be improving, but complications set in and she died in a few hours.*

'…sickle cell chest syndrome is a common complication of sickle cell disease, presenting with chest pain, fever and leucocytosis' [*British Medical Journal*]

'…venous air embolism is a potentially fatal complication of percutaneous venous catheterization' [*Southern Medical Journal*]

**compos mentis** /,kɒmpɒs 'mentɪs/ *adjective* not affected by a mental disorder (NOTE: The phrase is from Latin and means 'of sound mind'.)

**compound** /'kɒmpaʊnd/ *noun* a chemical substance made up of two or more components **■** *adjective* made up of two or more components

**compound fracture** /,kɒmpaʊnd 'fræktʃə/ *noun* a fracture where the skin surface is damaged or where the broken bone penetrates the surface of the skin. Also called **open fracture**

**compress** *noun* /'kɒmpres/ a wad of cloth soaked in hot or cold liquid and applied to the skin to relieve pain or swelling, or to force pus out of an infected wound **■** *verb* /kəm'pres/ to squeeze or press something

**compressed air sickness** /kəm,prest 'eə ,sɪknəs/ *noun* same as **caisson disease**

**compression** /kəm'preʃ(ə)n/ *noun* **1.** the act of squeezing or pressing ○ *The first-aider applied compression to the chest of the casualty.* **2.** a serious condition in which the brain is compressed by blood or cerebrospinal fluid accumulating in it or by a fractured skull

**compression stocking** /kəm,preʃ(ə)n 'stɒkɪŋ/ *noun* a strong elastic stocking worn to support a weak joint in the knee or to hold varicose veins tightly

**compression syndrome** /kəm'preʃ(ə)n ,sɪndrəʊm/ *noun* pain in muscles after strenuous exercise

**compulsion** /kəm'pʌlʃən/ *noun* **1.** an act of forcing someone to do something, or the fact of being forced to do something ○ *You are under no compulsion to treat a violent patient.* **2.** a strong psychological force which makes someone do something, often unwillingly ○ *She felt a sudden compulsion to wash her hands again.*

**compulsive** /kəm'pʌlsɪv/ *adjective* referring to a feeling which cannot be stopped ○ *She has a compulsive desire to steal.*

**compulsive eating** /kəm,pʌlsɪv 'iːtɪŋ/ *noun* a psychological condition in which someone has a continual desire to eat. ◊ **bulimia**

**compulsive–obsessive disorder** /kəm ,pʌlsɪv əb'sesɪv dɪs,ɔːdə/ *noun* same as **obsessive–compulsive disorder**

**compulsory admission** /kəm,pʌlsəri əd 'mɪʃ(ə)n/ *noun* the process of admitting someone who is mentally ill to hospital for treatment whether or not they consent

**computed tomography** /kəm,pjuːtɪd tə 'mɒɡrəfi/ *noun* same as **computerised axial tomography**. Abbr **CT**

**computerised axial tomography** /kəm ,pjuːtəraɪzd ,æksiəl tə'mɒɡrəfi/ *noun* a system of examining the body in which a narrow X-ray beam, guided by a computer, photographs a thin section of the body or of an organ from several angles, using the computer to build up an image of the section. Abbr **CAT**. Also called **computed tomography**

**-conazole** /kɒnəzəʊl/ *suffix* used in the names of antifungal drugs ○ *fluconazole*

**concave** /'kɒnkeɪv/ *adjective* curving towards the inside ○ *a concave lens*

**conceive** /kən'siːv/ *verb* **1.** (*of a woman*) to become pregnant with a child. ♦ **conception 2.** □ **to be conceived** (*of a child*) to come into existence through the fertilisation of an ovum ○ *Our son was conceived during our holiday in Italy.*

**concentrate** /'kɒnsəntreɪt/ *noun* a solution from which water has been removed **■** *verb* **1.**

to give full attention to something **2.** □ **to concentrate on** to examine something in particular **3.** to reduce a solution and increase its strength by evaporation

**concept** /'kɒnsept/ *noun* a thought or idea, or something which someone might be able to imagine

**conception** /kən'sepʃən/ *noun* the point at which a woman becomes pregnant and the development of a baby starts

COMMENT: Conception is usually taken to be either the moment when the sperm cell fertilises the ovum, or a few days later, when the fertilised ovum attaches itself to the wall of the uterus.

**conceptual framework** /kən,septʃuəl 'freɪmwɜːk/ *noun* the theoretical basis on which something is formed

**conceptus** /kən'septəs/ *noun* an embryo or fetus together with all the tissues that surround it during pregnancy (NOTE: The plural is **conceptuses.**)

**concha** /'kɒŋkə/ *noun* a part of the body shaped like a shell (NOTE: The plural is **conchae.**)

**concha auriculae** /,kɒŋkə ɔː'rɪkjuliː/ *noun* the depressed part of the outer ear that leads to the inner ear

**concordance** /kən'kɔːd(ə)ns/ *noun* **1.** a state in which two or more things are in the correct or expected relationship to each other. For example, the atrioventricular concordance is the relationship between the atria and the ventricles in the heart. **2.** the fact of two related people sharing the same genetic characteristic ○ *the concordance of schizophrenia in identical twins* **3.** an agreement between a professional and a patient on a course of treatment, especially related to use of medicines

**concretion** /kən'kriːʃ(ə)n/ *noun* a mass of hard material which forms in the body, e.g. a gallstone or deposits on bone in arthritis

**concussed** /kən'kʌst/ *adjective* referring to someone who has been hit on the head and has lost and then regained consciousness ○ *He was walking around in a concussed state.*

**concussion** /kən'kʌʃ(ə)n/ *noun* **1.** the act of applying force to any part of the body **2.** loss of consciousness for a short period, caused by a blow to the head

**concussive** /kən'kʌsɪv/ *adjective* causing concussion

**condensed** /kən'denst/ *adjective* made compact or more dense

**condition** /kən'dɪʃ(ə)n/ *noun* **1.** the particular state of someone or something ○ *in poor condition* ○ *Her condition is getting worse.* ○ *The conditions in the hospital are very good.* **2.** a particular illness, injury or disorder ○ *He is being treated for a heart condition.*

**conditioned reflex** /kən,dɪʃ(ə)nd 'riːfleks/ *noun* an automatic reaction by a person to a stimulus, or an expected reaction to a stimulus which comes from past experience

**conditioned response** /kən,dɪʃ(ə)nd rɪ 'spɒns/ *noun* a response to a stimulus as a result of associating it with an earlier stimulus

COMMENT: The classic example of a conditioned response is Pavlov's experiment with dogs in which they produced saliva, ready to eat their food, when a bell rang, because on previous occasions they had been fed when the bell was rung.

**condom** /'kɒndɒm/ *noun* a rubber sheath worn on the penis during intercourse as a contraceptive and also as a protection against sexually transmitted disease

**conducting system** /kən'dʌktɪŋ ,sɪstəm/ *noun* the nerve system in the heart which links an atrium to a ventricle, so that the two beat at the same rate

**conduction** /kən'dʌkʃən/ *noun* the process of passing heat, sound or nervous impulses from one part of the body to another

**conduction fibre** /kən'dʌkʃən ,faɪbə/ *noun* a fibre which transmits impulses, e.g. in the bundle of His

**conductive** /kən'dʌktɪv/ *adjective* referring to conduction

**conductive deafness** /kən,dʌktɪv 'defnəs/, **conductive hearing loss** /kən,dʌktɪv 'hɪərɪŋ lɒs/ *noun* deafness caused by inadequate conduction of sound into the inner ear

**conductor** /kən'dʌktə/ *noun* **1.** a substance or object which allows heat, electricity, light or sound to pass along it or through it **2.** a tube with a groove in it along which a knife is slid to cut open a sinus

**condyle** /'kɒndaɪl/ *noun* a rounded end of a bone which articulates with another

**condyloid process** /'kɒndɪlɔɪd ,prəʊses/ *noun* a projecting part at each end of the lower jaw which forms the head of the jaw, joining the jaw to the skull

**condyloma** /,kɒndɪ'ləʊmə/ *noun* a growth usually found on the vulva (NOTE: The plural is **condylomas** or **condylomata.**)

**cone** /kəʊn/ *noun* **1.** a shape with a circular base or top and a part that tapers to a point, or an object with this shape **2.** one of two types of cell in the retina of the eye which is sensitive to light, used especially in the perception of bright light and colour. ◊ **rod** ■ *verb* to show a rapid change for the worse in neurological condition due to herniation of the midbrain through the foramen magnum in the skull, caused by raised pressure inside the brain (NOTE: **cones – coning – coned**)

**cone biopsy** /'kəʊn baɪ,ɒpsi/ *noun* the removing of a cone of tissue from the cervix for examination

**confabulation** /kən,fæbjʊ'leɪʃ(ə)n/ *noun* the act of making up plausible stories to cover up loss of memory

**confidentiality** /ˌkɒnfɪdenʃiˈælɪti/ *noun* an obligation not to reveal professional information about a person or organisation

**confined** /kənˈfaɪnd/ *adjective* kept in a place ○ *She was confined to bed with pneumonia.* ○ *Since his accident he has been confined to a wheelchair.*

**confinement** /kənˈfaɪnmənt/ *noun* the period when a woman giving birth stays in hospital, from the beginning of labour until some time after the birth of her baby. This period is very short nowadays.

**confounding factor** /kənˈfaʊndɪŋ ˌfæktə/ *noun* a factor which has an association with both a disease and a risk factor and thus complicates the nature of the relationship between them

**confused** /kənˈfjuːzd/ *adjective* unable to think clearly or act rationally ○ *Many severely confused patients do not respond to spoken communication.*

**confusion** /kənˈfjuːʒ(ə)n/ *noun* the state of being confused

**congeal** /kənˈdʒiːl/ *verb* (*of fat or blood*) to become solid

**congenita** /kənˈdʒenɪtə/ ♦ **amyotonia congenita**

**congenital** /kənˈdʒenɪt(ə)l/ *adjective* existing at or before birth

**congenital aneurysm** /kənˌdʒenɪt(ə)l ˈænjərɪz(ə)m/ *noun* a weakening of the arteries at the base of the brain, present at birth

**congenital anomaly** /kənˌdʒenɪt(ə)l əˈnɒməli/ *noun* a medical condition arising during development of the fetus and present at birth. Also called **congenital defect**

COMMENT: A congenital condition is not always inherited from a parent through the genes, as it may be due to factors such as a disease which the mother had during pregnancy, e.g. German measles, or a drug which she has taken.

**congenital cataract** /kənˌdʒenɪt(ə)l ˈkætərækt/ *noun* a cataract which is present at birth

**congenital defect** /kənˌdʒenɪt(ə)l ˈdiːfekt/ *noun* same as **congenital anomaly** (NOTE: The word 'defect' is now avoided.)

**congenital dislocation of the hip** /kən ˌdʒenɪt(ə)l dɪsləˌkeɪʃ(ə)n əv ðə ˈhɪp/ *noun* a condition in which a person is born with weak ligaments in the hip, so that the femur does not stay in the pelvis

**congenital heart disease** /kənˌdʒenɪt(ə)l ˈhɑːt dɪˌziːz/, **congenital heart defect** /kən ˌdʒenɪt(ə)l ˈhɑːt ˌdiːfekt/ *noun* a heart condition existing at birth

**congenital hyperthyroidism** *noun* a disease caused by a malfunction of the thyroid before birth or in early life

**congenitally** /kənˈdʒenɪtli/ *adverb* at or before birth ○ *The baby is congenitally incapable of absorbing gluten.*

**congenital malformation** /kənˌdʒenɪt(ə)l ˌmælfɔːˈmeɪʃ(ə)n/ *noun* a malformation which is present at birth, e.g. a cleft palate

**congenital syphilis** /kənˌdʒenɪt(ə)l ˈsɪfɪlɪs/ *noun* syphilis which is passed on from a mother to her unborn child

**congenital toxoplasmosis** /kənˌdʒenɪt(ə)l ˌtɒksəʊplæzˈməʊsɪs/ *noun* a condition in which a baby has been infected with toxoplasmosis by its mother while still in the uterus

**congested** /kənˈdʒestɪd/ *adjective* with blood or fluid inside □ **congested face** a red face, caused by blood rushing to the face

**congestion** /kənˈdʒestʃən/ *noun* an accumulation of blood in an organ. ◊ **nasal congestion**

**congestive** /kənˈdʒestɪv/ *adjective* referring to congestion

**congestive heart failure** /kənˌdʒestɪv ˈhɑːt ˌfeɪljə/ *noun* a condition in which the heart is unable to pump away the blood returning to it fast enough, causing congestion in the veins

**coni** /ˈkəʊni/ plural of **conus**

**conisation** /ˌkɒnaɪˈzeɪʃ(ə)n/, **conization** *noun* the surgical removal of a cone-shaped piece of tissue

**conjoined twins** /kənˌdʒɔɪnd ˈtwɪnz/ *plural noun* twins who are joined together at birth. Also called **Siamese twins**

COMMENT: Conjoined twins are always identical and can be joined at the head, chest or hip. In some cases they can be separated by surgery, but this is not possible if they share a single important organ such as the heart.

**conjugate** /ˈkɒndʒʊgət/, **conjugate diameter** /ˌkɒndʒʊgət daɪˈæmɪtə/ *noun* a measurement of space in a woman's pelvis, used to calculate if it is large enough for a child to be delivered

**conjunctiva** /ˌkɒndʒʌŋkˈtaɪvə/ *noun* a membrane which covers the front of the eyeball and the inside of the eyelids. See illustration at EYE in Supplement (NOTE: The plural is **conjunctivas** or **conjunctivae**.)

**conjunctival** /ˌkɒndʒʌŋkˈtaɪv(ə)l/ *adjective* referring to the conjunctiva

**conjunctivitis** /kənˌdʒʌŋktɪˈvaɪtɪs/ *noun* inflammation of the conjunctiva from a range of causes

**connective tissue** /kəˌnektɪv ˈtɪʃuː/ *noun* tissue which forms the main part of bones and cartilage, ligaments and tendons, in which a large proportion of fibrous material surrounds the tissue cells

**Conn's syndrome** /ˈkɒnz ˌsɪndrəʊm/ *noun* a condition in which excessive production of the hormone aldosterone causes fluid retention and high blood pressure

**consanguinity** /ˌkɒnsæŋˈgwɪnɪti/ *noun* a blood relationship between people

**conscious** /ˈkɒnʃəs/ *adjective* **1.** awake and aware of what is happening ○ *He became conscious in the recovery room two hours after the operation.* **2.** deliberate and intended ○ *a conscious choice*

**-conscious** /kɒnʃəs/ *suffix* giving importance to ○ *health-conscious* ○ *safety-conscious*

**consciously** /ˈkɒnʃəsli/ *adverb* in a deliberate and knowing way

**consciousness** /ˈkɒnʃəsnəs/ *noun* the state of being mentally alert and knowing what is happening □ **to lose consciousness** to become unconscious □ **to regain consciousness** to become conscious after being unconscious

**consensus management** /kənˈsensəs ˌmænɪdʒmənt/ *noun* a form of management which aims to get everyone to agree on what actions should be taken

**consent** /kənˈsent/ *noun* agreement to allow someone to do something ○ *The parents gave their consent for their son's heart to be used in the transplant operation.*

**consent form** /kənˈsent fɔːm/ *noun* a form which a patient signs to show that he or she agrees to have a particular operation

**conservative** /kənˈsɜːvətɪv/ *adjective* **1.** reluctant to accept new things **2.** (*of a treatment*) designed to help relieve symptoms or preserve health with a minimum of medical intervention or risk ○ *Symptoms usually resolve with conservative treatment.*

**consolidation** /kənˌsɒlɪˈdeɪʃ(ə)n/ *noun* **1.** a stage in mending a broken bone in which the callus formed at the break changes into bone **2.** a condition in which part of the lung becomes solid, e.g. in pneumonia

**constipated** /ˈkɒnstɪpeɪtɪd/ *adjective* unable to pass faeces often enough

**constipation** /ˌkɒnstɪˈpeɪʃ(ə)n/ *noun* difficulty in passing faeces

COMMENT: Constipated bowel movements are hard and may cause pain in the anus. Constipation may be caused by worry or by a diet which does not contain enough roughage or by lack of exercise, as well as by more serious diseases of the intestine.

**constituent** /kənˈstɪtjuənt/ *noun* a substance which forms part of something ○ *the chemical constituents of nerve cells*

**constitution** /ˌkɒnstɪˈtjuːʃ(ə)n/ *noun* the general health and strength of a person ○ *She has a strong constitution* or *a healthy constitution.* ○ *He has a weak constitution and is often ill.*

**constitutional** /ˌkɒnstɪˈtjuːʃ(ə)nəl/ *adjective* referring to a person's constitution ■ *noun* a short walk taken for health reasons

**constitutionally** /ˌkɒnstɪˈtjuːʃ(ə)n(ə)li/ *adverb* because of a person's constitution

**constrict** /kənˈstrɪkt/ *verb* **1.** to make a passage narrower ○ *a constricted bowel* **2.** to slow down or stop the flow of something such as blood

**constriction** /kənˈstrɪkʃən/ *noun* the process of becoming narrow, or the state of being narrow. ◊ **stenosis**

**constrictive** /kənˈstrɪktɪv/ *adjective* restricting

**constrictive pericarditis** /kənˌstrɪktɪv perɪkɑːˈdaɪtɪs/ *noun* same as **chronic pericarditis**

**constrictor** /kənˈstrɪktə/ *noun* a muscle which squeezes an organ or which makes an organ contract

**consult** /kənˈsʌlt/ *verb* to ask someone for his or her opinion ○ *He consulted an eye specialist.*

**consultancy** /kənˈsʌltənsi/ *noun* the post of consultant ○ *She was appointed to a consultancy at a London hospital.*

**consultant** /kənˈsʌltənt/ *noun* a doctor who is a senior specialist in a particular branch of medicine and who is consulted by GPs ○ *She was referred to a consultant at the orthopaedic hospital.*

**consultation** /ˌkɒnsəlˈteɪʃ(ə)n/ *noun* **1.** a discussion between two doctors about a case **2.** a meeting between a doctor and a patient, in which the doctor may examine the patient, discuss his or her condition and prescribe treatment

**consulting room** /kənˈsʌltɪŋ ruːm/ *noun* a room where a doctor sees his or her patients

**consumption** /kənˈsʌmpʃən/ *noun* **1.** the act of taking food or liquid into the body ○ *the patient's increased consumption of alcohol* **2.** a former name for pulmonary tuberculosis

**contact** /ˈkɒntækt/ *noun* **1.** an act of touching someone or something, or the state of touching □ **to have (physical) contact with someone** *or* **something** to actually touch someone or something □ **to be in** *or* **come into contact with someone** to be near to or touching someone ○ *The hospital is anxious to trace anyone who may have come into contact with the patient.* **2.** an act of getting in touch or communicating with someone **3.** a person who has been in contact with a person suffering from an infectious disease ○ *Now that Lassa fever has been diagnosed, the authorities are anxious to trace all contacts which the patient may have met.* ■ *verb* to meet or get in touch with someone

**contact dermatitis** /ˌkɒntækt ˌdɜːmə ˈtaɪtɪs/ *noun* inflammation of the skin caused by touch, e.g. by touching some types of plant, soap or chemical. Also called **irritant dermatitis**

**contact lens** /ˈkɒntækt lenz/ *noun* a tiny plastic lens which fits over the eyeball and is worn instead of spectacles to improve eyesight

**contact tracing** /ˈkɒntækt ˌtreɪsɪŋ/ *noun* the process of tracing people with whom someone with an infectious disease has been in contact

**contagion** /kənˈteɪdʒən/ *noun* **1.** the process of spreading a disease by touching an infected person or objects which an infected person has touched **2.** a disease spread by touch ○ *The contagion spread through the whole school.*

**contagious** /kənˈteɪdʒəs/ *adjective* able to be transmitted by touching an infected person or objects which an infected person has touched □ **contagious stage** the period when a disease such as chickenpox is contagious and can be transmitted to someone else

**contagious disease** /kənˌteɪdʒəs dɪˈziːz/ *noun* a disease which can be transmitted by touching an infected person or objects which an infected person has touched. ◊ **communicable disease, infectious disease**

**containment** /kənˈteɪnmənt/ *noun* **1.** action taken to restrict the spread of something undesirable or dangerous such as a disease ○ *government policy of containment of the SARS virus* **2.** the eradication of a global disease such as smallpox by removing it region by region

**contaminant** /kənˈtæmɪnənt/ *noun* a substance which contaminates something

**contaminate** /kənˈtæmɪneɪt/ *verb* **1.** to make something impure by touching it or by adding something to it ○ *Supplies of drinking water were contaminated by refuse from the factories.* ○ *The whole group of tourists fell ill after eating contaminated food.* **2.** to spread infection to someone or something

**contamination** /kənˌtæmɪˈneɪʃ(ə)n/ *noun* the action of contaminating something, or the state of being contaminated ○ *The contamination resulted from polluted water.*

**continence** /ˈkɒntɪnəns/ *noun* **1.** the ability to control the discharge of urine and faeces **2.** self-restraint

**continent** /ˈkɒntɪnənt/ *adjective* able to exercise control over the discharge of urine and faeces

**continuing education** /kənˌtɪnjuɪŋ edjʊ ˈkeɪʃ(ə)n/ *noun* regular courses or training designed to bring professional people up to date with the latest developments in their particular field

**continuous ambulatory peritoneal dialysis** /kənˌtɪnjuəs ˌæmbjʊlət(ə)ri perɪtəˌniːəl daɪˈæləsɪs/ *noun* a method of dialysis of people while they are walking about. Abbr **CAPD**

**continuous positive airways pressure** /kənˌtɪnjuəs ˌpɒzɪtɪv ˈeəweɪz ˌpreʃə/ *noun* a method used in intensive care which forces air into the lungs of someone with lung collapse. Abbr **CPAP**

**contra-** /kɒntrə/ *prefix* against, opposite, contrasting

**contraception** /ˌkɒntrəˈsepʃən/ *noun* the prevention of pregnancy, e.g. by using devices such as a condom or an IUD, or drugs in the form of contraceptive pills or injections at regular intervals. Also called **birth control**

**contraceptive** /ˌkɒntrəˈseptɪv/ *adjective* preventing conception ○ *a contraceptive device* or *drug* ■ *noun* a drug or device which prevents pregnancy

**contraceptive sheath** /ˌkɒntrəˈseptɪv ʃiːθ/ *noun* same as **condom**

**contraceptive sponge** /ˌkɒntrəˈseptɪv spʌndʒ/ *noun* a piece of synthetic sponge impregnated with spermicide, which is inserted into the vagina before intercourse

**contract** /kənˈtrækt/ *verb* **1.** to become smaller and tighter, or make a muscle or part of the body smaller and tighter ○ *As the muscle contracts the limb moves.* ○ *The diaphragm acts to contract the chest.* **2.** to catch a disease ○ *He contracted Lassa fever.* **3.** to make a formal or legally binding agreement with someone to do something ○ *An outside firm is contracted to do the hospital cleaning.* ■ *noun* a formal or legally binding agreement

**contractibility** /ˈkɒntræktɪbɪlɪti/ *noun* the capacity to contract

**contractile tissue** /kənˌtræktaɪl ˈtɪʃuː/ *noun* the tissue in muscle which makes the muscle contract

**contraction** /kənˈtrækʃən/ *noun* **1.** the act of making something smaller or of becoming smaller ○ *the contraction of dental services* **2.** a tightening movement which makes a muscle shorter, which makes the pupil of the eye smaller or which makes the skin wrinkle **3.** a movement of the muscles of the uterus occurring during childbirth ○ *Her contractions began at one o'clock.*

**contracture** /kənˈtræktʃə/ *noun* a permanent tightening of a muscle caused by fibrosis

**contraindication** /ˌkɒntrəɪndɪˈkeɪʃ(ə)n/ *noun* something which suggests that someone should not be treated with a specific drug or not continue with a specific treatment because circumstances make that treatment unsuitable

**contralateral** /ˌkɒntrəˈlætərəl/ *adjective* located on or affecting the opposite side of the body. Opposite **ipsilateral**

**contrast medium** /ˈkɒntrɑːst ˌmiːdiəm/ *noun* a radio-opaque dye, or sometimes gas, put into an organ or part of the body so that it will show clearly in an X-ray photograph ○ *In an MRI scan no contrast medium is required; in a CAT scan iodine-based contrast media are often required.*

**contrecoup** /ˈkɒntrəkuː/ *noun* an injury to one point of an organ such as the brain, caused by a blow received on an opposite point of the organ

**control** *verb* **1.** to have the ability or authority to direct someone or something ○ *Sometimes* *we need help to control people who think they have waited too long.* **2.** to limit or restrain something ○ *administered drugs to control the pain* ■ *noun* **1.** the ability or authority to control something ○ *After her stroke she had no control over her left arm.* ○ *The administrators are in control of the admissions policy.* **2.** a person or group whose test data are used as a comparison in a study **3.** a comparison in a study

**control group** /kən'trəʊl gruːp/ *noun* a group of people who are not being treated but whose test data are used as a comparison in a study

**controlled drug** /kən,trəʊld 'drʌg/ *noun* a drug which is not freely available, which is restricted by law and classified as A, B, or C and of which possession may be an offence. Also called **controlled substance**

**controlled respiration** /kən,trəʊld ,respə'reɪʃ(ə)n/ *noun* the control of a person's breathing by an anaesthetist during an operation, when regular breathing has stopped

**controlled substance** /kən,trəʊld 'sʌbstəns/ *noun* same as **controlled drug**

**controlled trial** /kən,trəʊld 'traɪəl/ *noun* a trial in which members of one group are treated with a test substance and those of another group are treated with a placebo as a control

**controls assurance** /kən'trəʊlz ə,ʃʊərəns/ *noun* a process designed to provide evidence that NHS organisations are doing their best to manage themselves both in order to meet their objectives and to protect patients, staff and the public against risks of all kinds

**contused wound** /kən,tjuːzd 'wuːnd/ *noun* a wound caused by a blow where the skin is bruised as well as torn and bleeding

**contusion** /kən'tjuːʒ(ə)n/ *noun* same as **bruise**

**conus** /'kəʊnəs/ *noun* a structure shaped like a cone (NOTE: The plural is **coni**.)

**convalesce** /,kɒnvə'les/ *verb* to get back to good health gradually after an illness or operation

**convalescence** /,kɒnvə'les(ə)ns/ *noun* a period of time when someone is convalescing

**convalescent** /,kɒnvə'les(ə)nt/ *adjective* referring to convalescence ■ *noun* someone who is convalescing

**convalescent home** /,kɒnvə'les(ə)nt həʊm/ *noun* a type of hospital where people can recover from illness or surgery

**convergent strabismus** /kən,vɜːdʒənt strə'bɪzməs/, **convergent squint** /kən,vɜːdʒənt 'skwɪnt/ *noun* a condition in which one or both of a person's eyes look towards the nose. Also called **cross eye**

**conversion** /kən'vɜːʃ(ə)n/ *noun* the process of changing one thing into another ○ *the conversion of nutrients into tissue*

**convex** /'kɒnveks/ *adjective* curving towards the outside ○ *a convex lens*

**convoluted** /'kɒnvəluːtɪd/ *adjective* folded and twisted

**convoluted tubule** /,kɒnvəluːtɪd 'tjuːbjuːl/ *noun* a coiled part of a nephron

**convolution** /,kɒnvə'luːʃ(ə)n/ *noun* a twisted shape ○ *the convolutions of the surface of the cerebrum*

**convulse** /kən'vʌls/ *verb* to shake violently and uncontrollably

**convulsion** /kən'vʌlʃən/ *noun* the rapid involuntary contracting and relaxing of the muscles in several parts of the body ○ *The child had convulsions.* ◊ **fit** (NOTE: Often used in the plural.)

COMMENT: Convulsions in children may be caused by brain disease such as meningitis but can also often be found at the beginning of a disease such as pneumonia which is marked by a sudden rise in body temperature. In adults, convulsions are usually associated with epilepsy.

**convulsive** /kən'vʌlsɪv/ *adjective* referring to convulsions ○ *He had a convulsive seizure.* ◊ **electroconvulsive therapy**

**Cooley's anaemia** /'kuːliz ə,niːmiə/ *noun* same as **thalassaemia** [Described 1927. After Thomas Benton Cooley (1871–1945), Professor of Paediatrics at Wayne College of Medicine, Detroit, USA.]

**Coombs' test** /'kuːmz test/ *noun* a test for antibodies in red blood cells, used as a test for erythroblastosis fetalis and other haemolytic syndromes [Described 1945. After Robin Royston Amos Coombs (1921– ), Quick Professor of Biology, and Fellow of Corpus Christi College, Cambridge, UK.]

**coordinate** /kəʊ'ɔːdɪneɪt/ *verb* **1.** to make things work together ○ *He was unable to coordinate the movements of his arms and legs.* **2.** to organise a complex procedure

'…there are four recti muscles and two oblique muscles in each eye, which coordinate the movement of the eyes and enable them to work as a pair' [*Nursing Times*]

**coordination** /kəʊ,ɔːdɪ'neɪʃ(ə)n/ *noun* **1.** the combining of two or more things as an effective unit, or the way things combine effectively ○ *requires coordination between nursing staff and doctors* **2.** the ability to use two or more parts of the body at the same time to carry out a movement or task ○ *The patient showed lack of coordination between eyes and hands.*

'Alzheimer's disease is a progressive disorder which sees a gradual decline in intellectual functioning and deterioration of physical coordination' [*Nursing Times*]

**COPD** *abbr* chronic obstructive pulmonary disease

**coping mechanism** /'kəʊpɪŋ ,mekənɪz(ə)m/ *noun* a method of dealing with situations which cause psychological stress

**copper** /'kɒpə/ *noun* a metallic trace element (NOTE: The chemical symbol is **Cu**.)

**copr-** /kɒpr/ *prefix* faeces

**coprolith** /'kɒprəlɪθ/ *noun* a lump of hard faeces in the bowel

**coproporphyrin** /ˌkɒprə'pɔːfərɪn/ *noun* porphyrin excreted by the liver

**copulate** /'kɒpjʊleɪt/ *verb* to have sexual intercourse

**copulation** /ˌkɒpjʊ'leɪʃ(ə)n/ *noun* same as **sexual intercourse**

**cor** /kɔː/ *noun* the heart

**coraco-acromial** /ˌkɒrəkəʊ ə'krəʊmiəl/ *adjective* referring to the coracoid process and the acromion

**coracobrachialis** /ˌkɒrəkəʊbræki'eɪlɪs/ *noun* a muscle on the medial side of the upper arm, below the armpit

**coracoid process** /'kɒrəkɔɪd ˌprəʊses/ *noun* a projecting part on the shoulder blade

**cord** /kɔːd/ *noun* a long flexible structure in the body like a thread

**cordectomy** /kɔː'dektəmi/ *noun* a surgical operation to remove a vocal cord (NOTE: The plural is **cordectomies**.)

**cordon sanitaire** /ˌkɔːdɒn ˌsænɪ'teə/ *noun* a restriction of movement to and from an area to control the spread of a disease

**cordotomy** /kɔː'dɒtəmi/ *noun* another spelling of **chordotomy**

**corectopia** /ˌkɔːrek'təʊpiə/ *noun* ectopia of the pupil of the eye

**corium** /'kɔːriəm/ *noun* same as **dermis**

**corn** /kɔːn/ *noun* a hard painful lump of skin usually on a foot, where something such as a tight shoe has rubbed or pressed on the skin. Also called **heloma**

**cornea** /'kɔːniə/ *noun* a transparent part of the front of the eyeball. See illustration at EYE in Supplement (NOTE: The plural is **corneae**. For other terms referring to the cornea, see words beginning with **kerat-, kerato-**.)

**corneal** /'kɔːniəl/ *adjective* relating to a cornea

**corneal abrasion** /ˌkɔːniəl ə'breɪʒ(ə)n/ *noun* a scratch on the cornea, caused by something sharp getting into the eye

**corneal bank** /'kɔːniəl bæŋk/ *noun* a place where eyes of dead donors can be kept ready for use in corneal grafts

**corneal graft** /ˌkɔːniəl 'grɑːft/ *noun* **1.** a surgical operation to graft corneal tissue from a donor or from a dead person to replace diseased tissue. Also called **corneal transplant, keratoplasty 2.** a piece of corneal tissue used in a graft

**corneal reflex** /ˌkɔːniəl 'riːfleks/ *noun* a reflex from touching or hitting the cornea which makes the eyelid close

**corneal transplant** /'kɔːniəl ˌtrænsplɑːnt/ *noun* same as **corneal graft**

**cornification** /ˌkɔːnɪfɪ'keɪʃ(ə)n/ *noun* same as **keratinisation**

**cornu** /'kɔːnjuː/ *noun* **1.** a structure in the body which is shaped like a horn **2.** each of the four processes of the thyroid cartilage (NOTE: The plural is **cornua**.)

**corona** /kə'rəʊnə/ *noun* a structure in the body which is shaped like a crown

**corona capitis** /kəˌrəʊnə 'kæpɪtɪs/ *noun* the crown of the head or top part of the skull

**coronal** /'kɒrən(ə)l, kə'rəʊn(ə)l/ *adjective* **1.** referring to a corona **2.** referring to the crown of a tooth

**coronal plane** /ˌkɒrən(ə)l 'pleɪn/ *noun* a plane at right angles to the median plane, dividing the body into dorsal and ventral halves. See illustration at ANATOMICAL TERMS in Supplement

**coronal suture** /ˌkɒrən(ə)l 'suːtʃə/ *noun* a horizontal joint across the top of the skull between the parietal and frontal bones

**coronary** /'kɒrən(ə)ri/ *noun* same as **coronary thrombosis** (*informal*) ■ *adjective* referring to any structure shaped like a crown, but especially to the arteries which supply blood to the heart muscles

**coronary artery** /'kɒrən(ə)ri ˌɑːtəri/ *noun* one of the two arteries which supply blood to the heart muscles

**coronary artery bypass graft** /ˌkɒrən(ə)ri ˌɑːtəri 'baɪpɑːs grɑːft/, **coronary artery bypass** /ˌkɒrən(ə)ri 'ɑːtəri ˌbaɪpɑːs/ *noun* a surgical operation to treat angina by grafting pieces of vein around the diseased part of a coronary artery

**coronary care unit** /ˌkɒrən(ə)ri 'keə ˌjuːnɪt/ *noun* the section of a hospital caring for people who have heart disorders or who have had heart surgery. Abbr **CCU**

**coronary circulation** /ˌkɒrən(ə)ri ˌsɜːkjʊ'leɪʃ(ə)n/ *noun* blood circulation through the arteries and veins of the heart muscles

**coronary heart disease** /ˌkɒrən(ə)ri 'hɑːt dɪˌziːz/ *noun* any disease affecting the coronary arteries, which can lead to strain on the heart or a heart attack. Abbr **CHD**

'…coronary heart disease (CHD) patients spend an average of 11.9 days in hospital. Among primary health care services, 1.5% of all GP consultations are due to CHD.' [*Health Services Journal*]

'…apart from death, coronary heart disease causes considerable morbidity in the form of heart attack, angina and a number of related diseases' [*Health Education Journal*]

**coronary ligament** /ˌkɒrən(ə)ri 'lɪgəmənt/ *noun* folds of peritoneum connecting the back of the liver to the diaphragm

**coronary obstruction** /ˌkɒrən(ə)ri əb'strʌkʃ(ə)n/, **coronary occlusion** /ˌkɒrən(ə)ri ə'kluːʒ(ə)n/ *noun* a thickening of the walls of the coronary arteries or a blood clot in the coronary arteries which prevents blood from reaching the heart muscles and leads to heart failure

**coronary sinus** /ˌkɒrən(ə)ri ˈsaɪnəs/ *noun* a vein which takes most of the venous blood from the heart muscles to the right atrium

**coronary thrombosis** /ˌkɒrən(ə)ri θrɒm ˈbəʊsɪs/ *noun* a blood clot which blocks the coronary arteries, leading to a heart attack. Also called **coronary**

**coronary vein** /ˈkɒrən(ə)ri veɪn/ *noun* a vein that drains blood from the muscles of the heart

**coronavirus** /kəˈrəʊnəˌvaɪrəs/ *noun* a type of virus which has been identified in people who have the common cold

**coroner** /ˈkɒrənə/ *noun* a public official, either a doctor or a lawyer, who investigates sudden or violent deaths

COMMENT: Coroners investigate deaths which are caused by poison, violence, neglect or deprivation, deaths from unnatural causes, during the post-operative recovery period and when the doctor feels unable to give a reliable cause of death. They also investigate deaths of prisoners and deaths involving the police.

**coronoid process** /ˈkɒrənɔɪd ˌprəʊses/ *noun* **1.** a projecting piece of bone on the ulna **2.** a projecting piece on each side of the lower jaw

**corpora** plural of **corpus**

**corpse** /kɔːps/ *noun* the body of a dead person

**cor pulmonale** /ˌkɔː ˌpʌlməˈneɪli/ *noun* pulmonary heart disease in which the right ventricle is enlarged

**corpus** /ˈkɔːpəs/ *noun* any mass of tissue (NOTE: The plural is **corpora**.)

**corpus albicans** /ˌkɔːpəs ˈælbɪkænz/ *noun* scar tissue which replaces the corpus luteum in the ovary

**corpus callosum** /ˌkɔːpəs kəˈləʊsəm/ *noun* the thick band of nerve fibres that connects the two hemispheres of the brain and allows them to communicate. See illustration at BRAIN in Supplement (NOTE: The plural is **corpora callosa**.)

**corpus cavernosum** /ˌkɔːpəs ˌkævə ˈnəʊsəm/ *noun* a part of the erectile tissue in the penis and clitoris. See illustration at URO-GENITAL SYSTEM (MALE) in Supplement (NOTE: The plural is **corpora cavernosa**.)

**corpuscle** /ˈkɔːpʌs(ə)l/ *noun* **1.** a small round mass **2.** a cell in blood or lymph

**corpus haemorrhagicum** /ˌkɔːpəs ˌhemə ˈrædʒɪkəm/ *noun* a blood clot formed in an ovary where a Graafian follicle has ruptured (NOTE: The plural is **corpora haemorrhagica**.)

**corpus luteum** /ˌkɔːpəs ˈluːtiəm/ *noun* a body which forms in each ovary after a Graafian follicle has ruptured. The corpus luteum secretes the hormone progesterone to prepare

the uterus for implantation of the fertilised ovum. (NOTE: The plural is **corpora lutea**.)

**corpus spongiosum** /ˌkɔːpəs spʌnˈʒɪ ˈəʊsəm/ *noun* the part of the penis round the urethra, forming the glans. See illustration at UROGENITAL SYSTEM (MALE) in Supplement (NOTE: The plural is **corpora spongiosa**.)

**corpus striatum** /ˌkɔːpəs ˌstraɪˈeɪtəm/ *noun* a mass of nervous tissue in each cerebral hemisphere (NOTE: The plural is **corpora striata**.)

**corrective** /kəˈrektɪv/ *adjective* intended to correct an irregularity or problem ○ *corrective lenses* ■ *noun* a drug which changes the harmful effect of another drug

**Corrigan's pulse** /ˌkɒrɪgənz ˈpʌls/ *noun* a condition occurring in the arterial pulse in the neck in which there is a visible rise in pressure followed by a sudden collapse, caused by aortic regurgitation. Also called **water-hammer pulse**

**corrosive** /kəˈrəʊsɪv/ *adjective* destroying tissue ■ *noun* a substance which destroys tissue, e.g. acid or alkali

**corrugator muscle** /ˈkɒrəgeɪtə ˌmʌs(ə)l/ *noun* one of the muscles which produce vertical wrinkles on the forehead when someone frowns

**corset** /ˈkɔːsɪt/ *noun* a piece of stiff clothing worn on the chest or over the trunk to support the body, e.g. after a back injury

**cortex** /ˈkɔːteks/ *noun* the outer layer of an organ, as opposed to the soft inner medulla (NOTE: The plural is **cortices** or **cortexes**.)

**Corti** /ˈkɔːti/ ♦ organ of Corti

**cortical** /ˈkɔːtɪk(ə)l/ *adjective* referring to a cortex

**cortical mastoidectomy** /ˌkɔːtɪk(ə)l ˌmæstɔɪˈdektəmi/ *noun* same as **atticotomy**

**cortices** plural of **cortex**

**corticospinal** /ˌkɔːtɪkəʊˈspaɪn(ə)l/ *adjective* referring to both the cerebral cortex and the spinal cord

**corticosteroid** /ˌkɔːtɪkəʊˈstɪərɔɪd/ *noun* **1.** any steroid hormone produced by the cortex of the adrenal glands **2.** a drug which reduces inflammation, used in asthma, gastro-intestinal disease and in adrenocortical insufficiency

**corticosterone** /ˌkɔːtɪkəʊˈstɪərəʊn/ *noun* a hormone secreted by the cortex of the adrenal glands

**corticotrophin** /ˌkɔːtɪkəʊˈtrəʊfɪn/ *noun* same as **adrenocorticotrophic hormone** (NOTE: The US spelling is **corticotropin**.)

**cortisol** /ˈkɔːtɪsɒl/ *noun* same as **hydrocortisone**

**cortisone** /ˈkɔːtɪzəʊn/ *noun* a hormone secreted in small quantities by the adrenal cortex ○ *The doctor gave her a cortisone injection in the ankle.*

COMMENT: Synthetic cortisone was used in the treatment of rheumatoid arthritis, asthma and skin disorders, but it is now replaced by other drugs.

**Corynebacterium** /kəʊ,raɪnɪbæk'tɪəriəm/ *noun* a genus of bacteria which includes the bacterium which causes diphtheria

**coryza** /kə'raɪzə/ *noun* an illness, with inflammation of the nasal passages, in which someone sneezes and coughs and has a blocked and running nose (*technical*) Also called **cold, common cold**

**cosmetic surgery** /kɒz,metɪk 's3:dʒəri/ *noun* a surgical operation to improve a person's appearance

COMMENT: Whereas plastic surgery may be prescribed by a doctor to correct skin or bone conditions or the effect of burns or after a disfiguring operation, cosmetic surgery is carried out on the instructions of the patient to remove wrinkles, enlarge breasts or make some other perceived improvement.

**cost-** /kɒst/ *prefix* same as **costo-** (*used before vowels*)

**costal** /'kɒst(ə)l/ *adjective* referring to the ribs

**costal cartilage** /,kɒst(ə)l 'kɑːtəlɪdʒ/ *noun* cartilage which forms the end of each rib and either joins the rib to the breastbone or to the rib above

**costal pleura** /,kɒst(ə)l 'plʊərə/ *noun* a part of the pleura lining the walls of the chest

**costive** /'kɒstɪv/ *adjective* same as **constipated** ■ *noun* a drug which causes constipation

**costo-** /kɒstəʊ/ *prefix* referring to the ribs

**costocervical trunk** /,kɒstəʊs3:vɪk(ə)l 'trʌŋk/ *noun* a large artery in the chest

**costodiaphragmatic** /,kɒstəʊdaɪəfræg 'mætɪk/ *adjective* referring to both the ribs and the diaphragm

**costovertebral joint** /,kɒstəʊv3:tɪbr(ə)l 'dʒɔɪnt/ *noun* a joint between the ribs and the vertebral column

**cot death** /'kɒt deθ/ *noun* ♦ sudden infant death syndrome (NOTE: The US term is **crib death**.)

**co-trimoxazole** /kəʊ traɪ'mɒksəzəʊl/ *noun* a drug used to combat bacteria in the urinary tract

**cottage hospital** /,kɒtɪdʒ 'hɒspɪt(ə)l/ *noun* a small local hospital that admits patients under the care of a general practitioner

**cotton bud** /'kɒtən bʌd/ *noun* a little stick with some cotton wool usually at both ends, used for cleaning cavities

**cotton wool** /,kɒtən 'wʊl/ *noun* purified fibres from the cotton plant used to clean the skin or as padding ○ *She dabbed the cut with cotton wool soaked in antiseptic.* (NOTE: The US term is **absorbent cotton**.)

**cotyledon** /,kɒtɪ'liːd(ə)n/ *noun* one of the divisions of a placenta

**cotyloid cavity** /'kɒtɪlɔɪd ,kævɪti/ *noun* same as **acetabulum**

**couch** /kaʊtʃ/ *noun* a long bed on which a person lies when being examined by a doctor in a surgery

**couching** /'kaʊtʃɪŋ/ *noun* a surgical operation to displace the opaque lens of an eye as a treatment for cataracts

**cough** /kɒf/ *noun* a reflex action, caused by irritation in the throat, when the glottis is opened and air is sent out of the lungs suddenly □ **barking cough** a loud noisy dry cough □ **dry cough** a cough where no phlegm is produced □ **hacking cough** a continuous short dry cough ■ an infection that causes coughing ○ *She has a bad cough and cannot make the speech.* ■ *verb* to send air out of the lungs suddenly because the throat is irritated ○ *The smoke made him cough.* ○ *She has a cold and keeps on coughing and sneezing.*

**coughing fit** /'kɒfɪŋ fɪt/ *noun* a sudden attack of coughing

**cough medicine** /'kɒf ,med(ə)sɪn/, **cough linctus** /'kɒf ,lɪŋktəs/, **cough mixture** *noun* a liquid taken to soothe the irritation which causes a cough

**cough suppressant** /'kɒf sə,presənt/ *noun* an opioid or sedative antihistamine drug such as pholcodine which suppresses the cough reflex

**cough up** /,kɒf 'ʌp/ *verb* to cough hard to expel a substance from the trachea ○ *He coughed up phlegm.* ○ *She became worried when the girl started coughing up blood.*

**counselling** /'kaʊnsəlɪŋ/ *noun* a method of treating especially psychiatric disorders in which a specialist talks with a person about his or her condition and how to deal with it

**counsellor** /'kaʊnsələ/ *noun* a person who advises and talks with someone about his or her problems

**counteract** /,kaʊntər'ækt/ *verb* to act against something or reduce the effect of something ○ *The lotion should counteract the irritant effect of the spray on the skin.*

**counteraction** /,kaʊntər'ækʃən/ *noun* the action of one drug which acts against another drug

**counterextension** /,kaʊntərɪk'stenʃən/ *noun* an orthopaedic treatment in which the upper part of a limb is kept fixed and traction is applied to the lower part of it

**counterirritant** /,kaʊntər'ɪrɪt(ə)nt/ *noun* a substance which alleviates the pain in an internal organ by irritating an area of skin whose sensory nerves are close to those of the organ in the spinal cord

**counterirritation** /,kaʊntərɪrɪ'teɪʃ(ə)n/ *noun* a skin irritant applied artificially to alleviate the pain in another part of the body

**counterstain** /ˈkaʊntəsteɪn/ *noun* a stain used to identify tissue samples, e.g. red dye used to identify Gram-negative bacteria after having first stained them with violet dye ■ *verb* to stain specimens with a counterstain

**coupling** /ˈkʌplɪŋ/ *noun* **1.** an act of joining together or linking two people, things or processes **2.** something which joins two things, especially a device for connecting two pieces of pipe, hose or tube

**course** /kɔːs/ *noun* **1.** a programme of study or training ○ *went on a course to update his nursing skills* **2.** a series of drugs to be taken, or a series of sessions of treatment ○ *We'll put you on a course of antibiotics.*

**course of treatment** /ˌkɔːs əv ˈtriːtmənt/ *noun* a series of applications of a treatment, e.g. a series of injections or physiotherapy

**cover test** /ˈkʌvə test/ *noun* a test for a squint in which an eye is covered and its movements are checked when the cover is taken off

**Cowper's glands** /ˈkuːpəz glændz/ *plural noun* two glands at the base of the penis which secrete into the urethra. Also called **bulbourethral glands** [Described 1700. After William Cowper (1666–1709), English surgeon.]

**cowpox** /ˈkaʊpɒks/ *noun* an infectious viral disease of cattle which can be transmitted to humans. It was used as a constituent of the first vaccines for smallpox.

**cox-** /kɒks/ *prefix* the hip joint

**coxa** /ˈkɒksə/ *noun* the hip joint (NOTE: The plural is **coxae**.)

**coxalgia** /kɒkˈsældʒə/ *noun* pain in the hip joint

**coxa vara** /ˌkɒksə ˈveərə/ *noun* an unusual development of the hip bone, making the legs bow

**Coxsackie virus** /kɒkˈsæki ˌvaɪrəs/ *noun* one of a group of enteroviruses which enter the cells of the intestines and can cause diseases such as aseptic meningitis and Bornholm disease [After Coxsackie, New York, where the virus was first identified]

**CPAP** *abbr* continuous positive airways pressure

**CPN** *abbr* community psychiatric nurse

**CPR** *abbr* cardiopulmonary resuscitation

**crab** /kræb/, **crab louse** /ˈkræb laʊs/ *noun* a louse, *Phthirius pubis*, which infests the pubic region and other parts of the body with coarse hair. Also called **pubic louse**

**crack** /kræk/ *noun* a thin break ○ *There's a crack in one of the bones in the skull.* ■ *verb* to make a thin break in something, or become split ○ *She cracked a bone in her leg.* □ **cracked lip** a lip where the skin has split because of cold or dryness

**cradle** /ˈkreɪd(ə)l/ *noun* a metal frame put over a person in bed to keep the weight of the bedclothes off the body ■ *verb* to carry a child with one arm under the thigh and the other under the upper back

**cradle cap** /ˈkreɪd(ə)l kæp/ *noun* a yellow deposit on the scalp of babies, caused by seborrhoea

**cramp** /kræmp/ *noun* a painful involuntary spasm in the muscles, in which the muscle may stay contracted for some time

**crani-** /kreɪni/ *prefix* same as **cranio-** (used before vowels)

**cranial** /ˈkreɪniəl/ *adjective* referring to the skull

**cranial bone** /ˈkreɪniəl bəʊn/ *noun* one of the bones in the skull

**cranial cavity** /ˈkreɪniəl ˌkævɪti/ *noun* a space inside the bones of the cranium, in which the brain is situated

**cranial nerve** /ˈkreɪniəl nɜːv/ *noun* each of the nerves, twelve on each side, which are connected directly to the brain, governing mainly the structures of the head and neck

COMMENT: The cranial nerves are the olfactory, optic, loculomotor, trochlear, trigeminal, (ophthalmic, maxillary and mandibular), abducent, facial, auditory (vestibular and cochlear), glossopharyngeal, vagus, accessory and hypoglossal.

**cranio-** /kreɪniəʊ/ *prefix* the skull

**craniometry** /ˌkreɪniˈɒmɪtri/ *noun* the process of measuring skulls to find differences in size and shape

**craniopharyngioma** /ˌkreɪniəʊfəˌrɪndʒiˈəʊmə/ *noun* a tumour in the brain originating in the hypophyseal duct (NOTE: The plural is **craniopharyngiomas** or **craniopharyngiomata**.)

**craniostenosis** /ˌkreɪniəʊstəˈnəʊsɪs/, **craniosynostosis** /ˌkreɪniəʊˌsɪnəʊstˈəʊsɪs/ *noun* the early closing of the bones in a baby's skull, so making the skull contract

**craniotabes** /ˌkreɪniəʊˈteɪbiːz/ *noun* thinness of the bones in the occipital region of a child's skull, caused by rickets, marasmus or syphilis

**craniotomy** /ˌkreɪniˈɒtəmi/ *noun* a surgical operation on the skull, especially one cutting away part of the skull (NOTE: The plural is **craniotomies**.)

**cranium** /ˈkreɪniəm/ *noun* same as **skull** (NOTE: The plural is **craniums** or **crania**.)

COMMENT: The cranium consists of the occipital bone, two parietal bones, two temporal bones and the frontal, ethmoid and sphenoid bones.

**cream** /kriːm/ *noun* a medicinal oily substance, used to rub on the skin

**creatine** /ˈkriːətiːn/ *noun* a compound of nitrogen found in the muscles, produced by protein metabolism and excreted as creatinine

**creatine phosphate** /ˌkriːətiːn ˈfɒsfeɪt/ *noun* a store of energy-giving phosphate in muscles

**creatinine** /kri'ætəni:n/ *noun* a substance which is the form in which creatine is excreted

**creatinine clearance** /kri,ætəni:n 'kliərəns/ *noun* removal of creatinine from the blood by the kidneys

**creatinuria** /kri,ætɪ'njʊəriə/ *noun* excess creatine in the urine

**creatorrhoea** /,kri:ətə'ri:ə/ *noun* the presence of undigested muscle fibre in the faeces, occurring in some pancreatic diseases

**Credé's method** /kre'deɪz ,meθəd/ *noun* 1. a method of extracting a placenta by massaging the uterus through the abdomen 2. the putting of silver nitrate solution into the eyes of a baby born to a mother who has gonorrhoea, in order to prevent gonococcal conjunctivitis [Described 1860. After Karl Sigmund Franz Credé (1819–92), German gynaecologist.]

**creeping eruption** /,kri:pɪŋ ɪ'rʌpʃən/ *noun* an itching skin complaint, caused by larvae of various parasites which creep under the skin

**crepitation** /,krepɪ'teɪʃ(ə)n/ *noun* an unusual soft crackling sound heard in the lungs through a stethoscope. Also called **rale**

**crepitus** /'krepɪtəs/ *noun* 1. a harsh crackling sound heard through a stethoscope in a person with inflammation of the lungs 2. a scratching sound made by a broken bone or rough joint

**crest** /krest/ *noun* a long raised part on a bone

**crest of ilium** /,krest əv 'ɪliəm/ *noun* same as **iliac crest**

**cretinism** /'kretɪnɪz(ə)m/ *noun* now called **congenital hyperthyroidism** (NOTE: This term is regarded as offensive.)

**Creutzfeldt-Jakob disease** /,krɔɪtsfelt 'jækɒb dɪ,ziːz/ *noun* a disease of the nervous system caused by a slow-acting prion which eventually affects the brain. It may be linked to BSE in cows. Abbr **CJD.** ◊ **variant CJD** [Described 1920 by H.G. Creutzfeldt (1885–1964); 1921 by A.M. Jakob (1884–1931), German psychiatrists.]

**cribriform** /'krɪbrɪfɔ:m/ *adjective* having small holes like a sieve

**cribriform plate** /'krɪbrɪfɔ:m pleɪt/ *noun* the top part of the ethmoid bone which forms the roof of the nasal cavity and part of the roof of the eye sockets

**crick** /krɪk/ *noun* a painful stiffness in the neck or back (*informal*)

**cricoid** /'kraɪkɔɪd/ *adjective* relating to the lowest part of the cartilage of the larynx

**cricoid cartilage** /,kraɪkɔɪd 'ka:təlɪdʒ/ *noun* ring-shaped cartilage in the lower part of the larynx. See illustration at **LUNGS** in Supplement

**cri-du-chat syndrome** /,kri: dju: 'ʃɑː ,sɪn drəʊm/ *noun* a congenital condition, caused by loss of part of chromosome 5, which is

characterised in babies by a cry suggestive of that of a cat

**Crigler-Najjar syndrome** /,krɪglə 'nædʒɑː ,sɪndrəʊm/ *noun* a genetically controlled condition in which bilirubin cannot be formed, leading to jaundice or even brain damage

**criminal abortion** /,krɪmɪn(ə)l ə'bɔ:ʃ(ə)n/ *noun* an abortion which is carried out illegally

**crisis** /'kraɪsɪs/ *noun* 1. a situation or period of difficulty demanding action ○ *Is there a crisis in the health service?* 2. a turning point in a disease, after which the person may start to become better or very much worse

COMMENT: Many diseases progress to a crisis and then the patient rapidly gets better. The opposite situation where the patient gets better very slowly is called lysis.

**crista** /'krɪstə/ *noun* 1. a ridge, e.g. the border of a bone 2. a fold in the inner membrane of a mitrochondrion (NOTE: The plural is **cristae**.)

**crista galli** /,krɪstə 'gælaɪ/ *noun* a projection from the ethmoid bone

**criterion** /kraɪ'tɪəriən/ *noun* an accepted standard used in making a decision or judgment about something (NOTE: The plural is **criteria**.)

**critical** /'krɪtɪk(ə)l/ *adjective* 1. referring to a crisis 2. extremely serious ○ *He was taken to hospital in a critical condition* 3. which criticises ○ *The report was critical of the state of aftercare provision.*

**critical list** /'krɪtɪk(ə)l lɪst/ *noun* the list of patients in a hospital whose condition is medically life-threatening

**CRNA** *abbr* certified registered nurse anaesthetist

**Crohn's disease** /'krəʊnz dɪ,ziːz/ *noun* a persistent inflammatory disease, usually of the lower intestinal tract, characterised by thickening and scarring of the intestinal wall and obstruction [Described 1932. After Burrill Bernard Crohn (1884–1983), New York physician.]

COMMENT: No certain cause has been found for Crohn's disease, where only one section of the intestine becomes inflamed and can be blocked.

**cromolyn sodium** /,krəʊməlɪn 'səʊdiəm/ *noun* a drug that helps to prevent the release of histamine and other substances which cause many of the symptoms of asthma and hay fever

**cross-dresser** *noun* someone who wears clothes usually worn by people of the opposite sex, e.g. a transvestite

**cross-dressing** /krɒs 'dresɪŋ/ *noun* the practice of wearing clothes usually worn by people of the opposite sex, e.g. by transvestites

**cross eye** /'krɒs aɪ/ *noun* same as **convergent strabismus** (*informal*)

**cross-eyed** /,krɒs 'aɪd/ *adjective* having convergent strabismus (*informal*)

**cross-infection** /ˌkrɒs ɪnˈfekʃən/ *noun* an infection passed from one patient to another in hospital, either directly or from nurses, visitors or equipment

**crossmatch** /ˌkrɒsˈmætʃ/ *verb* (*in transplant surgery*) to match a donor to a recipient as closely as possible to avoid tissue rejection. ◊ **blood group**

**crossmatching** /ˌkrɒsˈmætʃɪŋ/ *noun* the process of matching a transplant donor to a recipient as closely as possible to avoid tissue rejection

**cross-resistance** /ˌkrɒs rɪˈzɪstəns/ *noun* the development by a disease agent of resistance to a number of similar drugs or chemicals of the same class

**cross-section** /ˈkrɒs ˌsekʃən/ *noun* **1.** a small part of something, taken to be representative of the whole ○ *The team consulted a cross-section of hospital ancillary staff.* **2.** a sample cut across a specimen for examination under a microscope ○ *He examined a cross-section of the lung tissue.*

**crotamiton** /krəˈtæmɪt(ə)n/ *noun* a chemical that kills mites, used to treat scabies

**crotch** /krɒtʃ/ *noun* the point where the legs meet the body, where the genitals are. Also called **crutch**

**croup** /kruːp/ *noun* acute infection of the upper respiratory passages which blocks the larynx, affecting children

COMMENT: The patient's larynx swells, and he or she breathes with difficulty and has a barking cough. Attacks usually occur at night. They can be fatal if the larynx becomes completely blocked.

**crown** /kraʊn/ *noun* **1.** the top part of a tooth above the level of the gums **2.** an artificial top attached to a tooth **3.** the top part of the head ■ *verb* to put an artificial crown on a tooth

**crowning** /ˈkraʊnɪŋ/ *noun* **1.** the act of putting an artificial crown on a tooth **2.** a stage in childbirth in which the top of the baby's head becomes visible

**cruciate** /ˈkruːʃiət/ *adjective* shaped like a cross

**cruciate ligament** /ˌkruːʃiət ˈlɪgəmənt/ *noun* any ligament shaped like a cross, especially either of two ligaments behind the knee which prevent the knee from bending forwards

**crude death rate** /kruːd ˈdeθ reɪt/ *noun* the number of deaths in a year, divided by the total population

**crura** /ˈkrʊərə/ plural of **crus**

**crural** /ˈkrʊərəl/ *adjective* referring to the thigh, leg or shin

**crura of the diaphragm** /ˌkrʊərə əv ðə ˈdaɪəfræm/ *plural noun* the long muscle fibres joining the diaphragm to the lumbar vertebrae

**crus** /krʌs/ *noun* a long projecting part (NOTE: The plural is **crura**.)

**crus cerebri** /krʌs ˈserɪbraɪ/ *noun* each of the nerve tracts between the cerebrum and the medulla oblongata (NOTE: The plural is **crura cerebri**.)

**crush fracture** /ˈkrʌʃ ˌfræktʃə/ *noun* a fracture by compression of the bone

**crush syndrome** /ˈkrʌʃ ˌsɪndrəʊm/ *noun* a condition in which a limb has been crushed, as in an accident, causing kidney failure and shock

**crus of penis** /ˌkrʌs əv ˈpiːnɪs/ *noun* a part of a corpus cavernosum attached to the pubic arch

**crust** /krʌst/ *noun* a dry layer of blood, pus or other secretion that forms over a cut or sore

**crutch** /krʌtʃ/ *noun* **1.** a strong support for someone with an injured leg, formed of a stick with a T-bar which fits under the armpit, especially formerly, or a holding bar and elbow clasp **2.** same as **crotch**

**cry-** /kraɪ/ *prefix* same as **cryo-** (*used before vowels*)

**cryaesthesia** /ˌkraɪiːsˈθiːziə/ *noun* the fact of being sensitive to cold

**cryo-** /kraɪəʊ/ *prefix* cold

**cryobank** /ˈkraɪəʊbæŋk/ *noun* a place where biological material such as semen and body tissue can be stored at extremely low temperatures

**cryoprecipitate** /ˌkraɪəʊprɪˈsɪpɪtət/ *noun* a precipitate such as from blood plasma, which separates out on freezing and thawing

COMMENT: Cryoprecipitate from blood plasma contains Factor VIII and is used to treat haemophilia.

**cryoprobe** /ˈkraɪəʊprəʊb/ *noun* an instrument used in cryosurgery with a tip that is kept very cold to destroy tissue

**cryosurgery** /ˌkraɪəʊˈsɜːdʒəri/ *noun* surgery which uses extremely cold instruments to destroy tissue

**cryotherapy** /ˌkraɪəʊˈθerəpi/ *noun* treatment using extreme cold, as in removing a wart with dry ice

**crypt** /krɪpt/ *noun* a small cavity in the body

**crypto-** /krɪptəʊ/ *prefix* hidden

**cryptocci** /ˌkrɪptəˈkɒki/ plural of **cryptococcus**

**cryptococcal meningitis** /ˌkrɪptəkɒk(ə)l menɪnˈdʒaɪtɪs/ *noun* a form of meningitis that is a feature of cryptococcosis

**cryptococcosis** /ˌkrɪptəʊkəˈkəʊsɪs/ *noun* an infection mainly affecting the brain or nervous system, caused by the fungus *Cryptococcus neoformans*. It occurs most often in people with HIV infection.

**cryptococcus** /ˌkrɪptəˈkɒkəs/ *noun* one of several single-celled yeasts which exist in the soil and can cause disease (NOTE: The plural is **cryptococci**.)

**cryptomenorrhoea** /ˌkrɪptəʊmenəˈriːə/ *noun* the retention of menstrual flow, usually caused by an obstruction

**cryptorchidism** /krɪpˈtɔːkɪdɪz(ə)m/, **cryptorchism** /krɪpˈtɔːkɪz(ə)m/ *noun* a condition in a young male in which the testicles do not move down into the scrotum

**cryptosporidia** /ˌkrɪptəʊspəˈrɪdiə/ *plural of* **cryptosporidium**

**cryptosporidiosis** /ˌkrɪptəʊspəˌrɪdiˈəʊsɪs/ *noun* an infectious condition of humans and domestic animals, spread by an intestinal parasite *Cryptosporidium parvum*. Its symptoms are fever, diarrhoea and stomach cramps.

**cryptosporidium** /ˌkrɪptəʊspəˈrɪdiəm/ *noun* a parasite which contaminates drinking water supplies, causing intestinal infection (NOTE: The plural is **cryptosporidia**.)

**crypts of Lieberkühn** /ˌkrɪpts əv ˈliːbəkuːn/ *plural noun* tubular glands found in the mucous membrane of the small and large intestine, especially those between the bases of the villi in the small intestine. Also called **Lieberkühn's glands** [Described 1745. After Johann Nathanial Lieberkuhn (1711–56), Berlin anatomist and physician.]

**crystal** /ˈkrɪst(ə)l/ *noun* a chemical formation of hard regular-shaped solids

**crystalline** /ˈkrɪstəlaɪn/ *adjective* clear like pure crystal

**crystal violet** /ˌkrɪst(ə)l ˈvaɪələt/ *noun* same as **gentian violet**

**CSF** *abbr* cerebrospinal fluid

**CT** *abbr* computed tomography

**CT scan** /ˌsiː ˈtiː skæn/ *noun* a computer picture of a slice of the body or an organ produced by a CT scanner. Also called **CAT scan**

**CT scanner** /ˌsiː ˈtiː ˌskænə/ *noun* a device which directs a narrow X-ray beam at a thin section of the body from various angles, using a computer to build up a complete picture of the cross-section. Also called **CAT scanner**

**cubital** /ˈkjuːbɪt(ə)l/ *adjective* referring to the ulna

**cubital fossa** /ˌkjuːbɪt(ə)l ˈfɒsə/ *noun* a depression in the front of the elbow joint

**cubitus** /ˈkjuːbɪtəs/ *noun* same as **ulna**

**cuboid** /ˈkjuːbɔɪd/, **cuboid bone** /ˈkjuːbɔɪd bəʊn/ *noun* one of the tarsal bones in the foot. See illustration at **FOOT** in Supplement

**cuboidal cell** /kjuːˈbɔɪd(ə)l sel/ *noun* a cube-shaped epithelial cell

**cuff** /kʌf/ *noun* **1.** an inflatable ring put round the arm and inflated when blood pressure is being measured **2.** an inflatable ring put round an endotracheal tube to close the passage

**cuirass respirator** /kwɪˌræs ˈrespɪreɪtə/ *noun* a type of artificial respirator which surrounds only the chest

**culdoscope** /ˈkʌldəʊskəʊp/ *noun* an instrument used to inspect the interior of a woman's pelvis, introduced through the vagina

**culdoscopy** /kʌlˈdɒskəpi/ *noun* an examination of the interior of a woman's pelvis using a culdoscope

**culture** /ˈkʌltʃə/ *noun* **1.** the shared values and behaviour of a group **2.** microooorganisms or tissues grown in a culture medium in a laboratory ■ *verb* to grow microorganisms or tissues in a culture medium

**culture medium** /ˈkʌltʃə ˌmiːdiəm/ *noun* a substance in which a culture of microorganisms or tissue is grown in a laboratory, e.g. agar

**cumulative** /ˈkjuːmjʊlətɪv/ *adjective* growing by adding

**cumulative action** /ˌkjuːmjʊlətɪv ˈækʃən/ *noun* an effect of a drug which is given more often than it can be excreted and so accumulates in the tissues

**cuneiform** /ˈkjuːnɪfɔːm/, **cuneiform bone** /ˈkjuːnɪfɔːm bəʊn/ *noun* one of the three tarsal bones in the foot. See illustration at **FOOT** in Supplement

**cupola** /ˈkjuːpələ/ *noun* **1.** a dome-shaped structure **2.** a piece of cartilage in a semicircular canal which is moved by the fluid in the canal and connects with the vestibular nerve

**curable** /ˈkjʊərəb(ə)l/ *adjective* able to be cured ○ *a curable form of cancer*

**curare** /kjʊˈrɑːri/ *noun* a drug derived from South American plants, antagonist to acetylcholine and used surgically to paralyse muscles during operations without causing unconsciousness (NOTE: Curare is the poison used to make poison arrows.)

**curative** /ˈkjʊərətɪv/ *adjective* able to cure

**cure** /kjʊə/ *noun* a particular way of making someone well or of stopping an illness ○ *Scientists are trying to develop a cure for the common cold.* ■ *verb* to make someone healthy ○ *She was completely cured.* ○ *Can the doctors cure his bad circulation?*

**curettage** /kjʊəˈretɪdʒ/ *noun* the procedure of scraping the inside of a hollow organ, often the uterus, to remove a growth or tissue for examination. Also called **curettement**

**curette** /kjʊəˈret/ *noun* a surgical instrument like a long thin spoon, used for scraping the inside of an organ (NOTE: The US spelling is **curet**.) ■ *verb* to scrape an organ with a curette (NOTE: **curettes – curetting – curetted**. The US spelling is **curet**.)

**curettement** same as **curettage**

**curie** /ˈkjʊəri/ *noun* a former unit of measurement of radioactivity, replaced by the becquerel. Symbol **Ci**

**Curling's ulcer** /ˌkɜːlɪŋz ˈʌlsə/ *noun* an ulcer of the duodenum following severe injury to the body

**curvature** /'kɜːvətʃə/ *noun* the way in which something bends from a straight line ○ *greater* or *lesser curvature of the stomach*

**curvature of the spine** /ˌkɜːvətʃər əv ðə 'spaɪn/ *noun* an unusual bending of the spine forwards or sideways

**cushingoid** /'kʊʃɪŋɔɪd/ *adjective* showing symptoms of Cushing's disease

**Cushing's disease** /'kʊʃɪŋz dɪˌziːz/, **Cushing's syndrome** /'kʊʃɪŋz ˌsɪndrəʊm/ *noun* a condition in which the adrenal cortex produces too many corticosteroids [Described 1932. After Harvey Williams Cushing (1869–1939), surgeon, Boston, USA.]

COMMENT: The syndrome is caused either by a tumour in the adrenal gland, by excessive stimulation of the adrenals by the basophil cells of the pituitary gland, or by a corticosteroid-secreting tumour. The syndrome causes swelling of the face and trunk, weakening of the muscles, raised blood pressure and retention of salt and water in the body.

**cusp** /kʌsp/ *noun* **1.** the pointed tip of a tooth **2.** a flap of membrane forming a valve in the heart

**cuspid** /'kʌspɪd/ *noun* same as **canine**

**cut** /kʌt/ *noun* **1.** a reduction in the number or amount of something **2.** a place where the skin has been penetrated by a sharp instrument ○ *She had a bad cut on her left leg.* ○ *The nurse will put a bandage on your cut.* ■ *verb* **1.** to make an opening in something using a knife, scissors or other sharp thing ○ *The surgeon cut the diseased tissue away with a scalpel.* ○ *She cut her finger on the broken glass.* **2.** to reduce the number or amount of something ○ *Accidents have been cut by 10%.* (NOTE: **cutting – cut**)

**cut-** *prefix* referring to the skin

**cutaneous** /kjuː'teɪniəs/ *adjective* referring to the skin

**cutaneous leishmaniasis** /kjuːˌteɪniəs liːʃməˈnaɪəsɪs/ *noun* a form of skin disease caused by the tropical parasite *Leishmania*. Also called **Delhi boil**

**cutdown** /'kʌtdaʊn/ *noun* the procedure of cutting a vein to insert a cannula or administer an intravenous drug

**cuticle** /'kjuːtɪk(ə)l/ *noun* **1.** same as **epidermis 2.** a strip of epidermis attached at the base of a nail

**cutis** /'kjuːtɪs/ *noun* the skin

**cutis anserina** /ˌkjuːtɪs 'ænseraɪnə/ *noun* a reaction of the skin when someone is cold or frightened, the skin being raised into many little bumps by the action of the arrector pili muscles. Also called **goose bumps**

**CVA** *abbr* cerebrovascular accident

**cyan-** /saɪən/ *prefix* same as **cyano-** (*used before vowels*)

**cyanide** /'saɪənaɪd/ *noun* a poison which kills very rapidly when drunk or inhaled

**cyano-** /saɪənəʊ/ *prefix* blue

**cyanocobalamin** /ˌsaɪənəʊkəʊ'bæləmɪn/ same as **Vitamin B$_{12}$**

**cyanosed** /'saɪənəʊst/ *adjective* with blue skin ○ *The patient was cyanosed round the lips.*

**cyanosis** /ˌsaɪə'nəʊsɪs/ *noun* a condition characterised by a blue colour of the peripheral skin and mucous membranes, a symptom of lack of oxygen in the blood, e.g. in heart or lung disease

**cyanotic** /ˌsaɪə'nɒtɪk/ *adjective* referring to or having cyanosis

**cyclandelate** /sɪ'klændəleɪt/ *noun* a drug used to treat cerebrovascular disease

**cycle** /'saɪk(ə)l/ *noun* a series of events which recur regularly

**cyclic** /'sɪklɪk, 'saɪklɪk/ *adjective* **1.** occurring or repeated in cycles **2.** referring to organic compounds composed of a closed ring of atoms

**cyclical** /'sɪklɪk(ə)l/ *adjective* referring to cycles

**cyclical vomiting** /ˌsɪklɪk(ə)l 'vɒmɪtɪŋ/ *noun* repeated attacks of vomiting

**-cycline** /saɪklɪn/ *suffix* used in names of antibiotics ○ *tetracycline*

**cyclitis** /sɪ'klaɪtɪs/ *noun* inflammation of the ciliary body in the eye

**cyclizine** /'saɪklɪziːn/ *noun* an antihistamine drug that can be used to control nausea and vomiting

**cyclo-** /saɪkləʊ/ *prefix* cycles

**cyclodialysis** /ˌsaɪkləʊdaɪ'æləsɪs/ *noun* a surgical operation to connect the anterior chamber of the eye and the choroid, as a treatment of glaucoma

**cyclopentolate** /ˌsaɪkləʊ'pentəleɪt/ *noun* a drug used to paralyse the ciliary muscle

**cyclophosphamide** /ˌsaɪkləʊ'fɒsfəmaɪd/ *noun* a drug which suppresses immunity, used in the treatment of leukaemia, lymphoma, Hodgkin's disease and tumours

**cycloplegia** /ˌsaɪkləʊ'pliːdʒə/ *noun* paralysis of the ciliary muscle which makes it impossible for the eye to focus properly

**cyclopropane** /ˌsaɪkləʊ'prəʊpeɪn/ *noun* a flammable hydrocarbon gas used as a general anaesthetic and in organic synthesis

**cyclothymia** /ˌsaɪkləʊ'θaɪmiə/ *noun* a mild form of bipolar disorder in which the person experiences alternating depression and excitement

**cyclotomy** /saɪ'klɒtəmi/ *noun* a surgical operation to make a cut in the ciliary body (NOTE: The plural is **cyclotomies**.)

**-cyclovir** /saɪkləʊvɪə/ *suffix* used in the names of antiviral drugs

**cyesis** /saɪ'iːsɪs/ *noun* same as **pregnancy** (*technical*)

**cylinder** /'sɪlɪndə/ *noun* ♦ **oxygen cylinder**

**cyst** /sɪst/ *noun* an unusual growth in the body shaped like a pouch, containing liquid or semi-liquid substances

**cyst-** /sɪst/ *prefix* the bladder

**cystadenoma** /ˌsɪstədɪˈnəʊmə/ *noun* an adenoma in which fluid-filled cysts form (NOTE: The plural is **cystadonomas** or **cystadonomata**.)

**cystalgia** /sɪˈstældʒə/ *noun* pain in the urinary bladder

**cystectomy** /sɪˈstektəmi/ *noun* a surgical operation to remove all or part of the urinary bladder (NOTE: The plural is **cystectomies**.)

**cystic** /ˈsɪstɪk/ *adjective* **1.** referring to cysts **2.** referring to a bladder

**cystic artery** /ˌsɪstɪk ˈɑːtəri/ *noun* an artery leading from the hepatic artery to the gall bladder

**cystic duct** /ˈsɪstɪk dʌkt/ *noun* a duct which takes bile from the gall bladder to the common bile duct

**cysticercosis** /ˌsɪstɪsɜːˈkəʊsɪs/ *noun* a disease caused by infestation of tapeworm larvae from pork

**cysticercus** /ˌsɪstɪˈsɜːkəs/ *noun* the larva of a tapeworm of the genus *Taenia*, found in pork, which is enclosed in a cyst (NOTE: The plural is **cysticerci**.)

**cystic fibrosis** /ˌsɪstɪk faɪˈbrəʊsɪs/ *noun* a hereditary disease in which there is malfunction of the exocrine glands such as the pancreas, in particular those which secrete mucus, causing respiratory difficulties, male infertility and malabsorption of food from the gastrointestinal tract. Also called **fibrocystic disease, mucoviscidosis**

COMMENT: The thick mucous secretions cause blockage of ducts and many serious secondary effects in the intestines and lungs. Symptoms include loss of weight, abnormal faeces and bronchitis. If diagnosed early, cystic fibrosis can be controlled with vitamins, physiotherapy and pancreatic enzymes.

**cystic vein** /ˈsɪstɪk veɪn/ *noun* a vein which drains the gall bladder

**cystine** /ˈsɪstiːn/ *noun* an amino acid. It can cause stones to form in the urinary system of people who have a rare inherited metabolic disorder.

**cystinosis** /ˌsɪstɪˈnəʊsɪs/ *noun* a disorder affecting the absorption of amino acids, resulting in excessive amounts of cystine accumulating in the kidneys

**cystinuria** /ˌsɪstɪˈnjʊəriə/ *noun* cystine in the urine

**cystitis** /sɪˈstaɪtɪs/ *noun* inflammation of the urinary bladder, which makes someone pass water often and with a burning sensation

**cystocele** /ˈsɪstəsiːl/ *noun* a hernia of the urinary bladder into the vagina

**cystogram** /ˈsɪstəɡræm/ *noun* an X-ray photograph of the urinary bladder

**cystography** /sɪˈstɒɡrəfi/ *noun* an examination of the urinary bladder by X-rays after radio-opaque dye has been introduced

**cystolithiasis** /ˌsɪstəlɪˈθaɪəsɪs/ *noun* a condition in which stones are formed in the urinary bladder

**cystometer** /sɪˈstɒmɪtə/ *noun* an apparatus which measures the pressure in the bladder

**cystometry** /sɪˈstɒmɪtri/ *noun* measurement of the pressure in the bladder

**cystopexy** /sɪˈstɒpeksi/ *noun* a surgical operation to fix the bladder in a different position. Also called **vesicofixation** (NOTE: The plural is **cystopexies**.)

**cystoplasty** /ˈsɪstəˌplæsti/ *noun* a surgical operation on the bladder (NOTE: The plural is **cystoplasties**.)

**cystoscope** /ˈsɪstəskəʊp/ *noun* an instrument made of a long tube with a light at the end, used to inspect the inside of the bladder

**cystoscopy** /sɪˈstɒskəpi/ *noun* an examination of the bladder using a cystoscope (NOTE: The plural is **cystoscopies**.)

**cystostomy** /sɪˈstɒstəmi/, **cystotomy** /sɪˈstɒtəmi/ *noun* a surgical operation to make an opening between the bladder and the abdominal wall to allow urine to pass without going through the urethra. Also called **vesicostomy** (NOTE: The plurals are **cystostomies** and **cystotomies**.)

**cystourethrography** /ˌsɪstəʊˌjʊəriˈθrɒɡrəfi/ *noun* X-ray examination of the bladder and urethra

**cystourethroscope** /ˌsɪstəʊjʊˈriːθrəskəʊp/ *noun* an instrument used to inspect the bladder and urethra

**cyt-** /saɪt/ *prefix* same as **cyto-** (*used before vowels*)

**cyto-** /saɪtəʊ/ *prefix* cell

**cytochemistry** /ˌsaɪtəʊˈkemɪstri/ *noun* the study of the chemical activity of cells

**cytodiagnosis** /ˌsaɪtəʊdaɪəɡˈnəʊsɪs/ *noun* diagnosis after examination of cells

**cytogenetics** /ˌsaɪtəʊdʒəˈnetɪks/ *noun* a branch of genetics which studies the function of cells, especially chromosomes, in heredity

**cytokine** /ˈsaɪtəʊkaɪn/ *noun* a protein secreted by cells of the lymph system which is involved in controlling response to inflammation

**cytokinesis** /ˌsaɪtəʊkɪˈniːsɪs/ *noun* changes in the cytoplasm of a cell during division

**cytological smear** /ˌsaɪtəlɒdʒɪk(ə)l ˈsmɪə/ *noun* a sample of tissue taken for examination under a microscope

**cytology** /saɪˈtɒlədʒi/ *noun* the study of the structure and function of cells

**cytolysis** /saɪˈtɒləsɪs/ *noun* the breaking down of cells

**cytomegalovirus** /ˌsaɪtəʊˈmeɡələʊˌvaɪrəs/ *noun* one of the herpesviruses which can cause serious congenital disorders in a fetus if it infects the pregnant mother. Abbr **CMV**

**cytometer** /saɪˈtɒmɪtə/ *noun* an instrument attached to a microscope, used for measuring and counting the number of cells in a specimen

**cytopenia** /ˌsaɪtəʊˈpiːniə/ *noun* a deficiency of cellular elements in blood or tissue

**cytoplasm** /ˈsaɪtəʊplæz(ə)m/ *noun* a substance inside the cell membrane which surrounds the nucleus of a cell

**cytoplasmic** /ˌsaɪtəʊˈplæzmɪk/ *adjective* referring to the cytoplasm of a cell

**cytosine** /ˈsaɪtəʊsiːn/ *noun* one of the four basic chemicals in DNA

**cytosome** /ˈsaɪtəʊsəʊm/ *noun* the body of a cell, not including the nucleus

**cytotoxic** /ˌsaɪtəʊˈtɒksɪk/ *adjective* **1.** referring to a drug or agent which prevents cell division **2.** referring to cells in the immune system which destroy other cells

**cytotoxic drug** /ˌsaɪtəʊtɒksɪk ˈdrʌg/ *noun* a drug which reduces the reproduction of cells, used to treat cancer

**cytotoxin** /ˌsaɪtəʊˈtɒksɪn/ *noun* a substance which has a toxic effect on cells

# D

**d** /diː/ *symbol* deci-

**da** *symbol* deca-

**dab** /dæb/ *verb* to touch something lightly ○ *He dabbed around the cut with a piece of cotton wool.*

**da Costa's syndrome** /dɑː ˈkɒstəz ˌsɪn drəʊm/ *noun* same as **disordered action of the heart** [Described 1871. After Jacob Mendes da Costa (1833–1900), Philadelphia surgeon, who described this condition in soldiers in the American Civil War.]

**dacryo-** /dækriəʊ/ *prefix* tears

**dacryoadenitis** /ˌdækriəʊædɪˈnaɪtɪs/ *noun* inflammation of the lacrimal gland

**dacryocystitis** /ˌdækriəʊsɪˈstaɪtɪs/ *noun* inflammation of the lacrimal sac when the tear duct, which drains into the nose, becomes blocked

**dacryocystography** /ˌdækriəʊsɪˈstɒɡrəfi/ *noun* contrast radiography to determine the site of an obstruction in the tear ducts

**dacryocystorhinostomy** /ˌdækriəʊ ˌsɪstəʊraɪˈnɒstəmi/ *noun* a surgical operation to bypass a blockage from the tear duct which takes tears into the nose. Abbr **DCR** (NOTE: The plural is **dacryocystorhinostomies**.)

**dacryolith** /ˈdækriəʊlɪθ/ *noun* a stone in the lacrimal sac

**dacryoma** /ˌdækriˈəʊmə/ *noun* a benign swelling in one of the tear ducts (NOTE: The plural is **dacryomas** or **dacryomata**.)

**dactyl** /ˈdæktɪl/ *noun* a finger or toe

**dactyl-** /ˈdæktɪl/ *prefix* same as **dactylo-** (*used before vowels*)

**dactylitis** /ˌdæktɪˈlaɪtɪs/ *noun* inflammation of the fingers or toes, caused by bone infection or rheumatic disease

**dactylo-** /ˈdæktɪləʊ/ *prefix* referring to the fingers or toes

**dactylology** /ˌdæktɪˈlɒlədʒi/ *noun* signs made with the fingers in place of words when talking to a person who is unable to hear, or when a person who is unable to hear or speak wants to communicate

**dactylomegaly** /ˌdæktɪləʊˈmeɡəli/ *noun* a condition in which a person has longer fingers than usual

**DAH** *abbr* disordered action of the heart

**daily** /ˈdeɪli/ *adverb* every day ○ *Take the medicine twice daily.*

**Daltonism** /ˈdɔːltənɪz(ə)m/ *noun* the commonest form of colour blindness, in which someone cannot see the difference between red and green. Also called **protanopia** [Described 1794. After John Dalton (1766–1844), English chemist and physician. Founder of the atomic theory, he himself was colour-blind.]

**damage** /ˈdæmɪdʒ/ *noun* harm done to things ○ *The disease caused damage to the brain cells.* ■ *verb* to harm something ○ *His hearing or his sense of balance was damaged in the accident.*

**damp** /dæmp/ *adjective* slightly wet ○ *You should put a damp compress on the bruise.*

**D & C** /diː ən/ *abbr* dilatation and curettage

**dander** /ˈdændə/ *noun* very small fragments that fall from the feathers, hair or skin of animals or people

**dandruff** /ˈdændrəf/ *noun* pieces of dead skin from the scalp which fall out when the hair is combed. Also called **pityriasis capitis, scurf**

**D and V** /ˌdiː ən ˈviː/ *abbr* diarrhoea and vomiting

**Dandy-Walker syndrome** /ˌdændi ˈwɔːkə ˌsɪndrəʊm/ *noun* a congenital condition in which there is no Magendie's foramen in the brain

**danger** /ˈdeɪndʒə/ *noun* the possibility of harm or death ○ *Unless the glaucoma is treated quickly, there's a danger that the patient will lose his eyesight* or *a danger of the patient losing his eyesight.* □ **out of danger** no longer likely to die

**dangerous** /ˈdeɪndʒərəs/ *adjective* causing harm or death

**dangerous drug** /ˌdeɪndʒərəs ˈdrʌɡ/ *noun* **1.** a drug which is harmful and is not available to the general public, e.g. morphine or heroin **2.** a poison which can only be sold to specific persons

**dark adaptation** /dɑːk ˌædæpˈteɪʃ(ə)n/ noun the reflex changes which enable the eye to continue to see in dim light. For example, the pupil becomes larger and the rods in the retina become more active than the cones.

**darkening** /ˈdɑːknɪŋ/ noun the act of becoming darker in colour ○ *Darkening of the tissue takes place after bruising.*

**data** /ˈdeɪtə/ plural noun information in words or figures about a particular subject, especially information which is available on computer (NOTE: In scientific usage, **data** is used with a plural verb: *The data are accurate.* In everyday language, **data** is often used with a singular verb: *The recent data supports our case.*)

**data bank** /ˈdeɪtə bæŋk/ noun a store of information in a computer ○ *The hospital keeps a data bank of information about possible kidney donors.*

**database** noun a structured collection of information in a computer that can be automatically retrieved and manipulated

**Data Protection Act** /ˌdeɪtə prəˈtekʃ(ə)n/ noun a parliamentary act intended to protect information about individuals that is held on computers. It ensures that all information is stored securely and allows people to have access to their entries.

**daughter** /ˈdɔːtə/ noun a female child of a parent ○ *They have two sons and one daughter.*

**daughter cell** /ˈdɔːtə sel/ noun any of the cells which develop by mitosis from a single parent cell

**day blindness** /ˈdeɪ ˌblaɪndnəs/ noun same as **hemeralopia**

**day care** /ˈdeɪ keə/ noun supervised recreation or medical care provided during the day for people who need special help, e.g. some elderly people or small children

**day case** /ˈdeɪ keɪs/ noun same as **day patient**

**day case surgery** /ˈdeɪ keɪs ˌsɜːdʒəri/ noun same as **day surgery**

**day centre** /ˈdeɪ ˌsentə/ noun a place providing day care

**day hospital** /ˈdeɪ ˌhɒspɪt(ə)l/ noun a hospital where people are treated during the day and go home in the evenings

**day nursery** /ˈdeɪ ˌnɜːs(ə)ri/ noun a place where small children can be looked after during the daytime while their parents or guardians are at work

**day patient** /ˈdeɪ ˌpeɪʃ(ə)nt/ noun a patient who is in hospital for treatment for a day and does not stay overnight. Also called **day case**

**day patient care** /ˈdeɪ peɪʃ(ə)nt keə/ noun care for patients who are resident in a hospital during the daytime only

**day recovery ward** /deɪ rɪˈkʌv(ə)ri wɔːd/ noun a ward where day patients who have had

minor operations can recover before going home

**day surgery** /ˈdeɪ ˌsɜːdʒəri/ noun a surgical operation which does not require the patient to stay overnight in hospital. Also called **day case surgery**

**dazed** /deɪzd/ adjective confused in the mind ○ *She was found walking about in a dazed condition.* ○ *He was dazed after the accident.*

**dB** abbr decibel

**DCR** abbr dacryocystorhinostomy

**DDS** abbr US doctor of dental surgery

**DDT** abbr dichlorodiphenyltrichloroethane

**de-** /diː/ prefix removal or loss

**dead** /ded/ adjective **1.** no longer alive ○ *My grandparents are both dead* ○ *The woman was rescued from the crash, but was certified dead on arrival at the hospital* **2.** not sensitive ○ *The nerve endings are dead.* ○ *His fingers went dead.*

**deaden** /ˈded(ə)n/ verb to make something such as pain or noise less strong ○ *The doctor gave him an injection to deaden the pain.*

**dead fingers** /ded ˈfɪŋgəz/ noun same as **Raynaud's disease**

**deadly nightshade** /ˌdedli ˈnaɪtʃeɪd/ noun same as **belladonna**

**dead man's fingers** /ˌded mænz ˈfɪŋgəz/ noun same as **Raynaud's disease**

**dead space** /ded speɪs/ noun a breath in the last part of the process of breathing in air which does not get further than the bronchial tubes

**deaf** /def/ adjective not able to hear in circumstances where most people would ○ *You have to speak slowly and clearly when you talk to Mr Jones because he's quite deaf.* ◊ **hearing-impaired** ■ plural noun □ **the deaf** people who are deaf

**deaf and dumb** /ˌdef ən ˈdʌm/ noun not able to hear or to speak (NOTE: This term is regarded as offensive.)

**deafen** /ˈdef(ə)n/ verb to make someone deaf for a time ○ *He was deafened by the explosion.*

**deafness** /ˈdefnəs/ noun the fact of being unable to hear in circumstances where most people would ◊ **partial deafness 1.** the condition of being able to hear some tones, but not all **2.** a general dulling of the whole range of hearing

COMMENT: Deafness has many degrees and many causes: old age, viruses, exposure to continuous loud noise or intermittent loud explosions, and diseases such as German measles.

**deaminate** /diːˈæmɪneɪt/ verb to remove an amino group from an amino acid, forming ammonia

**deamination** /diːˌæmɪˈneɪʃ(ə)n/ noun the process by which amino acids are broken down in the liver and urea is formed

COMMENT: After deamination, the ammonia which is formed is converted to urea by the liver, while the remaining carbon and hydrogen from the amino acid provide the body with heat and energy.

**death** /deθ/ *noun* the permanent end of all natural functions

**death certificate** /'deθ sə,tɪfɪkət/ *noun* an official document signed by a doctor stating that a person has died and giving details of the person and the cause of death

**death rate** /'deθ reɪt/ *noun* the number of deaths per year per thousand of population ○ *The death rate from cancer of the liver has remained stable.*

**debilitate** /dɪ'bɪlɪteɪt/ *verb* to make someone or something weak ○ *He was debilitated by a long illness.*

**debilitating disease** /dɪ,bɪlɪteɪtɪŋ dɪ'ziːz/ *noun* a disease which makes the person weak

**debility** /dɪ'bɪlɪti/ *noun* general weakness

**debridement** /dɪ'briːdmənt/ *noun* the removal of dirt or dead tissue from a wound to help healing

**deca-** /dekə/ *prefix* ten. Symbol **da**

**Decadron** /'dekədrɒn/ a trade name for dexamethasone

**decalcification** /diː,kælsɪfɪ'keɪʃ(ə)n/ *noun* the loss of calcium salts from teeth and bones

**decannulation** /diː,kænjʊ'leɪʃ(ə)n/ *noun* the removal of a tracheostomy tube

**decapitation** /dɪ,kæpɪ'teɪʃ(ə)n/ *noun* the act or process of cutting off the head of a person or animal

**decapsulation** /diː,kæpsjʊ'leɪʃ(ə)n/ *noun* a surgical operation to remove a capsule from an organ, especially from a kidney

**decay** /dɪ'keɪ/ *noun* **1.** the process by which tissues become rotten, caused by the action of microorganisms and oxygen **2.** damage caused to tissue or a tooth by the action of microorganisms, especially bacteria ■ *verb* (*of tissue*) to rot ○ *The surgeon removed decayed matter from the wound.*

**deci-** /desi/ *prefix* one tenth ($10^{-1}$) ○ *decigram* Symbol **d**

**decibel** /'desɪbel/ *noun* a unit of measurement of the loudness of sound, used to compare different levels of sound. Symbol **dB**

COMMENT: Normal conversation is at about 50dB. Very loud noise with a value of over 120dB, e.g. that of aircraft engines, can cause pain.

**decidua** /dɪ'sɪdjuə/ *noun* a membrane which lines the uterus after fertilisation (NOTE: The plural is **deciduas** or **deciduae**.)

COMMENT: The decidua is divided into several parts: the **decidua basalis**, where the embryo is attached, the **decidua capsularis**, which covers the embryo and the **decidua vera** which is the rest of the decidua not touching the embryo. It is expelled after the birth of the baby.

**decidual** /dɪ'sɪdjuəl/ *adjective* referring to the decidua

**deciduoma** /dɪ,sɪdju'əʊmə/ *noun* a mass of decidual tissue remaining in the uterus after birth (NOTE: The plural is **deciduomas** or **deciduomata**.)

**deciduous** /dɪ'sɪdjuəs/ *adjective* referring to teeth discarded at a later stage of development

**deciduous dentition** /dɪ,sɪdjuəs den'tɪʃ(ə)n/ *noun* the set of twenty teeth which are gradually replaced by the permanent teeth as a child grows older

**deciduous tooth** /dɪ'sɪdjuəs tuːθ/ *noun* same as **primary tooth**

**decilitre** /'desɪliːtə/ *noun* a unit of measurement of liquid equal to one tenth of a litre. Symbol **dl** (NOTE: The US spelling is **deciliter**.)

**decimetre** /'desɪmiːtə/ *noun* a unit of measurement of length equal to one tenth of a metre. Symbol **dm** (NOTE: The US spelling is **decimeter**.)

**decompensation** /diː,kɒmpən'seɪʃ(ə)n/ *noun* a condition in which an organ such as the heart cannot cope with extra stress placed on it and so is unable to perform its function properly

**decompose** /,diːkəm'pəʊz/ *verb* to rot or become putrefied (NOTE: **decomposing – decomposed**)

**decomposition** /,diːkɒmpə'zɪʃ(ə)n/ *noun* the process where dead matter is rotted by the action of bacteria or fungi

**decompression** /,diːkəm'preʃ(ə)n/ *noun* **1.** reduction of pressure **2.** a controlled reduction of atmospheric pressure which occurs as a diver returns to the surface

**decompression sickness** /,diːkəm,preʃ(ə)n 'sɪknəs/ *noun* same as **caisson disease**

**decongest** /,diːkən'dʒest/ *verb* to loosen or disperse mucus in the nasal passages, sinuses or bronchi

**decongestant** /,diːkən'dʒestənt/ *adjective* reducing congestion and swelling ■ *noun* a drug which reduces congestion and swelling, sometimes used to unblock the nasal passages

**decontamination** /,diːkəntæmɪ'neɪʃ(ə)n/ *noun* the removal of a contaminating substance such as radioactive material

**decortication** /diː,kɔːtɪ'keɪʃ(ə)n/ *noun* the surgical removal of the cortex of an organ □ **decortication of a lung** a surgical operation to remove part of the pleura which has been thickened or made stiff by chronic empyema

**decrudescence** /,diːkruː'des(ə)ns/ *noun* a reduction in the symptoms of a disease

**decubitus** /dɪ'kjuːbɪtəs/ *noun* the position of a person who is lying down

**decubitus ulcer** /dɪ,kjuːbɪtəs 'ʌlsə/ *noun* same as **bedsore**

**decussation** /,diːkʌ'seɪʃ(ə)n/ *noun* the crossing of nerve fibres in the central nervous system. Also called **chiasm**

**deep** /diːp/ *adjective* located, coming from or reaching relatively far inside the body. Opposite **superficial**

**deep cervical vein** /diːp 'sɜːvɪk(ə)l veɪn/ *noun* a vein in the neck which drains into the vertebral vein

**deep dermal burn** /diːp 'dɜːm(ə)l bɜːn/ *noun* a burn which is so severe that a graft will be necessary to repair the skin damage. Also called **full thickness burn**

**deep facial vein** /diːp 'feɪʃ(ə)l veɪn/ *noun* a small vein which drains from the pterygoid process behind the cheek into the facial vein

**deeply** /'diːpli/ *adverb* so as to take in a large amount of air ○ *He was breathing deeply.*

**deep plantar arch** /diːp 'plæntər ɑːtʃ/ *noun* a curved artery crossing the sole of the foot

**deep vein** /diːp 'veɪn/ *noun* a vein which is inside the body near a bone, as opposed to a superficial vein near the skin

**deep-vein thrombosis** /ˌdiːp veɪn θrɒm 'bəʊsɪs/ *noun* a condition arising when a thrombus formed in the deep veins of a leg or the pelvis travels to a lung where it may cause death. The condition may affect anyone who is inactive for long periods. Also called **phlebothrombosis**. Abbr **DVT**

**defecate** /'defəkeɪt/, **defaecate** *verb* to pass faeces out from the bowels through the anus (NOTE: **defecating – defecated**)

**defecation** /ˌdefə'keɪʃ(ə)n/, **defaecation** *noun* the act of passing out faeces from the bowels

**defect** /'diːfekt/ *noun* **1.** an unsatisfactory or imperfect feature of something **2.** a lack of something which is necessary

**defective** /dɪ'fektɪv/ *adjective* working badly or wrongly formed ○ *The surgeons operated to repair a defective heart valve.* ■ *noun* a person suffering from severe mental impairment (NOTE: The noun use is regarded as offensive.)

**defence** /dɪ'fens/ *noun* **1.** resistance against an attack of a disease **2.** behaviour of a person which is aimed at protecting him or her from harm (NOTE: The US spelling is **defense**.)

**defence mechanism** /dɪ'fens ˌmekənɪz(ə)m/ *noun* a subconscious reflex by which a person prevents himself or herself from showing emotion

**defense** /dɪ'fens/ *noun US* same as **defence**

**defensive medicine** /dɪˌfensɪv 'med(ə)s(ə)n/ *noun* extensive diagnostic testing before treatment to minimise the likelihood of a patient suing the doctor or hospital for negligence

**deferent** /'defərənt/ *adjective* **1.** going away from the centre **2.** referring to the vas deferens

**defervescence** /ˌdefə'ves(ə)ns/ *noun* a period during which a fever is subsiding

**defibrillation** /diːˌfɪbrɪ'leɪʃ(ə)n/ *noun* a procedure to correct an irregular heartbeat by applying a large electrical impulse to the chest wall, especially in potentially life-threatening circumstances. Also called **cardioversion**

**defibrillator** /diːˈfɪbrɪleɪtə/ *noun* an apparatus used to apply an electric impulse to the heart to make it beat regularly

**defibrination** /diːˌfaɪbrɪ'neɪʃ(ə)n/ *noun* the removal of fibrin from a blood sample to prevent clotting

**deficiency** /dɪ'fɪʃ(ə)nsi/ *noun* a lack of something necessary

**deficiency disease** /dɪ'fɪʃ(ə)nsi dɪˌziːz/ *noun* a disease caused by lack of an essential element in the diet such as vitamins or essential amino and fatty acids

**deficient** /dɪ'fɪʃ(ə)nt/ *adjective* not meeting the required standard □ **deficient in something** not containing the necessary amount of something ○ *His diet is deficient in calcium* or *he has a calcium-deficient diet.*

**deficit** /'defɪsɪt/ *noun* the amount by which something is less than it should be

**defloration** /ˌdiːflɔː'reɪʃ(ə)n/ *noun* the act of breaking the hymen of a virgin, usually at the first sexual intercourse

**deflorescence** /ˌdiːflɔː'res(ə)ns/ *noun* the disappearance of a rash

**deformans** /diː'fɔːmənz/ ♦ **osteitis deformans**

**deformation** /ˌdiːfɔː'meɪʃ(ə)n/ *noun* the process of becoming deformed, or the state of being deformed ○ *The later stages of the disease are marked by bone deformation.*

**deformed** /dɪ'fɔːmd/ *adjective* not shaped or formed in the expected way

**deformity** /dɪ'fɔːmɪti/ *noun* an unusual shape of part of the body

**degenerate** /dɪ'dʒenəreɪt/ *verb* to change so as not to be able to function ○ *His health degenerated so much that he was incapable of looking after himself.*

**degeneration** /dɪˌdʒenə'reɪʃ(ə)n/ *noun* a change in the structure of a cell or organ so that it no longer works properly

**degenerative disease** /dɪˌdʒen(ə)rətɪv dɪ 'ziːz/, **degenerative disorder** /dɪ ˌdʒen(ə)rətɪv dɪs'ɔːdə/ *noun* a disease or disorder in which there is progressive loss of function of a part of the body, or in which a part of the body fails to repair itself

**degenerative joint disease** /dɪ ˌdʒen(ə)rətɪv 'dʒɔɪnt dɪˌziːz/ *noun* same as **osteoarthritis**

**deglutition** /ˌdiːgluː'tɪʃ(ə)n/ *noun* the action of passing food or liquid, and sometimes also air, from the mouth into the oesophagus (*technical*) Also called **swallowing**

**dehisced** /dɪ'hɪst/ *adjective* referring to a wound which has split open after being closed

**dehiscence** /dɪˈhɪs(ə)ns/ *noun* the act of opening wide

**dehydrate** /ˌdiːhaɪˈdreɪt/ *verb* to lose water, or cause someone or something to lose water ○ *During strenuous exercise it's easy to become dehydrated.* (NOTE: **dehydrating – dehydrated**)

**dehydration** /ˌdiːhaɪˈdreɪʃ(ə)n/ *noun* loss of water

'…an estimated 60–70% of diarrhoeal deaths are caused by dehydration' [*Indian Journal of Medical Sciences*]

COMMENT: Water is more essential than food for a human being's survival. If someone drinks during the day less liquid than is passed out of the body in urine and sweat, he or she begins to dehydrate.

**dehydrogenase** /ˌdiːhaɪˈdrɒdʒəneɪz/ *noun* an enzyme that transfers hydrogen between chemical compounds

**déjà vu** /ˌdeɪʒɑː ˈvuː/ *noun* an illusion that a new situation is a previous one being repeated, usually caused by a disease of the brain

**Déjerine-Klumpke's syndrome** *noun* same as **Klumpke's paralysis**

**deleterious** /ˌdelɪˈtɪəriəs/ *adjective* damaging or harmful

**Delhi boil** /ˌdeli ˈbɔɪl/ *noun* same as **cutaneous leishmaniasis**

**delicate** /ˈdelɪkət/ *adjective* **1.** easily broken or harmed ○ *The bones of a baby's skull are very delicate.* ○ *The eye is covered by a delicate membrane.* **2.** easily falling ill ○ *His delicate state of health means that he is not able to work long hours.* **3.** requiring great care or sensitivity ○ *The surgeons carried out a delicate operation to join the severed nerves.*

**delirious** /dɪˈlɪriəs/ *adjective* affected by delirium. A person can become delirious because of shock, fear, drugs or fever.

**delirium** /dɪˈlɪriəm/ *noun* a mental state in which someone is confused, excited and restless and has hallucinations

**delirium tremens** /dɪˌlɪriəm ˈtriːmenz/, **delirium alcoholicum** /dɪˌlɪriəm ˌælkəˈhɒlɪkəm/ *noun* a state of mental illness usually found in long-term alcoholics who attempt to give up alcohol consumption. It includes hallucinations about insects, trembling and excitement. Abbr **DTs**

**delivery** /dɪˈlɪv(ə)ri/ *noun* the birth of a child

**delivery bed** /dɪˈlɪv(ə)ri bed/ *noun* a special bed on which a mother lies to give birth

**delivery room** /dɪˈlɪv(ə)ri ruːm/ *noun* a room in a hospital specially equipped for women to give birth

**delta** /ˈdeltə/ *noun* the fourth letter of the Greek alphabet

**delta hepatitis** /ˌdeltə ˌhepəˈtaɪtɪs/ *noun* a severe form of hepatitis caused by an RNA virus in conjunction with the hepatitis B virus. Also called **hepatitis delta**

**delta virus** /ˌdeltə ˈvaɪrəs/ *noun* the RNA virus which causes delta hepatitis

**delta wave** /ˈdeltə weɪv/ *noun* a slow brain wave which is produced in the front of the brain by adults in deep sleep, registering a frequency of 3.5 hertz

**deltoid** /ˈdeltɔɪd/, **deltoid muscle** /ˈdeltɔɪd ˌmʌs(ə)l/ *noun* a big triangular muscle covering the shoulder joint and attached to the humerus, which lifts the arm sideways

**deltoid tuberosity** /ˌdeltɔɪd ˌtjuːbəˈrɒsɪti/ *noun* a raised part of the humerus to which the deltoid muscle is attached

**delusion** /dɪˈluːʒ(ə)n/ *noun* a false belief which a person holds which cannot be changed by reason ○ *He suffered from the delusion that he was wanted by the police.*

**dementia** /dɪˈmenʃə/ *noun* the loss of mental ability and memory due to organic disease of the brain, causing disorientation and personality changes

'AIDS dementia is a major complication of HIV infection, occurring in 70–90% of patients' [*British Journal of Nursing*]

**dementia of the Alzheimer's type** /dɪˌmenʃə əv ði ˈæltshaɪməz ˌtaɪp/ *noun* a form of mental degeneration probably due to Alzheimer's disease

**dementia paralytica** /dɪˌmenʃə ˌpærəˈlɪtɪkə/ *noun* mental degeneration due to the tertiary stage of syphilis

**dementia praecox** /dɪˌmenʃə ˈpriːkɒks/ *noun* same as **schizophrenia** (*old*)

**dementing** /dɪˈmentɪŋ/ *adjective* referring to someone with dementia

**demi-** /demi/ *prefix* half

**demographic forecast** /ˌdeməgræfɪk ˈfɔːkɑːst/ *noun* a forecast of the numbers of people of different ages and sexes in an area at some time in the future

**demography** /dɪˈmɒgrəfi/ *noun* the study of populations and environments or changes affecting populations

**demulcent** /dɪˈmʌlsənt/ *noun* a soothing substance which relieves irritation in the stomach

**demyelinating** /diːˈmaɪəlɪneɪtɪŋ/ *adjective* relating to the destruction of the myelin sheath round nerve fibres

**demyelination** /diːˌmaɪəlɪˈneɪʃ(ə)n/ *noun* the destruction of the myelin sheath round nerve fibres, caused, e.g. by injury to the head, or as the main result of multiple sclerosis

**denatured alcohol** /diːˌneɪtʃəd ˈælkəhɒl/ *noun* ethyl alcohol such as methylated spirit, rubbing alcohol or surgical spirit with an additive, usually methyl alcohol, to make it unpleasant to drink

**dendrite** /ˈdendraɪt/ *noun* a branched structure growing out from a nerve cell, which receives impulses from the nerve endings of oth-

# dendritic

**104**

er nerve cells at synapses. See illustration at **NEURONE** in Supplement. Also called **dendron**

**dendritic** /den'drɪtɪk/ *adjective* referring to a dendrite

**dendritic ulcer** /den,drɪtɪk 'ʌlsə/ *noun* a branching ulcer on the cornea, caused by a herpesvirus

**dendron** /'dendrɒn/ *noun* same as **dendrite**

**denervation** /,diːnə'veɪʃ(ə)n/ *noun* the stopping or cutting of the nerve supply to a part of the body

**dengue** /'deŋgi/ *noun* a tropical disease caused by an arbovirus transmitted by mosquitoes, characterised by high fever, pains in the joints, headache and rash. Also called **breakbone fever**

**denial** /dɪ'naɪəl/ *noun* a person's refusal to accept that he or she has a serious medical problem

**Denis Browne splint** /,denɪs braun 'splɪnt/ *noun* a metal splint used to correct a club foot [Described 1934. After Sir Denis John Wolko Browne (1892–1967), Australian orthopaedic and general surgeon working in Britain.]

**dens** /denz/ *noun* a tooth, or something shaped like a tooth

**dent-** /dent/ *prefix* referring to a tooth or teeth

**dental** /'dent(ə)l/ *adjective* referring to teeth or to the treatment of teeth ○ *dental caries* ○ *dental surgeon*

**dental care** /'dent(ə)l keə/ *noun* the examination and treatment of teeth

**dental caries** /,dent(ə)l 'keəriz/ *noun* the rotting of a tooth. Also called **dental decay**

**dental cyst** /,dent(ə)l 'sɪst/ *noun* a cyst near the root of a tooth

**dental decay** /,dent(ə)l dɪ'keɪ/ *noun* same as **dental caries**

**dental floss** /'dent(ə)l flɒs/ *noun* a soft thread which can be pulled between the teeth to help keep them clean

**dental hygiene** /,dent(ə)l 'haɪdʒiːn/ *noun* procedures to keep the teeth clean and healthy

**dental impaction** /,dent(ə)l ɪm'pækʃ(ə)n/ *noun* a condition in which a tooth is closely pressed against other teeth and cannot grow normally

**dental plaque** /,dent(ə)l 'plæk/ *noun* a hard smooth bacterial deposit on teeth, which is the probable cause of caries

**dental plate** /'dent(ə)l pleɪt/ *noun* a prosthesis made to the shape of the mouth, which holds artificial teeth

**dental prosthesis** /,dent(ə)l prɒs'θiːsɪs/ *noun* one or more false teeth

**dental pulp** /,dent(ə)l 'pʌlp/ *noun* soft tissue inside a tooth

**dental surgeon** /'dent(ə)l ,sɜːdʒən/ *noun* a person who is qualified to practise surgery on teeth

**dental surgery** /'dent(ə)l ,sɜːdʒəri/ *noun* **1.** the office and operating room of a dentist **2.** surgery carried out on teeth

**dentine** /'dentiːn/ *noun* a hard substance which surrounds the pulp of teeth, beneath the enamel (NOTE: The US spelling is **dentin**.)

**dentist** /'dentɪst/ *noun* a person who is qualified to look after teeth and gums

**dentistry** /'dentɪstri/ *noun* the profession of a dentist, or the branch of medicine dealing with teeth and gums

**dentition** /den'tɪʃ(ə)n/ *noun* the number, arrangement and special characteristics of all the teeth in a person's jaws

COMMENT: Children have incisors, canines and molars, which are replaced over a period of years by the permanent teeth: eight incisors, four canines, eight premolars and twelve molars, the last four molars being called the wisdom teeth.

**dentoid** /'dentɔɪd/ *adjective* shaped like a tooth

**denture** /'dentʃə/ *noun* a set of false teeth, fixed to a device which fits inside the mouth

**deodorant** /diː'əud(ə)rənt/ *noun* a substance which hides or prevents unpleasant smells ■ *adjective* hiding or preventing odours

**deontology** /,diːɒn'tɒlədʒi/ *noun* the ethics of duty and of what is morally right or wrong

**deoxygenate** /diː'ɒksɪdʒəneɪt/ *verb* to remove oxygen from something

**deoxygenated blood** /diː,ɒksɪdʒəneɪt 'blʌd/ *noun* blood from which most of the oxygen has been removed by the tissues. It is darker than arterial oxygenated blood. Also called **venous blood**. Compare **deoxygenated blood**

**deoxyribonucleic acid** /diː,ɒksɪ,raɪbəu njuː,kliːɪk 'æsɪd/ *noun* full form of **DNA**

**Department of Health** /dɪ,pɑːtmənt əv 'helθ/ *noun* in the UK, the government department in charge of health services. Abbr **DH**

**dependant** /dɪ'pendənt/ *noun* a person who is looked after or supported by someone else ○ *He has to support a family of six children and several dependants.*

**dependence** /dɪ'pendəns/, **dependency** /dɪ'pendənsi/ *noun* the fact of needing the support of something or someone such as a carer, nurse or doctor, or of being addicted to a drug

**dependent** /dɪ'pendənt/ *adjective* **1.** needing the support of someone or something **2.** addicted to a drug **3.** referring to a part of the body which is hanging down

**dependent relative** /dɪ,pendənt 'relətɪv/ *noun* a person who is looked after by another member of the family

**depersonalisation** /diː,pɜːs(ə)n(ə)laɪ 'zeɪʃ(ə)n/, **depersonalization** *noun* a psychiatric state in which someone does not believe he or she is real

**depilation** /ˌdepɪˈleɪʃ(ə)n/ *noun* the removal of hair

**depilatory** /dɪˈpɪlət(ə)ri/ *noun* a substance which removes hair ■ *adjective* removing hair

**depletion** /dɪˈpliːʃ(ə)n/ *noun* the act or process of something being reduced

**Depo-Provera** a trademark for a progesterone derivative used in birth control and the treatment of endometriosis which is administered by three-monthly injection

**deposit** /dɪˈpɒzɪt/ *noun* a substance which is attached to part of the body ○ *Some foods leave a hard deposit on teeth.* ○ *A deposit of fat forms on the walls of the arteries.* ■ *verb* to attach a substance to part of the body ○ *Fat is deposited on the walls of the arteries.*

**depressant** /dɪˈpres(ə)nt/ *noun* a drug which reduces the activity of part of the body, e.g. a tranquilliser

**depressed** /dɪˈprest/ *adjective* 1. experiencing a mental condition that prevents someone from carrying out the normal activities of life in the usual way □ **clinically depressed** Same as **depressed** 2. feeling miserable and worried (*informal*) ○ *He was depressed after his exam results.* 3. referring to something such as a metabolic rate which is below the usual level

**depressed fracture** /dɪˌprest ˈfræktʃə/ *noun* a fracture of a flat bone such as those in the skull where part of the bone has been pushed down lower than the surrounding parts

**depression** /dɪˈpreʃ(ə)n/ *noun* 1. a mental condition that prevents someone from carrying out the normal activities of life in the usual way 2. a hollow on the surface of a part of the body

**depressive** /dɪˈpresɪv/ *adjective* relating to, causing, or experiencing mental depression ○ *He is in a depressive state.* ■ *noun* 1. a substance which causes depression 2. someone experiencing depression

**depressor** /dɪˈpresə/ *noun* 1. a muscle which pulls part of the body downwards 2. a nerve which reduces the activity of an organ such as the heart and lowers blood pressure

**deprivation** /ˌdeprɪˈveɪʃ(ə)n/ *noun* 1. the fact of not being able to have something that you need or want ○ *sleep deprivation* 2. the lack of basic necessities of life

**deradenitis** /dɪˌrædɪˈnaɪtɪs/ *noun* inflammation of the lymph nodes in the neck

**Dercum's disease** /ˈdɜːkəmz dɪˌziːz/ *noun* same as **adiposis dolorosa** [Described 1888. After François Xavier Dercum (1856–1931), Professor of Neurology at Jefferson Medical College, Philadelphia, USA.]

**derealisation** /diːˌrɪəlaɪˈzeɪʃ(ə)n/, **derealization** *noun* a psychological state in which someone feels the world around him or her is not real

**derivative** /dɪˈrɪvətɪv/ *noun* a substance which is derived from another substance

**derm-** /dɜːm/ *prefix* same as **derma-** (*used before vowels*)

**-derm** /dɜːm/ *suffix* skin

**derma-** /dɜːmə/ *prefix* skin

**dermal** /ˈdɜːm(ə)l/ *adjective* referring to the skin

**dermatitis** /ˌdɜːməˈtaɪtɪs/ *noun* inflammation of the skin

'…various types of dermal reaction to nail varnish have been noted. Also contact dermatitis caused by cosmetics such as toothpaste, soap, shaving creams.' [*Indian Journal of Medical Sciences*]

**dermatitis artefacta** /ˌdɜːmətaɪtɪs ˌɑːtɪˈfæktə/ *noun* injuries caused by someone to their own skin

**dermatitis herpetiformis** /ˌdɜːmətaɪtɪs hə ˌpetɪˈfɔːmɪs/ *noun* a type of dermatitis where large itchy blisters form on the skin

**dermato-** /dɜːmətəʊ/ *prefix* referring to the skin

**dermatochalasis** /ˌdɜːmətəʊkəˈlæsɪs/ *noun* a condition where a fold of skin moves down over the eyelid, common in older people

**dermatographia** /ˌdɜːmətəʊˈgræfiə/ *noun* same as **dermographia**

**dermatological** /ˌdɜːmətəˈlɒdʒɪk(ə)l/ *adjective* referring to dermatology

**dermatologist** /ˌdɜːməˈtɒlədʒɪst/ *noun* a doctor who specialises in the study and treatment of the skin and its diseases

**dermatology** /ˌdɜːməˈtɒlədʒi/ *noun* the study and treatment of the skin and its diseases

**dermatome** /ˈdɜːmətəʊm/ *noun* 1. a special knife used for cutting thin sections of skin for grafting 2. an area of skin supplied by one spinal nerve

**dermatomycosis** /ˌdɜːmətəʊmaɪˈkəʊsɪs/ *noun* a skin infection caused by a fungus that is not a dermatophyte

**dermatomyositis** /ˌdɜːmətəʊmaɪəʊˈsaɪtɪs/ *noun* a collagen disease with a wasting inflammation of the skin and muscles

**dermatophyte** /ˈdɜːmətəʊfaɪt/ *noun* a fungus belonging to one of three genera which affect the skin or hair, causing tinea

**dermatophytosis** /ˌdɜːmətəʊfaɪˈtəʊsɪs/ *noun* a fungal infection of the skin caused by a *dermatophyte*

**dermatoplasty** /ˈdɜːmətəʊplæsti/ *noun* a skin graft, replacing damaged skin by skin taken from another part of the body or from a donor

**dermatosis** /ˌdɜːməˈtəʊsɪs/ *noun* a disease of the skin

**dermis** /ˈdɜːmɪs/ *noun* a thick layer of living skin beneath the epidermis. Also called **corium**

**dermo-** /dɜːməʊ/ *prefix* same as **derma-**

**dermographia** /,dɜːməˈgræfiə/ *noun* a swelling on the skin produced by pressing with a blunt instrument, usually an allergic reaction. Also called **dermatographia**

**dermoid** /ˈdɜːmɔɪd/ *adjective* **1.** referring to the skin **2.** like skin

**dermoid cyst** /ˈdɜːmɔɪd sɪst/ *noun* a cyst found under the skin, usually in the midline, containing hair, sweat glands and sebaceous glands

**Descemet's membrane** /deˈʃəˈmets ˌmembreɪn/ *noun* one of the deep layers of the cornea [Described 1785. After Jean Descemet (1732–1810), French physician; Professor of Anatomy and Surgery in Paris.]

**descending aorta** /dɪˌsendɪŋ eɪˈɔːtə/ *noun* the second section of the aorta, which turns downwards. Compare **ascending aorta**

**descending colon** /dɪˌsendɪŋ ˈkəʊlɒn/ *noun* the third section of the colon which goes down the left side of the body. Compare **ascending colon**. See illustration at DIGESTIVE SYSTEM in Supplement

**descending tract** /dɪˌsendɪŋ ˈtrækt/ *noun* a set of nerves which takes impulses away from the head

**desensitisation** /diːˌsensɪtaɪˈzeɪʃ(ə)n/, **desensitization** *noun* **1.** the act of making someone or something no longer sensitive to something such as an allergen **2.** the treatment of an allergy by giving a person injections of small quantities of the substance to which he or she is allergic over a period of time until they become immune to it

**desensitise** /diːˈsensətaɪz/, **desensitize** *verb* **1.** to deaden a nerve and remove sensitivity ○ *The patient was prescribed a course of desensitising injections.* **2.** to treat someone suffering from an allergy by giving graduated injections of the substance to which he or she is allergic over a period of time until they become immune to it

**designer drug** /dɪˈzaɪnə drʌg/ *noun* a drug that has been modified to enhance its properties (*informal*)

**desogestrel** /ˌdesəˈdʒestrəl/ *noun* a hormone used an as oral contraceptive

**desquamate** /ˈdeskwəmeɪt/ *verb* (*of skin*) to peel off, or be removed in layers

**desquamation** /ˌdeskwəˈmeɪʃ(ə)n/ *noun* **1.** the continual process of losing the outer layer of dead skin **2.** peeling off of the epithelial part of a structure

**detach** /dɪˈtætʃ/ *verb* to separate one thing from another ○ *an operation to detach the cusps of the mitral valve*

**detached retina** /dɪˌtætʃt ˈretɪnə/ *noun* a condition in which the retina becomes partially separated from the eyeball, causing loss of vision. Also called **retinal detachment**

COMMENT: A detached retina can be caused by a blow to the eye, or simply is a condition occurring in old age. If left untreated the eye will become blind. A detached retina can sometimes be attached to the choroid again using lasers.

**detect** /dɪˈtekt/ *verb* to sense or to notice, usually something which is very small or difficult to see ○ *an instrument to detect microscopic changes in cell structure* ○ *The nurses detected a slight improvement in the patient's condition.*

**detection** /dɪˈtekʃən/ *noun* the action of detecting something ○ *the detection of sounds by nerves in the ears* ○ *the detection of a cyst using an endoscope*

**detergent** /dɪˈtɜːdʒənt/ *noun* a cleaning substance which removes grease and bacteria

COMMENT: Most detergents are not allergenic but some biological detergents which contain enzymes to remove protein stains can cause dermatitis.

**deteriorate** /dɪˈtɪəriəreɪt/ *verb* to become worse ○ *The patient's condition deteriorated rapidly.*

**deterioration** /dɪˌtɪəriəˈreɪʃ(ə)n/ *noun* the fact of becoming worse ○ *The nurses were worried by the deterioration in the patient's reactions.*

**determine** /dɪˈtɜːmɪn/ *verb* to find out something by examining the evidence ○ *Health inspectors are trying to determine the cause of the outbreak of Salmonella poisoning.*

**detox** /ˈdiːtɒks/ *noun* same as **detoxication** (*informal*)

**detoxication** /diːˌtɒksɪˈkeɪʃ(ə)n/, **detoxification** /diːˌtɒksɪfɪˈkeɪʃ(ə)n/ *noun* the removal of toxic substances to make a poisonous substance harmless

**detrition** /dɪˈtrɪʃ(ə)n/ *noun* the fact of wearing away by rubbing or use

**detritus** /dɪˈtraɪtəs/ *noun* rubbish produced when something disintegrates

**detrusor muscle** /dɪˈtruːzə ˌmʌs(ə)l/ *noun* the muscular coat of the urinary bladder

**Dettol** /ˈdetɒl/ *noun* a trade name for a disinfectant containing chloroxylenol

**detumescence** /ˌdiːtjuːˈmes(ə)ns/ *noun* **1.** (*of the penis or clitoris after an erection or orgasm*) the process of becoming limp **2.** (*of a swelling*) the process of disappearing

**deuteranopia** /ˌdjuːtərəˈnəʊpiə/ *noun* a form of colour blindness in which someone cannot see green

**develop** /dɪˈveləp/ *verb* **1.** to become larger and stronger, or more complex ○ *The embryo is developing normally.* ○ *A swelling developed under the armpit.* ○ *The sore throat developed into an attack of meningitis.* **2.** to make something start to happen ○ *We're developing a new system for dealing with admission to A & E.* **3.** to make something start to grow or become larger, stronger or more complex ○ *He does exercises to develop his muscles.* **4.** to start to have an illness ○ *The baby* *may be developing a cold.* ○ *He developed complications and was rushed to hospital.*

'…rheumatoid arthritis is a chronic inflammatory disease which can affect many systems in the body, but mainly the joints. 70% of sufferers develop the condition in the metacarpophalangeal joints.' [*Nursing Times*]

**development** /dɪˈveləpmənt/ *noun* **1.** the process of growing, or of becoming larger and stronger, or more complex ○ *The development of the embryo takes place in the uterus.* **2.** something which happens and causes a change in a situation ○ *Report any developments to me at once.*

**developmental** /dɪˌveləpˈment(ə)l/ *adjective* referring to the development of an embryo

**developmental delay** /dɪˈveləpmənt(ə)l dɪˌleɪ/ *noun* the fact of being later than usual in developing, either physically or psychologically

**deviance** /ˈdiːviəns/ *noun* sexual behaviour which is considered unusual

**deviated nasal septum** /ˌdiːvieɪtɪd ˌneɪz(ə)l ˈseptəm/, **deviated septum** /ˌdiːvieɪtɪd ˈseptəm/ *noun* an unusual position of the septum of the nose which may block the nose and cause nosebleeds

**deviation** /ˌdiːviˈeɪʃ(ə)n/ *noun* **1.** the fact of being different from what is usual or expected or something which is different from what is usual or expected **2.** an unusual position of a joint or of the eye, as in strabismus

**Devic's disease** /ˈdiːvɪks dɪˌziːz/ *noun* same as **neuromyelitis optica** [Described 1894. After Devic, a French physician who died in 1930.]

**dexamethasone** /ˌdeksəˈmeθəsəun/ *noun* a synthetic steroid drug that is used to treat inflammation and hormonal imbalances

**Dexa scan** *noun* a technique to assess changes in someone's bone density, as in osteoporosis or in Paget's disease. Full form **Dual Energy X-Ray Absorptiometry**

**dextro-** /dekstrəu/ *prefix* referring to the right, or the right side of the body

**dextrocardia** /ˌdekstrəuˈkɑːdiə/ *noun* a congenital condition in which the apex of the heart is towards the right of the body instead of the left. Compare **laevocardia**

**dextromoramide** /ˌdekstrəˈmɔːrəmaɪd/ *noun* an opioid drug used to reduce pain

**dextrose** /ˈdekstrəuz/ *noun* same as **glucose**

**DH** *abbr* Department of Health

**dhobie itch** /ˌdəubi ˈɪtʃ/ *noun* same as **tinea cruris**

**DI** *abbr* donor insemination

**di-** /daɪ/ *prefix* two, double

**dia-** /daɪə/ *prefix* **1.** through or throughout **2.** across **3.** in different or opposite directions **4.** apart

**diabetes** /ˌdaɪəˈbiːtiːz/ *noun* **1.** one of a group of diseases which cause the body to pro-

duce large amounts of urine. ◊ **gestational diabetes 2.** same as **diabetes mellitus**

**diabetes insipidus** /ˌdaɪəˌbiːtiːz ɪnˈsɪpɪdəs/ *noun* a rare disorder of the pituitary gland causing an inadequate amount of the hormone vasopressin, which controls urine production, to be produced, leading to excessive passing of urine and extreme thirst

**diabetes mellitus** /ˌdaɪəˌbiːtiːz ˈmelɪtəs/ *noun* a disease where the body cannot control sugar absorption because the pancreas does not secrete enough insulin

COMMENT: Diabetes mellitus has two forms: Type I may have a viral trigger caused by an infection which affects the cells in the pancreas which produce insulin; Type II is caused by a lower sensitivity to insulin, is common in older people, and is associated with obesity. Symptoms of diabetes mellitus are tiredness, unusual thirst, frequent passing of water and sweet-smelling urine. Blood and urine tests show high levels of sugar. Treatment for Type II diabetes involves keeping to a strict diet and reducing weight, and sometimes the use of oral hypoglycaemic drugs such as glibenclamide. Type II diabetes is treated with regular injections of insulin.

**diabetic** /ˌdaɪəˈbetɪk/ *adjective* **1.** referring to diabetes mellitus **2.** referring to food which contains few carbohydrates and sugar ○ *diabetic chocolate* ■ *noun* a person who has diabetes

**diabetic cataract** /ˌdaɪəbetɪk ˈkætərækt/ *noun* a cataract which develops in people who have diabetes

**diabetic coma** /ˌdaɪəbetɪk ˈkəumə/ *noun* a state of unconsciousness caused by untreated diabetes

**diabetic diet** /ˌdaɪəbetɪk ˈdaɪət/ *noun* a diet which is low in carbohydrates and sugar

**diabetic retinopathy** /ˌdaɪəbetɪk retɪˈnɒpəθi/ *noun* a disease of the retina, caused by diabetes

**diabetogenic** /ˌdaɪəbetəˈdʒenɪk/ *adjective* which causes diabetes

**diabetologist** /ˌdaɪəbeˈtɒlədʒɪst/ *noun* a doctor specialising in the treatment of diabetes mellitus

**diaclasia** /ˌdaɪəˈkleɪziə/ *noun* a fracture made by a surgeon to repair an earlier fracture which has set badly, or to correct a deformity

**diadochokinesis** /daɪˌædəkəukaɪˈniːsɪs/ *noun* the natural ability to make muscles move limbs in opposite directions

**diagnose** /ˈdaɪəgnəuz/ *verb* to identify a condition or illness, by examining the person and noting symptoms ○ *The doctor diagnosed appendicitis.* ○ *The patient was diagnosed with rheumatism.*

**diagnosis** /ˌdaɪəgˈnəusɪs/ *noun* the act of diagnosing a condition or illness ○ *The doctor's diagnosis was a viral infection, but the child's parents asked for a second opinion.* ○ *They* *found it difficult to make a diagnosis.* Compare **prognosis** (NOTE: The plural is **diagnoses**.)

**diagnostic** /ˌdaɪəgˈnɒstɪk/ *adjective* referring to diagnosis

**diagnostic and treatment centre** /ˌdaɪəgnɒstɪk ən ˈtriːtmənt ˌsentə/ *noun* a facility mainly for day surgery or short-term stay, where a range of planned operations such as joint replacements, hernia repair and cataract removal can be undertaken. Abbr **DTC**

**diagnostic imaging** /ˌdaɪəgnɒstɪk ˈɪmɪdʒɪŋ/ *noun* scanning for the purpose of diagnosis, e.g. of a pregnant woman to see if the fetus is healthy

**diagnostic process** /ˌdaɪəgˌnɒstɪk ˈprəʊses/ *noun* the series of steps taken in making a diagnosis

**diagnostic radiographer** *noun* ♦ **radiographer**

**diagnostic test** /ˌdaɪəgnɒstɪk ˈtest/ *noun* a test which helps a doctor diagnose an illness

**dialysate** /daɪˈælɪsət/ *noun* material which is subjected to dialysis

**dialyse** /ˈdaɪəlaɪz/ *verb* to treat someone using a kidney machine

**dialyser** /ˈdaɪəlaɪzə/ *noun* an apparatus which uses a membrane to separate solids from liquids, e.g. a kidney machine

**dialysis** /daɪˈæləsɪs/ *noun* **1.** a procedure in which a membrane is used as a filter to separate soluble waste substances from the blood **2.** same as **renal dialysis**

**diapedesis** /ˌdaɪəpɪˈdiːsɪs/ *noun* the movement of white blood cells through the walls of the capillaries into tissues in the development of inflammation

**diaphoresis** /ˌdaɪəfəˈriːsɪs/ *noun* excessive perspiration

**diaphoretic** /ˌdaɪəfəˈretɪk/ *noun* a drug which causes sweating ■ *adjective* causing sweating

**diaphragm** /ˈdaɪəfræm/ *noun* **1.** a thin layer of tissue stretched across an opening, especially the flexible sheet of muscle and fibre which separates the chest from the abdomen and moves to pull air into the lungs in respiration **2.** same as **vaginal diaphragm**

COMMENT: The diaphragm is a muscle which, in breathing, expands and contracts with the walls of the chest. The average rate of respiration is about 16 times a minute.

**diaphragmatic** /ˌdaɪəfrægˈmætɪk/ *adjective* referring to a diaphragm, or like a diaphragm

**diaphragmatic hernia** /ˌdaɪəfrægmætɪk ˈhɜːniə/ *noun* a condition in which a membrane and organ in the abdomen pass through an opening in the diaphragm into the chest

**diaphragmatic pleura** /ˌdaɪəfrægmætɪk ˈplʊərə/ *noun* part of the pleura which covers the diaphragm

**diaphragmatic pleurisy** /ˌdaɪəfrægmætɪk ˈplʊərɪsi/ *noun* inflammation of the pleura which covers the diaphragm

**diaphyseal** /ˌdaɪəˈfɪziəl/ *adjective* referring to a diaphysis

**diaphysis** /daɪˈæfəsɪs/ *noun* the long central part of a long bone. Also called **shaft**. See illustration at **BONE MARROW** in Supplement

**diaphysitis** /ˌdaɪəfəˈsaɪtɪs/ *noun* inflammation of the diaphysis, often associated with rheumatic disease

**diarrhoea** /ˌdaɪəˈriːə/ *noun* a condition in which someone frequently passes liquid faeces ○ *attack of diarrhoea* ○ *mild/severe diarrhoea* (NOTE: The US spelling is **diarrhea**.)

COMMENT: Diarrhoea can have many causes: types of food or allergy to food; contaminated or poisoned food; infectious diseases, such as dysentery; sometimes worry or other emotions.

**diarrhoeal** /ˌdaɪəˈriːəl/ *adjective* referring to or caused by diarrhoea

**diarthrosis** /ˌdaɪɑːˈθrəʊsɪs/ *noun* same as **synovial joint**

**diastase** /ˈdaɪəsteɪz/ *noun* an enzyme which breaks down starch and converts it into sugar

**diastasis** /ˌdaɪəˈsteɪsɪs/ *noun* **1.** a condition in which a bone separates into parts **2.** dislocation of bones at an immovable joint

**diastema** /ˌdaɪəˈstiːmə/ *noun* **1.** an unusually wide space between adjacent teeth **2.** an unusual gap in any body part or organ

**diastole** /daɪˈæstəli/ *noun* the part of the process involved in each beat of the heart when its chambers expand and fill with blood. The period of diastole (usually 95 mmHg) lasts about 0.4 seconds in an average heart rate. Compare **systole**

**diastolic** /ˌdaɪəˈstɒlɪk/ *adjective* relating to the diastole

**diastolic pressure** /ˌdaɪəstɒlɪk ˈpreʃə/ *noun* blood pressure taken at the diastole (NOTE: Diastolic pressure is always lower than systolic.)

**diathermy** /ˌdaɪəˈθɜːmi/ *noun* the use of high-frequency electric current to produce heat in body tissue

COMMENT: The difference between medical and surgical uses of diathermy is in the size of the electrodes used. Two large electrodes will give a warming effect over a large area (**medical diathermy**); if one of the electrodes is small, the heat will be concentrated enough to coagulate tissue (**surgical diathermy**).

**diathermy knife** /ˌdaɪəˈθɜːmi naɪf/ *noun* a knife used in surgical diathermy

**diathermy needle** /daɪəˌθɜːmi ˈniːd(ə)l/ *noun* a needle used in surgical diathermy

**diathermy snare** /ˌdaɪəˈθɜːmi sneə/ *noun* a snare which is heated by electrodes and burns away tissue

**diathesis** /daɪˈæθəsɪs/ *noun* the general inherited constitution of a person in relation to their susceptibility to specific diseases or allergies

**diazepam** /daɪˈæzəpæm/ *noun* a tranquilliser used in the short term to treat anxiety and as a muscle relaxant. In the long term it is potentially addictive.

**diazoxide** /ˌdaɪəˈzɒksaɪd/ *noun* a drug used as a vasodilator, to reduce hypertension

**DIC** *abbr* disseminated intravascular coagulation

**dicephalus** /daɪˈsefələs/ *noun* a fetus with two heads

**dichlorphenamide** /ˌdaɪklɔːˈfenəmaɪd/ *noun* a drug used to treat glaucoma

**dichromatism** /ˌdaɪkrəʊˈmætɪz(ə)m/ *noun* colour blindness in which only two of the three primary colours can be seen. Compare **monochromatism, trichromatism**

**diclofenac sodium** /ˌdaɪkləʊfenæk ˈsəʊdiəm/ *noun* an anti-inflammatory drug used to treat rheumatic disease

**dicrotic pulse** /daɪˌkrɒtɪk ˈpʌls/, **dicrotic wave** /daɪˌkrɒtɪk ˈweɪv/ *noun* a pulse which occurs twice with each heartbeat

**dicrotism** /ˈdaɪkrətɪz(ə)m/ *noun* a condition in which the pulse occurs twice with each heartbeat

**die** /daɪ/ *verb* to stop living ○ *His father died last year.* ○ *She died in a car crash.* (NOTE: **dying – died**)

**diencephalon** /ˌdaɪenˈsefələn, ˌdaɪenˈkefəlɒn/ *noun* the central part of the forebrain, formed of the thalamus, hypothalamus, pineal gland and third ventricle

**diet** /ˈdaɪət/ *noun* the amount and type of food eaten ○ *a balanced diet* ■ *verb* to reduce the quantity of food you eat, or to change the type of food you eat, in order to become thinner or healthier ○ *He is dieting to try to lose weight.*

**dietary** /ˈdaɪət(ə)ri/ *noun* a system of nutrition and energy ○ *The nutritionist supervised the dietaries for the patients.* ■ *adjective* referring to a diet

**dietary fibre** /ˈdaɪət(ə)ri ˌfaɪbə/ *noun* fibrous matter in food, which cannot be digested. Also called **roughage**

> COMMENT: Dietary fibre is found in cereals, nuts, fruit and some green vegetables. There are two types of fibre in food: insoluble fibre, e.g. in bread and cereals, which is not digested, and soluble fibre, e.g. in vegetables and pulses. Foods with the highest proportion of fibre include wholemeal bread, beans and dried apricots. Fibre is thought to be necessary to help digestion and avoid developing constipation, obesity and appendicitis.

**dietetic** /ˌdaɪəˈtetɪk/ *adjective* referring to diets

**dietetic principles** /ˌdaɪətetɪk ˈprɪnsəp(ə)lz/ *noun* rules concerning the body's needs in food, vitamins or trace elements

**dietetics** /ˌdaɪəˈtetɪks/ *noun* the study of food, nutrition and health, especially when applied to people's food intake

**dieting** /ˈdaɪətɪŋ/ *noun* the act of attempting to reduce weight by reducing the amount of food eaten ○ *Eat sensibly and get plenty of exercise, then there should be no need for dieting.*

**dietitian** /ˌdaɪəˈtɪʃ(ə)n/ *noun* someone who specialises in the study of diet, especially someone in a hospital who supervises dietaries as part of the medical treatment of patients. ◊ **nutritionist**

**Dietl's crisis** /ˈdiːt(ə)lz ˌkraɪsɪs/ *noun* a painful blockage of the ureter, causing back pressure on the kidney which fills with urine and swells [After Joseph Dietl (1804–78), Polish physician]

**diet sheet** /ˈdaɪət ʃiːt/ *noun* a list of suggestions for quantities and types of food given to someone to follow

**differential** /ˌdɪfəˈrenʃəl/ *adjective* referring to a difference

**differential blood count** /ˌdɪfərenʃəl ˈblʌd ˌkaʊnt/, **differential white cell count** /ˌdɪfərenʃəl ˈwaɪt sel ˌkaʊnt/ *noun* a test that shows the amounts of different types of white blood cell in a blood sample

**differential diagnosis** /ˌdɪfəˌrenʃ(ə)l ˌdaɪəgˈnəʊsɪs/ *noun* the identification of one disease from a number of other similar diseases by comparing the range of symptoms of each

**differentiation** /ˌdɪfərenʃiˈeɪʃ(ə)n/ *noun* the development of specialised cells during the early embryo stage

**diffuse** *verb* /dɪˈfjuːz/ to spread through tissue, or cause something to spread ○ *Some substances easily diffuse through the walls of capillaries.* ■ *adjective* /dɪˈfjuːs/ referring to a disease which is widespread in the body, or which affects many organs or cells

**diffusion** /dɪˈfjuːʒ(ə)n/ *noun* **1.** the process of mixing a liquid with another liquid, or a gas with another gas **2.** the passing of a liquid or gas through a membrane

**digest** /daɪˈdʒest/ *verb* to break down food in the alimentary canal and convert it into components which are absorbed into the body

**digestible** /daɪˈdʒestɪb(ə)l/ *adjective* able to be digested ○ *Glucose is an easily digestible form of sugar.*

**digestion** /daɪˈdʒestʃən/ *noun* the process by which food is broken down in the alimentary canal into components which can be absorbed by the body

**digestive** /daɪˈdʒestɪv/ *adjective* relating to digestion

**digestive enzyme** /daɪˌdʒestɪv ˈenzaɪm/ *noun* an enzyme which encourages digestion

**digestive juice** /daɪˈdʒestɪv juːs/ *noun* ♦ gastric juice, intestinal juice (*usually plural*)

**digestive system** /daɪˈdʒestɪv ˌsɪstəm/ *noun* the set of organs such as the stomach, liver and pancreas which are associated with the digestion of food. Also called **alimentary system**

**digestive tract** /daɪˈdʒestɪv trækt/ *noun* same as **alimentary canal**

**digestive tube** /daɪˈdʒestɪv tjuːb/ *adjective US* same as **alimentary canal**

**digit** /ˈdɪdʒɪt/ *noun* **1.** a finger or a toe **2.** a number

**digital** /ˈdɪdʒɪt(ə)l/ *adjective* **1.** referring to fingers or toes **2.** representing data or physical quantities in numerical form

**digitalin** /ˌdɪdʒɪˈteɪlɪn/, **digitalis** /ˌdɪdʒɪˈteɪlɪs/ *noun* a drug derived from foxglove leaves, used in small doses to treat heart conditions

**digitalise** /ˈdɪdʒɪtəlaɪz/, **digitalize** *verb* to treat someone who has heart failure with digoxin

**digital palpation** /ˌdɪdʒɪt(ə)l pælˈpeɪʃ(ə)n/ *noun* an examination of part of the body by feeling it with the fingers

**digital vein** /ˈdɪdʒɪt(ə)l veɪn/ *noun* a vein draining the fingers or toes

**digitoxin** /ˌdɪdʒɪˈtɒksɪn/ *noun* an extract of foxglove leaves, used as a drug to stimulate the heart in cases of heart failure or irregular heartbeat

**digoxin** /daɪˈdʒɒksɪn/ *noun* an extract of foxglove leaves, which acts more rapidly than digitoxin when used as a heart stimulant

**dihydrocodeine tartrate** /daɪˌhaɪdrəʊ ˌkəʊdiːn ˈtɑːtreɪt/ *noun* an analgesic used to treat severe pain

**dilatation** /ˌdaɪleɪˈteɪʃ(ə)n/, **dilation** /daɪ ˈleɪʃ(ə)n/ *noun* **1.** the act of making a hollow space or a passage in the body bigger or wider ○ *dilatation of the cervix during labour* **2.** expansion of the pupil of the eye as a reaction to bad light or to drugs

**dilatation and curettage** /daɪleɪˌteɪʃ(ə)n ən kjʊəˈretɪdʒ/ *noun* a surgical operation to scrape the interior of the uterus to obtain a tissue sample or to remove products of miscarriage. Abbr **D & C**

**dilate** /daɪˈleɪt, dɪˈleɪt/ *verb* to become wider or larger, or make something become wider or larger ○ *The veins in the left leg have become dilated.* ○ *The drug is used to dilate the pupil of the eye.*

**dilator** /daɪˈleɪtə/ *noun* **1.** an instrument used to widen the entrance to a cavity **2.** a drug used to make part of the body expand

**dilator pupillae muscle** /daɪˌleɪtə pjuːˈpɪli: ˌmʌs(ə)l/ *noun* a muscle in the iris which pulls the iris back and so makes the pupil expand

**diltiazem hydrochloride** /dɪlˌtaɪəzəm ˌhaɪdrəˈklɔːraɪd/ *noun* a calcium channel blocker used to treat hypertension

**diluent** /ˈdɪljuənt/ *noun* a substance which is used to dilute a liquid, e.g. water

**dilute** /daɪˈluːt/ *adjective* with water added ■ *verb* to add water to a liquid to make it less concentrated ○ *Dilute the disinfectant in four parts of water.*

**dilution** /daɪˈluːʃ(ə)n/ *noun* **1.** the action of diluting **2.** a liquid which has been diluted

**dimenhydrinate** /ˌdaɪmenˈhaɪdrəneɪt/ *noun* an antihistamine drug that relieves travel sickness

**dimetria** /daɪˈmiːtriə/ *noun* a condition in which a woman has a double uterus

**dioptre** /daɪˈɒptə/ *noun* a unit of measurement of the refraction of a lens (NOTE: The US spelling is **diopter**.)

COMMENT: A one dioptre lens has a focal length of one metre; the greater the dioptre, the shorter the focal length.

**dioxide** /daɪˈɒksaɪd/ ♦ **carbon dioxide**

**dioxin** /daɪˈɒksɪn/ *noun* an extremely poisonous gas

**DIP** *abbr* distal interphalangeal joint

**diphenoxalate** /ˌdaɪfenˈɒksɪleɪt/ *noun* a drug related to pethidine that is used to treat diarrhoea, sometimes mixed with a little atropine in commercial preparations

**diphtheria** /dɪfˈθɪəriə/ *noun* a serious infectious disease of children, caused by the bacillus *Corynebacterium diphtheriae*, characterised by fever and the formation of a fibrous growth like a membrane in the throat which restricts breathing

COMMENT: Symptoms of diphtheria are a sore throat, followed by a slight fever, rapid pulse and swelling of glands in the neck. The 'membrane' which forms can close the air passages, and the disease is often fatal, either because the patient is asphyxiated or because the heart becomes fatally weakened. The disease is also highly infectious, and all contacts of the patient must be tested. The Schick test is used to test if a person is immune or susceptible to diphtheria. In countries where infants are immunised the disease is rare.

**diphtheroid** /ˈdɪfθərɔɪd/ *adjective* referring to a bacterium similar to the diphtheria bacterium

**-dipine** /dɪpɪn/ *suffix* used in the names of calcium channel blockers ○ *nifedipine*

**dipl-** /dɪpl/ *prefix* same as **diplo-** (*used before vowels*)

**diplacusis** /ˌdɪpləˈkjuːsɪs/ *noun* a disorder of the cochlea in which a person hears one sound as two sounds of different pitch

**diplegia** /daɪˈpliːdʒə/ *noun* paralysis of a similar part on both sides of the body, e.g. paralysis of both arms. Compare **hemiplegia**

**diplegic** /daɪˈpliːdʒɪk/ *adjective* referring to diplegia

**diplo-** /ˈdɪpləʊ/ *prefix* double

**diplococcus** /ˌdɪpləʊˈkɒkəs/ *noun* a bacterium which usually occurs in pairs as a result of incomplete cell division, e.g. a pneumococcus (NOTE: The plural is **diplococci.**)

**diploe** /ˈdɪpləʊiː/ *noun* a layer of spongy bone tissue filled with red bone marrow, between the inner and outer layers of the skull

**diploid** /ˈdɪplɔɪd/ *adjective* referring to a cell where there are two copies of each chromosome, except the sex chromosome. In humans the diploid number of chromosomes is 46.

**diplopia** /dɪˈpləʊpiə/ *noun* a condition in which someone sees single objects as double. Also called **double vision**

**dipsomania** /ˌdɪpsəʊˈmeɪniə/ *noun* an uncontrollable desire to drink alcohol

**direct contact** /dɪˌrekt ˈkɒntækt/ *noun* a situation where someone or something physically touches an infected person or object

**directions** /daɪˈrekʃənz/ *noun* □ **directions for use** (*on a bottle of medicine, etc.*) instructions showing how to use something and how much of it to use

**director** /daɪˈrektə/ *noun* an instrument used to limit the incision made with a surgical knife

**dis-** /dɪs/ *prefix* **1.** undoing or reversal **2.** removal from **3.** lacking or deprived of

**disability** /ˌdɪsəˈbɪlɪti/ *noun* a condition in which part of the body does not function in the usual way and makes some activities difficult or impossible. ◊ **learning disability**

'…disability – any restriction or lack (resulting from an impairment) of ability to perform an activity in the manner or within the range considered normal for a human being' [WHO]

**disable** /dɪsˈeɪb(ə)l/ *verb* to make someone unable to do some activity ○ *He was disabled by a lung disease.*

**disabled** /dɪsˈeɪb(ə)ld/ *noun* people suffering from a physical or mental condition which makes some activities difficult or impossible

**Disabled Living Foundation** /dɪsˌeɪb(ə)ld ˈlɪvɪŋ faʊnˌdeɪʃ(ə)n/ *noun* a charity which aims to help disabled people live independently

**disablement** /dɪsˈeɪb(ə)lmənt/ *noun* a condition which makes some activities difficult or impossible

**disabling disease** /dɪsˌeɪblɪŋ dɪˈziːz/ *noun* a disease which makes some activities difficult or impossible

**disarticulation** /ˌdɪsɑːtɪkjʊˈleɪʃ(ə)n/ *noun* the amputation of a limb at a joint, which does not involve dividing a bone

**disc** /dɪsk/ *noun* a flat round structure. ◊ **intervertebral disc**

**discharge** *noun* /ˈdɪstʃɑːdʒ/ **1.** the secretion of liquid from an opening **2.** the process of sending a patient away from a hospital because the treatment has ended ■ *verb* /dɪsˈtʃɑːdʒ/ **1.** to secrete liquid out of an opening ○ *The*

wound discharged a thin stream of pus. **2.** to send a patient away from hospital because the treatment has ended ○ *He was discharged from hospital last week.* □ **to discharge yourself** to decide to leave hospital and stop taking the treatment provided

**discharge planning** /ˈdɪstʃɑːdʒ ˌplænɪŋ/ *noun* the work of making a plan for when a patient leaves hospital to live at home

**discharge rate** /ˈdɪstʃɑːdʒ reɪt/ *noun* the number of patients with a particular type of disorder who are sent home from hospitals in a particular area (shown as the number per 10,000 of population)

**discoloration** /dɪsˌkʌləˈreɪʃ(ə)n/ *noun* a change in colour

**discolour** /dɪsˈkʌlə/ *verb* to change the colour of something ○ *His teeth were discoloured from smoking cigarettes.* (NOTE: The US spelling is **discolor.**)

COMMENT: Teeth can be discoloured in fluorosis. If the skin on the lips is discoloured it may indicate that the person has swallowed a poison.

**discomfort** /dɪsˈkʌmfət/ *noun* a feeling of mild pain ○ *You may experience some discomfort after the operation.*

**discrete** /dɪˈskriːt/ *adjective* separate, not joined together

**discrete rash** /dɪˌskriːt ˈræʃ/ *noun* a rash which is formed of many separate spots, which do not join together into one large red patch

**disease** /dɪˈziːz/ *noun* a condition that stops the body from functioning in the usual way ○ *an infectious disease* ○ *She is suffering from a very serious disease of the kidneys* or *from a serious kidney disease.* ○ *He is a specialist in occupational diseases.* (NOTE: The term **disease** is applied to all physical and mental reactions which make a person ill. Diseases with distinct characteristics have individual names. For other terms referring to disease, see words beginning with **path-**, **patho-**.)

**diseased** /dɪˈziːzd/ *adjective* affected by a disease ○ *The surgeon cut away the diseased tissue.*

**disfigure** /dɪsˈfɪgə/ *verb* to change someone's appearance so as to make it less pleasant to look at ○ *Her legs were disfigured by scars.*

**dish** /dɪʃ/ *noun* a shallow open container

**disinfect** /ˌdɪsɪnˈfekt/ *verb* to make the surface of something or somewhere free from microorganisms ○ *She disinfected the skin with surgical spirit.* ○ *All the patient's clothes have to be disinfected.*

**disinfectant** /ˌdɪsɪnˈfektənt/ *noun* a substance used to kill microorganisms on the surface of something

**disinfection** /ˌdɪsɪnˈfekʃən/ *noun* the removal of microorganisms on the surface of something

COMMENT: The words **disinfect, disinfectant,** and **disinfection** are used for substances which destroy microorganisms on instruments, objects or the skin. Substances used to kill microorganisms inside infected people are **antibiotics.**

**disinfest** /ˌdɪsɪnˈfest/ *verb* to free a place, person or animal from insects or other pests

**disinfestation** /ˌdɪsɪnfeˈsteɪʃ(ə)n/ *noun* the removal of insects or other pests from a place, person or animal

**dislocate** /ˈdɪsləkeɪt/ *verb* to displace a bone from its usual position at a joint, or to become displaced ○ *He fell and dislocated his elbow.* ○ *The shoulder joint dislocates easily.*

**dislocation** /ˌdɪsləˈkeɪʃ(ə)n/ *noun* a condition in which a bone is displaced from its usual position at a joint. Also called **luxation**

**dismember** /dɪsˈmembə/ *verb* to cut off or pull off someone's arms or legs, often violently or in an accident

**dismemberment** /dɪsˈmembəmənt/ *noun* the state of being dismembered

**disorder** /dɪsˈɔːdə/ *noun* a condition in which part of the body is not functioning correctly ○ *The doctor specialises in disorders of the kidneys* or *in kidney disorders.*

**disordered** /dɪsˈɔːdəd/ *adjective* not functioning correctly

**disordered action of the heart** /dɪs,ɔːdəd ˈækʃən əv ðiː hɑːt/ *noun* a condition in which someone has palpitations, breathlessness and dizziness, caused by effort or worry. Also called **da Costa's syndrome, cardiac neurosis.** Abbr **DAH**

**disorientated** /dɪsˈɔːriən,teɪtɪd/ *adjective* referring to someone who is confused and does not know where he or she is

**disorientation** /ˌdɪsɔːriənˈteɪʃ(ə)n/ *noun* a condition in which someone is confused and does not know where he or she is

**dispensary** /dɪˈspensəri/ *noun* a place where drugs are prepared or mixed and given out according to a doctor's prescription, e.g. part of a chemist's shop or a department in a hospital

**dispense** /dɪˈspens/ *verb* to supply medicine according to a prescription

**dispenser** /dɪˈspensə/ *noun* someone who supplies medicine according to a prescription, especially in a hospital

**dispensing optician** /dɪˈspensɪŋ ɒp,tɪʃ(ə)n/ *noun* a person who fits and sells glasses but does not test eyes

**dispensing practice** /dɪˈspensɪŋ ,præktɪs/ *noun* a doctor's practice which dispenses prescribed medicines to its patients

**displace** /dɪsˈpleɪs/ *verb* to put something out of its usual place

**displaced intervertebral disc** /dɪs,pleɪsd ɪntə,vɜːtɪbr(ə)l ˈdɪsk/ *noun* a disc which has moved slightly, so that the soft interior passes through the tougher exterior and causes pressure on a nerve

**displacement** /dɪsˈpleɪsmənt/ *noun* the fact of being moved out of the usual position ○ *fracture of the radius together with displacement of the wrist*

**disposable** /dɪˈspəʊzəb(ə)l/ *adjective* designed to be thrown away after use ○ *disposable syringes*

**disposition** /ˌdɪspəˈzɪʃ(ə)n/ *noun* a person's general character or tendency to act in a particular way

**disproportion** /ˌdɪsprəˈpɔːʃ(ə)n/ *noun* a lack of proper relationships between two things

**dissecans** /ˈdɪsəkænz/ **♦ osteochondritis dissecans**

**dissect** /daɪˈsekt/ *verb* to cut and separate tissues in a body to examine them

**dissecting aneurysm** /ˌdaɪsektɪŋ ˈænjə,rɪz(ə)m/ *noun* an aneurysm which occurs when the inside wall of the aorta is torn and blood enters the membrane

**dissection** /daɪˈsekʃən/ *noun* the action of cutting and separating parts of a body or an organ as part of a surgical operation, an autopsy or a course of study

'…renal dissection usually takes from 40–60 minutes, while liver and pancreas dissections take from one to three hours. Cardiac dissection takes about 20 minutes and lung dissection takes 60 to 90 minutes.' [*Nursing Times*]

**disseminated** /dɪˈsemɪneɪtɪd/ *adjective* occurring in every part of an organ or in the whole body

**disseminated intravascular coagulation** /dɪ,semɪneɪtɪd ɪntrə,væskʊlə kəʊ,ægjʊˈleɪʃ(ə)n/ *noun* a disorder that causes extensive clot formation in the blood vessels, followed by severe bleeding. Abbr **DIC**

**disseminated lupus erythematosus** /dɪ,semɪneɪtd ,luːpəs ,erɪθiːməˈtəʊsɪs/ *noun* an inflammatory disease where a skin rash is associated with widespread changes in the central nervous system, the cardiovascular system and many organs. Abbr **DLE**

**disseminated sclerosis** /dɪ,semɪneɪtd skləˈrəʊsɪs/ *noun* same as **multiple sclerosis**

**dissemination** /dɪ,semɪˈneɪʃ(ə)n/ *noun* the fact of being widespread throughout the body

**dissociate** /dɪˈsəʊsieɪt/ *verb* **1.** to separate parts or functions **2.** in psychiatry, to separate part of the conscious mind from the rest

**dissociated anaesthesia** /dɪ,səʊsi,eɪtɪd ,ænəsˈθiːziə/ *noun* a loss of sensitivity to heat, pain or cold

**dissociation** /dɪ,səʊʃiˈeɪʃ(ə)n/ *noun* **1.** the separation of parts or functions **2.** (*in psychiatry*) a condition in which part of the consciousness becomes separated from the rest and becomes independent

**dissociative disorder** /dɪˈsəʊsiətɪv dɪs
ˌɔːdə/ *noun* a type of hysteria in which someone shows psychological changes such as a
split personality or amnesia rather than physical ones

**dissolve** /dɪˈzɒlv/ *verb* to absorb or disperse
something in liquid ○ *The gut used in sutures
slowly dissolves in the body fluids.*

**distal** /ˈdɪst(ə)l/ *adjective* further away from
the centre of a body

**distal convoluted tubule** /ˌdɪst(ə)l
ˌkɒnvəluːtɪd ˈtjuːbjuːl/ *noun* a part of the
kidney filtering system before the collecting
ducts

**Distalgesic** /ˌdɪst(ə)lˈdʒiːzɪk/ a trade name
for the analgesic co-proxamol

**distal interphalangeal joint** /ˌdɪst(ə)l
ˌɪntəfəˈlændʒiəl ˌdʒɔɪnt/ *noun* a joint nearest
the end of the finger or toe. Abbr **DIP**

**distally** /ˈdɪst(ə)li/ *adverb* placed further
away from the centre or point of attachment.
Opposite **proximally.** See illustration at **ANA-
TOMICAL TERMS** in Supplement

**distal phalanges** /ˌdɪst(ə)l fəˈlændʒiːz/
*noun* bones nearest the ends of the fingers and
toes

**distended** /dɪˈstendɪd/ *adjective* made larger
by gas such as air, by liquid such as urine, or
by a solid

**distended bladder** /dɪˌstendɪd ˈblædə/
*noun* a bladder which is full of urine

**distension** /dɪsˈtenʃən/ *noun* a condition in
which something is swollen ○ *Distension of
the veins in the abdomen is a sign of blocking
of the portal vein.*

**distichiasis** /ˌdɪstɪˈkaɪəsɪs/ *noun* the presence of extra eyelashes, sometimes growing on
the meibomian glands

**distil** /dɪˈstɪl/ *verb* to separate the component
parts of a liquid by boiling and collecting the
condensed vapour

**distillation** /ˌdɪstɪˈleɪʃ(ə)n/ *noun* the action
of distilling a liquid

**distilled water** /dɪˌstɪld ˈwɔːtə/ *noun* water
which has had impurities by distillation

**distort** /dɪˈstɔːt/ *verb* to twist something into
an unusual shape ○ *His lower limbs were distorted by the disease.*

**distortion** /dɪˈstɔːʃ(ə)n/ *noun* the act of
twisting part of the body out of its usual shape

**distraction** /dɪˈstrækʃən/ *noun* 1. something
that takes a person's attention away from
something else 2. a state where someone is
very emotionally and mentally troubled

**distress** /dɪˈstres/ *noun* unhappiness caused
by pain or worry ○ *mental distress*

**district general hospital** /ˌdɪstrɪkt
ˌdʒen(ə)rəl ˈhɒspɪt(ə)l/ *noun* a hospital
which serves the needs of the population of a
specific district

**district nurse** /ˌdɪstrɪkt ˈnɜːs/ *noun* a nurse
who visits and treats people in their homes

**disturb** /dɪˈstɜːb/ *verb* 1. to interrupt what
someone is doing ○ *Her sleep was disturbed
by the other patients in the ward.* 2. to upset or
worry someone

**disturbed** /dɪˈstɜːbd/ *adjective* affected by a
psychiatric disorder ○ *severely disturbed children*

**disulfiram** /daɪˈsʌlfɪræm/ *noun* a drug used
to treat alcoholism by causing severe nausea if
alcohol is consumed with it

**dithranol** /ˈdɪθrənɒl/ *noun* an anti-inflammatory drug used to treat dermatitis and psoriasis

**diuresis** /ˌdaɪjʊˈriːsɪs/ *noun* an increase in
the production of urine

**diuretic** /ˌdaɪjʊˈretɪk/ *adjective* causing the
kidneys to produce more urine ■ *noun* a substance which makes the kidneys produce more
urine and, in the treatment of oedema and hypertension

**diurnal** /daɪˈɜːn(ə)l/ *adjective* 1. happening in
the daytime 2. happening every day

**divarication** /daɪˌværɪˈkeɪʃ(ə)n/ *noun* 1.
separation into widely spread branches 2. the
point at which a structure forks or divides

**divergence** /daɪˈvɜːdʒəns/ *noun* 1. a condition in which one eye points directly at the object of interest but the other does not 2. the
process of moving apart to follow different
courses 3. the amount of difference between
two quantities, especially where the difference
is unexpected 4. a deviation from a typical behaviour pattern or expressed wish

**divergent strabismus** /daɪˌvɜːdʒənt strə
ˈbɪzməs/, **divergent squint** /daɪˌvɜːdʒənt
ˈskwɪnt/ *noun* a condition in which a person's
eyes both look away from the nose. Opposite
**convergent strabismus**

**diverticula** /ˌdaɪvəˈtɪkjʊlə/ plural of **diverticulum**

**diverticular disease** /ˌdaɪvəˈtɪkjʊlə dɪ
ˌziːz/ *noun* a disease of the large intestine,
where the colon thickens and diverticula form
in the walls, causing pain in the lower abdomen

**diverticulitis** /ˌdaɪvətɪkjʊˈlaɪtɪs/ *noun* inflammation of diverticula formed in the wall of
the colon

**diverticulosis** /ˌdaɪvətɪkjʊˈləʊsɪs/ *noun* a
condition in which diverticula form in the intestine but are not inflamed. In the small intestine, this can lead to blind loop syndrome.

**diverticulum** /ˌdaɪvəˈtɪkjʊləm/ *noun* a little
sac or pouch which develops in the wall of the
intestine or another organ (NOTE: The plural is
**diverticula.**)

**division** /dɪˈvɪʒ(ə)n/ *noun* the action of cutting or splitting into parts

**divulsor** /dɪˈvʌlsə/ *noun* a surgical instrument used to expand a passage in the body

**dizygotic** /ˌdaɪzaɪˈɡɒtɪk/ *adjective* developed from two separately fertilised eggs

**dizygotic twins** /ˌdaɪzaɪɡɒtɪk ˈtwɪnz/ *plural noun* twins who are not identical and not always of the same sex because they come from two different ova fertilised at the same time. Also called **fraternal twins**

**dizziness** /ˈdɪzinəs/ *noun* the feeling that everything is going round because the sense of balance has been affected

**dizzy** /ˈdɪzi/ *adjective* feeling that everything is going round because the sense of balance has been affected ○ *The ear infection made her feel dizzy for some time afterwards.* ○ *He experiences dizzy spells.*

**dl** *abbr* decilitre

**DLE** *abbr* disseminated lupus erythematosus

**dm** *abbr* decimetre

**DMD** *abbr US* doctor of dental medicine

**DNA** /ˌdi: en ˈeɪ/ *noun* one of the nucleic acids, the basic genetic material present in the nucleus of each cel. Full form **deoxyribonucleic acid**

**DNA fingerprint** /ˌdi: en eɪ ˈfɪŋɡəprɪnt/ *noun* same as **genetic fingerprint**

**DNA fingerprinting** /ˌdi: en eɪ ˈfɪŋɡə ˌprɪntɪŋ/ *noun* same as **genetic fingerprinting**

**DNR** *abbr* do not resuscitate

**DOA** *abbr* dead on arrival

**dobutamine** /dəʊˈbjuːtəmiːn/ *noun* a drug used to stimulate the heart

**doctor** /ˈdɒktə/ *noun* **1.** a person who has trained in medicine and is qualified to examine people when they are ill to find out what is wrong with them and to prescribe a course of treatment **2.** a title given to a qualified person who is registered with the General Medical Council (NOTE: **Doctor** is shortened to **Dr** when written before a name.)

COMMENT: In the UK surgeons are traditionally not called 'Doctor', but are addressed as 'Mr', 'Mrs', etc. The title 'doctor' is also applied to persons who have a higher degree from a university in a non-medical subject. So 'Dr Jones' may have a degree in music, or in any other subject without a connection with medicine.

**doctor-assisted suicide** /ˌdɒktə əˌsɪstɪd ˈsuːɪsaɪd/ *noun* the suicide of someone with an incurable disease carried out with the help of a doctor (NOTE: Doctor-assisted suicide is illegal in most countries.)

**Döderlein's bacillus** /ˈdɜːdəlaɪnz bə ˌsɪlʌs/ *noun* a bacterium usually found in the vagina [After Albert Siegmund Gustav Döderlein (1860–1941), German obstetrician and gynaecologist]

**dolicho-** /dɒlɪkəʊ/ *prefix* long

**dolichocephalic** /ˌdɒlɪkəʊseˈfælɪk/ *adjective* referring to a person with an unusually long skull

**dolichocephaly** /ˌdɒlɪkəʊˈsefəli/ *noun* a condition of a person who has a skull which is

longer than usual, the measurement across the skull being less than 75% of the length of the head from front to back

**dolor** /ˈdɒlə/ *noun* pain

**dolorimetry** /ˌdɒləˈrɪmətri/ *noun* the measurement of pain

**dolorosa** /ˌdɒləˈrəʊsə/ ♦ **adiposis dolorosa**

**domiciliary** /ˌdɒmɪˈsɪliəri/ *adjective* at home or in the home

**domiciliary care** /ˌdɒmɪˈsɪliəri keə/ *noun* personal, domestic, or nursing care provided at home for people who need it

**domiciliary midwife** /ˌdɒmɪsɪliəri ˈmɪdwaɪf/ *noun* a nurse with special qualification in midwifery, who can assist in childbirth at home

**domiciliary services** /ˌdɒmɪˈsɪliəri ˌsɜːvɪ sɪz/ *plural noun* nursing services which are available to people in their homes

**domiciliary visit** /ˌdɒmɪsɪliəri ˈvɪzɪt/ *noun* a visit to the patient's home

**dominance** /ˈdɒmɪnəns/ *noun* the characteristic of a gene form (**allele**) that leads to the trait which it controls being shown in any individual carrying it

**dominant** /ˈdɒmɪnənt/ *adjective* important or powerful ■ *noun* (*of an allele*) having the characteristic that leads to the trait which it controls being shown in any individual carrying it. Compare **recessive**

COMMENT: Since each physical trait is governed by two genes, if one is recessive and the other dominant, the resulting trait will be that of the dominant gene.

**domino booking** /ˈdɒmɪnəʊ ˌbʊkɪŋ/ *noun* an arrangement for the delivery of a baby, where the baby is delivered in hospital by a midwife and the mother and child return home soon afterwards

**Donald-Fothergill operation** /ˌdɒnəld ˈfɒðəɡɪl ɒpəˌreɪʃ(ə)n/ *noun* an operation to close the neck of the vagina

**donate** /dəʊˈneɪt/ *verb* to agree to give blood, tissue, organs, or reproductive material to be used to treat another person

**donor** /ˈdəʊnə/ *noun* a person who gives blood, tissue, organs or reproductive material to be used to treat another person

**donor card** /ˈdəʊnə kɑːd/ *noun* a card carried by people stating that they give permission for their organs to be transplanted into other people after they have died

**donor insemination** /ˌdəʊnə ɪnsemɪ ˈneɪʃ(ə)n/ *noun* artificial insemination using the sperm of an anonymous donor. Abbr **DI**

**dopa** /ˈdəʊpə/ *noun* a chemical related to adrenaline and dopamine. It occurs naturally in the body and in the form levodopa is used to treat Parkinson's disease.

**dopamine** /ˈdəʊpəmiːn/ *noun* a substance found in the medulla of the adrenal glands, which also acts as a neurotransmitter. Lack of dopamine is associated with Parkinson's disease.

**dopaminergic** /ˌdəʊpəmɪˈnɜːdʒɪk/ *adjective* referring to a neurone or receptor stimulated by dopamine

**Doppler transducer** /ˈdɒplə trænzˌdjuːsə/ *noun* a device to measure blood flow, commonly used to monitor fetal heart rate

**Doppler ultrasound** /ˌdɒplə ˈʌltrəsaʊnd/ *noun* the use of the Doppler effect in ultrasound to detect red blood cells

**Doppler ultrasound flowmeter** /ˌdɒplə ˌʌltrəsaʊnd ˈfləʊmiːtə/ *noun* a device which measures the flow of blood and detects steady or irregular flow, allowing abnormalities or blockages to be detected

**dormant** /ˈdɔːmənt/ *adjective* inactive for a time ○ *The virus lies dormant in the body for several years.*

**dorsa** /ˈdɔːsə/ plural of **dorsum**

**dorsal** /ˈdɔːs(ə)l/ *adjective* **1.** referring to the back. Opposite **ventral 2.** referring to the back of the body

**dorsal vertebrae** /ˌdɔːs(ə)l ˈvɜːtɪbreɪ/ *plural noun* the twelve vertebrae in the back between the cervical vertebrae and the lumbar vertebrae

**dorsi-** /dɔːsi/ *prefix* referring to the back

**dorsiflexion** /ˌdɔːsɪˈflekʃən/ *noun* flexion towards the back of part of the body, e.g. raising the foot at the ankle. Compare **plantar flexion**

**dorso-** /dɔːsəʊ/ *prefix* same as **dorsi-**

**dorsoventral** /ˌdɔːsəʊˈventrəl/ *adjective* **1.** referring to both the front and the back of the body **2.** extending from the back of the body to the front

**dorsum** /ˈdɔːsəm/ *noun* the back of any part of the body (NOTE: The plural is **dorsa.**)

**dosage** /ˈdəʊsɪdʒ/ *noun* a measured quantity of a drug calculated to be necessary for someone ○ *a low dosage* ○ *The doctor decided to increase the dosage of antibiotics.* ○ *The dosage for children is half that for adults.*

**dose** /dəʊs/ *noun* **1.** a measured quantity of a drug or radiation which is to be given to someone at one time ○ *It is dangerous to exceed the prescribed dose.* **2.** a short period of experiencing a minor illness (*informal*) ○ *a dose of flu* **3.** an infection with a sexually transmitted disease (*informal*) ■ *verb* to provide someone with medication (*informal*) ○ *She has been dosing herself with laxatives.*

**dosimeter** /dəʊˈsɪmɪtə/ *noun* an instrument which measures the amount of X-rays or other radiation received

**dosimetry** /dəʊˈsɪmətri/ *noun* the act of measuring the amount of X-rays or radiation received, using a dosimeter

**double-blind randomised controlled trial** /ˌdʌb(ə)l blaɪnd ˌrændəmaɪzd kənˌtrəʊld

ˈtraɪəl/ *noun* a trial used to test new treatments in which patients are randomly placed in either the treatment or the control group without either the patient or doctor knowing which group any particular patient is in

**double blind study** /ˌdʌb(ə)l ˈblaɪnd ˌstʌdi/ *noun* an investigation to test an intervention in which neither the patient nor the doctor knows if the patient is receiving active medication or a placebo

**double-jointed** /ˌdʌb(ə)l ˈdʒɔɪntɪd/ *adjective* able to bend joints to an unusual degree (*informal*)

**double pneumonia** /ˌdʌb(ə)l njuːˈməʊniə/ *noun* same as **bilateral pneumonia**

**double uterus** /ˌdʌb(ə)l ˈjuːt(ə)rəs/ *noun* a condition in which the uterus is divided into two sections by a membrane. Also called **uterus didelphys.** ◊ **dimetria**

**double vision** /ˌdʌb(ə)l ˈvɪʒ(ə)n/ *noun* same as **diplopia** (*informal*)

**douche** /duːʃ/ *noun* a liquid forced into the body to wash out a cavity, or a device used for washing out a cavity

**Douglas bag** /ˈdʌɡləs bæɡ/ *noun* a bag used for measuring the volume of air breathed out of the lungs

**Douglas' pouch** /ˈdʌɡləsɪz paʊtʃ/ *noun* the rectouterine peritoneal recess

**down below** /daʊn bɪˈləʊ/ *adverb* used to refer politely to the genital area (*informal*)

**Down's syndrome** /ˈdaʊnz ˌsɪndrəʊm/ *noun* a condition due to the existence of an extra copy of chromosome 21, in which a baby is born with slanting eyes, a wide face, speech difficulties and usually some degree of learning difficulty [Described 1866. After John Langdon Haydon Down (1828–96), British physician at Normansfield Hospital, Teddington, UK.]

**downstairs** /daʊnˈsteəz/ *adverb* used to refer politely to the genital area (*informal*)

**down there** /daʊn ðeə/ *adverb* used to refer politely to the genital area (*informal*)

**doxepin** /ˈdɒksɪpɪn/ *noun* a drug used as a sedative and antidepressant

**doxycycline** /ˌdɒksiˈsaɪkliːn/ *noun* a widely used antibiotic derived from tetracycline

**doze** /dəʊz/ *verb* to sleep lightly for a short time

**dozy** /ˈdəʊzi/ *adjective* sleepy ○ *These antihistamines can make you feel dozy.*

**DPT** *abbr* diphtheria, whooping cough, tetanus

**DPT vaccine** /ˌdiː piː ˈtiː ˌvæksiːn/, **DPT immunisation** /ˌdiː piː ˈtiː ɪmjʊnaɪˌzeɪʃ(ə)n/ *noun* a combined vaccine or immunisation against the three diseases, diphtheria, whooping cough and tetanus

**Dr** *abbr* doctor (NOTE: used when writing someone's name: *Dr Smith*)

**drachm** /dræm/ *noun* a measure used in pharmacy, equal to 3.8 g dry weight or 3.7 ml liquid measure

**dracontiasis** /ˌdrækɒnˈtaɪəsɪs/, **dracunculiasis** /drəˌkʌŋkjʊˈlaɪəsɪs/ *noun* a tropical disease caused by the guinea worm *Dracunculus medinensis* which enters the body from infected drinking water and forms blisters on the skin, frequently leading to secondary arthritis, fibrosis and cellulitis

**Dracunculus** /drəˈkʌŋkjʊləs/ *noun* a parasitic worm which enters the body and rises to the skin to form a blister. The infection frequently leads to secondary arthritis, fibrosis and cellulitis. Also called **guinea worm**

**dragee** /dræˈʒeɪ/ *noun* a sugar-coated tablet or pill

**drain** /dreɪn/ *noun* a tube to remove liquid from the body ■ *verb* to remove liquid from the body ○ *an operation to drain the sinus* ○ *They drained the pus from the abscess.*

**drainage** /ˈdreɪnɪdʒ/ *noun* the removal of liquid from the site of an operation or pus from an abscess by means of a tube or wick left in the body for a time

**drape** /dreɪp/ *noun* a thin material used to place over someone about to undergo surgery, leaving the operation site uncovered

**draw** /drɔː/ *verb* to drain a liquid such as blood, pus or water from a wound or incision

**drawn** /drɔːn/ *adjective* appearing tired and careworn, usually as a result of anxiety, grief or illness

**draw-sheet** /ˈdrɔː ʃiːt/ *noun* a sheet under a person in bed, folded so that it can be pulled out as it becomes soiled

**drepanocyte** /ˈdrepənəʊsaɪt/ *noun* same as **sickle cell**

**drepanocytosis** /ˌdrepənəʊsaɪˈtəʊsɪs/ *noun* same as **sickle-cell anaemia**

**dress** /dres/ *verb* 1. to put on clothes, or put clothes on someone 2. to clean a wound and put a covering over it ○ *Nurses dressed the wounds of the accident victims.*

**dresser** /ˈdresə/ *noun* someone who assists a surgeon during operations

**dressing** /ˈdresɪŋ/ *noun* a covering or bandage applied to a wound to protect it ○ *The patient's dressings need to be changed regularly.*

**dribble** /ˈdrɪb(ə)l/ *verb* to let liquid flow slowly out of an opening, especially saliva out of the mouth

**dribbling** /ˈdrɪblɪŋ/ *noun* 1. the act of letting saliva flow out of the mouth 2. same as **incontinence** (*informal*)

**drill** /drɪl/ *noun* a tool which rotates very rapidly to make a hole, especially a surgical instrument used in dentistry to remove caries ■ *verb* to make a hole with a drill ○ *A small hole is drilled in the skull.* ○ *The dentist drilled one of her molars.*

**Drinker respirator** /ˈdrɪŋkə ˌrespɪreɪtə/ *noun* a machine which encloses the whole of the body except the head, and in which air pressure is increased and decreased, so forcing the person to breathe in and out. Also called **iron lung**

**drip** /drɪp/ *noun* a system for introducing liquid slowly and continuously into the body, by which a bottle of liquid is held above a person and the fluid flows slowly down a tube into a needle in a vein or into the stomach ○ *After her operation, the patient was put on a drip.*

**drip feed** /ˈdrɪp fiːd/ *noun* a drip containing nutrients

**drop** /drɒp/ *noun* 1. a small quantity of liquid 2. a sudden reduction or fall in the quantity of something ○ *a drop in pressure* ■ *plural noun* **drops** liquid medicine for the eye, nose, or ear administered with a dropper ■ *verb* 1. to fall or let something fall ○ *Pressure in the artery dropped suddenly.* 2. to reduce suddenly

**drop attack** /ˈdrɒp əˌtæk/ *noun* a condition in which a person suddenly falls down, though he or she is not unconscious, caused by sudden weakness of the spine

**droperidol** /drɒˈperɪdɒl/ *noun* a drug used to keep someone in a calm state before an operation

**drop foot** /ˈdrɒp fʊt/ *noun* a condition, caused by a muscular disorder, in which the ankle is not strong and the foot hangs limp

**droplet** /ˈdrɒplət/ *noun* a very small quantity of liquid

**droplet infection** /ˈdrɒplət ɪnˌfekʃən/ *noun* an infection developed by inhaling droplets containing a virus, e.g. from a sneeze

**drop off** /ˌdrɒp ˈɒf/ *verb* (*informal*) 1. to fall asleep 2. to get less

**dropper** /ˈdrɒpə/ *noun* a small glass or plastic tube with a rubber bulb at one end, used to suck up and expel liquid in drops

**dropsy** /ˈdrɒpsi/ *noun* same as **oedema** (*dated*)

**drop wrist** /drɒp ˈrɪst/ *noun* a condition caused by a muscular disorder, in which the wrist is not strong and the hand hangs limp

**drown** /draʊn/ *verb* to die by inhaling liquid

**drowning** /ˈdraʊnɪŋ/ *noun* death as a result of inhaling liquid

**drowsiness** /ˈdraʊzinəs/ *noun* sleepiness ○ *The medicine is likely to cause drowsiness.*

**drowsy** /ˈdraʊzi/ *adjective* sleepy ○ *The injection will make you feel drowsy.*

**drug** /drʌg/ *noun* 1. a natural or synthetic chemical substance which is used in medicine and affects the way in which organs or tissues function ○ *She was prescribed a course of pain-killing drugs.* ○ *The drug is being monitored for possible side-effects.* 2. a substance taken by choice which produces a strong effect on a person's feelings and state of mind ○ *recreational drug* ○ *controlled drugs*

COMMENT: There are three classes of controlled drugs: **Class 'A' drugs** such as cocaine, heroin, crack and LSD; **Class 'B' drugs** such as amphetamines and codeine; and **Class 'C' drugs** such as cannabis and benzphetamine. The drugs are covered by five schedules under the Misuse of Drugs Regulations: **Schedule 1:** drugs which are not used medicinally, such as cannabis and LSD, for which possession and supply are prohibited. **Schedule 2:** drugs which can be used medicinally such as heroin, morphine, cocaine, and amphetamines: these are fully controlled as regards prescriptions by doctors, safe custody in pharmacies, registering of sales, etc. **Schedule 3:** barbiturates, which are controlled as regards prescriptions, but need not be kept in safe custody; **Schedule 4:** benzodiazepines, which are controlled as regards registers of purchasers; **Schedule 5:** other substances for which invoices showing purchasers; **Schedule 5:** other substances for which invoices showing purchase must be kept.

**drug abuse** /ˈdrʌg əˌbjuːs/ *noun* ♦ **substance abuse**

**drug abuser** /ˈdrʌg əˌbjuːzə/ *noun* a person who regularly uses drugs for non-medical purposes

**drug addict** /ˈdrʌg ˌædɪkt/ *noun* a person who is physically and mentally dependent on taking a particular drug regularly ○ *a heroin addict* ○ *a morphine addict*

**drug addiction** /ˈdrʌg əˌdɪkʃən/ *noun* the fact of being mentally and physically dependent on taking a particular drug regularly. Also called **drug dependence**

**drug allergy** /ˈdrʌg ˌælədʒi/ *noun* a reaction to a particular drug

**drug dependence** /ˈdrʌg dɪˌpendəns/ *noun* same as **drug addiction**

**drug-related** /ˈdrʌg rɪˌleɪtɪd/ *adjective* associated with the taking of drugs

**drug tolerance** /ˈdrʌg ˌtɒlərəns/ *noun* a condition in which a drug has been given to someone for so long that his or her body no longer reacts to it, and the dosage has to be increased

**drunk** /drʌŋk/ *adjective* intoxicated with too much alcohol

**dry** /draɪ/ *adjective* **1.** not wet ○ *The surface of the wound should be kept dry.* **2.** containing only a small amount of moisture ○ *She uses a cream to soften her dry skin.* (NOTE: **drier – driest**) ■ *verb* to remove moisture from something (NOTE: **dries – drying – dried**)

**dry beriberi** /ˌdraɪ beriˈberi/ *noun* beriberi associated with loss of feeling and paralysis

**dry burn** /ˌdraɪ ˈbɜːn/ *noun* an injury to the skin caused by touching a very hot dry surface

**dry drowning** /ˌdraɪ ˈdraʊnɪŋ/ *noun* death in which someone's air passage has been constricted by being under water, though he or she does not inhale any water

**dry-eye syndrome** /draɪ ˈaɪ ˌsɪndrəʊm/ *noun* same as **xerosis**

**dry gangrene** /ˌdraɪ ˈgæŋgriːn/ *noun* a condition in which the blood supply to a limb has been cut off and the tissue becomes black

**dry ice** /ˌdraɪ ˈaɪs/ *noun* solid carbon dioxide

**dryness** /ˈdraɪnəs/ *noun* the state of being dry ○ *dryness in the eyes, accompanied by rheumatoid arthritis* ○ *She complained of dryness in her mouth.*

**dry out** /ˌdraɪ ˈaʊt/ *verb* **1.** same as **dry 2. 2.** to treat someone for alcoholism, or undergo treatment for alcoholism (*informal*)

**dry socket** /draɪ ˈsɒkɪt/ *noun* inflammation of the socket of a tooth which has just been removed

**DTC** *abbr* diagnostic and treatment centre

**DTs** *abbr* delirium tremens

**Duchenne muscular dystrophy** /duːˌʃen ˌmʌskjʊlə ˈdɪstrəfi/, **Duchenne's muscular dystrophy** /duːˌʃenz ˌmʌskjʊlə ˈdɪstrəfi/, **Duchenne** /duːˈʃen/ *noun* an inherited form of muscular dystrophy that weakens the muscles of the upper respiratory and pelvic areas. It usually affects boys and causes early death. [Described 1849. After Guillaume Benjamin Arnaud Duchenne (1806–75), French neurologist.]

**Ducrey's bacillus** /duːˌkreɪz bəˈsɪləs/ *noun* a type of bacterium found in the lungs, causing chancroid [Described 1889. After Augusto Ducrey (1860–1940), Professor of Dermatology in Pisa, then Rome, Italy.]

**duct** /dʌkt/ *noun* a tube which carries liquids, especially one which carries secretions

**duct gland** /ˈdʌkt glænd/ *noun* same as **exocrine gland**

**ductless** /ˈdʌktləs/ *adjective* without a duct

**ductless gland** /ˌdʌktləs ˈglænd/ *noun* same as **endocrine gland**

**ductule** /ˈdʌktjuːl/ *noun* a very small duct

**ductus** /ˈdʌktəs/ *noun* same as **duct**

**ductus arteriosus** /ˌdʌktəs ɑːˌtɪəriˈəʊsəs/ *noun* in a fetus, the blood vessel connecting the left pulmonary artery to the aorta so that blood does not pass through the lungs

**ductus deferens** /ˌdʌktəs ˈdefərənz/ *noun* one of two tubes along which sperm pass from the epididymus to the seminal vesicles near the prostate gland. Also called **vas deferens**. See illustration at UROGENITAL SYSTEM (MALE) in Supplement

**ductus venosus** /ˌdʌktəs vɪˈnəʊsəs/ *noun* in a fetus, the blood vessel connecting the portal sinus to the inferior vena cava

**dull** /dʌl/ *adjective* referring to pain which is not strong but which is continuously present ○ *She complained of a dull throbbing pain in her head.* ○ *He felt a dull pain in the chest.* ■ *verb* to make a sensation or awareness of a sensation less sharp ○ *The treatment dulled the pain for a while.* ○ *The drug had dulled her senses.*

**dumb** /dʌm/ *adjective* not able to speak

**dumbness** /'dʌmnəs/ *noun* same as **mutism**

**dumping syndrome** /'dʌmpɪŋ ˌsɪndrəʊm/ *noun* same as **postgastrectomy syndrome**

**duo-** /djuːəʊ/ *prefix* two

**duoden-** /djuːəʊdiːn/ *prefix* referring to the duodenum

**duodenal** /ˌdjuːəʊ'diːn(ə)l/ *adjective* referring to the duodenum

**duodenal papillae** /djuːəʊˌdiːn(ə)l pə'pɪliː/ *plural noun* small projecting parts in the duodenum where the bile duct and pancreatic duct open

**duodenal ulcer** /djuːəʊˌdiːn(ə)l 'ʌlsə/ *noun* an ulcer in the duodenum

**duodenoscope** /ˌdjuːəʊ'diːnəʊskəʊp/ *noun* an instrument used to examine the inside of the duodenum

**duodenostomy** /ˌdjuːəʊdɪ'nɒstəmi/ *noun* a permanent opening made between the duodenum and the abdominal wall

**duodenum** /ˌdjuːə'diːnəm/ *noun* the first part of the small intestine, going from the stomach to the jejunum. See illustration at DIGESTIVE SYSTEM in Supplement

COMMENT: The duodenum is the shortest part of the small intestine, about 250 mm long. It takes bile from the gall bladder and pancreatic juice from the pancreas and continues the digestive processes started in the mouth and stomach.

**duplex imaging** /ˌdjuːpleks 'ɪmɪdʒɪŋ/ *noun* a type of ultrasonic imaging where the speed of the flow of blood is measured

**Dupuytren's contracture** /duːˌpwiːtrənz kən'træktʃə/ *noun* a condition in which the palmar fascia becomes thicker, causing the fingers, usually the middle and fourth fingers, to bend forwards [Described 1831. After Baron Guillaume Dupuytren (1775–1835), French surgeon.]

**dura** /'djʊərə/ *noun* same as **dura mater**

**dural** /'djʊər(ə)l/ *adjective* referring to the dura mater

**dura mater** /ˌdjʊərə 'meɪtə/ *noun* the thicker outer membrane of the three covering the brain. Also called **dura, pachymeninx.** ◊ **arachnoid**

**duty** /'djuːti/ *noun* the activities which a person has to do as part of their job ○ *What are the duties of a night sister?* (NOTE: The plural is **duties**.) □ **to be on duty** to be working ○ *She's on duty from 2 p.m. till 10 p.m.* □ **a duty of care** the requirement to treat a patient in an appropriate way, as part of the work of being a health professional

**duty nurse** /'djuːti nɜːs/ *noun* a nurse who is on duty

**duty rota** /'djuːti ˌrəʊtə/ *noun* a list of duties which have to be done and the names of the people who will do them

**d.v.t., DVT** *abbr* deep-vein thrombosis

**dwarfism** /'dwɔːfɪz(ə)m/ *noun* a condition in which the growth of a person has stopped, leaving him or her much smaller than average

COMMENT: Dwarfism may be caused by achondroplasia, where the long bones in the arms and legs do not develop fully but the trunk and head are of average size. Dwarfism can have other causes such as rickets or deficiency in the pituitary gland.

**dynamic splint** /daɪˌnæmɪk 'splɪnt/ *noun* a splint which uses springs to help the person move

**dynamometer** /ˌdaɪnə'mɒmɪtə/ *noun* an instrument for measuring the force of muscular contraction

**-dynia** /dɪniə/ *suffix* pain

**dys-** /dɪs/ *prefix* difficult or impaired

**dysaesthesia** /ˌdɪsiːs'θiːziə/ *noun* **1.** the impairment of a sense, in particular the sense of touch **2.** an unpleasant feeling of pain experienced when the skin is touched lightly

**dysarthria** /dɪs'ɑːθriə/, **dysarthrosis** /ˌdɪsɑː'θrəʊsɪs/ *noun* difficulty in speaking words clearly, caused by damage to the central nervous system

**dysbarism** /'dɪsbɑːrɪz(ə)m/ *noun* any disorder caused by differences between the atmospheric pressure outside the body and the pressure inside

**dysbasia** /dɪs'beɪziə/ *noun* difficulty in walking, especially when caused by a lesion to a nerve

**dyschezia** /dɪs'kiːziə/ *noun* difficulty in passing faeces

**dyschondroplasia** /ˌdɪskɒndrəʊ'pleɪziə/ *noun* a condition in which the long bones are shorter than usual

**dyschromatopsia** /ˌdɪskrəʊmə'tɒpsiə/ *noun* a condition where someone cannot distinguish colours

**dyscoria** /dɪs'kɔːriə/ *noun* **1.** an unusually shaped pupil of the eye **2.** an unusual reaction of the pupil

**dyscrasia** /dɪs'kreɪziə/ *noun* any unusual body condition (*dated*)

**dysdiadochokinesia** /ˌdɪsdaɪˌædəkəʊkaɪ'niːsiə/, **dysdiadochokinesis** /ˌdɪsdaɪˌædəkəʊkaɪ'niːsɪs/ *noun* the inability to carry out rapid movements, caused by a disorder or lesion of the cerebellum

**dysenteric** /ˌdɪsən'terɪk/ *adjective* referring to dysentery

**dysentery** /'dɪs(ə)ntri/ *noun* an infection and inflammation of the colon, causing bleeding and diarrhoea

COMMENT: Dysentery occurs mainly in tropical countries. The symptoms include diarrhoea, discharge of blood and pain in the intestines. There are two main types of dysentery: **bacillary dysentery**, caused by the bacterium *Shigella* in contaminated food, and **amoebic dysentery** or amoebiasis, caused by a parasitic amoeba *Entamoeba histolytica* spread through contaminated drinking water.

**dysfunction** /dɪsˈfʌŋkʃən/ *noun* an unusual functioning of an organ

**dysfunctional** /dɪsˈfʌŋkʃən(ə)l/ *adjective* **1.** not working properly **2.** unable to relate to other people emotionally or socially

**dysfunctional uterine bleeding** /dɪs ˌfʌŋkʃən(ə)l ˌjuːtəraɪn ˈbliːdɪŋ/ *noun* bleeding in the uterus not caused by a menstrual period

**dysgenesis** /dɪsˈdʒenəsɪs/ *noun* unusual development

**dysgerminoma** /dɪsˌdʒɜːmɪˈnəʊmə/ *noun* a malignant tumour of the ovary or testicle

**dysgraphia** /dɪsˈɡræfiə/ *noun* difficulty in writing caused by a brain lesion

**dyskariosis** /dɪsˌkæriˈəʊsɪs/ *noun* the fact of becoming mature in an unusual way

**dyskinesia** /ˌdɪskaɪˈniːziə/ *noun* the inability to control voluntary movements

**dyslalia** /dɪsˈleɪliə/ *noun* a disorder of speech, caused by an unusual development of the tongue

**dyslexia** /dɪsˈleksiə/ *noun* a disorder of development, where a person is unable to read or write properly and confuses letters

**dyslexic** /dɪsˈleksɪk/ *adjective* referring to dyslexia ∎ *noun* a person suffering from dyslexia

**dyslipidaemia** /ˌdɪslɪpɪˈdiːmiə/ *noun* an imbalance of lipids

**dyslogia** /dɪsˈləʊdʒə/ *noun* difficulty in putting ideas into words

**dysmaturity** /ˌdɪsməˈtʃʊərɪti/ *noun* a condition affecting newborn babies, shown by wrinkled skin, long fingernails and toenails and relatively little body fat

**dysmenorrhoea** /ˌdɪsmenəˈriːə/ *noun* pain experienced at menstruation

**dysostosis** /ˌdɪsɒsˈtəʊsɪs/ *noun* unusual formation of bones

**dyspareunia** /ˌdɪspæˈruːniə/ *noun* difficult or painful sexual intercourse in a woman

**dyspepsia** /dɪsˈpepsiə/ *noun* a condition in which a person feels pains or discomfort in the stomach, caused by indigestion

**dyspeptic** /dɪsˈpeptɪk/ *adjective* referring to dyspepsia

**dysphagia** /dɪsˈfeɪdʒiə/ *noun* difficulty in swallowing

**dysphasia** /dɪsˈfeɪziə/ *noun* difficulty in speaking and putting words into the correct order

**dysphemia** /dɪsˈfiːmiə/ *noun* same as **stammering**

**dysphonia** /dɪsˈfəʊniə/ *noun* difficulty in speaking caused by impairment of the vocal cords, or by laryngitis

**dysplasia** /dɪsˈpleɪziə/ *noun* an unusual development of tissue

**dyspnoea** /dɪspˈniːə/ *noun* difficulty or pain in breathing

**dyspnoeic** /dɪspˈniːɪk/ *adjective* difficult or painful when breathing

**dyspraxia** /dɪsˈpræksiə/ *noun* difficulty in carrying out coordinated movements

**dysrhythmia** /dɪsˈrɪðmiə/ *noun* an unusual rhythm, either in speaking or in electrical impulses in the brain

**dyssocial** /dɪsˈsəʊʃ(ə)l/ *adjective* same as **antisocial**

**dyssynergia** /ˌdɪsɪˈnɜːdʒiə/ *noun* same as **asynergia**

**dystaxia** /dɪsˈtæksiə/ *noun* an inability to coordinate the muscles

**dystocia** /dɪsˈtəʊsiə/ *noun* difficult childbirth

**dystonia** /dɪsˈtəʊniə/ *noun* disordered muscle tone, causing involuntary contractions which make the limbs deformed

**dystrophia** /dɪsˈtrəʊfiə/ *noun* the wasting of an organ, muscle or tissue due to lack of nutrients in that part of the body. Also called **dystrophy**

**dystrophia adiposogenitalis** /dɪsˌtrəʊfiə ædɪˌpəʊsəʊdʒenɪˈteɪlɪs/ *noun* same as **Fröhlich's syndrome**

**dystrophia myotonica** /dɪsˌtrəʊfiə ˌmaɪəʊˈtɒnɪkə/ *noun* same as **myotonic dystrophy**

**dystrophy** /ˈdɪstrəfi/ *noun* same as **dystrophia**

**dysuria** /dɪsˈjʊəriə/ *noun* difficulty in passing urine

# E

**ear** /ɪə/ *noun* an organ on the side of the head which is used for hearing (NOTE: For other terms referring to ears, see **auricular** and words beginning with **ot-, oto-.**)

COMMENT: The outer ear is shaped in such a way that it collects sound and channels it to the eardrum. Behind the eardrum, the three ossicles in the middle ear vibrate with sound and transmit the vibrations to the cochlea in the inner ear. From the cochlea, the vibrations are passed by the auditory nerve to the brain.

**Ear, Nose & Throat** /ˌɪə ˌnəʊz ən ˈθrəʊt/ *noun* the study of the ear, nose and throat. Abbr **ENT**. Also called **otorhinolaryngology**

**earache** /ˈɪəreɪk/ *noun* pain in the ear. Also called **otalgia**

**ear canal** /ˈɪə kəˌnæl/ *noun* one of several passages in or connected to the ear, especially the external auditory meatus, the passage from the outer ear to the eardrum

**eardrum** /ˈɪədrʌm/ *noun* the membrane at the end of the external auditory meatus leading from the outer ear, which vibrates with sound and passes the vibrations on to the ossicles in the middle ear. Also called **myringa, tympanum** (NOTE: For other terms referring to the eardrum, see words beginning with **tympan-, tympano-**.)

**early** /ˈɜːli/ *adjective* **1.** happening at the beginning of a period of time □ **early diagnosis** diagnosis made at the onset of an illness □ **early treatment** treatment given almost as soon as the illness has started **2.** (*of a condition or illness*) in its first stage ○ *early synovitis* □ **during early pregnancy** within the first months of pregnancy ■ *adverb* at the beginning of a period of time ○ *The treatment is usually successful if the condition is diagnosed early.*

**early onset pre-eclampsia** /ˌɜːli ˌɒnset ˌpriː ɪˈklæmpsiə/ *noun* pre-eclampsia which appears earlier than the 37th week of the pregnancy

**ear ossicle** /ˈɪə ˌɒsɪk(ə)l/ *noun* ♦ **auditory ossicles**

**earwax** /ˈɪəwæks/ *noun* same as **cerumen**

**ease** /iːz/ *verb* to make pain or worry less ○ *She had an injection to ease the pain in her leg.*

○ *The surgeon tried to ease the patient's fears about the results of the scan.*

**eating disorder** /ˈiːtɪŋ dɪsˌɔːdə/ *noun* an illness that causes the usual pattern of eating to be disturbed, e.g. anorexia or bulimia

**eating habits** /ˈiːtɪŋ ˌhæbɪts/ *plural noun* the types and quantities of food regularly eaten by a person ○ *The dietitian advised her to change her eating habits.*

**Ebola virus** /ɪˈbəʊlə ˌvaɪrəs/ *noun* a highly contagious virus found in West Africa. Patients who are affected with it vomit, have bloody diarrhoea and blood seeps through their skin.

**eburnation** /ˌiːbəˈneɪʃ(ə)n/ *noun* the conversion of cartilage into a hard mass with a shiny surface like bone

**ecbolic** /ekˈbɒlɪk/ *noun* a substance which produces contraction of the uterus and so induces childbirth or abortion ■ *adjective* causing contraction of the uterus

**ecchondroma** /ˌekənˈdrəʊmə/ *noun* a benign tumour on the surface of cartilage or bone

**ecchymosis** /ˌekɪˈməʊsɪs/ *noun* a dark area on the skin made by blood which has escaped into the tissues after a blow. Also called **bruise, contusion**

**eccrine** /ˈekrɪn/ *adjective* referring to a gland, especially a sweat gland, which does not disintegrate and remains intact during secretion. Also called **merocrine**

**eccyesis** /ˌeksaɪˈiːsɪs/ *noun* same as **ectopic pregnancy**

**ecdysis** /ˈekdɪsɪs/ *noun* same as **desquamation**

**ECG** *abbr* electrocardiogram

**echinococciasis** /ɪˌkaɪnəʊkɒˈkaɪəsɪs/, **echinococcosis** /ɪˌkaɪnəʊkəˈkəʊsɪs/ *noun* a disorder caused by a tapeworm *Echinococcus granulosus* which forms hydatid cysts in the lungs, liver, kidneys or brain

**Echinococcus granulosus** /ɪˌkaɪnəʊkɒkəs ˌgrænjʊˈləʊsəs/ *noun* a type of tapeworm, usually found in animals, but sometimes transmitted to humans, causing hydatid cysts in the lungs, liver, kidneys or brain

**echo-** /ekəʊ/ *prefix* referring to sound

**echocardiogram** /ˌekəʊˈkɑːdɪəgræm/ *noun* a record of heart movements made using ultrasound

**echocardiography** /ˌekəʊkɑːdiˈɒgrəfi/ *noun* the use of ultrasound to examine the heart

**echoencephalography** /ˌekəʊenˌkefəˈlɒgrəfi/ *noun* the use of ultrasound to examine the brain

**echography** /eˈkɒgrəfi/ *noun* same as **ultrasonography**

**echokinesis** /ˌekəʊkaɪˈniːsɪs/ *noun* same as **echopraxia**

**echolalia** /ˌekəʊˈleɪliə/ *noun* the repetition of words spoken by another person

**echopraxia** /ˌekəʊˈpræksiə/ *noun* the meaningless imitation of another person's actions

**echovirus** /ˈekəʊˌvaɪrəs/ *noun* one of a group of viruses which can be isolated from the intestine and which can cause serious illnesses such as aseptic meningitis, gastroenteritis and respiratory infection in small children. Compare **reovirus**

**eclabium** /ɪˈkleɪbiəm/ *noun* the turning outwards of the lips. ◊ **eversion**

**eclampsia** /ɪˈklæmpsiə/ *noun* a serious condition of pregnant women at the end of pregnancy, caused by toxaemia, in which the woman has high blood pressure and may go into a coma. ◊ **pre-eclampsia**

**ecmnesia** /ekˈniːziə/ *noun* a condition in which someone is not able to remember recent events, while remembering clearly events which happened some time ago

**E. coli** /ˌiː ˈkəʊlaɪ/ *noun* same as **Escherichia coli**

**economy class syndrome** /ɪˈkɒnəmi klɑːs ˌsɪndrəʊm/ *noun* same as **deep-vein thrombosis** (*informal*)

**écraseur** /ˌeɪkrɑːˈzɜː/ *noun* a surgical instrument, usually with a wire loop, used to cut a part or a growth off at its base

**ecstasy** /ˈekstəsi/ *noun* **1.** feeling of extreme happiness **2.** a powerful stimulant and hallucinatory illegal drug (*informal*) Also called **methylenedioxymethamphetamine**

**ECT** *abbr* electroconvulsive therapy

**ect-** /ekt/ *prefix* same as **ecto-** (*used before vowels*)

**ectasia** /ekˈteɪziə/ *noun* the dilatation of a passage

**ecthyma** /ekˈθaɪmə/ *noun* a skin disorder that is a serious form of impetigo which penetrates deep under the skin and leaves scars

**ecto-** /ektəʊ/ *prefix* outside

**ectoderm** /ˈektəʊdɜːm/ *noun* the outer layer of an early embryo. Also called **embryonic ectoderm**

**ectodermal** /ˌektəʊˈdɜːm(ə)l/ *adjective* referring to the ectoderm

**-ectomy** /ektəmi/ *suffix* referring to the removal of a part by surgical operation

**ectoparasite** /ˌektəʊˈpærəsaɪt/ *noun* a parasite which lives on the skin. Compare **endoparasite**

**ectopia** /ekˈtəʊpiə/ *noun* a condition in which an organ or part of the body is not in its usual position

**ectopic** /ekˈtɒpɪk/ *adjective* not in the usual position. Opposite **entopic**

**ectopic heartbeat** /ekˌtɒpɪk ˈhɑːtbiːt/ *noun* an unusual extra beat of the heart which originates from a point other than the sinoatrial node. Also called **extrasystole, premature beat**

**ectopic pacemaker** /ekˌtɒpɪk ˈpeɪsmeɪkə/ *noun* an unusual focus of the heart muscle which takes the place of the sinoatrial node

**ectopic pregnancy** /ekˌtɒpɪk ˈpregnənsi/ *noun* a pregnancy where the fetus develops outside the uterus, often in one of the Fallopian tubes. Also called **extrauterine pregnancy, eccyesis**

**ectro-** /ektrəʊ/ *prefix* referring to a usually congenital absence or lack of something

**ectrodactyly** /ˌektrəʊˈdæktɪli/ *noun* a congenital absence of all or part of a finger

**ectrogeny** /ekˈtrɒdʒəni/ *noun* a congenital absence of a part at birth

**ectromelia** /ˌektrəʊˈmiːliə/ *noun* a congenital absence of one or more limbs

**ectropion** /ekˈtrəʊpiən/ *noun* a turning of the edge of an eyelid outwards. ◊ **eversion**

**eczema** /ˈeksɪmə/ *noun* a non-contagious inflammation of the skin, with an itchy rash and blisters

**eczematous** /ekˈsemətəs/ *adjective* referring to eczema

**eczematous dermatitis** /ekˌsemətəs ˌdɜːməˈtaɪtɪs/ *noun* an itchy inflammation or irritation of the skin due to an allergic reaction to a substance which a person has touched or absorbed

**EDD** *abbr* expected date of delivery

**edema** /ɪˈdiːmə/ *noun US* same as **oedema**

**edentulous** /ɪˈdentjʊləs/ *adjective* having lost all teeth

**edible** /ˈedɪb(ə)l/ *adjective* able to be eaten without causing harm

**EDTA** *noun* a colourless chemical that can bind to heavy metals to remove them from the bloodstream. Full form **ethylene diamine tetra-acetate**

**Edwards' syndrome** /ˈedwədz ˌsɪndrəʊm/ *noun* a severe genetic disorder that results in malformations of the brain, kidney, heart, hands and feet. It is caused by an extra copy of chromosome 18 and those people who have it usually die within six months.

**EEG** *abbr* electroencephalogram

**EFA** *abbr* essential fatty acid

**effacement** /ɪˈfeɪsmənt/ *noun* the thinning of the cervix before it dilates in childbirth

# effect

# effect

# effect

# effect

**effect** /ɪˈfekt/ noun a result of a drug, treatment, disease or action ○ *The antiseptic cream has had no effect on the rash.* ■ verb to make something happen (*formal*) ○ *They will have to effect a change in procedures.* ○ *In some circumstances these drugs can effect surprising cures.*

**effective** /ɪˈfektɪv/ adjective having an effect ○ *Embolisation is an effective treatment for severe haemoptysis.*

**effective dose** /ɪˌfektɪv ˈdəʊs/ noun a size of dose which will produce the effect required

**effector** /ɪˈfektə/ noun a nerve ending in muscles or glands which is activated to produce contraction or secretion

**efferens** /ˈefərəns/ ♦ vas efferens

**efferent** /ˈefərənt/ adjective carrying something away from part of the body or from the centre. Opposite **afferent**

**efferent duct** /ˈefərənt dʌkt/ noun a duct which carries a secretion away from a gland

**efferent nerve** /ˈefərənt nɜːv/ noun same as **motor nerve**

**efferent vessel** /ˈefərənt ˌves(ə)l/ noun a vessel which drains lymph from a gland

**effleurage** /ˌeflɜːˈrɑːʒ/ noun a form of massage where the skin is stroked in one direction to increase blood flow

**effort syndrome** /ˈefət ˌsɪndrəʊm/ noun same as **disordered action of the heart**

**effusion** /ɪˈfjuːʒ(ə)n/ noun **1.** a discharge of blood, fluid or pus into or out of an internal cavity **2.** fluid, blood or pus which is discharged

**egg** /eg/ noun **1.** a reproductive cell produced in the female body by an ovary, and which, if fertilised by the male sperm, becomes an embryo **2.** an egg with a hard shell, laid by a hen or other bird, which is used for food

**egg cell** /ˈeg sel/ noun an immature ovum or female cell

**ego** /ˈiːgəʊ, ˈegəʊ/ noun (*in psychology*) the part of the mind which is consciously in contact with the outside world and is influenced by experiences of the world

**Egyptian ophthalmia** /ɪˌdʒɪpʃ(ə)n ɒf ˈθælmiə/ noun same as **trachoma**

**EHO** abbr Environmental Health Officer

**EIA** abbr exercise-induced asthma

**eidetic imagery** /aɪˌdetɪk ˈɪmɪdʒəri/ noun the recall of extremely clear pictures in the mind

**Eisenmenger syndrome** /ˈaɪzənmeŋə ˌsɪndrəʊm/ noun heart disease caused by a septal defect between the ventricles, with pulmonary hypertension [Described 1897. After Victor Eisenmenger (1864–1932), German physician.]

**ejaculate** /ɪˈdʒækjʊˌleɪt/ verb to send out semen from the penis

**ejaculation** /ɪˌdʒækjʊˈleɪʃ(ə)n/ noun the sending out of semen from the penis

**ejaculatio praecox** /ɪdʒækjʊˌleɪʃiəʊ ˈpriːkɒks/ noun a situation where a man ejaculates too early during sexual intercourse

**ejaculatory** /ɪˈdʒækjʊlətri/ adjective referring to ejaculation

**ejaculatory duct** /ɪˈdʒækjʊlətri dʌkt/ noun one of two ducts leading from the seminal vesicles through the prostate gland to the urethra. See illustration at **UROGENITAL SYSTEM (MALE)** in Supplement

**eject** /ɪˈdʒekt/ verb to send out something with force ○ *Blood is ejected from the ventricle during systole.*

**ejection** /ɪˈdʒekʃən/ noun the act of sending out something with force

**EKG** abbr US electrocardiogram

**elastic** /ɪˈlæstɪk/ adjective which can be stretched and compressed and return to its former shape

**elastic bandage** /ɪˌlæstɪk ˈbændɪdʒ/ noun a stretchy bandage used to support a weak joint or for the treatment of a varicose vein

**elastic cartilage** /ɪˌlæstɪk ˈkɑːtəlɪdʒ/ noun flexible cartilage, e.g. in the ear and epiglottis

**elastic fibre** /ɪˌlæstɪk ˈfaɪbə/ noun fibre which can expand easily and is found in elastic cartilage, the skin and the walls of arteries and the lungs. Also called **yellow fibre**

**elastic hose** /ɪˈlæstɪk həʊz/ noun same as **surgical hose**

**elasticity** /ˌɪlæˈstɪsɪti/ noun the ability to expand and be compressed and to return to its former shape

**elastic tissue** /ɪˌlæstɪk ˈtɪʃuː/ noun connective tissue which contains elastic fibres, e.g. in the walls of arteries or of the alveoli in the lungs

**elastin** /ɪˈlæstɪn/ noun a protein which occurs in elastic fibres

**elation** /ɪˈleɪʃ(ə)n/ noun the state of being happy, stimulated and excited

**elbow** /ˈelbəʊ/ noun a hinged joint where the upper arm bone (**humerus**) joins the forearm bones (**radius** and **ulna**)

**elbow crutch** /ˈelbəʊ krʌtʃ/ noun a crutch which surrounds the arms at the elbows and has a handle to hold lower down the shaft

**elderly** /ˈeldəli/ adjective older than 65 ○ *a home for elderly single women* ○ *She looks after her two elderly parents.* ■ noun □ the elderly people aged over 65

**elective** /ɪˈlektɪv/ adjective **1.** referring to a chemical substance which tends to combine with one substance rather others **2.** referring to surgery or treatment which someone can choose to have but is not urgently necessary to save their life

**elective care** /ɪˌlektɪv ˈkeə/ *noun* hospital care which is planned in advance, rather than a response to an emergency

**Electra complex** /ɪˈlektrə ˌkɒmpleks/ *noun* (*in psychology*) a condition in which a girl feels sexually attracted to her father and sees her mother as an obstacle

**electric shock** /ɪˌlektrɪk ˈʃɒk/ *noun* a sudden passage of electricity into the body, causing a nervous spasm or, in severe cases, death

**electric shock treatment** /ɪˌlektrɪk ˈʃɒk ˌtriːtmənt/ *noun* same as **electroconvulsive therapy** (*informal*)

**electro-** /ɪˈlektrəʊ/ *prefix* referring to electricity

**electrocardiogram** /ɪˌlektrəʊˈkɑːdiəgræm/ *noun* a chart which records the electrical impulses in the heart muscle. Abbr **ECG, EKG**

**electrocardiograph** /ɪˌlektrəʊˈkɑːdiəgrɑːf/ *noun* an apparatus for measuring and recording the electrical impulses of the muscles of the heart as it beats

**electrocardiography** /ɪˌlektrəʊkɑːdiˈɒgrəfi/ *noun* the process of recording the electrical impulses of the heart

**electrocardiophonography** /ɪˌlektrəʊkɑːdiəʊfəˈnɒgrəfi/ *noun* the process of electrically recording the sounds of the heartbeats

**electrocautery** /ɪˌlektrəʊˈkɔːtəri/ *noun* same as **galvanocautery**

**electrochemical** /ɪˌlektrəʊˈkemɪk(ə)l/ *adjective* referring to electricity and chemicals and their interaction

**electrocoagulation** /ɪˌlektrəʊkəʊæɡjʊˈleɪʃ(ə)n/ *noun* the control of haemorrhage in surgery by passing a high-frequency electric current through divided blood vessels

**electroconvulsive therapy** /ɪˌlektrəʊkən ˌvʌlsɪv ˈθerəpi/ *noun* the treatment of severe depression and some mental disorders by giving someone who has been anaesthetised small electric shocks in the brain to make him or her have convulsions. Abbr **ECT**. Also called **electroplexy**

**electrode** /ɪˈlektrəʊd/ *noun* the conductor of an electrical apparatus which touches the body and carries an electric shock

**electrodesiccation** /ɪˌlektrəʊdesɪˈkeɪʃ(ə)n/ *noun* same as **fulguration**

**electroencephalogram** /ɪˌlektrəʊɪnˈsefələgræm/ *noun* a chart on which the electrical impulses in the brain are recorded. Abbr **EEG**

**electroencephalograph** /ɪˌlektrəʊɪnˈsefələgrɑːf/ *noun* an apparatus which records the electrical impulses in the brain

**electroencephalography** /ɪˌlektrəʊɪnsefəˈlɒgrəfi/ *noun* the process of recording the electrical impulses in the brain

**electrolysis** /ɪlekˈtrɒləsɪs/ *noun* the destruction of tissue such as unwanted hair by applying an electric current

**electrolyte** /ɪˈlektrəlaɪt/ *noun* a chemical solution which can conduct electricity

**electrolyte mixture** /ɪˈlektrəlaɪt ˌmɪkstʃə/ *noun* a pint (0.56 litres) of boiled water with a teaspoonful of sugar and a generous pinch of table salt used for the prevention of diarrhoea

**electrolytic** /ɪˌlektrəˈlɪtɪk/ *adjective* referring to electrolytes or to electrolysis

**electromyogram** /ɪˌlektrəˈmaɪəʊgræm/ *noun* a chart showing the electric currents in active muscles. Abbr **EMG**

**electromyography** /ɪˌlektrəʊmaɪˈɒgrəfi/ *noun* the study of electric currents in active muscles

**electronic stethoscope** /ˌelektrɒnɪk ˈsteθəskəʊp/ *noun* a stethoscope with an amplifier which makes sounds louder

**electronystagmography** /eˌlektrəʊ ˌnɪstæɡˈmɒgrəfi/ *noun* measuring of nystagmus

**electrooculogram** /ɪˌlektrəʊˈɒkjʊləgræm/ *noun* a record of the electric currents round the eye, induced by eye movements

**electrooculography** /ɪˌlektrəʊˌɒkjʊˈlɒ grəfi/ *noun* recording the electric currents round the eye, induced by eye movements, especially for use in remote control

**electrophoresis** /ɪˌlektrəʊfəˈriːsɪs/ *noun* the analysis of a substance by the movement of charged particles towards an electrode in a solution

**electroplexy** /ɪˈlektrəpleksi/ *noun* same as **electroconvulsive therapy**

**electroretinogram** /ɪˌkektrəʊˈretɪnəgræm/ *noun* the printed result of electroretinography. Abbr **ERG**

**electroretinography** /ɪˌlektrəʊretɪˈnɒ grəfi/ *noun* the process of recording electrical changes in the retina when stimulated by light

**electrosurgery** /ɪˌlektrəʊˈsɜːdʒəri/ *noun* an operation in which the surgeon uses an electrical current to cut or cauterise tissue

**electrotherapy** /ɪˌlektrəʊˈθerəpi/ *noun* the treatment of a disorder such as some forms of paralysis by using low-frequency electric current to try to revive the muscles

**element** /ˈelɪmənt/ *noun* a basic simple chemical substance which cannot be broken down into simpler substances. ◊ **trace element**

**elephantiasis** /ˌelɪfənˈtaɪəsɪs/ *noun* a condition in which parts of the body swell and the skin becomes hardened, frequently caused by infestation with various species of the parasitic worm *Filaria*

**elevate** /ˈelɪveɪt/ *verb* to raise something or to lift something up ○ *To control bleeding, apply pressure and elevate the part.*

**elevation** /ˌeləˈveɪʃ(ə)n/ *noun* a raised part

**elevation sling** /ˌelɪˈveɪʃ(ə)n slɪŋ/ *noun* a sling tied round the neck, used to hold an injured hand or arm in a high position to control bleeding

**elevator** /ˈelɪveɪtə/ *noun* **1.** a muscle which raises part of the body **2.** a surgical instrument used to lift part of a broken bone

**eliminate** /ɪˈlɪmɪneɪt/ *verb* to remove waste matter from the body ○ *The excess salts are eliminated through the kidneys.*

**elimination** /ɪˌlɪmɪˈneɪʃ(ə)n/ *noun* the removal of waste matter from the body

**elimination diet** /ɪˌlɪmɪˈneɪʃ(ə)n ˌdaɪət/ *noun* a structured diet where different foods are eliminated one at a time in order to see the effect on symptoms, used in conditions such as allergies and attention deficit hyperactivity disorder

**ELISA** /ɪˈlaɪzə/ *noun* a process in which an enzyme binds to an antibody or antigen and causes a colour change that shows the presence or amount of protein in a sample of biological material. Full form **enzyme-linked immunosorbent assay**

**elixir** /ɪˈlɪksə/ *noun* a sweet liquid which hides the unpleasant taste of a drug

**elliptocytosis** /ɪˌlɪptəʊsaɪˈtəʊsɪs/ *noun* a condition in which unusual oval-shaped red cells appear in the blood

**emaciated** /ɪˈmeɪʃieɪtɪd/ *adjective* very thin and extremely underweight

**emaciation** /ɪˌmeɪsiˈeɪʃ(ə)n/ *noun* **1.** the fact of being extremely thin and underweight **2.** the loss of body tissue

**emaculation** /ɪˌmækjʊˈleɪʃ(ə)n/ *noun* the removal of spots from the skin

**emasculation** /ɪˌmæskjʊˈleɪʃ(ə)n/ *noun* **1.** the removal of the penis **2.** the loss of male characteristics

**embalm** /ɪmˈbɑːm/ *verb* to preserve a dead body by using special antiseptic chemicals to prevent decay

**embolectomy** /ˌembəˈlektəmi/ *noun* a surgical operation to remove a blood clot

**emboli** /ˈembəli/ plural of **embolus**

**embolisation** /ˌembəlaɪˈzeɪʃ(ə)n/, **embolization** *noun* the use of emboli inserted down a catheter into a blood vessel to treat internal bleeding

'…once a bleeding site has been located, a catheter is manipulated as near as possible to it, so that embolization can be carried out. Many different materials are used as the embolus.' [*British Medical Journal*]

**embolism** /ˈembəlɪz(ə)m/ *noun* the blocking of an artery by a mass of material, usually a blood clot, preventing the flow of blood

**embolus** /ˈembələs/ *noun* **1.** a mass of material which blocks a blood vessel, e.g. a blood clot, air bubble or fat globule **2.** material inserted into a blood vessel down a catheter to treat internal bleeding (NOTE: The plural is **emboli**.)

**embrocation** /ˌembrəˈkeɪʃ(ə)n/ *noun* same as **liniment**

**embryo** /ˈembriəʊ/ *noun* an unborn baby during the first eight weeks after conception (NOTE: After eight weeks, the unborn baby is called a **fetus**.)

**embryological** /ˌembriəˈlɒdʒɪk(ə)l/ *adjective* referring to embryology

**embryology** /ˌembriˈɒlədʒi/ *noun* the study of the early stages of the development of an embryo

**embryonic** /ˌembriˈɒnɪk/ *adjective* **1.** referring to an embryo **2.** in an early stage of development

**embryonic ectoderm** /ˌembriɒnɪk ˈektəʊdɜːm/ *noun* ♦ **ectoderm**

**embryonic membrane** /ˌembriɒnɪk ˈmembreɪn/ *noun* one of the two layers around an embryo providing protection and food supply, i.e. the **amnion** and the **chorion**

**embryonic mesoderm** /ˌembriɒnɪk ˈmesəʊdɜːm/ *noun* ♦ **mesoderm**

**emergency** /ɪˈmɜːdʒənsi/ *noun* a situation where urgent immediate action has to be taken

**emergency medical technician** /ɪˌmɜːdʒənsi ˌmedɪk(ə)l tekˈnɪʃ(ə)n/ *noun* US a trained paramedic who gives care to victims at the scene of an accident or in an ambulance. Abbr **EMT**

**emergency medicine** /ɪˌmɜːdʒənsi ˈmed(ə)s(ə)n/ *noun* the treatment of patients whose condition is serious and requires urgent immediate action

**emergency room** /ɪˈmɜːdʒənsi ruːm/ *noun* US the part of a hospital where people who need urgent immediate treatment are dealt with

**emergency ward** /ɪˈmɜːdʒənsi wɔːd/ *noun* the part of a hospital where people who need urgent immediate treatment are dealt with

**emesis** /ˈeməsɪs/ *noun* same as **vomiting**

**emetic** /ɪˈmetɪk/ *noun* a substance which causes vomiting ■ *adjective* causing vomiting

**EMG** *abbr* electromyogram

**eminence** /ˈemɪnəns/ *noun* something which protrudes from a surface, e.g. a lump on a bone or swelling on the skin

**emissary vein** /ˈemɪsəri ˌveɪn/ *noun* a vein through the skull which connects the venous sinuses with the scalp veins

**emission** /ɪˈmɪʃ(ə)n/ *noun* a discharge or release of fluid

**emmenagogue** /ɪˈmenəgɒg/ *noun* a drug which will help increase menstrual flow

**emmetropia** /ˌemɪˈtrəʊpiə/ *noun* the correct focusing of light rays by the eye onto the retina giving normal vision. Compare **ametropia**

**emollient** /ɪˈmɒliənt/ *noun* a substance which soothes or smooths the skin, e.g. to prevent the development of eczema ■ *adjective* smoothening

**emotion** /ɪ'məʊʃ(ə)n/ *noun* a strong feeling

**emotional disorder** /ɪ,məʊʃ(ə)nəl dɪs'ɔːdə/ *noun* a disorder due to worry, stress, grief or other strong emotion

**emotional immaturity** /ɪ,məʊʃ(ə)nəl ɪmə'tʃʊətɪ/ *noun* lacking in emotional development

**empathy** /'empəθi/ *noun* the ability to understand the problems and feelings of another person

**emphysema** /,emfɪ'siːmə/ *noun* a condition in which the walls of the alveoli of the lungs break down, reducing the surface available for gas exchange and resulting in a lower oxygen level in the blood and shortness of breath. It can be caused by smoking, living in a polluted environment, old age, asthma or whooping cough. ◊ **surgical emphysema**

**empirical treatment** /ɪm,pɪrɪk(ə)l 'triːtmənt/ *noun* treatment which is based on symptoms and clinical experience rather than on a thorough knowledge of the cause of the disorder

**empowerment** /ɪm'paʊəmənt/ *noun* the act of giving someone authority and power to make decisions that will affect them

**empyema** /,empaɪ'iːmə/ *noun* the collection of pus in a cavity, especially in the pleural cavity. Also called **pyothorax**

**EMS** *abbr* Emergency Medical Services

**EMT** *abbr US* emergency medical technician

**emulsion** /ɪ'mʌlʃən/ *noun* a combination of liquids such as oil and water which do not usually mix

**EN** *abbr* enrolled nurse

**EN(G)** *abbr* enrolled nurse (general)

**EN(M)** *abbr* enrolled nurse (mental)

**EN(MH)** *abbr* enrolled nurse (mental handicap)

**en-** /en, ɪn/ *prefix* **1.** in, into **2.** to provide with **3.** to cause to be **4.** to put into or cover with **5.** to go into

**enalapril** /e'næləprɪl/ *noun* a drug used for the short-term management of high blood pressure

**enamel** /ɪ'næm(ə)l/ *noun* the hard white shiny outer covering of the crown of a tooth

**enanthema** /,enən'θiːmə/ *noun* a rash on a mucous membrane, such as that of the mouth or vagina, produced by the action of toxic substances on small blood vessels

**enarthrosis** /,enɑː'θrəʊsɪs/ *noun* a ball and socket joint, e.g. the hip joint

**encapsulated** /ɪn'kæpsjʊleɪtɪd/ *adjective* enclosed in a capsule or in a sheath of tissue

**encefalin** /en'kefəlɪn/ *noun* another spelling of **encephalin**

**encephal-** /enkefəl/ *prefix* same as **encephalo-** (*used before vowels*)

**encephalin** /en'kefəlɪn/ *noun* a peptide produced in the brain which acts as a natural pain-killer. ◊ **endorphin** (NOTE: The US spelling is **enkephalin**.)

**encephalitis** /en,kefə'laɪtɪs, en,sefə'laɪtɪs/ *noun* inflammation of the brain

COMMENT: Encephalitis is caused by any of several viruses (**viral encephalitis**) and is also associated with infectious viral diseases such as measles or mumps. The variant **St Louis encephalitis** is transmitted by mosquitoes.

**encephalitis lethargica** /,enkefəlaɪtɪs lɪ'θɑːdʒɪkə/ *noun* same as **lethargic encephalitis**

**encephalo-** /enkefələ/ *prefix* referring to the brain

**encephalocele** /en'kefələʊsiːl/ *noun* a condition in which the brain protrudes through a congenital or traumatic gap in the skull bones

**encephalogram** /en'kefələgræm/, **encephalograph** /en'kefələgrɑːf/ *noun* an X-ray photograph of the ventricles and spaces of the brain taken after air has been injected into the cerebrospinal fluid by lumbar puncture

**encephalography** /en,kefə'lɒgrəfi/ *noun* an X-ray examination of the ventricles and spaces of the brain taken after air has been injected into the cerebrospinal fluid by lumbar puncture

COMMENT: The air takes the place of the cerebrospinal fluid and makes it easier to photograph the ventricles clearly. This technique has been superseded by CT and MRI.

**encephaloid** /en'kefələɪd/ *adjective* like brain tissue

**encephaloma** /en,kefə'ləʊmə/ *noun* a tumour of the brain

**encephalomalacia** /en,kefələʊmə'leɪʃiə/ *noun* softening of the brain

**encephalomyelitis** /en,kefələʊmaɪə'laɪtɪs/ *noun* a group of diseases which cause inflammation of the brain and the spinal cord

**encephalomyelopathy** /en,kefələʊmaɪə'lɒpəθi/ *noun* any condition where the brain and spinal cord are diseased

**encephalon** /en'kefəlɒn/ *noun* same as **brain** (NOTE: The plural is **encephala**.)

**encephalopathy** /en,kefə'lɒpəθi/ *noun* any disease of the brain

**enchondroma** /,enkən'drəʊmə/ *noun* a tumour formed of cartilage growing inside a bone

**enchondromatosis** /,enkəndrɒmə'təʊsɪs/ *noun* a condition in which a tumour formed of cartilage grows inside a bone

**encopresis** /,enkəʊ'priːsɪs/ *noun* faecal incontinence not associated with a physical condition or disease

**encounter group** /ɪn'kaʊntə gruːp/ *noun* a form of treatment of psychological disorders, where people meet and talk about their problems in a group

**encysted** /en'sɪstɪd/ *adjective* enclosed in a capsule like a cyst

**end-** /end/ *prefix* same as **endo-** (*used before vowels*)

**endanger** /ɪn'deɪndʒə/ *verb* to put someone or something at risk ○ *The operation may endanger the life of the patient.*

**endarterectomy** /ˌendɑːtə'rektəmi/ *noun* the surgical removal of the lining of a blocked artery. Also called **rebore**

**endarteritis** /ˌendɑːtə'raɪtɪs/ *noun* inflammation of the inner lining of an artery

**endarteritis obliterans** /ˌendɑːt ̩raɪtɪs ə 'blɪtərænz/ *noun* a condition where inflammation in an artery is so severe that it blocks the artery

**end artery** /'end ̩ɑːtəri/ *noun* the last section of an artery which does not divide into smaller arteries and does not join to other arteries

**endaural** /end'ɔːrəl/ *adjective* inside the ear

**endemic** /en'demɪk/ *adjective* referring to any disease which is very common in specific places ○ *This disease is endemic to Mediterranean countries.*

**endemic haemoptysis** /enˌdemɪk hiː 'mɒptəsɪs/ *noun* same as **paragonimiasis**

**endemic syphilis** /enˌdemɪk 'sɪfəlɪs/ *adjective* same as **bejel**

**endemic typhus** /enˌdemɪk 'taɪfəs/ *noun* fever transmitted by fleas from rats

**endemiology** /enˌdiːmi'ɒlədʒi/ *noun* the study of endemic diseases

**end-expiratory** /ˌend ɪk'spaɪrətri/ *noun* ♦ **positive end-expiratory pressure**

**endo-** /endəʊ/ *prefix* inside

**endobronchial** /endəʊ'brɒŋkiəl/ *adjective* inside the bronchi

**endocardial** /ˌendəʊ'kɑːdiəl/ *adjective* referring to the endocardium

**endocardial pacemaker** /ˌendəʊkɑːdiəl 'peɪsmeɪkə/ *noun* a pacemaker attached to the lining of the heart

**endocarditis** /ˌendəʊkɑː'daɪtɪs/ *noun* inflammation of the membrane lining of the heart

**endocardium** /ˌendəʊ'kɑːdiəm/ *noun* a membrane which lines the heart. See illustration at **HEART** in Supplement

**endocervicitis** /ˌendəʊsɜːvɪ'saɪtɪs/ *noun* inflammation of the membrane in the neck of the uterus

**endocervix** /ˌendəʊ'sɜːvɪks/ *noun* a membrane which lines the neck of the uterus

**endochondral** /ˌendəʊ'kɒndrəl/ *adjective* inside a cartilage

**endocrine** /'endəʊkraɪn/ *adjective* relating to the endocrine glands or the hormones they secrete

**endocrine gland** /'endəʊkraɪn glænd/ *noun* a gland without a duct which produces hormones which are introduced directly into the bloodstream, e.g. the pituitary gland, thyroid gland, the adrenal gland and the gonads. Also called **ductless gland**. Compare **exocrine gland**

**endocrine system** /'endəʊkraɪn ˌsɪstəm/ *noun* a system of related ductless glands

**endocrinologist** /ˌendəʊkrɪ'nɒlədʒɪst/ *noun* a doctor who specialises in the study of endocrinology

**endocrinology** /ˌendəʊkrɪ'nɒlədʒi/ *noun* the study of the endocrine system, its function and effects

**endoderm** /'endəʊdɜːm/ *noun* the inner of three layers surrounding an embryo. Also called **entoderm**

COMMENT: The endoderm gives rise to most of the epithelium of the respiratory system, the alimentary canal, some of the ductless glands the bladder and part of the urethra.

**endodermal** /ˌendəʊ'dɜːm(ə)l/ *adjective* referring to the endoderm. Also called **entodermal**

**endodontia** /ˌendəʊ'dɒnʃiə/ *noun* treatment of chronic toothache by removing the roots of a tooth

**endogenous** /en'dɒdʒənəs/ *adjective* developing or being caused by something inside an organism. Compare **exogenous**

**endogenous depression** /enˌdɒdʒənəs dɪ'preʃ(ə)n/ *noun* depression caused by no obvious external factor

**endogenous eczema** /enˌdɒdʒənəs 'eksɪmə/ *noun* eczema which is caused by no obvious external factor

**endolymph** /'endəʊlɪmf/ *noun* a fluid inside the membranous labyrinth in the inner ear

**endolymphatic duct** /ˌendəʊlɪmfætɪk 'dʌkt/ *noun* a duct which carries the endolymph inside the membranous labyrinth

**endolysin** /en'dɒlɪsɪn/ *noun* a substance present in cells, which kills bacteria

**endometria** /ˌendəʊ'miːtriə/ plural of **endometrium**

**endometrial** /ˌendəʊ'miːtriəl/ *adjective* referring to the endometrium

**endometrial laser ablation** /ˌendəʊmiːtriəl 'leɪzə əbˌleɪʃ(ə)n/ *noun* a gynaecological surgical procedure using a laser to treat fibroids or other causes of thickening of the lining of the uterus

**endometriosis** /ˌendəʊmiːtri'əʊsɪs/ *noun* a condition affecting women, in which tissue similar to the tissue of the uterus is found in other parts of the body

**endometritis** /ˌendəʊmɪ'traɪtɪs/ *noun* inflammation of the lining of the uterus

**endometrium** /ˌendəʊ'miːtriəm/ *noun* the mucous membrane lining the uterus, part of which is shed at each menstruation (NOTE: The plural is **endometria**.)

**endomyocarditis** /ˌendəʊmaɪəʊkɑːˈdaɪtɪs/ *noun* inflammation of the muscle and inner membrane of the heart

**endomysium** /ˌendəʊˈmɪsiəm/ *noun* connective tissue around and between muscle fibres

**endoneurium** /ˌendəʊˈnjʊəriəm/ *noun* fibrous tissue between the individual fibres in a nerve

**endoparasite** /ˌendəʊˈpærəsaɪt/ *noun* a parasite which lives inside its host, e.g. in the intestines. Compare **ectoparasite**

**endophthalmitis** /ˌendɒfθælˈmaɪtɪs/ *noun* inflammation of the interior of the eyeball

**end organ** /ˈend ˌɔːɡən/ *noun* a nerve ending with encapsulated nerve filaments

**endorphin** /enˈdɔːfɪn/ *noun* a peptide produced by the brain which acts as a natural painkiller. ◊ **encephalin**

**endoscope** /ˈendəskəʊp/ *noun* an instrument used to examine the inside of the body, made of a thin tube which is passed into the body down a passage. The tube has a fibre optic light, and may have small surgical instruments attached.

**endoscopic retrograde cholangiopancreatography** /ˌendəʊskɒpɪk ˌretrəɡreɪd kəˈlændʒiəʊpæŋkriəˈtɒɡrəfi/ *noun* a method used to examine the pancreatic duct and bile duct for possible obstructions. Abbr **ERCP**

**endoscopy** /enˈdɒskəpi/ *noun* an examination of the inside of the body using an endoscope

**endoskeleton** /ˈendəʊˌskelɪt(ə)n/ *noun* the inner structure of bones and cartilage in an animal

**endosteum** /enˈdɒstiəm/ *noun* a membrane lining the bone marrow cavity inside a long bone

**endothelial** /ˌendəʊˈθiːliəl/ *adjective* referring to the endothelium

**endothelioma** /ˌendəʊθiːliˈəʊmə/ *noun* a malignant tumour originating inside the endothelium

**endothelium** /ˌendəʊˈθiːliəm/ *noun* a membrane of special cells which lines the heart, the lymph vessels, the blood vessels and various body cavities. Compare **epithelium, mesothelium**

**endotoxin** /ˌendəʊˈtɒksɪn/ *noun* a toxic substance released after the death of some bacterial cells

**endotracheal** /ˌendəʊˈtreɪkiəl/ *adjective* same as **intratracheal**

**endotracheal tube** /ˌendəʊˈtreɪkiəl tjuːb/ *noun* a tube passed down the trachea, through either the nose or mouth, in anaesthesia or to help a person breathe

**end plate** /ˈend pleɪt/ *noun* the end of a motor nerve, where it joins muscle fibre

**end stage renal disease** /ˌend steɪdʒ ˈriːn(ə)l dɪˌziːz/ *noun* the stage of kidney disease at which uraemia occurs and dialysis needs to start. Abbr **ESRD**

**enema** /ˈenɪmə/ *noun* a liquid substance put into the rectum to introduce a drug into the body, to wash out the colon before an operation or for diagnosis

**enema bag** /ˈenəmə bæɡ/ *noun* a bag containing the liquid for an enema, attached to a tube into the rectum

**energy** /ˈenədʒi/ *noun* the force or strength to carry out activities ○ *You need to eat certain types of food to give you energy.*

**enervation** /ˌenəˈveɪʃ(ə)n/ *noun* **1.** general nervous weakness **2.** a surgical operation to remove a nerve

**engagement** /ɪnˈɡeɪdʒmənt/ *noun* (*in obstetrics*) the moment where part of the fetus, usually the head, enters the pelvis at the beginning of labour

**engorged** /ɪnˈɡɔːdʒd/ *adjective* excessively filled with liquid, usually blood

**engorgement** /ɪnˈɡɔːdʒmənt/ *noun* the excessive filling of a vessel, usually with blood

**enkephalin** /enˈkefəlɪn/ *noun* US same as **encephalin**

**enophthalmos** /ˌenɒfˈθælməs/ *noun* a condition in which the eyes are very deep in their sockets

**enostosis** /ˌenəˈstəʊsɪs/ *noun* a harmless growth inside a bone, usually in the skull or in a long bone

**enrolled** /ɪnˈrəʊld/ *adjective* registered on an official list

**Enrolled Nurse** /ɪnˌrəʊld ˈnɜːs/ *noun* ♦ **second-level nurse**

**ensiform** /ˈensifɔːm/ *adjective* shaped like a sword

**ensiform cartilage** /ˌensifɔːm ˈkɑːtəlɪdʒ/ *noun* same as **xiphoid process**

**ENT** *abbr* Ear, Nose & Throat

**Entamoeba coli** /ˌentamiːbə ˈkəʊlaɪ/ *noun* a harmless intestinal parasite

**Entamoeba gingivalis** /ˌentamiːbə ˌdʒɪndʒɪˈvælɪs/ *noun* an amoeba that lives in the gums and tonsils, and causes gingivitis

**Entamoeba histolytica** /ˌentamiːbə ˌhɪstəˈlɪtɪkə/ *noun* an intestinal amoeba which causes amoebic dysentery

**ENT department** /ˌiː en ˈtiː dɪˌpɑːtmənt/ *noun* a department of otorhinolaryngology

**ENT doctor** /ˌiː en ˈtiː ˌdɒktə/ *noun* same as **otorhinolaryngologist**

**enter-** /entə/ *prefix* same as **entero-** (*used before vowels*)

**enteral** /ˈentərəl/ *adjective* **1.** referring to the intestine. Compare **parenteral 2.** referring to medication or food which is taken by mouth or through a nasogastric tube

**enteral feeding** /ˌentərəl ˈfiːdɪŋ/ *noun* the feeding of a person by a nasogastric tube or by the infusion of liquid food directly into the intestine. Also called **enteral nutrition**

'Standard nasogastric tubes are usually sufficient for enteral feeding in critically ill patients' [*British Journal of Nursing*]

**enteralgia** /ˌentərˈældʒə/ *noun* same as **colic**

**enterally** /ˈentərəli/ *adverb* referring to a method of feeding a person by nasogastric tube or directly into the intestine

'All patients requiring nutrition are fed enterally, whether nasogastrically or directly into the small intestine' [*British Journal of Nursing*]

**enteral nutrition** /ˌentərəl njuːˈtrɪʃ(ə)n/ *noun* same as **enteral feeding**

**enterectomy** /ˌentərˈektəmi/ *noun* the surgical removal of part of the intestine

**enteric** /enˈterɪk/ *adjective* referring to the intestine

**enteric-coated** /enˌterɪk ˈkəʊtɪd/ *adjective* referring to a capsule with a coating which prevents it from being digested and releasing the drug until it reaches the intestine

**enteric fever** /enˌterɪk ˈfiːvə/ *noun* US **1.** any one of three fevers (typhoid, paratyphoid A and paratyphoid B) **2.** any febrile disease of the intestines

**enteritis** /ˌentəˈraɪtɪs/ *noun* inflammation of the mucous membrane of the intestine

**entero-** /entərəʊ/ *prefix* referring to the intestine

**Enterobacteria** /ˌentərəʊbækˈtɪəriə/ *noun* a family of Gram-negative bacteria, including Salmonella, Shigella, Escherichia and Klebsiella

**enterobiasis** /ˌentərəʊˈbaɪəsɪs/ *noun* a common children's disease, caused by threadworms in the large intestine which cause itching round the anus. Also called **oxyuriasis**

**Enterobius** /ˌentəˈrəʊbiəs/ *noun* a small thin nematode worm, one species of which, *Enterobius vermicularis*, infests the large intestine and causes itching round the anus. Also called **threadworm, pinworm**

**enterocele** /ˈentərəʊsiːl/, **enterocoele** /ˈentərəʊsiːl/ *noun* a hernia of the intestine

**enterocentesis** /ˌentərəʊsenˈtiːsɪs/ *noun* surgical puncturing of the intestines where a hollow needle is pushed through the abdominal wall into the intestine to remove gas or fluid

**enterococcus** /ˌentərəʊˈkɒkəs/ *noun* a streptococcal bacterium that lives in the intestine (NOTE: The plural is **enterococci**.)

**enterocoele** /ˈentərəʊsiːl/ *noun* another spelling of **enterocele**

**enterocolitis** /ˌentərəʊkəˈlaɪtɪs/ *noun* inflammation of the colon and small intestine

**enterogastrone** /ˌentərəʊˈgæstrəʊn/ *noun* a hormone released in the duodenum, which controls secretions of the stomach

**enterogenous** /ˌentərəʊˈdʒiːnəs/ *adjective* originating in the intestine

**enterolith** /ˈentərəʊlɪθ/ *noun* a stone in the intestine

**enteron** /ˈentərɒn/ *noun* the whole intestinal tract

**enteropathy** /ˌentəˈrɒpəθi/ *noun* any disorder of the intestine. ◊ **gluten-induced enteropathy**

**enteropeptidase** /ˌentərəʊˈpeptɪdeɪz/ *noun* an enzyme produced by glands in the small intestine

**enteroptosis** /ˌentərɒpˈtəʊsɪs/ *noun* a condition in which the intestine is lower than usual in the abdominal cavity

**enterorrhaphy** /ˌentərˈɔːrəfi/ *noun* a surgical operation to stitch up a perforated intestine

**enteroscope** /ˈentərəskəʊp/ *noun* an instrument for inspecting the inside of the intestine

**enterospasm** /ˈentərəʊˌspæz(ə)m/ *noun* an irregular painful contraction of the intestine

**enterostomy** /ˌentəˈrɒstəmi/ *noun* a surgical operation to make an opening between the small intestine and the abdominal wall

**enterotomy** /ˌentəˈrɒtəmi/ *noun* a surgical incision in the intestine

**enterotoxin** /ˌentərəʊˈtɒksɪn/ *noun* a bacterial exotoxin which particularly affects the intestine

**enterovirus** /ˌentərəʊˈvaɪrəs/ *noun* a virus which prefers to live in the intestine. Enteroviruses include poliomyelitis virus, Coxsackie viruses and the echoviruses.

**enterozoon** /ˌentərəʊˈzəʊɒn/ *noun* a parasite which infests the intestine (NOTE: The plural is **enterozoa**.)

**entoderm** /ˈentəʊdɜːm/ *noun* same as **endoderm**

**entodermal** /ˌentəʊˈdɜːm(ə)l/ *adjective* same as **endodermal**

**Entonox** /ˈentɒnɒks/ *noun* a gas consisting of 50% oxygen and 50% nitrous oxide that is used as a painkiller during childbirth

**entopic** /ɪnˈtɒpɪk/ *adjective* located or taking place in the usual position. Opposite **ectopic**

**entropion** /ɪnˈtrəʊpiən/ *noun* a turning of the edge of the eyelid towards the inside

**enucleate** /ɪˈnjuːklieɪt/ *verb* to remove something completely

**enucleation** /ɪˌnjuːkliˈeɪʃ(ə)n/ *noun* **1.** the surgical removal of all of a tumour **2.** the surgical removal of the whole eyeball

**enuresis** /ˌenjʊˈriːsɪs/ *noun* the involuntary passing of urine

**enuretic** /ˌenjʊˈretɪk/ *adjective* referring to enuresis, or causing enuresis

**envenomation** /ɪnˌvenəˈmeɪʃ(ə)n/ *noun* the use of snake venom as part of a therapeutic treatment

**environment** /ɪn'vaɪrənmənt/ *noun* the conditions and influences under which an organism lives

**environmental** /ɪn,vaɪrən'ment(ə)l/ *adjective* referring to the environment

**Environmental Health Officer** /ɪn ,vaɪrənmənt(ə)l 'helθ ,ɒfɪsə/ *noun* an official of a local authority who examines the environment and tests for air pollution, bad sanitation, noise pollution and similar threats to public health. Abbr **EHO**

**environmental temperature** /ɪn,vaɪrən ment(ə)l 'temprɪtʃə/ *noun* the temperature of the air outside the body

**enzymatic** /,enzaɪ'mætɪk/ *adjective* referring to enzymes

**enzyme** /'enzaɪm/ *noun* a protein substance produced by living cells which aids a biochemical reaction in the body (NOTE: The names of enzymes mostly end with the suffix -**ase**.)
COMMENT: Many different enzymes exist in the body, working in the digestive system, in the metabolic processes and helping the synthesis of certain compounds.

**enzyme-linked immunosorbent assay** /,enzaɪm lɪŋkt ,ɪmjʊnəʊ,sɔːbənt 'æseɪ/ *noun* full form of **ELISA**

**eonism** /'iːənɪz(ə)m/ *noun* cross-dressing, when a male wears female dress

**eosin** /'iːəʊsɪn/ *noun* a red crystalline solid used as a biological staining dye

**eosinopenia** /,iːəʊsɪnə'piːniə/ *noun* a reduction in the number of eosinophils in the blood

**eosinophil** /,iːəʊ'sɪnəfɪl/ *noun* a type of cell that can be stained with eosin

**eosinophilia** /,iːəʊsɪnə'fɪliə/ *noun* an excess of eosinophils in the blood

**eparterial** /,epɑː'tɪəriəl/ *adjective* situated over or on an artery

**ependyma** /ɪ'pendɪmə/ *noun* a thin membrane which lines the ventricles of the brain and the central canal of the spinal cord

**ependymal** /ɪ'pendɪm(ə)l/ *adjective* referring to the ependyma

**ependymal cell** /ɪ'pendɪm(ə)l sel/ *noun* one of the cells which form the ependyma

**ependymoma** /ɪ,pendɪ'məʊmə/ *noun* a tumour in the brain originating in the ependyma

**ephedrine** /'efɪdriːn/ *noun* a drug that relieves asthma and blocked noses by causing the air passages to widen

**ephidrosis** /,efɪ'drəʊsɪs/ *noun* an unusual amount of sweat

**epi-** /epɪ/ *prefix* on or over

**epiblepharon** /,epɪ'blefərɒn/ *noun* an unusual fold of skin over the eyelid, which may press the eyelashes against the eyeball

**epicanthus** /,epɪ'kænθəs/, **epicanthic fold** / ,epɪkænθɪk 'fəʊld/ *noun* a large fold of skin in the inner corner of the eye, common in babies and also found in adults of some groups such as the Chinese

**epicardial** /,epɪ'kɑːdiəl/ *adjective* referring to the epicardium

**epicardial pacemaker** /,epɪkɑːdiəl 'peɪs meɪkə/ *noun* a pacemaker attached to the surface of the ventricle

**epicardium** /,epɪ'kɑːdiəm/ *noun* the inner layer of the pericardium which lines the walls of the heart, outside the myocardium. See illustration at **HEART** in Supplement

**epicondyle** /,epɪ'kɒndaɪl/ *noun* a projecting part of the round end of a bone above the condyle

**epicondylitis** /,epɪkɒndɪ'laɪtɪs/ *noun* same as **tennis elbow**

**epicranium** /,epɪ'kreɪniəm/ *noun* the five layers of the scalp, the skin and hair on the head covering the skull

**epicranius** /,epɪ'kreɪniəs/ *noun* a scalp muscle

**epicritic** /,epɪ'krɪtɪk/ *adjective* referring to the nerves which govern the fine senses of touch and temperature

**epidemic** /,epɪ'demɪk/ *adjective* spreading quickly through a large part of the population ○ *The disease rapidly reached epidemic proportions.* ■ *noun* an outbreak of an infectious disease which spreads very quickly and affects a large number of people

**epidemic pleurodynia** /,epɪdemɪk ,plʊərə 'dɪniə/ *noun* a viral disease affecting the intestinal muscles, with symptoms like influenza, such as fever, headaches and pains in the chest. Also called **Bornholm disease**

**epidemic typhus** /,epɪdemɪk 'taɪfəs/ *noun* fever with headaches, mental disorder and a rash, caused by lice which come from other humans

**epidemiological** /,epɪ,diːmɪə'lɒdʒɪk(ə)l/ *adjective* concerning epidemiology

**epidemiologist** /,epɪ,diːmɪ'ɒlədʒɪst/ *noun* a person who specialises in the study of diseases in groups of people

**epidemiology** /,epɪ,diːmɪ'ɒlədʒi/ *noun* the study of diseases in the community, in particular how they spread and how they can be controlled

**epidermal** /,epɪ'dɜːm(ə)l/ *adjective* referring to the epidermis

**epidermis** /,epɪ'dɜːmɪs/ *noun* the outer layer of the skin, including the dead skin on the surface. Also called **cuticle**

**epidermoid cyst** /,epɪdɜːmɔɪd 'sɪst/ *noun* same as **sebaceous cyst**

**epidermolysis** /,epɪdɜː'mɒləsɪs/ *noun* separation of the epidermis from the tissue underneath, usually forming a blister

**epidermolysis bullosa** /ˌepɪdɜːˌmɒləsɪs bʊˈləʊsə/ *noun* a group of disorders where blisters form on the skin

**Epidermophyton** /ˌepɪdɜːˈmɒfɪtən/ *noun* a fungus which grows on the skin and causes athlete's foot, among other disorders

**epidermophytosis** /ˌepɪˌdɜːməʊfaɪˈtəʊsɪs/ *noun* a fungus infection of the skin, e.g. athlete's foot

**epididymal** /ˌepɪˈdɪdɪm(ə)l/ *adjective* referring to the epididymis

**epididymectomy** /ˌepɪdɪdɪˈmektəmi/ *noun* the removal of the epididymis

**epididymis** /ˌepɪˈdɪdɪmɪs/ *noun* a long twisting thin tube at the back of the testis, which forms part of the efferent duct of the testis, and in which spermatozoa are stored before ejaculation. See illustration at **UROGENITAL SYSTEM (MALE)** in Supplement

**epididymitis** /ˌepɪdɪdɪˈmaɪtɪs/ *noun* inflammation of the epididymis

**epididymo-orchitis** /epɪˌdɪdɪməʊ ɔːˈkaɪtɪs/ *noun* inflammation of the epididymis and the testes

**epidural** /ˌepɪˈdjʊərəl/ *adjective* on the outside of the dura mater. Also called **extradural** ■ *noun* same as **epidural anaesthesia**

**epidural anaesthesia** /epɪˌdjʊərəl ˌænəsˈθiːziə/ *noun* a local anaesthesia in which anaesthetic is injected into the space between the vertebral canal and the dura mater

**epidural block** /ˌepɪdjʊərəl ˈblɒk/ *noun* analgesia produced by injecting an analgesic solution into the space between the vertebral canal and the dura mater

**epidural space** /ˌepɪdjʊərəl ˈspeɪs/ *noun* a space in the spinal cord between the vertebral canal and the dura mater

**epigastric** /ˌepɪˈɡæstrɪk/ *adjective* referring to the upper abdomen ○ *The patient complained of pains in the epigastric area.*

**epigastrium** /ˌepɪˈɡæstriəm/ *noun* the part of the upper abdomen between the ribcage and the navel. Also called **the pit of the stomach**

**epigastrocele** /ˌepɪˈɡæstrəʊsiːl/ *noun* a hernia in the upper abdomen

**epiglottis** /ˌepɪˈɡlɒtɪs/ *noun* a flap of cartilage at the root of the tongue which moves to block the windpipe when food is swallowed, so that the food does not go down the trachea

**epiglottitis** /ˌepɪɡlɒˈtaɪtɪs/ *noun* inflammation and swelling of the epiglottis

**epilation** /ˌepɪˈleɪʃ(ə)n/ *noun* the process of removing hair by destroying the hair follicles

**epilepsy** /ˈepɪlepsi/ *noun* a disorder of the nervous system in which there are convulsions and loss of consciousness due to a disordered discharge of cerebral neurones

COMMENT: The commonest form of epilepsy is major epilepsy or 'grand mal', where a person loses consciousness and falls to the ground with convulsions. A less severe form is minor epilepsy or 'petit mal', where attacks last only a few seconds, and the person appears simply to be hesitating or thinking deeply.

**epileptic** /ˌepɪˈleptɪk/ *adjective* having epilepsy, or relating to epilepsy ■ *noun* a person with epilepsy (NOTE: The word 'epileptic' to describe a person is now avoided.)

**epileptic fit** /ˌepɪleptɪk ˈfɪt/ *noun* an attack of convulsions, and sometimes unconsciousness, due to epilepsy

**epileptiform** /ˌepɪˈleptɪfɔːm/ *adjective* being similar to epilepsy

**epileptogenic** /ˌepɪˌleptəʊˈdʒenɪk/ *adjective* causing epilepsy

**epiloia** /ˌepɪˈlɔɪə/ *noun* a hereditary disease of the brain associated with learning disabilities, epilepsy and tumours on the kidney and heart. Also called **tuberose sclerosis**

**epimenorrhagia** /ˌepɪmenəˈreɪdʒə/ *noun* very heavy bleeding during menstruation occurring at very short intervals

**epimenorrhoea** /ˌepɪmenəˈriːə/ *noun* menstruation at shorter intervals than twenty-eight days

**epimysium** /ˌepɪˈmaɪsiəm/ *noun* a connective tissue binding striated muscle fibres

**epinephrine** /ˌepɪˈnefrɪn/ *noun US* same as **adrenaline**

**epineurium** /ˌepɪˈnjʊəriəm/ *noun* a sheath of connective tissue round a nerve

**epiphenomenon** /ˌepɪfəˈnɒmɪnən/ *noun* an unusual symptom which may not be caused by a disease

**epiphora** /eˈpɪfərə/ *noun* a condition in which the eye fills with tears either because the lacrimal duct is blocked or because excessive tears are being secreted

**epiphyseal** /ˌepɪˈfɪziəl/ *adjective* referring to an epiphysis

**epiphyseal cartilage** /epɪˌfɪziəl ˈkɑːtəlɪdʒ/ *noun* a type of cartilage in the bones of children and adolescents which expands and hardens as the bones grow to full size

**epiphyseal line** /epɪˈfɪziəl laɪn/ *noun* a plate of epiphyseal cartilage separating the epiphysis and the diaphysis of a long bone

**epiphysis** /eˈpɪfəsɪs/ *noun* the area of growth in a bone which is separated from the main part of the bone by cartilage until bone growth stops. See illustration at **BONE STRUCTURE** in Supplement. Compare **diaphysis, metaphysis**

**epiphysis cerebri** /eˌpɪfəsɪs səˈriːbri/ *noun* the pineal gland. See illustration at **BONE STRUCTURE** in Supplement

**epiphysitis** /ˌepɪfɪˈsaɪtɪs/ *noun* inflammation of an epiphysis

**epiplo-** /epɪpləʊ/ *prefix* referring to the omentum

**epiplocele** /eˈpɪpləʊsiːl/ *noun* a hernia containing part of the omentum

**epiploic** /ˌepɪˈpləʊik/ *adjective* referring to the omentum

**epiploon** /eˈpɪpləʊɒn/ *noun* same as **omentum**

**episclera** /ˈepɪsklɪərə/ *noun* the outer surface of the sclera of the eyeball

**episcleritis** /ˌepɪskləˈraɪtɪs/ *noun* inflammation of the outer surface of the sclera in the eyeball

**episi-** /əpɪziəʊ/, **episio-** /əpɪzi/ *prefix* referring to the vulva

**episiorrhaphy** /əˌpɪziˈɔːrəfi/ *noun* a procedure for stitching torn labia majora

**episiotomy** /əˌpɪziˈɒtəmi/ *noun* a surgical cut of the perineum near the vagina to prevent tearing during childbirth

**episode** /ˈepɪsəʊd/ *noun* a separate occurrence of an illness

**episodic** /ˌepɪˈsɒdɪk/ *adjective* happening in separate but related incidents, e.g. asthma which occurs in separate attacks

**epispadias** /ˌepɪˈspeɪdiəs/ *noun* a congenital condition where the urethra opens on the top of the penis and not at the end. Compare **hypospadias**

**epispastic** /ˌepɪˈspæstɪk/ *noun* same as **vesicant**

**epistaxis** /ˌepɪˈstæksɪs/ *noun* same as **nosebleed**

**epithalamus** /ˌepɪˈθæləməs/ *noun* the part of the forebrain containing the pineal body

**epithelial** /ˌepɪˈθiːliəl/ *adjective* referring to the epithelium

**epithelialisation** /ˌepɪˌθiːliəlaɪˈzeɪʃ(ə)n/, **epithelialization** *noun* the growth of skin over a wound

**epithelial layer** /epɪˌθiːliəl ˈleɪə/ *noun* the epithelium

**epithelial tissue** /epɪˌθiːliəl ˈtɪʃuː/ *noun* epithelial cells arranged as a continuous sheet consisting of one or several layers

**epithelioma** /epɪθiːliˈəʊmə/ *noun* a tumour arising from epithelial cells

**epithelium** /ˌepɪˈθiːliəm/ *noun* the layer or layers of cells covering an organ, including the skin and the lining of all hollow cavities except blood vessels, lymphatics and serous cavities. Compare **endothelium, mesothelium**

COMMENT: Epithelium is classified according to the shape of the cells and the number of layers of cells which form it. The types of epithelium according to the number of layers are: **simple epithelium** (epithelium formed of a single layer of cells) and **stratified epithelium** (epithelium formed of several layers of cells). The main types of epithelial cells are: **columnar epithelium** (simple epithelium with long narrow cells, forming the lining of the intestines); **ciliated epithelium** (simple epithelium where the cells have little hairs, forming the lining of air passages); **cuboidal epithelium** (with cube-shaped cells, forming the lining of glands and intestines) and **squamous epi-**

**thelium** or **pavement epithelium** (with flat cells like scales, forming the lining of the pericardium, peritoneum and pleura).

**epituberculosis** /ˌepɪtjuːˌbɜːkjʊˈləʊsɪs/ *noun* swelling of the lymph node in the thorax, due to tuberculosis

**eponym** /ˈepənɪm/ *noun* a procedure, disease or condition such as Dupuytren's contracture, or part of the body which is named after a person

COMMENT: An eponym can refer to a disease or condition such as Dupuytren's contracture, or Guillain–Barré syndrome, a part of the body such as circle of Willis, an organism such as Leishmania, a surgical procedure such as Trendelenburg's operation or an appliance such as Kirschner wire.

**Epsom salts** /ˌepsəm ˈsɔːlts/ *noun* same as **magnesium sulphate**

**Epstein–Barr virus** /ˌepstaɪn ˈbɑː ˌvaɪrəs/ *noun* a virus which probably causes glandular fever. Also called **EB virus** [Isolated and described 1964. After Michael Anthony Epstein (b. 1921), Bristol pathologist; Murray Llewellyn Barr (1908–95), Canadian anatomist and cytologist, head of the Department of Anatomy at the University of Western Ontario, Canada.]

**epulis** /ɪˈpjuːlɪs/ *noun* a small fibrous swelling on a gum

**equi-** /iːkwɪ, ekwɪ/ *prefix* equal

**equilibrium** /ˌiːkwɪˈlɪbriəm/ *noun* a state of balance

**equinovarus** /ɪˌkwaɪnəʊˈveərəs/ ♦ **talipes**

**equipment** /ɪˈkwɪpmənt/ *noun* apparatus or tools which are required to do something ○ *The centre urgently needs surgical equipment.* ○ *The surgeons complained about the out-of-date equipment in the hospital.* (NOTE: No plural: for one item say *a piece of equipment*.)

**ER** *abbr* **1.** *US* emergency room **2.** endoplasmic reticulum

**eradicate** /ɪˈrædɪkeɪt/ *verb* to remove something completely ○ *international action to eradicate tuberculosis*

**eradication** /ɪˌrædɪˈkeɪʃ(ə)n/ *noun* the act of removing something completely

**Erb's palsy** /ˌɜːbz ˈpɔːlzi/, **Erb's paralysis** /ˌɜːbz pəˈræləsɪs/ *noun* a condition in which an arm is paralysed because of birth injuries to the brachial plexus. ◊ **Bell's palsy**

**ERCP** *abbr* endoscopic retrograde cholangiopancreatography

**erect** /ɪˈrekt/ *adjective* stiff and straight

**erectile** /ɪˈrektaɪl/ *adjective* able to become erect

**erectile dysfunction** /ɪˌrektaɪl dɪsˈfʌŋkʃən/ *noun* a condition in which a man finds it difficult or impossible to have or maintain an erection during intercourse

**erectile tissue** /ɪˈrektaɪl ˌtɪʃuː/ *noun* vascular tissue which can become erect and stiff when engorged with blood, e.g. the corpus cavernosum in the penis

**erection** /ɪ'rekʃən/ *noun* a state where a body part such as the penis becomes swollen because of engorgement with blood

**erector** /ɪ'rektə/ *noun* a small muscle which raises a body part

**erector spinae** /ɪ,rektə 'spaɪniː/ *noun* a large muscle starting at the base of the spine, and dividing as it runs up the spine

**erepsin** /ɪ'repsɪn/ *noun* a mixture of enzymes produced by the glands in the intestine, used in the production of amino acids

**erethism** /'erəθɪz(ə)m/ *noun* unusual irritability

**ERG** *abbr* electroretinogram

**ergograph** /'ɜːɡəʊɡrɑːf/ *noun* apparatus which records the work of one or several muscles

**ergometrine maleate** /,ɜːɡəʊmetriːn 'mælieɪt/ *noun* a drug used to speed up the delivery of the placenta in childbirth and to control postnatal bleeding

**ergonomics** /,ɜːɡə'nɒmɪks/ *noun* the study of humans at work

**ergot** /'ɜːɡət/ *noun* a disease of rye caused by the fungus *Clariceps purpurea*

**ergotamine** /ɜː'ɡɒtəmiːn/ *noun* a drug that causes narrowing of blood vessels and alleviates migraine, derived from the ergot fungus

**ergotism** /'ɜːɡətɪz(ə)m/ *noun* poisoning caused by eating rye which has been contaminated with the ergot fungus

COMMENT: The symptoms of ergotism are muscle cramps and dry gangrene in the fingers and toes.

**erogenous** /ɪ'rɒdʒənəs/ *adjective* producing sexual excitement

**erogenous zone** /ɪ'rɒdʒənəs zəʊn/ *noun* a part of the body which, if stimulated, produces sexual arousal, e.g. the penis, clitoris or nipples

**erosion** /ɪ'rəʊʒ(ə)n/ *noun* the action of wearing away tissue or breaking down tissue

**erotic** /ɪ'rɒtɪk/ *adjective* relating to or arousing the feeling of sexual desire

**ERPC** *abbr* evacuation of retained products of conception

**eructation** /,iːrʌk'teɪʃ(ə)n/ *noun* same as **belching**

**erupt** /ɪ'rʌpt/ *verb* to break through the skin ○ *The permanent incisors erupt before the premolars.*

**eruption** /ɪ'rʌpʃən/ *noun* **1.** something which breaks through the skin, e.g. a rash or pimple **2.** the appearance of a new tooth in a gum

**ery-** /erɪ/ *prefix* same as **erythro-**

**erysipelas** /,erɪ'sɪpələs/ *noun* a contagious skin disease, where the skin on the face becomes hot, red and painful, caused by *Streptococcus pyogenes*

**erysipeloid** /,erɪ'sɪpəlɔɪd/ *noun* a bacterial skin infection caused by touching infected fish or meat

**erythema** /,erɪ'θiːmə/ *noun* redness on the skin, caused by hyperaemia of the blood vessels near the surface

**erythema ab igne** /,erɪθiːmə æb 'ɪɡneɪ/ *noun* a pattern of red lines on the skin caused by exposure to heat

**erythema induratum** /,erɪθiːmə ,ɪndjʊ 'reɪtəm/ *noun* a tubercular disease where ulcerating nodules appear on the legs of young women. Also called **Bazin's disease**

**erythema multiforme** /,erɪθiːmə 'mʌltiɔːmi/ *noun* the sudden appearance of inflammatory red patches and sometimes blisters on the skin

**erythema nodosum** /,erɪθiːmə nəʊ 'dəʊsəm/ *noun* an inflammatory disease where red swellings appear on the front of the legs

**erythema pernio** /,erɪθiːmə 'pɜːniəʊ/ *noun* same as **chilblain**

**erythema serpens** /,erɪθiːmə 'sɜːpens/ *noun* a bacterial skin infection caused by touching infected fish or meat

**erythematosus** /,erɪ,θiːmə'təʊsɪs/ ♦ **lupus**

**erythematous** /,erɪ'θiːmətəs/ *adjective* referring to erythema

**erythr-** /erɪθr/ *prefix* same as **erythro-** (*used before vowels*)

**erythraemia** /,erɪ'θriːmiə/ *noun* a blood disorder where the number of red blood cells increases sharply, together with an increase in the number of white cells, making the blood thicker and slower to flow. Also called **polycythaemia vera**

**erythrasma** /,erɪ'θræzmə/ *noun* a persistent bacterial skin infection occurring in a fold in the skin or where two skin surfaces touch, such as between the toes. It is caused by *Corynebacterium*.

**erythro-** /ɪrɪθrəʊ/ *prefix* red

**erythroblast** /ɪ'rɪθrəblæst/ *noun* a cell which forms an erythrocyte or red blood cell

**erythroblastosis** /ɪ,rɪθrəʊblæ'stəʊsɪs/ *noun* the presence of erythroblasts in the blood, usually found in haemolytic anaemia

COMMENT: Usually erythroblastosis occurs where the mother is rhesus negative and has developed rhesus positive antibodies, which are passed into the blood of a rhesus positive fetus.

**erythroblastosis fetalis** /ɪ,rɪθrəʊblæ ,stəʊsɪs fiː'tɑːlɪs/ *noun* a blood disease affecting newborn babies, caused by a reaction between the rhesus factor of the mother and the fetus

**erythrocyanosis** /ɪ,rɪθrəsaɪə'nəʊsɪs/ *noun* red and purple patches on the skin of the thighs, often accompanied by chilblains and made worse by cold

**erythrocyte** /ɪˈrɪθrəsaɪt/ *noun* a mature red blood cell

'...anemia may be due to insufficient erythrocyte production, in which case the corrected reticulocyte count will be low, or it may be due to hemorrhage or hemolysis, in which cases there should be reticulocyte response' [*Southern Medical Journal*]

**erythrocyte sedimentation rate** /ɪˌrɪθrə saɪt sedɪmenˈteɪʃ(ə)n reɪt/ *noun* a test that measures how fast erythrocytes settle in a sample of blood plasma, used to confirm whether various blood conditions are present. Abbr **ESR**

**erythrocytosis** /ɪˌrɪθrəsaɪˈtəʊsɪs/ *noun* an increase in the number of red blood cells in the blood

**erythroderma** /ɪˌrɪθrəˈdɜːmə/ *noun* a condition in which the skin becomes red and flakes off

**erythroedema** /ɪˌrɪθrɔɪˈdiːmə/ *noun* same as **acrodynia**

**erythrogenesis** /ɪˌrɪθrəˈdʒenəsɪs/, **erythropoiesis** /ɪˌrɪθrəpɔɪˈiːsɪs/ *noun* the formation of red blood cells in red bone marrow

**erythromelalgia** /ɪˌrɪθrəmelˈældʒə/ *noun* a painful swelling of blood vessels in the extremities

**erythromycin** /ɪˌrɪθrəˈmaɪsɪn/ *noun* a antibacterial drug suitable for people who are sensitive to penicillin

**erythropenia** /ɪrɪθrəˈpiːniə/ *noun* a condition in which a person has a low number of erythrocytes in their blood

**erythroplasia** /ɪˌrɪθrəˈpleɪziə/ *noun* the formation of lesions on the mucous membrane

**erythropoiesis** /ɪˌrɪθrəpɔɪˈiːsɪs/ *noun* same as **erythrogenesis**

**erythropoietin** /ɪˌrɪθrəˈpɔɪətɪn/ *noun* a hormone which regulates the production of red blood cells

COMMENT: Erythropoietin can now be produced by genetic techniques and is being used to increase the production of red blood cells in anaemia.

**erythropsia** /ˌerɪˈθrɒpsiə/ *noun* a condition in which someone sees things as if coloured red

**Esbach's albuminometer** /ˌesbɑːks ˌæl bjuːmɪˈnɒmɪtə/ *noun* a glass for measuring albumin in urine, using Esbach's method

**eschar** /ˈeskɑː/ *noun* a dry scab, e.g. one forming on a burn

**escharotic** /ˌeskəˈrɒtɪk/ *noun* a substance which produces an eschar

**Escherichia** /ˌeʃəˈrɪkiə/ *noun* a bacterium commonly found in faeces

**Escherichia coli** /eʃəˌrɪkiə ˈkəʊlaɪ/ *noun* a Gram-negative bacterium associated with acute gastroenteritis. Also called **E. coli**

**escort nurse** /ˈeskɔːt ˌnɜːs/ *noun* a nurse who goes with patients to the operating theatre and back again to the ward

**Esmarch's bandage** /ˈesmɑːks ˌbændɪdʒ/ *noun* a rubber band wrapped round a limb as a tourniquet before a surgical operation and left in place during the operation so as to keep the site free of blood [Described 1869. After Johann Friedrich August von Esmarch (1823–1908), Professor of Surgery at Kiel, Germany.]

**esophagus** /iːˈsɒfəgəs/ *noun* US spelling of **oesophagus**

**esotropia** /esəˈtrəʊpiə/ *noun* a type of squint, where the eyes both look towards the nose. Also called **convergent strabismus**

**espundia** /ɪˈspuːndiə/ ♦ **leishmaniasis**

**ESR** *abbr* erythrocyte sedimentation rate

**ESRD** *abbr* end-stage renal disease

**essence** /ˈes(ə)ns/ *noun* a concentrated oil from a plant, used in cosmetics, and sometimes as analgesics or antiseptics

**essential** /ɪˈsenʃəl/ *adjective* **1.** extremely important ○ *It is essential to keep accurate records.* **2.** necessary for health ○ *essential nutrients* **3.** without obvious cause ○ *essential hypertension* Also called **idiopathic 4.** extracted from a plant ○ *essential oil*

**essential amino acid** /ɪˌsenʃəl əˌmiːnəʊ ˈæsɪd/ *noun* an amino acid which is necessary for growth but which cannot be synthesised in the body and has to be obtained from the food supply

COMMENT: The essential amino acids are: isoleucine, leucine, lysine, methionine, phenylalanine, threonine, tryptophan and valine.

**essential dysmenorrhoea** /ɪˌsenʃəl dɪs menəˈriːə/ *noun* same as **primary dysmenorrhoea**

**essential element** /ɪˌsenʃəl ˈelɪmənt/ *noun* a chemical element which is necessary to the body's growth or function, e.g. carbon, oxygen, hydrogen and nitrogen

**essential fatty acid** /ɪˌsenʃəl ˌfæti ˈæsɪd/ *noun* an unsaturated fatty acid which is necessary for growth and health. Abbr **EFA**

COMMENT: The essential fatty acids are linoleic acid, linolenic acid and arachidonic acid.

**essential hyperkinesia** /ɪˌsenʃəl ˌhaɪpəkɪ ˈniːziə/ *noun* a condition of children where their movements are excessive and repeated

**essential hypertension** /ɪˌsenʃəl ˈhaɪpə ˌtenʃən/ *noun* high blood pressure without any obvious cause

**essential oil** /ɪˌsenʃəl ˈɔɪl/ *noun* a medicinal or fragrant oil distilled from some part of a plant

**essential tremor** /ɪˌsenʃəl ˈtremə/ *noun* an involuntary slow trembling movement of the hands often seen in elderly people

**essential uterine haemorrhage** /ɪˌsenʃəl ˌjuːtəraɪn ˈhem(ə)rɪdʒ/ *noun* heavy uterine bleeding for which there is no obvious cause

**estrogen** /ˈiːstrədʒən/ *noun* US same as **oestrogen**

**ethambutol** /ɪˈθæmbjʊtɒl/ *noun* a drug that is part of the treatment for bacterial infections such as tuberculosis

**ethanol** /ˈeθənɒl/ *noun* a colourless liquid, present in alcoholic drinks such as whisky, gin and vodka, and also used in medicines and as a disinfectant. Also called **ethyl alcohol**. ◊ **pure alcohol**

**ethene** /ˈiːθiːn/ *noun* same as **ethylene**

**ether** /ˈiːθə/ *noun* an anaesthetic substance, now rarely used

**ethical** /ˈeθɪk(ə)l/ *adjective* **1.** concerning ethics **2.** referring to a drug available on prescription only

**ethical committee** /ˈeθɪk(ə)l kəˌmɪti/ *noun* a group of specialists who monitor experiments involving human beings or who regulate the way in which members of the medical profession conduct themselves

**ethinyloestradiol** /ˌeθɪn(ə)lˌiːstrəˈdaɪɒl/ *noun* an artificial hormone related to oestrogen that is effective in small doses. It forms part of hormone replacement therapy.

**ethmoid** /eθˈmɔɪd/, **ethmoidal** /eθˈmɔɪd(ə)l/ *adjective* referring to the ethmoid bone or near to the ethmoid bone

**ethmoidal sinuses** /eθˌmɔɪd(ə)l ˈsaɪnəsɪz/ *plural noun* air cells inside the ethmoid bone

**ethmoid bone** /ˈeθmɔɪd bəʊn/ *noun* a bone which forms the top of the nasal cavity and part of the orbits

**ethmoidectomy** /ˌeθmɔɪˈdektəmi/ *noun* an operation to remove the lining between the sinuses

**ethmoiditis** /ˌeθmɔɪˈdaɪtɪs/ *noun* inflammation of the ethmoid bone or of the ethmoidal sinuses

**ethnic** /ˈeθnɪk/ *adjective* relating to a culturally or racially distinctive group of people

**ethyl alcohol** /ˌiθaɪl ˈælkəhɒl/ *noun* same as **ethanol**

**ethylene** /ˈeθəliːn/ *noun* a gas used as an anaesthetic

**ethylestrenol** /ˌeθ(ə)lˈestrənɒl/ *noun* an anabolic steroid

**etiology** /ˌiːtiˈɒlədʒi/ *noun US* same as **aetiology**

**eu-** /juː/ *prefix* good, well

**eubacteria** /ˌjuːbækˈtɪəriə/ *noun* true bacteria with rigid cell walls

**eucalyptol** /ˌjuːkəˈlɪptəl/ *noun* a substance obtained from eucalyptus oil

**eucalyptus** /ˌjuːkəˈlɪptəs/ *noun* a genus of tree growing mainly in Australia, from which a strongly smelling oil is distilled

**eucalyptus oil** /ˌjuːkəˈlɪptəs ɔɪl/ *noun* an aromatic medicinal oil distilled from the leaves of various species of tree in the genus *Eucalyptus*

COMMENT: Eucalyptus oil is used in pharmaceutical products especially to relieve congestion in the respiratory passages.

**eugenics** /juːˈdʒenɪks/ *noun* the study of how to improve the human race by genetic selection

**eunuch** /ˈjuːnək/ *noun* a castrated male

**eupepsia** /juːˈpepsiə/ *noun* good digestion

**euphoria** /juːˈfɔːriə/ *noun* a feeling of extreme happiness

**euplastic** /juːˈplæstɪk/ *adjective* referring to tissue which heals well

**Eustachian canal** /juːˈsteɪʃ(ə)n kəˌnæl/ *noun* a passage through the porous bone forming the outside part of the Eustachian tube

**Eustachian tube** /juːˈsteɪʃ(ə)n tjuːb/ *noun* the tube which connects the pharynx to the middle ear. See illustration at EAR in Supplement [Described 1562, but actually named after Eustachio by Valsalva a century later. Bartolomeo Eustachio (1520–74), physician to the Pope and Professor of Anatomy in Rome.]

COMMENT: The Eustachian tubes balance the air pressure on each side of the eardrum. When a person swallows or yawns, air is allowed into the Eustachian tubes and equalises the pressure with the normal atmospheric pressure outside the body. The tubes can be blocked by an infection, as in a cold, or by pressure differences, as inside an aircraft, and if they are blocked, the hearing is impaired.

**euthanasia** /ˌjuːθəˈneɪziə/ *noun* the painless killing of an incurably ill person or someone in a permanent coma in order to end their distress. Also called **mercy killing** (NOTE: This practice is illegal in most countries.)

**euthanise** /ˈjuːθənaɪz/, **euthanize** *verb* to kill an incurably ill person or someone in a permanent coma

**euthyroid** /juːˈθaɪrɔɪd/ *noun* a condition where the thyroid is functioning normally

**euthyroidism** /juːˈθaɪrɔɪdɪz(ə)m/, **euthyroid state** /juːˈθaɪrɔɪd ˌsteɪt/ *noun* the fact of having a healthy thyroid gland

**eutocia** /juːˈtəʊsiə/ *noun* a standard childbirth

**evacuant** /ɪˈvækjuənt/ *noun* a medicine which makes a person have a bowel movement

**evacuate** /ɪˈvækjueɪt/ *verb* to discharge faeces from the bowel, or to have a bowel movement

**evacuation** /ɪˌvækjuˈeɪʃ(ə)n/ *noun* the act of removing the contents of something, especially discharging faeces from the bowel

**evacuation of retained products of conception** /ɪˌvækjuˌeɪʃ(ə)n əv rɪˌteɪnd ˌprɒdʌkts əv kənˈsepʃən/ *noun* a D & C operation performed after an abortion or miscarriage to ensure the uterus is left empty. Abbr **ERPC**

**evacuator** /ɪˈvækjueɪtə/ *noun* an instrument used to empty a cavity such as the bladder or bowel

**evaluate** /ɪˈvæljueɪt/ *verb* **1.** to examine and calculate the quantity or level of something ○ *The laboratory is still evaluating the results of the tests.* **2.** to examine someone and calculate the treatment required

'…all patients were evaluated and followed up at the hypertension unit' [*British Medical Journal*]

**evaluation** /ɪˌvæljuˈeɪʃ(ə)n/ *noun* the act of examining and calculating the quantity or level of something ○ *In further evaluation of these patients no side-effects of the treatment were noted.*

'…evaluation of fetal age and weight has proved to be of value in the clinical management of pregnancy, particularly in high-risk gestations' [*Southern Medical Journal*]

**eventration** /ˌiːvenˈtreɪʃ(ə)n/ *noun* the pushing of the intestine through the wall of the abdomen

**eversion** /ɪˈvɜːʃ(ə)n/ *noun* the act of turning towards the outside or turning inside out. See illustration at ANATOMICAL TERMS in Supplement □ **eversion of the cervix** a condition after laceration during childbirth, where the edges of the cervix sometimes turn outwards

**evertor** /ɪˈvɜːtə/ *noun* a muscle which makes a limb turn outwards

**evidence-based** /ˈevɪdəns beɪst/ *adjective* based on the results of well-designed trials of specific types of treatment for specific conditions ○ *evidence-based practice*

**evidence-based medicine** /ˈevɪd(ə)ns beɪst ˌmed(ə)sɪn/ *noun* medical practice where findings from research are used as the basis for decisions

**evisceration** /ɪˌvɪsəˈreɪʃ(ə)n/ *noun* **1.** the surgical removal of the abdominal viscera. Also called **exenteration 2.** removal of the contents of an organ □ **evisceration of the eye** surgical removal of the contents of an eyeball

**evolution** /ˌiːvəˈluːʃ(ə)n/ *noun* a process of change in organisms which takes place over a very long period involving many generations

**evulsion** /ɪˈvʌlʃən/ *noun* the act of extracting something by force

**Ewing's tumour** /ˈjuːɪŋz ˈtjuːmə/, **Ewing's sarcoma** /ˌjuːɪŋz sɑːˈkəʊmə/ *noun* a malignant tumour in the marrow of a long bone [Described 1922. After James Ewing (1866–1943), Professor of Pathology at Cornell University, New York, USA.]

**ex-** /eks/ *prefix* same as **exo-** (*used before vowels*)

**exacerbate** /ɪɡˈzæsəˌbeɪt/ *verb* to make a condition more severe ○ *The cold damp weather will only exacerbate his chest condition.*

**exacerbation** /ɪɡˌzæsəˈbeɪʃ(ə)n/ *noun* **1.** the fact of making a condition worse **2.** a period when a condition becomes worse

'…patients were re-examined regularly or when they felt they might be having an exacerbation. Exacerbation rates were calculated from the number of exacerbations during the study' [*Lancet*]

**examination** /ɪɡˌzæmɪˈneɪʃ(ə)n/ *noun* **1.** an act of looking at someone or something carefully ○ *From the examination of the X-ray photographs, it seems that the tumour has not spread.* **2.** the act of looking at someone to find out what is wrong with him or her ○ *The surgeon carried out a medical examination before operating.* **3.** a written or oral test to see if a student is progressing satisfactorily (NOTE: In this sense, often abbreviated to **exam**.)

**examine** /ɪɡˈzæmɪn/ *verb* **1.** to look at or to investigate someone or something carefully ○ *The tissue samples were examined in the laboratory.* **2.** to look at and test someone to find out what is wrong with him or her ○ *The doctor examined the patient's heart.*

**exanthem** /ɪɡˈzænθəm/ *noun* a skin rash found with infectious diseases like measles or chickenpox

**exanthematous** /ˌeksænˈθemətəs/ *adjective* referring to an exanthem or like an exanthem

**exanthem subitum** /ɪɡˌzænθəm ˈsʊbɪtəm/ *noun* same as **roseola infantum**

**excavator** /ˈekskəveɪtə/ *noun* a surgical instrument shaped like a spoon

**excavatum** /ˈekskəveɪtəm/ ♦ **pectus excavatum**

**exception** /ɪkˈsepʃən/ *noun* **1.** something that does not fit into or is excluded from a general rule or pattern **2.** the act or condition of being excluded

**excess** /ɪkˈses/ *noun* too much of a substance ○ *The gland was producing an excess of hormones.* ○ *The body could not cope with an excess of blood sugar.* □ **in excess of** more than ○ *Short men who weigh in excess of 100 kilos are very overweight.*

**excessive** /ɪkˈsesɪv/ *adjective* more than normal ○ *The patient was passing excessive quantities of urine.* ○ *The doctor noted an excessive amount of bile in the patient's blood.*

**excessively** /ɪkˈsesɪvli/ *adverb* too much ○ *She has an excessively high blood pressure.* ○ *If the patient sweats excessively, it may be necessary to cool his body with cold compresses.*

**exchange transfusion** /ɪksˌtʃeɪndʒ trænsˈfjuːʒ(ə)n/ *noun* a method of treating leukaemia or erythroblastosis in newborn babies, where almost all the blood is removed from the body and replaced with healthy blood

**excipient** /ɪkˈsɪpiənt/ *noun* a substance added to a drug so that it can be made into a pill

**excise** /ɪkˈsaɪz/ *verb* to cut something out

**excision** /ɪkˈsɪʒ(ə)n/ *noun* an operation by a surgeon to cut and remove part of the body such as a growth. Compare **incision**

**excitation** /ˌeksɪˈteɪʃ(ə)n/ *noun* the state of being mentally or physically aroused

**excitatory** /ɪkˈsaɪtətri/ *adjective* tending to excite

**excite** /ɪkˈsaɪt/ *verb* **1.** to stimulate someone or something **2.** to give an impulse to a nerve or muscle

**excited** /ɪkˈsaɪtɪd/ *adjective* **1.** very lively and happy **2.** aroused

**excitement** /ɪkˈsaɪtmənt/ *noun* **1.** the act of being excited **2.** the second stage of anaesthesia

**excoriation** /ɪksˌkɔːriˈeɪʃ(ə)n/ *noun* a raw skin surface or mucous membrane after rubbing or burning

**excrement** /ˈekskrɪmənt/ *noun* same as **faeces**

**excrescence** /ɪkˈskres(ə)ns/ *noun* a growth on the skin

**excreta** /ɪkˈskriːtə/ *plural noun* waste material from the body, especially faeces

**excrete** /ɪkˈskriːt/ *verb* to pass waste matter out of the body, especially to discharge faeces ○ *The urinary system separates waste liquids from the blood and excretes them as urine.*

**excretion** /ɪkˈskriːʃ(ə)n/ *noun* the act of passing waste matter, e.g. faeces, urine or sweat, out of the body

**excruciating** /ɪkˈskruːʃieɪtɪŋ/ *adjective* extremely painful ○ *He had excruciating pains in his head.*

**exenteration** /ekˌsentəˈreɪʃ(ə)n/ *noun* same as **evisceration**

**exercise** /ˈeksəsaɪz/ *noun* **1.** physical or mental activity, especially the active use of the muscles as a way of keeping fit, correcting a deformity or strengthening a part ○ *Regular exercise is good for your heart.* ○ *He doesn't do* or *take enough exercise.* **2.** a particular movement or action designed to use and strengthen the muscles ■ *verb* to take exercise, or exert part of the body in exercise ○ *He exercises twice a day to keep fit.*

**exercise cycle** /ˈeksəsaɪz ˌsaɪk(ə)l/ *noun* a type of cycle which is fixed to the floor, so that someone can pedal on it for exercise

**exercise-induced asthma** /ˌeksəsaɪz ɪn ˌdjuːst ˈæsmə/ *noun* asthma which is caused by exercise such as running or cycling. Abbr **EIA**

**exertion** /ɪgˈzɜːʃ(ə)n/ *noun* physical activity

**exfoliation** /eksˌfəʊliˈeɪʃ(ə)n/ *noun* the loss of layers of tissue such as sunburnt skin

**exfoliative** /eksˈfəʊlieɪtɪv/ *adjective* referring to exfoliation

**exfoliative dermatitis** /eksˌfəʊliətɪv ˌdɜːməˈtaɪtɪs/ *noun* a typical form of dermatitis where the skin becomes red and comes off in flakes

**exhalation** /ˌekshəˈleɪʃ(ə)n/ *noun* **1.** the act of breathing out **2.** air which is breathed out ▶ opposite **inhalation**

**exhale** /eksˈheɪl/ *verb* to breathe out. Opposite **inhale**

**exhaust** /ɪgˈzɔːst/ *verb* to tire someone out

**exhaustion** /ɪgˈzɔːstʃən/ *noun* extreme tiredness or fatigue

**exhibitionism** /ˌeksɪˈbɪʃ(ə)nɪz(ə)m/ *noun* a desire to show the genitals to a person of the opposite sex

**exo-** /eksəʊ/ *prefix* out of, outside

**exocrine** /ˈeksəkraɪn/ *adjective* □ **exocrine secretions of the pancreas** enzymes carried from the pancreas to the second part of the duodenum

**exocrine gland** /ˈeksəkraɪn glænd/ *noun* a gland with ducts which channel secretions to particular parts of the body such as the liver, the sweat glands, the pancreas and the salivary glands. Compare **endocrine gland**

**exogenous** /ekˈsɒdʒənəs/ *adjective* developing or caused by something outside the organism. Compare **endogenous**

**exomphalos** /ekˈsɒmfələs/ *noun* same as **umbilical hernia**

**exophthalmic goitre** /ˌeksɒfˈθælmɪk ˈgɔɪtə/ *noun* a form of hyperthyroidism, in which the neck swells and the eyes protrude. Also called **Graves' disease**

**exophthalmos** /ˌeksɒfˈθælməs/ *noun* protruding eyeballs

**exoskeleton** /ˈeksəʊˌskelɪt(ə)n/ *noun* the outer skeleton of some animals such as insects. Compare **endoskeleton**

**exostosis** /ˌeksəˈstəʊsɪs/ *noun* a benign growth on the surface of a bone

**exotic** /ɪgˈzɒtɪk/ *adjective* referring to a disease which occurs in a foreign country

**exotoxin** /ˌeksəʊˈtɒksɪn/ *noun* a poison, produced by bacteria, which affects parts of the body away from the place of infection, e.g. the toxins which cause botulism or tetanus

COMMENT: Diphtheria is caused by a bacillus. The exotoxin released causes the generalised symptoms of the disease such as fever and rapid pulse while the bacillus itself is responsible for the local symptoms in the upper throat.

**exotropia** /ˌeksəʊˈtrəʊpiə/ *noun* same as **divergent strabismus**

**expectant mother** /ɪkˌspektənt ˈmʌðə/ *noun* a pregnant woman

**expected date of delivery** /ɪkˌspektɪd ˌdeɪt əv dɪˈlɪv(ə)ri/ *noun* the day on which a doctor calculates that the birth of a baby will take place

**expectorant** /ɪkˈspekt(ə)rənt/ *noun* a drug which helps someone to cough up phlegm

**expectorate** /ɪk'spektəreɪt/ *verb* to cough up phlegm or sputum from the respiratory passages

**expectoration** /ɪkˌspektə'reɪʃ(ə)n/ *noun* the act of coughing up fluid or phlegm from the respiratory tract

**expel** /ɪk'spel/ *verb* to send something out of the body ○ *Air is expelled from the lungs when a person breathes out.*

**experiential learning** /ɪkˌspɪərienʃəl 'lɜːnɪŋ/ *noun* the process of learning from experience

**experiment** /ɪk'sperɪmənt/ *noun* a scientific test conducted under set conditions ○ *The scientists did some experiments to try the new drug on a small sample of people.*

**expert patient** /ˌekspɜːt 'peɪʃ(ə)nt/ *noun* a patient with a long-term illness who has been taught how to manage his or her own medical care

**expiration** /ˌekspə'reɪʃ(ə)n/ *noun* **1.** the act of breathing out, or pushing air out of the lungs ○ *Expiration takes place when the chest muscles relax and the lungs become smaller.* Opposite **inspiration 2.** death **3.** dying

**expiratory** /ek'spɪrət(ə)ri/ *adjective* referring to the process of breathing out

**expire** /ɪk'spaɪə/ *verb* **1.** to breathe out **2.** to die

**explant** /eks'plɑːnt/ *noun* tissue taken from a body and grown in a culture in a laboratory ■ *verb* **1.** to take tissue from a body and grow it in a culture in a laboratory **2.** to remove an implant

**explantation** /ˌeksplɑːn'teɪʃ(ə)n/ *noun* **1.** the act of taking tissue from a body and growing it in a culture in a laboratory **2.** the removal of an implant

**exploration** /ˌeksplə'reɪʃ(ə)n/ *noun* a procedure or surgical operation where the aim is to discover the cause of symptoms or the nature and extent of an illness

**exploratory** /ɪk'splɒrət(ə)ri/ *adjective* referring to an exploration

**exploratory surgery** /ɪkˌsplɒrət(ə)ri 'sɜːdʒəri/ *noun* a surgical operation in which the aim is to discover the cause of a person's symptoms or the nature and extent of an illness

**explore** /ɪk'splɔː/ *verb* to examine a part of the body in order to make a diagnosis

**expose** /ɪk'spəʊz/ *verb* **1.** to show something which was hidden ○ *The operation exposed a generalised cancer.* ○ *The report exposed a lack of medical care on the part of some of the hospital staff.* **2.** to place something or someone under the influence of something ○ *He was exposed to the disease for two days.* ○ *She was exposed to a lethal dose of radiation.*

**exposure** /ɪk'spəʊʒə/ *noun* **1.** the fact of being exposed to something ○ *his exposure to radiation* **2.** the fact of being damp, cold and with

no protection from the weather ○ *The survivors of the crash were all suffering from exposure after spending a night in the snow.*

**express** /ɪk'spres/ *verb* to squeeze liquid or air out of something, especially to squeeze out breast milk for a baby to feed on later

**expression** /ɪk'spreʃ(ə)n/ *noun* **1.** the look on a person's face which shows what he or she thinks and feels ○ *His expression showed that he was annoyed.* **2.** the act of pushing something out of the body ○ *the expression of the fetus and placenta during childbirth*

**exquisitely tender** /ɪkˌskwɪzɪtli 'tendə/ *adjective* producing a sharp localised pain or tenderness when touched

**exsanguinate** /ɪk'sæŋgwɪneɪt/ *verb* to drain blood from the body

**exsanguination** /ɪkˌsæŋgwɪ'neɪʃ(ə)n/ *noun* the removal of blood from the body

**exsufflation** /ˌeksə'fleɪʃ(ə)n/ *noun* an act of forcing breath out of the body

**extend** /ɪk'stend/ *verb* to stretch out, or cause something to stretch out ○ *The patient is unable to extend his arms fully.*

**extension** /ɪk'stenʃən/ *noun* **1.** the stretching or straightening out of a joint **2.** the stretching of a joint by traction

**extensor** /ɪk'stensə/, **extensor muscle** /ɪk 'stensə ˌmʌs(ə)l/ *noun* a muscle which makes a joint become straight. Compare **flexor**

**exterior** /ɪk'stɪəriə/ *noun* the outside of something

**exteriorisation** /ɪkˌstɪəriəraɪ'zeɪʃ(ə)n/, **exteriorization** *noun* a surgical operation to bring an internal organ to the outside surface of the body

**externa** /ɪk'stɜːnə/ ♦ **otitis externa**

**external** /ɪk'stɜːn(ə)l/ *adjective* on the outside, especially outside the surface of the body. Opposite **internal** □ **the lotion is for external use only** it should only be used on the outside of the body

**external auditory canal** /ɪkˌstɜːn(ə)l 'ɔːdɪt(ə)ri kəˌnæl/, **external auditory meatus** /ɪkˌstɜːn(ə)l ˌɔːdɪt(ə)ri mɪ'eɪtəs/ *noun* a tube in the skull leading from the outer ear to the eardrum. See illustration in **EAR** in Supplement

**external cardiac massage** /ɪkˌstɜːn(ə)l ˌkɑːdiæk 'mæsɑːʒ/ *noun* a method of making someone's heart start beating again by rhythmic pressing on the breastbone

**external ear** /ɪkˌstɜːn(ə)l 'ɪə/ *noun* same as **outer ear**

**external haemorrhoids** /ɪkˌstɜːn(ə)l 'hemərɔɪdz/ *plural noun* haemorrhoids in the skin just outside the anus

**external iliac artery** /ɪkˌstɜːn(ə)l 'ɪliæk ˌɑːtəri/ *noun* an artery which branches from the aorta in the abdomen and leads to the leg

**external jugular** /ɪkˌstɜːn(ə)l ˈdʒæɡjʊlə/ noun the main jugular vein in the neck, leading from the temporal vein

**externally** /ɪkˈstɜːn(ə)li/ adverb on the outside of the body ○ *The ointment should only be used externally.*

**external nares** plural noun same as **anterior nares**

**external oblique** /ɪkˌstɜːn(ə)l əˈbliːk/ noun an outer muscle covering the abdomen

**external otitis** /ɪkˌstɜːn(ə)l əˈtaɪtɪs/ noun same as **otitis externa**

**external respiration** /ɪkˌstɜːn(ə)l ˌrespɪˈreɪʃ(ə)n/ noun the part of respiration concerned with oxygen in the air being exchanged in the lungs for carbon dioxide from the blood

**exteroceptor** /ˈekstərəʊˌseptə/ noun a sensory nerve which is affected by stimuli from outside the body, e.g. in the eye or ear

**extinction** /ɪkˈstɪŋkʃən/ noun 1. the destruction or stopping of something 2. the lessening or stopping of a conditioned behavioural response through lack of reinforcement

**extirpate** /ˈekstɜːˌpeɪt/ verb to remove something by surgery

**extirpation** /ekstɜːˈpeɪʃ(ə)n/ noun the total removal of a structure, an organ or growth by surgery

**extra-** /ekstrə/ prefix outside

**extracapsular** /ˌekstrəˈkæpsjʊlə/ adjective outside a capsule

**extracapsular fracture** /ˌekstrəˌkæpsjʊlə ˈfræktʃə/ noun a fracture of the upper part of the femur, which does not involve the capsule round the hip joint

**extracellular** /ˌekstrəˈseljʊlə/ adjective outside cells

**extracellular fluid** /ˌekstrəseljʊlə ˈfluːɪd/ noun a fluid which surrounds cells

**extract** noun /ˈekstrækt/ a preparation made by removing water or alcohol from a substance, leaving only the essence □ **liver extract** concentrated essence of liver ■ verb /ɪkˈstrækt/ to take out something ○ *Adrenaline extracted from the animal's adrenal glands is used in the treatment of asthma.*

'…all the staff are RGNs, partly because they do venesection, partly because they work in plasmapheresis units which extract plasma and return red blood cells to the donor' [*Nursing Times*]

**extraction** /ɪkˈstrækʃən/ noun 1. the removal of part of the body, especially a tooth 2. in obstetrics, delivery, usually a breech presentation, which needs medical assistance

**extradural** /ˌekstrəˈdjʊərəl/ adjective same as **epidural**

**extradural haematoma** /ˌekstrəˌdjʊərəl hiːməˈtəʊmə/ noun a blood clot which forms in the head outside the dura mater, caused by a blow

**extradural haemorrhage** /ˌekstrəˌdjʊərəl ˈhem(ə)rɪdʒ/ noun a serious condition where

bleeding occurs between the dura mater and the skull

**extraembryonic** /ˌekstrəembriˈɒnɪk/ adjective referring to part of a fertilised ovum, such as the amnion, allantois and chorion which is not part of the embryo

**extraembryonic membranes** /ˌekstrə embriˌɒnɪk ˈmembreɪnz/ plural noun membranes which are not part of the embryo

**extrapleural** /ˌekstrəˈplʊərəl/ adjective outside the pleural cavity

**extrapyramidal** /ˌekstrəpɪˈræmɪd(ə)l/ adjective outside the pyramidal tracts

**extrapyramidal system** /ˌekstrəpɪ ˌræmɪd(ə)l ˈsɪstəm/ noun a motor system which carries motor nerves outside the pyramidal system

**extrapyramidal tracts** /ˌekstrəpɪ ˌræmɪd(ə)l ˈtrækts/ plural noun same as **extrapyramidal system**

**extrasensory** /ˌekstrəˈsensəri/ adjective involving perception by means other than the usual five senses

**extrasystole** /ˌekstrəˈsɪstəli/ noun same as **ectopic heartbeat**

**extrauterine** /ˌekstrəˈjuːtəraɪn/ adjective occurring or developing outside the uterus

**extrauterine pregnancy** /ˌekstrəjuːtəraɪn ˈpregnənsi/ noun same as **ectopic pregnancy**

**extravasation** /ekˌstrævəˈseɪʃ(ə)n/ noun a situation where a bodily fluid, such as blood or secretions, escapes into tissue

**extraversion** /ˌekstrəˈvɜːʃ(ə)n/ noun same as **extroversion**

**extravert** /ˈekstrəvɜːt/ noun same as **extrovert**

**extremities** /ɪkˈstremətiz/ plural noun the parts of the body at the ends of limbs, e.g. fingers, toes, nose and ears

**extremity** /ɪkˈstremɪti/ noun 1. a limb 2. the part of a limb farthest away from the body, especially the hand and foot 3. a situation or state of great distress or danger 4. the greatest intensity of something

**extrinsic** /eksˈtrɪnsɪk/ adjective external, originating outside a structure

**extrinsic allergic alveolitis** /eksˌtrɪnsɪk ə ˌlɜːdʒɪk ˌælviəˈlaɪtɪs/ noun a condition in which the lungs are allergic to fungus and other allergens

**extrinsic factor** /eksˌtrɪnsɪk ˈfæktə/ noun a former term for vitamin $B_{12}$, which is necessary for the production of red blood cells

**extrinsic ligament** /eksˌtrɪnsɪk ˈlɪgəmənt/ noun a ligament between the bones in a joint which is separate from the joint capsule

**extrinsic muscle** /eksˌtrɪnsɪk ˈmʌs(ə)l/ noun a muscle which is some way away from the part of the body which it operates

**extroversion** /ˌekstrəˈvɜːʃ(ə)n/ noun 1. (in psychology) a condition in which a person is interested in people and things other than themselves **2.** a congenital turning of an organ inside out

**extrovert** /'ekstrəvɜːt/ *noun* a person who is interested in people and things in the external world

**extroverted** /'ekstrəʊ,vɜːtɪd/ *adjective* **1.** (*of a person*) interested in people and things other than oneself **2.** (*of an organ*) turned inside out

**extubation** /,ekstjuː'beɪʃ(ə)n/ *noun* the removal of a tube after intubation

**exudate** /'eksjudeɪt/ *noun* fluid which is deposited on the surface of tissue as the result of a condition or disease

**exudation** /,eksjuː'deɪʃ(ə)n/ *noun* the escape of material such as fluid or cells into tissue as a defence mechanism

**eye** /aɪ/ *noun* the part of the body with which a person sees (NOTE: For other terms referring to the eye, see **ocular**, **optic** and words beginning with **oculo-, ophth-, ophthalm-, ophthalmo-**.)

**eyeball** /'aɪbɔːl/ *noun* the round ball of tissue through which light passes, located in the eye socket and controlled by various muscles

COMMENT: Light rays enter the eye through the cornea, pass through the pupil and are refracted through the aqueous humour onto the lens, which then focuses the rays through the vitreous humour onto the retina at the back of the eyeball. Impulses from the retina pass along the optic nerve to the brain.

**eye bank** /'aɪ bæŋk/ *noun* a place where parts of eyes given by donors can be kept for use in grafts

**eyebath** /'aɪbɑːθ/ *noun* a small dish into which a solution can be put for bathing the eye

**eyebrow** /'aɪbraʊ/ *noun* an arch of skin with a line of hair above the eye

**eye drops** /'aɪ drɒps/ *plural noun* medicine in liquid form which is put into the eye in small amounts

**eyeglasses** /'aɪ,glɑːsɪz/ *plural noun US* glasses or spectacles for correcting vision

**eyelash** /'aɪlæʃ/ *noun* a small hair which grows out from the edge of the eyelid

**eyelid** /'aɪlɪd/ *noun* a piece of skin which covers the eye. Also called **blepharon, palpebra** (NOTE: For other terms referring to the eyelids, see words beginning with **blephar-, blepharo-**.)

**eye ointment** /'aɪ ,ɔɪntmənt/ *noun* an ointment in a special tube to be used in eye treatment

**eyesight** /'aɪsaɪt/ *noun* the ability to see ○ *He has got very good eyesight.* ○ *Failing eyesight is common in elderly people.*

**eye socket** /'aɪ ,sɒkɪt/ *noun* same as **orbit**

**eye specialist** /'aɪ ,speʃəlɪst/ *noun* same as **ophthalmologist**

**eyestrain** /'aɪstreɪn/ *noun* tiredness in the muscles of the eye with a headache, which may be caused by an activity such as reading in bad light or working on a computer screen. Also called **asthenopia**

**eye surgeon** /'aɪ ,sɜːdʒ(ə)n/ *noun* a surgeon who specialises in operations on eyes

**eye test** /'aɪ test/ *noun* an examination of the inside of an eye to see if it is working correctly, and if the person needs glasses

**eyetooth** /'aɪtuːθ/ *noun* a canine tooth, one of two pairs of pointed teeth next to the incisors (NOTE: The plural is **eyeteeth**.)

# F

**F** *abbr* Fahrenheit

**face** /feɪs/ *noun* the front part of the head, where the eyes, nose and mouth are placed ■ *verb* to have your face towards or to look towards something ○ *Please face the screen.*

**face delivery** /'feɪs dɪ,lɪv(ə)ri/ *noun* a birth where the baby's face appears first

**face lift** /'feɪs lɪft/, **face-lifting operation** /'feɪs ,lɪftɪŋ ɒpə,reɪʃ(ə)n/ *noun* a surgical operation to remove wrinkles on the face and neck

**face mask** /'feɪs mɑːsk/ *noun* **1.** a rubber mask that fits over the nose and mouth and is used to administer an anaesthetic **2.** a piece of gauze which fits over the mouth and nose to prevent droplet infection

**face presentation** /'feɪs prez(ə)n,teɪʃ(ə)n/ *noun* a position of a baby in the uterus where the face will appear first at birth

**facet** /'fæsɪt/ *noun* a flat surface on a bone

**facet syndrome** /'fæsɪt ,sɪndrəʊm/ *noun* a condition in which a joint in the vertebrae becomes dislocated

**facial** /'feɪʃ(ə)l/ *adjective* relating to, or appearing on, the face ○ *The psychiatrist examined the patient's facial expression.*

**facial artery** /'feɪʃ(ə)l ,ɑːtəri/ *noun* an artery which branches off the external carotid into the face and mouth

**facial bone** /'feɪʃ(ə)l bəʊn/ *noun* one of the fourteen bones which form the face

COMMENT: The bones which make up the face are: two maxillae forming the upper jaw; two nasal bones forming the top part of the nose; two lacrimal bones on the inside of the orbit near the nose; two zygomatic or malar bones forming the sides of the cheeks; two palatine bones forming the back part of the top of the mouth; two nasal conchae or turbinate bones which form the sides of the nasal cavity; the mandible or lower jaw; and the vomer in the centre of the nasal septum.

**facial nerve** /'feɪʃ(ə)l nɜːv/ *noun* the seventh cranial nerve, which governs the muscles of the face, the taste buds on the front of the tongue and the salivary and lacrimal glands

**facial paralysis** /,feɪʃ(ə)l pə'ræləsɪs/ *noun* same as **Bell's palsy**

**facial vein** /'feɪʃ(ə)l veɪn/ *noun* a vein which drains down the side of the face into the internal jugular vein

**-facient** /feɪʃənt/ *suffix* making or causing ○ *abortifacient*

**facies** /'feɪʃiiːz/ *noun* someone's facial appearance, used as a guide to diagnosis

**facilitation** /fə,sɪlɪ'teɪʃ(ə)n/ *noun* an act where several slight stimuli help a neurone to be activated

**facilities** /fə'sɪlɪtiz/ *plural noun* something such as equipment, accommodation, treatment or help that is provided for people who need them ○ *the provision of aftercare facilities*

**factor** /'fæktə/ *noun* **1.** something which has an influence or which makes something else take place **2.** a substance, variously numbered, e.g. Factor I, Factor II, in the plasma, which makes the blood coagulate when a blood vessel is injured

**Factor II** /,fæktə 'tuː/ same as **prothrombin**

**Factor IX** /,fæktə 'naɪn/ *noun* a protein in plasma which promotes the clotting of blood and is lacking in people with haemophilia B. Also called **Christmas factor**

**Factor VIII** /,fæktər 'eɪt/ *noun* a protein in plasma which promotes the clotting of blood and is lacking in people with haemophilia A

**Factor XI** /,fæktər ɪ'lev(ə)n/ *noun* a protein in plasma which promotes the clotting of blood and is lacking in people with haemophilia C

**Factor XII** /,fæktə 'twelv/ *noun* a protein in plasma which promotes the clotting of blood and is lacking in people with haemophilia. Also called **Hageman factor**

**faculty** /'fæk(ə)lti/ *noun* the ability to do something

**fade away** /feɪd ə'weɪ/ *verb* to be in the process of dying (*informal*)

**faecal** /'fiːk(ə)l/ *adjective* referring to faeces

**faecal impaction** /,fiːkl(ə)l ɪm'pækʃən/ *noun* a condition in which a hardened mass of faeces stays in the rectum

**faecal incontinence** /ˌfiːk(ə)l ɪnˈkɒntɪnəns/ *noun* an inability to control the bowel movements

**faecalith** /ˈfiːkəlɪθ/ *noun* same as **coprolith**

**faecal matter** /ˈfiːk(ə)l ˌmætə/ *noun* solid waste matter from the bowels

**faeces** /ˈfiːsiːz/ *plural noun* solid waste matter passed from the bowels through the anus. Also called **stools, bowel movement** (NOTE: For other terms referring to faeces, see words beginning with **sterco-**.)

**Fahrenheit** /ˈfærənhaɪt/, **Fahrenheit scale** /ˈfærənhaɪt skeɪl/ *noun* a scale of temperatures where the freezing and boiling points of water are 32° and 212° under standard atmospheric pressure (NOTE: Used in the US, but less common in the UK. Usually written as an **F** after the degree sign: **32°F** (say: 'thirty-two degrees Fahrenheit').)

COMMENT: To convert degrees Fahrenheit into degrees Celsius, subtract 32 and divide the remainder by 1.8.

**fail** /feɪl/ *verb* **1.** not to be successful in doing something ○ *The doctor failed to see the symptoms.* ○ *She has failed her pharmacy exams.* ○ *He failed his medical and was rejected by the police force.* **2.** to become weaker and less likely to recover

**failing** /ˈfeɪlɪŋ/ *adjective* weakening, or becoming closer to death

**failure to thrive** /ˌfeɪljə tə ˈθraɪv/ *noun* same as **marasmus**

**faint** /feɪnt/ *verb* to stop being conscious for a short time and, usually, fall down ■ *noun* a loss of consciousness for a short period, caused by a temporary reduction in the blood flow to the brain

**fainting fit** /ˈfeɪntɪŋ fɪt/, **fainting spell** /ˈfeɪntɪŋ spel/ *noun* same as **syncope** ○ *She often had fainting fits when she was dieting.*

**Fairbanks' splint** /ˈfeəbæŋks splɪnt/ *noun* a special splint used for correcting Erb's palsy

**faith healing** /ˈfeɪθ ˌhiːlɪŋ/ *noun* the treatment of pain or illness by a person who prays and may also lay his or her hands on the patient

**falciform** /ˈfælsɪfɔːm/ *adjective* in the shape of a sickle

**falciform ligament** /ˌfælsɪfɔːm ˈlɪɡəmənt/ *noun* a piece of tissue which separates the two lobes of the liver and attaches it to the diaphragm

**fall** /fɔːl/ *verb* □ **to fall pregnant, to fall for a baby** to become pregnant

**fall asleep** /ˌfɔːl əˈsliːp/ *verb* to go to sleep

**fallen arches** /ˌfɔːlən ˈɑːtʃɪz/ *plural noun* a condition in which the arches in the sole of the foot are not high

**fall ill** /ˌfɔːl ˈɪl/ *verb* to get ill or to start to have an illness ○ *He fell ill while on holiday and had to be flown home.*

**Fallopian tube** /fəˈləʊpiən tjuːb/ *noun* one of two tubes which connect the ovaries to the uterus. See illustration at UROGENITAL SYSTEM (FEMALE) in Supplement. Also called **oviduct, salpinx** (NOTE: For other terms referring to Fallopian tubes, see words beginning with **salping-, salpingo-**.) [Described 1561. After Gabriele Fallopio (1523–63), Italian man of medicine. He was Professor of Surgery and Anatomy at Padua, where he was also Professor of Botany.]

COMMENT: Once a month, ova (unfertilised eggs) leave the ovaries and move down the Fallopian tubes to the uterus. At the point where the Fallopian tubes join the uterus an ovum may be fertilised by a sperm cell. Sometimes fertilisation and development of the embryo take place in the Fallopian tube itself. This is called an ectopic pregnancy, and can be life-threatening if not detected early.

**Fallot's tetralogy** /ˌfæləʊz teˈtrælədʒi/ *noun* same as **tetralogy of Fallot** [Described 1888. After Etienne-Louis Arthur Fallot (1850–1911), Professor of Hygiene and Legal Medicine at Marseilles, France.]

**false** /fɔːls/ *adjective* not true or not real

**false pains** /ˌfɔːls ˈpeɪnz/ *plural noun* pains which appear to be labour pains but are not

**false pregnancy** /ˌfɔːls ˈpreɡnənsi/ *noun* a condition in which a woman believes wrongly that she is pregnant and displays symptoms and signs of pregnancy

**false rib** /ˌfɔːls ˈrɪb/ *noun* one of the bottom five ribs on each side which are not directly attached to the breastbone

**false teeth** /ˌfɔːls ˈtiːθ/ *plural noun* dentures, artificial teeth made of plastic, which fit in the mouth and take the place of teeth which have been extracted

**false vocal cords** /ˌfɔːls ˈvəʊk(ə)l ˌkɔːdz/ *plural noun* same as **vestibular folds**

**falx** /fælks/, **falx cerebri** /ˌfælks ˈserəbri/ *noun* a fold of the dura mater between the two hemispheres of the cerebrum

**familial** /fəˈmɪliəl/ *adjective* referring to a family

**familial adenomatous polyposis** /fəˌmɪliəl ædəˌnɒmətəs pɒlɪˈpəʊsɪs/ *noun* a hereditary disorder where polyps develop in the small intestine. Abbr **FAP**

**familial disorder** /fəˌmɪliəl dɪsˈɔːdə/ *noun* a hereditary disorder which affects several members of the same family

**family** /ˈfæm(ə)li/ *noun* a group of people who are related to each other, especially mother, father and children

**family doctor** /ˌfæm(ə)li ˈdɒktə/ *noun* a general practitioner

**family planning** /ˌfæm(ə)li ˈplænɪŋ/ *noun* the use of contraception to control the number of children in a family

**family planning clinic** /ˌfæm(ə)li ˈplænɪŋ ˌklɪnɪk/ *noun* a clinic which gives advice on contraception

**family therapy** /ˌfæm(ə)li ˈθerəpi/ *noun* a type of psychotherapy where members of the family of a person with a disorder meet a therapist to discuss the condition and try to come to terms with it

**famotidine** /fəˈmɒtɪdiːn/ *noun* a histamine which reduces the secretion of gastric acid and is used to treat ulcers

**Fanconi syndrome** /fænˈkəʊni ˌsɪndrəʊm/ *noun* a kidney disorder where amino acids are present in the urine [Described 1927. After Guido Fanconi (b.1892), Professor of Paediatrics at the University of Zurich, Switzerland.]

**fantasise** /ˈfæntəsaɪz/, **fantasize** *verb* to imagine that things have happened

**fantasy** /ˈfæntəsi/ *noun* a series of imaginary events which someone believes really took place

**FAP** *abbr* familial adenomatous polyposis

**farcy** /ˈfɑːsi/ *noun* a form of glanders which affects the lymph nodes

**farinaceous** /ˌfærɪˈneɪʃəs/ *adjective* referring to flour, or containing starch

**farmer's lung** /ˌfɑːməz ˈlʌŋ/ *noun* a type of asthma caused by an allergy to rotting hay

**FAS** *abbr* fetal alcohol syndrome

**fascia** /ˈfeɪʃə/ *noun* fibrous tissue covering a muscle or an organ (NOTE: The plural is **fasciae**.)

**fascia lata** /ˌfeɪʃə ˈlætə/ *noun* a wide sheet of tissue covering the thigh muscles

**fasciculation** /fəˌsɪkjʊˈleɪʃ(ə)n/ *noun* small muscle movements which appear as trembling skin

**fasciculus** /fəˈsɪkjʊləs/ *noun* a bundle of nerve fibres (NOTE: The plural is **fasciculi**.)

**fasciitis** /ˌfæʃiˈaɪtɪs/ *noun* an inflammation of the connective tissue between muscles or around organs

**fascioliasis** /fəˌsiəˈlaɪəsɪs/ *noun* a disease caused by parasitic liver flukes

**Fasciolopsis** /ˌfæsiəʊˈlɒpsɪs/ *noun* a type of liver fluke, often found in the Far East, which is transmitted to humans through contaminated waterplants

**fast** /fɑːst/ *noun* a period of going without food, e.g. to lose weight or for religious reasons ■ *verb* to go without food ○ *The patient should fast from midnight of the night before an operation.*

**fastigium** /fæˈstɪdʒiəm/ *noun* the highest temperature during a bout of fever

**fat** /fæt/ *adjective* big and round in the body ○ *You ought to eat less – you're getting too fat.* (NOTE: **fatter – fattest**) ■ *noun* **1.** a white oily substance in the body, which stores energy and protects the body against cold **2.** a type of food which supplies protein and Vitamins A and D, especially that part of meat which is white, and solid substances like lard or butter produced from animals and used for cooking, or liquid substances like oil ○ *If you don't like the fat on the meat, cut it off.* ○ *Fry the eggs in some fat.*

(NOTE: **Fat** has no plural when it means the substance; the plural **fats** is used to mean different types of fat. For other terms referring to fats, see also **lipid** and words beginning with **steato-**.)

COMMENT: Fat is a necessary part of the diet because of the vitamins and energy-giving calories which it contains. Fat in the diet comes from either animal fats or vegetable fats. Animal fats such as butter, fat meat or cream, are saturated fatty acids. It is believed that the intake of unsaturated and polyunsaturated fats, mainly vegetable fats and oils, and fish oil, in the diet, rather than animal fats, helps keep down the level of cholesterol in the blood and so lessens the risk of atherosclerosis. A low-fat diet does not always help to reduce body weight.

**fatal** /ˈfeɪt(ə)l/ *adjective* causing or resulting in death ○ *He had a fatal accident.* ○ *Cases of bee stings are rarely fatal.*

**fatality** /fəˈtælɪti/ *noun* a death as the result of something other than natural causes ○ *There were three fatalities during the flooding.*

**fatally** /ˈfeɪt(ə)li/ *adverb* in a way which causes death ○ *His heart was fatally weakened by the lung disease.*

**father** /ˈfɑːðə/ *noun* a biological or adoptive male parent

**fatigue** /fəˈtiːg/ *noun* very great tiredness ■ *verb* to tire someone out ○ *He was fatigued by the hard work.*

**fatigue fracture** /fəˈtiːg ˌfræktʃə/ *noun* ♦ **stress fracture**

**fat-soluble** /ˌfæt ˈsɒljʊb(ə)l/ *adjective* able to dissolve in fat ○ *Vitamin D is fat-soluble.*

**fatty** /ˈfæti/ *adjective* containing fat

**fatty acid** /ˌfæti ˈæsɪd/ *noun* an organic acid belonging to a group that occurs naturally as fats, oils and waxes. ◊ **essential fatty acid**

**fatty degeneration** /ˌfæti dɪˌdʒenəˈreɪʃ(ə)n/ *noun* same as **adipose degeneration**

**fauces** /ˈfɔːsiːz/ *noun* an opening between the tonsils at the back of the throat, leading to the pharynx

**favism** /ˈfeɪvɪz(ə)m/ *noun* a type of inherited anaemia caused by an allergy to beans

**favus** /ˈfeɪvəs/ *noun* a highly contagious type of ringworm caused by a fungus which attacks the scalp

**FDA** *abbr US* Food and Drug Administration

**fear** /fɪə/ *noun* a state where a person is afraid of something ○ *fear of flying*

**febricula** /feˈbrɪkjʊlə/ *noun* a low fever

**febrifuge** /ˈfebrɪfjuːdʒ/ *noun* a drug which prevents or lowers a fever, e.g. aspirin ■ *adjective* preventing or lowering fever

**febrile** /ˈfiːbraɪl/ *adjective* referring to a fever, or caused by a fever

**febrile convulsion** /ˌfiːbraɪl kənˈvʌlʃ(ə)n/ *noun* a convulsion in a child, lasting a short time, associated with a fever

**febrile disease** /ˈfiːbraɪl dɪˌziːz/ *noun* a disease which is accompanied by fever

**fecal** /ˈfiːk(ə)l/ *adjective US* same as **faecal**

**fecundation** /ˌfekənˈdeɪʃ(ə)n/ *noun* the act of bringing male and female reproductive matter together. Also called **fertilisation**

**feeble** /ˈfiːb(ə)l/ *adjective* very weak

**feed** /fiːd/ *verb* to give food to someone ○ *He has to be fed with a spoon.* ○ *The baby has reached the stage when she can feed herself.* (NOTE: **feeding – fed**)

**feed back** /ˌfiːd ˈbæk/ *verb* to give information or comments on something that has been done ○ *The patients' responses were fed back to the students.*

**feedback** /ˈfiːdbæk/ *noun* **1.** information or comments about something which has been done ○ *The initial feedback from patients on the new service was encouraging.* **2.** the linking of the result of an action back to the action itself

**feeding** /ˈfiːdɪŋ/ *noun* the action of giving someone something to eat. ◊ **breast feeding, bottle feeding, intravenous feeding**

**feeding cup** /ˈfiːdɪŋ kʌp/ *noun* a special cup with a spout, used for feeding people who cannot feed themselves

**feel** /fiːl/ *verb* **1.** to touch someone or something, usually with your fingers ○ *The midwife felt the abdomen gently.* □ **to feel someone's pulse** to establish someone's pulse rate, usually by holding the inner wrist **2.** to give a sensation ○ *My skin feels hot and itchy.* **3.** to have a sensation ○ *When she got the results of her test, she felt relieved.* ○ *He felt ill after eating the fish.* **4.** to believe or think something ○ *The doctor feels the patient is well enough to be moved out of intensive care.* (NOTE: **feeling – felt**)

**feeling** /ˈfiːlɪŋ/ *noun* **1.** a sensation ○ *a prickling feeling* **2.** an emotional state or attitude to something

**Fehling's solution** /ˈfeɪlɪŋz səˌluːʃ(ə)n/ *noun* a solution used in Fehling's test to detect sugar in urine [Described 1848. After Hermann Christian von Fehling (1812–85), Professor of Chemistry at Stuttgart, Germany.]

**Fehling's test** /ˈfeɪlɪŋ test/ *noun* a test for the presence of aldehydes and sugars in a biological sample by means of Fehling's solution

**felon** /ˈfelən/ *noun* same as **whitlow**

**Felty's syndrome** /ˈfeltiːz ˌsɪndrəʊm/ *noun* a condition, associated with rheumatoid arthritis, in which the spleen is enlarged and the number of white blood cells increases [Described 1924. After Augustus Roi Felty (1895–1963), physician at Hartford Hospital, Connecticut, USA.]

**female condom** /ˌfiːmeɪl ˈkɒndɒm/ *noun* a rubber sheath inserted into the vagina before intercourse, covering the walls of the vagina and the cervix

**female sex hormone** /ˌfiːmeɪl ˈseks ˌhɔːməʊn/ *noun* same as **oestrogen**

**feminisation** /ˌfemɪnaɪˈzeɪʃ(ə)n/, **feminization** *noun* the development of female characteristics in a male

**femora** /ˈfemərə/ plural of **femur**

**femoral** /ˈfemərəl/ *adjective* referring to the femur or to the thigh

**femoral artery** /ˌfemərəl ˈɑːtəri/ *noun* a continuation of the external iliac artery, which runs down the front of the thigh and then crosses to the back of the thigh

**femoral canal** /ˌfemərəl kəˈnæl/ *noun* the inner tube of the sheath surrounding the femoral artery and vein

**femoral head** /ˌfemərəl ˈhed/ *noun* the head of the femur, the rounded projecting end part of the thigh bone which joins the acetabulum at the hip

**femoral hernia** /ˌfemərəl ˈhɜːniə/ *noun* a hernia of the bowel at the top of the thigh

**femoral neck** /ˌfemərəl ˈnek/ *noun* the narrow part between the head and the diaphysis of the femur. Also called **neck of the femur**

**femoral nerve** /ˈfemərəl nɜːv/ *noun* a nerve which governs the muscle at the front of the thigh

**femoral pulse** /ˌfemərəl ˈpʌls/ *noun* a pulse taken in the groin

**femoral triangle** /ˌfemərəl ˈtraɪæŋgəl/ *noun* a slight hollow in the groin which contains the femoral vessels and nerve. Also called **Scarpa's triangle**

**femoral vein** /ˈfemərəl veɪn/ *noun* a vein running up the upper leg, a continuation of the popliteal vein

**femoris** /ˈfemərɪs/ *noun* ♦ **rectus femoris**

**femur** /ˈfiːmə/ *noun* the bone in the top part of the leg which joins the acetabulum at the hip and the tibia at the knee. Also called **thighbone**. See illustration at PELVIS in Supplement (NOTE: The plural is **femora**.)

**-fen** /fen/ *suffix* used in names of non-steroidal anti-inflammatory drugs ○ *ibuprofen*

**fenestra** /fəˈnestrə/ *noun* a small opening in the ear

**fenestra ovalis** /fəˌnestrə əʊˈvɑːlɪs/ *noun* same as **oval window**

**fenestra rotunda** /fəˌnestrə rəʊˈtʌndə/ *noun* same as **round window**

**fenestration** /ˌfenəˈstreɪʃ(ə)n/ *noun* a surgical operation to relieve deafness by making a small opening in the inner ear

**fenoprofen** /ˌfenəʊˈprəʊfen/ *noun* a nonsteroidal, anti-inflammatory drug that is used to manage the pain of arthritis

**fentanyl** /ˈfentənɪl/ *noun* a narcotic drug that is a powerful painkiller

**fermentation** /ˌfɜːmenˈteɪʃ(ə)n/ *noun* a process where carbohydrates are broken down by enzymes from yeast and produce alcohol. Also called **zymosis**

**ferric** /'ferɪk/ *adjective* containing iron with a valency of three

**ferritin** /'ferɪtɪn/ *noun* a protein found in the liver that binds reversibly to iron and stores it for later use in making haemoglobin in red blood cells

**ferrous** /'ferəs/ *adjective* containing iron with a valency of two

**ferrous sulphate** /ˌferəs 'sʌlfeɪt/ *noun* a white or pale green iron salt that is used in the treatment of iron-deficient anaemia

**ferrule** /'feruːl/ *noun* a metal or rubber cap or ring that strengthens and protects the lower end of a crutch or walking stick ■ *verb* to fit a ferrule onto a crutch or walking stick

**fertile** /'fɜːtaɪl/ *adjective* able to produce children. Opposite **sterile**

**fertilisation** /ˌfɜːtɪlaɪ'zeɪʃ(ə)n/, **fertilization** *noun* the joining of an ovum and a sperm to form a zygote and so start the development of an embryo

**fertilise** /'fɜːtəlaɪz/, **fertilize** *verb* (*of a sperm*) to join with an ovum

**fertility** /fɜː'tɪlɪti/ *noun* the fact of being fertile. Opposite **sterility**

**fertility drug** /fɜː'tɪlɪti drʌg/ *noun* a drug that stimulates ovulation, given to women undergoing in vitro fertilisation

**fertility rate** /fɜː'tɪlɪti reɪt/ *noun* the number of births per year calculated per 1000 females aged between 15 and 44

**FESS** *abbr* functional endoscopic sinus surgery

**fester** /'festə/ *verb* (*of an infected wound*) to become inflamed and produce pus ○ *His legs were covered with festering sores.*

**festination** /ˌfestɪ'neɪʃ(ə)n/ *noun* a way of walking in which a person takes short steps, seen in people who have Parkinson's disease

**fetal** /'fiːt(ə)l/ *adjective* referring to a fetus

**fetal alcohol syndrome** /ˌfiːt(ə)l 'ælkəhɒl ˌsɪndrəʊm/ *noun* damage caused to the fetus by alcohol in the blood of the mother, which affects the growth of the embryo, including its facial and brain development. Abbr **FAS**

**fetal distress** /ˌfiːt(ə)l dɪ'stres/ *noun* a condition, e.g. a heart or respiratory problem, in which a fetus may not survive if the condition is not monitored and corrected

**fetal dystocia** /ˌfiːt(ə)l dɪs'təʊsiə/ *noun* a difficult childbirth caused by a malformation or malpresentation of the fetus

**fetal heart** /ˌfiːt(ə)l 'hɑːt/ *noun* the heart of the fetus

**fetalis** /fiː'tɑːlɪs/ **♦ erythroblastosis fetalis**

**fetal monitor** /ˌfiːt(ə)l 'mɒnɪtə/ *noun* an electronic device which monitors the fetus in the uterus

**fetal position** /'fiːt(ə)l pəˌzɪʃ(ə)n/ *noun* a position where a person lies curled up on his or her side, like a fetus in the uterus

**fetishism** /'fetɪʃɪz(ə)m/, **fetichism** *noun* a psychological disorder in which someone gets sexual satisfaction from touching objects

**fetishist** /'fetɪʃɪst/, **fetichist** *noun* a person who has fetishism

**feto-** /'fiːtəʊ/ *prefix* fetus

**fetoprotein** /ˌfiːtəʊ'prəʊtiːn/ *noun* **♦ alpha-fetoprotein**

**fetor** /'fiːtə/ *noun* a bad smell

**fetoscope** /'fiːtəskəʊp/ *noun* a stethoscope used in fetoscopy

**fetoscopy** /fɪ'tɒskəpi/ *noun* an examination of a fetus inside the uterus, taking blood samples to diagnose blood disorders

**fetus** /'fiːtəs/ *noun* an unborn baby from two months after conception until birth, before which it is called an embryo

**FEV** *abbr* forced expiratory volume

**fever** /'fiːvə/ *noun* **1.** a rise in body temperature ○ *She is running a slight fever.* ○ *You must stay in bed until the fever has gone down.* **2.** a condition when the temperature of the body is higher than usual ▶ also called **pyrexia**

COMMENT: Average oral body temperature is about 98.6°F or 37°C and rectal temperature is about 99°F or 37.2°C. A fever often makes the patient feel cold, and is accompanied by pains in the joints. Most fevers are caused by infections. Infections which result in fever include cat-scratch fever, dengue, malaria, meningitis, psittacosis, Q fever, rheumatic fever, Rocky Mountain spotted fever, scarlet fever, septicaemia, typhoid fever, typhus and yellow fever.

**fever blister** /'fiːvə ˌblɪstə/ *noun* same as **fever sore**

**feverfew** /'fiːvəfjuː/ *noun* a herb, formerly used to reduce fevers, but now used to relieve migraine

**feverish** /'fiːvərɪʃ/ *adjective* with a fever ○ *He felt feverish and took an aspirin.* ○ *She is in bed with a feverish chill.*

**fever sore** /'fiːvə sɔː/ *noun* a cold sore or burning sore, usually on the lips

**fiber** /'faɪbə/ *noun US* same as **fibre**

**fibr-** /faɪbr/ *prefix* referring to fibres, fibrous (*used before vowels*)

**-fibrate** /faɪbreɪt/ *suffix* used in names of lipid-lowering drugs

**fibre** /'faɪbə/ *noun* **1.** a structure in the body shaped like a thread **2.** same as **dietary fibre**

**fibre optics** /ˌfaɪbər 'ɒptɪks/, **fibreoptics** *noun* the use of thin fibres which conduct light and images to examine internal organs

**fibrescope** /'faɪbəskəʊp/ *noun* a device made of bundles of optical fibres which is passed into the body, used for examining internal organs

**fibril** /'faɪbrɪl/ *noun* a very small fibre

**fibrillate** /'faɪbrɪleɪt/ *verb* to undergo rapid irregular uncontrolled contractions, or make the heart or muscles undergo this type of contraction

**fibrillating** /'faɪbrɪleɪtɪŋ/ *adjective* with fluttering of a muscle ○ *They applied a defibrillator to correct a fibrillating heartbeat.*

**fibrillation** /ˌfaɪbrɪ'leɪʃ(ə)n/ *noun* the fluttering of a muscle

'Cardiovascular effects may include atrial arrhythmias but at 30°C there is the possibility of spontaneous ventricular fibrillation' [*British Journal of Nursing*]

**fibrin** /'fɪbrɪn/ *noun* a protein produced by fibrinogen, which helps make blood coagulate

COMMENT: Removal of fibrin from a blood sample is called defibrination.

**fibrin foam** /'fɪbrɪn fəʊm/ *noun* a white material made artificially from fibrinogen, used to prevent bleeding

**fibrinogen** /fɪ'brɪnədʒən/ *noun* a substance in blood plasma which produces fibrin when activated by thrombin

**fibrinolysin** /ˌfɪbrɪ'nɒləsɪn/ *noun* an enzyme which digests fibrin. Also called **plasmin**

**fibrinolysis** /ˌfɪbrɪ'nɒləsɪs/ *noun* the removal of blood clots from the system by the action of fibrinolysin on fibrin. Also called **thrombolysis**

**fibrinolytic** /ˌfɪbrɪnə'lɪtɪk/ *adjective* referring to fibrinolysis ○ *fibrinolytic drugs* Also called **thrombolytic**

**fibro-** /faɪbrəʊ/ *prefix* referring to fibres

**fibroadenoma** /ˌfaɪbrəʊˌædɪ'nəʊmə/ *noun* a benign tumour formed of fibrous and glandular tissue

**fibroblast** /'faɪbrəʊblæst/ *noun* a long flat cell found in connective tissue, which develops into collagen

**fibrocartilage** /ˌfaɪbrəʊ'kɑːtəlɪdʒ/ *noun* cartilage and fibrous tissue combined

COMMENT: Fibrocartilage is found in the discs of the spine. It is elastic like cartilage and pliable like fibre.

**fibrochondritis** /ˌfaɪbrəʊkɒn'draɪtɪs/ *noun* inflammation of the fibrocartilage

**fibrocyst** /'faɪbrəʊsɪst/ *noun* a benign tumour of fibrous tissue

**fibrocystic** /ˌfaɪbrəʊ'sɪstɪk/ *adjective* referring to a fibrocyst

**fibrocystic disease** /ˌfaɪbrəʊ'sɪstɪk dɪˈziːz/, **fibrocystic disease of the pancreas** /ˌfaɪbrəʊˌsɪstɪk dɪˌziːz əv ðə 'pæŋkriəs/ *noun* same as **cystic fibrosis**

**fibrocyte** /'faɪbrəʊsaɪt/ *noun* a cell which derives from a fibroblast and is found in connective tissue

**fibroelastosis** /ˌfaɪbrəʊˌiːlæ'stəʊsɪs/ *noun* a deformed growth of the elastic fibres, especially in the ventricles of the heart

**fibroid** /'faɪbrɔɪd/ *adjective* like fibre ■ *noun* same as **fibroid tumour**

**fibroid degeneration** /ˌfaɪbrɔɪd dɪˌdʒenə'reɪʃ(ə)n/ *noun* the change of healthy tissue to fibrous tissue, e.g. as in cirrhosis of the liver

**fibroid tumour** /ˌfaɪbrɔɪd 'tjuːmə/ *noun* a benign tumour in the muscle fibres of the uterus. Also called **uterine fibroid**, **fibromyoma**

**fibroma** /faɪ'brəʊmə/ *noun* a small benign tumour formed in connective tissue

**fibromuscular** /ˌfaɪbrəʊ'mʌskjʊlə/ *adjective* referring to fibrous tissue and muscular tissue

**fibromyoma** /ˌfaɪbrəʊmaɪ'əʊmə/ *noun* same as **fibroid tumour**

**fibroplasia** /ˌfaɪbrəʊ'pleɪziə/ *noun* ♦ **retrolental fibroplasia**

**fibrosa** /faɪ'brəʊsə/ ♦ **osteitis fibrosa cystica**

**fibrosarcoma** /ˌfaɪbrəʊsɑː'kəʊmə/ *noun* a malignant tumour of the connective tissue, most common in the legs

**fibrosis** /faɪ'brəʊsɪs/ *noun* the process of replacing damaged tissue by scar tissue

**fibrositis** /ˌfaɪbrə'saɪtɪs/ *noun* a painful inflammation of the fibrous tissue which surrounds muscles and joints, especially the muscles of the back

**fibrous** /'faɪbrəs/ *adjective* made of fibres, or like fibre

**fibrous capsule** /ˌfaɪbrəs 'kæpsjuːl/ *noun* fibrous tissue surrounding a kidney. Also called **renal capsule**

**fibrous joint** /'faɪbrəs dʒɔɪnt/ *noun* a joint where fibrous tissue holds two bones together so that they cannot move, as in the bones of the skull

**fibrous pericardium** /ˌfaɪbrəs ˌperɪ'kɑːdiəm/ *noun* the outer part of the pericardium which surrounds the heart, and is attached to the main blood vessels

**fibrous tissue** /ˌfaɪbrəs 'tɪʃuː/ *noun* strong white tissue which makes tendons and ligaments and also scar tissue

**fibula** /'fɪbjʊlə/ *noun* the thinner of the two bones in the lower leg between the knee and the ankle. Compare **tibia** (NOTE: The plural is **fibulae**.)

**fibular** /'fɪbjʊlə/ *adjective* referring to the fibula

**field** /fiːld/ *noun* an area of interest ○ *He specialises in the field of community medicine.* ○ *Don't see that specialist with your breathing problems – his field is obstetrics.*

**field of vision** /ˌfiːld əv 'vɪʒ(ə)n/ *noun* same as **visual field**

**fight or flight reaction** /ˌfaɪt ɔː 'flaɪt riˌækʃən/ *noun* the theory that an organism which is faced with a threat reacts either by preparing to fight or to escape

**fil-** /fɪl/ *prefix* referring to a thread

**filament** /'fɪləmənt/ *noun* a long thin structure like a thread

**filamentous** /ˌfɪləˈmentəs/ *adjective* like a thread

**Filaria** /fɪˈleəriə/ *noun* a thin parasitic worm which is found especially in the lymph system, and is passed to humans by mosquitoes (NOTE: The plural is **Filariae**.)

COMMENT: Infestation with Filariae in the lymph system causes elephantiasis.

**filariasis** /ˌfɪləˈraɪəsɪs/ *noun* a tropical disease caused by parasitic threadworms in the lymph system, transmitted by mosquito bites

**filiform** /ˈfɪlɪfɔːm/ *adjective* shaped like a thread

**filiform papillae** /ˌfɪlɪfɔːm pəˈpɪliː/ *plural noun* papillae on the tongue which are shaped like threads, and have no taste buds

**filipuncture** /ˈfɪlɪpʌŋktʃə/ *noun* the procedure of putting a wire into an aneurysm to cause blood clotting

**fill** /fɪl/ *verb* □ **to fill a tooth** to put metal into a hole in a tooth after it has been drilled

**filling** /ˈfɪlɪŋ/ *noun* **1.** a surgical operation carried out by a dentist to fill a hole in a tooth with amalgam **2.** amalgam, metallic mixture put into a hole in a tooth by a dentist

**film** /fɪlm/ *noun* a very thin layer of a substance covering a surface

**filter** /ˈfɪltə/ *noun* a piece of paper or cloth through which a liquid is passed to remove any solid substances in it ■ *verb* to pass a liquid through a membrane, piece of paper or cloth to remove solid substances ○ *Impurities are filtered from the blood by the kidneys.*

**filtrate** /ˈfɪltreɪt/ *noun* a substance which has passed through a filter

**filtration** /fɪlˈtreɪʃ(ə)n/ *noun* the action of passing a liquid through a filter

**filum** /ˈfaɪləm/ *noun* a structure which is shaped like a thread

**filum terminale** /ˌfaɪləm ˌtɜːmɪˈneɪli/ *noun* the thin end section of the pia mater in the spinal cord

**FIM** *abbr* functional independence measure

**fimbria** /ˈfɪmbriə/ *noun* a fringe, especially the fringe of hair-like processes at the end of a Fallopian tube near the ovaries (NOTE: The plural is **fimbriae**.)

**final common pathway** /ˌfaɪn(ə)l ˌkɒmən ˈpɑːθweɪ/ *noun* linked neurones which take all impulses from the central nervous system to a muscle

**fine** /faɪn/ *adjective* **1.** healthy ○ *He was ill last week, but he's feeling fine now.* **2.** referring to something such as hair or thread which is very thin ○ *There is a growth of fine hair on the back of her neck.* ○ *Fine sutures are used for delicate operations.*

**finger** /ˈfɪŋgə/ *noun* one of the five parts at the end of the hand, but usually not including the thumb (NOTE: The names of the fingers are: lit-tle finger, third finger or ring finger, middle finger, forefinger or index finger.)

COMMENT: Each finger is formed of three finger bones (the **phalanges**), but the thumb has only two.

**fingernail** /ˈfɪŋgəneɪl/ *noun* a hard thin growth covering the end of a finger ○ *ridged and damaged fingernails*

**finger-nose test** /ˌfɪŋgə ˈnəʊz test/ *noun* a test of coordination, where the person is asked to close their eyes, stretch out their arm and then touch their nose with their index finger

**fingerprint** /ˈfɪŋgəprɪnt/ *noun* a mark left by a finger when something is touched. ◊ **genetic**

**fingerstall** /ˈfɪŋgəstɔːl/ *noun* a cover for an infected finger, attached to the hand with strings

**fireman's lift** /ˌfaɪəmənz ˈlɪft/ *noun* a way of carrying an injured person by putting their body over one shoulder

**firm** /fɜːm/ *noun* a group of doctors and consultants in a hospital, especially one to which a trainee doctor is attached during clinical studies (*informal*)

**first aid** /ˌfɜːst ˈeɪd/ *noun* help given by a non-medical person to someone who is suddenly ill or injured before full-scale medical treatment can be given ○ *She gave him first aid in the street until the ambulance arrived.*

**first-aider** /ˌfɜːst ˈeɪdə/ *noun* a person who gives first aid to someone who is suddenly ill or injured

**first-aid kit** /ˌfɜːst ˈeɪd ˌkɪt/ *noun* a box with bandages and dressings kept ready to be used in an emergency

**first-aid post** /ˌfɜːst ˈeɪd ˌpəʊst/, **first-aid station** /ˌfɜːst ˈeɪd ˌsteɪʃ(ə)n/ *noun* a place where injured people can be taken for immediate care

**first-degree burn** /ˌfɜːst dɪˌgriː ˈbɜːn/ *noun* a former classification of the severity of a burn, where the skin turns red

**first-degree haemorrhoids** /ˌfɜːst dɪˌgriː ˈhemərɔɪdz/ *plural noun* haemorrhoids which remain in the rectum

**first-degree relative** /ˌfɜːst dɪˌgriː ˈrelətɪv/ *noun* a relative with whom an individual shares 50% of their genes, e.g. a father, mother, sibling or child

**first-ever stroke** /ˌfɜːst ˌevə ˈstrəʊk/ *noun* a stroke which someone has for the first time in his or her life

**first intention** /fɜːst ɪnˈtenʃən/ *noun* the healing of a clean wound where the tissue forms again rapidly and no prominent scar is left

**first-level nurse** /ˌfɜːst ˌlev(ə)l ˈnɜːs/, **first-level Registered Nurse** /ˌfɜːst ˌlev(ə)l ˌredʒɪstəd ˈnɜːs/ *noun* a nurse who has passed qualifying examinations, is registered as such with the Nursing and Midwifery Council and can act in an independent decision-making role. Compare **second-level nurse**

**fissile** /'fɪsaɪl/ *adjective* able to split or be split

**fission** /'fɪʃ(ə)n/ *noun* the act of dividing into two or more parts

**fissure** /'fɪʃə/ *noun* a crack or groove in the skin, tissue or an organ □ **horizontal and oblique fissures** grooves between the lobes of the lungs. See illustration at LUNGS in Supplement

**fist** /fɪst/ *noun* a hand which is tightly closed

**fistula** /'fɪstjʊlə/ *noun* a passage or opening which has been made unusually between two organs, often near the rectum or anus

**fistula in ano** /ˌfɪstjʊlə ɪn 'ænəʊ/ *noun* same as **anal fistula**

**fit** /fɪt/ *adjective* strong and physically healthy ○ *She exercises every day to keep fit.* ○ *The doctors decided the patient was not fit for surgery.* (NOTE: **fitter – fittest**) □ **he isn't fit enough to work** he is still too ill to work ■ *noun* a sudden attack of a disorder, especially convulsions and epilepsy ○ *She had a fit of coughing.* ○ *He had an epileptic fit.* ○ *The baby had a series of fits.* ■ *verb* **1.** to attach an appliance correctly ○ *The surgeons fitted the artificial hand to the patient's arm* or *fitted the patient with an artificial hand.* **2.** to provide a piece of equipment for someone to wear ○ *She was fitted with temporary support.* **3.** to have convulsions ○ *The patient has fitted twice.* (NOTE: **fitting – fitted**. Note also: you fit someone **with** an appliance.)

**fitness** /'fɪtnəs/ *noun* the fact of being strong and healthy ○ *Being in the football team demands a high level of physical fitness.* ○ *He had to pass a fitness test to join the police force.*

**fixated** /fɪk'seɪtɪd/ *adjective* referring to a person who has too close an attachment to another person, often to a parent

**fixation** /fɪk'seɪʃ(ə)n/ *noun* a psychological disorder where a person does not develop beyond a particular stage

**fixative** /'fɪksətɪv/ *noun* a chemical used in the preparation of samples on slides

**fixator** /fɪk'seɪtə/ *noun* a metal rod placed through a bone to keep a part of the body rigid

**fixed oil** /ˌfɪkst 'ɔɪl/ *noun* **1.** an oil which is liquid at 20°C **2.** liquid fats, especially those used as food

**flab** /flæb/ *noun* soft fat flesh (*informal*) ○ *He's doing exercises to try to fight the flab.*

**flabby** /'flæbi/ *adjective* with soft flesh ○ *She has got flabby from sitting at her desk all day.*

**flaccid** /'flæksɪd, 'flæsɪd/ *adjective* soft or flabby

**flaccidity** /flæk'sɪdɪti, flæ'sɪdɪti/ *noun* the state of being flaccid

**flagellate** /'flædʒələt/ *noun* a type of parasitic protozoan which uses whip-like hairs to swim, e.g. *Leishmania*

**flagellum** /flə'dʒeləm/ *noun* a tiny growth on a microorganism, shaped like a whip (NOTE: The plural is **flagella**.)

**Flagyl** /'flædʒaɪl/ a trade name for metronidazole

**flail** /fleɪl/ *verb* to thrash around with uncontrollable or violent movements, particularly of the arms

**flail chest** /'fleɪl tʃest/ *noun* a condition in which the chest is not stable, because several ribs have been broken

**flake** /fleɪk/ *noun* a thin piece of tissue ○ *Dandruff is formed of flakes of dead skin on the scalp.*

**flake fracture** /'fleɪk ˌfræktʃə/ *noun* a fracture where thin pieces of bone come off

**flake off** /ˌfleɪk 'ɒf/ *verb* to fall off as flakes

**flap** /flæp/ *noun* a flat piece attached to something, especially a piece of skin or tissue still attached to the body at one side and used in grafts

**flare** /fleə/ *noun* red colouring of the skin at an infected spot or in urticaria

**flashback** /'flæʃbæk/ *noun* a repeated and very vivid memory of a traumatic event

**flash burn** /'flæʃ bɜːn/ *noun* a burn caused when a body part is briefly exposed to a source of intense heat

**flat foot** /ˌflæt 'fʊt/, **flat feet** /ˌflæt 'fiːt/ *noun* a condition in which the soles of the feet lie flat on the ground instead of being arched as usual. Also called **pes planus**

**flatline** /'flætlaɪn/ *verb* to fail to show on a monitor any of the electrical currents associated with heart or brain activity ■ *noun* a monitor readout on an EEG or ECG indicating total cessation of brain or cardiac activity, respectively

**flatulence** /'flætjʊləns/ *noun* gas or air which collects in the stomach or intestines causing discomfort

COMMENT: Flatulence is generally caused by indigestion, but can be made worse if the person swallows air (**aerophagy**).

**flatulent** /'flætjʊlənt/ *adjective* having flatulence, or caused by flatulence

**flatus** /'fleɪtəs/ *noun* air and gas which collects in the intestines and is painful

**flatworm** /'flætwɜːm/ *noun* any of several types of parasitic worm with a flat body, e.g. a tapeworm. Compare **roundworm**

**flea** /fliː/ *noun* a tiny insect which sucks blood and is a parasite on animals and humans

COMMENT: Fleas can transmit disease, most especially bubonic plague which is transmitted by infected rat fleas.

**flecainide** /fle'keɪnaɪd/ *noun* a drug that helps to correct an irregular heartbeat

**flesh** /fleʃ/ *noun* tissue containing blood, forming the part of the body which is not skin, bone or organs

**flesh wound** /'fleʃ wuːnd/ *noun* a wound which only affects the fleshy part of the body ○ *She had a flesh wound in her leg.*

**fleshy** /'fleʃi/ *adjective* **1.** made of flesh **2.** fat

**flex** /fleks/ *verb* to bend something □ **to flex a joint** to use a muscle to make a joint bend

**flexibilitas cerea** /fleksɪˌbɪlɪtəs 'sɪəriə/ *noun* a condition in which, if someone's arms or legs are moved, they remain in that set position for some time

**flexion** /'flekʃən/ *noun* the act of bending a joint

**Flexner's bacillus** /ˌfleksnəz bə'sɪləs/ *noun* a bacterium which causes bacillary dysentery

**flexor** /'fleksə/, **flexor muscle** /'fleksə ˌmʌs(ə)l/ *noun* a muscle which makes a joint bend. Compare **extensor**

**flexure** /'flekʃə/ *noun* **1.** a bend in an organ **2.** a fold in the skin

**floaters** /'fləʊtəz/ *plural noun* same as **muscae volitantes**

**floating kidney** /ˌfləʊtɪŋ 'kɪdni/ *noun* same as **nephroptosis**

**floating rib** /ˌfləʊtɪŋ 'rɪb/ *noun* one of the two lowest ribs on each side, which are not attached to the breastbone

**floccillation** /ˌflɒksɪ'leɪʃ(ə)n/ *noun* the action of constantly touching the bedclothes, a sign that someone is approaching death

**floccitation** /ˌflɒksɪ'teɪʃ(ə)n/ *noun* same as **carphology**

**flooding** /'flʌdɪŋ/ *noun* same as **menorrhagia**

**floppy baby syndrome** /ˌflɒpi 'beɪbi ˌsɪndrəʊm/ *noun* same as **amyotonia congenita**

**flora** /'flɔːrə/ *noun* bacteria which exist in a particular part of the body

**florid** /'flɒrɪd/ *adjective* with an unhealthily glowing pink or red complexion

**floss** /flɒs/ *noun* same as **dental floss** ■ *verb* to clean the teeth with dental floss

**flow** /fləʊ/ *noun* **1.** a movement of liquid or gas ○ *They used a tourniquet to try to stop the flow of blood.* **2.** the amount of liquid or gas which is moving ○ *The meter measures the flow of water through the pipe.*

**flowmeter** /'fləʊmiːtə/ *noun* a meter attached to a pipe, e.g. as in anaesthetic equipment, to measure the speed at which a liquid or gas moves in the pipe

**flu** /fluː/ *noun* **1.** same as **influenza 2.** a very bad cold (*informal*) (NOTE: Sometimes written **'flu** to show it is a short form of **influenza**.)

**flucloxacillin** /fluːˈklɒksəsɪlɪn/ *noun* a drug related to penicillin and effective against streptococcal infections and pneumonia

**fluconazole** /fluːˈkɒnəzəʊl/ *noun* a drug used to treat fungal infections such as candidiasis

**fluctuation** /ˌflʌktʃuˈeɪʃ(ə)n/ *noun* the feeling of movement of liquid inside part of the body or inside a cyst when pressed by the fingers

**fluid** /'fluːɪd/ *noun* **1.** a liquid **2.** any gas, liquid or powder which flows

**fluid balance** /'fluːɪd ˌbæləns/ *noun* the maintenance of the balance of fluids in the body during dialysis or other treatment

**fluke** /fluːk/ *noun* a parasitic flatworm which settles inside the liver, in the bloodstream and in other parts of the body

**flunitrazepam** /ˌfluːnaɪˈtræzɪpæm/ *noun* a tranquilliser that, because of its association with 'date rape' cases, is a controlled drug in the UK

**fluorescence** /fluəˈres(ə)ns/ *noun* the sending out of light from a substance which is receiving radiation

**fluorescent** /fluəˈres(ə)nt/ *adjective* referring to a substance which sends out light

**fluoridate** /'flɔːrɪdeɪt/ *verb* to add fluoride to a substance, usually to drinking water, in order to help prevent tooth decay

**fluoride** /'fluəraɪd/ *noun* a chemical compound of fluorine and sodium, potassium or tin ○ *fluoride toothpaste*

COMMENT: Fluoride will reduce decay in teeth and is often added to drinking water or to toothpaste. Some people object to fluoridation and it is thought that too high a concentration, such as that achieved by highly fluoridated water and the use of a highly fluoridated toothpaste, may discolour the teeth of children.

**fluorine** /'fluəriːn/ *noun* a chemical element found in bones and teeth (NOTE: The chemical symbol is **F**.)

**fluoroscope** /'fluərəskəʊp/ *noun* an apparatus which projects an X-ray image of a part of the body onto a screen, so that the part of the body can be examined as it moves

**fluoroscopy** /fluəˈrɒskəpi/ *noun* an examination of the body using X-rays projected onto a screen

**fluorosis** /flɔːˈrəʊsɪs/ *noun* a condition caused by excessive fluoride in drinking water

COMMENT: At a low level, fluorosis causes discoloration of the teeth, and as the level of fluoride rises, ligaments can become calcified.

**fluoxetine** /fluːˈɒksətiːn/ *noun* a drug that increases serotonin in the brain and is used to treat anxiety and depression

**flush** /flʌʃ/ *noun* a red colour in the skin ■ *verb* **1.** to wash a wound with liquid **2.** (*of person*) to turn red

**flushed** /flʌʃt/ *adjective* with red skin, e.g. due to heat, emotion or overeating ○ *Her face was flushed and she was breathing heavily.*

**flutter** /'flʌtə/, **fluttering** /'flʌtərɪŋ/ *noun* a rapid movement, especially of the atria of the heart, which is not controlled by impulses from the sinoatrial node

**flux** /flʌks/ *noun* an excessive production of liquid from the mouth

**focal** /'fəʊk(ə)l/ *adjective* referring to a focus

**focal distance** /ˌfəʊk(ə)l 'dɪstəns/, **focal length** /ˌfəʊk(ə)l 'leŋθ/ *noun* the distance between the lens of the eye and the point behind the lens where light is focused

**focal epilepsy** /ˌfəʊk(ə)l 'epɪlepsi/ *noun* epilepsy arising from a localised area of the brain

**focal myopathy** /ˌfəʊk(ə)l maɪ'ɒpəθi/ *noun* destruction of muscle tissue caused by a substance injected in an intramuscular injection

**focus** /'fəʊkəs/ *noun* **1.** the point where light rays converge through a lens **2.** the centre of an infection (NOTE: The plural is **foci.**) ■ *verb* **1.** to adjust a lens until an image is clear and sharp **2.** to see clearly ○ *He has difficulty in focusing on the object.*

**focus group** /'fəʊkəs gruːp/ *noun* a discussion group of lay people brought together under professional guidance to discuss issues such as care

**foetal** /'fiːt(ə)l/ *adjective* another spelling of **fetal** (NOTE: The spelling **foetal** is common in general use in British English, but the spelling **fetal** is the accepted international spelling for technical use.)

**foetor** /'fiːtə/ *noun* another spelling of **fetor**

**foetoscope** /'fiːtəskəʊp/ *noun* another spelling of **fetoscope**

**foetoscopy** /fɪ'tɒskəpi/ *noun* another spelling of **fetoscopy**

**foetus** /'fiːtəs/ *noun* another spelling of **fetus** (NOTE: The spelling **foetus** is common in general use in British English, but the spelling **fetus** is the accepted international spelling for technical use.)

**folacin** /'fəʊləsɪn/ *noun* same as **folic acid**

**fold** /fəʊld/ *noun* a part of the body which is bent so that it lies on top of another part

**folic acid** /ˌfəʊlɪk 'æsɪd/ *noun* a vitamin in the Vitamin B complex found in milk, liver, yeast and green vegetables such as spinach, which is essential for creating new blood cells
COMMENT: Lack of folic acid can cause anaemia and neural tube disorders in the developing fetus. It can also be caused by alcoholism.

**folie à deux** /ˌfɒli æ 'dɜː/ *noun* a rare condition where a psychological disorder is communicated between two people who live together

**follicle** /'fɒlɪk(ə)l/ *noun* a tiny hole or sac in the body
COMMENT: An ovarian follicle goes through several stages in its development. The first stage is called a primordial follicle, which then develops into a primary follicle and becomes a mature follicle by the sixth day of the period. This follicle secretes oestrogen until the ovum has developed to the point when it can break out, leaving the corpus luteum behind.

**follicle-stimulating hormone** /ˌfɒlɪk(ə)l ˌstɪmjʊleɪtɪŋ 'hɔːməʊn/ *noun* a hormone produced by the pituitary gland which stimulates ova in the ovaries and sperm in the testes. Abbr **FSH**

**follicular** /fə'lɪkjʊlə/, **folliculate** /fə'lɪkjʊlət/ *adjective* referring to follicles

**follicular tumour** /fəˌlɪkjʊlə 'tjuːmə/ *noun* a tumour in a follicle

**folliculin** /fə'lɪkjʊlɪn/ *noun* an oestrone, a type of oestrogen ○ *She is undergoing folliculin treatment.*

**folliculitis** /fəˌlɪkjʊ'laɪtɪs/ *noun* inflammation of the hair follicles, especially where hair has been shaved

**follow** /'fɒləʊ/, **follow up** /ˌfɒləʊ 'ʌp/ *verb* to check on someone who has been examined before in order to assess the progress of a disease or the results of treatment

**follow-up** /'fɒləʊ ʌp/ *noun* a check on someone who has been examined before
'…length of follow-ups varied from three to 108 months. Thirteen patients were followed for less than one year, but the remainder were seen regularly for periods from one to nine years' [*New Zealand Medical Journal*]

**fomentation** /ˌfəʊmen'teɪʃ(ə)n/ *noun* same as **poultice**

**fomites** /'fəʊmɪtiːz/ *plural noun* objects touched by someone with a communicable disease which can then be the means of passing on the disease to others

**fontanelle** /ˌfɒntə'nel/, **fontanel** *noun* the soft cartilage between the bony sections of a baby's skull
COMMENT: The fontanelles gradually harden over a period of months and by the age of 18 months the bones of the baby's skull are usually solid.

**food allergen** /'fuːd ˌælədʒen/ *noun* a substance in food which produces an allergy

**food allergy** /'fuːd 'ælədʒi/ *noun* an allergy to a specific food such as nuts, which causes a severe reaction that may lead to life-threatening anaphylactic shock

**food canal** /'fuːd kə,næl/ *noun* the passage from the mouth to the rectum through which food passes and is digested

**food intolerance** /'fuːd ɪn'tɒlərəns/ *noun* an adverse reaction to some foods such as oranges, eggs, tomatoes and strawberries

**food poisoning** /'fuːd ˌpɔɪz(ə)nɪŋ/ *noun* an illness caused by eating food which is contaminated with bacteria

**foot** /fʊt/ *noun* the end part of the leg on which a person stands
COMMENT: The foot is formed of 26 bones: 14 phalanges in the toes, five metatarsals in the main part of the foot and seven tarsals in the heel.

**footpump** /'fʊtpʌmp/ *noun* a device to reduce the risk of post-operative deep-vein thrombosis by mechanical use of leg muscles

**foramen** /fə'reɪmən/ *noun* a natural opening inside the body, e.g. the opening in a bone through which veins or nerves pass (NOTE: The plural is **foramina**.)

**foramen magnum** /fə,reɪmən 'mægnəm/ *noun* the hole at the bottom of the skull where the brain is joined to the spinal cord

**foramen ovale** /fə,reɪmən əʊ'vɑːleɪ/ *noun* an opening between the two parts of the heart in a fetus

COMMENT: The foramen ovale usually closes at birth, but if it stays open the blood from the veins can mix with the blood going to the arteries, causing cyanosis.

**foramina** /fə'reɪmɪnə/ plural of **foramen**

**forced expiratory volume** /,fɔːst ek'spɪrət(ə)ri ,vɒljuːm/ *noun* the maximum amount of air that can be expelled in a given time. Abbr **FEV**

**force-feed** /,fɔːs 'fiːd/ *verb* to make someone swallow food against their will, e.g. by using a tube to put it directly down their throat

**forceps** /'fɔːseps/ *noun* a surgical instrument with handles like a pair of scissors, made in different sizes and with differently shaped ends, used for holding and pulling

**forceps delivery** /'fɔːseps dɪ,lɪv(ə)ri/ *noun* childbirth where the doctor uses forceps to help the baby out of the mother's uterus

**fore-** /fɔː/ *prefix* in front

**forearm** /'fɔːrɑːm/ *noun* the lower part of the arm from the elbow to the wrist

**forearm bones** /'fɔːrɑːm bəʊnz/ *plural noun* the ulna and the radius

**forebrain** /'fɔːbreɪn/ *noun* the front part of the brain in an embryo

**forefinger** /'fɔːfɪŋgə/ *noun* the first finger on the hand, next to the thumb

**foregut** /'fɔːgʌt/ *noun* the front part of the gut in an embryo

**forehead** /'fɔːhed/ *noun* the part of the face above the eyes

**foreign** /'fɒrɪn/ *adjective* **1.** not belonging to your own country ○ *foreign visitors* ○ *a foreign language* **2.** referring to something that is found where it does not naturally belong, especially something found in the human body that comes from a source outside the body ○ *a foreign object* ○ *foreign matter*

**foreign body** /,fɒrɪn 'bɒdi/ *noun* a piece of material which is not part of the surrounding tissue and should not be there, e.g. sand in a cut, dust in the eye or a pin which has been swallowed ○ *The X-ray showed the presence of a foreign body.* □ **swallowed foreign bodies** something which should not have been swallowed, e.g. a pin, coin or button

**foremilk** /'fɔːmɪlk/ *noun* the relatively low-fat milk with a high sugar content that is produced by a woman at the beginning of a breast feed

**forensic** /fə'rensɪk/ *adjective* relating to the use of science in solving criminal investigations or settling legal cases

**forensic medicine** /fə,rensɪk 'med(ə)sɪn/ *noun* the branch of medical science concerned with finding solutions to crimes against people and which involves procedures such as conducting autopsies on murdered people or taking blood samples from clothes

**foreskin** /'fɔːskɪn/ *noun* the skin covering the top of the penis, which can be removed by circumcision. Also called **prepuce**

**forewaters** /'fɔːwɔːtəz/ *plural noun* fluid which comes out of the vagina at the beginning of childbirth when the amnion bursts

**forgetful** /fə'getf(ə)l/ *adjective* referring to someone who often forgets things ○ *She became very forgetful, and had to be looked after by her sister.*

**forgetfulness** /fə'getf(ə)lnəs/ *noun* a condition in which someone often forgets things ○ *Increasing forgetfulness is a sign of old age.*

**form** /fɔːm/ *noun* **1.** shape **2.** a piece of paper with blank spaces which you have to write in ○ *You have to fill in a form when you are admitted to hospital.* **3.** a state or condition ○ *in good form* □ **he's in good form today** he is very amusing, he is doing things well ■ *verb* to make or to be the main part of something ○ *Calcium is one the elements which form bones* or *bones are mainly formed of calcium.* ○ *An ulcer formed in his duodenum.* ○ *In diphtheria a membrane forms across the larynx.*

**formaldehyde** /fɔː'mældɪhaɪd/ *noun* a gas with an unpleasant smell that is a strong disinfectant. When dissolved in water to make **formalin**, it is also used to preserve medical specimens

**formalin** /'fɔːməlɪn/ *noun* a solution of formaldehyde in water, used to preserve medical specimens

**formation** /fɔː'meɪʃ(ə)n/ *noun* the action of forming something ○ *Drinking milk helps the formation of bones.*

**formication** /,fɔːmɪ'keɪʃ(ə)n/ *noun* an itching feeling where the skin feels as if it were covered with insects

**formula** /'fɔːmjʊlə/ *noun* **1.** a way of indicating a chemical compound using letters and numbers, e.g. $H_2SO_4$ **2.** instructions on how to prepare a drug **3.** *US* powdered milk for babies (NOTE: The plural is **formulas** or **formulae**.)

**formulary** /'fɔːmjʊləri/ *noun* a book that lists medicines together with their formulae

**fornix** /'fɔːnɪks/ *noun* an arch (NOTE: The plural is **fornices**.) □ **fornix of the vagina** space between the cervix of the uterus and the vagina

**fornix cerebri** /,fɔːnɪks 'serɪbraɪ/ *noun* a section of white matter in the brain between the hippocampus and the hypothalamus. See illustration at BRAIN in Supplement

**fortification figures** /ˌfɔːtɪfɪˈkeɪʃ(ə)n ˈfɪɡəz/ *plural noun* patterns of coloured light, seen as part of the aura before a migraine attack occurs

**foscarnet** /fɒsˈkɑːnət/ *noun* an antiviral drug administered by intravenous injection that is effective against herpesviruses that are resistant to acyclovir. It is especially used for people with AIDS.

**fossa** /ˈfɒsə/ *noun* a shallow hollow in a bone or the skin

**foster children** /ˈfɒstə ˌtʃɪldrən/ *plural noun* children brought up by people who are not their own parents

**foster parent** /ˈfɒstə ˌpeərənt/ *noun* a woman or man who brings up a child born to other parents

**Fothergill's operation** /ˈfɒðəɡɪlz ɒpəˌreɪʃ(ə)n/ *noun* a surgical operation to correct prolapse of the uterus [After W. E. Fothergill (1865–1926), British gynaecologist.]

**foundation hospital** /faʊnˌdeɪʃ(ə)n ˈhɒspɪt(ə)l/ *noun* in the UK, a proposed type of hospital that would be independent of its Local Health Authority in financial matters

**fourchette** /fʊəˈʃet/ *noun* a fold of skin at the back of the vulva

**fovea** /ˈfəʊviə/, **fovea centralis** /ˌfəʊviə sen ˈtrɑːlɪs/ *noun* a depression in the retina which is the point where the eye sees most clearly. See illustration at EYE in Supplement

**FP10** /ˌef piː ˈten/ *noun* in the UK, an NHS prescription from a GP

**fracture** /ˈfræktʃə/ *verb* 1. (*of bone*) to break ○ *The tibia fractured in two places.* 2. to break a bone ○ *He fractured his wrist.* ■ *noun* a break in a bone ○ *rib fracture* or *fracture of a rib*

**fractured** /ˈfræktʃəd/ *adjective* broken ○ *He had a fractured skull.* ○ *She went to hospital to have her fractured leg reset.*

**fragile** /ˈfrædʒaɪl/ *adjective* easily broken ○ *Elderly people's bones are more fragile than those of adolescents.*

**fragile-X syndrome** /ˌfrædʒaɪl ˈeks ˌsɪn drəʊm/ *noun* a hereditary condition in which part of an X chromosome is constricted, causing mental impairment

**fragilitas** /frəˈdʒɪlɪtəs/ *noun* fragility or brittleness

**fragilitas ossium** /frəˌdʒɪlɪtəs ˈɒsiəm/ *noun* a hereditary condition where the bones are brittle and break easily, similar to osteogenesis imperfecta

**frail** /freɪl/ *adjective* weak, easily broken ○ *Grandfather is getting frail, and we have to look after him all the time.* ○ *The baby's bones are still very frail.*

**framboesia** /fræmˈbiːziə/ *noun* same as **yaws**

**frame** /freɪm/ *noun* 1. the particular size and shape of someone's body 2. a solid support for something. ◊ **walking frame, Zimmer frame**

**framework** /ˈfreɪmwɜːk/ *noun* the main bones which make up the structure of part of the body

**framycetin** /fræˈmaɪsətɪn/ *noun* an antibiotic

**fraternal twins** /frəˌtɜːn(ə)l ˈtwɪnz/ *plural noun* same as **dizygotic twins**

**freckle** /ˈfrek(ə)l/ *noun* a harmless small brownish patch on the skin that becomes more noticeable after exposure to the sun. Freckles are often found in people with fair hair. Also called **lentigo** ■ *verb* to mark something, or become marked with freckles

**freckled** /ˈfrek(ə)ld/ *adjective* with brown spots on the skin

**freeze** /friːz/ *verb* to anaesthetise part of the body (*informal*) ○ *They froze my big toe to remove the nail.*

**freeze dry** /ˌfriːz ˈdraɪ/ *verb* to freeze something rapidly then dry it in a vacuum

**freeze drying** /ˈfriːz ˌdraɪɪŋ/ *noun* a method of preserving food or tissue specimens by freezing rapidly and drying in a vacuum

**Freiberg's disease** /ˈfraɪbɜːɡz dɪˌziːz/ *noun* osteochondritis of the head of the second metatarsus [Described 1914. After Albert Henry Freiberg (1869–1940), US surgeon.]

**Frei test** /ˈfraɪ test/ *noun* a test for the venereal disease lymphogranuloma inguinale [Described 1925. After Wilhelm Siegmund Frei (1885–1943), Professor of Dermatology at Berlin, Germany. He settled in New York, USA.]

**fremitus** /ˈfremɪtəs/ *noun* vibrations or trembling in part of someone's body, felt by the doctor's hand or heard through a stethoscope

**French letter** /ˌfrentʃ ˈletə/ *noun* ♦ **condom** (*informal*)

**frenectomy** /frəˈnektəmi/ *noun* an operation to remove a frenum

**Frenkel's exercises** /ˈfrenkəlz ˌeksəsaɪzɪz/ *plural noun* exercises for people who have locomotor ataxia, to teach coordination of the muscles and limbs

**frenotomy** /frəˈnɒtəmi/ *noun* an operation to split a frenum

**frenum** /ˈfriːnəm/, **frenulum** /ˈfrenjʊləm/ *noun* a fold of mucous membrane under the tongue or by the clitoris

**frequency** /ˈfriːkwənsi/ *noun* 1. the number of times something takes place in a given time ○ *the frequency of micturition* 2. the rate of vibration in oscillations

**fresh air** /ˌfreʃ ˈeə/ *noun* open air ○ *They came out of the hospital into the fresh air.*

**fresh frozen plasma** /ˌfreʃ ˌfrəʊz(ə)n ˈplæzmə/ *noun* plasma made from freshly donated blood, and kept frozen

**fretful** /ˈfretf(ə)l/ *adjective* referring to a baby that cries, cannot sleep or seems unhappy

**Freudian** /ˈfrɔɪdiən/ *adjective* understandable in terms of Freud's theories, especially with regard to human sexuality ■ *noun* someone who is influenced by or follows Freud's theories or methods of psychoanalysis

**friable** /ˈfraɪəb(ə)l/ *adjective* easily broken up into small pieces

**friar's balsam** /ˌfraɪəz ˈbɔːlsəm/ *noun* a mixture of various plant oils, including benzoin and balsam, which can be inhaled as a vapour to relieve bronchitis or congestion

**friction** /ˈfrɪkʃən/ *noun* the rubbing together of two surfaces

**friction fremitus** /ˌfrɪkʃən ˈfremɪtəs/ *noun* a scratching sensation felt when the hand is placed on the chest of someone who has pericarditis

**friction murmur** /ˌfrɪkʃən ˈmɜːmə/ *noun* the sound of two serous membranes rubbing together, heard with a stethoscope in someone who has pericarditis or pleurisy

**Friedländer's bacillus** /ˈfriːdlendəz bəˌsɪləs/ *noun* the bacterium *Klebsiella pneumoniae* which can cause pneumonia [Described 1882. After Carl Friedländer (1847–87), pathologist at the Friedrichshain Hospital, Berlin, Germany.]

**Friedman's test** /ˈfriːdmənz test/ *noun* a test for pregnancy [After Maurice H. Friedman (b. 1903), US physician.]

**Friedreich's ataxia** /ˌfriːdraɪks əˈtæksiə/ *noun* an inherited nervous disease which affects the spinal cord and is associated with club foot, an unsteady walk and speech difficulties. Also called **dystrophia adiposogenitalis** [Described 1863. After Nicholaus Friedreich (1825–82), Professor of Pathological Anatomy at Würzburg, later Professor of Pathology and Therapy at Heidelberg, Germany.]

**frigidity** /frɪˈdʒɪdɪti/ *noun* the fact of being unable to experience orgasm, sexual pleasure or sexual desire

**fringe medicine** /ˈfrɪnʒ ˌmed(ə)sɪn/ *noun* types of medical practice which are not usually taught in medical schools, e.g. homeopathy or acupuncture (*informal*)

**frog plaster** /ˈfrɒg ˌplɑːstə/ *noun* a plaster cast made to keep the legs in an open position after an operation to correct a dislocated hip

**Fröhlich's syndrome** /ˈfrɜːlɪks ˌsɪndrəʊm/ *noun* a condition in which someone becomes obese and the genital system does not develop, caused by an adenoma of the pituitary gland [Described 1901. After Alfred Fröhlich (1871–1953), Professor of Pharmacology at the University of Vienna, Austria.]

**frontal** /ˈfrʌnt(ə)l/ *adjective* referring to the forehead or to the front of the head. Opposite **occipital**

**frontal bone** /ˈfrʌnt(ə)l bəʊn/ *noun* a bone forming the front of the upper part of the skull behind the forehead

**frontal lobe** /ˈfrʌnt(ə)l ləʊb/ *noun* the front lobe of each cerebral hemisphere

**frontal lobotomy** /ˌfrʌnt(ə)l ləʊˈbɒtəmi/ *noun* formerly, a surgical operation on the brain to treat mental illness by removing part of the frontal lobe

**frontal sinus** /ˌfrʌnt(ə)l ˈsaɪnəs/ *noun* one of two sinuses in the front of the face above the eyes and near the nose

**front passage** /frʌnt ˈpæsɪdʒ/ (*informal*) **1.** same as **urethra 2.** same as **vagina**

**frostbite** /ˈfrɒstbaɪt/ *noun* an injury caused by very severe cold which freezes tissue

**frostbitten** /ˈfrɒstbɪt(ə)n/ *adjective* having frostbite

COMMENT: In very cold conditions, the outside tissue of the fingers, toes, ears and nose can freeze, becoming white and numb. Thawing of frostbitten tissue can be very painful and must be done very slowly. Severe cases of frostbite may require amputation because the tissue has died and gangrene has set in.

**frozen shoulder** /ˌfrəʊz(ə)n ˈʃəʊldə/ *noun* stiffness and pain in the shoulder, caused by inflammation of the membranes of the shoulder joint after injury or a period of immobility, when deposits may form in the tendons

**frozen watchfulness** /ˌfrəʊz(ə)n ˈwɒtʃfəlnəs/ *noun* an expression of petrified fear on a child's face, especially in children who have been abused

**fructose** /ˈfrʌktəʊs/ *noun* fruit sugar found in honey and some fruit, which together with glucose forms sucrose

**fructosuria** /ˌfrʌktəʊˈsjʊəriə/ *noun* the presence of fructose in the urine

**frusemide** /ˈfruːsəmaɪd/ *noun* same as **furosemide**

**FSH** *abbr* follicle-stimulating hormone

**fugax** /ˈfjuːgæks/ ♦ **amaurosis fugax**

**-fuge** /fjuːdʒ/ *suffix* driving away

**fugue** /fjuːg/ *noun* a condition in which someone loses his or her memory and leaves home

**fulguration** /ˌfʌlgəˈreɪʃ(ə)n/ *noun* the removal of a growth such as a wart by burning with an electric needle. Also called **electrodesiccation**

**full term** /ˌfʊl ˈtɜːm/ *noun* a complete pregnancy of forty weeks ○ *She has had several pregnancies but none has reached full term.*

**full thickness burn** /fʊl ˈθɪknəs bɜːn/ *noun* same as **deep dermal burn**

**fulminant** /ˈfʊlmɪnənt/, **fulminating** /ˈfʊlmɪˌneɪtɪŋ/ *adjective* referring to a dangerous disease which develops very rapidly

'…the major manifestations of pneumococcal infection in sickle-cell disease are septicaemia, meningitis and pneumonia. The illness is frequently fulminant' [*The Lancet*]

**fumes** /fjuːmz/ *plural noun* gas or smoke

**fumigate** /'fjuːmɪgeɪt/ *verb* to kill insects in an area by using gas or smoke

**fumigation** /ˌfjuːmɪ'geɪʃ(ə)n/ *noun* the process of killing insects in an area with gas or smoke

**function** /'fʌŋkʃən/ *noun* the particular work done by an organ ○ *What is the function of the pancreas?* ○ *The function of an ovary is to form ova.* ■ *verb* to work in a particular way ○ *The heart and lungs were functioning normally.* ○ *His kidneys suddenly stopped functioning.*

'…insulin's primary metabolic function is to transport glucose into muscle and fat cells, so that it can be used for energy' [*Nursing '87*]

'…the AIDS virus attacks a person's immune system and damages the ability to fight other disease. Without a functioning immune system to ward off other germs, the patient becomes vulnerable to becoming infected' [*Journal of American Medical Association*]

**functional** /'fʌŋkʃən(ə)l/ *adjective* referring to a disorder or illness which does not have a physical cause and may have a psychological cause, as opposed to an organic disorder

**functional endoscopic sinus surgery** /ˌfʌŋkʃən(ə)l ˌendəskɒpɪk 'saɪnəs ˌsɜːdʒəri/ *noun* the removal of soft tissue in the sinuses using an endoscope. Abbr **FESS**

**functional enuresis** /ˌfʌŋkʃən(ə)l ˌenjʊ'riːsɪs/ *noun* bedwetting which has a psychological cause

**functional independence measure** /ˌfʌŋkʃən(ə)l ˌɪndɪ'pendəns ˌmeʒə/ *noun* a measure of disability. Abbr **FIM**

**fundus** /'fʌndəs/ *noun* 1. the bottom of a hollow organ such as the uterus 2. the top section of the stomach, above the body of the stomach

**fungal** /'fʌŋɡəl/ *adjective* relating to, or caused by, fungi ○ *a fungal skin infection*

**fungate** /'fʌŋɡeɪt/ *verb* (*of some skin cancers*) to increase rapidly at a late stage of tumour formation

**fungicide** /'fʌŋɡɪsaɪd/ *noun* a substance used to kill fungi

**fungiform papillae** /ˌfʌŋɡɪfɔːm pə'pɪliː/ *noun* rounded papillae on the tip and sides of the tongue, which have taste buds

**fungoid** /'fʌŋɡɔɪd/ *adjective* like a fungus

**fungus** /'fʌŋɡəs/ *noun* an organism such as yeast or mould, some of which cause disease (NOTE: The plural is **fungi**. For other terms referring to fungi, see words beginning with **myc-**, **myco-**.)

COMMENT: Some fungi can become parasites of man, and cause diseases such as thrush.

Other fungi, such as yeast, react with sugar to form alcohol. Some antibiotics, such as penicillin, are derived from fungi.

**fungus disease** /'fʌŋɡəs dɪˌziːz/ *noun* a disease caused by a fungus

**fungus poisoning** /'fʌŋɡəs ˌpɔɪz(ə)nɪŋ/ *noun* poisoning by eating a poisonous fungus

**funiculitis** /fjuːnɪkjʊ'laɪtɪs/ *noun* inflammation of the spermatic cord

**funiculus** /fjuː'nɪkjʊləs/ *noun* one of the three parts of the white matter in the spinal cord ○ *The three parts are called the lateral, anterior and posterior funiculus.*

**funis** /'fjuːnɪs/ *noun* an umbilical cord

**funnel chest** /ˌfʌn(ə)l 'tʃest/ *noun* same as **pectus excavatum**

**funny bone** /'fʌni bəʊn/ *noun* same as **olecranon** (*informal*)

**funny turn** /'fʌni tɜːn/ *noun* a dizzy spell (*informal*)

**furfuraceous** /ˌfɜːfjə'reɪʃəs/ *adjective* referring to skin which is scaly

**Furley stretcher** /'fɜːli ˌstretʃə/ *noun* a stretcher made of a folding frame with a canvas bed, with carrying poles at each side and small feet underneath

**furor** /'fjʊərɔː/ *noun* an attack of wild violence, especially in someone who is mentally unwell

**furosemide** a drug which causes an increase in urine production, used to relieve water retention in the body. Also called **frusemide**

**furred tongue** /fɜːd 'tʌŋ/ *noun* a condition when the papillae of the tongue are covered with a whitish coating. Also called **coated tongue**

**furuncle** /'fjʊərʌŋkəl/ *noun* same as **boil**

**furunculosis** /fjʊəˌrʌŋkjʊ'ləʊsɪs/ *noun* a condition in which several boils appear at the same time

**fuse** /fjuːz/ *verb* to join together to form a single structure, or to join two or more things together ○ *The bones of the joint fused.*

**fusidic acid** /fjuːˌsɪdɪk 'æsɪd/ *noun* an antibiotic used to prevent protein synthesis

**fusiform** /'fjuːzɪfɔːm/ *adjective* referring to muscles which are shaped like a spindle, with a wider middle section which becomes narrower at each end

**fusion** /'fjuːʒ(ə)n/ *noun* the act of joining, especially a surgical operation to relieve pain in the joint by joining the bones at the joint permanently so that they cannot move

**Fybogel** /'faɪbəʊdʒel/ a trade name for ispaghula

# G

**g** *abbr* gram

**GABA** /ˈɡæbə/ *abbr* gamma aminobutyric acid

**gag** /ɡæɡ/ *noun* an instrument placed between the teeth to stop the mouth from closing ■ *verb* to experience a reaction similar to that of vomiting ○ *Every time the doctor tries to examine her throat, she gags.* ○ *He started gagging on the endotracheal tube.*

**gain** /ɡeɪn/ *noun* an act of adding or increasing something ○ *The baby showed a gain in weight of 25g* or *showed a weight gain of 25g.* ■ *verb* to obtain something, or to increase ○ *to gain in weight* or *to gain weight*

**gait** /ɡeɪt/ *noun* a way of walking

**galact-** /ɡəlækt/ *prefix* same as **galacto-** (*used before vowels*)

**galactagogue** /ɡəˈlæktəɡɒɡ/ *noun* a substance which stimulates the production of milk

**galacto-** /ɡəlæktəʊ/ *prefix* referring to milk

**galactocele** /ɡəˈlæktəsiːl/ *noun* a breast tumour which contains milk

**galactorrhoea** /ɡəˌlæktəˈrɪə/ *noun* the excessive production of milk

**galactosaemia** /ɡəˌlæktəˈsiːmiə/ *noun* a congenital condition where the liver is incapable of converting galactose into glucose, with the result that a baby's development may be affected (NOTE: The treatment is to remove galactose from the diet.)

**galactose** /ɡəˈlæktəʊs/ *noun* a sugar which forms part of milk, and is converted into glucose by the liver

**galea** /ˈɡeɪliə/ *noun* **1.** any part of the body shaped like a helmet, especially the loose band of tissue in the scalp (NOTE: The plural is **galeae**.) **2.** a type of bandage wrapped round the head

**gall** /ɡɔːl/ *noun* same as **bile**

**gall bladder** /ˈɡɔːl ˌblædə/ *noun* a sac situated underneath the liver, in which bile produced by the liver is stored. See illustration at **DIGESTIVE SYSTEM** in Supplement

COMMENT: Bile is stored in the gall bladder until required by the stomach. If fatty food is present in the stomach, bile moves from the gall bladder along the bile duct to the stomach. Since the liver also secretes bile directly into the duodenum, the gall bladder is not an essential organ and can be removed by surgery.

**Gallie's operation** /ˈɡæliz ɒpəˌreɪʃ(ə)n/ *noun* a surgical operation where tissues from the thigh are used to hold a hernia in place [Described 1921. After William Edward Gallie (1882–1959), Professor of Surgery at the University of Toronto, Canada.]

**gallipot** /ˈɡælɪpɒt/ *noun* a little container for ointment

**gallium** /ˈɡæliəm/ *noun* a metallic element a radioisotope of which is used to detect tumours or other tissue disorders (NOTE: The chemical symbol is **Ga.**)

**gallop rhythm** /ˈɡæləp ˌrɪð(ə)m/ *noun* the rhythm of heart sounds, three to each cycle, when someone is experiencing tachycardia

**gallstone** /ˈɡɔːlstəʊn/ *noun* a small stone formed from insoluble deposits from bile in the gall bladder. ◊ **calculus**

COMMENT: Gallstones can be harmless, but some cause pain and inflammation and a serious condition can develop if a gallstone blocks the bile duct. Sudden pain going from the right side of the stomach towards the back indicates that a gallstone is passing through the bile duct.

**galvanism** /ˈɡælvənɪz(ə)m/ *noun* a treatment using low voltage electricity

**galvanocautery** /ˌɡælvənəʊˈkɔːtəri/ *noun* the removal of diseased tissue using an electrically heated needle or loop of wire. Also called **electrocautery**

**gamete** /ˈɡæmiːt/ *noun* a sex cell, either a spermatozoon or an ovum

**gamete intrafallopian transfer** /ˌɡæmiːt ɪntrəfəˌləʊpiən ˈtrænsfɜː/ *noun* a technique to combine eggs and sperm outside the body and then insert them into the Fallopian tubes. Abbr **GIFT**

**gametocide** /ɡəˈmiːtəʊsaɪd/ *noun* a drug which kills gametocytes

**gametocyte** /ɡəˈmiːtəʊsaɪt/ *noun* a cell which is developing into a gamete

**gametogenesis** /ɡəˌmiːtəʊˈdʒenəsɪs/ *noun* the process by which a gamete is formed

**gamgee tissue** /'gæmdʒiː ˌtɪʃuː/ *noun* a surgical dressing, formed of a layer of cotton wool between two pieces of gauze

**gamma** /'gæmə/ *noun* the third letter of the Greek alphabet

**gamma aminobutyric acid** /ˌgæmə ə ˌmiːnəʊbjuːˌtɪrɪk 'æsɪd/ *noun* an amino acid neurotransmitter. Abbr **GABA**

**gamma camera** /'gæmə ˌkæm(ə)rə/ *noun* a camera for taking photographs of parts of the body into which radioactive isotopes have been introduced

**gamma globulin** /ˌgæmə 'glɒbjʊlɪn/ *noun* a protein found in plasma, forming antibodies as protection against infection

COMMENT: Gamma globulin injections are sometimes useful as a rapid source of protection against a wide range of diseases.

**gamma ray** /'gæmə reɪ/ *noun* a ray which is shorter than an X-ray and is given off by radioactive substances

**gangli-** /gæŋgli/ *prefix* referring to ganglia

**ganglion** /'gæŋgliən/ *noun* **1.** a mass of nerve cell bodies and synapses usually covered in connective tissue, found along the peripheral nerves with the exception of the basal ganglia **2.** a cyst of a tendon sheath or joint capsule, usually at the wrist, which results in a painless swelling containing fluid (NOTE: [all senses] The plural is **ganglia**.)

**ganglionectomy** /ˌgæŋgliə'nektəmi/ *noun* the surgical removal of a ganglion

**ganglionic** /ˌgæŋgli'ɒnɪk/ *adjective* referring to a ganglion. ◊ **postganglionic**

**gangrene** /'gæŋgriːn/ *noun* a condition in which tissues die and decay, as a result of bacterial action, because the blood supply has been lost through injury or disease of the artery ○ *After she had frostbite, gangrene set in and her toes had to be amputated.*

**gangrenous** /'gæŋgrɪnəs/ *adjective* referring to, or affected by, gangrene

**Ganser state** /'gænsə ˌsteɪt/ *noun* same as **pseudodementia** [After Sigbert Joseph Maria Ganser (1853–1931), psychiatrist at Dresden and Munich, Germany]

**gargle** /'gɑːg(ə)l/ *noun* a mildly antiseptic solution used to clean the mouth ■ *verb* to put some antiseptic liquid solution into the back of the mouth and then breathe out air through it

**gargoylism** /'gɑːgɔɪlɪz(ə)m/ *noun* a congenital condition of the metabolism which causes polysaccharides and fat cells to accumulate in the body, resulting in mental impairment, swollen liver and coarse features. Also called **Hurler's syndrome**

**gas** /gæs/ *noun* **1.** a substance such as nitrogen, carbon dioxide or air, which is neither solid nor fluid at ordinary temperatures and can expand infinitely (NOTE: The plural **gases** is used only when referring to different types of gas.) **2.** gas which accumulates in the stomach or alimentary canal and causes pain

**gas and air analgesia** /ˌgæs ənd 'eə æn(ə)lˌdʒiːziə/ *noun* a form of analgesia used when giving birth, in which a mixture of air and gas is given

**gas chromatography** /ˌgæs ˌkrəʊmə'tɒgrəfi/ *noun* a method of separating chemicals by passing them through a gas, used in analysing compounds and mixtures

**gas exchange** /'gæs ɪks,tʃeɪndʒ/ *noun* the process by which oxygen in the air is exchanged in the lungs for waste carbon dioxide carried by the blood

**gas gangrene** /gæs 'gæŋgriːn/ *noun* a complication of severe wounds in which the bacterium *Clostridium welchii* breeds in the wound and then spreads to healthy tissue which is rapidly decomposed with the formation of gas

**gash** /gæʃ/ *noun* a long deep cut made accidentally by something sharp ○ *She had to have three stitches in the gash in her thigh.* ■ *verb* to make a long deep cut in something accidentally ○ *She gashed her hand on the broken glass.*

**gasp** /gɑːsp/ *noun* a short breath taken with difficulty ○ *His breath came in short gasps.* ■ *verb* to breathe with difficulty taking quick breaths ○ *She was gasping for breath.*

**gas pain** /'gæs peɪn/ *noun* a pain caused by excessive formation of gas in the stomach or intestine. ◊ **flatus**

**gas poisoning** /'gæs ˌpɔɪz(ə)nɪŋ/ *noun* poisoning by breathing in carbon monoxide or other toxic gas

**Gasserian ganglion** /gə,sɪəriən 'gæŋgliən/ *noun* same as **trigeminal ganglion** [After Johann Laurentius Gasser (1723–65), Professor of Anatomy in Vienna, Austria. He left no writings, and the ganglion was given his name by Anton Hirsch, one of his students, in his thesis of 1765.]

**gastr-** /gæstr/ *prefix* same as **gastro-** (*used before vowels*)

**gastralgia** /gæ'strældʒə/ *noun* pain in the stomach

**gastrectomy** /gæ'strektəmi/ *noun* the surgical removal of the stomach

**gastric** /'gæstrɪk/ *adjective* referring to the stomach

**gastric acid** /ˌgæstrɪk 'æsɪd/ *noun* hydrochloric acid secreted into the stomach by acid-forming cells

**gastric artery** /ˌgæstrɪk 'ɑːtəri/ *noun* an artery leading from the coeliac trunk to the stomach

**gastric flu** /ˌgæstrɪk 'fluː/ *noun* any mild stomach disorder (*informal*)

**gastric juice** /'gæstrɪk dʒuːs/ *noun* the mixture of hydrochloric acid, pepsin, intrinsic factor and mucus secreted by the cells of the lining membrane of the stomach to help the digestion of food (NOTE: Often used in the plural.)

**gastric lavage** /ˌgæstrɪk 'lævɪdʒ/ noun a lavage of the stomach, usually to remove a poisonous substance which has been absorbed. Also called **stomach washout**

**gastric pit** /ˌgæstrɪk 'pɪt/ noun a deep hollow in the mucous membrane forming the walls of the stomach

**gastric ulcer** /ˌgæstrɪk 'ʌlsə/ noun an ulcer in the stomach. Abbr **GU**

**gastric vein** /ˌgæstrɪk 'veɪn/ noun a vein which follows the gastric artery

**gastrin** /'gæstrɪn/ noun a hormone which is released into the bloodstream from cells in the lower end of the stomach, stimulated by the presence of protein, and which in turn stimulates the flow of acid from the upper part of the stomach

**gastrinoma** /ˌgæstrɪ'nəʊmə/ noun a tumour of the islet cells, leading to excessive gastric acid

**gastritis** /gæ'straɪtɪs/ noun inflammation of the stomach

**gastro-** /gæstrəʊ/ prefix referring to the stomach

**gastrocele** /'gæstrəʊsiːl/ noun a condition in which part of the stomach wall becomes weak and bulges out. Also called **stomach hernia**

**gastrocnemius** /ˌgæstrɒk'niːmiəs/ noun a large calf muscle

**gastrocolic** /ˌgæstrəʊ'kɒlɪk/ adjective referring to the stomach and colon

**gastrocolic reflex** /ˌgæstrəʊkɒlɪk 'riːfleks/ noun a sudden peristalsis of the colon produced when food is taken into an empty stomach

**gastroduodenal** /ˌgæstrəʊˌdjuːəʊ'diːn(ə)l/ adjective referring to the stomach and duodenum

**gastroduodenal artery** /ˌgæstrəʊdↄ djuːəʊdiːn(ə)l 'ɑːtəri/ noun an artery leading from the gastric artery towards the pancreas

**gastroduodenoscopy** /ˌgæstrəʊˌdjuːəʊ dɪ'nɒskəpi/ noun an examination of the stomach and duodenum

**gastroduodenostomy** /ˌgæstrəʊˌdjuːəʊ dɪ'nɒstəmi/ noun a surgical operation to join the duodenum to the stomach so as to bypass a blockage in the pylorus

**gastroenteritis** /ˌgæstrəʊentə'raɪtɪs/ noun inflammation of the membrane lining the intestines and the stomach, caused by a viral infection and resulting in diarrhoea and vomiting

**gastroenterologist** /ˌgæstrəʊentə'rɒlə dʒɪst/ noun a doctor who specialises in the digestive system and its disorders

**gastroenterology** /ˌgæstrəʊentə'rɒlədʒi/ noun the study of the digestive system and its disorders

**gastroenterostomy** /ˌgæstrəʊentə'rɒstəmi/ noun a surgical operation to join the small intestine directly to the stomach so as to bypass a peptic ulcer

**gastroepiploic** /ˌgæstrəʊepɪ'plɒɪk/ adjective referring to the stomach and greater omentum

**gastroepiploic artery** /ˌgæstrəʊepɪˌplɒɪk 'ɑːtəri/ noun an artery linking the gastroduodenal artery to the splenic artery

**Gastrografin** /ˌgæstrəʊ'græfɪn/ a trade name for an enema used in bowel X-rays

**gastroileac reflex** /ˌgæstrəʊˌɪliæk 'riːfleks/ noun automatic relaxation of the ileocaecal valve when food is present in the stomach

**gastrointestinal** /ˌgæstrəʊɪn'testɪn(ə)l/ adjective referring to the stomach and intestine ○ gastrointestinal bleeding. Abbr **GI**

**gastrojejunostomy** /ˌgæstrəʊdʒɪdʒuː 'nɒstəmi/ noun a surgical operation to join the jejunum to the stomach

**gastrolith** /'gæstrəʊlɪθ/ noun a calculus in the stomach

**gastrology** /gæ'strɒlədʒi/ noun the study of the stomach and diseases of the stomach

**gastro-oesophageal reflux** /ˌgæstrəʊ ɪ ˌsɒfədʒiəl 'riːflʌks/, **gastro-oesophageal reflux disease** /ˌgæstrəʊ ɪˌsɒfədʒiəl 'riːflʌks dɪˌziːz/ noun the return of bitter-tasting, partly digested food from the stomach to the oesophagus

**gastropexy** /'gæstrəʊpeksi/ noun a surgical operation to attach the stomach to the wall of the abdomen

**gastroplasty** /'gæstrəʊplæsti/ noun surgery to correct a deformed stomach

**gastroptosis** /ˌgæstrəʊ'təʊsɪs/ noun a condition in which the stomach hangs down

**gastrorrhoea** /ˌgæstrə'rɪə/ noun an excessive flow of gastric juices

**gastroschisis** /ˌgæstrəʊ'saɪsɪs/ noun a split in the wall of the abdomen, with viscera passing through it

**gastroscope** /'gæstrəskəʊp/ noun an instrument formed of a tube or bundle of glass fibres with a lens attached, which a doctor can pass down into the stomach through the mouth to examine the inside of the stomach

**gastroscopy** /gæ'strɒskəpi/ noun an examination of the stomach using a gastroscope

**gastrostomy** /gæ'strɒstəmi/ noun a surgical operation to create an opening into the stomach from the wall of the abdomen, so that food can be introduced without passing through the mouth and throat

**gastrotomy** /gæ'strɒtəmi/ noun a surgical operation to open up the stomach

**gastrula** /ˈgæsˈtruːlə/ *noun* the second stage of the development of an embryo

**gathering** /ˈgæðərɪŋ/ *noun* a swelling that is filled with pus

**Gaucher's disease** /ˈgəʊʃeɪz dɪˌziːz/ *noun* an enzyme disease where fatty substances accumulate in the lymph glands, spleen and liver, causing anaemia, a swollen spleen and darkening of the skin. The disease can be fatal in children. [Described 1882. After Philippe Charles Ernest Gaucher (1854–1918), French physician and dermatologist.]

**gauze** /gɔːz/ *noun* a thin light material used to make dressings

**gauze dressing** /gɔːz ˈdresɪŋ/ *noun* a dressing of thin light material

**gavage** /gæˈvɑːʒ/ *noun* the forced feeding of someone who cannot eat or who refuses to eat

**gay** /geɪ/ *adjective* relating to sexual activity among people of the same sex

**GDC** *abbr* General Dental Council

**Gehrig's disease** /ˈgeɪrɪgz dɪˌziːz/ *noun* same as **amyotrophic lateral sclerosis**

**Geiger counter** /ˈgaɪgə ˌkaʊntə/ *noun* an instrument for the detection and measurement of radiation [Described 1908. After Hans Geiger (1882–1945), German physicist who worked with Rutherford at Manchester University, UK.]

**gel** /dʒel/ *noun* a suspension that sets into a jelly-like solid

**gelatin** /ˈdʒelətɪn/ *noun* a protein found in collagen which is soluble in water, used to make capsules for medicines

**gelatinous** /dʒəˈlætɪnəs/ *adjective* referring to gelatin or something with a texture like jelly

**gemellus** /dʒɪˈmeləs/ *noun* either of the two muscles arising from the ischium. Also called **gemellus superior muscle, gemellus inferior muscle**

**gender** /ˈdʒendə/ *noun* the fact of being of the male or female sex

**gender identity disorder** /ˌdʒendə aɪˈden↓tɪtɪ dɪsˌɔːdə/ *noun* a condition in which someone experiences strong discomfort with his or her birth gender

**gender reassignment surgery** /ˌdʒendə riːəˈsaɪnmənt ˌsɜːdʒəri/ *noun* surgery to change someone's sex

**gender reorientation** /ˌdʒendə riːˌɔːriən ˈteɪʃ(ə)n/ *noun* the alteration of a person's sex through surgical and drug treatment

**gene** /dʒiːn/ *noun* a unit of DNA on a chromosome which governs the synthesis of a protein sequence and determines a particular characteristic

COMMENT: A gene may be dominant, in which case the characteristic it controls is always passed on to the child, or recessive, in which case the characteristic only appears if both parents have contributed the same form of the gene.

**general amnesia** /ˌdʒen(ə)rəl æmˈniːziə/ *noun* a sudden and complete loss of memory, to the extent that a person does not even remember who he or she is

**general anaesthesia** /ˌdʒen(ə)rəl ˌænəs ˈθiːziə/ *noun* loss of feeling and loss of sensation throughout the body, after being given an anaesthetic

**general anaesthetic** /ˌdʒen(ə)rəl ˌænəs ˈθetɪk/ *noun* a substance given to make someone lose consciousness so that a major surgical operation can be carried out

**General Dental Council** /ˌdʒen(ə)rəl ˈdent(ə)l ˌkaʊnsəl/ *noun* in the UK, the official body that registers and supervises dentists. Abbr **GDC**

**general hospital** /ˌdʒen(ə)rəl ˈhɒspɪt(ə)l/ *noun* a hospital which does not specialise in particular types of illness or particular age groups

**generalise** /ˈdʒen(ə)rəlaɪz/, **generalize** *verb* to spread to other parts of the body

**generalised** /ˈdʒen(ə)rəlaɪzd/, **generalized** *adjective* **1.** spreading throughout the body. Opposite **localised 2.** not having a specific cause

**generalised anxiety disorder** /ˌdʒen(ə)rəlaɪzd æŋˈzaɪəti dɪsˌɔːdə/ *noun* a state of continual anxiety for which there is no specific cause

**General Medical Council** /ˌdʒen(ə)rəl ˈmedɪk(ə)l ˌkaʊnsəl/ *noun* in the UK, the official body that licenses qualified doctors to practise medicine. Abbr **GMC**

**General Optical Council** /ˈdʒenrəl ˈɒp↓tɪk(ə)l ˈkaʊnsəl/ *noun* in the UK, the official body that registers and supervises opticians

**general practice** /ˌdʒen(ə)rəl ˈpræktɪs/ *noun* a medical practice where doctors offer first-line medical care for all types of illness to people who live locally, refer them to hospital if necessary and encourage health promotion

**general practitioner** /ˌdʒen(ə)rəl præk ˈtɪʃ(ə)nə/ *noun* a doctor who provides first-line medical care for all types of illness to people who live locally, refers them to hospital if necessary and encourages health promotion. Abbr **GP**

**gene replacement therapy** /ˌdʒiːn rɪ ˈpleɪsmənt ˌθerəpi/ *noun* the replacement of missing genes or damaging gene variations in cells by the insertion of appropriate genes to treat a genetic disorder. Also called **gene therapy**

COMMENT: Gene replacement therapy has been used successfully in animals, and is in the early stages of research in humans, but may be useful in the future treatment of cystic fibrosis, thalassaemia and other genetic disorders.

**generic** /dʒəˈnerɪk/ *adjective* **1.** referring to medicine which does not have a special trademark or brand name given to it by its manufacturer **2.** referring to a genus ○ *The generic name of this type of bacterium is Staphylococcus.*

**-genesis** /dʒenəsɪs/ *suffix* production or origin

**gene therapy** /'dʒiːn ˌθerəpi/ *noun* same as **gene replacement therapy**

**genetic** /dʒə'netɪk/ *adjective* referring to genes

**genetic code** /dʒə,netɪk 'kəʊd/ *noun* the characteristics of the DNA of a cell which are passed on when the cell divides and so are inherited by a child from its parents

**genetic counselling** /dʒə,netɪk 'kaʊnsəlɪŋ/ *noun* advice and support given to people if they or their children might be affected by inherited genetic disorders

**genetic disorder** /dʒə,netɪk dɪs'ɔːdə/ *noun* a disorder or disease caused by a damaging gene variation that may be inherited

**genetic engineering** /dʒə,netɪk endʒɪ'nɪərɪŋ/ *noun* same as **genetic modification** (*informal*)

**genetic fingerprint** /dʒə,netɪk 'fɪŋɡəprɪnt/ *noun* the pattern of sequences of genetic material unique to an individual. Also called **DNA fingerprint**

**genetic fingerprinting** /dʒə,netɪk 'fɪŋɡəˌprɪntɪŋ/ *noun* a method of revealing an individual's genetic profile, used in paternity queries and criminal investigations. Also called **DNA fingerprinting**

**geneticist** /dʒə'netɪsɪst/ *noun* a person who specialises in the study of the way in which characteristics and diseases are inherited through the genes

**genetic modification, genetic manipulation** *noun* the combination of genetic material from different sources to produce organisms with altered characteristics

**genetics** /dʒə'netɪks/ *noun* the study of genes, and of the way characteristics and diseases are inherited through the genes

**genetic screening** /dʒə,netɪk 'skriːnɪŋ/ *noun* the process of testing large numbers of people to see if anyone has a particular genetic disorder

**gene tracking** /'dʒiːn ˌtrækɪŋ/ *noun* the method used to trace throughout a family the inheritance of a gene such as those causing cystic fibrosis or Huntington's Chorea, in order to diagnose and predict genetic disorders

**-genic** /dʒenɪk/ *suffix* referring to a product or something which produces

**genicular** /dʒe'nɪkjʊlə/ *adjective* referring to the knee

**genital** /'dʒenɪt(ə)l/ *adjective* referring to the reproductive organs ■ *plural noun* **genitals** same as **genital organs**

**genitalia** /ˌdʒenɪ'teɪliə/ *noun* the genital organs

**genital organs** /ˌdʒenɪt(ə)l 'ɔːɡənz/ *plural noun* the external organs for reproduction, i.e. the penis and testicles in males and the vulva in females. Also called **genitals, genitalia**

**genital wart** /ˌdʒenɪt(ə)l 'wɔːt/ *noun* a wart in the genital or anal area, caused by a sexually transmitted virus

**genito-** /dʒenɪtəʊ/ *prefix* referring to the reproductive system

**genitourinary** /ˌdʒenɪtəʊ'jʊərɪnəri/ *adjective* referring to both the reproductive and urinary systems. Abbr **GU**

**genitourinary system** /ˌdʒenɪtəʊ'jʊərɪnəri ˌsɪstəm/ *noun* the organs of reproduction and urination, including the kidneys

**genome** /'dʒiːnəʊm/ *noun* the set of all the genes of an individual

**genotype** /'dʒenətaɪp/ *noun* the genetic makeup of an individual. Compare **phenotype**

**gentamicin** /ˌdʒentə'maɪsɪn/ *noun* an antibiotic that is effective against a variety of different disease-causing organisms. Patients usually receive it by injection and it can cause serious side effects.

**gentian violet** /ˌdʒenʃən 'vaɪələt/ *noun* an antiseptic blue dye, used to paint on skin infections and also to stain specimens. Also called **crystal violet**

**genu** /'dʒenjuː/ *noun* the knee

**genual** /'dʒenjuəl/ *adjective* referring to the knee

**genucubital position** /ˌdʒenjuː'kjuːbɪt(ə)l pəˌzɪʃ(ə)n/ *noun* the position of someone resting on their knees and elbows

**genupectoral position** /ˌdʒenjuː'pektər(ə)l pəˌzɪʃ(ə)n/ *noun* the position of someone resting on their knees and upper chest

**genus** /'dʒiːnəs/ *noun* a category of related living organisms ○ *A genus is divided into different species.* (NOTE: The plural is **genera**.)

**genu valgum** /ˌdʒenjuː 'vælɡəm/ *noun* same as **knock-knee**

**genu varum** /ˌdʒenjuː 'veərəm/ *noun* same as **bow legs**

**geri-** /dʒeri/ *prefix* referring to old age

**geriatric** /ˌdʒeri'ætrɪk/ *adjective* **1.** referring to old people **2.** specialising in the treatment of old people ○ *geriatric unit*

**geriatrician** /ˌdʒeriə'trɪʃ(ə)n/ *noun* a doctor who specialises in the treatment or study of diseases of old people

**geriatrics** /ˌdʒeri'ætrɪks/ *noun* the study of the diseases and disorders of old people. Compare **paediatrics**

**germ** /dʒɜːm/ *noun* **1.** a microorganism which causes a disease, e.g. a virus or bacterium (*informal*) ○ *Germs are not visible to the naked* *eye*. **2.** a part of an organism capable of developing into a new organism

**German measles** /ˌdʒɜːmən ˈmiːz(ə)lz/ *noun* same as **rubella**

**germ cell** /ˈdʒɜːm sel/ *noun* a cell which is capable of developing into a spermatozoon or ovum. Also called **gonocyte**

**germinal** /ˈdʒɜːmɪn(ə)l/ *adjective* referring to an embryo

**germinal epithelium** /ˌdʒɜːmɪn(ə)l epɪ ˈθiːliəm/ *noun* the outer layer of the ovary

**germ layer** /ˈdʒɜːm ˌleɪə/ *noun* one of two or three layers of cells in animal embryos that form the organs of the body

**gerontologist** /ˌdʒerənˈtɒlədʒɪst/ *noun* a specialist in gerontology

**gerontology** /ˌdʒerənˈtɒlədʒi/ *noun* the study of the process of ageing and the diseases of old people

**Gerstmann's syndrome** /ˈɡɜːstmænz ˌsɪndrəʊm/ *noun* a condition in which someone no longer recognises his or her body image, cannot tell the difference between left and right, cannot recognise his or her different fingers and is unable to write

**Gesell's developmental chart** /ɡəˌzelz dɪ ˌveləpˈment(ə)l tʃɑːt/ *noun* a chart showing the development of motor reactions and growth patterns in children

**gestate** /dʒeˈsteɪt/ *verb* to carry a baby in the womb from conception to birth

**gestation** /dʒeˈsteɪʃ(ə)n/ *noun* **1.** the process of development of a baby from conception to birth in the mother's womb **2.** same as **gestation period**

'…evaluation of fetal age and weight has proved to be of value in the clinical management of pregnancy, particularly in high-risk gestations' [*Southern Medical Journal*]

**gestational age** /dʒeˌsteɪʃ(ə)n(ə)l ˈeɪdʒ/ *noun* the age of a fetus, calculated from the mother's last period to the date of birth

**gestational diabetes** /dʒeˌsteɪʃ(ə)n(ə)l ˌdaɪəˈbiːtiːz/ *noun* a form of diabetes mellitus which develops in a pregnant woman

**gestation period** /dʒeˈsteɪʃ(ə)n ˌpɪəriəd/ *noun* the period, usually of 266 days, from conception to birth, during which the baby develops in the mother's womb. Also called **pregnancy**

**gestodene** /ˈdʒestədiːn/ *noun* an oral contraceptive

**get around** /ˌɡet əˈraʊnd/ *verb* to move about ○ *Since she had the accident she gets around using crutches.*

**get better** /ˌɡet ˈbetə/ *verb* **1.** to become healthy again after being ill ○ *He was seriously ill, but seems to be getting better.* **2.** (*of an illness*) to stop or become less severe ○ *Her cold has got better.*

**get dressed** /ˌɡet ˈdrest/ *verb* to put your clothes on ○ *This patient still needs helps to get dressed.*

**get on with** /ˌɡet ˈɒn wɪð/ *verb* to continue to do some work ○ *I must get on with the blood tests.*

**get over** /ˌɡet ˈəʊvə/ *verb* to become better after an illness or a shock ○ *He got over his cold.* ○ *She never got over her mother's death.*

**getting on** /ˌɡetɪŋ ˈɒn/ *adjective* becoming elderly ○ *Her parents are getting on.*

**get up** /ˌɡet ˈʌp/ *verb* **1.** to stand up ○ *Try to get up from your chair slowly and walk across the room.* **2.** to get out of bed ○ *What time did you get up this morning?*

**get well** /ˌɡet ˈwel/ *verb* to become healthy again after being ill ○ *We hope your mother will get well soon.*

**GFR** *abbr* glomerular filtration rate

**GH** *abbr* growth hormone

**Ghon's focus** /ˌɡɒnz ˈfəʊkəs/ *noun* a spot on the lung produced by the tuberculosis bacillus [Described 1912. After Anton Ghon (1866–1936), Professor of Pathological Anatomy at Prague, Czech Republic.]

**GI** *abbr* gastrointestinal

**giant cell** /ˌdʒaɪənt ˈsel/ *noun* a very large cell, e.g. an osteoclast or megakaryocyte

**giant-cell arteritis** /ˌdʒaɪənt sel ˌɑːtə ˈraɪtɪs/ *noun* a disease of old people, which often affects the arteries in the scalp

**giant hives** /ˌdʒaɪənt ˈhaɪvz/ *noun* a large flat white blister caused by an allergic reaction

**Giardia** /dʒiːˈɑːdiə/ *noun* a microscopic protozoan parasite which causes giardiasis

**giardiasis** /ˌdʒiːɑːˈdaɪəsɪs/ *noun* a disorder of the intestine caused by the parasite *Giardia lamblia*, usually with no symptoms, but in heavy infections the absorption of fat may be affected, causing diarrhoea. Also called **lambliasis**

**gibbosity** /ɡɪˈbɒsəti/ *noun* a sharp angle in the curvature of the spine caused by the weakening of a vertebra as a result of tuberculosis of the backbone

**gibbus** /ˈɡɪbəs/ *noun* same as **gibbosity**

**giddiness** /ˈɡɪdɪnəs/ *noun* a condition in which someone has difficulty in standing up and keeping their balance because of a feeling that everything is turning around ○ *He began to experience attacks of giddiness.*

**giddy** /ˈɡɪdi/ *adjective* feeling that everything is turning round ○ *She has had several giddy spells.*

**GIFT** /ɡɪft/ *noun* a procedure in which a surgeon removes eggs from a woman's ovary, mixes them with sperm and places them in one of her Fallopian tubes to help her conceive a child. Full form **gamete intrafallopian transfer**

**gigantism** /dʒaɪˈɡæntɪz(ə)m/ *noun* a condition in which someone grows very tall, caused by excessive production of growth hormone by the pituitary gland

**Gilbert's syndrome** /ˈɡɪlbəts ˌsɪndrəʊm/ *noun* an inherited disorder where the liver does not deal with bilirubin correctly

**Gilles de la Tourette syndrome** /ˌʒiː də læ tʊəˈret ˌsɪndrəʊm/ *noun* same as **Tourette's syndrome**

**Gilliam's operation** /ˈɡɪliəmz ɒpəˌreɪʃ(ə)n/ *noun* a surgical operation to correct retroversion of the uterus [After David Tod Gilliam (1844–1923), physician, Columbus, Ohio, USA]

**gingiv-** /dʒɪndʒɪv/ *prefix* referring to the gums

**gingiva** /dʒɪnˈdʒaɪvə/ *noun* same as **gum** (NOTE: The plural is **gingivae**.)

**gingival** /ˈdʒɪndʒɪv(ə)l/ *adjective* relating to the gums

**gingivectomy** /ˌdʒɪndʒɪˈvektəmi/ *noun* the surgical removal of excess gum tissue

**gingivitis** /ˌdʒɪndʒɪˈvaɪtɪs/ *noun* inflammation of the gums as a result of bacterial infection

**ginglymus** /ˈdʒɪŋɡlɪməs/ *noun* a joint which allows movement in two directions only, e.g. the knee or elbow. Also called **hinge joint**. Compare **ball and socket joint**

**ginseng** /ˈdʒɪnseŋ/ *noun* a plant root widely used as a tonic and a traditional Chinese herbal remedy

**gippy tummy** /ˌdʒɪpi ˈtʌmi/ *noun* same as **diarrhoea** (*informal*)

**girdle** /ˈɡɜːd(ə)l/ *noun* a set of bones making a ring or arch

**Girdlestone's operation** /ˈɡɜːdəlstəʊnz ɒpəˌreɪʃ(ə)n/ *noun* a surgical operation to relieve osteoarthritis of the hip [After Gathorne Robert Girdlestone (1881–1950), Nuffield Professor of Orthopaedics at Oxford, UK]

**give up** /ˌɡɪv ˈʌp/ *verb* not to do something any more ○ *He was advised to give up smoking.*

**glabella** /ɡləˈbelə/ *noun* a flat area of bone in the forehead between the eyebrows

**gladiolus** /ˌɡlædiˈəʊləs/ *noun* the middle section of the sternum

**gland** /ɡlænd/ *noun* an organ in the body containing cells that secrete substances such as hormones, sweat or saliva which act elsewhere

**glanders** /ˈɡlændəz/ *noun* a bacterial disease of horses, which can be caught by humans, with symptoms of high fever and inflammation of the lymph nodes

**glandular** /ˈɡlændjʊlə/ *adjective* referring to glands

**glandular fever** /ˌɡlændjʊlə ˈfiːvə/ *noun* same as **infectious mononucleosis**

**glans** /ɡlænz/ *noun* a rounded part at the end of the penis or clitoris. See illustration at **UROGENITAL SYSTEM (MALE)** in Supplement

**glare** /ɡleə/ *noun* **1.** a long stare that expresses a negative emotion such as anger **2.** an uncomfortably or dazzlingly bright light **3.** scattered bright light when examining something with a microscope ■ *verb* **1.** to stare angrily **2.** to shine uncomfortably brightly **3.** to be very obvious or conspicuous

**Glasgow coma scale** /ˌɡlɑːsɡəʊ ˈkəʊmə ˌskeɪl/, **Glasgow scoring system** /ˌɡlɑːsɡəʊ ˈskɔːrɪŋ ˌsɪstəm/ *noun* a seven-point scale for evaluating someone's level of consciousness

**glass eye** /ɡlɑːs ˈaɪ/ *noun* an artificial eye made of glass

**glaucoma** /ɡlɔːˈkəʊmə/ *noun* a condition of the eyes, caused by unusually high pressure of fluid inside the eyeball, resulting in disturbances of vision and blindness

**gleet** /ɡliːt/ *noun* a thin discharge from the vagina, penis, a wound or an ulcer

**glenohumeral** /ˌɡliːnəʊˈhuːmərəl/ *adjective* referring to both the glenoid cavity and the humerus

**glenohumeral joint** /ˌɡliːnəʊˈhuːmərəl dʒɔɪnt/ *noun* the shoulder joint

**glenoid** /ˈɡliːnɔɪd/ *adjective* shaped like a small shallow cup or socket

**glenoid cavity** /ˌɡliːnɔɪd ˈkævɪti/, **glenoid fossa** /ˌɡliːnɔɪd ˈfɒsə/ *noun* a socket in the shoulder joint into which the head of the humerus fits

**glia** /ˈɡliːə/ *noun* connective tissue of the central nervous system, surrounding cell bodies, axons and dendrites. Also called **neuroglia**

**glial cell** /ˈɡliːəl sel/ *noun* a cell in the glia

**glial tissue** /ˌɡliːəl ˈtɪʃuː/ *noun* same as **glia**

**glibenclamide** /ɡlɪˈbeŋkləmaɪd/ *noun* a sulphonylurea drug used to treat Type II diabetes mellitus

**gliclazide** /ˈɡlɪkləzaɪd/ *noun* an antibacterial drug used to treat Type II diabetes mellitus

**glio-** /ɡlaɪəʊ/ *prefix* referring to brain tissue

**glioblastoma** /ˌɡlaɪəʊblæˈstəʊmə/ *noun* a rapidly developing malignant tumour of the glial tissue in the brain or spinal cord. Also called **spongioblastoma**

**glioma** /ɡlaɪˈəʊmə/ *noun* any tumour of the glial tissue in the brain or spinal cord

**gliomyoma** /ˌɡlaɪəʊmaɪˈəʊmə/ *noun* a tumour of both the nerve and muscle tissue

**glipizide** /ˈɡlɪpɪzaɪd/ *noun* a drug used to reduce the glucose level in the blood

**Glisson's capsule** /ˌɡlɪs(ə)nz ˈkæpsjuːl/ *noun* a tissue sheath in the liver containing the blood vessels [After Francis Glisson (1597–1677), philosopher, physician and anatomist at Cambridge and London, UK]

**globin** /'gləʊbɪn/ *noun* a protein which combines with other substances to form compounds such as haemoglobin and myoglobin

**globule** /'glɒbjuːl/ *noun* a round drop, especially of fat

**globulin** /'glɒbjʊlɪn/ *noun* a protein, present in blood, belonging to a group that includes antibodies

**globulinuria** /ˌglɒbjʊlɪ'njʊəriə/ *noun* the presence of globulins in the urine

**globus** /'gləʊbəs/ *noun* any ball-shaped part of the body

**globus hystericus** /ˌgləʊbəs hɪ'sterɪkəs/ *noun* a feeling of not being able to swallow, caused by worry or embarrassment

**glomangioma** /gləˌmændʒi'əʊmə/ *noun* a tumour of the skin at the ends of the fingers and toes

**glomerular** /glɒ'merʊlə/ *adjective* referring to a glomerulus

**glomerular capsule** /glɒˌmerʊlə 'kæpsjuːl/ *noun* same as **Bowman's capsule**

**glomerular filtration rate** /glɒˌmerʊlə fɪl'treɪʃ(ə)n reɪt/ *noun* the rate at which the kidneys filter blood and remove waste matter

**glomerular tuft** /glɒˌmerʊlə 'tʌft/ *noun* a group of blood vessels in the kidney which filter the blood

**glomeruli** /glɒ'merʊli/ plural of **glomerulus**

**glomerulitis** /glɒˌmerʊ'laɪtɪs/ *noun* inflammation causing lesions of glomeruli in the kidney

**glomerulonephritis** /glɒˌmerʊləʊnɪ'fraɪtɪs/ *noun* same as **Bright's disease**

**glomerulus** /glɒ'merʊləs/ *noun* a group of blood vessels which filter waste matter from the blood in a kidney (NOTE: The plural is **glomeruli**.)

**gloss-** /glɒs/ *prefix* same as **glosso-** (used before vowels)

**glossa** /'glɒsə/ *noun* same as **tongue**

**glossal** /'glɒs(ə)l/ *adjective* relating to the tongue

**glossectomy** /glɒ'sektəmi/ *noun* the surgical removal of the tongue

**Glossina** /glɒ'saɪnə/ *noun* a genus of African flies which cause trypanosomiasis, e.g. the tsetse fly

**glossitis** /glɒ'saɪtɪs/ *noun* inflammation of the surface of the tongue

**glosso-** /'glɒsəʊ/ *prefix* referring to the tongue

**glossodynia** /ˌglɒsəʊ'dɪniə/ *noun* pain in the tongue

**glossopharyngeal** /ˌglɒsəʊfærɪn'dʒiːəl/ *adjective* relating to the tongue and pharynx

**glossopharyngeal nerve** /ˌglɒsəʊfærɪn'dʒiːəl nɜːv/ *noun* the ninth cranial nerve which controls the pharynx, the salivary glands and part of the tongue

**glossoplegia** /ˌglɒsəʊ'pliːdʒə/ *noun* paralysis of the tongue

**glossotomy** /glɒ'sɒtəmi/ *noun* a surgical incision into the tongue

**glottis** /'glɒtɪs/ *noun* an opening in the larynx between the vocal cords, which forms the entrance to the main airway from the pharynx

**gluc-** /gluːk/ *prefix* referring to glucose

**glucagon** /'gluːkəgɒn/ *noun* a hormone secreted by the islets of Langerhans in the pancreas, which increases the level of blood sugar by stimulating the breakdown of glycogen

**glucagonoma** /ˌgluːkəgɒ'nəʊmə/ *noun* a tumour of the cells of the pancreas that produces glucagon

**glucocorticoid** /ˌgluːkəʊ'kɔːtɪkɔɪd/ *noun* any corticosteroid which breaks down carbohydrates and fats for use by the body, produced by the adrenal cortex

**gluconeogenesis** /ˌgluːkəʊˌniːəʊ'dʒenəsɪs/ *noun* the production of glucose in the liver from protein or fat reserves

**glucose** /'gluːkəʊz/ *noun* a simple sugar found in some fruit, but also broken down from white sugar or carbohydrate and absorbed into the body or secreted by the kidneys. Also called **dextrose**

COMMENT: Combustion of glucose with oxygen to form carbon dioxide and water is the body's main source of energy.

**glucose tolerance test** /'gluːkəʊz ˌtɒlərəns test/ *noun* a test for diabetes mellitus, in which someone eats glucose and his or her urine and blood are tested at regular intervals. Abbr **GTT**

**glucosuria** /ˌgluːkəʊ'sjʊəriə/ *noun* same as **glycosuria**

**glucuronic acid** /ˌgluːkjʊrɒnɪk 'æsɪd/ *noun* an acid formed by glucose that acts on bilirubin

**glue ear** /gluː 'ɪə/ *noun* a condition in which fluid forms behind the eardrum and causes deafness. Also called **secretory otitis media**

**glue-sniffing** /'gluː ˌsnɪfɪŋ/ *noun* ♦ **solvent abuse**

**glutamic acid** /gluːˌtæmɪk 'æsɪd/ *noun* an amino acid

**glutamic oxaloacetic transaminase** /gluːˌtæmɪk ɒksələʊəˌsiːtɪk træns'æmɪneɪz/ *noun* an enzyme used to test for viral hepatitis

**glutamic pyruvic transaminase** /gluːˌtæmɪk paɪˌruːvɪk træns'æmɪneɪz/ *noun* an enzyme produced in the liver and released into the blood if the liver is damaged

**glutaminase** /gluː'tæmɪneɪz/ *noun* an enzyme in the kidneys that helps to break down glutamine

**glutamine** /'gluːtəmiːn/ *noun* an amino acid

**gluteal** /'gluːtiəl/ *adjective* referring to the buttocks

**gluteal artery** /ˈgluːtɪəl ˈɑːtəri/ *noun* one of the two arteries supplying the buttocks, the **inferior gluteal artery** or the **superior gluteal artery**

**gluteal muscle** /ˈgluːtɪəl ˌmʌs(ə)l/ *noun* a muscle in the buttock. ◊ **gluteus**

**gluteal vein** /ˈgluːtɪəl veɪn/ *noun* one of two veins draining the buttocks, the **inferior gluteal vein** and the **superior gluteal vein**

**gluten** /ˈgluːt(ə)n/ *noun* a protein found in some cereals, which makes the grains form a sticky paste when water is added

**gluten enteropathy** same as **gluten-induced enteropathy**

**gluten-free diet** /ˌgluːt(ə)n friː ˈdaɪət/ *noun* a diet containing only food containing no gluten

**gluten-induced enteropathy** /ˌgluːt(ə)n ɪnˌdjuːst ˌentəˈrɒpəθi/ *noun* **1.** an allergic disease mainly affecting children, in which the lining of the intestine is sensitive to gluten, preventing the small intestine from digesting fat **2.** a condition in adults where the villi in the intestine become smaller and so reduce the surface which can absorb nutrients (NOTE: Symptoms include a swollen abdomen, pale diarrhoea, abdominal pains and anaemia.) ▶ also called **coeliac disease**

**gluteus** /ˈgluːtɪəs/ *noun* one of three muscles in the buttocks, responsible for movements of the hip. The largest is the **gluteus maximus**, while the **gluteus medius** and **gluteus minimus** are smaller.

**glyc-** /glaɪk/ *prefix* same as **glyco-** (*used before vowels*)

**glycaemia** /glaɪˈsiːmiə/ *noun* the level of glucose found in the blood. ◊ **hypoglycaemia**, **hyperglycaemia**

**glycerin** /ˈglɪsərɪn/, **glycerine**, **glycerol** /ˈglɪsərɒl/ *noun* a colourless viscous sweet-tasting liquid present in all fats (NOTE: Synthetic glycerin is used in various medicinal preparations and also as a lubricant in items such as toothpaste and cough medicines.)

**glycine** /ˈglaɪsiːn/ *noun* an amino acid

**glyco-** /glaɪkəʊ/ *prefix* referring to sugar

**glycocholic acid** /ˌglaɪkəʊkɒlɪk ˈæsɪd/ *noun* one of the bile acids

**glycogen** /ˈglaɪkədʒən/ *noun* a type of starch, converted from glucose by the action of insulin, and stored in the liver as a source of energy

**glycogenesis** /ˌglaɪkəʊˈdʒenəsɪs/ *noun* the process by which glucose is converted into glycogen in the liver

**glycogenolysis** /ˌglaɪkəʊdʒəˈnɒləsɪs/ *noun* the process by which glycogen is broken down to form glucose

**glycolysis** /glaɪˈkɒləsɪs/ *noun* the metabolic breakdown of glucose to release energy

**glycoside** /ˈglaɪkəʊsaɪd/ *noun* a chemical compound of a type which is formed from a simple sugar and another compound (NOTE: Many of the drugs produced from plants are glycosides.)

**glycosuria** /ˌglaɪkəʊˈsjʊəriə/ *noun* a high level of sugar in the urine, a symptom of diabetes mellitus

**GMC** *abbr* General Medical Council

**gnathic** /ˈnæθɪk/ *adjective* referring to the jaw

**gnathoplasty** /ˈnæθəʊˌplæsti/ *noun* surgery on the jaw

**gnawing** /ˈnɔːɪŋ/ *adjective* referring to a physical or emotional feeling that is persistent and uncomfortable ○ *a gnawing pain*

**goblet cell** /ˈgɒblət sel/ *noun* a tube-shaped cell in the epithelium which secretes mucus

**GOC** *abbr* General Optical Council

**go down** /ˌgəʊ ˈdaʊn/ *verb* to become smaller ○ *The swelling has started to go down*

**goitre** /ˈgɔɪtə/ *noun* an excessive enlargement of the thyroid gland, seen as a swelling round the neck, caused by a lack of iodine (NOTE: The US spelling is **goiter**.)

**goitrogen** /ˈgɔɪtrədʒən/ *noun* a substance which causes goitre

**gold** /gəʊld/ *noun* a soft yellow-coloured precious metal, used as a compound in various drugs, and sometimes as a filling for teeth

**golden eye ointment** /ˌgəʊld(ə)n ˈaɪ ˌɔɪntmənt/ *noun* a yellow ointment, made of an oxide of mercury, used to treat inflammation of the eyelids

**golden hour** /ˈgəʊldən ˌaʊə/ *noun* the first hour after a serious injury when the most difference can be made to the patient's health

**gold injection** /ˈgəʊld ɪnˌdʒekʃən/ *noun* an injection of a solution containing gold, used to relieve rheumatoid arthritis

**golfer's elbow** /ˌgɒlfəz ˈelbəʊ/ *noun* inflammation of the tendons of the elbow

**Golgi apparatus** /ˈgɒldʒi æpəˌreɪtəs/ *noun* a folded membranous structure inside the cell cytoplasm which stores and transports enzymes and hormones [Described 1898. After Camillo Golgi (1843–1926), Professor of Histology and later Rector of the University of Pavia, Italy. In 1906 he shared the Nobel Prize with Santiago Ramón y Cajal for work on the nervous system.]

**Golgi cell** /ˈgɒldʒi ˌsel/ *noun* a type of nerve cell in the central nervous system, either with long axons (Golgi Type 1) or without axons (Golgi Type 2)

**gomphosis** /gɒmˈfəʊsɪs/ *noun* a joint which cannot move, like that between a tooth and the jaw

**gonad** /ˈgəʊnæd/ *noun* a sex gland which produces gametes and also sex hormones, e.g. a testicle in males or an ovary in females

**gonadotrophic hormone** /ˌɡəʊnədəʊˌtrɒ fɪk ˈhɔːməʊn/ *noun* one of two hormones, the follicle-stimulating hormone and the luteinising hormone, produced by the anterior pituitary gland which have an effect on the ovaries in females and on the testes in males

**gonadotrophin** /ˌɡəʊnədəʊˈtrəʊfɪn/ *noun* any of a group of hormones produced by the pituitary gland which stimulates the sex glands at puberty. ◊ **human chorionic gonadotrophin** (NOTE: The US spelling is **gonadotropin**.)

**gonagra** /ɡɒˈnæɡrə/ *noun* a form of gout which occurs in the knees

**goni-** /ɡəʊni/ *prefix* same as **gonio-** (*used before a vowel*)

**gonio-** /ɡəʊniəʊ/ *prefix* referring to an angle

**gonion** /ˈɡəʊniɒn/ *noun* the outer point at which the lower jawbone angles upwards

**goniopuncture** /ˈɡəʊniəʊˌpʌŋktʃə/ *noun* a surgical operation for draining fluid from the eyes of someone who has glaucoma

**gonioscope** /ˈɡəʊniəskəʊp/ *noun* a lens for measuring the angle of the front part of the eye

**goniotomy** /ˌɡəʊniˈɒtəmi/ *noun* a surgical operation to treat glaucoma by cutting Schlemm's canal

**gonococcal** /ˌɡɒnəˈkɒk(ə)l/ *adjective* referring to gonococcus

**gonococcus** /ˌɡɒnəˈkɒkəs/ *noun* a type of bacterium, *Neisseria gonorrhoea,* which causes gonorrhoea (NOTE: The plural is **gonococci**.)

**gonocyte** /ˈɡɒnəsaɪt/ *noun* same as **germ cell**

**gonorrhoea** /ˌɡɒnəˈriːə/ *noun* a sexually transmitted disease which produces painful irritation of the mucous membrane and a watery discharge from the vagina or penis

**gonorrhoeal** /ˌɡɒnəˈriːəl/ *adjective* referring to gonorrhoea

**Goodpasture's syndrome** /ɡʊdˈpɑːstʃəz ˌsɪndrəʊm/ *noun* a rare lung disease in which someone coughs up blood, is anaemic, and may have kidney failure [Described 1919. After Ernest William Goodpasture (1886–1960), US pathologist.]

**goose bumps** /ˈɡuːs bʌmps/, **goose flesh** / ˈɡuːs fleʃ/, **goose pimples** /ˈɡuːs ˌpɪmp(ə)lz/ *noun* a reaction of the skin when someone is cold or frightened, the skin being raised into many little bumps by the action of the arrector pili muscles. Also called **cutis anserina**

**Gordh needle** /ˈɡɔːd ˌniːd(ə)l/ *noun* a needle with a bag attached, so that several injections can be made one after the other

**gorget** /ˈɡɔːdʒɪt/ *noun* a surgical instrument used to remove stones from the bladder

**gouge** /ɡaʊdʒ/ *noun* a surgical instrument like a chisel, used to cut bone

**goundou** /ˈɡuːnduː/ *noun* a condition caused by yaws, in which growths form on either side of the nose

**gout** /ɡaʊt/ *noun* a disease in which unusual quantities of uric acid are produced and form crystals in the cartilage round joints. Also called **podagra**

COMMENT: Gout was formerly associated with drinking strong wines such as port, but is now believed to arise in three ways: excess uric acid in the diet, overproduction of uric acid in the body and inadequate excretion of uric acid. It is likely that both overproduction and inadequate excretion are due to inherited biochemical developments. Excess intake of alcohol can provoke an attack by interfering with the excretion of uric acid.

**gown** /ɡaʊn/ *noun* a long robe worn over other clothes to protect them ○ *The surgeons were wearing green gowns.* ○ *The patient was dressed in a theatre gown, ready to go to the operating theatre.*

**GP** *abbr* general practitioner

**GP co-op** /ˌdʒiː ˈpiː kəʊ ˌɒp/ *noun* a group of GPs who work together to provide out-of-hours care without making any profit

**gr** *symbol* grain

**Graafian follicle** /ˌɡræfiən ˈfɒlɪk(ə)l/ *noun* same as **ovarian follicle** [After Reijnier de Graaf (1641–73), Dutch physician]

**gracilis** /ˈɡreɪsɪlɪs/ *noun* a thin muscle running down the inside of the leg from the top of the leg down to the top of the tibia

**graduated** /ˈɡrædʒueɪtɪd/ *adjective* with marks showing various degrees or levels ○ *a graduated measuring jar*

**Graefe's knife** /ˈɡrefəz ˌnaɪf/ *noun* a sharp knife used in operations on cataracts [After Friedrich Wilhelm Ernst Albrecht von Graefe (1828–70), Professor of Ophthalmology in Berlin, Germany]

**graft** /ɡrɑːft/ *noun* **1.** the act of transplanting an organ or tissue to replace one which is not functioning or which is diseased ○ *a skin graft* **2.** an organ or tissue which is transplanted ○ *The corneal graft was successful.* ○ *The patient was given drugs to prevent the graft being rejected.* ■ *verb* to take a healthy organ or tissue and transplant it in place of diseased or malfunctioning organ or tissue ○ *The surgeons grafted a new section of bone at the side of the skull.* ◊ **autograft, homograft**

**graft versus host disease** /ˌɡrɑːft ˌvɜːsəs ˈhəʊst dɪˌziːz/ *noun* a condition which develops when cells from the grafted tissue react against the person's own tissue, causing skin disorders. Abbr **GVHD**

**grain** /ɡreɪn/ *noun* **1.** a very small piece of something hard such as salt **2.** a measure of weight equal to 0.0648 grams. Symbol **gr**

**-gram** /ɡræm/ *suffix* a record in the form of a picture

**Gram-negative bacterium** /ɡræm ˈneɡətɪv bækˌtɪəriəm/ *noun* a bacterium which takes up the red counterstain, after the alcohol has washed out the first violet dye

**Gram-positive bacterium** /ˌgræm ˈpɒzɪtɪv bækˌtɪəriəm/ *noun* a bacterium which retains violet dye and appears blue-black when viewed under the microscope

**Gram's stain** /ˌgræmz ˈsteɪn/ *noun* a method of staining bacteria so that they can be identified [Described 1884. After Hans Christian Joachim Gram (1853–1938), Professor of Medicine in Copenhagen, Denmark. He discovered the stain by accident as a student in Berlin, Germany.]

COMMENT: The tissue sample is first stained with a violet dye, treated with alcohol, and then counterstained with a red dye.

**grand mal** /ˌgrɒn ˈmæl/ *noun* a type of epilepsy, in which someone becomes unconscious and falls down, while the muscles become stiff and twitch violently

**grand multiparity** /ˌgræn ˌmʌltiˈpærɪti/ *noun* the fact of having given birth to more than four children

**granular** /ˈgrænjʊlə/ *adjective* made up of granules

**granular cast** /ˌgrænjʊlə ˈkɑːst/ *noun* a cast composed of cells filled with protein and fatty granules

**granular leucocyte** /ˌgrænjʊlə ˈluːkəsaɪt/ *noun* same as **granulocyte**

**granulation** /ˌgrænjʊˈleɪʃ(ə)n/ *noun* the formation of rough red tissue on the surface of a wound or site of infection, the first stage in the healing process

**granulation tissue** /ˌgrænjʊˈleɪʃ(ə)n ˌtɪʃuː/ *noun* soft tissue, consisting mainly of tiny blood vessels and fibres, which forms over a wound

**granule** /ˈgrænjuːl/ *noun* a very small piece of something hard

**granulocyte** /ˈgrænjʊləsaɪt/ *noun* a type of leucocyte or white blood cell which contains granules, e.g. a basophil, eosinophil or neutrophil

**granulocytopenia** /ˌgrænjʊləʊˌsaɪtəʊˈpiːniə/ *noun* a usually fatal disease caused by the lowering of the number of granulocytes in the blood due to bone marrow malfunction

**granuloma** /ˌgrænjʊˈləʊmə/ *noun* a mass of granulation tissue which forms at the site of bacterial infections (NOTE: The plural is **granulomata** or **granulomas**.)

**granuloma inguinale** /ˌgrænjʊˌləʊmə ˌɪŋgwɪˈneɪli/ *noun* a sexually transmitted disease affecting the anus and genitals in which the skin becomes covered with ulcers, usually occurring in the tropics

**granulomatosis** /ˌgrænjʊləʊməˈtəʊsɪs/ *noun* persistent inflammation leading to the formation of nodules

**granulopoiesis** /ˌgrænjuːləʊpɔɪˈiːsɪs/ *noun* the normal production of granulocytes in the bone marrow

**graph** /grɑːf/ *noun* a diagram which shows the relationship between quantities as a line

**graph-** /græf/ *prefix* writing

**-graph** /grɑːf/ *suffix* a machine which records something as pictures

**-grapher** /grəfə/ *suffix* a technician who operates a machine which records

**-graphy** /grəfi/ *suffix* the technique of study through pictures

**grattage** /græˈtɑːʒ/ *noun* a procedure that involves scraping the surface of an ulcer which is healing slowly to make it heal more rapidly

**gravel** /ˈgræv(ə)l/ *noun* small stones which pass from the kidney to the urinary system, causing pain in the ureter

**Graves' disease** /ˈgreɪvz dɪˌziːz/ *noun* same as **exophthalmic goitre** [Described 1835. After Robert James Graves (1796–1853), Irish physician at the Meath Hospital, Dublin, Ireland, where he was responsible for introducing clinical ward work for medical students.]

**gravid** /ˈgrævɪd/ *adjective* pregnant

**gravides multiparae** /ˌgrævɪdiːz ˌmʌlti ˈpɑːriː/ *plural noun* women who have given birth to at least four live babies

**gravity** /ˈgrævɪti/ *noun* the importance or potential danger of a disease or situation

**Grawitz tumour** /ˈgrɑːvɪts ˌtjuːmə/ *noun* a malignant tumour in kidney cells [Described 1883. After Paul Albert Grawitz (1850–1932), Professor of Pathology at Greifswald, Germany.]

**gray** /greɪ/ *noun* an SI unit of measurement of absorbed radiation equal to 100 rads. Symbol **Gy**. ◊ **rad**

**graze** /greɪz/ *noun* a scrape on the skin surface, making some blood flow ■ *verb* to scrape the skin surface accidentally

**great cerebral vein** /ˌgreɪt ˈserəbrəl veɪn/ *noun* a median vein draining the choroid plexuses of the lateral and third ventricles

**greater curvature** /ˌgreɪtə ˈkɜːvətʃə/ *noun* a convex line of the stomach

**greater vestibular glands** /ˌgreɪtə veˈstɪbjʊlə glændz/ *noun* same as **Bartholin's glands**

**great toe** /ˈgreɪt təʊ/ *noun* same as **big toe**

**green monkey disease** /ˌgriːn ˈmʌŋki dɪ ˌziːz/ *noun* same as **Marburg disease**

**greenstick fracture** /ˈgriːnstɪk ˌfræktʃə/ *noun* a type of fracture occurring in children, where a long bone bends, but is not completely broken

**grey commissure** /greɪ ˈkɒmɪsjʊə/ *noun* part of the grey matter nearest to the central canal of the spinal cord, where axons cross over each other

**grey matter** /ˈgreɪ ˌmætə/ *noun* nerve tissue which is of a dark grey colour and forms part of the central nervous system

COMMENT: In the brain, grey matter encloses the white matter, but in the spinal cord, white matter encloses the grey matter.

**grief counsellor** /ˈgriːf ˌkaʊns(ə)lə/ *noun* a person who helps someone to cope with the feelings they have when someone such as a close relative dies

**Griffith's types** /ˈgrɪfɪθs ˌtaɪps/ *noun* various types of haemolytic streptococci, classified according to the antigens present in them

**gripe water** /ˈgraɪp ˌwɔːtə/ *noun* a solution of glucose and alcohol, used to relieve abdominal pains in babies

**griping** /ˈgraɪpɪŋ/ *adjective* referring to stomach pains that are sudden, sharp and intense

**grocer's itch** /ˌgrəʊsəz ˈɪtʃ/ *noun* a form of dermatitis on the hands caused by handling flour and sugar

**groin** /grɔɪn/ *noun* a junction at each side of the body where the lower abdomen joins the top of the thighs ○ *He had a dull pain in his groin.* (NOTE: For other terms referring to the groin, see **inguinal**.)

**grommet** /ˈgrɒmɪt/ *noun* a tube which can be passed from the external auditory meatus into the middle ear, usually to allow fluid to drain off, as in someone who has glue ear

**gross anatomy** /ˌgrəʊs əˈnætəmi/ *noun* the study of the structure of the body that can be seen without the use of a microscope

**ground substance** /ˌgraʊnd ˈsʌbstəns/ *noun* same as **matrix**

**group** /gruːp/ *noun* several people, animals or things which are all close together ○ *A group of patients were waiting in the surgery.* ■ *verb* to bring things or people together in a group, or come together in a group ○ *The drugs are grouped under the heading 'antibiotics'.*

**group practice** /ˌgruːp ˈpræktɪs/ *noun* a medical practice where several doctors or dentists share the same office building and support services

**group therapy** /ˌgruːp ˈθerəpi/ *noun* a type of psychotherapy where a group of people with the same disorder meet together with a therapist to discuss their condition and try to help each other

**growing pains** /ˈgrəʊɪŋ peɪnz/ *plural noun* pains associated with adolescence, which can be a form of rheumatic fever

**growth** /grəʊθ/ *noun* **1.** the process of increasing in size ○ *the growth in the population since 1960* ○ *The disease stunts children's growth.* **2.** a cyst or tumour ○ *The doctor found a cancerous growth on the left breast.* ○ *He had an operation to remove a small growth from his chin.*

**growth factor** /ˈgrəʊθ ˌfæktə/ *noun* a chemical, especially a polypeptide, produced in the body which encourages particular cells to grow ○ *a nerve growth factor*

**growth hormone** /ˈgrəʊθ ˌhɔːməʊn/ *noun* a hormone secreted by the pituitary gland during deep sleep, which stimulates growth of the

long bones and protein synthesis. Also called **somatropin**

**grumbling appendix** /ˌgrʌmblɪŋ əˈpendɪks/ *noun* a vermiform appendix that is always slightly inflamed (*informal*) ▷ **chronic appendicitis**

**GTT** *abbr* glucose tolerance test

**GU** *abbr* **1.** gastric ulcer **2.** genitourinary

**guanine** /ˈgwɑːniːn/ *noun* one of the four basic chemicals in DNA

**guardian ad litem** /ˌgɑːdiən æd ˈliːtəm/ *noun* a person who acts on behalf of a minor who is a defendant in a court case

**guardian Caldicott** /ˌgɑːdiən ˈkɔːldɪkɒt/ *noun* in the UK, a person appointed by a hospital or Health Trust to make sure that information about patients is kept confidential, following the Caldicott Report of 1997

**gubernaculum** /ˌguːbəˈnækjʊləm/ *noun* in a fetus, fibrous tissue connecting the testes (the gonads) to the groin

**Guillain-Barré syndrome** /ˌgiːjæn ˈbæreɪ ˌsɪndrəʊm/ *noun* a nervous disorder in which, after a non-specific infection, demyelination of the spinal roots and peripheral nerves takes place, leading to generalised weakness and sometimes respiratory paralysis. Also called **Landry's paralysis** [Described 1916. After Georges Guillain (1876–1961), Professor of Neurology in Paris, France, Jean Alexandre Barré (1880–1967), Professor of Neurology in Strasbourg, France.]

**guillotine** /ˈgɪlətiːn/ *noun* a surgical instrument for cutting out tonsils

**guinea worm** /ˈgɪni wɜːm/ *noun* same as **Dracunculus**

**Gulf War syndrome** /gʌlf ˈwɔː ˌsɪndrəʊm/ *noun* a collection of unexplained symptoms, including fatigue, skin disorders, and muscle pains, affecting some soldiers who fought in the Gulf War in 1991

**gullet** /ˈgʌlɪt/ *noun* same as **oesophagus**

**gum** /gʌm/ *noun* the soft tissue covering the part of the jaw which surrounds the teeth ○ *Her gums are red and inflamed.* ○ *A build-up of tartar can lead to gum disease.* Also called **gingiva** (NOTE: For other terms referring to the gums, see words beginning with **gingiv-**.)

**gumboil** /ˈgʌmbɔɪl/ *noun* an abscess on the gum near a tooth

**gumma** /ˈgʌmə/ *noun* an abscess of dead tissue and overgrown scar tissue, which develops in the later stages of syphilis

**gustation** /gʌˈsteɪʃ(ə)n/ *noun* the act of tasting

**gustatory** /ˈgʌstət(ə)ri/ *adjective* referring to the sense of taste

**gut** /gʌt/ *noun* **1.** the tubular organ for the digestion and absorption of food. Also called **intestine 2.** a type of thread, made from the intestines of sheep. It is used to sew up internal incisions and dissolves slowly so does not need to be removed. ◊ **catgut**

**Guthrie test** /ˈgʌθri test/ *noun* a test used on babies to detect the presence of phenylketonuria [After R. Guthrie (b. 1916), US paediatrician.]

**gutta** /ˈgʌtə/ *noun* a drop of liquid, as used in treatment of the eyes (NOTE: The plural is **guttae**.)

**gutter splint** /ˈgʌtə splint/ *noun* a shaped container in which a broken limb can rest without being completely surrounded

**GVHD** *abbr* graft versus host disease

**gyn-** /gaɪn/ *prefix* same as **gynae-** (*used before a vowel*)

**gynae-** /gaɪni/ *prefix* referring to women (NOTE: In US English words beginning with **gynae-** are spelled **gyne-**.)

**gynaecological** /ˌgaɪnɪkəˈlɒdʒɪk(ə)l/ *adjective* referring to the treatment of diseases of women

**gynaecologist** /ˌgaɪnɪˈkɒlədʒɪst/ *noun* a doctor who specialises in the treatment of diseases of women

**gynaecology** /gaɪnɪˈkɒlədʒi/ *noun* the study of female sex organs and the treatment of diseases of women in general

**gynaecomastia** /ˌgaɪnɪkəˈmæstiə/ *noun* the unusual development of breasts in a male

**gyne** /ˈgaɪni/ same as **gynaecology, gynaecological** (*informal*) ○ *a gyne appointment*

**gypsum** /ˈdʒɪpsəm/ *noun* calcium sulphate, used as plaster of Paris

**gyrus** /ˈdʒaɪərəs/ *noun* a raised part of the cerebral cortex between the sulci

# H

**H2-receptor antagonist** /ˌeɪtʃ tuː rɪ ˈseptər ænˌtægənɪst/ *noun* a drug that inhibits the production of stomach acid and so relieves indigestion and gastric ulcers

**HA** *abbr* health authority

**habit** /ˈhæbɪt/ *noun* **1.** an action which is an automatic response to a stimulus **2.** a regular way of doing something ○ *He got into the habit of swimming every day before breakfast.* ○ *She's got out of the habit of taking any exercise.* □ **from force of habit** because you do it regularly ○ *I wake up at 6 o'clock from force of habit.*

**habit-forming** /ˈhæbɪt ˌfɔːmɪŋ/ *adjective* making someone addicted

**habit-forming drug** /ˈhæbɪt ˌfɔːmɪŋ drʌg/ *noun* a drug which is addictive

**habitual** /həˈbɪtʃuəl/ *adjective* done frequently or as a matter of habit

**habitual abortion** /həˌbɪtʃuəl əˈbɔːʃ(ə)n/ *noun* a condition in which a woman has abortions with successive pregnancies

**habituation** /həˌbɪtʃuˈeɪʃ(ə)n/ *noun* the fact of being psychologically but not physically addicted to or dependent on a drug, alcohol or other substance

**habitus** /ˈhæbɪtəs/ *noun* the general physical appearance of a person, including build and posture

**hacking cough** /ˌhækɪŋ ˈkɒf/ *noun* a continuous short dry cough

**haem** /hiːm/ *noun* a molecule containing iron which binds proteins to form haemoproteins such as haemoglobin and myoglobin

**haem-** /hiːm/ *prefix* same as **haemo-** (*used before vowels*) (NOTE: In US English, words beginning with the prefix **haem-** are spelled **hem-** .)

**haemagglutination** /ˌhiːməgluːtɪˈneɪʃ(ə)n/ *noun* the clumping of red blood cells, often used to test for the presence of antibodies

**haemangioma** /ˌhiːmændʒiˈəʊmə/ *noun* a harmless tumour which forms in blood vessels and appears on the skin as a birthmark

**haemarthrosis** /ˌhiːmɑːˈθrəʊsɪs/ *noun* pain and swelling caused by blood leaking into a joint

**haematemesis** /ˌhiːməˈteməsɪs/ *noun* a condition in which someone vomits blood, usually because of internal bleeding

**haematic** /hiːˈmætɪk/ *adjective* referring to blood

**haematin** /ˈhiːmətɪn/ *noun* a substance which forms from haemoglobin when bleeding takes place

**haematinic** /ˌhiːməˈtɪnɪk/ *noun* a drug which increases haemoglobin in blood, used to treat anaemia, e.g. an iron compound

**haemato-** /hiːmətəʊ/ *prefix* referring to blood

**haematocoele** /ˈhiːmətəʊsiːl/, **haematocele** *noun* a swelling caused by blood leaking into a cavity, especially the scrotum

**haematocolpos** /ˌhiːmətəʊˈkɒlpəs/ *noun* a condition in which the vagina is filled with blood at menstruation because the hymen has no opening

**haematocrit** /ˈhiːmətəʊkrɪt/ *noun* **1.** same as **packed cell volume 2.** an instrument for measuring haematocrit

**haematocyst** /ˈhiːmətəʊsɪst/ *noun* a cyst which contains blood

**haematogenous** /ˌhiːməˈtɒdʒənəs/ *adjective* **1.** producing blood **2.** produced by blood

**haematological** /ˌhiːmətəʊˈlɒdʒɪk(ə)l/ *adjective* referring to haematology

**haematologist** /ˌhiːməˈtɒlədʒɪst/ *noun* a doctor who specialises in haematology

**haematology** /ˌhiːməˈtɒlədʒi/ *noun* the scientific study of blood, its formation and its diseases

**haematoma** /ˌhiːməˈtəʊmə/ *noun* a mass of blood under the skin caused by a blow or by the effects of an operation

**haematometra** /ˌhiːməˈtɒmɪtrə/ *noun* **1.** excessive bleeding in the uterus **2.** a swollen uterus, caused by haematocolpos

**haematomyelia** /ˌhiːmətəʊmaɪˈiːliə/ *noun* a condition in which blood leaks into the spinal cord

**haematopoiesis** /ˌhiːmətəʊpɔɪˈiːsɪs/ *noun* same as **haemopoiesis**

**haematoporphyrin** /ˌhiːmətəʊˈpɔːfərɪn/ noun porphyrin produced from haemoglobin

**haematosalpinx** /ˌhiːmətəʊˈsælpɪŋks/ noun same as **haemosalpinx**

**haematospermia** /ˌhiːmætəʊˈspɜːmiə/ noun the presence of blood in the sperm

**haematozoon** /ˌhiːmətəʊˈzəʊɒn/ noun a parasite living in the blood (NOTE: The plural is **haematozoa**.)

**haematuria** /ˌhiːməˈtjʊəriə/ noun the unusual presence of blood in the urine, as a result of injury or disease of the kidney or bladder

**haemin** /ˈhiːmɪn/ noun a salt derived from haemoglobin, used in the treatment of porphyria

**haemo-** /hiːməʊ/ prefix referring to blood

**haemochromatosis** /ˌhiːməʊkrəʊməˈtəʊsɪs/ noun an inherited disease in which the body absorbs and stores too much iron, causing cirrhosis of the liver and giving the skin a dark colour. Also called **bronze diabetes**

**haemoconcentration** /ˌhiːməʊˌkɒnsənˈtreɪʃ(ə)n/ noun an increase in the percentage of red blood cells because the volume of plasma is reduced. Compare **haemodilution**

**haemocytoblast** /ˌhiːməʊˈsaɪtəʊblæst/ noun an embryonic blood cell in the bone marrow from which red and white blood cells and platelets develop

**haemocytometer** /ˌhiːməʊsaɪˈtɒmɪtə/ noun a glass jar in which a sample of blood is diluted and the blood cells counted

**haemodialyse** /ˌhiːməʊˈdaɪəlaɪz/ verb to remove waste matter from the blood using a dialyser (kidney machine)

**haemodialysed patient** /ˌhiːməʊ daɪəlaɪzd ˈpeɪʃ(ə)nt/ noun someone who has undergone haemodialysis

**haemodialysis** /ˌhiːməʊdaɪˈæləsɪs/ noun same as **kidney dialysis**

**haemodilution** /ˌhiːməʊdaɪˈluːʃ(ə)n/ noun a decrease in the percentage of red blood cells because the volume of plasma has increased. Compare **haemoconcentration**

**haemoglobin** /ˌhiːməʊˈɡləʊbɪn/ noun a red respiratory pigment formed of haem and globin in red blood cells which gives blood its red colour. It absorbs oxygen in the lungs and carries it in the blood to the tissues. Abbr **Hb**. ◊ **oxyhaemoglobin, carboxyhaemoglobin**

**haemoglobinaemia** /ˌhiːməʊɡləʊbɪˈniːmiə/ noun a condition in which haemoglobin is found in blood plasma

**haemoglobinopathy** /ˌhiːməʊɡləʊbɪˈnɒpəθi/ noun an inherited disease of a group which result from damaging variations in the production of haemoglobin, e.g. sickle-cell anaemia

**haemoglobinuria** /ˌhiːməʊɡləʊbɪˈnjʊəriə/ noun a condition in which haemoglobin is found in the urine

**haemogram** /ˈhiːməʊɡræm/ noun the printed result of a blood test

**haemolysin** /ˌhiːməʊˈlaɪsɪn/ noun a protein which destroys red blood cells

**haemolysis** /hiːˈmɒləsɪs/ noun the destruction of red blood cells

**haemolytic** /ˌhiːməʊˈlɪtɪk/ adjective destroying red blood cells ■ noun a substance which destroys red blood cells, e.g. snake venom

**haemolytic anaemia** /ˌhiːməlɪtɪk əˈniːmiə/ noun a condition in which the destruction of red blood cells is about six times the usual rate, and the supply of new cells from the bone marrow cannot meet the demand

**haemolytic disease of the newborn** /ˌhiːməʊlɪtɪk dɪˌziːz əv ðə ˈnjuːbɔːn/ noun a condition in which the red blood cells of the fetus are destroyed because antibodies in the mother's blood react against them

**haemolytic jaundice** /ˌhiːməʊlɪtɪk ˈdʒɔːndɪs/ noun jaundice caused by haemolysis of the red blood cells. Also called **prehepatic jaundice**

**haemolytic uraemic syndrome** /ˌhiːməʊlɪtɪk jʊˈriːmɪk ˌsɪndrəʊm/ noun a condition in which haemolytic anaemia damages the kidneys

**haemopericardium** /ˌhiːməʊperɪˈkɑːdiəm/ noun a condition in which blood is found in the pericardium

**haemoperitoneum** /ˌhiːməʊperɪtəˈniːəm/ noun a condition in which blood is found in the peritoneal cavity

**haemophilia** /ˌhiːməˈfɪliə/ noun a disorder linked to a recessive gene on the X-chromosome in which the blood clots much more slowly than usual, resulting in extensive bleeding from even minor injuries. The gene is passed by women to their male children and the disorder is seen almost exclusively in boys.

**haemophilia A** /ˌhiːməʊfɪliə ˈeɪ/ noun the most common type of haemophilia, in which the inability to synthesise Factor VIII, a protein that promotes blood clotting, means that the blood clots very slowly

**haemophilia B** /ˌhiːməfɪliə ˈbiː/ noun a less common type of haemophilia, in which the inability to synthesise Factor IX, a protein that promotes blood clotting, means that the blood clots very slowly. Also called **Christmas disease**

**haemophiliac** /ˌhiːməˈfɪliæk/ noun a person who has haemophilia

**haemophilic** /ˌhiːməʊˈfɪlɪk/ adjective referring to haemophilia

**Haemophilus** /hiːˈmɒfɪləs/ noun a genus of bacteria which needs specific factors in the blood to grow

**Haemophilus influenzae** /hiːˌmɒfɪləs ˌɪn↓ fluˈenzə/ noun a bacterium which lives in healthy throats, but which can cause pneumonia if a person's resistance is lowered by a bout of flu

**Haemophilus influenzae type b** /hi:ˌmɒ fɪləs ɪnfluˌenzə taɪp 'bi:/ *noun* a bacterium which causes meningitis. Abbr **Hib**

**haemophthalmia** /ˌhi:mɒf'θælmiə/ *noun* a condition in which blood is found in the vitreous humour of the eye

**haemopneumothorax** /ˌhi:məʊˌnju:məʊ 'θɔːræks/ *noun* same as **pneumohaemothorax**

**haemopoiesis** /ˌhi:məʊpɔɪ'i:sɪs/ *noun* the continual production of blood cells and blood platelets in the bone marrow. Also called **blood formation**

**haemopoietic** /ˌhi:məʊpɔɪ'etɪk/ *adjective* referring to the formation of blood in the bone marrow

**haemoptysis** /hi:'mɒptəsɪs/ *noun* a condition in which someone coughs blood from the lungs, caused by a serious illness such as anaemia, pneumonia, tuberculosis or cancer

**haemorrhage** /'hem(ə)rɪdʒ/ *noun* the loss of a large quantity of blood, especially from a burst blood vessel ○ *He died of a brain haemorrhage.* ■ *verb* to bleed heavily ○ *The injured man was haemorrhaging from the mouth.*

**haemorrhagic** /ˌhemə'rædʒɪk/ *adjective* referring to heavy bleeding

**haemorrhagic disease of the newborn** /ˌhemərædʒɪk dɪˌzi:z əv ðə 'nju:bɔːn/ *noun* a disease of newly born babies, which makes them haemorrhage easily, caused by temporary lack of prothrombin

**haemorrhagic disorder** /ˌheməˌrædʒɪk dɪs'ɔːdə/ *noun* a disorder in which haemorrhages occur, e.g. haemophilia

**haemorrhagic fever** /ˌhemərædʒɪk 'fi:və/ *noun* a viral infection that results in profuse internal bleeding from the capillaries, e.g. dengue or Ebola

**haemorrhagic stroke** /ˌhemərædʒɪk 'strəʊk/ *noun* a stroke caused by a burst blood vessel

**haemorrhoidal** /ˌhemə'rɔɪdəl/ *adjective* referring to haemorrhoids

**haemorrhoidectomy** /ˌhemərɔɪ'dektəmi/ *noun* the surgical removal of haemorrhoids

**haemorrhoids** /'hemərɔɪdz/ *plural noun* swollen veins in the anorectal passage. Also called **piles**

**haemosalpinx** /hi:məʊ'sælpɪŋks/ *noun* the accumulation of blood in the Fallopian tubes

**haemosiderosis** /ˌhi:məʊsɪdə'rəʊsɪs/ *noun* a disorder in which iron forms large deposits in the tissue, causing haemorrhaging and destruction of red blood cells

**haemostasis** /ˌhi:məʊ'steɪsɪs/ *noun* the process of stopping bleeding or slowing the movement of blood

**haemostat** /'hi:məʊstæt/ *noun* a device which stops bleeding, e.g. a clamp

**haemostatic** /ˌhi:məʊ'stætɪk/ *adjective* stopping bleeding ■ *noun* a drug which stops bleeding

**haemothorax** /ˌhi:məʊ'θɔːræks/ *noun* a condition in which blood is found in the pleural cavity

**Hageman factor** /'hɑːɡəmən ˌfæktə/ *noun* same as **Factor XII**

**HAI** *abbr* Hospital Acquired Infection

**hair cell** /'heə sel/ *noun* a receptor cell which converts fluid pressure changes into nerve impulses carried in the auditory nerve (NOTE: For other terms referring to hair, see words beginning with **pilo-, trich-, tricho-**.)

**hair follicle** /'heə ˌfɒlɪk(ə)l/ *noun* the cells and tissue that surround the root of a hair

**hairline fracture** /'heəlaɪn ˌfræktʃə/ *noun* a very slight crack in a bone caused by injury

**hair papilla** /heə pə'pɪlə/ *noun* a part of the skin containing capillaries which feed blood to the hair

**hairy cell leukaemia** /ˌheəri sel lu: 'ki:miə/ *noun* a form of leukaemia in which white blood cells have fine projections

**half-life** /'hɑːf laɪf/ *noun* **1.** a measurement of the period of time taken before the concentration of a drug has reached half of what it was when it was administered **2.** the time taken for half the atoms in a radioactive isotope to decay

**halitosis** /ˌhælɪ'təʊsɪs/ *noun* a condition in which a person has breath which smells unpleasant. Also called **bad breath**

COMMENT: Halitosis can have several causes: caries in the teeth, infection of the gums, and indigestion are the most usual. The breath can also have an unpleasant smell during menstruation, or in association with certain diseases such as diabetes mellitus and uraemia.

**halluces** /'hælusi:z/ *plural of* **hallux**

**hallucinate** /hə'lu:sɪneɪt/ *verb* to have hallucinations ○ *The patient was hallucinating.*

**hallucination** /həˌlu:sɪ'neɪʃ(ə)n/ *noun* an experience of seeing an imaginary scene or hearing an imaginary sound as clearly as if it were really there

**hallucinatory** /hə'lu:sɪnət(ə)ri/ *adjective* referring to a drug which causes hallucinations

**hallucinogen** /ˌhælu:'sɪnədʒən/ *noun* a drug which causes hallucinations, e.g. cannabis or LSD

**hallucinogenic** /həˌlu:sɪnə'dʒenɪk/ *adjective* referring to a substance which produces hallucinations ○ *a hallucinogenic fungus*

**hallux** /'hæləks/ *noun* the big toe (NOTE: The plural is **halluces**.)

**hallux valgus** /ˌhæləks 'vælɡəs/ *noun* a condition of the foot, where the big toe turns towards the other toes and a bunion is formed

**haloperidol** /ˌhæləʊˈperɪdɒl/ *noun* a tranquilliser used in the treatment of schizophrenia, mania and psychoses

**halo splint** /ˈheɪləʊ splɪnt/ *noun* a device used to keep the head and neck still so that they can recover from injury or an operation

**halothane** /ˈhæləʊθeɪn/ *noun* a general anaesthetic that is given by inhalation

**hamamelis** /ˌhæməˈmiːlɪs/ ♦ **witch hazel**

**hamartoma** /ˌhæmɑːˈtəʊmə/ *noun* a benign tumour containing tissue from any organ

**hamate** /ˈheɪmeɪt/, **hamate bone** /ˈheɪmeɪt bəʊn/ *noun* one of the eight small carpal bones in the wrist, shaped like a hook. Also called **unciform bone**. See illustration at HAND in Supplement

**hammer** /ˈhæmə/ *noun* same as **malleus**

**hammer toe** /ˈhæmə təʊ/ *noun* a toe which has the middle joint permanently bent downwards

**hamstring** /ˈhæmstrɪŋ/ *noun* one of a group of tendons behind the knee, which link the thigh muscles to the bones in the lower leg

**hamstring muscles** /ˈhæmstrɪŋ ˌmʌs(ə)lz/ *plural noun* a group of muscles at the back of the thigh, which flex the knee and extend the gluteus maximus

**hand** /hænd/ *noun* the part at the end of the arm, beyond the wrist, which is used for holding things ○ *He injured his hand with a saw.* ■ *verb* to pass something to someone

COMMENT: The hand is formed of 27 bones: 14 phalanges in the fingers, 5 metacarpals in the main part of the hand, and 8 carpals in the wrist.

**hand, foot and mouth disease** /ˌhænd fʊt ən ˈmaʊθ dɪˌziːz/ *noun* a mild viral infection in children, causing small blisters

**handicap** /ˈhændikæp/ *noun* a physical or mental condition which prevents someone from doing some everyday activities ■ *verb* to prevent someone from doing an everyday activity (NOTE: The word 'handicap' is now usually avoided.)

'…handicap – disadvantage for a given individual, resulting from an impairment or a disability, that limits or prevents the fulfilment of a role that is normal for that individual' [WHO]

**handicapped** /ˈhændikæpt/ *adjective* referring to a person who has a disability (NOTE: The word 'handicapped' is now usually avoided.)

**Hand-Schüller Christian disease** /ˌhænt ˌʃʊlə ˈkrɪʃən dɪˌziːz/ *noun* a disturbance of cholesterol metabolism in young children which causes disorders in membranous bone, mainly in the skull, exophthalmos, diabetes insipidus, and a yellow-brown colour of the skin [First described 1893 then 1915 by Schüller and 1920 by Christian. After Alfred Hand Jr. (1868–1949), US paediatrician; Artur Schüller (1874–1958), Austrian neurologist; Henry Asbury Christian (1876–1951), Professor of Medicine at Harvard, USA.]

**hangnail** /ˈhæŋneɪl/ *noun* a piece of torn skin at the side of a nail

**hangover** /ˈhæŋəʊvə/ *noun* a condition occurring after a person has drunk too much alcohol, with dehydration caused by inhibition of the antidiuretic hormone in the kidneys. The symptoms include headache, inability to stand noise and trembling of the hands.

**Hansen's bacillus** /ˌhænsənz bəˈsɪləs/ *noun* the bacterium which causes leprosy, *Mycobacterium leprae* [Discovered 1873. After Gerhard Henrik Armauer Hansen (1841–1912), Norwegian physician.]

**Hansen's disease** /ˈhænsənz dɪˌziːz/ *noun* same as **leprosy**

**haploid** /ˈhæplɔɪd/ *adjective* referring to a cell such as a gamete where each chromosome occurs only once. In humans the haploid number of chromosomes is 23.

**hapt-** /hæpt/ *prefix* relating to the sense of touch

**hapten** /ˈhæpten/ *noun* a substance which causes an allergy, probably by changing a protein so that it becomes antigenic

**hardening of the arteries** /ˌhɑːd(ə)nɪŋ əv ðə ˈɑːtəriz/ *noun* same as **atherosclerosis**

**hard of hearing** /ˌhɑːd əv ˈhɪərɪŋ/ *adjective* same as **hearing-impaired**

**hard palate** /ˌhɑːd ˈpælət/ *noun* the front part of the roof of the mouth between the upper teeth

**harelip** /ˈheəlɪp/ *noun* same as **cleft lip**

**harm** /hɑːm/ *noun* injury or damage as a result of something that you do ○ *Walking to work every day won't do you any harm.* □ **there's no harm in taking the tablets only for one week** there will be no side effects from taking the tablets for a week ■ *verb* to damage or hurt someone or something ○ *Walking to work every day won't harm you.*

**harmful** /ˈhɑːmf(ə)l/ *adjective* causing injury or damage ○ *Bright light can be harmful to your eyes.* ○ *Sudden violent exercise can be harmful.*

**harmless** /ˈhɑːmləs/ *adjective* causing no injury or damage ○ *These herbal remedies are quite harmless.*

**Harrison's sulcus** /ˌhærɪsənz ˈsʌlk(ə)s/, **Harrison's groove** /ˌhærɪs(ə)nz ˈgruːv/ *noun* a hollow on either side of the chest which develops in children who have difficulty in breathing, seen especially in cases of rickets

**Harris's operation** /ˈhærɪsɪz ɒpəˌreɪʃ(ə)n/ *noun* the surgical removal of the prostate gland [After S.H. Harris (1880–1936), Australian surgeon]

**Hartmann's solution** /ˈhɑːtmənz səˌluːʃ(ə)n/ *noun* a chemical solution used in drips to replace body fluids lost in dehydration, particularly as a result of infantile gastroenteritis [Described 1932. After Alexis Frank

Hartmann (1898–1964), paediatrician, St Louis, Missouri, USA.]

**Hartnup disease** /ˈhɑːtnəp dɪˌziːz/ *noun* an inherited condition affecting amino acid metabolism and producing thick skin and impaired mental development [After the name of the family in which this hereditary disease was first recorded]

**harvest** /ˈhɑːvɪst/ *verb* to take something for use elsewhere, e.g. a piece of skin for a graft or eggs for IVF

**Hashimoto's disease** /hæʃɪˈməʊtəz dɪ ˌziːz/ *noun* a type of goitre in middle-aged women, where the woman is sensitive to secretions from her own thyroid gland, and, in extreme cases, the face swells and the skin turns yellow [Described 1912. After Hakuru Hashimoto (1881–1934), Japanese surgeon.]

**hashish** /ˈhæʃɪʃ/ *noun* ♦ cannabis

**haustrum** /ˈhɔːstrəm/ *noun* a sac on the outside of the colon (NOTE: The plural is **haustra**.)

**HAV** *abbr* hepatitis A virus

**Haversian canal** /həˈvɜːʃ(ə)n kəˌnæl/ *noun* a fine canal which runs vertically through the Haversian systems in compact bone, containing blood vessels and lymph ducts [Described 1689. After Clopton Havers (1657–1702), English surgeon.]

**Haversian system** /həˈvɜːʃ(ə)n ˌsɪstəm/ *noun* a unit of compact bone built around a Haversian canal, made of a series of bony layers which form a cylinder. Also called **osteon**

**hayfever** /ˈheɪˌfiːvə/ *noun* inflammation in the nasal passage and eyes caused by an allergic reaction to plant pollen. ♦ allergic rhinitis

**HAZ** *abbr* health action zone

**Hb** *abbr* haemoglobin

**HBV** *abbr* hepatitis B virus

**hCG** *abbr* human chorionic gonadotrophin

**HCHS** *abbr* Health and Community Health Services

**HDL** *abbr* high density lipoprotein

**head** /hed/ *noun* **1.** the round top part of the body, which contains the eyes, nose, mouth, brain, etc (NOTE: For other terms referring to the head, see words beginning with **cephal-, cephalo-**.) **2.** a rounded top part of a bone which fits into a socket ○ *head of humerus* ○ *head of femur*

**headache** /ˈhedeɪk/ *noun* a pain in the head, caused by changes in pressure in the blood vessels feeding the brain which act on the nerves. Also called **cephalalgia**

COMMENT: Headaches can be caused by a blow to the head, by lack of sleep or food, by eye strain, sinus infections and many other causes. Mild headaches can be treated with an analgesic and rest. Severe headaches which recur may be caused by serious disorders in the head or nervous system.

**head cold** /hed kəʊld/ *noun* a minor illness, with inflammation of the nasal passages, excess mucus in the nose and sneezing

**head louse** /ˈhed laʊs/ *noun* a small insect of the *Pediculus* genus, which lives on the scalp and sucks blood. Also called **Pediculus capitis** (NOTE: The plural is **head lice**.)

**Heaf test** /ˈhiːf test/ *noun* a test in which tuberculin is injected into the skin to find out whether a person is immune to tuberculosis. ♦ **Mantoux test**

**heal** /hiːl/ *verb* **1.** (*of wound*) to return to a healthy state ○ *After six weeks, her wound had still not healed.* ○ *A minor cut will heal faster if it is left without a bandage.* **2.** to make someone or something get better

**healing** /ˈhiːlɪŋ/ *noun* the process of getting better ○ *a substance which will accelerate the healing process*

**healing by first intention** /ˌhiːlɪŋ baɪ ˌfɜːst ɪnˈtenʃən/ *noun* the healing of a clean wound where the tissue reforms quickly

**healing by second intention** /ˌhiːlɪŋ baɪ ˌsekənd ɪnˈtenʃən/ *noun* the healing of an infected wound or ulcer, which takes place slowly and may leave a permanent scar

**health** /helθ/ *noun* the general condition of the mind or body ○ *He's in good health.* ○ *She had suffered from bad health for some years.* ○ *The council said that fumes from the factory were a danger to public health.* ○ *All cigarette packets carry a government health warning.*

**health action zone** /ˌhelθ ˈækʃən zəʊn/ *noun* in the UK, an area in which the government has funded specific actions to redress health inequalities. Abbr **HAZ**

**Health and Safety at Work Act** /ˌhelθ ən ˌseɪfti ət ˈwɜːk ækt/ *noun* in the UK, an Act of Parliament which rules how the health of workers should be protected by the companies they work for

**Health and Safety Executive** /ˌhelθ ən ˈseɪfti ɪɡˌzekjʊtɪv/ *noun* in the UK, a government organisation responsible for overseeing the health and safety of workers

**health authority** /helθ ɔːˈθɒrəti/ *noun* ♦ **Strategic Health Authority**

**healthcare** /ˈhelθkeə/, **health care** *noun* the general treatment of people with medical disorders, especially the use of measures to stop a disease from occurring

**healthcare assistant** /ˈhelθkeər əˌsɪstənt/ *noun* someone who assists health professionals in looking after a sick or dependent person

**healthcare delivery** /ˈhelθkeə dɪˌlɪv(ə)ri/ *noun* the provision of care and treatment by the health service

**healthcare professional** /ˈhelθkeə prəˌfeʃ(ə)n(ə)l/ *noun* a qualified person who works in an occupation related to health care, e.g. a nurse

**healthcare system** /ˈhelθkeə ˌsɪstəm/ noun any organised set of health services

**health centre** /ˈhelθ ˌsentə/ noun a public building in which a group of doctors practise

**health education** /helθ ˌedjʊˈkeɪʃ(ə)n/ noun the process of teaching people, both school children and adults, to do things to improve their health, e.g. to take more exercise

**Health Education Authority** /ˌhelθ ˌedjʊ ˈkeɪʃ(ə)n ɔːˌθɒrɪti/ noun a government health promotion agency in England designed to help people make aware of how they can improve their health. Abbr **HEA**

**health food** /ˈhelθ fuːd/ noun food that is regarded as good for health, especially containing ingredients such as cereals, dried fruit and nuts and without additives

**health inequality** /helθ ˌɪnɪˈkwɒlɪti/ noun the differences that exist in health across the social classes, with poorer people tending to experience poorer health

**health information service** /ˌhelθ ɪnfə ˈmeɪʃ(ə)n ˌsɜːvɪs/ noun a nation-wide information service delivered via a free telephone helpline. Abbr **HIS**

**health insurance** /ˈhelθ ɪnˌʃʊərəns/ noun insurance which pays the cost of treatment for illness

**Health Ombudsman** /ˈhelθ ˌɒmbʊdzmən/ noun same as **Health Service Commissioner**

'…the HA told the Health Ombudsman that nursing staff and students now received full training in the use of the nursing process' [*Nursing Times*]

**health promotion** /ˈhelθ prəˌməʊʃ(ə)n/ noun the act of improving the health of a particular community or of the public generally, e.g. using health education, immunisation and screening

**Health Protection Agency** /ˌhelθ prə ˈtekʃ(ə)n ˌeɪdʒənsi/ noun a national organisation for England and Wales, established in 2003, dedicated to the protection of people's health, especially by reducing the impact of infectious diseases, chemicals, poisons and radiation. It brings together existing sources of expertise in public health, communicable diseases, emergency planning, infection control, poisons and radiation hazards.

**health service** /ˈhelθ ˌsɜːvɪs/ noun an organisation which is in charge of providing health care to a particular community

**Health Service Commissioner** /ˌhelθ ˌsɜːvɪs kəˈmɪʃ(ə)nə/, **Health Service Ombudsman** /ˈhelθ ˌsɜːvɪs ˌɒmbʊdzmən/ noun in the UK, an official who investigates complaints from the public about the National Health Service

**health service manager** /ˌhelθ ˌsɜːvɪs ˈmænɪdʒə/ noun someone who is responsible for the provision of local health care, through the management of hospital, GP, and community health services

**health service planning** /ˌhelθ ˌsɜːvɪs ˈplænɪŋ/ noun the process of deciding what the health care needs of a community are, with the help of statistics, and what resources can be provided for that community

**health visitor** /ˈhelθ ˌvɪzɪtə/ noun a registered nurse with qualifications in midwifery or obstetrics and preventive medicine, who visits mothers and babies and sick people in their homes and advises on treatment

'…in the UK, the main screen is carried out by health visitors at 6–10 months' [*Lancet*]

**healthy** /ˈhelθi/ adjective **1.** in good physical condition **2.** helping you to stay in good physical condition ○ *People are healthier than they were fifty years ago.* ○ *This town is the healthiest place in England.* ○ *If you eat a healthy diet and take plenty of exercise there is no reason why you should fall ill.* (NOTE: **healthier – healthiest**)

**hear** /hɪə/ verb to sense sounds with the ears ○ *I can't hear what you're saying.* (NOTE: **hearing – heard**)

**hearing** /ˈhɪərɪŋ/ noun the ability to hear, or the function performed by the ear of sensing sounds and sending sound impulses to the brain ○ *His hearing is failing.* (NOTE: For other terms referring to hearing, see words beginning with **audi-, audio-**.)

**hearing aid** /ˈhɪərɪŋ eɪd/ noun a small electronic device fitted into or near the ear, to improve someone's hearing by making the sounds louder

**hearing-impaired** /ˌhɪərɪŋ ɪmˈpeəd/ adjective having a degree of hearing loss

**hearing loss** /ˈhɪərɪŋ lɒs/ noun partial or complete loss of the ability to hear

**heart** /hɑːt/ noun the main organ in the body, which maintains the circulation of the blood around the body by its pumping action ○ *The doctor listened to his heart.* ○ *She has heart trouble.* (NOTE: For other terms referring to the heart, see also words beginning with **cardi-, cardio-**.)

COMMENT: The heart is situated slightly to the left of the central part of the chest, between the lungs. It is divided into two parts by a vertical septum; each half is itself divided into an upper chamber (the atrium) and a lower chamber (the ventricle). The veins bring blood from the body into the right atrium; from there it passes into the right ventricle and is pumped into the pulmonary artery which takes it to the lungs. Oxygenated blood returns from the lungs to the left atrium, passes to the left ventricle and from there is pumped into the aorta for circulation round the arteries. The heart expands and contracts by the force of the heart muscle (the myocardium) under impulses from the sinoatrial node, and an average heart beats about 70 times a minute. The contracting beat as it pumps blood out (the systole) is followed by a weaker diastole, where the muscles relax to allow blood to flow back into the heart. In a heart attack, part of the myocardium is deprived of blood because of a clot in a coronary artery. This has an effect on the rhythm of the heartbeat and can be fatal. In heart block, impulses from the sinoatrial node fail to reach the ventricles properly.

**heart attack** /'hɑːt ə,tæk/ *noun* a condition in which the heart has a reduced blood supply because one of the arteries becomes blocked by a blood clot, causing myocardial ischaemia and myocardial infarction (*informal*)

**heartbeat** /'hɑːtbiːt/ *noun* the regular noise made by the heart as it pumps blood

**heart block** /'hɑːt blɒk/ *noun* the slowing of the action of the heart because the impulses from the sinoatrial node to the ventricles are delayed or interrupted. There are either longer impulses (first degree block) or missing impulses (second degree block) or no impulses at all (complete heart block), in which case the ventricles continue to beat slowly and independently of the sinoatrial node.

**heartburn** /'hɑːtbɜːn/ *noun* indigestion which causes a burning feeling in the stomach and oesophagus, and a flow of acid saliva into the mouth (*informal*)

**heart bypass** /,hɑːt 'baɪpɑːs/, **heart bypass operation** /,hɑːt 'baɪpɑːs ɒpə,reɪʃ(ə)n/ *noun* same as **coronary artery bypass graft**

**heart disease** /'hɑːt dɪ,ziːz/ *noun* any disease of the heart in general

**heart failure** /'hɑːt ,feɪljə/ *noun* the failure of the heart to maintain the output of blood to meet the demands of the body. It may affect the left or right sides of the heart, or both sides.
◊ congestive heart failure

**heart-lung machine** /hɑːt 'lʌŋ mə,ʃiːn/ *noun* a machine used to pump blood round the body and maintain the supply of oxygen to the blood during heart surgery

**heart-lung transplant** /hɑːt 'lʌŋ ,trɑːns plɑːnt/ *noun* an operation to transplant a new heart and lungs into someone

**heart massage** /'hɑːt ,mæsɑːʒ/ *noun* a treatment which involves pressing on the chest to make a heart which has stopped beating start working again

**heart murmur** /'hɑːt ,mɜːmə/ *noun* an unusual sound made by turbulent blood flow, sometimes as a result of valve disease

**heart rate** /'hɑːt reɪt/ *noun* the number of times the heart beats per minute

**heart sounds** /'hɑːt saʊndz/ *plural noun* two different sounds made by the heart as it beats.
♦ lubb-dupp

**heart stoppage** /'hɑːt ,stɒpɪdʒ/ *noun* a situation where the heart has stopped beating

**heart surgeon** /'hɑːt ,sɜːdʒən/ *noun* a surgeon who specialises in operations on the heart

**heart surgery** /'hɑːt ,sɜːdʒəri/ *noun* a surgical operation to remedy a condition of the heart

**heart tamponade** /hɑːt tæmpə'neɪd/ *noun* same as **cardiac tamponade**

**heart transplant** /'hɑːt ,trænsplɑːnt/ *noun* a surgical operation to transplant a heart into someone

**heat cramp** /'hiːt kræmp/ *noun* cramp produced by loss of salt from the body in very hot conditions

**heat exhaustion** /'hiːt ɪg,zɔːstʃ(ə)n/ *noun* collapse caused by physical exertion in hot conditions, involving loss of salt and body fluids

**heat rash** /'hiːt ræʃ/ *noun* same as **miliaria**

**heat spots** /'hiːt spɒts/ *plural noun* little red spots which develop on the face in very hot weather

**heatstroke** /'hiːtstrəʊk/ *noun* a condition in which someone becomes too hot and his or her body temperature rises abnormally, leading to headaches, stomach cramps and sometimes loss of consciousness

**heat therapy** /'hiːt ,θerəpi/, **heat treatment** /'hiːt ,triːtmənt/ *noun* same as **thermotherapy**

**heavy period** /,hevi 'pɪəriəd/ *noun* a monthly period during which a woman loses an unusually large amount of blood. It is often painful and sometimes indicates possible health problems, such as fibroids or hypothyroidism.

**hebephrenia** /,hiːbɪ'friːniə/, **hebephrenic schizophrenia** /,hiːbɪfrenɪk skɪtsəʊ'friːniə/ *noun* a condition in which someone, usually an adolescent, has hallucinations, delusions and deterioration of personality, talks rapidly and generally acts in a strange manner

**Heberden's node** /,hiːbədənz 'nəʊd/ *noun* a small bony lump which develops on the end joints of fingers in osteoarthritis [Described 1802. After William Heberden (1767–1845), British physician, specialist in rheumatic diseases.]

**hebetude** /'hebɪtjuːd/ *noun* dullness of the senses during acute fever, which makes the person uninterested in his or her surroundings and unable to respond to stimuli

**hectic** /'hektɪk/ *adjective* recurring regularly

**hectic fever** /,hektɪk 'fiːvə/ *noun* an attack of fever which occurs each day in someone who has tuberculosis

**heel** /hiːl/ *noun* the back part of the foot

**heel bone** /'hiːl bəʊn/ *noun* the bone forming the heel, beneath the talus. Also called **calcaneus**

**Hegar's sign** /'heɪgəz ,saɪn/ *noun* a way of detecting pregnancy, by inserting the fingers into the uterus and pressing with the other hand on the pelvic cavity to feel if the neck of the uterus has become soft [After Alfred Hegar (1830–1914), Professor of Obstetrics and Gynaecology at Freiburg, Germany]

**Heimlich manoeuvre** /'haɪmlɪk mə,nuːvə/ *noun* an emergency treatment for choking, in which a strong upward push beneath the breastbone of a patient clasped from behind forces the blockage out of the windpipe

**helco-** /ˈhelkəʊ/ prefix relating to an ulcer

**helcoplasty** /ˈhelkəʊplæsti/ noun a skin graft to cover an ulcer to aid healing

**Helicobacter pylori** /ˌhelɪkəʊbæktə paɪ ˈlɔːriː/ noun a bacterium found in gastric secretions, strongly associated with duodenal ulcers and gastric carcinoma

**helicopter-based emergency medical services** /ˌhelɪkɒptə beɪst ɪˌmɜːdʒənsi ˈmedɪk(ə)l ˌsɜːvɪsɪz/ plural noun full form of **HEMS**

**helio-** /ˈhiːliəʊ/ prefix relating to the sun

**heliotherapy** /ˌhiːliəʊˈθerəpi/ noun treatment by sunlight or sunbathing

**helium** /ˈhiːliəm/ noun a very light gas used in combination with oxygen, especially to relieve asthma or sickness caused by decompression (NOTE: The chemical symbol is **He**.)

**helix** /ˈhiːlɪks/ noun the curved outer edge of the ear

**Heller's operation** /ˈheləz ɒpəˌreɪʃ(ə)n/ noun same as **cardiomyotomy** [After E. Heller (1877–1964), German surgeon.]

**Heller's test** /ˈheləz test/ noun a test for protein in the urine [After Johann Florenz Heller (1813–71), Austrian physician]

**Hellin's law** /ˌhelɪnz ˈlɔː/ noun a finding which states that twins should occur naturally once in 90 live births, triplets once in 8,100 live births, quadruplets once in 729, 000 live births, and quintuplets once in 65, 610, 000 live births (NOTE: Since the 1960s the numbers have changed due to fertility treatment. For example, twins now occur once in only 38 births.)

**HELLP syndrome** /ˈhelp ˌsɪndrəʊm/ noun a serious pre-eclamptic disorder which makes it necessary to terminate a pregnancy. Full form **haemolysis-elevated liver enzymes–low platelet count syndrome**

**helminth** /ˈhelmɪnθ/ noun a parasitic worm, e.g. a tapeworm or fluke

**helminthiasis** /ˌhelmɪnˈθaɪəsɪs/ noun infestation with parasitic worms

**heloma** /hɪˈləʊmə/ noun same as **corn**

**helper** /ˈhelpə/ noun a person who helps someone to do something, especially without payment

**helper T-cell** /ˌhelpə ˈtiː sel/ noun a type of white blood cell that stimulates the production of cells that destroy antigens

**hemeralopia** /ˌhemərəˈləʊpiə/ noun a usually congenital condition in which someone is able to see better in bad light than in ordinary daylight. Also called **day blindness**

**hemi-** /hemi/ prefix half

**hemianopia** /ˌhemiəˈnəʊpiə/ noun a state of partial blindness in which someone has only half the usual field of vision in each eye

**hemiarthroplasty** /ˌhemiˈɑːθrəʊplæsti/ noun an operation to repair a joint which replaces one of its surfaces with an artificial substance, often metal

**hemiatrophy** /ˌhemiˈætrəfi/ noun a condition in which half of the body or half of an organ or part is atrophied

**hemiballismus** /ˌhemibəˈlɪzməs/ noun a sudden movement of the limbs on one side of the body, caused by a disease of the basal ganglia

**hemicolectomy** /ˌhemikəˈlektəmi/ noun the surgical removal of part of the colon

**hemicrania** /ˌhemiˈkreɪniə/ noun a headache in one side of the head, as in migraine

**hemimelia** /ˌhemiˈmiːliə/ noun a congenital condition in which someone has absent or extremely short arms or legs

**hemiparesis** /ˌhemipəˈriːsɪs/ noun slight paralysis of the muscles of one side of the body

**hemiplegia** /ˌhemiˈpliːdʒə/ noun severe paralysis affecting one side of the body due to damage of the central nervous system. Compare **diplegia**

**hemiplegic** /ˌhemiˈpliːdʒɪk/ adjective referring to paralysis of one side of the body

**hemisphere** /ˈhemɪsfɪə/ noun half of a sphere

**hemo-** /hiːməʊ/ prefix US spelling of **haemo-**

**HEMS** /hemz/ plural noun a system of delivering a paramedic crew to the scene of an accident or medical emergency by helicopter and then transporting patients to the nearest major hospital or specialist unit. Full form **helicopter-based emergency medical services**

**Henderson's model** /ˈhendəs(ə)nz ˌmɒd(ə)l/ noun a model of nurse–patient relationships based on 14 basic principles of nursing. The main idea is that 'the nurse does for others what they would do for themselves if they had the strength, the will, and the knowledge…but that the nurse makes the patient independent of him or her as soon as possible'.

**Henle's loop** /ˌhenliːz ˈluːp/ noun same as **loop of Henle** [Described 1862. After Friedrich Gustav Jakob Henle (1809–85), Professor of Anatomy at Göttingen, Germany.]

**Henoch-Schönlein purpura** /ˌhenək ˌʃɜːnlaɪn ˈpɜːpjʊrə/, **Henoch's purpura** /ˌhenəks ˈpɜːpjʊrə/ noun a condition in which blood vessels become inflamed and bleed into the skin, causing a rash called purpura and also pain in the stomach and the joints, vomiting and diarrhoea. It often occurs after an upper respiratory infection, mostly in children aged two to 11. [Described 1832 by Schönlein and 1865 by Henoch. Eduard Heinrich Henoch (1820–1910), Professor of Paediatrics at Berlin, Germany; Johannes Lukas Schönlein (1793–1864), physician and pathologist at Würzburg, Zürich and Berlin.]

**hep** /hep/ *noun* same as **hepatitis** (*informal*)

**heparin** /'hepərɪn/ *noun* an anticoagulant substance found in the liver and lungs, and also produced artificially for use in the treatment of thrombosis

**hepat-** /hɪpæt/ *prefix* same as **hepato-** (*used before vowels*)

**hepatalgia** /ˌhepə'tældʒə/ *noun* pain in the liver

**hepatectomy** /ˌhepə'tektəmi/ *noun* the surgical removal of part of the liver

**hepatic** /hɪ'pætɪk/ *adjective* referring to the liver

**hepatic artery** /hɪˌpætɪk 'ɑːtəri/ *noun* an artery which takes the blood to the liver

**hepatic cell** /hɪˌpætɪk 'sel/ *noun* an epithelial cell of the liver acini

**hepatic duct** /hɪˌpætɪk 'dʌkt/ *noun* a duct which links the liver to the bile duct leading to the duodenum

**hepatic flexure** /hɪˌpætɪk 'flekʃə/ *noun* a bend in the colon, where the ascending and transverse colons join

**hepaticostomy** /hɪˌpætɪ'kɒstəmi/ *noun* a surgical operation to make an opening in the hepatic duct taking bile from the liver

**hepatic portal system** /hɪˌpætɪk 'pɔːt(ə)l ˌsɪstəm/ *noun* a group of veins linking to form the portal vein, which brings blood from the pancreas, spleen, gall bladder and the abdominal part of the alimentary canal to the liver

**hepatic vein** /hɪˌpætɪk 'veɪn/ *noun* a vein which takes blood from the liver to the inferior vena cava

**hepatis** /'hepətɪs/ ♦ **porta hepatis**

**hepatitis** /ˌhepə'taɪtɪs/ *noun* inflammation of the liver through disease or drugs

COMMENT: Infectious hepatitis and serum hepatitis are caused by different viruses called A and B, and having had one does not give immunity against an attack of the other. Hepatitis A is less serious than the B form, which can cause severe liver failure and death. Other hepatitis viruses have also been identified.

**hepatitis A** /ˌhepətaɪtɪs 'eɪ/ *noun* a relatively mild form of viral hepatitis that is transmitted through contaminated food and water

**hepatitis A virus** /ˌhepətaɪtɪs 'eɪ ˌvaɪrəs/ *noun* a virus which causes hepatitis A. Abbr **HAV**

**hepatitis B** /ˌhepətaɪtɪs 'biː/ *noun* a severe form of viral hepatitis that is transmitted by contact with infected blood or other body fluids

**hepatitis B virus** /ˌhepətaɪtɪs 'biː ˌvaɪrəs/ *noun* a virus which causes hepatitis B. Abbr **HBV**

**hepatitis C** *noun* a form of viral hepatitis that is transmitted by contact with infected blood or other body fluids but is often without symptoms (NOTE: It was formerly called non-A, non-B hepatitis.)

**hepatitis C virus** *noun* a virus which causes hepatitis C. Abbr **HCV**

**hepatitis delta** /ˌhepəˌtaɪtɪs 'deltə/ *noun* same as **delta hepatitis**

**hepato-** /hepətəʊ/ *prefix* referring to the liver

**hepatoblastoma** /ˌhepətəʊblæ'stəʊmə/ *noun* a malignant tumour in the liver, made up of epithelial-type cells often with areas of immature cartilage and embryonic bone

**hepatocele** /'hepətəʊsiːl/ *noun* a hernia of the liver through the diaphragm or the abdominal wall

**hepatocellular** /ˌhepətəʊ'seljʊlə/ *adjective* referring to liver cells

**hepatocellular jaundice** /ˌhepətəʊˌseljʊlə 'dʒɔːndɪs/ *noun* jaundice caused by injury to or disease of the liver cells

**hepatocirrhosis** /ˌhepətəʊsɪ'rəʊsɪs/ *noun* same as **cirrhosis**

**hepatocolic ligament** /ˌhepətəʊkɒlɪk 'lɪgəmənt/ *noun* a ligament which links the gall bladder and the right bend of the colon

**hepatocyte** /'hepətəʊsaɪt, hɪ'pætəsaɪt/ *noun* a liver cell which synthesises and stores substances, and produces bile

**hepatogenous** /ˌhepə'tɒdʒənəs/ *noun* referring to or originating in the liver ○ *hepatogenous jaundice*

**hepatolenticular degeneration** /ˌhepətəʊ len,tɪkjʊlə dɪˌdʒenə'reɪʃ(ə)n/ *noun* same as **Wilson's disease**

**hepatoma** /ˌhepə'təʊmə/ *noun* a malignant tumour of the liver formed of mature cells, especially found in people with cirrhosis

**hepatomegaly** /ˌhepətəʊ'megəli/ *noun* a condition in which the liver becomes very large

**hepatosplenomegaly** /ˌhepətəʊˌspliːnəʊ 'megəli/ *noun* enlargement of both the liver and the spleen, as occurs in leukaemia or lymphoma

**hepatotoxic** /ˌhepətəʊ'tɒksɪk/ *adjective* destroying the liver cells

**herald patch** /'herəld ˌpætʃ/ *noun* a small spot of a rash such as pityriasis rosea which appears some time before the main rash

**herb** /hɜːb/ *noun* a plant which can be used in preparing medicines

**herbal** /'hɜːb(ə)l/ *adjective* referring to plants which are used as medicines

**herbalism** /'hɜːbəlɪz(ə)m/ *noun* ♦ **herbal medicine**

**herbalist** /'hɜːbəlɪst/ *noun* a person who treats illnesses or disorders with substances extracted from plants

**herbal medicine** /ˌhɜːb(ə)l 'med(ə)sɪn/ *noun* a system of medical treatment involving the use of substances extracted from plants

**herbal remedy** /ˌhɜːb(ə)l 'remədi/ *noun* a medicine made from plants, e.g. an infusion made from dried leaves or flowers in hot water

**herd immunity** /ˈhɜːd ɪˌmjuːnɪti/ *noun* the fact of a group of people being resistant to a specific disease, because many individuals in the group are immune to or immunised against the microorganism which causes it

**hereditary** /həˈredɪt(ə)ri/ *adjective* passed as from parents to children through the genes

**hereditary spherocytosis** /həˌredɪt(ə)ri ˌsfɪərəʊsaɪˈtəʊsɪs/ *noun* same as **acholuric jaundice**

**heredity** /həˈredɪti/ *noun* the process by which genetically controlled characteristics pass from parents to children

**Hering-Breuer reflexes** /ˌherɪŋ ˈbrɔɪə ˌriːfleksɪz/ *plural noun* the reflexes which maintain the usual rhythmic inflation and deflation of the lungs

**hermaphrodite** /hɜːˈmæfrədaɪt/ *noun* a person with both male and female characteristics

**hermaphroditism** /hɜːˈmæfrədaɪtɪz(ə)m/ *noun* a condition in which a person has both male and female characteristics

**hernia** /ˈhɜːniə/ *noun* a condition in which an organ bulges through a hole or weakness in the wall which surrounds it. Also called **rupture** □ **reduction of a hernia** putting a hernia back into the correct position

**hernial** /ˈhɜːniəl/ *adjective* referring to a hernia

**hernial sac** /ˌhɜːniəl ˈsæk/ *noun* a sac formed where a membrane has pushed through a cavity in the body

**herniated** /ˈhɜːnieɪtɪd/ *adjective* referring to an organ which has developed a hernia

**herniated disc** /ˌhɜːnieɪtɪd ˈdɪsk/ *noun* ♦ displaced intervertebral disc

**herniation** /ˌhɜːniˈeɪʃ(ə)n/ *noun* the development of a hernia

**hernio-** /hɜːniəʊ/ *prefix* relating to a hernia

**hernioplasty** /ˈhɜːniəʊˌplæsti/ *noun* a surgical operation to reduce a hernia

**herniorrhaphy** /ˌhɜːniˈɔːrəfi/ *noun* a surgical operation to remove a hernia and repair the organ through which it protruded

**herniotomy** /ˌhɜːniˈɒtəmi/ *noun* a surgical operation to remove a hernial sac

**heroin** /ˈherəʊɪn/ *noun* a narcotic drug in the form of a white powder derived from morphine

**herpangina** /ˌhɜːpænˈdʒaɪnə/ *noun* an infectious disease of children, where the tonsils and back of the throat become inflamed and ulcerated, caused by a Coxsackie virus

**herpes** /ˈhɜːpiːz/ *noun* inflammation of the skin or mucous membrane, caused by a virus, where small blisters are formed

**herpes simplex** /ˌhɜːpiːz ˈsɪmpleks/ *noun* **1.** (*Type I*) a virus that produces a painful blister, called a cold sore, usually on the lips **2.** (*Type II*) a sexually transmitted disease which

forms blisters in the genital region. Also called **genital herpes**

**herpesvirus** /ˈhɜːpiːzˌvaɪrəs/ *noun* one of a group of viruses which cause herpes and chickenpox (herpesvirus Type I), and genital herpes (herpesvirus Type II)

COMMENT: Because the same virus causes herpes and chickenpox, anyone who has had chickenpox as a child carries the dormant herpesvirus in his or her bloodstream and can develop shingles in later life. It is not known what triggers the development of shingles, though it is known that an adult suffering from shingles can infect a child with chickenpox.

**herpes zoster** /ˌhɜːpiːz ˈzɒstə/ *noun* inflammation of a sensory nerve, characterised by pain along the nerve and causing a line of blisters to form on the skin, usually found mainly on the abdomen or back, or on the face. Also called **shingles, zona**

**herpetic** /hɜːˈpetɪk/ *adjective* referring to herpes

**herpetiformis** /hɜːˌpetɪˈfɔːmɪs/ ♦ **dermatitis herpetiformis**

**hetero-** /hetərəʊ/ *prefix* different

**heterochromia** /ˌhetərəʊˈkrəʊmiə/ *noun* a condition in which the irises of the eyes are different colours

**heterogametic** /ˌhetərəʊɡəˈmetɪk/ *adjective* producing gametes with different sex chromosomes, as in the human male

**heterogeneous** /ˌhetərəʊˈdʒiːniəs/ *adjective* having different characteristics or qualities (NOTE: Do not confuse with **heterogenous**.)

**heterogenous** /ˌhetəˈrɒdʒɪnəs/ *adjective* coming from a different source (NOTE: Do not confuse with **heterogeneous**.)

**heterograft** /ˈhetərəʊɡrɑːft/ *noun* tissue taken from one species and grafted onto an individual of another species. Compare **homograft**

**heterologous** /hetəˈrɒləɡʌs/ *adjective* of a different type

**heterophoria** /ˌhetərəʊˈfɔːriə/ *noun* a condition in which if an eye is covered it tends to squint

**heteroplasty** /ˈhetərəʊplæsti/ *noun* same as **heterograft**

**heteropsia** /ˌhetəˈrɒpsiə/ *noun* a condition in which the two eyes see differently

**heterosexual** /ˌhetərəʊˈsekʃuəl/ *adjective* attracted to people of the opposite sex or relating to relations between males and females ■ *noun* a person who is sexually attracted to people of the opposite sex. Compare **bisexual, homosexual**

**heterosexuality** /ˌhetərəʊsekʃuˈælɪti/ *noun* sexual attraction towards persons of the opposite sex

**heterotopia** /ˌhetərəʊˈtəʊpiə/ *noun* **1.** a state where an organ is placed in a different position from usual or is malformed or deformed

**2.** the development of tissue which is not natural to the part in which it is produced

**heterotropia** /ˌhetərəʊ'trəʊpiə/ *noun* same as **strabismus**

**heterozygous** /ˌhetərəʊ'zaɪɡəs/ *adjective* having two or more different versions of a specific gene. Compare **homozygous**

**hex-** /heks/ *prefix* same as **hexa-** (NOTE: used before vowels)

**hexa-** /heksə/ *prefix* six

**HFEA** *abbr* Human Fertilization and Embryology Authority

**hGH** *abbr* human growth hormone

**HGPRT** *abbr* hypoxanthine guanine phosphoribosyl transferase. ♦ **HPRT**

**HI** *abbr* hearing-impaired

**hiatus** /haɪ'eɪtəs/ *noun* an opening or space

**hiatus hernia** /haɪˌeɪtəs 'hɜːniə/, **hiatal hernia** /haɪˌeɪt(ə)l 'hɜːniə/ *noun* a hernia where the stomach bulges through the opening in the diaphragm muscle through which the oesophagus passes

**Hib** /hɪb/ *abbr Haemophilus influenzae* type B

**Hib vaccine** /'hɪb ˌvæksiːn/ *noun* a vaccine used to inoculate against the bacterium *Haemophilius influenzae* that causes meningitis

**hiccup** /'hɪkʌp/, **hiccough** *noun* a spasm in the diaphragm which causes a sudden inhalation of breath followed by sudden closure of the glottis which makes a characteristic sound ○ *She had an attack of hiccups* or *had a hiccupping attack* or *got the hiccups.* Also called **singultus** ■ *verb* to make a hiccup

COMMENT: Many cures have been suggested for hiccups, but the main treatment is to try to get the patient to think about something else. A drink of water, holding the breath and counting, breathing into a paper bag, are all recommended.

**Hickman catheter** /ˌhɪkmən 'kæθɪtə/, **Hickman line** /ˌhɪkmən 'laɪn/ *noun* a plastic tube which is put into the large vein above the heart so that drugs can be given and blood samples can be taken easily

**hidr-** /haɪdr/ *prefix* referring to sweat

**hidradenitis** /ˌhaɪdrədə'naɪtɪs/ *noun* inflammation of the sweat glands

**hidrosis** /haɪ'drəʊsɪs/ *noun* sweating, especially when it is excessive

**hidrotic** /haɪ'drɒtɪk/ *adjective* referring to sweating ■ *noun* a substance which makes someone sweat

**Higginson's syringe** /'hɪɡɪnsənz sɪˌrɪnʒ/ *noun* a syringe with a rubber bulb in the centre that allows flow in one direction only, used mainly to give enemas [After Alfred Higginson (1808–84), British surgeon]

**high-altitude sickness** /haɪ 'æltɪtjuːd ˌsɪknəs/ *noun* same as **altitude sickness**

**high blood pressure** /ˌhaɪ 'blʌd ˌpreʃə/ *noun* same as **hypertension**

**high-calorie diet** /haɪ ˌkæləri 'daɪət/ *noun* a diet containing over 4000 calories per day

**high-density lipoprotein** /haɪ ˌdensɪti lɪpəʊ'prəʊtin/ *noun* a lipoprotein with a low percentage of cholesterol. Abbr **HDL**

**high-energy food** /ˌhaɪ ˌenədʒi 'fuːd/ *noun* food such as fats or carbohydrates which contain a large number of calories and give a lot of energy when they are broken down in the body

**high-fibre diet** /haɪ ˌfaɪbə 'daɪət/ *noun* a diet which contains a high percentage of cereals, nuts, fruit and vegetables

**high-protein diet** /haɪ ˌprəʊtiːn 'daɪət/ *noun* a diet containing mostly foods high in protein and low in carbohydrates and saturated fat, adopted by people who are trying to lose weight

**high-risk** /ˌhaɪ 'rɪsk/ *adjective* referring to someone who is very likely to catch or develop a disease, develop a cancer or have an accident

**high-risk patient** /ˌhaɪ rɪsk 'peɪʃ(ə)nt/ *noun* a patient who has a high risk of catching an infection or developing a disease

**hilar** /'haɪlə/ *adjective* referring to a hilum

**hilum** /'haɪləm/ *noun* a hollow where blood vessels or nerve fibres enter an organ such as a kidney or lung (NOTE: The plural is **hila.**)

**hindbrain** /'haɪndbreɪn/ *noun* the part of brain of an embryo from which the medulla oblongata, the pons and the cerebellum eventually develop

**hindgut** /'haɪndɡʌt/ *noun* part of an embryo which develops into the colon and rectum

**hinge joint** /'hɪndʒ dʒɔɪnt/ *noun* same as **ginglymus**

**hip** /hɪp/ *noun* a ball and socket joint where the thigh bone or femur joins the acetabulum of the hip bone

**hip bone** /'hɪp bəʊn/ *noun* a bone made of the ilium, the ischium and the pubis which are fused together, forming part of the pelvic girdle. Also called **innominate bone**

**hip fracture** /'hɪp ˌfræktʃə/ *noun* a fracture of the ball at the top of the femur

**hip girdle** /'hɪp ˌɡɜːd(ə)l/ *noun* same as **pelvic girdle**

**hip joint** /'hɪp dʒɔɪnt/ *noun* the place where the hip is joined to the upper leg. See illustration at **PELVIS** in Supplement

**Hippel-Lindau** /ˌhɪpəl 'lɪndaʊ/ ♦ **von Hippel-Lindau syndrome**

**hippocampal formation** /ˌhɪpəkæmp(ə)l fɔː'meɪʃ(ə)n/ *noun* curved pieces of cortex inside each part of the cerebrum

**hippocampus** /ˌhɪpəʊ'kæmpəs/ *noun* a long rounded elevation projecting into the lateral ventricle in the brain

**Hippocratic oath** /ˌhɪpəkrætɪk 'əʊθ/ *noun* an ethical code observed by doctors, by which they will treat patients equally, put patients'

welfare first and not discuss openly the details of a patient's case

**hippus** /'hɪpəs/ *noun* alternating rapid contraction and dilatation of the pupil of the eye

**hip replacement** /'hɪp rɪ,pleɪsmənt/ *noun* a surgical operation to replace the whole ball and socket joint at the hip with an artificial one

**Hirschsprung's disease** /'hɪəʃsprʌŋz dɪ ,ziːz/ *noun* a congenital condition where parts of the lower colon lack nerve cells, making peristalsis impossible, so that food accumulates in the upper colon which becomes swollen [Described 1888. After Harald Hirschsprung (1830–1916), Professor of Paediatrics in Copenhagen, Denmark.]

**hirsute** /'hɜːsjuːt/ *adjective* with a lot of hair

**hirsutism** /'hɜːsjuːtɪz(ə)m/ *noun* the condition of having excessive hair, especially a condition in which a woman grows hair on the body in the same way as a man

**hirudin** /hɪ'ruːdɪn/ *noun* an anticoagulant substance produced by leeches, which is injected into the bloodstream while the leech is feeding on a body

**HIS** *abbr* Health Information Service

**hist-** /hɪst/ same as **histo-** (NOTE: used before vowels)

**histamine** /'hɪstəmiːn/ *noun* a substance released in response to allergens from mast cells throughout the body. Histamines dilate blood vessels, constrict the cells of smooth muscles and cause an increase in acid secretions in the stomach.

**histamine headache** /'hɪstəmiːn ,hedeɪk/ *noun* ♦ Horton's syndrome

**histamine receptor** /'hɪstəmiːn rɪ,septə/ *noun* a cell which is stimulated by histamine. H1 receptors in blood vessels are involved in allergic reactions, H2 receptors in the stomach are involved in gastric acid secretion.

**histamine test** /'hɪstəmiːn test/ *noun* a test to determine the acidity of gastric juice

**histaminic** /,hɪstə'mɪnɪk/ *adjective* referring to histamines

**histaminic headache** /,hɪstəmɪnɪk 'hel deɪk/ *noun* ♦ Horton's syndrome

**histidine** /'hɪstədiːn/ *noun* an amino acid from which histamine is derived

**histiocyte** /'hɪstiəʊsaɪt/ *noun* a macrophage of the connective tissue, involved in tissue defence

**histiocytoma** /,hɪstiəʊsaɪ'təʊmə/ *noun* a tumour containing histiocytes

**histiocytosis** /hɪstiəʊsaɪ'təʊsɪs/ *noun* a condition in which histiocytes are present in the blood

**histiocytosis X** /,hɪstiəʊsaɪ,təʊsɪs 'eks/ *noun* any form of histiocytosis where the cause is not known, e.g. Hand-Schüller-Christian disease

**histo-** /hɪstəʊ/ *prefix* relating to the body's tissue ○ *histology*

**histochemistry** /,hɪstəʊ'kemɪstri/ *noun* the study of the chemical constituents of cells and tissues and also their function and distribution, using a light or electron microscope to evaluate the stains

**histocompatibility** /,hɪstəʊkəmpætə'bɪlɪ ti/ *noun* compatibility between the antigens of tissues from two individuals, important in transplants

**histocompatible** /,hɪstəʊkəm'pætɪb(ə)l/ *adjective* referring to tissues from two individuals which have compatible antigens

**histogenesis** /,hɪstəʊ'dʒenəsɪs/ *noun* the formation and development of tissue from the embryological germ layer

**histogram** /'hɪstəɡræm/ *noun* a way of displaying frequency values as columns whose height is proportional to the corresponding frequency ○ *a histogram showing numbers of patients with the condition in each age group*

**histoid** /'hɪstɔɪd/ *adjective* **1.** made of or developed from a particular tissue **2.** like standard tissue

**histological** /,hɪstə'lɒdʒɪk(ə)l/ *adjective* referring to histology

**histological grade** /,hɪstəlɒdʒɪk(ə)l 'ɡreɪd/ *noun* a system of classifying tumours according to how malignant they are

**histology** /hɪ'stɒlədʒi/ *noun* the study of the anatomy of tissue cells and minute cellular structure

**histolysis** /hɪ'stɒləsɪs/ *noun* the disintegration of tissue

**histolytica** /,hɪstə'lɪtɪkə/ ♦ Entamoeba histolytica

**histoplasmosis** /,hɪstəʊplæz'məʊsɪs/ *noun* a lung disease caused by infection with the fungus *Histoplasma*

**history** /'hɪst(ə)ri/ *noun* the background information on someone's illness. ◊ **case history, medical history** □ **to take a patient's history** to ask someone to tell what has happened to them in their own words on being admitted to hospital

'…these children gave a typical history of exercise-induced asthma' [*Lancet*]

'…the need for evaluation of patients with a history of severe heart disease' [*Southern Medical Journal*]

**histotoxic** /,hɪstəʊ'tɒksɪk/ *adjective* referring to a substance which is poisonous to tissue

**HIV** *abbr* human immunodeficiency virus

'HIV-associated dementia is characterized by psychomotor slowing and inattentiveness' [*British Journal of Nursing*]

COMMENT: HIV is the virus which causes AIDS. Three strains of HIV virus have been identified: HIV-1, HIV-2 and HIV-3.

**hives** /haɪvz/ *noun* same as **urticaria** (NOTE: Takes a singular verb.)

**HIV-negative** /ˌeɪtʃ aɪ ˌviː ˈnegətɪv/ *adjective* referring to someone who has been tested and shown not to have HIV

**HIV-positive** /ˌeɪtʃ aɪ ˌviː ˈpɒzɪtɪv/ *adjective* referring to someone who has been tested and shown to have HIV

**HLA** *abbr* human leucocyte antigen

**HLA system** /ˌeɪtʃ el ˈeɪ ˌsɪstəm/ *noun* a system of HLA antigens on the surface of cells which need to be histocompatible to allow transplants to take place

COMMENT: HLA-A is the most important of the antigens responsible for rejection of transplants.

**HMO** *abbr US* Health Maintenance Organization

**hoarse** /hɔːs/ *adjective* referring to a voice which is harsh and rough

**hoarseness** /ˈhɔːsnəs/ *noun* a harsh and rough sound of the voice, often caused by laryngitis

**hobnail liver** /ˌhɒbneɪl ˈlɪvə/ *noun* same as **atrophic cirrhosis**

**Hodgkin's disease** /ˈhɒdʒkɪn dɪˌziːz/ *noun* a malignant disease in which the lymph glands are enlarged and there is an increase in the lymphoid tissues in the liver, spleen and bone marrow. It is frequently fatal if not treated early. [Described 1832. After Thomas Hodgkin (1798–1866), British physician.]

**hoist** /hɔɪst/ *noun* a device with pulleys and wires for raising a bed or a patient

**hole in the heart** /ˌhəʊl ɪn ðə ˈhɑːt/ *noun* same as **septal defect** (*informal*)

**Holger-Nielsen method** /ˌhɒlgə ˈniːlsən ˌmeθəd/ *noun* a formerly used method of giving artificial respiration by pressing a person's back and raising their arms backwards

**holism** /ˈhəʊlɪz(ə)m/ *noun* the theory that all of a person's physical, mental and social conditions should be considered in the treatment of his or her illness

**holistic** /həʊˈlɪstɪk/ *adjective* referring to a method of treatment involving all of someone's mental and family circumstances rather than just dealing with the condition from which he or she is suffering

**holistic care** /həʊˌlɪstɪk ˈkeə/ *noun* the care and treatment of a whole person rather than just of his or her medical symptoms

**holo-** /hɒləʊ/ *prefix* entire, complete

**holocrine** /ˈhɒləkrɪn/ *adjective* referring to a gland where the secretions are made up of disintegrated cells of the gland itself

**Homans' sign** /ˈhəʊmənz saɪn/ *noun* pain in the calf when the foot is bent back, a sign of deep-vein thrombosis [Described 1941. After John Homans (1877–1954), Professor of Clinical Surgery at Harvard, USA.]

**homeo-** /həʊmiəʊ/ *prefix* like or similar

**homeopathic** /ˌhəʊmiəˈpæθɪk/, **homoeopathic** /həʊmiəˈpæθɪk/ *adjective* **1.** referring to homeopathy ○ *a homeopathic clinic* ○ *She is having a course of homeopathic treatment.* **2.** referring to a drug which is given in very small quantities

**homeopathist** /ˌhəʊmiˈɒpəθɪst/, **homoeopathist** /həʊmiˈɒpəθɪst/ *noun* a person who practises homeopathy

**homeopathy** /ˌhəʊmiˈɒpəθi/, **homoeopathy** /həʊmiˈɒpəθi/ *noun* the treatment of a condition by giving the person very small quantities of a substance which, when given to a healthy person, would cause symptoms like those of the condition being treated. Compare **allopathy**

**homeostasis** /ˌhəʊmiəʊˈsteɪsɪs/ *noun* the process by which the functions and chemistry of a cell or internal organ are kept stable, even when external conditions vary greatly

**homo-** /həʊməʊ/ *prefix* the same

**homoeo-** /həʊmiəʊ/ *prefix* another spelling of **homeo-** (*used before vowels*)

**homogenise** /həˈmɒdʒənaɪz/, **homogenize** *verb* to give something a uniform nature

**homograft** /ˈhɒməgrɑːft/ *noun* the graft of an organ or tissue from a donor to a recipient of the same species, e.g. from one person to another. Also called **allograft**. Compare **heterograft**

**homolateral** /ˌhɒməˈlæt(ə)rəl/ *adjective* same as **ipsilateral**

**homologous** /hɒˈmɒləgəs/ *adjective* **1.** of the same type **2.** referring to chromosomes which form a pair

**homonymous** /həˈmɒnɪməs/ *adjective* affecting the two eyes in the same way

**homonymous hemianopia** /həˌmɒnɪməs hemiəˈnəʊpiə/ *noun* a condition in which the same half of the field of vision is lost in each eye

**homoplasty** /ˈhəʊməʊplæsti/ *noun* surgery to replace lost tissues by grafting similar tissues from another person

**homosexual** /ˌhəʊməʊˈsekʃuəl/ *adjective* referring to homosexuality ■ *noun* a person who is sexually attracted to people of the same sex. Compare **bisexual, heterosexual** (NOTE: Although **homosexual** can apply to both males and females, it is commonly used for males only, and **lesbian** is used for females.)

**homosexuality** /ˌhəʊməʊsekʃuˈælɪti/ *noun* sexual attraction to people of the same sex or sexual relations with people of the same sex

**homozygous** /ˌhəʊməʊˈzaɪgəs/ *adjective* having two identical versions of a specific gene. Compare **heterozygous**

**hook** /hʊk/ *noun* a surgical instrument with a bent end used for holding structures apart in operations

**hookworm** /ˈhʊkwɜːm/ noun a parasitic worm

**hookworm disease** /ˈhʊkwɜːm dɪˌziːz/ noun ♦ ancylostomiasis

**hordeolum** /hɔːˈdiːələm/ noun an infection of the gland at the base of an eyelash. Also called **stye**

**horizontal** /ˌhɒrɪˈzɒnt(ə)l/ adjective lying flat or at a right angle to the vertical

**horizontal fissure** /ˌhɒrɪˌzɒnt(ə)l ˈfɪʃə/ noun ANAT a horizontal groove between the superior and middle lobes of a lung. See illustration at LUNGS in Supplement

**horizontal plane** /ˌhɒrɪzɒnt(ə)l ˈpleɪn/ adjective same as **transverse plane**. see illustration at ANATOMICAL TERMS in Supplement

**hormonal** /hɔːˈməʊn(ə)l/ adjective referring to hormones

**hormone** /ˈhɔːməʊn/ noun a substance which is produced by one part of the body, especially the endocrine glands and is carried to another part of the body by the bloodstream where it has particular effects or functions

**hormone replacement therapy** /ˌhɔːməʊn rɪˈpleɪsmənt ˌθerəpi/, **hormone therapy** / ˈhɔːməʊn ˌθerəpi/ noun **1.** treatment for someone whose endocrine glands have been removed **2.** treatment to relieve the symptoms of the menopause by supplying oestrogen and reducing the risk of osteoporosis ▸ Abbr **HRT**

**horn** /hɔːn/ noun **1.** (in humans) tissue which grows out of an organ **2.** (in humans) one of the H-shaped limbs of grey matter seen in a cross-section of the spinal cord **3.** (in humans) an extension of the pulp chamber of a tooth towards the cusp

**Horner's syndrome** /ˈhɔːnəz ˌsɪndrəʊm/ noun a condition caused by paralysis of the sympathetic nerve in one side of the neck, making the eyelids hang down and the pupils contract [Described 1869. After Johann Friedrich Horner (1831–86), Professor of Ophthalmology in Zürich, Switzerland.]

**horny** /ˈhɔːni/ adjective referring to skin which is very hard (NOTE: For terms referring to horny tissue, see words beginning with **kerat-, kerato-**.)

**horseshoe kidney** /ˌhɔːsʃuː ˈkɪdni/ noun a congenital condition of the kidney, where sometimes the upper but usually the lower parts of both kidneys are joined together

**Horton's syndrome** /ˈhɔːt(ə)nz ˌsɪndrəʊm/ noun a severe headache, often with constant pain around one eye, which starts usually within a few hours of going to sleep. It is caused by the release of histamine in the body. [After Bayard Taylor Horton (b. 1895), US physician]

**hose** /həʊz/ noun **1.** a long rubber or plastic tube **2.** ♦ support hose

**hospice** /ˈhɒspɪs/ noun a hospital which offers palliative care for terminally ill people

**hospital** /ˈhɒspɪt(ə)l/ noun a place where sick or injured people are looked after ◇ **hospital bed 1.** a special type of bed used in hospitals, usually adjustable in many ways for the comfort of the patient ○ A hospital bed is needed if the patient has to have traction. **2.** a place in a hospital which can be occupied by a patient ○ There will be no reduction in the number of hospital beds.

**hospital-acquired infection** /ˌhɒspɪt(ə)l ə ˌkwaɪəd ɪnˈfekʃən/ noun a disease caught during a stay in hospital

**Hospital Activity Analysis** /ˌhɒspɪt(ə)l ækˈtɪvɪti əˌnæləsɪs/ noun a regular detailed report on patients in hospitals, including information about treatment, length of stay and outcome

**hospital care** /ˈhɒspɪt(ə)l keə/ noun treatment in a hospital

**hospital chaplain** /ˌhɒspɪt(ə)l ˈtʃæplɪn/ noun a religious minister attached to a hospital, who visits and comforts patients and their families and gives them the sacraments if necessary

**hospital corner** /ˌhɒspɪt(ə)l ˈkɔːnə/ noun a way of folding the overlapping bedding at each corner of a bed that keeps it tight

**hospital doctor** /ˌhɒspɪt(ə)l ˈdɒktə/ noun a doctor who works only in a hospital and does not receive people in his or her own surgery

**hospital gangrene** /ˌhɒspɪt(ə)l ˈgæŋgriːn/ noun gangrene caused by insanitary hospital conditions

**hospital infection** /ˈhɒspɪt(ə)l ɪnˌfekʃən/ noun an infection which someone gets during a hospital visit, or one which develops among hospital staff

COMMENT: Hospital infection is an increasingly common problem due to growing antimicrobial resistance and inappropriate antibiotic use. Strains of bacteria such as MRSA have evolved which seem to be more easily transmitted between patients and are difficult to treat.

**hospitalisation** /ˌhɒspɪt(ə)laɪˈzeɪʃ(ə)n/, **hospitalization** noun the act of sending someone to hospital ○ The doctor recommended immediate hospitalisation.

**hospitalise** /ˈhɒspɪt(ə)laɪz/, **hospitalize** verb to send someone to hospital ○ He is so ill that he has had to be hospitalised.

**hospital orderly** /ˌhɒspɪt(ə)l ˈɔːdəli/ noun a person who does heavy work in a hospital, such as wheeling patients into the operating theatre or moving equipment about

**hospital trust** /ˈhɒspɪt(ə)l trʌst/ noun same as **self-governing hospital**

**host** /həʊst/ noun a person or animal on which a parasite lives

**hot** /hɒt/ *adjective* very warm or having a high temperature

**hot flush** /ˌhɒt 'flʌʃ/ *noun* a condition in menopausal women, in which the woman becomes hot and sweats, and which is often accompanied by redness of the skin

**hotpack** /'hɒtpæk/ *noun* a cloth bag or a pad filled with gel or grains which can be heated and applied to the skin to relieve pain or stiffness

**hot wax treatment** /ˌhɒt 'wæks ˌtriːtmənt/ *noun* a treatment for arthritis in which the joints are painted with hot liquid wax

**hourglass contraction** /'auəglɑːs kən ˌtrækʃən/ *noun* a condition in which an organ such as the stomach is constricted in the centre

**hourglass stomach** /'auəglɑːs ˌstʌmək/ *noun* a condition in which the wall of the stomach is pulled in so that it is divided into two cavities, cardiac and pyloric

**hourly** /'auəli/ *adjective, adverb* happening every hour

**houseman** /'hausmən/ *noun* same as **house officer**

**house mite** /haus mait/, **house dust mite** /'haus dʌst ˌmait/ *noun* a tiny insect living mainly in bedding and soft furnishings, that can cause an allergic reaction

**house officer** /'haus ˌɒfɪsə/ *noun* a doctor who works in a hospital as a house surgeon or house physician during the final year of training before registration by the General Medical Council (NOTE: The US term is **intern**.)

**HPRT** *noun* an enzyme that is lacking in children, usually boys, who have Lesch-Nyhan disease. Full form **hypoxanthine phosphoribosyl transferase**. Also called **HGPRT (hypoxanthine guanine phosphoribosyl transferase)**

**HPV** *abbr* human papillomavirus

**HRT** *abbr* hormone replacement therapy

**Huhner's test** /'huːnəz ˌtest/ *noun* a test carried out several hours after sexual intercourse to determine the number and motility of spermatozoa [After Max Huhner (1873–1947), US urologist]

**human** /'hjuːmən/ *adjective* referring to any man, woman or child ■ *noun* a person ○ *Most animals are afraid of humans.*

**human anatomy** /ˌhjuːmən ə'nætəmi/ *noun* the structure, shape and functions of the human body

**human being** /ˌhjuːmən 'biːɪŋ/ *noun* a person

**human chorionic gonadotrophin** /ˌhjuːmən kɔːriˌɒnɪk ˌgəunədə'trəufɪn/ *noun* a hormone produced by the placenta, which suppresses the mother's usual menstrual cycle during pregnancy. It is found in the urine during pregnancy, and can be given by injection to encourage ovulation and help a woman to become pregnant. Abbr **hCG**

**human crutch** /ˌhjuːmən 'krʌtʃ/ *noun* a method of helping an injured person to walk, where they rest one arm over the shoulders of the person helping

**human immunodeficiency virus** /ˌhjuːmən ˌɪmjunəudɪˈfɪʃ(ə)nsi ˌvairəs/ *noun* a virus which causes AIDS. Abbr **HIV**

**human leucocyte antigen** /ˌhjuːmən 'luːkəsait ˌæntidʒ(ə)n/ *noun* any of the system of antigens on the surface of cells which need to be histocompatible to allow transplants to take place. Abbr **HLA**. ♦ **HLA system**

**human nature** /ˌhjuːmən 'neitʃə/ *noun* the general behavioural characteristics of human beings

**human papillomavirus** /ˌhjuːmən pæpɪ'ləumə ˌvairəs/ *noun* a virus that causes genital warts in humans. Abbr **HPV**

**humectant** /hjuːˈmektənt/ *adjective* able to absorb or retain moisture ■ *noun* a substance that can absorb or retain moisture, e.g. a skin lotion

**humeroulnar joint** /ˌhjuːmərəu'ʌlnə dʒɔɪnt/ *noun* part of the elbow joint, where the trochlea of the humerus and the trochlear notch of the ulna move next to each other

**humerus** /'hjuːmərəs/ *noun* the top bone in the arm, running from the shoulder to the elbow (NOTE: The plural is **humeri**.)

**humid** /'hjuːmɪd/ *adjective* damp, containing moisture vapour

**humoral** /'hjuːmərəl/ *adjective* relating to human body fluids, in particular blood serum

**humour** /'hjuːmə/, **humor** *noun* a fluid in the body

**hunchback** /'hʌntʃbæk/ *noun* ♦ **kyphosis**

**hunger** /'hʌŋgə/ *noun* a need to eat

**hunger pains** /'hʌŋgə peinz/ *plural noun* pains in the abdomen when a person feels hungry, sometimes a sign of a duodenal ulcer

**Hunter's syndrome** /'hʌntəz ˌsɪndrəum/ *noun* an inherited disorder caused by an enzyme deficiency, which leads to learning difficulties

**Huntington's chorea** /ˌhʌntɪŋtənz kɔː 'riːə/ *noun* a progressive hereditary disease which affects adults, where the outer layer of the brain degenerates and the person makes involuntary jerky movements and develops progressive dementia [Described 1872. After George Sumner Huntington (1850–1916), US physician.]

**Hurler's syndrome** /'hɜːləz ˌsɪndrəum/ *noun* same as **gargoylism** [Described 1920. After Gertrud Hurler, German paediatrician.]

**hurt** /hɜːt/ *noun* **1.** emotional pain **2.** a painful area (*used by children*) ○ *She has a hurt on her knee.* ■ *verb* **1.** to have pain ○ *He's hurt his hand.* **2.** to cause someone pain ○ *His arm is* *hurting so much he can't write.* ○ *She fell down and hurt herself.* (NOTE: **hurting – hurt**) ■ *adjective* 1. feeling physical pain ○ *He was slightly hurt in the car crash.* ○ *Two players got hurt in the football game.* 2. feeling emotional pain ○ *Her parents' divorce hurt her deeply.*

**husky** /ˈhʌski/ *adjective* slightly hoarse

**Hutchinson's tooth** /ˈhʌtʃɪnsənz ˌtuːθ/ *noun* a narrow upper incisor tooth, with notches along the cutting edge, a symptom of congenital syphilis but also occurring naturally (NOTE: The plural is **Hutchinson's teeth**.) [After Sir Jonathan Hutchinson (1828–1913), British surgeon]

**hyal-** /haɪəl/ *prefix* like glass (*used before vowels*)

**hyalin** /ˈhaɪəlɪn/ *noun* a transparent substance produced from collagen and deposited around blood vessels and scars when some tissues degenerate

**hyaline** /ˈhaɪəlɪn/ *adjective* nearly transparent like glass

**hyaline cartilage** /ˌhaɪəlɪn ˈkɑːtɪlɪdʒ/ *noun* a type of cartilage found in the nose, larynx and joints. It forms most of the skeleton of the fetus. See illustration at CARTILAGINOUS JOINT in Supplement

**hyaline membrane disease** /ˌhaɪəlɪn ˈmembreɪn dɪˌziːz/ *noun* same as **respiratory distress syndrome**

**hyalitis** /ˌhaɪəˈlaɪtɪs/ *noun* inflammation of the vitreous humour or the hyaloid membrane in the eye. Also called **vitritis**

**hyaloid membrane** /ˈhaɪəlɔɪd ˌmembreɪn/ *noun* a transparent membrane round the vitreous humour in the eye

**hyaluronic acid** /ˌhaɪəlʊrɒnɪk ˈæsɪd/ *noun* a substance which binds connective tissue and is found in the eyes

**hyaluronidase** /ˌhaɪəlʊˈrɒnɪdeɪz/ *noun* an enzyme which destroys hyaluronic acid

**hybrid** /ˈhaɪbrɪd/ *noun* an organism that is a result of a cross between individuals that are not genetically the same as each other

**HYCOSY** *abbr* hysterosalpingo-contrast sonography

**hydatid** /ˈhaɪdətɪd/ *noun* any cyst-like structure

**hydatid cyst** /ˌhaɪdətɪd ˈsɪst/ *noun* the larval form of the tapeworms of the genus *Echinococcus*

**hydatid disease** /ˈhaɪdətɪd dɪˌziːz/, **hydatidosis** /ˌhaɪdətɪˈdəʊsɪs/ *noun* an infection, usually in the lungs or liver, caused by expanding hydatid cysts that destroy the tissues of the infected organ

**hydatid mole** /ˌhaɪdətɪd ˈməʊl/ *noun* an abnormal pregnancy from a pathologic ovum, resulting in a mass of cysts shaped like a bunch of grapes

**hydr-** /haɪdr/ *prefix* same as **hydro-** (*used before vowels*)

**hydraemia** /haɪˈdriːmiə/ *noun* an excess of water in the blood

**hydragogue** /ˈhaɪdrəgɒg/ *noun* a laxative or substance which produces watery faeces

**hydralazine** /haɪˈdræləziːn/ *noun* a drug that lowers blood pressure. People usually receive it in combination with other drugs that increase the output of urine.

**hydramnios** /haɪˈdræmnɪɒs/ *noun* an unusually large amount of amniotic fluid surrounding the fetus

**hydrarthrosis** /ˌhaɪdrɑːˈθrəʊsɪs/ *noun* swelling caused by excess synovial liquid at a joint

**hydrate** /ˈhaɪdreɪt/ *verb* to give water to someone so as to re-establish or maintain fluid balance ■ *noun* a chemical compound containing water molecules that can usually be driven off by heat without altering the compound's structure

**hydro-** /haɪdrəʊ/ *prefix* referring to water

**hydroa** /haɪˈdrəʊə/ *noun* an eruption of small itchy blisters, e.g. those caused by sunlight

**hydrocalycosis** /ˌhaɪdrəʊˌkælɪˈkəʊsɪs/ *noun* same as **caliectasis**

**hydrocele** /ˈhaɪdrəʊsiːl/ *noun* the collection of watery liquid found in a cavity such as the scrotum

**hydrocephalus** /ˌhaɪdrəʊˈkefələs/ *noun* an excessive quantity of cerebrospinal fluid in the brain

**hydrochloric acid** /haɪdrəʊˈklɒrɪk ˈæsɪd/ *noun* an acid found in the gastric juices which helps to break apart the food

**hydrocolloid strip** /ˌhaɪdrəʊkɒlɔɪd ˈstrɪp/ *noun* a waterproof gel dressing that seals a wound, retaining moisture and preventing access to germs and dirt

**hydrocolpos** /ˌhaɪdrəʊˈkɒlpəs/ *noun* a cyst in the vagina containing clear fluid

**hydrocortisone** /ˌhaɪdrəʊˈkɔːtɪzəʊn/ *noun* a steroid hormone secreted by the adrenal cortex or produced synthetically, used in the treatment of rheumatoid arthritis and inflammatory and allergic conditions

**hydrocyanic acid** /ˌhaɪdrəʊsaɪænɪk ˈæsɪd/ *noun* an acid which forms cyanide. Abbr **HCN**

**hydrogen** /ˈhaɪdrədʒən/ *noun* a chemical element, a gas which combines with oxygen to form water, and with other elements to form acids, and is present in all animal tissue (NOTE: The chemical symbol is **H**.)

**hydrogen peroxide** /ˌhaɪdrədʒən pəˈrɒksaɪd/ *noun* a solution used as a disinfectant

**hydrolysis** /haɪˈdrɒləsɪs/ *noun* the breaking down of a chemical compound when it reacts with water to produce two or more different compounds, as in the conversion of starch to glucose

**hydroma** /haɪˈdrəʊmə/ *noun* same as **hygroma**

**hydrometer** /haɪˈdrɒmɪtə/ *noun* an instrument which measures the density of a liquid

**hydromyelia** /ˌhaɪdrəʊmaɪˈiːliə/ *noun* a condition in which fluid swells the central canal of the spinal cord

**hydronephrosis** /ˌhaɪdrəʊneˈfrəʊsɪs/ *noun* swelling of the pelvis of a kidney caused by accumulation of water due to infection or a kidney stone blocking the ureter

**hydropathy** /haɪˈdrɒpəθi/ *noun* the treatment of injuries or disease by bathing in water or drinking mineral waters

**hydropericarditis** /ˌhaɪdrəʊˌperikɑːˈdaɪtɪs/, **hydropericardium** /ˌhaɪdrəʊˌperiˈkɑːdiəm/ *noun* an accumulation of liquid round the heart

**hydroperitoneum** /ˌhaɪdrəʊˌperɪtəˈniːəm/ *noun* a build-up of fluid in the peritoneal cavity (NOTE: The plural is **hydroperitoneums** or **hydroperitonea**.)

**hydrophobia** /ˌhaɪdrəˈfəʊbiə/ *noun* same as **rabies**

COMMENT: Hydrophobia affects the mental balance, and the symptoms include difficulty in breathing or swallowing and a horror of water.

**hydropneumoperitoneum** /ˌhaɪdrəʊˌnjuːməʊˌperɪtəˈniːəm/ *noun* a condition in which watery fluid and gas collect in the peritoneal cavity

**hydropneumothorax** /ˌhaɪdrəʊˌnjuːməʊˈθɔːræks/ *noun* a condition in which watery fluid and gas collect in the pleural cavity (NOTE: The plural is **hydropneumothoraxes** or **hydropneumothoraces**.)

**hydrops** /ˈhaɪdrɒps/ *noun* same as **oedema** (NOTE: The plural is **hydropses**.)

**hydrorrhoea** /ˌhaɪdrəʊˈriːə/ *noun* a discharge of watery fluid (NOTE: The US spelling is **hydrorrhea**.)

**hydrosalpinx** /ˌhaɪdrəʊˈsælpɪŋks/ *noun* an occasion when watery fluid collects in one or both of the Fallopian tubes, causing swelling (NOTE: The plural is **hydrosalpinges**.)

**hydrotherapy** /ˌhaɪdrəʊˈθerəpi/ *noun* a type of physiotherapy involving treatment in water, where people are put in hot baths or are encouraged to swim

**hydrothorax** /ˌhaɪdrəʊˈθɔːræks/ *noun* the collection of liquid in the pleural cavity

**hydrotubation** /ˌhaɪdrəʊtjuːˈbeɪʃ(ə)n/ *noun* an act of putting a fluid through the neck of the uterus and the Fallopian tubes under pressure to check whether the tubes are blocked

**hydroureter** /ˌhaɪdrəʊjuˈriːtə/ *noun* a condition in which water or urine collect in the ureter because it is blocked

**hydroxide** /haɪˈdrɒksaɪd/ *noun* a chemical compound containing a hydroxyl group

**hydroxyproline** /haɪˌdrɒksiˈprəʊliːn/ *noun* an amino acid present in some proteins, especially in collagen

**hygiene** /ˈhaɪdʒiːn/ *noun* **1.** the procedures and principles designed to keep things clean and to keep conditions healthy ○ *Nurses have to maintain a strict personal hygiene.* **2.** the science of health

**hygienic** /haɪˈdʒiːnɪk/ *adjective* **1.** clean ○ *Don't touch the food with dirty hands – it isn't hygienic.* **2.** producing healthy conditions

**hygienist** /ˈhaɪdʒiːnɪst/ *noun* a person who specialises in hygiene and its application

**hygr-** /haɪgr/ *prefix* same as **hygro-** (*used before vowels*)

**hygro-** /haɪgrəʊ/ *prefix* relating to moisture

**hygroma** /haɪˈgrəʊmə/ *noun* a kind of cyst which contains a thin fluid

**hymen** /ˈhaɪmen/ *noun* a membrane which partially covers the vaginal passage in a female who has never had sexual intercourse

**hymenectomy** /ˌhaɪməˈnektəmi/ *noun* **1.** the surgical removal of the hymen, or an operation to increase the size of the opening of the hymen **2.** the surgical removal of any membrane

**hymenotomy** /ˌhaɪməˈnɒtəmi/ *noun* an incision of the hymen during surgery

**hyo-** /haɪəʊ/ *prefix* relating to the hyoid bone

**hyoglossus** /ˌhaɪəʊˈglɒsəs/ *noun* a muscle which is attached to the hyoid bone and depresses the tongue

**hyoid** /ˈhaɪɔɪd/ *adjective* relating to the hyoid bone

**hyoid bone** /ˈhaɪɔɪd bəʊn/ *noun* a small U-shaped bone at the base of the tongue

**hyoscine** /ˈhaɪəʊsiːn/ *noun* a drug used as a sedative, in particular for treatment of motion sickness

**hyp-** /haɪp/ *prefix* same as **hypo-** (*used before vowels*)

**hypaemia** /haɪˈpiːmiə/ *noun* an insufficient amount of blood in the body

**hypalgesia** /ˌhaɪpælˈdʒiːziə/ *noun* low sensitivity to pain

**hyper-** /haɪpə/ *prefix* higher or too much. Opposite **hypo-**

**hyperacidity** /ˌhaɪpərəˈsɪdɪti/ *noun* the production of more acid in the stomach than is usual. Also called **acidity, acid stomach**

**hyperacousia** /ˌhaɪpərəˈkjuːziə/ *noun* same as **hyperacusis**

**hyperactive** /haɪpərˈæktɪv/ *adjective* very or unusually active

**hyperactivity** /haɪpərækˈtɪvəti/ *noun* a condition in which something or someone, e.g. a gland or a child, is too active

**hyperacusis** /ˌhaɪpərəˈkjuːsɪs/ *noun* a condition in which someone is very sensitive to sounds

**hyperadrenalism** /ˌhaɪpərəˈdriːn(ə)lɪz(ə)m/ *noun* a disorder in which too many adrenal hormones are produced, e.g. because of pituitary gland malfunction, a tumour of the adrenal gland or high doses of steroids

**hyperaemia** /ˌhaɪpərˈiːmiə/ *noun* excess blood in any part of the body

**hyperaesthesia** /ˌhaɪpəriːsˈθiːziə/ *noun* an extremely high sensitivity in the skin

**hyperalgesia** /ˌhaɪpərælˈdʒiːziə/ *noun* an increased sensitivity to pain

**hyperalimentation** /ˌhaɪpərˌælɪmenˈteɪʃ(ə)n/ *noun* the feeding of large amounts of nutrients by mouth or intravenously to someone with serious nutritional deficiency

**hyperandrogenism** /ˌhaɪpərəˈdrɒdʒənɪz(ə)m/ *noun* a condition in which a woman produces too many androgens, associated with many problems such as hirsutism, acne, infertility and polycystic ovarian disease

**hyperbaric** /ˌhaɪpəˈbærɪk/ *adjective* referring to a treatment in which someone is given oxygen at high pressure, used to treat carbon monoxide poisoning

**hypercalcaemia** /ˌhaɪpəkælˈsiːmiə/ *noun* an excess of calcium in the blood

**hypercalcinuria** /ˌhaɪpəkælsɪˈnjʊəriə/ *noun* a condition in which an unusually high amount of calcium occurs in the urine

**hypercapnia** /ˌhaɪpəˈkæpniə/ *noun* an unusually high concentration of carbon dioxide in the bloodstream

**hypercatabolism** /ˌhaɪpəkəˈtæbəlɪz(ə)m/ *noun* a condition in which the body breaks down its own tissues or a particular substance too much. It causes weight loss and wasting.

**hyperchloraemia** /ˌhaɪpəklɔːˈriːmiə/ *noun* a condition in which there is too much chloride in the blood

**hyperchlorhydria** /ˌhaɪpəklɔːˈhaɪdriə/ *noun* an excess of hydrochloric acid in the stomach

**hyperdactylism** /ˌhaɪpəˈdæktɪlɪz(ə)m/ *noun* the condition of having more than the usual number of fingers or toes. Also called **polydactylism**

**hyperemesis** /ˌhaɪpərˈemɪsɪs/ *noun* excessive vomiting (NOTE: The plural is **hyperemeses**.)

**hyperemesis gravidarum** /ˌhaɪpəremɪsɪs ˌɡrævɪˈdeərəm/ *noun* uncontrollable vomiting in pregnancy

**hyperextension** /ˌhaɪpərɪkˈstenʃən/ *noun* the act of stretching an arm or leg beyond its usual limits of movement

**hyperflexion** /ˌhaɪpəˈflekʃən/ *noun* the act of flexing a joint beyond the usual limit ○ *a hyperflexion injury*

**hyperfunction** /ˈhaɪpəˌfʌŋkʃ(ə)n/ *noun* excessive activity of a gland or other organ of the body

**hypergalactia** /ˌhaɪpəɡəˈlæktiə/, **hypergalactosis** /ˌhaɪpəˌɡæləkˈtəʊsɪs/ *noun* a condition in which too much milk is secreted

**hyperglycaemia** /ˌhaɪpəɡlaɪˈsiːmiə/ *noun* an excess of glucose in the blood

**hyperhidrosis** /ˌhaɪpəhaɪˈdrəʊsɪs/ *noun* a condition in which too much sweat is produced

**hyperinsulinism** /ˌhaɪpərˈɪnsjʊlɪnɪz(ə)m/ *noun* the reaction of a diabetic to an excessive dose of insulin or to hypoglycaemia

**hyperkalaemia** /ˌhaɪpəkæˈliːmiə/ *noun* a condition in which too much potassium occurs in the blood, which can result in cardiac arrest. Various possible causes include kidney failure and chemotherapy.

**hyperkeratosis** /ˌhaɪpəkerəˈtəʊsɪs/ *noun* a condition in which the outer layer of the skin becomes unusually thickened

**hyperkinesia** /ˌhaɪpəkɪˈniːziə/ *noun* a condition in which there is unusually great strength or movement

**hyperkinetic syndrome** /ˌhaɪpəkɪˈnetɪk ˌsɪndrəʊm/ *noun* a condition in which someone experiences fatigue, shortness of breath, pain under the heart and palpitation

**hyperlipidaemia** /ˌhaɪpəlɪpɪˈdiːmiə/ *noun* the pathological increase of the amount of lipids, or fat, in the blood

**hypermenorrhoea** /ˌhaɪpəmenəˈriːə/ *noun* menstruation in which the flow is excessive

**hypermetropia** /ˌhaɪpəmɪˈtrəʊpiə/, **hyperopia** /ˌhaɪpəˈrəʊpiə/ *noun* a condition in which someone sees more clearly objects which are a long way away, but cannot see objects which are close. Also called **longsightedness**, **hyperopia**

**hypernatraemia** /ˌhaɪpənæˈtriːmiə/ *noun* a serious condition occurring most often in babies or elderly people, in which too much sodium is present in the blood as a result of loss of water and electrolytes through diarrhoea, excessive sweating, not drinking enough or excessive salt intake

**hypernephroma** /ˌhaɪpənəˈfrəʊmə/ *noun* same as **Grawitz tumour**

**hyperopia** /ˌhaɪpəˈrəʊpiə/ *noun* same as **hypermetropia**

**hyperostosis** /ˌhaɪpərɒˈstəʊsɪs/ *noun* excessive overgrowth on the outside surface of a bone, especially the frontal bone

**hyperparathyroidism** /ˌhaɪpəˌpærəˈθaɪrɔɪdɪz(ə)m/ *noun* an unusually high concentration of parathyroid hormone in the body. It causes various medical problems including damage to the kidneys.

**hyperphagia** /ˌhaɪpəˈfeɪdʒiə/ *noun* long-term compulsive overeating

**hyperpiesia** /ˌhaɪpəpaɪˈiːziə/ *noun* same as **hypertension**

**hyperpiesis** /ˌhaɪpəpaɪˈiːsɪs/ *noun* unusually high pressure, especially of the blood

**hyperpituitarism** /ˌhaɪpəˈpɪtjuːɪtərˌɪz(ə)m/ *noun* a condition in which the pituitary gland is overactive

**hyperplasia** /ˌhaɪpəˈpleɪzɪə/ *noun* a condition in which there is an increase in the number of cells in an organ

**hyperpnoea** /ˌhaɪpəˈpniːə/ *noun* unusually deep or fast breathing, e.g. after physical exercise

**hyperpyrexia** /ˌhaɪpəpaɪˈreksɪə/ *noun* a body temperature of above 41.1°C

**hypersecretion** /ˌhaɪpəsɪˈkriːʃ(ə)n/ *noun* a condition in which too much of a substance is secreted

**hypersensitive** /ˌhaɪpəˈsensɪtɪv/ *adjective* referring to a person who reacts more strongly than usual to an antigen

**hypersensitivity** /ˌhaɪpəsensɪˈtɪvɪti/ *noun* a condition in which someone reacts very strongly to something such as an allergic substance ○ *her hypersensitivity to dust* ○ *Anaphylactic shock shows hypersensitivity to an injection.*

**hypersplenism** /ˌhaɪpəˈsplɪnɪz(ə)m/ *noun* a condition in which too many red blood cells are destroyed by the spleen, which is often enlarged

**hypertelorism** /ˌhaɪpəˈtelərɪz(ə)m/ *noun* a condition in which there is too much space between two organs or parts of the body

**hypertension** /ˌhaɪpəˈtenʃən/ *noun* arterial blood pressure that is higher than the usual range for gender and age. Also called **high blood pressure, hyperpiesia**. Compare **hypotension**

> COMMENT: Hypertension is without a specific cause in more than 50% of cases (**essential hypertension**) but may be associated with other diseases. It is treated with drugs such as beta blockers, ACE inhibitors, diuretics and calcium channel blockers.

**hypertensive** /ˌhaɪpəˈtensɪv/ *adjective* referring to high blood pressure

**hypertensive headache** /ˌhaɪpətensɪv ˈhedeɪk/ *noun* a headache caused by high blood pressure

**hypertensive retinopathy** /ˌhaɪpətensɪv ˌretɪnˈɒpəθi/ *noun* changes in the retina caused by local bleeding and a restricted blood supply that threaten eyesight, as the condition indicates that the blood pressure is excessively high

**hyperthermia** /ˌhaɪpəˈθɜːmiə/ *noun* a very high body temperature

**hyperthyroidism** /ˌhaɪpəˈθaɪrɔɪdɪz(ə)m/ *noun* a condition in which the thyroid gland is too active and releases unusual amounts of thyroid hormones into the blood, giving rise to a rapid heartbeat, sweating and trembling. It

can be treated with carbimazole. Also called **thyrotoxicosis**

**hypertonia** /ˌhaɪpəˈtəʊniə/ *noun* an increased rigidity and spasticity of the muscles

**hypertonic** /ˌhaɪpəˈtɒnɪk/ *adjective* **1.** referring to a solution which has a higher osmotic pressure than another specified solution **2.** referring to a muscle which is under unusually high tension

**hypertrichosis** /ˌhaɪpətrɪˈkəʊsɪs/ *noun* a condition in which someone has excessive growth of hair on the body or on part of the body

**hypertrophic** /ˌhaɪpəˈtrɒfɪk/ *adjective* associated with hypertrophy

**hypertrophic rhinitis** /ˌhaɪpətrɒfɪk raɪˈnaɪtɪs/ *noun* a condition in which the mucous membranes in the nose become thicker

**hypertrophy** /haɪˈpɜːtrəfi/ *noun* an increase in the number or size of cells in a tissue

**hypertropia** /ˌhaɪpəˈtrəʊpiə/ *noun* US same as **hypermetropia**

**hyperventilate** /ˌhaɪpəˈventɪleɪt/ *verb* to breathe very fast ○ *We hyperventilate as an expression of fear or excitement.*

**hyperventilation** /ˌhaɪpəventɪˈleɪʃ(ə)n/ *noun* very fast breathing which can be accompanied by dizziness or tetany

**hypervitaminosis** /ˌhaɪpəˌvɪtəmɪˈnəʊsɪs/ *noun* a condition caused by taking too many synthetic vitamins, especially Vitamins A and D

**hypervolaemia** /ˌhaɪpəvɒˈliːmiə/ *noun* a condition in which there is too much plasma in the blood

**hyphaema** /haɪˈfiːmiə/ *noun* bleeding into the front chamber of the eye

**hypn-** /hɪpn/ *prefix* referring to sleep

**hypnosis** /hɪpˈnəʊsɪs/ *noun* a state like sleep, but caused artificially, where a person can remember forgotten events in the past and will do whatever the hypnotist tells him or her to do

**hypnotherapist** /ˌhɪpnəʊˈθerəpɪst/ *noun* a person who practises hypnotherapy

**hypnotherapy** /ˌhɪpnəʊˈθerəpi/ *noun* treatment by hypnosis, used in treating some addictions

**hypnotic** /hɪpˈnɒtɪk/ *adjective* **1.** relating to hypnosis and hypnotism **2.** referring to a state which is like sleep but which is caused artificially **3.** referring to a drug which causes sleep

**hypnotise** /ˈhɪpnətaɪz/, **hypnotize** *verb* to make someone go into a state where he or she appears to be asleep, and will do whatever the hypnotist suggests ○ *He hypnotises his patients, and then persuades them to reveal their hidden problems.*

**hypnotism** /ˈhɪpnətɪz(ə)m/ *noun* the techniques used to induce hypnosis

**hypnotist** /'hɪpnətɪst/ *noun* a person who hypnotises other people ○ *The hypnotist passed his hand in front of her eyes and she went immediately to sleep.*

**hypo** /'haɪpəʊ/ *noun* (*informal*) **1.** same as **hypodermic syringe 2.** an attack of hypoglycaemia, experienced, e.g., by people who are diabetic

**hypo-** /haɪpəʊ/ *prefix* less, too little or beneath

**hypoacidity** /ˌhaɪpəʊə'sɪdɪti/ *noun* unusually low acidity, especially in the stomach

**hypoaesthesia** /ˌhaɪpəʊiːs'θiːziə/ *noun* a condition in which someone has a diminished sense of touch

**hypoallergenic** /ˌhaɪpəʊələ'dʒenɪk/ *adjective* not likely to cause an allergic reaction

**hypocalcaemia** /ˌhaɪpəʊkæl'siːmiə/ *noun* an unusually low amount of calcium in the blood, which can cause tetany

**hypocapnia** /ˌhaɪpəʊ'kæpniə/ *noun* a condition in which there is not enough carbon dioxide in the blood

**hypochloraemia** /ˌhaɪpəʊklɔː'riːmiə/ *noun* a condition in which there are not enough chlorine ions in the blood

**hypochlorhydria** /ˌhaɪpəʊklɔː'haɪdriə/ *noun* a condition in which there is not enough hydrochloric acid in the stomach

**hypochondria** /ˌhaɪpəʊ'kɒndriə/ *noun* a condition in which a person is too worried about his or her own health and believes he or she is ill

**hypochondriac** /ˌhaɪpəʊ'kɒndriæk/ *noun* a person who worries about his or her health too much

**hypochondriac region** /ˌhaɪpəʊ'kɒndriæk ˌriːdʒən/ *noun* one of two parts of the upper abdomen, on either side of the epigastrium below the floating ribs

**hypochondrium** /ˌhaɪpəʊ'kɒndriəm/ *noun* one of the two hypochondriac regions in the upper part of the abdomen

**hypochromic** /ˌhaɪpəʊ'krəʊmɪk/ *adjective* referring to blood cells or body tissue which do not have the usual amount of pigmentation ○ *hypochromic scars*

**hypochromic anaemia** /ˌhaɪpəʊkrəʊmɪk ə'niːmiə/ *noun* anaemia where haemoglobin is reduced in proportion to the number of red blood cells, which then appear very pale

**hypodermic** /ˌhaɪpə'dɜːmɪk/ *adjective* beneath the skin ■ *noun* a hypodermic syringe, needle or injection (*informal*)

**hypodermic injection** /ˌhaɪpədɜːmɪk ɪn'dʒekʃən/ *noun* an injection of a liquid, e.g. a painkilling drug, beneath the skin. Also called **subcutaneous injection**

**hypodermic needle** /ˌhaɪpədɜːmɪk 'niːd(ə)l/ *noun* a needle for injecting liquid under the skin

**hypodermic syringe** /ˌhaɪpədɜːmɪk sɪ'rɪndʒ/ *noun* a syringe fitted with a hypodermic needle for injecting liquid under the skin

**hypofibrinogenaemia** /ˌhaɪpəʊˌfɪbrɪnəʊdʒə'niːmiə/ *noun* a condition in which there is not enough fibrinogen in the blood, e.g. because of several blood transfusions or as an inherited condition

**hypogammaglobulinaemia** /ˌhaɪpəʊgæməˌglɒbjʊlɪn'iːmiə/ *noun* an unusually low concentration of gamma globulin in the blood that causes an immune deficiency. It may be present from birth or acquired later in life.

**hypogastrium** /ˌhaɪpə'gæstriəm/ *noun* the part of the abdomen beneath the stomach

**hypoglossal** /ˌhaɪpəʊ'glɒsəl/ *adjective* **1.** underneath or on the lower side of the tongue **2.** relating to the hypoglossal nerve

**hypoglossal nerve** /haɪpə'glɒs(ə)l nɜːv/ *noun* the twelfth cranial nerve which governs the muscles of the tongue

**hypoglycaemia** /ˌhaɪpəʊglaɪ'siːmiə/ *noun* a low concentration of glucose in the blood

   COMMENT: Hypoglycaemia affects diabetics who feel weak from lack of sugar. A hypoglycaemic attack can be prevented by eating glucose or a lump of sugar when feeling faint.

**hypoglycaemic** /ˌhaɪpəʊglaɪ'siːmɪk/ *adjective* having hypoglycaemia

**hypoglycaemic coma** /ˌhaɪpəʊglaɪˌsiːmɪk 'kəʊmə/ *noun* a state of unconsciousness affecting diabetics after taking an overdose of insulin

**hypohidrosis** /ˌhaɪpəʊhaɪ'drəʊsɪs/, **hypoidrosis** /haɪpɔɪ'drəʊsɪs/ *noun* a condition in which someone produces too little sweat

**hypoinsulinism** /ˌhaɪpəʊ'ɪnsjʊlɪnɪz(ə)m/ *noun* a condition in which the body does not have enough insulin, often because of a problem with the pancreas

**hypokalaemia** /ˌhaɪpəʊkæ'liːmiə/ *noun* a deficiency of potassium in the blood

**hypomania** /ˌhaɪpəʊ'meɪniə/ *noun* a state of mild mania or overexcitement, especially when part of a manic-depressive cycle

**hypomenorrhoea** /ˌhaɪpəmenə'riːə/ *noun* the production of too little blood at menstruation

**hypometropia** /ˌhaɪpəʊmɪ'trəʊpiə/ *noun* same as **myopia**

**hyponatraemia** /ˌhaɪpəʊnæ'triːmiə/ *noun* a lack of sodium in the body

**hypoparathyroidism** /ˌhaɪpəʊˌpærə'θaɪrɔɪdɪz(ə)m/ *noun* a condition in which the parathyroid glands do not secrete enough parathyroid hormone, leading to low blood calcium and muscle spasms

**hypopharynx** /ˌhaɪpəʊ'færɪŋks/ *noun* the part of the pharynx between the hyoid bone and the bottom of the cricoid cartilage (NOTE: The plural is **hypopharynxes** or **hypopharynges.**)

**hypophyseal** /ˌhaɪpəˈfɪziəl/ adjective referring to the pituitary gland

**hypophyseal stalk** /ˌhaɪpəfɪziəl ˈstɔːk/ noun a funnel-shaped stem which attaches the pituitary gland to the hypothalamus

**hypophysectomy** /haɪˌpɒfɪˈsektəmi/ noun the surgical removal of the pituitary gland

**hypophysis cerebri** /haɪˌpɒfəsɪs ˈserəbri/ noun same as **pituitary gland**

**hypopiesis** /ˌhaɪpəʊpaɪˈiːsɪs/ noun a condition in which the blood pressure is too low

**hypopituitarism** /ˌhaɪpəʊpɪˈtjuːɪtərˌɪz(ə)m/ noun a condition in which the pituitary gland is underactive

**hypoplasia** /ˌhaɪpəʊˈpleɪziə/ noun a lack of development or incorrect formation of a body tissue or an organ

**hypoplastic left heart** /haɪpəʊˌplæstɪk left ˈhɑːt/ noun a serious heart disorder in which the left side of the heart does not develop properly, leading to death within six weeks of birth unless surgery is performed

**hypopnoea** /ˌhaɪpəʊˈpniːə/ noun unusually shallow and slow breathing

**hypoproteinaemia** /ˌhaɪpəʊprəʊtɪˈniːmiə/ noun a condition in which there is not enough protein in the blood

**hypoprothrombinaemia** /ˌhaɪpəʊprəʊˌθrɒmbɪˈniːmiə/ noun a condition in which there is not enough prothrombin in the blood, so that the person bleeds and bruises easily

**hypopyon** /ˌhaɪpəˈpaɪən/ noun an accumulation of pus in the aqueous humour in the front chamber of the eye

**hyposensitise** /ˌhaɪpəʊˈsensɪtaɪz/, **hyposensitize** verb to reduce someone's sensitivity to something, e.g. in the treatment of allergies

**hyposensitive** /ˌhaɪpəʊˈsensɪtɪv/ adjective being less sensitive than usual

**hyposensitivity** /ˌhaɪpəʊˌsensɪˈtɪvɪti/ noun an unusually low sensitivity to stimuli such as allergens

**hypospadias** /ˌhaɪpəˈspeɪdiəs/ noun a congenital condition of the wall of the male urethra or the vagina, so that the opening occurs on the under side of the penis or in the vagina. Compare **epispadias**

**hypostasis** /haɪˈpɒstəsɪs/ noun a condition in which fluid accumulates in part of the body because of poor circulation

**hypostatic** /ˌhaɪpəʊˈstætɪk/ adjective referring to hypostasis

**hypostatic eczema** /ˌhaɪpəʊstætɪk ˈeksɪmə/ noun same as **varicose eczema**

**hypostatic pneumonia** /ˌhaɪpəʊstætɪk njuːˈməʊniə/ noun pneumonia caused by fluid accumulating in the lungs of a bedridden person with a weak heart

**hyposthenia** /ˌhaɪpɒsˈθiːniə/ noun a condition of unusual bodily weakness

**hypotension** /ˌhaɪpəʊˈtenʃən/ noun a condition in which the pressure of the blood is unusually low. Also called **low blood pressure**. Compare **hypertension**

**hypotensive** /ˌhaɪpəˈtensɪv/ adjective having low blood pressure

**hypothalamic** /ˌhaɪpəʊθəˈlæmɪk/ adjective referring to the hypothalamus

**hypothalamic hormone** /ˌhaɪpəʊθəˌlæmɪk ˈhɔːməʊn/ noun same as **releasing hormone**

**hypothalamus** /ˌhaɪpəʊˈθæləməs/ noun the part of the brain above the pituitary gland, which controls the production of hormones by the pituitary gland and regulates important bodily functions such as hunger, thirst and sleep. See illustration at **BRAIN** in Supplement

**hypothalmus** /ˌhaɪpəʊˈθælməs/ noun same as **hypothalamus** (NOTE: The plural is **hypothalmuses** or **hypothalmi**.)

**hypothenar** /haɪˈpɒθɪnə/ adjective referring to the soft fat part of the palm beneath the little finger

**hypothenar eminence** /haɪˌpɒθɪnə ˈemɪnəns/ noun a lump on the palm beneath the little finger. Compare **thenar**

**hypothermal** /ˌhaɪpəʊˈθɜːm(ə)l/ adjective referring to hypothermia

**hypothermia** /ˌhaɪpəʊˈθɜːmiə/ noun a reduction in body temperature below normal, for medical purposes taken to be below 35°C

'…inadvertent hypothermia can readily occur in patients undergoing surgery when there is reduced heat production and a greater potential for heat loss to the environment' [British Journal of Nursing]

**hypothermic** /ˌhaɪpəˈθɜːmɪk/ adjective suffering from hypothermia ○ Examination revealed that she was hypothermic, with a rectal temperature of only 29.4°C.

**hypothermic perfusion** /ˌhaɪpəθɜːmɪk pəˈfjuːʒ(ə)n/ noun a method of preserving a donor organ by introducing a preserving solution and storing the organ at a low temperature

**hypothesis** /haɪˈpɒθəsɪs/ noun a suggested explanation for an observation or experimental result, which is then refined or disproved by further investigation

**hypothyroidism** /ˌhaɪpəʊˈθaɪrɔɪdɪz(ə)m/ noun underactivity of the thyroid gland

**hypotonia** /ˌhaɪpəʊˈtəʊniə/ noun reduced tone of the skeletal muscles

**hypotonic** /ˌhaɪpəʊˈtɒnɪk/ adjective 1. showing hypotonia 2. referring to a solution with a lower osmotic pressure than plasma

**hypotrichosis** /ˌhaɪpəʊtrɪˈkəʊsɪs/ noun a condition in which less hair develops than usual. Compare **alopecia** (NOTE: The plural is **hypotrichoses**.)

**hypotropia** /ˌhaɪpəʊˈtrəʊpiə/ noun a form of squint where one eye looks downwards

**hypoventilation** /ˌhaɪpəʊventɪˈleɪʃ(ə)n/ noun very slow breathing

**hypovitaminosis** /ˌhaɪpəʊˌvɪtəmɪˈnəʊsɪs/ *noun* a lack of vitamins

**hypoxaemia** /ˌhaɪpɒkˈsiːmiə/ *noun* an inadequate supply of oxygen in the arterial blood

**hypoxanthine phosphoribosyl transferase** *noun* full form of **HPRT**

**hypoxia** /haɪˈpɒksiə/ *noun* **1.** an inadequate supply of oxygen to tissue as a result of a lack of oxygen in the arterial blood **2.** same as **hypoxaemia**

**hyster-** /hɪstə/ *prefix* same as **hystero-** (*used before vowels*)

**hysteralgia** /ˌhɪstərˈældʒə/ *noun* pain in the uterus

**hysterectomy** /ˌhɪstəˈrektəmi/ *noun* the surgical removal of the uterus, often either to treat cancer or because of the presence of fibroids

**hysteria** /hɪˈstɪəriə/ *noun* a term formerly used in psychiatry, but now informally used for a condition in which the person appears unstable, and may scream and wave their arms about, but also is repressed, and may be slow to react to outside stimuli (*dated*)

**hysterical** /hɪˈsterɪk(ə)l/ *adjective* referring to a reaction showing hysteria (*informal*)

**hysterically** /hɪˈsterɪkli/ *adverb* in a hysterical way (*informal*)

**hysterical personality** /hɪˌsterɪk(ə)l ˌpɜːsəˈnælɪti/ *noun* the mental condition of a person who is unstable, lacks usual feelings and is dependent on others (*dated*)

**hysterics** /hɪˈsterɪks/ *noun* an attack of hysteria (*dated*)

**hystericus** /hɪˈsterɪkəs/ ♦ **globus hystericus**

**hystero-** /hɪstərəʊ/ *prefix* referring to the uterus

**hysterocele** /ˈhɪstərəʊsiːl/ *noun* same as **uterocele**

**hystero-oöphorectomy** /ˌhɪstərəʊ ˌəʊəfəˈrektəmi/ *noun* the surgical removal of the uterus, the uterine tubes and the ovaries

**hysteroptosis** /ˌhɪstərɒpˈtəʊsɪs/ *noun* prolapse of the uterus

**hysterosalpingo-contrast sonography** /ˌhɪstərəʊˌsælpɪŋgəʊ ˌkɒntrɑːst sɒnˈɒgrəfi/ *noun* examination of the uterus and Fallopian tubes by ultrasound. Abbr **HYCOSY**

**hysterosalpingography** /ˌhɪstərəʊˌsælpɪŋˈgɒgrəfi/ *noun* an X-ray examination of the uterus and Fallopian tubes following injection of radio-opaque material. Also called **uterosalpingography**

**hysterosalpingostomy** /ˌhɪstərəʊˌsælpɪŋˈgɒstəmi/ *noun* an operation to remake an opening between the uterine tube and the uterus, to help with infertility problems

**hysteroscope** /ˈhɪstərəskəʊp/ *noun* a tube for inspecting the inside of the uterus

**hysteroscopy** /ˌhɪstəˈrɒskəpi/ *noun* an examination of the uterine cavity using a hysteroscope or fibrescope

**hysterotomy** /ˌhɪstəˈrɒtəmi/ *noun* a surgical incision into the uterus, as in caesarean section or for some types of abortion

**hysterotrachelorrhaphy** /ˌhɪstərəʊˌtrækiəˈlɒrəfi/ *noun* an operation to repair a tear in the cervix

# I

**-iasis** /aɪəsɪs/ *suffix* disease caused by something ○ *amoebiasis*

**iatro-** /aɪætrəʊ/ *prefix* relating to medicine or doctors

**iatrogenesis** /aɪˌætrəʊˈdʒenəsɪs/ *noun* any condition caused by the actions of doctors or other healthcare professionals

**iatrogenic** /aɪˌætrəˈdʒenɪk/ *adjective* referring to a condition which is caused by a doctor's treatment for another disease or condition ○ *an iatrogenic infection*

COMMENT: An iatrogenic condition can be caused by a drug, i.e. a side effect, by infection from the doctor or simply by worry about possible treatment.

**IBS** *abbr* irritable bowel syndrome

**ibuprofen** /ˌaɪbjuːˈprəʊfən/ *noun* a nonsteroidal anti-inflammatory drug that relieves pain and swelling, especially in arthritis and rheumatism. It is also widely used as a household painkiller.

**ice bag** /ˈaɪs bæg/, **icebag, ice pack** /ˈaɪs pæk/ *noun* a cold compress made of lumps of ice wrapped in a cloth or put in a special bag and held against an injured part of the body to reduce pain or swelling

**ichthamol** /ˈɪkˈθæmɒl/ *noun* a thick dark red liquid which is a mild antiseptic and analgesic, used in the treatment of skin diseases

**ichthyosis** /ˌɪkθɪˈəʊsɪs/ *noun* a hereditary condition in which the skin does not form properly, resulting in a dry, non-inflammatory and scaly appearance

**ICM** *abbr* International Confederation of Midwives

**ICN** *abbr* 1. International Council of Nurses 2. infection control nurse

**ICP** *abbr* intracranial pressure

**ICRC** *abbr* International Committee of the Red Cross

**ICSH** *abbr* interstitial cell stimulating hormone

**icteric** /ɪkˈterɪk/ *adjective* referring to someone with jaundice

**icterus** /ˈɪktərəs/ *noun* same as **jaundice**

**icterus gravis neonatorum** /ˌɪktərəs ˌɡrævɪs ˌniːəʊnəˈtɔːrəm/ *noun* jaundice associated with erythroblastosis fetalis

**ictus** /ˈɪktəs/ *noun* a stroke or fit

**ICU** *abbr* intensive care unit

**id** /ɪd/ *noun* (*in Freudian psychology*) the basic unconscious drives which exist in hidden forms in a person

**ideation** /ˌaɪdiˈeɪʃ(ə)n/ *noun* the act or process of imagining or forming thoughts and ideas

**identical twins** /aɪˈdentɪk(ə)l twɪnz/ *plural noun* twins who are exactly the same in appearance because they developed from the same ovum. Also called **monozygotic twins, uniovular twins**

**identification** /aɪˌdentɪfɪˈkeɪʃ(ə)n/ *noun* the act of discovering or stating who someone is or what something is □ **identification with someone** the act of associating with and unconsciously taking on the viewpoints and behaviours of one or more other people

**identity bracelet** /aɪˈdentɪti ˌbreɪslət/, **identity label** /aɪˈdentɪti ˌleɪb(ə)l/ *noun* a label attached to the wrist of a newborn baby or patient in hospital, so that he or she can be identified

**ideo-** /aɪdiəʊ/ *prefix* involving ideas

**idio-** /ɪdiəʊ/ *prefix* referring to one particular person

**idiopathic** /ˌɪdiəˈpæθɪk/ *adjective* 1. referring to a disease with no obvious cause 2. referring to idiopathy

**idiopathic epilepsy** /ˌɪdiəpæθɪk ˈepɪˌlepsi/ *noun* epilepsy not caused by a brain disorder, beginning during childhood or adolescence

**idiopathy** /ˌɪdiˈɒpəθi/ *noun* a condition which develops without any known cause

**idiosyncrasy** /ˌɪdiəʊˈsɪŋkrəsi/ *noun* a way of behaving which is particular to one person

**idiot savant** /ˌɪdiəʊ ˈsævɒŋ/ *noun* a person with learning difficulties who also possesses a single particular mental ability, such as the ability to play music by ear, to draw remembered objects or to do mental calculations, which is very highly developed

**idioventricular** /ˌɪdiəʊvenˈtrɪkjʊlə/ *adjective* relating to the ventricles of the heart

**idioventricular rhythm** /ˌɪdiəʊvenˌtrɪkjʊlə ˈrɪð(ə)m/ *noun* a slow natural rhythm in the ventricles of the heart, but not in the atria

**IDK** *abbr* internal derangement of the knee

**Ig** *abbr* immunoglobulin

**Ig A antiendomysial antibody** /ˌaɪ dʒiː eɪ ˌæntiendəʊˌmaɪsiəl ˈæntɪbɒdi/ *noun* a serological screening test for coeliac disease

**IHD** *abbr* ischaemic heart disease

**IL-1** *abbr* interleukin-1

**IL-2** *abbr* interleukin-2

**ile-** /ɪli/ *prefix* same as **ileo-** (*used before vowels*)

**ilea** /ˈɪliə/ plural of **ileum**

**ileac** /ˈɪliæk/ *adjective* **1.** relating to an ileus **2.** relating to the ileum

**ileal** /ˈɪliəl/ *adjective* referring to the ileum

**ileal bladder** /ˌɪliəl ˈblædə/, **ileal conduit** /ˌɪliəl ˈkɒndjuɪt/ *noun* an artificial tube formed when the ureters are linked to part of the ileum, and that part is linked to an opening in the abdominal wall

**ileal pouch** /ˌɪliəl ˈpaʊtʃ/ *noun* a part of the small intestine which is made into a new rectum in a surgical operation, freeing someone from the need for an ileostomy after their colon is removed

**ileectomy** /ˌɪliˈektəmi/ *noun* the surgical removal of all or part of the ileum

**ileitis** /ˌɪliˈaɪtɪs/ *noun* inflammation of the ileum

**ileo-** /ɪliəʊ/ *prefix* relating to the ileum

**ileocaecal** /ˌɪliəʊˈsiːk(ə)l/ *adjective* referring to the ileum and the caecum

**ileocaecal orifice** /ˌɪliəʊsiːk(ə)l ˈɒrɪfɪs/ *noun* an opening where the small intestine joins the large intestine

**ileocaecal valve** /ˌɪliːəʊsiːk(ə)l ˈvælv/ *noun* a valve at the end of the ileum, which allows food to pass from the ileum into the caecum

**ileocaecocystoplasty** /ˌɪliəʊˌsiːkəʊˈsaɪtəʊplæsti/ *noun* an operation to reconstruct the bladder using a piece of the combined ileum and caecum

**ileocolic** /ˌɪliəʊˈkɒlɪk/ *adjective* referring to both the ileum and the colon

**ileocolic artery** /ˌɪliːəʊkɒlɪk ˈɑːtəri/ *noun* a branch of the superior mesenteric artery

**ileocolitis** /ˌɪliəʊkəˈlaɪtɪs/ *noun* inflammation of both the ileum and the colon

**ileocolostomy** /ˌɪliəʊkəˈlɒstəmi/ *noun* a surgical operation to make a link directly between the ileum and the colon

**ileoproctostomy** /ˌɪliəʊprɒkˈtɒstəmi/ *noun* a surgical operation to create a link between the ileum and the rectum

**ileorectal** /ˌɪliəʊˈrekt(ə)l/ *adjective* referring to both the ileum and the rectum

**ileosigmoidostomy** /ˌɪliəʊsɪgmɔɪˈdɒstəmi/ *noun* a surgical operation to create a link between the ileum and the sigmoid colon

**ileostomy** /ˌɪliˈɒstəmi/ *noun* a surgical operation to make an opening between the ileum and the abdominal wall to act as an artificial opening for excretion of faeces

**ileostomy bag** /ɪliˈɒstəmi bæg/ *noun* a bag attached to the opening made by an ileostomy, to collect faeces as they are passed out of the body

**ileum** /ˈɪliəm/ *noun* the lower part of the small intestine, between the jejunum and the caecum. Compare **ilium**. See illustration at **DIGESTIVE SYSTEM** in Supplement (NOTE: The plural is **ilea**.)

> COMMENT: The ileum is the longest section of the small intestine, being about 2.5 metres long.

**ileus** /ˈɪliəs/ *noun* obstruction of the intestine, usually distension caused by loss of muscular action in the bowel. ♦ **paralytic ileus**

**ili-** /ɪli/ *prefix* same as **ilio-** (*used before vowels*)

**ilia** /ˈɪliə/ plural of **ilium**

**iliac** /ˈɪliæk/ *adjective* referring to the ilium

**iliac crest** /ˌɪliæk ˈkrest/ *noun* a curved top edge of the ilium. See illustration at **PELVIS** in Supplement

**iliac fossa** /ˌɪliæk ˈfɒsə/ *noun* a depression on the inner side of the hip bone

**iliac region** /ˈɪliæk ˌriːdʒən/ *noun* one of two regions of the lower abdomen, on either side of the hypogastrium

**iliac spine** /ˈɪliæk spaɪn/ *noun* a projection at the posterior end of the iliac crest

**iliacus** /ɪliˈækəs/ *noun* a muscle in the groin which flexes the thigh

**ilio-** /ɪliəʊ/ *prefix* relating to the ilium

**iliococcygeal** /ˌɪliəʊkɒkˈsɪdʒiəl/ *adjective* referring to both the ilium and the coccyx

**iliolumbar** /ˌɪliəʊˈlʌmbə/ *adjective* referring to the iliac and lumbar regions

**iliopectineal** /ˌɪliəʊpekˈtɪniəl/ *adjective* referring to both the ilium and the pubis

**iliopectineal eminence** /ˌɪliəʊpektɪniəl ˈemɪnəns/ *noun* a raised area on the inner surface of the innominate bone

**iliopsoas** /ˌɪliəʊˈsəʊəs/ *noun* a muscle formed from the iliacus and psoas muscles

**iliopubic** /ˌɪliəʊˈpjuːbɪk/ *adjective* same as **iliopectineal**

**iliopubic eminence** /ˌɪliəʊˌpjuːbɪk ˈemɪnəns/ *noun* same as **iliopectineal eminence**

**iliotibial tract** /ˌɪliəʊˈtɪbiəl ˌtrækt/ *noun* a thick fascia which runs from the ilium to the tibia

**ilium** /ˈɪliəm/ *noun* the top part of each of the hip bones, which form the pelvis. Compare **ileum**. See illustration at **PELVIS** in Supplement (NOTE: The plural is **ilia**.)

**ill** /ɪl/ *adjective* not well ○ *If you feel very ill you ought to see a doctor.*

**illegal abortion** /ɪ,liːg(ə)l ə'bɔːʃ(ə)n/ *noun* same as **criminal abortion**

**ill health** /,ɪl 'helθ/ *noun* the fact of not being well ○ *He has been in ill health for some time.* ○ *She has a history of ill health.* ○ *He had to retire early for reasons of ill health.*

**illness** /'ɪlnəs/ *noun* **1.** a state of not being well ○ *Most of the children stayed away from school because of illness.* **2.** a type of disease ○ *Scarlet fever is no longer considered to be a very serious illness.* ○ *He is in hospital with an infectious tropical illness.*

**illusion** /ɪ'luːʒ(ə)n/ *noun* a condition in which a person has a wrong perception of external objects

**i.m., IM** *abbr* intramuscular

**image** /'ɪmɪdʒ/ *noun* a sensation, e.g. a smell, sight or taste, which is remembered clearly

**imagery** /'ɪmɪdʒəri/ *noun* visual sensations clearly produced in the mind

**imaginary** /ɪ'mædʒɪn(ə)ri/ *adjective* referring to something which does not exist but is imagined

**imaginary playmate** /ɪ,mædʒɪnəri 'pleɪˌmeɪt/ *noun* a friend who does not exist but who is imagined by a small child to exist

**imagination** /ɪ,mædʒɪ'neɪʃ(ə)n/ *noun* the ability to see or invent things in your mind ○ *In her imagination she saw herself sitting on a beach in the sun.*

**imagine** /ɪ'mædʒɪn/ *verb* to see, hear or feel something in your mind ○ *Imagine yourself sitting on the beach in the sun.* ○ *I thought I heard someone shout, but I must have imagined it because there is no one there.* □ **to imagine things** to have delusions ○ *She keeps imagining things.* ○ *Sometimes he imagines he is swimming in the sea.*

**imaging** /'ɪmɪdʒɪŋ/ *noun* a technique for creating pictures of sections of the body, using scanners attached to computers

**imbalance** /ɪm'bæləns/ *noun* a situation in which things are unequal or in the wrong proportions to one another, e.g. in the diet

**imipramine** /ɪ'mɪprəmiːn/ *noun* a drug that is used as a treatment for depression

**immature** /,ɪmə'tjʊə/ *adjective* not mature, lacking insight and emotional stability

**immature cell** /,ɪmətjʊə 'sel/ *noun* a cell which is still developing

**immaturity** /,ɪmə'tʃʊərɪti/ *noun* behaviour which is lacking in maturity

**immersion foot** /ɪ,mɜːʃ(ə)n 'fʊt/ *noun* same as **trench foot**

**immiscible** /ɪ'mɪsəb(ə)l/ *adjective* (of liquids) not able to be mixed

**immobile** /ɪ'məʊbaɪl/ *adjective* not moving, which cannot move

**immobilisation** /ɪ,məʊbɪlaɪ'zeɪʃ(ə)n/, **immobilization** *noun* the act of preventing somebody or something from being able to move

**immobilise** /ɪ'məʊbɪlaɪz/, **immobilize** *verb* **1.** to keep someone from moving **2.** to attach a splint to a joint or fractured limb to prevent the bones from moving

**immovable** /ɪ'muːvəb(ə)l/ *adjective* referring to a joint which cannot be moved

**immune** /ɪ'mjuːn/ *adjective* protected against an infection or allergic disease ○ *She seems to be immune to colds.* ○ *The injection should make you immune to yellow fever.*

**immune deficiency** /ɪ,mjuːn dɪ'fɪʃ(ə)nsi/ *noun* a lack of immunity to a disease. ◊ **AIDS**

**immune reaction** /ɪ,mjuːn ri'ækʃ(ə)n/, **immune response** /ɪ,mjuːn rɪ'spɒns/ *noun* a reaction of a body to an antigen

**immune system** /ɪ'mjuːn ,sɪstəm/ *noun* a complex network of cells and cell products, which protects the body from disease. It includes the thymus, spleen, lymph nodes, white blood cells and antibodies.

'…the reason for this susceptibility is a profound abnormality of the immune system in children with sickle-cell disease' [*Lancet*]

'…the AIDS virus attacks a person's immune system and damages his or her ability to fight other diseases' [*Journal of the American Medical Association*]

**immunisation** /,ɪmjʊnaɪ'zeɪʃ(ə)n/, **immunization** *noun* the process of making a person immune to an infection, either by injecting an antiserum, passive immunisation or by inoculation

'…vaccination is the most effective way to prevent children getting the disease. Children up to 6 years old can be vaccinated if they missed earlier immunization' [*Health Visitor*]

**immunise** /'ɪmjʊnaɪz/, **immunize** *verb* to give someone immunity from an infection. ◊ **vaccinate** (NOTE: You immunise someone **against** a disease.)

COMMENT: In the UK, infants are immunised routinely against diphtheria, pertussis, polio, tetanus, Hib, mumps, measles and rubella, unless there are contra-indications or the parents object.

**immunity** /ɪ'mjuːnɪti/ *noun* the ability to resist attacks of a disease because antibodies are produced ○ *The vaccine gives immunity to tuberculosis.*

**immuno-** /ɪmjʊnəʊ, ɪmjuːnəʊ/ *prefix* immune, immunity

**immunoassay** /,ɪmjʊnəʊæˈseɪ/ *noun* a test for the presence and strength of antibodies

**immunocompetence** /,ɪmjʊnəʊ'kɒmpɪtəns/ *noun* the ability to develop an immune response following exposure to an antigen

**immunocompromised** /,ɪmjʊnəʊ'kɒmprəmaɪzd/ *adjective* not able to offer resistance to infection

**immunodeficiency** /ˌɪmjʊnəʊdɪˈfɪʃ(ə)nsi/
*noun* a lack of immunity to a disease

**immunodeficiency virus** /ˌɪmjʊnəʊdɪ
ˈfɪʃ(ə)nsi ˌvaɪrəs/ *noun* a retrovirus which attacks the immune system

**immunodeficient** /ˌɪmjʊnəʊdɪˈfɪʃ(ə)nt/,
*adjective* lacking immunity to a disease ○ *This
form of meningitis occurs in persons who are
immunodeficient.*

**immunoelectrophoresis** /ˌɪmjʊnəʊɪˌlektrəʊfə
ˈriːsɪs/ *noun* a method of identifying antigens in
a laboratory, using electrophoresis

**immunogenic** /ˌɪmjʊnəʊˈdʒenɪk/ *adjective*
producing an immune response

**immunogenicity** /ˌɪmjʊnəʊdʒəˈnɪsɪti/
*noun* the property which makes a substance
able to produce an immune response in an organism

**immunoglobulin** /ˌɪmjʊnəʊˈglɒbjʊlɪn/
*noun* an antibody, a protein produced in blood
plasma as protection against infection, the
commonest being gamma globulin. Abbr **Ig**
(NOTE: The five main classes are called: **immunoglobulin G, A, D, E and M** or **IgG, IgA, IgD,
IgE and IgM**.)

**immunological** /ˌɪmjʊnəˈlɒdʒɪk(ə)l/ *adjective* referring to immunology

**immunological staining** /ˌɪmjʊnə
ˈlɒdʒɪk(ə)l ˈsteɪnɪŋ/ *noun* the process of
checking if cancer is likely to return after
someone has been declared free of the disease,
by staining cells

**immunological tolerance** /ˌɪmjʊnə
ˈlɒdʒɪk(ə)l ˈtɒlərəns/ *noun* tolerance of the
lymphoid tissues to an antigen

**immunologist** /ˌɪmjʊˈnɒlədʒɪst/ *noun* a
specialist in immunology

**immunology** /ˌɪmjʊˈnɒlədʒi/ *noun* the study
of immunity and immunisation

**immunosuppressant** /ˌɪmjʊnəʊsə
ˈpres(ə)nt/ *noun* a drug used to act against the
response of the immune system to reject a
transplanted organ

**immunosuppression** /ˌɪmjʊnəʊsə
ˈpreʃ(ə)n/ *noun* the suppression of the body's
natural immune system so that it will not reject
a transplanted organ

**immunosuppressive** /ˌɪmjʊnəʊsəˈpresɪv/
*adjective* counteracting the immune system

**immunotherapy** /ˌɪmjʊnəʊˈθerəpi/ *noun* ♦
adoptive immunotherapy

**immunotransfusion** /ˌɪmjʊnəʊtræns
ˈfjuːʒ(ə)n/ *noun* a transfusion of blood, serum
or plasma containing immune bodies

**Imodium** /ɪˈməʊdiəm/ a trade name for Ioperamide hydrochloride

**impacted** /ɪmˈpæktɪd/ *adjective* tightly
pressed or firmly lodged against something

**impacted faeces** /ɪmˌpæktɪd ˈfiːsiːz/ *plural
noun* extremely hard dry faeces which cannot

pass through the anus and have to be surgically
removed

**impacted fracture** /ɪmˌpæktɪd ˈfræktʃə/
*noun* a fracture where the broken parts of the
bones are pushed into each other

**impacted tooth** /ɪmˌpæktɪd ˈtuːθ/ *noun* a
tooth which is held against another tooth and
so cannot grow normally

**impacted ureteric calculus** /ɪmˌpæktɪd
ˌjʊərɪterɪk ˈkælkjʊləs/ *noun* a small hard
mass of mineral salts which is lodged in a ureter

**impaction** /ɪmˈpækʃən/ *noun* a condition in
which two things are impacted

**impair** /ɪmˈpeə/ *verb* to harm a sense or function so that it does not work properly

**impaired hearing** /ɪmˌpeəd ˈhɪərɪŋ/ *noun*
hearing which is not clear and sharp

**impaired vision** /ɪmˌpeəd ˈvɪʒ(ə)n/ *noun*
eyesight which is not fully clear

**impairment** /ɪmˈpeəmənt/ *noun* a condition
in which a sense or function is harmed so that
it does not work properly ○ *His hearing impairment does not affect his work.* ○ *The impairment that her eyesight was getting worse.*

'…impairment – any loss or abnormality of psychological, physical or anatomical structure or function'
[*WHO*]

**impalpable** /ɪmˈpælpəb(ə)l/ *adjective* not
able to be felt when touched

**impediment** /ɪmˈpedɪmənt/ *noun* an obstruction

**imperforate** /ɪmˈpɜːf(ə)rət/ *adjective* without an opening

**imperforate anus** /ɪmˌpɜːf(ə)rət ˈeɪnəs/
*noun* same as **proctatresia**

**imperforate hymen** /ɪmˌpɜːf(ə)rət ˈhaɪmen/
*noun* a membrane in the vagina which is missing the opening for the menstrual flow

**impermeable** /ɪmˈpɜːmiəb(ə)l/ *adjective* not
allowing liquids or gases to pass through

**impetigo** /ˌɪmpɪˈtaɪgəʊ/ *noun* an irritating
and very contagious skin disease caused by
staphylococci, which spreads rapidly and is
easily passed from one child to another, but
can be treated with antibiotics

**implant** *noun* /ˈɪmplɑːnt/ something grafted
or inserted into a person, e.g. tissue, a drug, inert material or a device such as a pacemaker ■
*verb* /ɪmˈplɑːnt/ **1.** to fix into something ○ *The
ovum implants in the wall of the uterus.* **2.** to
graft or insert tissue, a drug, inert material or a
device ○ *The site was implanted with the biomaterial.*

**implantation** /ˌɪmplɑːnˈteɪʃ(ə)n/ *noun* **1.**
the act of grafting or inserting tissue, a drug,
inert material or a device into a person, or the
introduction of one tissue into another surgically **2.** same as **nidation**

**implant material** /'ɪmplɑːnt mə,tɪərɪəl/ noun a substance grafted or inserted into a person

**implant site** /'ɪmplɑːnt saɪt/ noun a place in or on the body where the implant is positioned

**impotence** /'ɪmpət(ə)ns/ noun the inability in a male to have an erection or to ejaculate, and so have sexual intercourse

**impotent** /'ɪmpət(ə)nt/ adjective (of a man) unable to have sexual intercourse

**impregnate** /'ɪmpregneɪt/ verb **1.** to make a female pregnant **2.** to soak a cloth with a liquid ○ a cloth impregnated with antiseptic

**impregnation** /,ɪmpreg'neɪʃ(ə)n/ noun the action of impregnating

**impression** /ɪm'preʃ(ə)n/ noun **1.** a mould of a person's jaw made by a dentist before making a denture **2.** a depression on an organ or structure into which another organ or structure fits ◇ **cardiac impression 1.** concave area near the centre of the upper surface of the liver under the heart **2.** depression on the mediastinal part of the lungs where they touch the pericardium

**improve** /ɪm'pruːv/ verb to get better, or make something better ○ She was very ill, but she is improving now.

**improvement** /ɪm'pruːvmənt/ noun the act of getting better ○ The patient's condition has shown a slight improvement. ○ Doctors have not detected any improvement in her asthma.

**impulse** /'ɪmpʌls/ noun **1.** a message transmitted by a nerve **2.** a sudden feeling of wanting to act in a specific way

**impure** /ɪm'pjuə/ adjective not pure

**impurity** /ɪm'pjuərɪti/ noun a substance which is not pure or clean ○ The kidneys filter impurities out of the blood.

**in-** /ɪn/ prefix **1.** in, into, towards **2.** not

**inaccessible** /,ɪnək'sesɪb(ə)l/ adjective **1.** physically difficult or impossible to reach **2.** very technical and difficult to understand

**inactive** /ɪn'æktɪv/ adjective **1.** not being active, not moving ○ Patients must not be allowed to become inactive. **2.** not working ○ The serum makes the poison inactive.

**inactivity** /,ɪnæk'tɪvɪti/ noun a lack of activity

**inanition** /,ɪnə'nɪʃ(ə)n/ noun a state of exhaustion caused by starvation

**inarticulate** /,ɪnɑː'tɪkjʊlət/ adjective **1.** without joints or segments, as in the bones of the skull **2.** unable to speak fluently or intelligibly **3.** not understandable as speech or language

**in articulo mortis** /ɪn ɑː,tɪkjʊləʊ 'mɔːtɪs/ adverb a Latin phrase meaning 'at the onset of death'

**inborn** /ɪn'bɔːn/ adjective congenital, which is in the body from birth ○ A body has an inborn tendency to reject transplanted organs.

**inbreeding** /'ɪnbriːdɪŋ/ noun a situation where closely related males and females, or those with very similar genetic make-up, have children together, so allowing congenital conditions to be passed on

**incapacitated** /,ɪnkə'pæsɪteɪtɪd/ adjective not able to act or work ○ He was incapacitated for three weeks by his accident.

**incarcerated** /ɪn'kɑːsəreɪtɪd/ adjective referring to a hernia which cannot be corrected by physical manipulation

**incest** /'ɪnsest/ noun an act of sexual intercourse or other sexual activity with so close a relative, that it is illegal or culturally not allowed

**incidence** /'ɪnsɪd(ə)ns/ noun the number of times something happens in a specific population over a period of time ○ the incidence of drug-related deaths ○ Men have a higher incidence of strokes than women.

**incidence rate** /'ɪnsɪd(ə)ns reɪt/ noun the number of new cases of a disease during a given period, per thousand of population

**incipient** /ɪn'sɪpɪənt/ adjective just beginning or in its early stages ○ He has an incipient appendicitis. ○ The tests detected incipient diabetes mellitus.

**incise** /ɪn'saɪz/ verb to cut into something

**incised wound** /ɪn'saɪzd wuːnd/ noun a wound with clean edges, caused by a sharp knife or razor

**incision** /ɪn'sɪʒ(ə)n/ noun a cut in a person's body made by a surgeon using a scalpel, or any cut made with a sharp knife or razor ○ The first incision is made two millimetres below the second rib. Compare **excision**

**incisional** /ɪn'sɪʒ(ə)n(ə)l/ adjective referring to an incision

**incisional hernia** /ɪn,sɪʒ(ə)n(ə)l 'hɜːnɪə/ noun a hernia which breaks through the abdominal wall at a place where a surgical incision was made during an operation

**incisor** /ɪn'saɪzə/, **incisor tooth** /ɪn'saɪzə tuːθ/ noun one of the front teeth, of which there are four each in the upper and lower jaws, which are used to cut off pieces of food. See illustration at TEETH in Supplement

**inclusion** /ɪn'kluːʒ(ə)n/ noun something enclosed inside something else

**inclusion bodies** /ɪn'kluːʒ(ə)n ,bɒdiz/ plural noun very small particles found in cells infected by a virus

**inclusive** /ɪn'kluːsɪv/ adjective (of health services) provided whether or not someone has a disability or special needs

**incoherent** /,ɪnkəʊ'hɪərənt/ adjective not able to speak in a way which makes sense

**incompatibility** /,ɪnkəmpætɪ'bɪlɪti/ noun the fact of being incompatible ○ the incompatibility of the donor's blood with that of the patient

**incompatible** /ˌɪnkəm'pætɪb(ə)l/ *adjective*
**1.** referring to something which does not go together with something else **2.** referring to drugs which must not be used together because they undergo chemical change and the therapeutic effect is lost or changed to something undesirable **3.** referring to tissue which is genetically different from other tissue, making it impossible to transplant into that tissue

**incompatible blood** /ˌɪnkəmpætəb(ə)l 'blʌd/ *noun* blood from a donor that does not match the blood of the person receiving the transfusion

**incompetence** /ɪn'kɒmpɪt(ə)ns/ *noun* the inability to do a particular act, especially a lack of knowledge or skill which makes a person unable to do particular job

**incompetent cervix** /ɪnˌkɒmpɪt(ə)nt 'sɜːvɪks/ *noun* a dysfunctional cervix of the uterus which is often the cause of spontaneous abortions and premature births and can be remedied by purse-string stitching

**incomplete abortion** /ˌɪnkəmpliːt ə'bɔːʃ(ə)n/ *noun* an abortion where part of the contents of the uterus is not expelled

**incomplete fracture** /ˌɪnkəmpliːt 'fræktʃə/ *noun* a fracture that does not go all the way through a bone

**incontinence** /ɪn'kɒntɪnəns/ *noun* the inability to control the discharge of urine or faeces (NOTE: Single incontinence is the inability to control the bladder. Double incontinence is the inability to control both the bladder and the bowels.)

**incontinence pad** /ɪn'kɒntɪnəns pæd/ *noun* a pad of material to absorb urine

**incontinent** /ɪn'kɒntɪnənt/ *adjective* unable to control the discharge of urine or faeces

**incoordination** /ˌɪnkəʊɔːdɪ'neɪʃ(ə)n/ *noun* a situation in which the muscles in various parts of the body do not act together, making it impossible to carry out some actions

**incubation** /ˌɪŋkjʊ'beɪʃ(ə)n/ *noun* **1.** the development of an infection inside the body before the symptoms of the disease appear **2.** the keeping of an ill or premature baby in a controlled environment in an incubator **3.** the process of culturing cells or microorganisms under controlled conditions

**incubation period** /ˌɪŋkjʊ'beɪʃ(ə)n ˌpɪəriəd/ *noun* the time during which a virus or bacterium develops in the body after contamination or infection, before the appearance of the symptoms of the disease. Also called **stadium invasioni**

**incubator** /'ɪŋkjʊbeɪtə/ *noun* **1.** an apparatus for growing bacterial cultures **2.** an enclosed container in which a premature baby can be kept, within which conditions such as temperature and oxygen levels can be controlled

**incudes** /ɪn'kjuːdiːz/ plural of **incus**

**incus** /'ɪŋkəs/ *noun* one of the three ossicles in the middle ear, shaped like an anvil. See illustration at **EAR**, in Supplement

**independent** /ˌɪndɪ'pendənt/ *adjective* not controlled by someone or something else

**independent nursing function** /ˌɪndɪ pendənt 'nɜːsɪŋ ˌfʌŋkʃən/ *noun* any part of the nurse's job for which the nurse takes full responsibility

**Inderal** /'ɪndəræl/ a trade name for propranolol

**index finger** /'ɪndeks ˌfɪŋgə/ *noun* the first finger next to the thumb

**indican** /'ɪndɪkæn/ *noun* potassium salt

**indication** /ˌɪndɪ'keɪʃ(ə)n/ *noun* a situation or sign which suggests that a specific treatment should be given or that a condition has a particular cause ○ *Sulpha drugs have been replaced by antibiotics in many indications.* ◊ **contraindication**

**indicator** /'ɪndɪkeɪtə/ *noun* **1.** a substance which shows something, e.g. a substance secreted in body fluids which shows which blood group a person belongs to **2.** something that serves as a warning or guide

**indigenous** /ɪn'dɪdʒɪnəs/ *adjective* **1.** natural or inborn **2.** native to or representative of a country or region

**indigestion** /ˌɪndɪ'dʒestʃən/ *noun* a disturbance of the normal process of digestion, where the person experiences pain or discomfort in the stomach ○ *He is taking tablets to relieve his indigestion* or *He is taking indigestion tablets.* ◊ **dyspepsia**

**indigo carmine** /ˌɪndɪgəʊ 'kɑːmaɪn/ *noun* a blue dye which is injected into a person to test how well their kidneys are working

**indirect contact** /ˌɪndaɪrekt 'kɒntækt/ *noun* the fact of catching a disease by inhaling germs or by being in contact with a vector

**indisposed** /ˌɪndɪ'spəʊzd/ *adjective* slightly ill ○ *My mother is indisposed and cannot see any visitors.*

**indisposition** /ˌɪndɪspə'zɪʃ(ə)n/ *noun* a slight illness

**individualise** /ˌɪndɪ'vɪdʒuəˌlaɪz/, **individualize** *verb* to provide something that matches the needs of a specific person or situation ○ *individualised care*

**individualised nursing care** /ˌɪndɪˌvɪdʒuəlaɪzd 'nɜːsɪŋ keə/ *noun* care which is designed to provide exactly what one particular patient needs ○ *The home's staff are specially trained to provide individualised nursing care.*

**Indocid** /'ɪndəsɪd/ a trade name for indomethacin

**indolent** /'ɪndələnt/ *adjective* **1.** causing little pain **2.** referring to an ulcer which develops slowly and does not heal

**indomethacin** /ˌɪndəʊ'meθəsɪn/ *noun* a drug that reduces pain, fever and inflammation, especially that caused by arthritis

**indrawing** /ɪn'drɔːɪŋ/ *noun* the act of pulling towards the inside

**indrawn** /ɪn'drɔːn/ *adjective* pulled inside

**induce** /ɪn'djuːs/ *verb* to make something happen □ **to induce labour** to make a woman go into labour

**induced abortion** /ɪnˌdjuːst ə'bɔːʃ(ə)n/ *noun* an abortion which is deliberately caused by drugs or by surgery

**induction** /ɪn'dʌkʃən/ *noun* **1.** the process of starting or speeding up the birth of a baby **2.** the stimulation of an enzyme's production when the substance on which it acts increases in concentration **3.** a process by which one part of an embryo influences another part's development **4.** information and support given to new employees in an organisation

**induction of labour** /ɪnˌdʌkʃən əv 'leɪbə/ *noun* the action of starting childbirth artificially

**induration** /ˌɪndjʊə'reɪʃ(ə)n/ *noun* the hardening of tissue or of an artery because of pathological change

**induratum** /ˌɪndjʊə'reɪtəm/ ♦ **erythema**

**industrial disease** /ɪn'dʌstriəl dɪˌziːz/ *noun* a disease which is caused by the type of work done by a worker or by the conditions in which he or she works, e.g. by dust produced or chemicals used in the factory

**indwelling catheter** /ɪnˌdwelɪŋ 'kæθɪtə/ *noun* a catheter left in place for a period of time after its introduction

**inebriation** /ɪˌniːbri'eɪʃ(ə)n/ *noun* a state where a person is drunk, especially habitually drunk

**inert** /ɪ'nɜːt/ *adjective* **1.** (*of person*) not moving **2.** (*of chemical, etc.*) not active or not producing a chemical reaction

**inertia** /ɪ'nɜːʃə/ *noun* a lack of activity in the body or mind

**in extremis** /ɪn ɪks'triːmɪs/ *adverb* at the moment of death

**infant** /'ɪnfənt/ *noun* a child under two years of age

**infanticide** /ɪn'fæntɪsaɪd/ *noun* **1.** the act of killing an infant **2.** a person who kills an infant

**infantile** /'ɪnfəntaɪl/ *adjective* **1.** referring to small children **2.** referring to a disease which affects children

**infantile convulsions** /ˌɪnfəntaɪl kən'vʌlʃənz/, **infantile spasms** /ˌɪnfəntaɪl 'spæzəmz/ *plural noun* convulsions or minor epileptic fits in small children

**infantile paralysis** /ˌɪnfəntaɪl pə'ræləsɪs/ *noun* a former name for poliomyelitis

**infantilism** /ɪn'fæntɪlɪz(ə)m/ *noun* a condition in which a person keeps some characteris-

tics of an infant when he or she becomes an adult

**infant mortality rate** /ˌɪnfənt mɔː'tælɪti reɪt/ *noun* the number of infants who die per thousand births

**infant respiratory distress syndrome** /ˌɪnfənt rɪˌspɪrət(ə)ri dɪ'stres ˌsɪndrəʊm/ *noun* a condition of newborn babies in which the lungs do not function properly. Abbr **IRDS**

**infarct** /'ɪnfɑːkt/ *noun* an area of tissue which is killed when the blood supply is cut off by the blockage of an artery

**infarction** /ɪn'fɑːkʃ(ə)n/ *noun* a condition in which tissue is killed by the cutting off of blood supply

'…cerebral infarction accounts for about 80% of first-ever strokes' [*British Journal of Hospital Medicine*]

**infect** /ɪn'fekt/ *verb* to contaminate someone or something with microorganisms that cause disease or toxins ○ *The disease infected her liver.* ○ *The whole arm soon became infected.*

**infected wound** /ɪnˌfektɪd 'wuːnd/ *noun* a wound into which bacteria have entered

**infection** /ɪn'fekʃən/ *noun* **1.** the entry or introduction into the body of microorganisms, which then multiply ○ *As a carrier he was spreading infection to other people in the office.* **2.** an illness which is caused by the entry of microbes into the body ○ *She is susceptible to minor infections.*

**infectious** /ɪn'fekʃəs/ *adjective* referring to a disease which is caused by microorganisms and can be transmitted to other persons by direct means ○ *This strain of flu is highly infectious.* ○ *Her measles is at the infectious stage.*

**infectious disease** /ɪnˌfekʃəs dɪ'ziːz/ *noun* a disease caused by microorganisms such as bacteria, viruses or fungi. ◊ **communicable disease, contagious disease**

**infectious hepatitis** /ɪnˌfekʃəs ˌhepə'taɪtɪs/ *noun* hepatitis A, transmitted by a carrier through food or drink. Also called **infective hepatitis**

**infectious mononucleosis** /ɪnˌfekʃəs ˌmɒnəʊˌnjuːkli'əʊsɪs/ *noun* an infectious disease where the body has an excessive number of white blood cells. Also called **glandular fever**

**infectious parotitis** /ɪnˌfekʃəs ˌpærə'taɪtɪs/ *noun* same as **mumps**

**infectious virus hepatitis** /ɪnˌfekʃəs 'vaɪrəs ˌhepətaɪtɪs/ *noun* hepatitis transmitted by a carrier through food or drink

**infective** /ɪn'fektɪv/ *adjective* referring to a disease caused by a microorganism, which can be caught from another person but which may not always be directly transmitted

**infective enteritis** /ɪnˌfektɪv ˌentə'raɪtɪs/ *noun* enteritis caused by bacteria

**infective hepatitis** /ɪnˌfektɪv ˌhepə'taɪtɪs/ *noun* same as **infectious hepatitis**

**infectivity** /ˌɪnfek'tɪvɪti/ *noun* the fact of being infective ○ *The patient's infectivity can last about a week.*

**inferior** /ɪn'fɪəriə/ *adjective* referring to a lower part of the body. Opposite **superior**

**inferior aspect** /ɪnˌfɪəriər 'æspekt/ *noun* a view of the body from below

**inferiority** /ɪnˌfɪəri'ɒrɪti/ *noun* the fact of being lower in value or quality, substandard. Opposite **superiority**

**inferiority complex** /ɪnˌfɪəri'ɒrɪti ˌkɒmpleks/ *noun* a mental disorder arising from a combination of wanting to be noticed and fear of humiliation. The resulting behaviour may either be aggression or withdrawal from the external world.

**inferior mesenteric artery** /ɪnˌfɪəriə mesenˌterɪk 'ɑːtəri/ *noun* one of the arteries which supply the transverse colon and rectum

**inferior vena cava** /ɪnˌfɪəriə ˌviːnə 'kɑːvə/ *noun* the main vein carrying blood from the lower part of the body to the heart. See illustration at **HEART** in Supplement, **KIDNEY** in Supplement

**infertile** /ɪn'fɜːtaɪl/ *adjective* not fertile, not able to reproduce

**infertility** /ˌɪnfə'tɪlɪti/ *noun* the fact of not being fertile, not able to reproduce

**infest** /ɪn'fest/ *verb* (*of parasites*) to be present somewhere in large numbers ○ *The child's hair was infested with lice.*

**infestation** /ˌɪnfe'steɪʃ(ə)n/ *noun* the fact of having large numbers of parasites, or an invasion of the body by parasites ○ *The condition is caused by infestation of the hair with lice.*

**infiltrate** /'ɪnfɪltreɪt/ *verb* (*of liquid or waste*) to pass from one part of the body to another through a wall or membrane and be deposited in the other part ■ *noun* a substance which has infiltrated a part of the body

'…the chest roentgenogram often discloses interstitial pulmonary infiltrates, but may occasionally be normal' [*Southern Medical Journal*]

**infiltration** /ˌɪnfɪl'treɪʃ(ə)n/ *noun* **1.** the process where a liquid passes through the walls of one part of the body into another part **2.** a condition in which waste is brought to and deposited around cells

'…the lacrimal and salivary glands become infiltrated with lymphocytes and plasma cells. The infiltration reduces lacrimal and salivary secretions which in turn leads to dry eyes and dry mouth' [*American Journal of Nursing*]

**infirm** /ɪn'fɜːm/ *adjective* old and weak

**infirmary** /ɪn'fɜːməri/ *noun* **1.** a room in a school or workplace where people can go if they are ill **2.** a former name for a hospital (NOTE: **Infirmary** is still used in the names of some hospitals: **the Glasgow Royal Infirmary.**)

**infirmity** /ɪn'fɜːmɪti/ *noun* a lack of strength and energy because of illness or age (*formal*)

**inflame** /ɪn'fleɪm/ *verb* to make an organ or a tissue react to an infection, an irritation or a blow by becoming sore, red and swollen

**inflamed** /ɪn'fleɪmd/ *adjective* sore, red and swollen ○ *The skin has become inflamed around the sore.*

**inflammation** /ˌɪnflə'meɪʃ(ə)n/ *noun* the fact of having become sore, red and swollen as a reaction to an infection, an irritation or a blow ○ *She has an inflammation of the bladder* or *a bladder inflammation.* ○ *The body's reaction to infection took the form of an inflammation of the eyelid.*

**inflammatory** /ɪn'flæmət(ə)ri/ *adjective* causing an organ or a tissue to become sore, red and swollen

**inflammatory bowel disease** /ɪn ˌflæmət(ə)ri 'baʊəl dɪˌziːz/ *noun* any condition, e.g. Crohn's disease, colitis or ileitis, in which the bowel becomes inflamed

**inflammatory response** /ɪnˌflæmət(ə)ri rɪ 'spɒns/, **inflammatory reaction** /ɪn ˌflæmət(ə)ri rɪ'ækʃən/ *noun* any condition where an organ or a tissue reacts to an external stimulus by becoming inflamed ○ *She showed an inflammatory response to the ointment.*

**inflate** /ɪn'fleɪt/ *verb* to fill something with air, or be filled with air ○ *The abdomen is inflated with air before a coelioscopy.* ○ *In valvuloplasty, a balloon is introduced into the valve and inflated.*

**influenza** /ˌɪnflu'enzə/ *noun* an infectious disease of the upper respiratory tract with fever and muscular aches, which is transmitted by a virus and can occur in epidemics. Also called **flu**

COMMENT: The influenza virus is spread by droplets of moisture in the air, so the disease can be spread by coughing or sneezing. Influenza can be quite mild, but virulent strains occur from time to time, such as Spanish influenza or Hong Kong flu, and can weaken the person so much that he or she becomes susceptible to pneumonia and other more serious infections.

**informal patient** /ɪnˌfɔːm(ə)l 'peɪʃ(ə)nt/ *noun* a patient who has admitted himself or herself to a hospital, without being referred by a doctor

**information** /ˌɪnfə'meɪʃ(ə)n/ *noun* facts about something ○ *Have you any information about the treatment of sunburn?* ○ *The police won't give us any information about how the accident happened.* ○ *You haven't given me enough information about when your symptoms started.* ○ *That's a very useful piece* or *bit of information.* (NOTE: No plural: **some information; a piece of information.**)

**informed** /ɪn'fɔːmd/ *adjective* having the latest information

**informed consent** /ɪnˌfɔːmd kən'sent/ *noun* an agreement to allow a procedure to be carried out, given by a patient, or the guardian of a patient, who has been provided with all the necessary information

**infra-** /'ɪnfrə/ *prefix* below

**infracostal** /ˌɪnfrə'kɒst(ə)l/ *adjective* lying below the ribs

**infraorbital nerve** /ˌɪnfrɔː'bɪt(ə)l 'nɜːv/ *noun* a continuation of the maxillary nerve below the orbit of the eye

**infraorbital vein** /ˌɪnfrɔː'bɪt(ə)l 'veɪn/ *noun* a vessel draining the face through the infraorbital canal to the pterygoid plexus

**infrared** /ˌɪnfrə'red/ *adjective* relating to infrared radiation ■ *noun* invisible electromagnetic radiation between light and radio waves

**infrared radiation** /ˌɪnfrəred ˌreɪdi'eɪʃ(ə)n/ *noun* same as **infrared rays**

**infrared rays** /ˌɪnfrəred 'reɪz/ *plural noun* long invisible rays, below the visible red end of the colour spectrum, used to produce heat in body tissues in the treatment of traumatic and inflammatory conditions. ◊ **light therapy**

**infundibulum** /ˌɪnfʌn'dɪbjʊləm/ *noun* any part of the body shaped like a funnel, especially the stem which attaches the pituitary gland to the hypothalamus

**infuse** /ɪn'fjuːz/ *verb* to introduce a solution such as saline, sucrose or glucose using a drip into a vein, body cavity or the intestinal tract in order to treat or feed someone

**infusion** /ɪn'fjuːʒ(ə)n/ *noun* **1.** a drink made by pouring boiling water on a dry substance such as herb tea or a powdered drug **2.** the process of putting of liquid into someone's body, using a drip

**ingesta** /ɪn'dʒestə/ *plural noun* food or liquid that enters the body via the mouth

**ingestion** /ɪn'dʒestʃən/ *noun* **1.** the act of taking in food, drink or medicine by the mouth **2.** the process by which a foreign body such as a bacillus is surrounded by a cell

**ingredient** /ɪn'griːdiənt/ *noun* a substance which is used with others to make something

**ingrowing toenail** /ˌɪngrəʊɪŋ 'təʊneɪl/, **ingrowing nail** /ˌɪngrəʊɪŋ 'neɪl/, **ingrown toenail** /ˌɪngrəʊn 'təʊneɪl/ *noun* a toenail which is growing into the skin at the side of the nail, causing pain and swelling. The toenail cuts into the tissue on either side of it, creating inflammation and sometimes sepsis and ulceration.

**inguinal** /'ɪŋgwɪn(ə)l/ *adjective* referring to the groin

**inguinal canal** /ˌɪŋgwɪn(ə)l kə'næl/ *noun* a passage in the lower abdominal wall, carrying the spermatic cord in the male and the round ligament of the uterus in the female

**inguinale** /ˌɪŋgwɪ'neɪli/ ♦ **granuloma inguinale**

**inguinal hernia** /ˌɪŋgwɪn(ə)l 'hɜːniə/ *noun* a hernia where the intestine bulges through the muscles in the groin

**inguinal ligament** /ˌɪŋgwɪn(ə)l 'lɪgəmənt/ *noun* a ligament in the groin, running from the spine to the pubis. Also called **Poupart's ligament**

**inguinal region** /ˌɪŋgwɪn(ə)l 'riːdʒən/ *noun* the part of the body where the lower abdomen joins the top of the thigh. ◊ **groin**

**INH** *abbr* isoniazid

**inhalant** /ɪn'heɪlənt/ *noun* a medicinal substance which is breathed in

**inhalation** /ˌɪnhə'leɪʃ(ə)n/ *noun* **1.** the act of breathing in. Opposite **exhalation 2.** the action of breathing in a medicinal substance as part of a treatment

**inhale** /ɪn'heɪl/ *verb* **1.** to breathe in, or breathe something in ○ *She inhaled some toxic gas fumes and was rushed to hospital.* **2.** to breathe in a medicinal substance as part of a treatment. Opposite **exhale**

**inhaler** /ɪn'heɪlə/ *noun* a small device for administering medicinal substances into the mouth or nose so that they can be breathed in

**inherent** /ɪn'hɪərənt/ *adjective* referring to a thing which is part of the essential character of a person or a permanent characteristic of an organism

**inherit** /ɪn'herɪt/ *verb* to receive genetically controlled characteristics from a parent ○ *She inherited her father's red hair.* ○ *Haemophilia is a condition which is inherited through the mother's genes.*

**inheritance** /ɪn'herɪt(ə)ns/ *noun* **1.** the process by which genetically controlled characteristics pass from parents to offspring ○ *the inheritance of chronic inflammatory bowel disease* **2.** all of the qualities and characteristics which are passed down from parents ○ *an unfortunate part of our genetic inheritance*

**inherited** /ɪn'herɪtɪd/ *adjective* passed on from a parent through the genes ○ *an inherited disorder of the lungs*

**inhibit** /ɪn'hɪbɪt/ *verb* to prevent an action happening, or stop a functional process ○ *Aspirin inhibits the clotting of blood.* □ **to have an inhibiting effect on something** to block something, to stop something happening

**inhibition** /ˌɪnhɪ'bɪʃ(ə)n/ *noun* **1.** the action of blocking or preventing something happening, especially of preventing a muscle or organ from functioning properly **2.** (*in psychology*) the suppression of a thought which is associated with a sense of guilt **3.** (*in psychology*) the blocking of a spontaneous action by some mental influence

**inhibitor** /ɪn'hɪbɪtə/ *noun* a substance which inhibits

**inhibitory nerve** /ɪn'hɪbɪtəri ˌnɜːv/ *noun* a nerve which stops a function taking place ○ *The vagus nerve is an inhibitory nerve which slows down the action of the heart.*

**inion** /ˈɪniən/ *noun* a part of the occipital bone that can be felt as a slight lump at the back of the skull just above the neck

**inject** /ɪnˈdʒekt/ *verb* to put a liquid into someone's body under pressure, by using a hollow needle inserted into the tissues ○ *He was injected with morphine.* ○ *She injected herself with a drug.*

**injected** /ɪnˈdʒektɪd/ *adjective* **1.** referring to a liquid or substance introduced into the body **2.** referring to surface blood vessels which are swollen

**injection** /ɪnˈdʒekʃən/ *noun* **1.** the act of injecting a liquid into the body ○ *He had a penicillin injection.* **2.** a liquid introduced into the body

**injure** /ˈɪndʒə/ *verb* to hurt someone or a part of the body ○ *Six people were injured in the accident.*

**injured** /ˈɪndʒəd/ *adjective* referring to someone who has been hurt ■ *plural noun* □ **the injured** people who have been injured ○ *All the injured were taken to the nearest hospital.*

**injury** /ˈɪndʒəri/ *noun* damage or a wound caused to a person's body ○ *His injuries required hospital treatment.* ○ *He received severe facial injuries in the accident.*

**injury scoring system** /ˈɪndʒəri ˈskɔːrɪŋ ˌsɪstəm/ *noun* any system used for deciding how severe an injury is ○ *a standard lung injury scoring system* Abbr **ISS**

**inlay** /ˈɪnleɪ/ *noun* (*in dentistry*) a type of filling for teeth

**inlet** /ˈɪnlet/ *noun* a passage or opening through which a cavity can be entered

**INN** *abbr* international nonproprietary name

**innards** /ˈɪnədz/ *plural noun* the internal organs of the body, especially the intestines

**innate** /ɪˈneɪt/ *adjective* inherited, which is present in a body from birth

**inner** /ˈɪnə/ *adjective* referring to a part which is inside

**inner ear** /ˌɪnər ˈɪə/ *noun* the part of the ear inside the head, behind the eardrum, containing the semicircular canals, the vestibule and the cochlea

**inner pleura** /ˌɪnə ˈplʊərə/ *noun* same as **visceral pleura**

**innervate** /ˈɪnɜːveɪt/ *verb* to cause a muscle, organ or other part of the body to act

**innervation** /ˌɪnɜːˈveɪʃ(ə)n/ *noun* the nerve supply to an organ, including both motor nerves and sensory nerves

**innocent** /ˈɪnəs(ə)nt/ *adjective* referring to a growth which is benign, not malignant

**innominate** /ɪˈnɒmɪnət/ *adjective* with no name

**innominate artery** /ɪˌnɒmɪnət ˈɑːtəri/ *noun* the largest branch of the arch of the aorta, which continues as the right common carotid and right subclavian arteries

**innominate bone** /ɪˌnɒmɪnət ˈbəʊn/ *noun* same as **hip bone**

**innominate vein** /ɪˌnɒmɪnət ˈveɪn/ *noun* same as **brachiocephalic vein**

**inoculant** /ɪˈnɒkjʊlənt/ *noun* same as **inoculum**

**inoculate** /ɪˈnɒkjʊleɪt/ *verb* to introduce vaccine into a person's body in order to make the body create its own antibodies, so making the person immune to the disease ○ *The baby was inoculated against diphtheria.* (NOTE: You inoculate someone **with** or **against** a disease.)

**inoculation** /ɪˌnɒkjʊˈleɪʃ(ə)n/ *noun* the action of inoculating someone ○ *Has the baby had a diphtheria inoculation?*

**inoculum** /ɪˈnɒkjʊləm/ *noun* a substance used for inoculation, e.g. a vaccine (NOTE: The plural is **inocula**.)

**inoperable** /ɪnˈɒpər(ə)b(ə)l/ *adjective* referring to a condition which cannot be operated on ○ *The surgeon decided that the cancer was inoperable.*

**inorganic** /ˌɪnɔːˈɡænɪk/ *adjective* referring to a substance which is not made from animal or vegetable sources

**inorganic acid** /ˌɪnɔːɡænɪk ˈæsɪd/ *noun* an acid which comes from minerals, used in dilute form to help indigestion

**inotropic** /ˌɪnəʊˈtrɒpɪk/ *adjective* affecting the way muscles contract, especially those of the heart

**inpatient** /ˈɪnˌpeɪʃ(ə)nt/ *noun* someone who stays overnight or for some time in a hospital for treatment or observation. Compare **outpatient**

**inquest** /ˈɪŋkwest/ *noun* an inquiry by a coroner into the cause of a death

COMMENT: An inquest has to take place where death is violent or not expected, where death could be murder or where a prisoner dies and when police are involved.

**insane** /ɪnˈseɪn/ *adjective* mentally unwell (*dated, informal*)

**insanitary** /ɪnˈsænɪt(ə)ri/ *adjective* not hygienic ○ *Cholera spread rapidly because of the insanitary conditions in the town.*

**insect** /ˈɪnsekt/ *noun* a small animal with six legs and a body in three parts

**insect bite** /ˈɪnsekt baɪt/ *noun* a sting caused by an insect which punctures the skin to suck blood, and in so doing introduces irritants

COMMENT: Most insect bites are simply irritating. Others can be more serious, as insects can carry the organisms which produce typhus, sleeping sickness, malaria, filariasis and many other diseases.

**insecticide** /ɪnˈsektɪsaɪd/ *noun* a substance which kills insects

**insemination** /ɪnˌsemɪˈneɪʃ(ə)n/ *noun* the introduction of sperm into the vagina

**insensible** /ɪnˈsensɪb(ə)l/ *adjective* **1.** lacking feeling or consciousness **2.** not aware of or responding to a stimulus **3.** too slight to be perceived by the senses

**insert** /ɪnˈsɜːt/ *verb* to put something into something ○ *The catheter is inserted into the passage.*

**insertion** /ɪnˈsɜːʃ(ə)n/ *noun* **1.** the point of attachment of a muscle to a bone **2.** the point where an organ is attached to its support **3.** a change in the structure of a chromosome, where a segment of the chromosome is introduced into another member of the complement

**insides** /ɪnˈsaɪdz/ *plural noun* internal organs, especially the stomach and intestines (*informal*) ○ *He says he has a pain in his insides.* ○ *You ought to see the doctor if you think there is something wrong with your insides.*

**insidious** /ɪnˈsɪdiəs/ *adjective* causing harm without showing any obvious signs

**insidious disease** /ɪnˌsɪdiəs dɪˈziːz/ *noun* a disease which causes damage before being detected

**insight** /ˈɪnsaɪt/ *noun* the ability of a person to realise that he or she is ill or has particular problems or characteristics

**insipidus** /ɪnˈsɪpɪdəs/ ⟶ **diabetes insipidus**

**in situ** /ˌɪn ˈsɪtjuː/ *adverb* in place

**insoluble** /ɪnˈsɒljʊb(ə)l/ *adjective* not able to be dissolved in liquid

**insoluble fibre** /ɪnˌsɒljʊb(ə)l ˈfaɪbə/ *noun* the fibre in bread and cereals, which is not digested but which swells inside the intestine

**insomnia** /ɪnˈsɒmniə/ *noun* the inability to sleep ○ *She experiences insomnia.* ○ *What does the doctor give you for your insomnia?* Also called **sleeplessness**

**insomniac** /ɪnˈsɒmniæk/ *noun* a person who has insomnia

**inspiration** /ˌɪnspɪˈreɪʃ(ə)n/ *noun* the act of taking air into the lungs. Opposite **expiration**

COMMENT: Inspiration takes place when the muscles of the diaphragm contract, allowing the lungs to expand.

**inspiratory** /ɪnˈspaɪrət(ə)ri/ *adjective* referring to breathing in

**inspire** /ɪnˈspaɪə/ *verb* to inhale air or a gas into the lungs

**inspissated** /ɪnˈspɪseɪtɪd/ *adjective* referring to a liquid which is thickened by removing water from it

**inspissation** /ˌɪnspɪˈseɪʃ(ə)n/ *noun* the act of removing water from a solution to make it thicker

**instep** /ˈɪnstep/ *noun* an arched top part of the foot

**instil** /ɪnˈstɪl/, **instill** *verb* to put a liquid in something drop by drop ○ *Instil four drops in each nostril twice a day.*

**instillation** /ˌɪnstɪˈleɪʃ(ə)n/ *noun* **1.** the process of putting a liquid in drop by drop **2.** a liquid put in drop by drop

**instinct** /ˈɪnstɪŋkt/ *noun* a tendency or ability which the body has from birth and does not need to learn ○ *The body has a natural instinct to protect itself from danger.*

**instinctive** /ɪnˈstɪŋktɪv/ *adjective* automatic or unconscious rather than planned ○ *an instinctive reaction*

**institution** /ˌɪnstɪˈtjuːʃ(ə)n/ *noun* a place where people are cared for, e.g. a hospital or clinic, especially a psychiatric hospital or children's home

**institutionalisation** /ˌɪnstɪˌtjuːʃ(ə)nəlaɪˈzeɪʃ(ə)n/, **institutionalization**, **institutional neurosis** /ˌɪnstɪtjuːʃən(ə)l njʊˈrəʊsɪs/ *noun* a condition in which someone has become so adapted to life in an institution that it is impossible for him or her to live outside it

**institutionalise** /ˌɪnstɪˈtjuːʃ(ə)nəlaɪz/, **institutionalize** *verb* to put someone into an institution

**instructions** /ɪnˈstrʌkʃənz/ *plural noun* spoken or written information which explains how something is used or how to do something ○ *She gave the taxi driver instructions on how to get to the hospital.* ○ *The instructions are written on the medicine bottle.* ○ *We can't use this machine because we have lost the book of instructions.*

**instrument** /ˈɪnstrʊmənt/ *noun* a piece of equipment or a tool ○ *The doctor had a box of surgical instruments.*

**instrumental** /ˌɪnstrʊˈment(ə)l/ *adjective* □ **instrumental in** helping to do something ○ *She was instrumental in developing the new technique.*

**instrumental delivery** /ˌɪnstrʊment(ə)l dɪˈlɪv(ə)ri/ *noun* childbirth where the doctor uses forceps to help the baby out of the mother's uterus

**insufficiency** /ˌɪnsəˈfɪʃ(ə)nsi/ *noun* **1.** the fact of not being strong or large enough to perform usual functions ○ *The patient is suffering from a renal insufficiency.* **2.** the incompetence of an organ

**insufflate** /ˈɪnsəfleɪt/ *verb* to blow gas, vapour or powder into the lungs or another body cavity as a treatment

**insufflation** /ˌɪnsəˈfleɪʃ(ə)n/ *noun* the act of blowing gas, vapour or powder into the lungs or another body cavity as a treatment

**insula** /ˈɪnsjʊlə/ *noun* part of the cerebral cortex which is covered by the folds of the sulcus

**insulin** /ˈɪnsjʊlɪn/ *noun* a hormone produced by the islets of Langerhans in the pancreas

COMMENT: Insulin controls the way in which the body converts sugar into energy and regulates the level of sugar in the blood. A lack of insulin caused by diabetes mellitus makes the level of glucose in the blood rise. Insulin injections are regularly used to treat diabetes mellitus, but care has to be taken not to exceed the dose as this will cause hyperinsulinism and hypoglycaemia.

**insulinase** /ˈɪnsjʊlɪneɪz/ *noun* an enzyme which breaks down insulin

**insulin dependence** /ˌɪnsjʊlɪn dɪˈpendəns/ *noun* the fact of being dependent on insulin injections

**insulin-dependent diabetes** /ˌɪnsjʊlɪn dɪˌpendənt daɪəˈbiːtiz/ *noun* same as **Type I diabetes mellitus**

**insulinoma** /ˌɪnsjʊlɪˈnəʊmə/ *noun* a tumour in the islets of Langerhans

**insulin-resistant** /ˌɪnsjʊlɪn rɪˈzɪst(ə)nt/ *adjective* referring to a condition in which the muscle and other tissue cells respond inadequately to insulin, as in Type II diabetes

**insulin shock** /ˈɪnsjʊlɪn ˌʃɒk/ *noun* a serious drop in blood sugar, caused by too much insulin accompanied by sweating, dizziness, trembling and eventually coma

**insuloma** /ˌɪnsjʊˈləʊmə/ *noun* same as **insulinoma**

**insult** /ˈɪnsʌlt/ *noun* **1.** a physical injury or trauma **2.** something that causes a physical injury or trauma

**intact** /ɪnˈtækt/ *adjective* having all body parts present and undamaged

**intake** /ˈɪnteɪk/ *noun* **1.** the amount of a substance taken in ○ *a high intake of alcohol* ○ *She was advised to reduce her intake of sugar.* **2.** the process of taking in a substance

**Intal** /ˈɪntæl/ a trade name for a preparation of cromolyn sodium

**integrated service** /ˌɪntɪɡreɪtɪd ˈsɜːvɪs/ *noun* a broad care service provided by health and social agencies acting together

**integrative medicine** /ˌɪntɪɡreɪtɪv ˈmed(ə)s(ə)n/ *noun* the combination of mainstream therapies and those complementary or alternative therapies for which there is scientific evidence of efficacy and safety

**integument** /ɪnˈteɡjʊmənt/ *noun* a covering layer, e.g. the skin

**intellect** /ˈɪntɪlekt/ *noun* a person's ability to think, reason and understand

**intelligence** /ɪnˈtelɪdʒəns/ *noun* the ability to learn and understand quickly

**intelligence quotient** /ɪnˈtelɪdʒəns ˌkwəʊʃ(ə)nt/ *noun* the ratio of the mental age, as given by an intelligence test, to the chronological age of the person. Abbr **IQ**

**intense** /ɪnˈtens/ *adjective* referring to a very strong pain ○ *She is suffering from intense post herpetic neuralgia.*

**intensity** /ɪnˈtensɪti/ *noun* the strength of e.g. pain

**intensive care** /ɪnˌtensɪv ˈkeə/ *noun* **1.** the continual supervision and treatment of an extremely ill person in a special section of a hospital ○ *The patient was put in intensive care.* ◊ **residential care 2.** same as **intensive care unit**

**intensive care unit** /ɪnˌtensɪv ˈkeə ˌjuːnɪt/ *noun* a section of a hospital equipped with life-saving and life-support equipment in which seriously ill people who need constant medical attention are cared for. Abbr **ICU**

**intention** /ɪnˈtenʃən/ *noun* a plan to do something

**intention tremor** /ɪnˈtenʃən ˌtremə/ *noun* a trembling of the hands seen when people suffering from particular brain diseases make voluntary movements to try to touch something

**inter-** /ɪntə/ *prefix* between

**interaction** /ˌɪntərˈækʃən/ *noun* an effect which two or more substances such as drugs have on each other

**interatrial septum** /ˌɪntərˈeɪtriəl ˌseptəm/ *noun* a membrane between the right and left atria in the heart

**intercalated** /ɪnˈtɜːkəleɪtɪd/ *adjective* inserted between other tissues

**intercalated disc** /ɪnˌtɜːkəleɪtɪd ˈdɪsk/ *noun* closely applied cell membranes at the end of adjacent cells in cardiac muscle, seen as transverse lines

**intercellular** /ˌɪntəˈseljʊlə/ *adjective* between the cells in tissue

**intercostal** /ˌɪntəˈkɒst(ə)l/ *adjective* between the ribs ■ *noun* same as **intercostal muscle**

**intercostal muscle** /ɪntəˌkɒst(ə)l ˈmʌs(ə)l/ *noun* one of the muscles between the ribs

COMMENT: The intercostal muscles expand and contract the thorax, so changing the pressure in the thorax and making the person breathe in or out. There are three layers of intercostal muscle: external, internal and innermost or intercostalis intimis.

**intercourse** /ˈɪntəkɔːs/ *noun* same as **sexual intercourse**

**intercurrent disease** /ˌɪntəkʌrənt dɪˈziːz/, **intercurrent infection** /ˌɪntəkʌrənt ɪnˈfekʃən/ *noun* a disease or infection which affects someone who has another disease

**interdigital** /ˌɪntəˈdɪdʒɪt(ə)l/ *adjective* referring to the space between the fingers or toes

**interdisciplinary** /ˌɪntəˌdɪsɪˈplɪnəri/ *adjective* combining two or more different areas of medical or scientific study

**interferon** /ˌɪntəˈfɪərɒn/ *noun* a protein produced by cells, usually in response to a virus, and which then reduces the spread of viruses

COMMENT: Although it is now possible to synthesise interferon outside the body, large-scale production is extremely expensive and the substance has not proved as successful at combating viruses as had been hoped, though it is used in multiple sclerosis with some success.

**interior** /ɪnˈtɪəriə/ *noun* a part which is inside ■ *adjective* inside

**interleukin** /ˌɪntəˈluːkɪn/ *noun* a protein produced by the body's immune system

**interleukin-1** /ˌɪntəluːkɪn ˈwʌn/ *noun* a protein which causes high temperature. Abbr **IL-1**

**interleukin-2** /ˌɪntəluːkɪn 'tuː/ noun a protein which stimulates T-cell production, used in the treatment of cancer. Abbr **IL-2**

**interlobar** /ˌɪntə'ləʊbə/ adjective between lobes

**interlobar artery** /ˌɪntələʊbər 'ɑːtəri/ noun an artery running towards the cortex on each side of a renal pyramid

**interlobular** /ɪntə'lɒbjʊlə/ adjective between lobules

**interlobular artery** /ɪntə'lɒbjʊlə ˌɑːtəri/ noun one of the arteries running to the glomeruli of the kidneys

**intermediate care** /ˌɪntəmiːdiət 'keə/ noun care following surgery or illness that can be delivered in special units attached to a hospital or in the person's home by a special multidisciplinary team

**intermedius** /ˌɪntə'miːdiəs/ ♦ **vastus intermedius**

**intermenstrual** /ˌɪntə'menstruəl/ adjective between the menstrual periods

**intermittent** /ˌɪntə'mɪt(ə)nt/ adjective occurring at intervals

**intermittent claudication** /ˌɪntəmɪt(ə)nt ˌklɔːdɪ'keɪʃ(ə)n/ noun a condition of the arteries causing severe pain in the legs which makes the person limp after having walked a short distance (NOTE: The symptoms increase with walking, stop after a short rest and recur when the person walks again.)

**intermittent fever** /ˌɪntəmɪt(ə)nt 'fiːvə/ noun fever which rises and falls regularly, as in malaria

**intermittent self-catheterisation** /ˌɪntəmɪt(ə)nt self ˌkæθɪtəraɪ'zeɪʃ(ə)n/ noun a procedure in which someone puts a catheter through the urethra into their own bladder from time to time to empty out the urine. Abbr **ISC**

**intern** /'ɪntɜːn/ noun US a medical graduate who is working in a hospital before being licensed to practise medicine. ♦ **house officer**

**interna** /ɪn'tɜːnə/ ♦ **otitis interna**

**internal** /ɪn'tɜːn(ə)l/ adjective inside the body or a body part. Opposite **external** □ **the drug is for internal use only** it should not be used on the outside of the body

**internal auditory meatus** /ɪnˌtɜːn(ə)l ɔːdɪt(ə)ri mi'eɪtəs/ noun a channel which takes the auditory nerve through the temporal bone

**internal bleeding** /ɪnˌtɜːn(ə)l 'bliːdɪŋ/ noun loss of blood inside the body, e.g. from a wound in the intestine

**internal capsule** /ɪnˌtɜːn(ə)l 'kæpsjuːl/ noun a bundle of fibres linking the cerebral cortex and other parts of the brain

**internal cardiac massage** /ɪnˌtɜːn(ə)l ˌkɑːdiæk 'mæsɑːʒ/ noun a method of making the heart start beating again by pressing on the heart itself

**internal carotid** /ɪnˌtɜːn(ə)l kæ'rɒtɪd/ noun an artery in the neck, behind the external carotid, which gives off the ophthalmic artery and ends by dividing into the anterior and middle cerebral arteries

**internal derangement of the knee** /ɪnˌtɜːn(ə)l dɪ'reɪnʒmənt əv ðə 'niː/ noun a condition in which the knee cannot function properly because of a torn meniscus. Abbr **IDK**

**internal ear** /ɪnˌtɜːn(ə)l 'ɪə/ noun the part of the ear inside the head, behind the eardrum, containing the semicircular canals, the vestibule and the cochlea

**internal haemorrhage** /ɪnˌtɜːn(ə)l 'hem(ə)rɪdʒ/ noun a haemorrhage which takes place inside the body

**internal haemorrhoids** /ɪnˌtɜːn(ə)l 'hemərɔɪdz/ plural noun swollen veins inside the anus

**internal iliac artery** /ɪnˌtɜːn(ə)l 'ɪliæk ˌɑːtəri/ noun an artery which branches from the aorta in the abdomen and leads to the pelvis

**internal injury** /ɪnˌtɜːn(ə)l 'ɪndʒəri/ noun damage to one of the internal organs

**internal jugular** /ɪnˌtɜːn(ə)l 'dʒʌɡjʊlə/ noun the largest jugular vein in the neck, leading to the brachiocephalic veins

**internally** /ɪn'tɜːn(ə)li/ adverb inside the body ○ He was bleeding internally.

**internal medicine** /ɪnˌtɜːn(ə)l 'med(ə)s(ə)n/ noun US the treatment of diseases of the internal organs by specialists

**internal nares** /ɪnˌtɜːn(ə)l 'neəriːz/ plural noun the two openings shaped like funnels leading from the nasal cavity to the pharynx. Also called **posterior nares**

**internal oblique** /ɪnˌtɜːn(ə)l ə'bliːk/ noun the middle layer of muscle covering the abdomen, beneath the external oblique

**internal organ** /ɪnˌtɜːn(ə)l 'ɔːɡən/ noun an organ situated inside the body

**internal respiration** /ɪnˌtɜːn(ə)l ˌrespɪ'reɪʃ(ə)n/ noun the part of respiration concerned with the passage of oxygen from the blood to the tissues, and the passage of carbon dioxide from the tissues to the blood

**International Committee of the Red Cross** /ˌɪntəˌnæʃ(ə)n(ə)l kəˌmɪti əv ðə ˌred 'krɒs/ noun an international organisation which provides mainly emergency medical help, but also relief to victims of earthquakes, floods and other disasters, or to prisoners of war. Abbr **ICRC**

**International Council of Nurses** /ˌɪntənæʃ(ə)n(ə)l ˌkaʊnsəl əv 'nɜːsɪz/ noun an organisation founded in 1899 which now represents nurses in more than 120 countries. Its aims are to bring nurses together, to advance nursing worldwide and to influence health policies. Abbr **ICN**

**international nonproprietary name** /ˌɪntənæʃ(ə)nəl ˌnɒnprəpraɪət(ə)ri ˈneɪm/ *noun* each of 8,000 names selected by the World Health Organization that are the legally required generic names for pharmaceutical product labelling for most countries in the world, including all EU countries. Abbr **INN**

**international unit** /ˌɪntənæʃ(ə)nəl ˈjuːnɪt/ *noun* an internationally agreed standard used in pharmacy as a measure of a substance such as a drug or hormone. Abbr **IU**

**interneurone** /ˌɪntəˈnjuːrəʊn/ *noun* a neurone with short processes which is a link between two other neurones in sensory or motor pathways

**internist** /ˈɪntɜːnɪst/ *noun* a specialist who treats diseases of the internal organs by non-surgical means

**internodal** /ˌɪntəˈnəʊd(ə)l/ *adjective* between two nodes

**internuncial neurone** /ˌɪntənʌnʃ(ə)l ˈnjuːrəʊn/ *noun* a neurone which links two other nerve cells

**internus** /ɪnˈtɜːnəs/ *noun* medial rectus muscle in the orbit of the eye

**interoceptor** /ˌɪntərəʊˈseptə/ *noun* a nerve cell which reacts to a change taking place inside the body

**interosseous** /ˌɪntərˈɒsiəs/ *adjective* between bones

**interparietal** /ˌɪntəpəˈraɪət(ə)l/ *adjective* between parietal parts, especially between the parietal bones ■ *noun* same as **interparietal bone**

**interparietal bone** /ˌɪntəpəˈraɪət(ə)l ˌbəʊn/ *noun* a triangular bone in the back of the skull, rarely present in humans

**interpeduncular cistern** /ˌɪntəpə ˈdʌŋkjʊlər ˌsɪstən/ *noun* subarachnoid space between the two cerebral hemispheres beneath the midbrain and the hypothalamus

**interphalangeal joint** /ˌɪntəfəˈlændʒɪəl dʒɔɪnt/ *noun* a joint between the phalanges. Also called **IP joint**

**interphase** /ˈɪntəfeɪz/ *noun* a stage of a cell between divisions

**interpubic joint** /ˌɪntəpjuːbɪk ˈdʒɔɪnt/ *noun* a piece of cartilage which joins the two sections of the pubic bone. Also called **pubic symphysis**

**interruptus** /ˌɪntəˈrʌptəs/ ♦ **coitus interruptus**

**intersex** /ˈɪntəseks/ *noun* an organism that has both male and female characteristics

**intersexuality** /ˌɪntəsekʃuˈælɪti/ *noun* a condition in which a baby has both male and female characteristics, as in Klinefelter's syndrome and Turner's syndrome

**interstice** /ɪnˈtɜːstɪs/ *noun* a small space between body parts or within a tissue

**interstitial** /ˌɪntəˈstɪʃ(ə)l/ *adjective* referring to tissue located in the spaces between parts of something, especially between the active tissues in an organ

**interstitial cell** /ˌɪntəˈstɪʃ(ə)l sel/ *noun* a testosterone-producing cell between the tubules in the testes. Also called **Leydig cell**

**interstitial cell stimulating hormone** /ˌɪntəˈstɪʃ(ə)l sel ˈstɪmjʊleɪtɪŋ ˌhɔːməʊn/ *noun* a hormone produced by the pituitary gland which stimulates the formation of corpus luteum in females and testosterone in males. Abbr **ICSH**. Also called **luteinising hormone**

**interstitial cystitis** /ˌɪntəstɪʃ(ə)l sɪˈstaɪtɪs/ *noun* a persistent nonbacterial condition in which someone has bladder pain and wants to pass urine frequently. It is often associated with Hunner's ulcer.

**intertrigo** /ˌɪntəˈtraɪgəʊ/ *noun* an irritation which occurs when two skin surfaces rub against each other, as in the armpit or between the buttocks

**intertubercular plane** /ˌɪntətjuˌbɜːkjʊlə ˈpleɪn/ *noun* same as **transtubercular plane**

**intervention** /ˌɪntəˈvenʃən/ *noun* a treatment

**interventional radiology** /ˌɪntəvenʃən(ə)l ˌreɪdiˈɒlədʒi/ *noun* the area of medicine which uses X-rays, ultrasound and computer-assisted tomography to guide small instruments into the body for procedures such as biopsies, draining fluids or widening narrow vessels

**interventricular** /ˌɪntəvenˈtrɪkjʊlə/ *adjective* between ventricles in the heart or brain

**interventricular foramen** /ˌɪntəven ˌtrɪkjʊlə fəˈreɪmən/ *noun* an opening in the brain between the lateral ventricle and the third ventricle, through which the cerebrospinal fluid passes

**interventricular septum** /ˌɪntəven ˌtrɪkjʊlə ˈseptəm/ *noun* a membrane between the right and left ventricles in the heart

**intervertebral** /ˌɪntəˈvɜːtɪbr(ə)l/ *adjective* between vertebrae

**intervertebral disc** /ˌɪntəˌvɜːtɪbrəl ˈdɪsk/ *noun* a round plate of cartilage which separates two vertebrae in the spinal column. See illustration at **CARTILAGINOUS JOINT** in Supplement. Also called **vertebral disc**

**intervertebral foramen** /ˌɪntəˌvɜːtɪbrəl fə ˈreɪmən/ *noun* a space between two vertebrae

**intestinal** /ɪnˈtestɪn(ə)l/ *adjective* referring to the intestine

**intestinal anastomosis** /ɪnˌtestɪn(ə)l ə ˌnæstəˈməʊsɪs/ *noun* a surgical operation to join one part of the intestine to another, after a section has been removed

**intestinal flora** /ɪnˌtestɪn(ə)l ˈflɔːrə/ *plural noun* beneficial bacteria which are always present in the intestine

**intestinal glands** /ɪnˈtestɪn(ə)l glændz/ *plural noun* tubular glands found in the mucous membrane of the small and large intestine, especially those between the bases of the villi in the small intestine. Also called **Lieberkühn's glands, crypts of Lieberkühn**

**intestinal infection** /ɪnˈtestɪn(ə)l ɪnˌfekʃ(ə)n/ *noun* an infection in the intestines

**intestinal juice** /ɪnˈtestɪn(ə)l dʒuːs/ *noun* alkaline liquid secreted by the small intestine which helps to digest food

**intestinal obstruction** /ɪnˌtestɪn(ə)l əbˈstrʌkʃən/ *noun* a blocking of the intestine

**intestinal villi** /ɪnˌtestɪn(ə)l ˈvɪlaɪ/ *plural noun* projections on the walls of the intestine which help in the digestion of food

**intestinal wall** /ɪnˌtestɪn(ə)l ˈwɔːl/ *noun* the layers of tissue which form the intestine

**intestine** /ɪnˈtestɪn/ *noun* the part of the digestive system between the stomach and the anus that digests and absorbs food. ◊ **large intestine, small intestine** (NOTE: For other terms referring to the intestines, see words beginning with **entero-**.)

**intima** /ˈɪntɪmə/ ♦ **tunica intima**

**intolerance** /ɪnˈtɒlərəns/ *noun* the fact of being unable to endure something such as pain or to take a medicine without an adverse reaction ○ *He developed an intolerance to penicillin.*

**intoxicant** /ɪnˈtɒksɪkənt/ *noun* a substance which induces a state of intoxication or poisoning, e.g. an alcoholic drink

**intoxicate** /ɪnˈtɒksɪkeɪt/ *verb* to make someone incapable of controlling his or her actions, because of the influence of alcohol on the nervous system ○ *He drank six glasses of whisky and became completely intoxicated.*

**intoxication** /ɪnˌtɒksɪˈkeɪʃ(ə)n/ *noun* a condition which results from the absorption and diffusion in the body of a substance such as alcohol ○ *She was driving in a state of intoxication.*

**intra-** /ɪntrə/ *prefix* inside

**intra-abdominal** /ˌɪntrə æbˈdɒmɪn(ə)l/ *adjective* inside the abdomen

**intra-articular** /ˌɪntrə ɑːˈtɪkjʊlə/ *adjective* inside a joint

**intracellular** /ˌɪntrəˈseljʊlə/ *adjective* inside a cell

**intracerebral haematoma** /ˌɪntrə ˌserəbrəl ˌhiːməˈtəʊmə/ *noun* a blood clot inside a cerebral hemisphere

**intracranial** /ˌɪntrəˈkreɪniəl/ *adjective* inside the skull

**intracranial pressure** /ˌɪntrəkreɪniəl ˈpreʃə/ *noun* the pressure of the subarachnoi-

dal fluid, which fills the space between the skull and the brain. Abbr **ICP**

**intractable** /ɪnˈtræktəb(ə)l/ *adjective* not able to be controlled ○ *an operation to relieve intractable pain*

**intracutaneous** /ˌɪntrəkjuːˈteɪniəs/ *adjective* inside layers of skin tissue

**intracutaneous injection** /ˌɪntrəkjuː ˌteɪniəs ɪnˈdʒekʃən/ *noun* an injection of a liquid between the layers of skin, as for a test for an allergy

**intradermal** /ˌɪntrəˈdɜːm(ə)l/ *adjective* within or introduced between the layers of the skin

**intradermal test** /ɪntrəˈdɜːm(ə)l test/ *noun* a test requiring an injection into the thickness of the skin, e.g. a Mantoux test or an allergy test

**intradermic** /ˌɪntrəˈdɜːmɪk/ *adjective* same as **intradermal**

**intradural** /ˌɪntrəˈdjʊərəl/ *adjective* inside the dura mater

**intramedullary** /ˌɪntrəmeˈdʌləri/ *adjective* inside the bone marrow or spinal cord

**intramural** /ˌɪntrəˈmjʊərəl/ *adjective* inside the wall of an organ

**intramuscular** /ˌɪntrəˈmʌskjʊlə/ *adjective* inside a muscle

**intramuscular injection** /ˌɪntrəˌmʌskjʊlə ɪnˈdʒekʃən/ *noun* an injection of liquid into a muscle, e.g. for a slow release of a drug

**intranasal** /ˌɪntrəˈneɪz(ə)l/ *adjective* inside or into the nose

**intraocular** /ˌɪntrəˈɒkjʊlə/ *adjective* inside the eye

**intraocular lens** /ˌɪntrəˌɒkjʊlə ˈlenz/ *noun* an artificial lens implanted inside the eye. Abbr **IOL**

**intraocular pressure** /ˌɪntrəˌɒkjʊlə ˈpreʃə/ *noun* the pressure inside the eyeball (NOTE: If the pressure is too high, it causes glaucoma.)

**intraoperative ultrasound** *noun* high-resolution imaging used in surgery. Abbr **IOUS**

**intraorbital** /ˌɪntrəˈɔːbɪt(ə)l/ *adjective* within the orbit of the eye

**intraosseous** /ˌɪntrəˈɒsiəs/ *adjective* within a bone

**intrathecal** /ˌɪntrəˈθiːk(ə)l/ *adjective* inside a sheath, especially inside the intradural or subarachnoid space

**intratracheal** /ˌɪntrətrəˈkiəl/ *adjective* within the trachea. Also called **endotracheal**

**intratubercular plane** /ˌɪntrətjuːbɜːkjʊlə ˈpleɪn/ *noun* a plane at right angles to the sagittal plane, passing through the tubercles of the iliac crests

**intrauterine** /ˌɪntrəˈjuːtəraɪn/ *adjective* inside the uterus

**intrauterine contraceptive device** /ˌɪntrə juːtəraɪn ˌkɒntrəˈseptɪv dɪˌvaɪs/, **intrauterine device** /ˌɪntrəjuːtəraɪn dɪˈvaɪs/ *noun* a plastic coil placed inside the uterus to prevent pregnancy. Abbr **IUCD, IUD**

**intravascular** /ˌɪntrəˈvæskjʊlə/ *adjective* inside the blood vessels

**intravenous** /ˌɪntrəˈviːnəs/ *adjective* into a vein. Abbr **IV**

**intravenous drip** /ˌɪntrəviːnəs ˈdrɪp/ *noun* a thin tube that is inserted into a vein and is used to very gradually give a person fluids, either for rehydration, feeding or medication purposes

**intravenous feeding** /ˌɪntrəviːnəs ˈfiːdɪŋ/ *noun* the procedure of giving someone liquid food by means of a tube inserted into a vein

**intravenous injection** /ˌɪntrəviːnəs ɪnˈdʒekʃən/ *noun* an injection of liquid into a vein, e.g. for the fast release of a drug

**intravenously** /ˌɪntrəˈviːnəsli/ *adverb* into a vein ○ *a fluid given intravenously*

**intravenous pyelogram** /ˌɪntrəviːnəs ˈpaɪələɡræm/, **intravenous urogram** /ˌɪntrəviːnəs ˈjʊərəɡræm/ *noun* a series of X-ray photographs of the kidneys using pyelography. Abbr **IVP, IVU**

**intravenous pyelography** /ˌɪntrəviːnəs ˌpaɪəˈlɒɡrəfi/, **intravenous urography** /ˌɪntrəviːnəs jʊˈrɒɡrəfi/ *noun* an X-ray examination of the urinary tract after opaque liquid has been injected intravenously into the body and taken by the blood into the kidneys

**intraventricular** /ˌɪntrəvenˈtrɪkjʊlə/ *adjective* inside or placed into a ventricle in the heart or the brain

**intra vitam** /ˌɪntrə ˈvaɪtəm/ *adverb* during life

**intrinsic** /ɪnˈtrɪnsɪk/ *adjective* belonging to the essential nature of an organism, or entirely within an organ or part

**intrinsic factor** /ɪnˌtrɪnsɪk ˈfæktə/ *noun* a protein produced in the gastric glands which reacts with the extrinsic factor, and which, if lacking, causes pernicious anaemia

**intrinsic ligament** /ɪnˌtrɪnsɪk ˈlɪɡəmənt/ *noun* a ligament which forms part of the capsule surrounding a joint

**intrinsic muscle** /ɪnˌtrɪnsɪk ˈmʌs(ə)l/ *noun* a muscle lying completely inside the part or segment, especially of a limb, which it moves

**intro-** /ɪntrəʊ/ *prefix* inward

**introduce** /ˌɪntrəˈdjuːs/ *verb* **1.** to put something into something ○ *He used a syringe to introduce a medicinal substance into the body.* ○ *The nurse introduced the catheter into the vein.* **2.** to present two people to one another when they have never met before ○ *Can I introduce my new assistant?* **3.** to start a new way of doing something ○ *The hospital has introduced a new screening process for cervical cancer.*

**introduction** /ˌɪntrəˈdʌkʃən/ *noun* **1.** the act of putting something inside something ○ *the*

introduction of semen into the woman's uterus ○ *the introduction of an endotracheal tube into the patient's mouth* **2.** the act of starting a new process

**introitus** /ɪnˈtrəʊɪtəs/ *noun* an opening into any hollow organ or canal

**introjection** /ˌɪntrəʊˈdʒekʃən/ *noun* a person's unconscious adoption of the attitudes or values of another person whom he or she wants to impress

**introspection** /ˌɪntrəˈspekʃən/ *noun* a detailed and sometimes obsessive mental self-examination of feelings, thoughts and motives

**introversion** /ˌɪntrəˈvɜːʃ(ə)n/ *noun* a condition in which a person is excessively interested in himself or herself and his or her own mental state. Compare **extroversion**

**introvert** /ˈɪntrəvɜːt/ *noun* a person who thinks only about himself or herself and his or her own mental state. Compare **extrovert**

**introverted** /ˈɪntrəʊˌvɜːtɪd/ *adjective* referring to someone who thinks only about himself or herself

**intubate** /ˈɪntjuːbeɪt/ *verb* to insert a tube into any organ or part of the body. Also called **catheterise**

**intubation** /ˌɪntjuːˈbeɪʃ(ə)n/ *noun* the therapeutic insertion of a tube into the larynx through the glottis to allow the passage of air. Also called **catheterisation**

**intumescence** /ˌɪntjuːˈmes(ə)ns/ *noun* the swelling of an organ

**intussusception** /ˌɪntəsəˈsepʃən/ *noun* a condition in which part of the gastrointestinal tract becomes folded down inside the part beneath it, causing an obstruction and strangulation of the folded part

**inunction** /ɪnˈʌŋkʃən/ *noun* **1.** the act of rubbing an ointment into the skin so that the medicine in it is absorbed **2.** an ointment which is rubbed into the skin

**in utero** /ˌɪn ˈjuːtərəʊ/ *adverb, adjective* in, or while still inside, a woman's womb

**invade** /ɪnˈveɪd/ *verb* to enter and spread gradually throughout a part of the body, e.g. the entry of a microorganism that causes disease

**invagination** /ɪnˌvædʒɪˈneɪʃ(ə)n/ *noun* **1.** same as **intussusception 2.** the surgical treatment of hernia, in which a sheath of tissue is made to cover the opening

**invalid** /ˈɪnvəlɪd/ (*dated*) *noun* someone who has had an illness and has not fully recovered from it or who has been permanently disabled ■ *adjective* weak or disabled

**invalidity** /ˌɪnvəˈlɪdɪti/ *noun* the condition of being disabled

**invasion** /ɪnˈveɪʒ(ə)n/ *noun* the entry of bacteria into a body, or the first attack of a disease

**invasive** /ɪnˈveɪsɪv/ *adjective* **1.** referring to cancer which tends to spread throughout the body **2.** referring to an inspection or treatment which involves entering the body by making an incision. ◊ **non-invasive**

**inverse care law** /ˌɪnvɜːs ˈkeə lɔː/ *noun* the idea that the people who most need care and services are least likely or able to access them

**inversion** /ɪnˈvɜːʃ(ə)n/ *noun* the fact of being turned towards the inside ○ *inversion of the foot* See illustration at **ANATOMICAL TERMS** in Supplement □ **inversion of the uterus** a condition in which the top part of the uterus touches the cervix, as if it were inside out, which may happen after childbirth

**invertase** /ɪnˈvɜːteɪz/ *noun* an enzyme in the intestine which splits sucrose

**investigation** /ɪnˌvestɪˈɡeɪʃ(ə)n/ *noun* an examination to find out the cause of something which has happened ○ *The Health Authority ordered an investigation into how the drugs were stolen.*

**investigative surgery** /ɪnˌvestɪɡətɪv ˈsɜːdʒəri/ *noun* surgery to investigate the cause of a condition

**in vitro** /ɪn ˈviːtrəʊ/ *adjective, adverb* a Latin phrase meaning 'in a glass', i.e. in a test tube or similar container used in a laboratory □ **in vitro activity**, **in vitro experiment** experiment which takes place in the laboratory

**in vitro fertilisation** /ɪn ˌviːtrəʊ ˌfɜːtəlaɪˈzeɪʃ(ə)n/ *noun* the fertilisation of an ovum in the laboratory. ◊ **test-tube baby**. Abbr **IVF**

**in vivo** *adjective, adverb* a Latin phrase meaning 'in living tissue', i.e. referring to an experiment which takes place on the living body

**in vivo experiment** /ɪn ˌviːvəʊ ɪkˈsperɪmənt/ *noun* an experiment on a living body, e.g. that of an animal

**involucrum** /ˌɪnvəˈluːkrəm/ *noun* a covering of new bone which forms over diseased bone

**involuntary** /ɪnˈvɒlənt(ə)ri/ *adjective* done automatically, without any conscious thought or decision-making being involved ○ *Patients are advised not to eat or drink, to reduce the risk of involuntary vomiting while on the operating table.*

**involuntary action** /ɪnˌvɒlənt(ə)ri ˈækʃən/ *noun* an action which someone does without thinking or making a conscious decision

**involuntary muscle** /ɪnˌvɒlənt(ə)ri ˈmʌs(ə)l/ *noun* a muscle supplied by the autonomic nervous system, and therefore not under voluntary control, e.g. the muscle which activates a vital organ such as the heart

**involution** /ˌɪnvəˈluːʃ(ə)n/ *noun* **1.** the return of an organ to its usual size, e.g. the shrinking of the uterus after childbirth **2.** a period of decline of organs which sets in after middle age

**involutional** /ˌɪnvəˈluːʃ(ə)n(ə)l/ *adjective* referring to involution

**involutional melancholia** /ɪnvə ˌluːʃ(ə)n(ə)l melənˈkəʊliə/ *noun* a depression

which occurs in people, mainly women, after middle age, probably caused by a change of endocrine secretions

**iodine** /ˈaɪədiːn/ *noun* a chemical element which is essential to the body, especially to the functioning of the thyroid gland (NOTE: Lack of iodine in the diet can cause goitre. The chemical symbol is I.)

**IOL** *abbr* intraocular lens

**ion** /ˈaɪən/ *noun* an atom that has an electric charge (NOTE: Ions with a positive charge are called cations and those with a negative charge are called anions.)

COMMENT: It is believed that living organisms, including human beings, react to the presence of ionised particles in the atmosphere. Hot dry winds contain a higher proportion of positive ions than usual and these winds cause headaches and other illnesses. If negative ionised air is introduced into an air-conditioning system, the incidence of headaches and nausea among people working in the building may be reduced.

**ionise** /ˈaɪənaɪz/, **ionize** *verb* to give an atom an electric charge

**ioniser** /ˈaɪənaɪzə/, **ionizer** *noun* a machine that increases the amount of negative ions in the atmosphere of a room, so counteracting the effect of positive ions

**ionotherapy** /aɪˌɒnəˈθerəpi/ *noun* treatment by ions introduced into the body via an electric current

**iontophoresis** /aɪˌɒntəʊfəˈriːsɪs/ *noun* the movement of ions through a biological material when an electric current passes through it

**IOUS** *abbr* intraoperative ultrasound

**IPAV** *abbr* intermittent positive airway ventilation. ◊ **positive pressure ventilation**

**ipecacuanha** /ˌɪpɪkækjuˈænə/ *noun* a drug made from the root of an American plant, used as a treatment for coughs, and also as an emetic (NOTE: The US term is **ipecac**.)

**IP joint** /ˌaɪ ˈpiː dʒɔɪnt/ *noun* same as **interphalangeal joint**

**IPPV** *abbr* intermittent positive pressure ventilation. ◊ **positive pressure ventilation**

**ipratropium** /ˌaɪprəˈtrəʊpiəm/, **ipratropium bromide** /ˌaɪprəˌtrəʊpiəm ˈbrəʊmaɪd/ *noun* a drug which helps to relax muscles in the airways, used in the treatment of conditions such as asthma, bronchitis and emphysema

**ipsilateral** /ˌɪpsɪˈlætərəl/ *adjective* located on or affecting the same side of the body. Also called **homolateral**. Opposite **contralateral**

**IQ** *abbr* intelligence quotient

**IRDS** *abbr* infant respiratory distress syndrome

**irid-** /ɪrɪd/ *prefix* referring to the iris

**iridectomy** /ˌɪrɪˈdektəmi/ *noun* the surgical removal of part of the iris

**iridencleisis** /ˌɪrɪdenˈklaɪsɪs/ *noun* an operation to treat glaucoma, where part of the iris is used as a drainage channel through a hole in the conjunctiva

**iridocyclitis** /ˌɪrɪdəʊsɪˈklaɪtɪs/ *noun* inflammation of the iris and the tissues which surround it

**iridodialysis** /ˌɪrɪdəʊdaɪˈæləsɪs/ *noun* the separation of the iris from its insertion

**iridoplegia** /ˌɪrɪdəʊˈpliːdʒə/ *noun* paralysis of the iris

**iridoptosis** /ˌɪrɪdəʊˈtəʊsɪs/ *noun* the pushing forward of the iris through a wound in the cornea

**iridotomy** /ˌɪrɪˈdɒtəmi/ *noun* a surgical incision into the iris

**iris** /ˈaɪrɪs/ *noun* a coloured ring in the eye, with the pupil at its centre. See illustration at EYE in Supplement

COMMENT: The iris acts like the aperture in a camera shutter, opening and closing to allow more or less light through the pupil into the eye.

**iritis** /aɪˈraɪtɪs/ *noun* inflammation of the iris

**iron** /ˈaɪən/ *noun* **1.** a chemical element essential to the body, present in foods such as liver and eggs **2.** a common grey metal (NOTE: The chemical symbol is **Fe**.)

COMMENT: Iron is an essential part of the red pigment in red blood cells. Lack of iron in haemoglobin results in iron-deficiency anaemia. Storage of too much iron in the body results in haemochromatosis.

**iron-deficiency anaemia** /ˌaɪən dɪˈfɪʃ(ə)nsi əˌniːmiə/ *noun* anaemia caused by a lack of iron in red blood cells

**iron lung** /ˌaɪən ˈlʌŋ/ *noun* same as **Drinker respirator**

**irradiation** /ɪˌreɪdɪˈeɪʃ(ə)n/ *noun* **1.** the process of spreading from a centre, as e.g., nerve impulses do **2.** the use of radiation to treat people or to kill bacteria in food

**irreducible hernia** /ɪrɪˌdjuːsəb(ə)l ˈhɜːniə/ *noun* a hernia where the organ cannot be returned to its usual position

**irregular** /ɪˈreɡjʊlə/ *adjective* not regular or normal ○ *The patient's breathing was irregular.* ○ *The nurse noted that the patient had developed an irregular pulse.* ○ *He has irregular bowel movements.*

**irrigate** /ˈɪrɪɡeɪt/ *verb* to wash out a cavity in the body

**irrigation** /ˌɪrɪˈɡeɪʃ(ə)n/ *noun* the washing out of a cavity in the body

**irritability** /ˌɪrɪtəˈbɪlɪti/ *noun* the state of being irritable

**irritable** /ˈɪrɪtəb(ə)l/ *adjective* **1.** easily able to become inflamed and painful **2.** feeling annoyed and impatient

**irritable bowel syndrome** /ˌɪrɪtəb(ə)l ˈbaʊəl ˌsɪndrəʊm/ *noun* ♦ **mucous colitis**. Abbr **IBS**

**irritable colon** /ˌɪrɪtəb(ə)l ˈkəʊlɒn/ *noun* ♦ **mucous colitis**

**irritable hip** /ˌɪrɪtəb(ə)l ˈhɪp/ *noun* a condition of pain in the hip which is caused by swelling of the synovium. Treatment involves bed rest, traction and anti-inflammatory drugs.

**irritant** /ˈɪrɪt(ə)nt/ *noun* a substance which can irritate

**irritant dermatitis** /ˌɪrɪt(ə)nt ˌdɜːmə ˈtaɪtɪs/ *noun* same as **contact dermatitis**

**irritate** /ˈɪrɪteɪt/ *verb* to cause a painful reaction in part of the body, especially to make it inflamed ○ *Some types of wool can irritate the skin.*

**irritation** /ˌɪrɪˈteɪʃ(ə)n/ *noun* a feeling of being irritated ○ *an irritation caused by the ointment*

**ISC** *abbr* intermittent self-catheterisation

**isch-** /ɪsk/ *prefix* too little

**ischaemia** /ɪˈskiːmiə/ *noun* a deficient blood supply to a part of the body

**ischaemic** /ɪˈskiːmɪk/ *adjective* lacking in blood

'…the term stroke does not refer to a single pathological entity. Stroke may be haemorrhagic or ischaemic: the latter is usually caused by thrombosis or embolism' [*British Journal of Hospital Medicine*]

**ischaemic heart disease** /ɪˌskiːmɪk ˈhɑːt dɪˌziːz/ *noun* a disease of the heart caused by a failure in the blood supply, as in coronary thrombosis. Abbr **IHD**

**ischi-** /ɪski/ *prefix* same as **ischio-** (*used before vowels*)

**ischia** /ˈɪskiə/ *plural of* **ischium**

**ischial** /ˈɪskiəl/ *adjective* referring to the ischium or hip joint

**ischial tuberosity** /ˌɪskiəl ˌtjuːbəˈrɒsɪti/ *noun* a lump of bone forming the ring of the ischium

**ischio-** /ɪskiəʊ/ *prefix* referring to the ischium

**ischiocavernosus muscle** /ˌɪskiəʊkævə ˈnəʊsəs ˌmʌs(ə)l/ *noun* a muscle along one side of the perineum

**ischiorectal** /ˌɪskiəʊˈrekt(ə)l/ *adjective* referring to both the ischium and the rectum

**ischiorectal abscess** /ˌɪskiəʊˌrekt(ə)l ˈæbses/ *noun* an abscess which forms in fat cells between the anus and the ischium

**ischiorectal fossa** /ˌɪskiəʊˌrekt(ə)l ˈfɒsə/ *noun* a space on either side of the lower end of the rectum and anal canal

**ischium** /ˈɪskiəm/ *noun* the lower part of the hip bone in the pelvis. See illustration at PELVIS in Supplement (NOTE: The plural is **ischia**.)

**Ishihara colour charts** /ˌɪʃɪhɑːrə ˈkʌlə ˌtʃɑːts/ *plural noun* charts used in a test for colour vision in which numbers or letters are shown in dots of primary colours with dots of other colours around them. People with normal colour vision can see them, but people who are colour-blind cannot.

**Ishihara test** /ˌɪʃɪˈhɑːrə test/ *noun* a test using **Ishihara colour charts**

**islets of Langerhans** /ˌaɪləts əv ˈlæŋəhæns/, **islands of Langerhans** /ˌaɪləndz əv ˈlæŋəhænz/, **islet cells** /ˈaɪlət selz/ *plural noun* groups of cells in the pancreas which secrete the hormones glucagon, insulin and gastrin [Described 1869. After Paul Langerhans (1847–88), Professor of Pathological Anatomy at Freiburg, Germany.]

**iso-** /aɪsəʊ/ *prefix* equal

**isoantibody** /ˌaɪsəʊˈæntɪbɒdi/ *noun* an antibody which forms in one person as a reaction to antigens from another person (NOTE: The plural is **isoantibodies**.)

**isograft** /ˈaɪsəʊɡrɑːft/ *noun* a graft of tissue from an identical twin. Also called **syngraft**

**isoimmunisation** /ˌaɪsəʊˌɪmjunaɪˈzeɪʃ(ə)n/, **isoimmunization** *noun* immunisation of a person with antigens derived from another person

**isolate** /ˈaɪsəleɪt/ *verb* **1.** to keep one person apart from others because he or she has a dangerous infectious disease **2.** to identify a single virus, bacterium or other pathogen among many ○ *Scientists have been able to isolate the virus which causes Legionnaires' disease.* ○ *Candida is easily isolated from the mouths of healthy adults.*

**isolation** /ˌaɪsəˈleɪʃ(ə)n/ *noun* the separation of a person, especially one with an infectious disease, from others

**isolation ward** /ˌaɪsəˈleɪʃ(ə)n wɔːd/ *noun* a special ward where people who have dangerous infectious diseases can be kept isolated from others

**isolator** /ˈaɪsəleɪtə/ *noun* **1.** a large clear plastic bag in which a person can be nursed, or operated on, in a sterile environment **2.** a room or piece of equipment which keeps people or substances separated from others which may contaminate them ○ *an isolator stretcher* ○ *an isolator cabinet*

**isoleucine** /aɪsəʊˈluːsiːn/ *noun* an essential amino acid

**isometric** /ˌaɪsəʊˈmetrɪk/ *adjective* **1.** involving equal measurement ○ *an isometric view of the system* **2.** referring to muscle contraction in which tension occurs with very little shortening of muscle fibres **3.** referring to exercises in which the muscles are put under tension but not contracted

**isometrics** /ˌaɪsəʊˈmetrɪks/ *plural noun* exercises to strengthen the muscles, in which the muscles contract but do not shorten

**isoniazid** /ˌaɪsəˈnaɪəzɪd/ *noun* a colourless crystalline compound that is used in the treatment of tuberculosis. Abbr **INH**

**isoprenaline** /ˌaɪsəʊˈprenəliːn/, **isoproterenol** *noun* a drug that relieves asthma by widening the bronchial tubes in the lungs

**isosorbide dinitrate** /ˌaɪsəʊˌsɔːbaɪd daɪˈnaɪtreɪt/ *noun* a compound which causes widening or relaxation of the blood vessels, used in the treatment of angina pectoris

**isotonic** /ˌaɪsəʊˈtɒnɪk/ *adjective* referring to a solution, e.g. a saline drip, which has the same osmotic pressure as blood serum and which can therefore be passed directly into the body. Compare **hypertonic, hypotonic**

**isotonicity** /ˌaɪsətɒˈnɪsɪti/ *noun* the equal osmotic pressure of two or more solutions

**isotonic solution** /ˌaɪsəʊtɒnɪk səˈluːʃ(ə)n/ *noun* a solution which has the same osmotic pressure as blood serum, or as another liquid it is compared with

**isotope** /ˈaɪsətəʊp/ *noun* a form of a chemical element which has the same chemical properties as other forms but a different atomic mass

**isotretinoin** /ˌaɪsəʊtreˈtɪnɔɪn/ *noun* a drug used in the treatment of severe acne and several other skin diseases

**ispaghula** /ˌɪspəˈɡuːlə/, **ispaghula husk** /ˌɪspəˈɡuːlə hʌsk/ *noun* a natural dietary fibre used to treat constipation, diverticulitis and irritable bowel syndrome

**ISS** *abbr* injury scoring system

**isthmus** /ˈɪsməs/ *noun* **1.** a short narrow canal or cavity **2.** a narrow band of tissue joining two larger masses of similar tissue, e.g. the section in the centre of the thyroid gland, which joins the two lobes (NOTE: The plural is **isthmi** or **isthmuses**.)

**itch** /ɪtʃ/ *noun* **1.** an irritated place on the skin which makes a person want to scratch **2. the itch** same as **scabies** (*informal*) ■ *verb* to produce an irritating sensation, making someone want to scratch

**itching** /ˈɪtʃɪŋ/ *noun* same as **pruritus**

**itchy** /ˈɪtʃi/ *adjective* making a person want to scratch ○ *The main symptom of the disease is an itchy red rash.*

**-itis** /aɪtɪs/ *suffix* inflammation

**ITU** *abbr* intensive therapy unit

**IU** *abbr* international unit

**IUCD** *abbr* intrauterine contraceptive device

**IUD** *abbr* **1.** intrauterine death **2.** intrauterine device

**IUS** *abbr* intrauterine system

**IV** *abbr* intravenous

**IVF** *abbr* in vitro fertilisation

**IVP** *abbr* intravenous pyelogram

**IVU** *abbr* intravenous urography

# J

**J** /dʒeɪ/ *abbr* joule

**jab** /dʒæb/ *noun* an injection or inoculation (*informal*) ○ *a tetanus jab*

**Jacksonian epilepsy** /dʒæk،səʊnɪən ˈepɪ↓lepsi/ *noun* a form of epilepsy in which the jerking movements start in one part of the body before spreading to others [Described 1863. After John Hughlings Jackson (1835–1911), British neurologist.]

**Jacquemier's sign** /ˈdʒækəmɪəz ،saɪn/ *noun* a sign of early pregnancy in which the vaginal mucosa becomes slightly blue due to an increased amount of blood in the arteries [After Jean Marie Jacquemier (1806–79), French obstetrician]

**jactitation** /،dʒæktɪˈteɪʃ(ə)n/ *noun* the action of constantly moving the body around in a restless way, especially because of mental illness

**jag** /dʒæg/ *noun* in Scotland, an injection or inoculation (*informal*)

**jargon** /ˈdʒɑːgən/ *noun* **1.** the words used by people who have a particular area of knowledge, which are usually only understood by those people ○ *medical jargon* **2.** a stream of words that makes no sense, produced by someone with aphasia or a severe mental disorder

**jaundice** /ˈdʒɔːndɪs/ *noun* a condition in which there is an excess of bile pigment in the blood, and in which the pigment is deposited in the skin and the whites of the eyes, which have a yellow colour. Also called **icterus**

COMMENT: Jaundice can have many causes, usually relating to the liver: the most common are blockage of the bile ducts by gallstones or by disease of the liver and Weil's disease.

**jaw** /dʒɔː/ *noun* the bones in the face which hold the teeth and form the mouth ○ *He fell down and broke his jaw.* ○ *The punch on his mouth broke his jaw.*

COMMENT: The jaw has two parts, the upper (the maxillae) being fixed parts of the skull, and the lower (the mandible) being attached to the skull with a hinge so that it can move up and down.

**jawbone** /ˈdʒɔːbəʊn/ *noun* one of the bones which form the jaw, especially the lower jaw or mandible

**jejun-** /dʒɪdʒuːn/ *prefix* same as **jejuno-** (*used before vowels*)

**jejunal** /dʒɪˈdʒuːn(ə)l/ *adjective* referring to the jejunum

**jejunal ulcer** /dʒɪ،dʒuːn(ə)l ˈʌlsə/ *noun* an ulcer in the jejunum

**jejunectomy** /،dʒɪdʒuːˈnektəmi/ *noun* a surgical operation to remove all or part of the jejunum (NOTE: The plural is **jejunectomies**.)

**jejuno-** /dʒiːdʒuːnəʊ/ *prefix* referring to the jejunum

**jejunoileostomy** /dʒɪ،dʒuːnəʊ،ɪliˈɒstəmi/ *noun* a surgical operation to make an artificial link between the jejunum and the ileum (NOTE: The plural is **jejunoileostomies**.)

**jejunostomy** /،dʒɪdʒuːˈnɒstəmi/ *noun* a surgical operation to make an artificial passage to the jejunum through the wall of the abdomen (NOTE: The plural is **jejunostomies**.)

**jejunotomy** /،dʒɪdʒuːˈnɒtəmi/ *noun* a surgical operation to cut into the jejunum (NOTE: The plural is **jejunotomies**.)

**jejunum** /dʒɪˈdʒuːnəm/ *noun* the part of the small intestine between the duodenum and the ileum, about 2 metres long. See illustration at DIGESTIVE SYSTEM in Supplement

**jerk** /dʒɜːk/ *noun* a sudden movement of part of the body which indicates that the local reflex arc is intact ■ *verb* to make sudden movements, or cause something to make sudden movements ○ *In some forms of epilepsy the limbs jerk.*

**jet lag** /ˈdʒet læg/ *noun* a condition suffered by people who travel long distances in planes, caused by rapid changes in time zones which affect sleep patterns and meal times and thus interfere with the body's metabolism ○ *We had jet lag when we flew from Australia.*

**jet-lagged** /ˈdʒet lægd/ *adjective* experiencing jet lag ○ *jet-lagged travellers* ○ *We were jet-lagged for a week.*

**joint** /dʒɔɪnt/ *noun* a structure at a point where two or more bones join, especially one which allows movement of the bones ○ *The elbow is a joint in the arm.* ○ *Arthritis is accompanied by stiffness in the joints.* ♦ **Charcot's**

**joint** (NOTE: For other terms referring to joints, see words beginning with **arthr-, arthro-**.)

**joint-breaker fever** /ˈdʒɔɪnt ˌbreɪkə ˌfiːvə/ *noun* same as **o'nyong-nyong fever**

**joint capsule** /ˈdʒɔɪnt ˌkæpsjuːl/ *noun* white fibrous tissue which surrounds and holds a joint together. See illustration at SYNOVIAL JOINT in Supplement

**joint investment plan** /ˌdʒɔɪnt ɪnˈvestmənt plæn/ *noun* a plan that health and social services draw up together for specific areas of care

**joint mouse** /ˈdʒɔɪnt maʊs/ *plural noun* a loose piece of bone or cartilage in the knee joint, making the joint lock

**joule** /dʒuːl/ *noun* the SI unit of measurement of work or energy. 4.184 joules equals one calorie. Symbol **J**

**jugular** /ˈdʒʌɡjʊlə/ *adjective* referring to the throat or neck ■ *noun* same as **jugular vein**

COMMENT: There are three jugular veins on each side: the **internal jugular** is large and leads to the brachiocephalic vein, the **external jugular** is smaller and leads to the subclavian vein and the **anterior jugular** is the smallest.

**jugular nerve** /ˈdʒʌɡjʊlə nɜːv/ *noun* one of the nerves in the neck

**jugular trunk** /ˈdʒʌɡjʊlə trʌŋk/ *noun* a terminal lymph vessel in the neck, draining into the subclavian vein

**jugular vein** /ˈdʒʌɡjʊlə veɪn/ *noun* one of the veins which pass down either side of the neck. Also called **jugular**

**juice** /dʒuːs/ *noun* **1.** liquid from a fruit or vegetable ○ *a glass of orange juice* or *tomato juice* **2.** a natural fluid of the body. ♦ **gastric juice**

**jumper's knee** /ˌdʒʌmpəz ˈniː/ *noun* a painful condition suffered by athletes and dancers in which inflammation develops in the knee joint

**junction** /ˈdʒʌŋkʃən/ *noun* a joining point

**junior doctor** /ˌdʒuːniə ˈdɒktə/ *noun* a doctor who is completing his or her training in hospital

**junk food** /ˈdʒʌŋk fuːd/ *noun* food of little nutritional value, e.g. high-fat processed snacks, eaten between or instead of meals

**juvenile** /ˈdʒuːvənaɪl/ *adjective* relating to or affecting children or adolescents

**juxta-** /dʒʌkstə/ *prefix* beside or near

**juxta-articular** /ˌdʒʌkstə ɑːˈtɪkjʊlə/ *adjective* occurring near a joint

**juxtaposition** /ˌdʒʌkstəpəˈzɪʃ(ə)n/ *noun* the placing of two or more things side by side so as to make their similarities or differences more obvious

# K

**k** *symbol* kilo-

**Kahn test** /ˈkɑːn test/ *noun* a test of blood serum to diagnose syphilis [Described 1922. After Reuben Leon Kahn, Lithuanian-born serologist who worked in the USA.]

**kala-azar** /ˌkɑːlə əˈzɑː/ *noun* an often fatal form of leishmaniasis caused by the infection of the intestines and internal organs by a parasite, *Leishmania*, spread by flies. Symptoms are fever, anaemia, general wasting of the body and swelling of the spleen and liver.

**kalium** /ˈkeɪliəm/ *noun* same as **potassium**

**kaolin** /ˈkeɪəlɪn/ *noun* a fine soft clay used in the making of medical preparations, especially for the treatment of diarrhoea

**Kaposi's sarcoma** /kəˌpəʊziz sɑːˈkəʊmə/ *noun* a cancer which takes the form of many haemorrhagic nodes affecting the skin, especially on the extremities [Described 1872. After Moritz Kohn Karposi (1837–1902), Professor of Dermatology at Vienna, Austria.]

COMMENT: Formerly a relatively rare disease, found mainly in tropical countries, Kaposi's sarcoma is now more common as it is one of the diseases associated with AIDS.

**Kartagener's syndrome** /ˌkɑːtəˈdʒiːnəz ˌsɪndrəʊm/ *noun* a hereditary condition in which all the organs in the chest and abdomen are positioned on the opposite side from the usual one, i.e. the heart and stomach are on the right

**karyo-** /kæriəʊ/ *prefix* relating to a cell nucleus

**karyotype** /ˈkæriəʊtaɪp/ *noun* the chromosome complement of a cell, shown as a diagram or as a set of letters and numbers

**Kawasaki disease** /ˌkɑːwəˈsɑːkiz dɪˌziːz/ *noun* a retrovirus infection that often occurs in small children and causes a high temperature, rash, reddened eyes, peeling skin and swollen lymph nodes

**Kayser-Fleischer ring** /ˌkaɪzə ˈflaɪʃə ˌrɪŋ/ *noun* a brown ring on the outer edge of the cornea, which is a diagnostic sign of hepatolenticular degeneration [Described 1902 by Kayser, 1903 by Fleischer. Bernard Kayser (1869–

1954), German ophthalmologist; Bruno Richard Fleischer (1848–1904), German physician.]

**kcal** *abbr* kilocalorie

**Kegel exercises** /ˈkeɪg(ə)l ˌeksəsaɪzɪz/ *plural noun* exercises which strengthen the muscles of the pelvic floor in women and help to prevent any accidental leakage of urine when they cough, sneeze or lift things

**Keller's operation** /ˈkeləz ɒpəˌreɪʃ(ə)n/ *noun* a surgical operation on the big toe to remove a bunion or to correct an ankylosed joint [Described 1904. After William Lordan Keller (1874–1959), US surgeon.]

**keloid** /ˈkiːlɔɪd/ *noun* an excessive amount of scar tissue at the site of a skin injury

**kerat-** /kerət/ *prefix* same as **kerato-** (*used before vowels*)

**keratalgia** /ˌkerəˈtældʒiə/ *noun* pain felt in the cornea

**keratectasia** /ˌkerətekˈteɪziə/ *noun* a condition in which the cornea bulges

**keratectomy** /ˌkerəˈtektəmi/ *noun* a surgical operation to remove the whole or part of the cornea (NOTE: The plural is **keratectomies**.)

**keratic** /kəˈrætɪk/ *adjective* **1.** relating to horny tissue or to keratin **2.** relating to the cornea

**keratin** /ˈkerətɪn/ *noun* a protein found in horny tissue such as fingernails, hair or the outer surface of the skin

**keratinisation** /ˌkerətɪnaɪˈzeɪʃ(ə)n/, **keratinization** *noun* the appearance of horny characteristics in tissue. Also called **cornification**

**keratinise** /ˈkerətɪnaɪz/, kəˈrætɪnaɪz/, **keratinize** *verb* to convert something into keratin or into horny tissue (NOTE: **keratinising – keratinised**)

**keratinocyte** /ˌkerəˈtɪnəʊsaɪt/ *noun* a cell which produces keratin

**keratitis** /ˌkerəˈtaɪtɪs/ *noun* inflammation of the cornea

**kerato-** /kerətəʊ/ *prefix* referring to horn, horny tissue or the cornea

**keratoacanthoma** /ˌkerətəʊˌækənˈθəʊmə/ *noun* a type of benign skin tumour which disappears after a few months (NOTE: The plural is **keratoacanthomas** or **keratoacanthomata**.)

**keratoconjunctivitis** /ˌkerətəʊkən ˌdʒʌŋktɪˈvaɪtɪs/ *noun* inflammation of the cornea with conjunctivitis

**keratoconus** /ˌkerətəʊˈkəʊnəs/ *noun* a cone-shaped lump on the cornea

**keratoglobus** /ˌkerətəʊˈgləʊbəs/ *noun* swelling of the eyeball

**keratoma** /ˌkerəˈtəʊmə/ *noun* a hard thickened growth due to hypertrophy of the horny zone of the skin (NOTE: The plural is **keratomas** or **keratomata**.)

**keratomalacia** /ˌkerətəʊməˈleɪʃə/ *noun* **1.** a softening of the cornea frequently caused by Vitamin A deficiency **2.** softening of the horny layer of the skin

**keratome** /ˈkerətəʊm/ *noun* a surgical knife used for operations on the cornea

**keratometer** /ˌkerəˈtɒmɪtə/ *noun* an instrument for measuring the curvature of the cornea

**keratometry** /ˌkerəˈtɒmɪtri/ *noun* the process of measuring the curvature of the cornea

**keratopathy** /ˌkerəˈtɒpəθi/ *noun* any non-inflammatory disorder of the cornea (NOTE: The plural is **keratopathies**.)

**keratoplasty** /ˈkerətəplæsti/ *noun* a surgical operation to graft corneal tissue from a donor in place of diseased tissue (NOTE: The plural is **keratoplasties**.)

**keratoprosthesis** /ˌkerətəʊprɒsˈθiːsɪs/ *noun* **1.** a surgical operation to replace the central area of a cornea with clear plastic, when it has become opaque **2.** a piece of clear plastic put into the cornea (NOTE: The plural is **keratoprostheses**.)

**keratoscope** /ˈkerətəskəʊp/ *noun* an instrument for examining the cornea to see if it has an unusual curvature. Also called **Placido's disc**

**keratosis** /ˌkerəˈtəʊsɪs/ *noun* a lesion of the skin (NOTE: The plural is **keratoses**.)

**keratotomy** /ˌkerəˈtɒtəmi/ *noun* a surgical operation to make a cut in the cornea, the first step in many intraocular operations (NOTE: The plural is **keratotomies**.)

**kerion** /ˈkɪərɪɒn/ *noun* a painful soft mass, usually on the scalp, caused by ringworm

**kernicterus** /kəˈnɪktərəs/ *noun* yellow pigmentation of the basal ganglia and other nerve cells in the spinal cord and brain, found in children with icterus

**Kernig's sign** /ˈkɜːnɪgz saɪn/ *noun* a symptom of meningitis in which the knee cannot be straightened if the person is lying down with the thigh brought up against the abdomen [Described 1882. After Vladimir Mikhailovich Kernig (1840–1917), Russian neurologist.]

**ketamine** /ˈketəmiːn/ *noun* a white crystalline powder that is a general anaesthetic, used in human and veterinary medicine

**ketoacidosis** /ˌkiːtəʊˌæsɪˈdəʊsɪs/ *noun* an accumulation of ketone bodies in tissue in diabetes, causing acidosis

**ketoconazole** /ˌkiːtəʊˈkɒnəzəʊl/ *noun* a drug which is effective against a wide range of fungal infections such as cryptococcosis and thrush

**ketogenesis** /ˌkiːtəʊˈdʒenəsɪs/ *noun* the production of ketone bodies

**ketogenic** /ˌkiːtəʊˈdʒenɪk/ *adjective* forming ketone bodies

**ketogenic diet** /ˌkiːtəʊdʒenɪk ˈdaɪət/ *noun* a diet with a high fat content, producing ketosis

**ketonaemia** /ˌkiːtəʊˈniːmiə/ *noun* a morbid state in which ketone bodies exist in the blood

**ketone** /ˈkiːtəʊn/ *noun* a chemical compound produced when glucose is unavailable for use as energy, as in untreated diabetes, and fats are used instead, leading to ketosis

**ketone bodies** /ˈkiːtəʊn ˌbɒdiz/ *plural noun* ketone compounds formed from fatty acids

**ketone group** /ˈkiːtəʊn gruːp/ *noun* a chemical group characteristic of ketones, with carbon atoms doubly bonded to an oxygen atom and to the carbon atoms of two other organic groups

**ketonuria** /ˌkiːtəʊˈnjʊəriə/ *noun* a state in which ketone bodies are excreted in the urine

**ketoprofen** /ˌkiːtəʊˈprəʊfən/ *noun* an anti-inflammatory drug used in the treatment of rheumatoid arthritis and osteoarthritis

**ketosis** /kiːˈtəʊsɪs/ *noun* a state in which ketone bodies such as acetone and acetic acid accumulate in the tissues, a late complication of Type I diabetes mellitus

**ketosteroid** /ˌkiːtəʊˈstɪərɔɪd/ *noun* a steroid such as cortisone which contains a ketone group

**keyhole surgery** /ˈkiːhəʊl ˌsɜːdʒəri/ *noun* surgery carried out by inserting tiny surgical instruments through an endoscope (*informal*) Also called **laparoscopic surgery**

**kg** *abbr* kilogram

**kidney** /ˈkɪdni/ *noun* either of two organs situated in the lower part of the back on either side of the spine behind the abdomen, whose function is to maintain the usual concentrations of the main constituents of blood, passing the waste matter into the urine. See illustration at KIDNEY in Supplement

COMMENT: A kidney is formed of an outer cortex and an inner medulla. The nephrons which run from the cortex into the medulla filter the blood and form urine. The urine is passed through the ureters into the bladder. Sudden sharp pain in back of the abdomen, going downwards, is an indication of a kidney stone passing into the ureter.

**kidney dialysis** /ˈkɪdni daɪˌæləsɪs/ *noun* the process of removing waste matter from blood by passing it through a kidney machine. Also called **haemodialysis**

**kidney donor** /'kɪdni ˌdəʊnə/ *noun* a person who gives one of his or her kidneys as a transplant

**kidney failure** /'kɪdni ˌfeɪljə/ *noun* a situation in which the kidneys do not function properly

**kidney machine** /'kɪdni məˌʃiːn/ *noun* an apparatus through which blood is passed to be cleaned by dialysis if the person's kidneys have failed

**kidney stone** /'kɪdni stəʊn/ *noun* a hard mass of calcium like a little piece of stone which forms in the kidney

**kidney transplant** /'kɪdni ˌtrænsplɑːnt/ *noun* a surgical operation to give someone with a diseased or damaged kidney from another person

**kill** /kɪl/ *verb* to make someone or something die ○ *She was killed in a car crash.* ○ *Heart attacks kill more people every year.* ○ *Antibodies are created to kill bacteria.*

**killer** /'kɪlə/ *noun* a person or disease which kills ○ *In the winter, bronchitis is the killer of hundreds of senior citizens.* ○ *Virulent typhoid fever can be a killer disease.* ◊ **painkiller**

**killer cell** /'kɪlə sel/, **killer T cell** *noun* a type of immune cell that recognises and destroys cells that have specific antigens on their surface, e.g. virus-infected or cancerous cells

**Killian's operation** /'kɪliənz ɒpəˌreɪʃ(ə)n/ *noun* a surgical operation to clear the frontal sinus by curetting in which the incision is made in the eyebrow [After Gustav Killian (1860–1921), German laryngologist]

**kilo-** /kɪləʊ/ *prefix* one thousand (10³). Symbol **k**

**kilogram** /'kɪləgræm/ *noun* an SI unit of measurement of weight equal to 1 000 grams ○ *She weighs 62 kilos (62 kg).* Symbol **kg**

**kilojoule** /'kɪləʊdʒuːl/ *noun* an SI unit of measurement of energy or heat equal to 1 000 joules. Symbol **kJ**

**kilopascal** /'kɪləʊpæskəl/ *noun* an SI unit of measurement of pressure equal to 1 000 pascals. Symbol **kPa**

**Kimmelstiel-Wilson disease** /ˌkɪməlstiːl ˈwɪlsən dɪˌziːz/, **Kimmelstiel-Wilson syndrome** /ˌkɪməlstiːl ˈwɪlsən ˌsɪndrəʊm/ *noun* a form of nephrosclerosis found in people with diabetes [Described 1936. After Paul Kimmelstiel (1900–70), US pathologist; Clifford Wilson (1906–98), Professor of Medicine, London University, UK.]

**kin** /kɪn/ *noun* relatives or close members of the family

**kin-** /kɪn/ *prefix* same as **kine-** (*used before vowels*)

**kinaesthesia** /ˌkɪniːsˈθiːziə/ *noun* the fact of being aware of the movement and position of parts of the body (NOTE: The US spelling is **kinesthesia**.)

COMMENT: Kinaesthesia is the result of information from muscles and ligaments which is passed to the brain and which allows the brain to recognise movements, touch and weight.

**kinanaesthesia** /ˌkɪnænɪːsˈθiːziə/ *noun* the fact of not being able to sense the movement and position of parts of the body (NOTE: The US spelling is **kinanesthesia**.)

**kinase** /'kaɪneɪz/ *noun* an enzyme belonging to a large family of related substances that bind to the energy-providing molecule ATP and regulate functions such as cell division and signalling between cells

**kine-** /kɪni/ *prefix* movement

**kinematics** /ˌkɪnɪˈmætɪks/ *noun* the science of movement, especially of body movements

**kineplasty** /'kɪnɪplæsti/ *noun* an amputation in which the muscles of the stump of the amputated limb are used to operate an artificial limb (NOTE: The plural is **kineplasties**.)

**kinesi-** /kaɪniːsi/ *prefix* movement (NOTE: used before vowels)

**kinesiology** /ˌkaɪniːsiˈɒlədʒi/ *noun* the study of human movements, particularly with regard to their use in treatment

**kinesis** *noun* the movement of a cell in response to a stimulus. Compare **taxis**

**-kinesis** /kɪniːsɪs/ *suffix* **1.** activity or motion **2.** a change in the movement of a cell, though not in any particular direction. Examples are a change in its speed or in its turning behaviour.

**kinesitherapy** /ˌkaɪniːsiˈθerəpi/ *noun* therapy involving movement of parts of the body

**kinetic** /kɪˈnetɪk, kaɪˈnetɪk/ *adjective* relating to movement

**King's Fund** /'kɪŋz fʌnd/ *noun* a major independent health charity in London

**King's model** /'kɪŋz ˌmɒd(ə)l/ *noun* a model of nurse–patient relationships based on ten principles: interaction, perception, communication, transaction, role, stress, growth and development, time, self and space. Through an exchange of information nurses and patients work together to help individuals and groups attain, maintain and restore health.

**kinin** /'kaɪnɪn/ *noun* a polypeptide that makes blood vessels widen and smooth muscles contract

**Kirschner wire** /ˌkɜːʃ(ə)nə ˈwaɪə/, **Kirschner's wire** *noun* a wire attached to a bone and tightened to provide traction to a fracture [Described 1909. After Martin Kirschner (1879–1942), Professor of Surgery at Heidelberg, Germany.]

**kiss of life** /ˌkɪs əv ˈlaɪf/ *noun* same as **cardiopulmonary resuscitation** (*informal*)

**kJ** *abbr* kilojoule

**Klebsiella** /ˌklebsiˈelə/ *noun* a Gram-negative bacterium, one form of which, *Klebsiella pneumoniae,* can cause pneumonia

**Klebs-Loeffler bacillus** /ˌklebz ˈleflə bəˌsɪləs/ *noun* the bacterium which causes diphtheria, *Corynebacterium diphtheriae* [After Theodor Albrecht Klebs (1834–1913), bacteriologist in Zürich, Switzerland, and Chicago, USA; Friedrich August Loeffler (1852–1915), bacteriologist in Berlin, Germany]

**Kleihauer test** /ˈklaɪhaʊə test/, **Kleihauer-Betke test** *noun* a test used to check whether there has been any blood loss from a fetus to the mother across the placenta. It is usually done immediately after delivery.

**klepto-** /kleptəʊ/ *prefix* stealing or theft

**kleptomania** /ˌkleptəʊˈmeɪniə/ *noun* a form of mental disorder in which someone has a compulsive desire to steal things, even things of little value

**kleptomaniac** /ˌkleptəʊˈmeɪniæk/ *noun* a person who has a compulsive desire to steal

**Klinefelter's syndrome** /ˈklaɪnfeltəz ˌsɪndrəʊm/ *noun* a genetic disorder in which a male has an extra female chromosome, making an XXY set, giving sterility and partial female characteristics [Described 1942. After Harry Fitch Klinefelter Jr. (b. 1912), Associate Professor of Medicine, John Hopkins Medical School, Baltimore, USA.]

**Klumpke's paralysis** /ˌkluːmpkəz pəˈræləsɪs/ *noun* a form of paralysis due to an injury during birth, affecting the forearm and hand. Also called **Déjerine-Klumpke's syndrome** [Described 1885. After Augusta Klumpke (Madame Déjerine-Klumpke) (1859–1937), French neurologist, one of the first women to qualify in Paris in 1888.]

**knee** /niː/ *noun* a joint in the middle of the leg, joining the femur and the tibia (NOTE: For other terms referring to the knee, see **genu**.)

**kneecap** /ˈniːkæp/ *noun* same as **patella**

**knee jerk** /ˈniː dʒɜːk/ *noun* same as **patellar reflex**

**knee joint** /niː dʒɔɪnt/ *noun* a joint where the femur and the tibia are joined, covered by the kneecap

**knit** /nɪt/ *verb* (*of broken bones*) to join together again ○ *Broken bones take longer to knit in elderly people than in children.* (NOTE: **knitting – knitted – knit**)

**knock-knee** /ˌnɒk ˈniː/ *noun* a state in which the knees touch and the ankles are apart when a person is standing straight. Also called **genu valgum**

**knock-kneed** /ˌnɒk ˈniːd/ *adjective* referring to a person whose knees touch when he or she stands straight with feet slightly apart

**knock out** /ˌnɒk ˈaʊt/ *verb* to hit someone so hard that he or she is no longer conscious ○ *He was knocked out by a blow on the head.*

**knuckle** /ˈnʌk(ə)l/ *noun* the back of each joint on a person's hand

**Kocher manoeuvre** /ˈkɒkə məˌnuːvə/ *noun* a method for realigning a dislocated shoulder in which the arm is raised and a sudden change is made between inward and outward rotation of the head of the joint

**Koch's bacillus** /ˌkɒks bəˈsɪləs/ *noun* the bacterium which causes tuberculosis, *Mycobacterium tuberculosis* [Described 1882. After Robert Koch (1843–1910), Professor of Hygiene in Berlin, Germany, later Director of the Institute for Infectious Diseases. (Nobel Prize 1905).]

**Koch-Weeks bacillus** /ˌkɒk ˈwiːks bəˌsɪləs/ *noun* the bacillus which causes conjunctivitis

**Köhler's disease** /ˈkɜːləz dɪˌsiːz/ *noun* a degeneration of the navicular bone in children. Also called **scaphoiditis** [Described 1908 and 1926. After Alban Köhler (1874–1947), German radiologist.]

**koilonychia** /ˌkɔɪləʊˈnɪkiə/ *noun* a condition in which the fingernails are brittle and concave, caused by iron-deficiency anaemia

**Koplik's spots** /ˈkɒplɪks spɒts/ *plural noun* small white spots with a blue tinge surrounded by a red areola, found in the mouth in the early stages of measles [Described 1896. After Henry Koplik (1858–1927), US paediatrician.]

**Korotkoff's method** /ˈkɒrətkɒfs ˌmeθəd/ *noun* a method of finding a person's blood pressure by inflating a cuff around his or her upper arm to a pressure well above the systolic blood pressure and then gradually decreasing it

**Korsakoff's syndrome** /ˈkɔːsəkɒfs ˌsɪndrəʊm/ *noun* a condition, caused usually by chronic alcoholism or disorders in which there is a deficiency of vitamin B, in which a person's memory fails and he or she invents things which have not happened and is confused [Described 1887. After Sergei Sergeyevich Korsakoff (1854–1900), Russian psychiatrist.]

**kraurosis penis** /krɔːˌrəʊsɪs ˈpiːnɪs/ *noun* a condition in which the foreskin becomes dry and shrivelled

**kraurosis vulvae** /krɔːˌrəʊsɪs ˈvʌlvə/ *noun* a condition in which the vulva becomes thin and dry due to lack of oestrogen, found usually in elderly women

**Krause corpuscles** /ˈkraʊzə ˌkɔːpʌs(ə)lz/ *plural noun* encapsulated nerve endings in the mucous membrane of the mouth, nose, eyes and genitals [Described 1860. After Wilhelm Johann Friedrich Krause (1833–1910), German anatomist.]

**Krebs cycle** /ˈkrebz ˌsaɪk(ə)l/ *noun* same as **citric acid cycle** [Described 1937. After Sir Hans Adolf Krebs (1900–81), German biochemist who emigrated to England in 1934. Shared the Nobel prize for Medicine 1953 with F.A. Lipmann.]

**Krukenberg tumour** /ˈkruːkənbɜːg ˌtjuːmə/ *noun* a malignant tumour in the ovary secondary to a tumour in the stomach [After Friedrich Krukenberg (1871–1946), German gynaecologist]

**Kuntscher nail** /'kʌntʃə neɪl/, **Küntscher nail** *noun* a long steel nail used in operations to pin fractures of long bones, especially the femur, through the bone marrow [Described 1940. After Gerhard Küntscher (1900–72), German surgeon.]

**Kupffer's cells** /'kʊpfəz selz/, **Kupffer cells** *plural noun* large specialised liver cells which break down haemoglobin into bile [Described 1876. After Karl Wilhelm von Kupffer (1829–1902), German anatomist.]

**Kveim test** /'kvaɪm test/ *noun* a skin test to confirm the presence of sarcoidosis [After Morten Ansgar Kveim (b. 1892), Swedish physician]

**kwashiorkor** /ˌkwɒʃi'ɔːkɔː/ *noun* malnutrition of small children, mostly in tropical countries, causing anaemia, wasting of the body and swollen liver

**kypho-** /kaɪfəʊ/ *prefix* a hump

**kyphoscoliosis** /ˌkaɪfəʊˌskɒli'əʊsɪs/ *noun* a condition in which someone has both backward and lateral curvature of the spine

**kyphosis** /kaɪ'fəʊsɪs/ *noun* an excessive backward curvature of the top part of the spine (NOTE: The plural is **kyphoses**.)

**kyphotic** /kaɪ'fɒtɪk/ *adjective* referring to kyphosis

# L

**I, L** symbol **litre**

**lab** /læb/ *noun* same as **laboratory** (*informal*) ○ *The samples have been returned by the lab.* ○ *We'll send the specimens away for a lab test.*

**lab-** /leɪb/ *prefix* same as **labio-** (*used before vowels*)

**label** /ˈleɪb(ə)l/ *noun* a piece of paper or card attached to an object or person for identification ■ *verb* to attach a label to an object ○ *The bottle is labelled 'poison'.* (NOTE: **labelling – labelled**. The US spellings are **labeling – labeled**.)

**labia** /ˈleɪbiə/ plural of **labium**

**labial** /ˈleɪbiəl/ *adjective* referring to the lips or to labia

**labia majora** /ˌleɪbiə məˈdʒɔːrə/ *plural noun* two large fleshy folds at the outside edge of the vulva. See illustration at UROGENITAL SYSTEM (FEMALE) in Supplement

**labia minora** /ˌleɪbiə mɪˈnɔːrə/ *plural noun* two small fleshy folds on the inside edge of the vulva. See illustration at UROGENITAL SYSTEM (FEMALE) in Supplement. Also called **nymphae**

**labile** /ˈleɪbaɪl/ *adjective* referring to a drug which is unstable and likely to change if heated or cooled

**lability of mood** /ləˌbɪlɪti əv ˈmuːd/ *noun* a tendency for a person's mood to change suddenly

**labio-** /leɪbiəʊ/ *prefix* referring to the lips or to labia

**labioplasty** /ˈleɪbiəʊˌplæsti/ *noun* a surgical operation to repair damaged or deformed lips (NOTE: The plural is **labioplasties**.)

**labium** /ˈleɪbiəm/ *noun* **1.** any of the four fleshy folds which surround the female genital organs **2.** a structure which looks like a lip (NOTE: The plural is **labia**.)

**labor** /ˈleɪbə/ *noun* US spelling of **labour**

**laboratory** /ləˈbɒrət(ə)ri/ *noun* a special room or place where scientists can do specialised work such as research, the testing of chemical substances or the growing of tissues in culture ○ *The samples of water from the hospital have been sent to the laboratory for testing.* ○ *The new drug has passed its laboratory tests.* (NOTE: The plural is **laboratories**.)

**laboratory officer** /ləˈbɒrət(ə)ri ˌɒfɪsə/ *noun* a qualified person in charge of a laboratory

**laboratory technician** /ləˌbɒrət(ə)ri tekˈnɪʃ(ə)n/ *noun* a person who does practical work in a laboratory and has particular care of equipment

**laboratory techniques** /ləˈbɒrət(ə)ri tek ˌniːkz/ *plural noun* the methods or skills needed to perform experiments in a laboratory

**laboratory test** /ləˈbɒrət(ə)ri test/ *noun* a test carried out in a laboratory

**labour** /ˈleɪbə/ *noun* childbirth, especially the contractions in the uterus which take place during childbirth □ **in labour** experiencing the physical changes such as contractions in the uterus which precede the birth of a child ○ *She was in labour for 14 hours.* □ **to go into labour** to start to experience the contractions which indicate the birth of a child is imminent ○ *She went into labour at 6 o'clock.*

COMMENT: Labour usually starts about nine months, or 266 days, after conception. The cervix expands and the muscles in the uterus contract, causing the amnion to burst. The muscles continue to contract regularly, pushing the baby into, and then through, the vagina.

**laboured breathing** /ˌleɪbəd ˈbriːðɪŋ/ *noun* difficult breathing, which can be due to various causes such as asthma

**labour pains** /ˈleɪbə peɪnz/ *plural noun* the pains felt at regular intervals by a woman as the muscles of the uterus contract during childbirth

**labrum** /ˈleɪbrəm/ *noun* a ring of cartilage around the rim of a joint (NOTE: The plural is **labra**.)

**labyrinth** /ˈlæbərɪnθ/ *noun* a series of interconnecting tubes, especially those in the inside of the ear

COMMENT: The labyrinth of the inner ear is in three parts: the three semicircular canals, the vestibule and the cochlea. The osseous labyrinth is filled with a fluid (perilymph) and the membranous labyrinth is a series of ducts and canals inside the osseous labyrinth. The membranous labyrinth contains a fluid (endolymph). As the endolymph moves about in the membranous labyrinth it stimulates the vestibular nerve which communicates the sense of movement of the head to the brain. If a person turns round and round and then stops, the endolymph continues to move and creates the sensation of giddiness.

**labyrinthectomy** /ˌlæbərɪnˈθektəmi/ *noun* a surgical operation to remove the labyrinth of the inner ear (NOTE: The plural is **labyrinthectomies.**)

**labyrinthitis** /ˌlæbərɪnˈθaɪtɪs/ *noun* same as **otitis interna**

**lacerated** /ˈlæsəreɪtɪd/ *adjective* torn or with a rough edge

**lacerated wound** /ˌlæsəreɪtɪd ˈwuːnd/ *noun* a wound where the skin is torn, as by a rough surface or barbed wire

**laceration** /ˌlæsəˈreɪʃ(ə)n/ *noun* **1.** a wound which has been cut or torn with rough edges, and is not the result of stabbing or pricking **2.** the act of tearing tissue

**lachrymal** /ˈlækrɪm(ə)l/ *adjective* same as **lacrimal**

**lacrimal** /ˈlækrɪm(ə)l/ *adjective* referring to tears, the tear ducts or the tear glands. ◊ **nasolacrimal**

**lacrimal apparatus** /ˌlækrɪm(ə)l ˌæpəˈreɪtəs/ *noun* the arrangement of glands and ducts which produce and drain tears. Also called **lacrimal system**

**lacrimal bone** /ˈlækrɪm(ə)l bəʊn/ *noun* one of two little bones which join with others to form the orbits

**lacrimal canaliculus** /ˌlækrɪm(ə)l kænəˈlɪkjʊləs/ *noun* a small canal draining tears into the lacrimal sac

**lacrimal caruncle** /ˌlækrɪm(ə)l kəˈrʌŋk(ə)l/ *noun* a small red point at the inner corner of each eye

**lacrimal duct** /ˈlækrɪm(ə)l dʌkt/ *noun* a small duct leading from the lacrimal gland. Also called **tear duct**

**lacrimal gland** /ˈlækrɪm(ə)l glænd/ *noun* a gland beneath the upper eyelid which secretes tears. Also called **tear gland**

**lacrimal puncta** /ˌlækrɪm(ə)l ˈpʌŋktə/ *plural noun* small openings of the lacrimal canaliculus at the corners of the eyes through which tears drain into the nose

**lacrimal sac** /ˌlækrɪm(ə)l ˈsæk/ *noun* a sac at the upper end of the nasolacrimal duct, linking it with the lacrimal canaliculus

**lacrimal system** /ˈlækrɪm(ə)l ˌsɪstəm/ *noun* same as **lacrimal apparatus**

**lacrimation** /ˌlækrɪˈmeɪʃ(ə)n/ *noun* the production of tears

**lacrimator** /ˈlækrɪmeɪtə/ *noun* a substance which irritates the eyes and makes tears flow

**lacrymal** /ˈlækrɪml/, **lachrymal** /ˈlækrɪm(ə)l/ *adjective* another spelling of **lacrimal**

**lact-** /lækt/ *prefix* same as **lacto-** (*used before vowels*)

**lactase** /ˈlækteɪz/ *noun* an enzyme, secreted in the small intestine, which converts milk sugar into glucose and galactose

**lactate** /lækˈteɪt/ *verb* to produce milk in the body (NOTE: **lactating – lactated**)

**lactation** /lækˈteɪʃ(ə)n/ *noun* **1.** the production of milk in the body **2.** the period during which a mother is breastfeeding a baby

COMMENT: Lactation is stimulated by the production of the hormone prolactin by the pituitary gland. It starts about three days after childbirth, before which period the breasts secrete colostrum.

**lacteal** /ˈlæktɪəl/ *adjective* referring to milk ■ *noun* a lymph vessel in a villus which helps the digestive process in the small intestine by absorbing fat

**lactic** /ˈlæktɪk/ *adjective* relating to milk

**lactic acid** /ˌlæktɪk ˈæsɪd/ *noun* a sugar which forms in cells and tissue, and also in sour milk, cheese and yoghurt

COMMENT: Lactic acid is produced as the body uses up sugar during exercise. Excessive amounts of lactic acid in the body can produce muscle cramp.

**lactiferous** /lækˈtɪfərəs/ *adjective* producing, secreting or carrying milk

**lactiferous duct** /lækˌtɪfərəs ˈdʌkt/ *noun* a duct in the breast which carries milk

**lactiferous sinus** /lækˌtɪfərəs ˈsaɪnəs/ *noun* a dilatation of the lactiferous duct at the base of the nipple

**lacto-** *prefix* referring to milk

**Lactobacillus** /ˌlæktəʊbəˈsɪləs/ *noun* a genus of Gram-positive bacteria which produces lactic acid from glucose and may be found in the digestive tract and the vagina

**lactogenic hormone** /ˌlæktəʊˌdʒenɪk ˈhɔːməʊn/ *noun* same as **prolactin**

**lactose** /ˈlæktəʊs/ *noun* a type of sugar found in milk

**lactose intolerance** /ˈlæktəʊs ɪnˌtɒlərəns/ *noun* a condition in which a person cannot digest lactose because lactase is absent in the intestine or because of an allergy to milk, causing diarrhoea

**lactosuria** /ˌlæktəʊˈsjʊəriə/ *noun* the excretion of lactose in the urine

**lactovegetarian** /ˌlæktəʊvedʒɪˈteəriən/ *noun* a person who does not eat meat, but eats vegetables, fruit, dairy produce and eggs and sometimes fish ○ *He has been a lactovegetarian for twenty years.* Compare **vegan, vegetarian**

**lactulose** /ˈlæktjʊləʊs/ *noun* an artificially produced sugar used as a laxative

**lacuna** /læˈkjuːnə/ *noun* a small hollow or cavity (NOTE: The plural is **lacunae.**)

**lacunar** /læˈkjuːnə/ *adjective* relating to hollows or cavities in tissue such as in bone or cartilage, especially ones that are unusual

**Laënnec's cirrhosis** /ˌleɪəneks səˈrəʊsɪs/ *noun* the commonest form of alcoholic cirrhosis of the liver [Described 1819. After René Théophile Hyacinthe Laennec (1781–1826), Professor of medicine at the Collège de France, and inventor of the stethoscope.]

**laevocardia** /ˌliːvəʊˈkɑːdiə/ *noun* the condition of having the heart in the usual position, with the apex towards the left side of the body. Compare **dextrocardia**

**-lalia** /leɪliə/ *suffix* speech or a speech disorder

**lambda** /ˈlæmdə/ *noun* **1.** the 11th letter of the Greek alphabet **2.** the point at the back of the skull where the sagittal suture and lambdoidal suture meet

**lambdoid** /ˈlæmdɔɪd/ *adjective* shaped like the capital Greek letter lambda, like an upside down V or y

**lambdoid suture** /ˌlæmˌdɔɪd ˈsuːtʃə/, **lambdoidal suture** /ˌlæmˌdɔɪd(ə)l ˈsuːtʃə/ *noun* a horizontal joint across the back of the skull between the parietal and occipital bones

**lamblia** /ˈlæmbliə/ *noun* same as **Giardia**

**lambliasis** /læmˈblaɪəsɪs/ *noun* same as **giardiasis**

**lame** /leɪm/ *adjective* not able to walk easily because of pain, stiffness or damage in a leg or foot (NOTE: This term is regarded as offensive.)

**lamella** /ləˈmelə/ *noun* **1.** a thin sheet of tissue **2.** a thin disc placed under the eyelid to apply a drug to the eye (NOTE: The plural is **lamellae**.)

**lameness** /ˈleɪmnəs/ *noun* the inability to walk normally because of pain, stiffness or damage in a leg or foot

**lamina** /ˈlæmɪnə/ *noun* **1.** a thin membrane **2.** a side part of the posterior arch in a vertebra (NOTE: The plural is **laminae**.)

**lamina propria** /ˌlæmɪnə ˈprəʊpriə/ *noun* the connective tissue of mucous membranes containing, e.g., blood vessels and lymphatic tissues

**laminectomy** /ˌlæmɪˈnektəmi/ *noun* a surgical operation to cut through the lamina of a vertebra in the spine to get to the spinal cord. Also called **rachiotomy** (NOTE: The plural is **laminectomies**.)

**lamotrigine** /ləˈmɒtrɪdʒiːn/ *noun* a drug that helps to control petit mal epilepsy

**lance** /lɑːns/ *verb* to make a cut in a boil or abscess to remove the pus

**lancet** /ˈlɑːnsɪt/ *noun* **1.** a sharp two-edged pointed knife formerly used in surgery **2.** a small pointed implement used to take a small capillary blood sample, e.g. to measure blood glucose levels

**lancinate** /ˈlɑːnsɪneɪt/ *verb* to lacerate or cut something (NOTE: **lancinating – lancinated**)

**lancinating** /ˈlɑːnsɪneɪtɪŋ/ *adjective* referring to pain which is sharp and cutting

**Landry's paralysis** /ˌlændrɪz pəˈræləsɪs/ *noun* same as **Guillain-Barré syndrome** (*see*)

[After Jean-Baptiste Octave Landry (1826–65), French physician]

**Landsteiner's classification** /ˌlændstaɪnəz ˌklæsɪfɪˈkeɪʃ(ə)n/ *noun* same as **ABO system**

**Langerhans' cells** /ˈlæŋəhæns selz/ *plural noun* cells on the outer layers of the skin

**Langer's lines** /ˈlæŋəz laɪnz/ *plural noun* the arrangement of collagen protein fibres which causes the usual skin creases. Cuts made along these lines sever fewer fibres and heal better than other cuts. Also called **cleavage lines**

**Lange test** /ˈlæŋə test/ *noun* a method of detecting globulin in the cerebrospinal fluid [Described 1912. After Carl Friedrich August Lange (b. 1883), German physician.]

**lanolin** /ˈlænəlɪn/ *noun* grease from sheep's wool which absorbs water and is used to rub on dried skin, or in the preparation of cosmetics

**lanugo** /ləˈnjuːɡəʊ/ *noun* **1.** soft hair on the body of a fetus or newborn baby **2.** soft hair on the body of an adult, except on the palms of the hands, the soles of the feet and the parts where long hair grows

**laparo-** /læpərəʊ/ *prefix* the lower abdomen

**laparoscope** /ˈlæpərəskəʊp/ *noun* a surgical instrument which is inserted through a hole in the abdominal wall to allow a surgeon to examine the inside of the abdominal cavity. Also called **peritoneoscope**

**laparoscopic** /ˌlæpərəˈskɒpɪk/ *adjective* using a laparoscope

**laparoscopic surgery** /ˌlæpərəˌskɒpɪk ˈsɜːdʒəri/ *noun* same as **keyhole surgery**

**laparoscopy** /ˌlæpəˈrɒskəpi/ *noun* a procedure in which a laparoscope is used to examine the inside of the abdominal cavity. Also called **peritoneoscopy** (NOTE: The plural is **laparoscopies**.)

**laparotomy** /ˌlæpəˈrɒtəmi/ *noun* a surgical operation to cut open the abdominal cavity (NOTE: The plural is **laparotomies**.)

**large intestine** /lɑːdʒ ɪnˈtestɪn/ *noun* the section of the digestive system from the caecum to the rectum

**Lariam** /ˈlæriəm/ a trade name for mefloquine hydrochloride

**larva** /ˈlɑːvə/ *noun* a stage in the development of an insect or tapeworm, after the egg has hatched but before the animal becomes adult (NOTE: The plural is **larvae**.)

**laryng-** /ləˈrɪndʒ/ *prefix* same as **laryngo-** (*used before vowels*)

**laryngeal** /ləˈrɪndʒiəl/ *adjective* referring to the larynx

**laryngeal inlet** /ləˌrɪndʒiəl ˈɪnlət/ *noun* the entrance from the laryngopharynx leading through the vocal cords to the trachea

**laryngeal prominence** /ləˌrɪndʒiəl ˈprɒmɪnəns/ *noun* same as **Adam's apple**

**laryngeal reflex** /ləˌrɪndʒɪəl ˈriːfleks/ *noun* the reflex that makes a person cough

**laryngectomy** /ˌlærɪnˈdʒektəmi/ *noun* a surgical operation to remove the larynx, usually as treatment for throat cancer (NOTE: The plural is **laryngectomies**.)

**larynges** /ləˈrɪndʒiːz/ plural of **larynx**

**laryngismus** /ˌlærɪnˈdʒɪzməs/, **laryngismus stridulus** /lærɪnˌdʒɪzməs ˈstrɪdjʊləs/ *noun* a spasm of the throat muscles with a sharp intake of breath which occurs when the larynx is irritated, as in children who have croup

**laryngitis** /ˌlærɪnˈdʒaɪtɪs/ *noun* inflammation of the larynx

**laryngo-** /lərɪŋgəʊ/ *prefix* larynx

**laryngofissure** /ləˌrɪŋgəʊˈfɪʃə/ *noun* a surgical operation to make an opening into the larynx through the thyroid cartilage

**laryngologist** /ˌlærɪnˈgɒlədʒɪst/ *noun* a doctor who specialises in diseases of the larynx, throat and vocal cords

**laryngology** /ˌlærɪnˈgɒlədʒi/ *noun* the study of diseases of the larynx, throat and vocal cords

**laryngomalacia** /ləˌrɪŋgəʊməˈleɪʃə/ *noun* a condition in which breathing is made difficult by softness of the larynx, occurring mainly in children under the age of two

**laryngopharyngeal** /ləˌrɪŋgəʊfəˈrɪndʒɪəl/ *adjective* referring to both the larynx and the pharynx

**laryngopharynx** /lərɪŋgəʊˈfærɪŋks/ *noun* the part of the pharynx below the hyoid bone

**laryngoscope** /ləˈrɪŋgəskəʊp/ *noun* an instrument for examining the inside of the larynx using a light and mirrors

**laryngoscopy** /ˌlærɪŋˈgɒskəpi/ *noun* an examination of the larynx with a laryngoscope (NOTE: The plural is **laryngoscopies**.)

**laryngospasm** /ləˈrɪŋgəspæzəm/ *noun* a muscular spasm which suddenly closes the larynx

**laryngostenosis** /ləˌrɪŋgəʊstəˈnəʊsɪs/ *noun* narrowing of the lumen of the larynx

**laryngostomy** /ˌlærɪnˈgɒstəmi/ *noun* a surgical operation to make a permanent opening from the neck into the larynx (NOTE: The plural is **laryngostomies**.)

**laryngotomy** /ˌlærɪnˈgɒtəmi/ *noun* a surgical operation to make an opening in the larynx through the membrane, especially in an emergency, when the throat is blocked (NOTE: The plural is **laryngotomies**.)

**laryngotracheal** /ləˌrɪŋgəʊˈtreɪkɪəl/ *adjective* relating to both the larynx and the trachea ○ *laryngotracheal stenosis*

**laryngotracheobronchitis** /ləˌrɪŋgəʊˌtreɪkɪəʊbrɒŋˈkaɪtɪs/ *noun* inflammation of the larynx, trachea and bronchi, as in croup

**larynx** /ˈlærɪŋks/ *noun* the organ in the throat which produces sounds. Also called **voice box** (NOTE: The plural is **larynges** or **larynxes**.)

COMMENT: The larynx is a hollow passage made of cartilage, containing the vocal cords, situated behind the Adam's apple. It is closed by the epiglottis when swallowing or before coughing.

**laser** /ˈleɪzə/ *noun* an instrument which produces a highly concentrated beam of light which can be used to cut or attach tissue, as in operations for a detached retina

**laser laparoscopy** /ˌleɪzə læpəˈrɒskəpi/ *noun* surgery performed through a laparoscope using a laser

**laser probe** /ˈleɪzə prəʊb/ *noun* a metal probe which is inserted into the body and through which a laser beam can be passed to remove a blockage in an artery

**laser surgery** /ˈleɪzə ˌsɜːdʒəri/ *noun* surgery using lasers, e.g. for the removal of tumours, sealing blood vessels, or the correction of shortsightedness

**Lasix** /ˈleɪzɪks/ a trade name for frusemide

**Lassa fever** /ˈlæsə ˌfiːvə/ *noun* a highly infectious and often fatal virus disease found in Central and West Africa, causing high fever, pains, and ulcers in the mouth [After a village in northern Nigeria where the fever was first reported]

**Lassar's paste** /ˈlæsəz ˌpeɪst/ *noun* an ointment made of zinc oxide, used to treat eczema [After Oskar Lassar (1849–1907), German dermatologist]

**lassitude** /ˈlæsɪtjuːd/ *noun* a state where a person does not want to do anything, sometimes because he or she is depressed

**lata** /ˈlætə/ ♦ **fascia lata**

**latent** /ˈleɪt(ə)nt/ *adjective* referring to a disease which is present in the body but does not show any signs ○ *The children were tested for latent viral infection.*

**lateral** /ˈlæt(ə)rəl/ *adjective* **1.** further away from the midline of the body **2.** referring to one side of the body

**lateral aspect** /ˌlæt(ə)rəl ˈæspekt/ *noun* a view of the side of part of the body. Also called **lateral view**. See illustration at ANATOMICAL TERMS in Supplement

**lateral epicondyle** /ˌlæt(ə)rəl ˌepɪˈkɒndaɪl/, **lateral epicondyle of the humerus** /ˌlæt(ə)rəl epɪˌkɒndaɪl əv ðə ˈhjuːmərəs/ *noun* a lateral projection on the rounded end of the humerus at the elbow joint

**lateral epicondylitis** /ˌlæt(ə)rəl ˌepɪkɒndɪˈlaɪtɪs/ *noun* same as **tennis elbow**

**lateral fissure** /ˌlæt(ə)rəl ˈfɪʃə/ *noun* a groove along the side of each cerebral hemisphere

**laterally** /ˈlætrəli/ *adverb* towards or on the side of the body. See illustration at ANATOMICAL TERMS in Supplement

**lateral malleolus** /ˌlæt(ə)rəl məˈliːələs/ noun the part of the end of the fibula which protrudes on the outside of the ankle

**lateral view** /ˌlæt(ə)rəl ˈvjuː/ noun same as **lateral aspect**

**lateroversion** /ˌlæt(ə)rəʊˈvɜːʃ(ə)n/ noun a condition in which an organ is turned to one side

**latissimus dorsi** /ləˌtɪsɪməs ˈdɔːsi/ noun a large flat triangular muscle covering the lumbar region and the lower part of the chest

**laudanum** /ˈlɔːd(ə)nəm/ noun a solution of opium in alcohol that was formerly in widespread use for pain relief

**laughing gas** /ˈlɑːfɪŋ gæs/ noun same as **nitrous oxide** (informal)

**lavage** /ˈlævɪdʒ, læˈvɑːʒ/ noun the act of washing out or irrigating an organ such as the stomach

**laxative** /ˈlæksətɪv/ adjective causing a bowel movement ■ noun a medicine which causes a bowel movement, e.g. bisacodyl, which stimulates intestinal motility, or lactulose which alters fluid retention in the bowel ▶ also called (all senses) **purgative**

COMMENT: Laxatives are very commonly used without prescription to treat constipation, although they should only be used as a short term solution. Change of diet and regular exercise are better ways of treating most types of constipation.

**lazy eye** /ˌleɪzi ˈaɪ/ noun an eye which does not focus properly without an obvious cause (informal) ◊ **amblyopia**

**LD** abbr lethal dose

**LDL** abbr low-density lipoprotein

**L-dopa** /el ˈdəʊpə/ noun same as **levodopa**

**LE** abbr lupus erythematosus

**lead** /led/ noun a very heavy soft metallic element, which is poisonous in compounds (NOTE: The chemical symbol is **Pb**.)

**lead-free** /ˌled ˈfriː/ adjective with no lead in it ○ lead-free paint ○ lead-free petrol

**lead line** /ˈled laɪn/ noun a blue line seen on the gums in cases of lead poisoning

**lead poisoning** /led ˈpɔɪz(ə)nɪŋ/ noun poisoning caused by taking in lead salts. Also called **plumbism**, **saturnism**

COMMENT: Lead salts are used externally to treat bruises or eczema, but if taken internally produce lead poisoning. Lead poisoning can also be caused by paint (children's toys must be painted in lead-free paint) or by lead fumes from car engines not using lead-free petrol.

**learning** /ˈlɜːnɪŋ/ noun the act of gaining knowledge of something or of how to do something

**learning disability** /ˈlɜːnɪŋ dɪsəˌbɪlɪti/, **learning difficulty** /ˈlɜːnɪŋ ˌdɪfɪk(ə)lti/ noun a condition that results in someone finding it difficult to learn skills or information at the same rate as others of similar age ○ children with learning disabilities

**LE cells** /ˌel ˈiː selz/ plural noun white blood cells which show that someone has lupus erythematosus

**lecithin** /ˈlesɪθɪn/ noun a chemical which is a constituent of all animal and plant cells and is involved in the transport and absorption of fats

**leech** /liːtʃ/ noun a blood-sucking parasitic worm which lives in water, occasionally used in specialist procedures

COMMENT: Leeches were formerly commonly used in medicine to remove blood from a patient. Today they are used in special cases, where it is necessary to make sure that blood does not build up in part of the body, e.g. in a severed finger which has been sewn back on.

**left-handed** /ˌleft ˈhændɪd/ adjective using the left hand in preference to the right in most everyday tasks

**left-handedness** /ˌleft ˈhændɪdnəs/ noun the fact of being left-handed

**leg** /leg/ noun a part of the body with which a person or animal walks and stands

COMMENT: The leg is formed of the thigh, with the thighbone or femur, the knee with the kneecap or patella, and the lower leg, with two bones – the tibia and fibula.

**legal abortion** /ˌliːg(ə)l əˈbɔːʃ(ə)n/ noun an abortion which is carried out legally

**Legg-Calvé disease** /ˌleg ˈkælveɪ dɪˌziːz/, **Legg-Calvé-Perthes disease** /ˌleg ˌkælveɪ ˈpɜːtɪz dɪˌziːz/ noun degeneration of the upper end of the thighbone in young boys, which prevents the bone growing properly and can result in a permanent limp [Described 1910 separately by all three workers. Arthur Thornton Legg (1874–1939), American orthopaedic surgeon; Jacques Calvé (1875–1954), French orthopaedic surgeon; Georg Clemens Perthes (1869–1927), German surgeon.]

**Legionnaires' disease** /ˌliːdʒəˈneəz dɪ ˌziːz/ noun a bacterial disease similar to pneumonia

COMMENT: The disease is thought to be transmitted in droplets of moisture in the air, and so the bacterium is found in central air-conditioning systems. It can be fatal to elderly or sick people, and so is especially dangerous if present in a hospital.

**leio-** /leɪəʊ/ prefix smooth or smoothness

**leiomyoma** /ˌlaɪəʊmaɪˈəʊmə/ noun a tumour of smooth muscle, especially the smooth muscle coating the uterus (NOTE: The plural is **leiomyomas** or **leiomyomata**.)

**leiomyosarcoma** /ˌlaɪəʊˌmaɪəʊsɑːˈkəʊmə/ noun a sarcoma in which large bundles of smooth muscle are found (NOTE: The plural is **leiomyosarcomas** or **leiomyosarcomata**.)

**Leishmania** /liːʃˈmeɪniə/ noun a tropical parasite which is passed to humans by the bites of sandflies and causes the group of infections known as leishmaniasis

**leishmaniasis** /ˌliːʃməˈnaɪəsɪs/ noun a disease caused by the parasite Leishmania, one form of which causes disfiguring ulcers, while another attacks the liver and bone marrow

**Lembert's suture** /'lɑːmbeəz ˌsuːtʃə/ *noun* a suture used to close a wound in the intestine which includes all the coats of the intestine [Described 1826. After Antoine Lembert (1802–51), French surgeon.]

**lens** /lenz/ *noun* **1.** the part of the eye behind the iris and pupil, which focuses light coming from the cornea onto the retina. See illustration at **EYE** in Supplement **2.** a piece of shaped glass or plastic which forms part of a pair of spectacles or microscope **3.** same as **contact lens**

> COMMENT: The lens in the eye is elastic, and can change its shape under the influence of the ciliary muscle, to allow the eye to focus on objects at different distances.

**lens implant** /lenz 'ɪmplɑːnt/ *noun* an artificial lens implanted in the eye when the natural lens is removed, as in the case of cataract

**lenticular** /len'tɪkjʊlə/ *adjective* referring to or like a lens

**lentigo** /len'taɪɡəʊ/ *noun* a small brown spot on the skin often caused by exposure to sunlight. Also called **freckle** (NOTE: The plural is **lentigines**.)

**leontiasis** /ˌliːɒn'taɪəsɪs/ *noun* a rare disorder in which the skull bones become enlarged and may give the appearance of a lion's head. It occurs if Paget's disease is not treated.

**lepidosis** /ˌlepɪ'dəʊsɪs/ *noun* a skin eruption in which pieces of skin fall off in flakes

**leproma** /le'prəʊmə/ *noun* a lesion of the skin caused by leprosy (NOTE: The plural is **lepromas** or **lepromata**.)

**leprosy** /'leprəsi/ *noun* an infectious bacterial disease of skin and peripheral nerves caused by *Mycobacterium leprae*, which destroys the tissues and causes severe disfigurement if left untreated. Also called **Hansen's disease**

> COMMENT: Leprosy attacks the nerves in the skin, and finally the patient loses all feeling in a limb, and parts such as fingers or toes can drop off.

**leptin** /'leptɪn/ *noun* a hormone produced by fat cells that signals the body's level of hunger to the hypothalamus of the brain

**lepto-** /leptəʊ/ *prefix* thin

**leptocyte** /'leptəsaɪt/ *noun* a thin red blood cell found in anaemia

**leptomeninges** /ˌleptəʊme'nɪndʒiːz/ *plural noun* the two inner meninges, the pia mater and arachnoid

**leptomeningitis** /ˌleptəʊmenɪn'dʒaɪtɪs/ *noun* inflammation of the leptomeninges

**Leptospira** /ˌleptəʊ'spaɪrə/ *noun* a genus of bacteria excreted continuously in the urine of rats and many domestic animals. It can infect humans, causing leptospirosis or Weil's disease.

**leptospirosis** /ˌleptəʊspaɪ'rəʊsɪs/ *noun* an infectious disease caused by the spirochaete *Leptospira*, transmitted to humans from rat urine, causing jaundice and kidney damage. Also called **Weil's disease**

**leresis** /lə'riːsɪs/ *noun* uncoordinated speech, a sign of dementia

**lesbian** /'lezbiən/ *noun* a woman who experiences sexual attraction towards other women ■ *adjective* referring to a lesbian

**lesbianism** /'lezbiənɪz(ə)m/ *noun* sexual attraction in one woman for another. Compare **homosexuality**

**Lesch-Nyhan disease** /ˌleʃ 'naɪhən dɪ ˌziːz/, **Lesch-Nyhan syndrome** /ˌleʃ 'naɪhən ˌsɪndrəʊm/ *noun* a rare genetic disorder in boys caused by a lack of the enzyme HPRT. Symptoms include uncontrolled muscle movements and learning disabilities, and life expectancy is 20 – 25.

**lesion** /'liːʒ(ə)n/ *noun* a wound, sore or damage to the body (NOTE: Used to refer to any damage to the body, from the fracture of a bone to a cut on the skin.)

**lesser** /'lesə/ *adjective* smaller

**lesser circulation** /ˌlesə ˌsɜːkjʊ'leɪʃ(ə)n/ *noun* same as **pulmonary circulation**

**lesser trochanter** /ˌlesə trə'kæntə/ *noun* a projection on the femur which is the insertion of the psoas major muscle

**lesser vestibular gland** /ˌlesə ve'stɪbjʊlə ɡlænd/ *noun* the more anterior of the vestibular glands

**lethal** /'liːθ(ə)l/ *adjective* killing or able to kill ○ *These fumes are lethal if inhaled.*

**lethal dose** /'liːθl dəʊs/ *noun* the amount of a drug or other substance which will kill the person who takes it ○ *She took a lethal dose of aspirin.* Abbr **LD**

**lethal gene** /ˌliːθ(ə)l 'dʒiːn/, **lethal mutation** /ˌliːθ(ə)l mjuː'teɪʃ(ə)n/ *noun* a gene, usually recessive, that results in the premature death of an individual who inherits it, e.g. the gene controlling sickle-cell anaemia

**lethargic** /lɪ'θɑːdʒɪk/ *adjective* showing lethargy

**lethargic encephalitis** /ləˌθɑːdʒɪk enˌkefə'laɪtɪs/ *noun* a common type of virus encephalitis occurring in epidemics in the 1920s. Also called **encephalitis lethargica, sleepy sickness**

**lethargy** /'leθədʒi/ *noun* a state in which someone is not mentally alert, has slow movements and is almost inactive

**Letterer-Siwe disease** /ˌletərə 'siːweɪ dɪ ˌziːz/ *noun* a usually fatal disease, most common in infants, caused by the overproduction of a specialised type of immune cell

**leucine** /'luːsiːn/ *noun* an essential amino acid

**leuco-** /'luːkəʊ/, **leuko-** /luːkəʊ/ *prefix* white

**leucocyte** /'lu:kəsaɪt/, **leukocyte** *noun* a white blood cell which contains a nucleus but has no haemoglobin

COMMENT: In average conditions the blood contains far fewer leucocytes than erythrocytes (red blood cells), but their numbers increase rapidly when infection is present in the body. Leucocytes are either granular (with granules in the cytoplasm) or nongranular. The main types of leucocyte are: lymphocytes and monocytes which are nongranular, and neutrophils, eosinophils and basophils which are granular (granulocytes). Granular leucocytes are produced by the bone marrow, and their main function is to remove foreign particles from the blood and fight infection by forming antibodies.

**leucocytolysis** /ˌluːkəʊsaɪˈtɒləsɪs/, **leukocytolysis** /luːkəsaɪˈtɒləsɪs/ *noun* destruction of leucocytes

**leucocytosis** /ˌluːkəʊsaɪˈtəʊsɪs/, **leukocytosis** /luːkəsaɪˈtəʊsɪs/ *noun* an increase in the numbers of leucocytes in the blood above the usual upper limit, in order to fight an infection

**leucodeplete** /ˌluːkəʊdɪˈpliːt/, **leukodeplete** *verb* to remove white cells from the blood (NOTE: **leucodepleting – leucodepleted**)

**leucoderma** /ˌluːkəʊˈdɜːmə/, **leukoderma** *noun* same as **vitiligo**

**leucolysin** /ˌluːkəʊˈlaɪsɪn/, **leukolysin** *noun* a protein which destroys white blood cells

**leucoma** /luˈkəʊmə/, **leukoma** *noun* a white scar of the cornea (NOTE: The plural is **leucomas** or **leucomata**.)

**leuconychia** /ˌluːkəʊˈnɪkiə/, **leukonychia** *noun* a condition in which white marks appear on the fingernails

**leucopenia** /ˌluːkəˈpiːniə/, **leukopenia** *noun* a reduction in the number of leucocytes in the blood, usually as the result of a disease

**leucoplakia** /ˌluːkəʊˈplækiə/, **leukoplakia** *noun* a condition in which white patches form on mucous membranes, e.g. on the tongue or inside of the mouth

**leucopoiesis** /ˌluːkəʊpɔɪˈiːsɪs/, **leukopoiesis** *noun* the production of leucocytes

**leucorrhoea** /ˌluːkəˈriːə/, **leukorrhoea** *noun* an excessive discharge of white mucus from the vagina. Also called **whites** (NOTE: The US spelling is **leukorrhea**.)

**leukaemia** /luːˈkiːmiə/ *noun* any of several malignant diseases where an unusual number of leucocytes form in the blood (NOTE: The US spelling is **leukemia**.)

COMMENT: Apart from the increase in the number of leucocytes, the symptoms include swelling of the spleen and the lymph glands. There are several forms of leukaemia: the commonest is acute lymphoblastic leukaemia which is the commonest cancer occurring in children and can be treated by radiotherapy.

**leuko-** /luːkəʊ/ *prefix* same as **leuco-**

**levator** /ləˈveɪtə/ *noun* **1.** a surgical instrument for lifting pieces of fractured bone **2.** a muscle which lifts a limb or a part of the body

**level of care** /ˌlev(ə)l əv ˈkeə/ *noun* any of the planned divisions within the system of health care which is offered by a particular organisation ○ *Our care homes offer six different levels of care to allow the greatest independence possible.*

**levodopa** /ˌliːvəˈdəʊpə/ *noun* a natural chemical that stimulates the production of dopamine in the brain and is used to treat Parkinson's disease

**levonorgestrel** /ˌliːvəʊnɔːˈdʒestrəl/ *noun* an artificially produced female sex hormone, used mostly in birth control pills or capsules

**Lewy body** /'luːwi ˌbɒdi/ *noun* an unusual deposit of protein in neurons in the brain

**Lewy body dementia** /ˌluːwi ˌbɒdi dɪˈmenʃə/ *noun* a disease characterised by the presence of Lewy bodies in the brain, which affects the mental processes. It is similar to Alzheimer's disease, but people with it are more prone to hallucinations and delusions.

**Leydig cells** /'laɪdɪɡ selz/ *plural noun* testosterone-producing cells between the tubules in the testes. Also called **interstitial cells** [Described 1850. After Franz von Leydig (1821–1908), Professor of Histology at Würzburg, Tübingen and then Bonn, Germany.]

**Leydig tumour** /'laɪdɪɡ ˌtjuːmə/ *noun* a tumour of the Leydig cells of the testis. It often releases testosterone, which makes young boys show early signs of maturing.

**l.g.v.** *abbr* lymphogranuloma venereum

**LH** *abbr* luteinising hormone

**libido** /lɪˈbiːdəʊ/ *noun* **1.** the sexual urge **2.** (*in psychology*) a force which drives the unconscious mind

**Librium** /'lɪbriəm/ a trade name for chlordiazepoxide

**lice** /laɪs/ plural of **louse**

**licence** /'laɪs(ə)ns/ *noun* an official document which allows someone to do something, e.g. one allowing a doctor to practise, a pharmacist to make and sell drugs or, in the USA, a nurse to practise ○ *He was practising as a doctor without a licence.* ○ *She is sitting her registered nurse licence examination.* (NOTE: The US spelling is **license**.)

**licensure** /'laɪsənʃə/ *noun US* the act of licensing a nurse to practise nursing

**licentiate** /laɪˈsenʃiət/ *noun* a person who has been given a licence to practise as a doctor

**lichen** /'laɪkən/ *noun* a type of skin disease with thick skin and small lesions

**lichenification** /laɪˌkenɪfɪˈkeɪʃ(ə)n/ *noun* a thickening of the skin at the site of a lesion

**lichenoid** /'laɪkənɔɪd/ *adjective* like lichen

**lichen planus** /ˌlaɪkən ˈpleɪnəs/ noun a skin disease where itchy purple spots appear on the arms and thighs

**lid** /lɪd/ noun the top which covers a container ○ *a medicine bottle with a child-proof lid*

**lidocaine** /ˈlaɪdəkeɪn/ noun US a drug used as a local anaesthetic. Also called **lignocaine**

**lie** /laɪ/ noun same as **lie of fetus** ■ verb to be in a flat position ○ *The accident victim was lying on the pavement.* ○ *Make sure the patient lies still and does not move.* (NOTE: **lying – lay – lain**)

**Lieberkühn's glands** /ˈliːbəkuːnz glændz/ plural noun same as **crypts of Lieberkühn**

**lien-** /laɪən/ prefix spleen

**lienal** /ˈlaɪən(ə)l/ adjective relating to or affecting the spleen ○ *the lienal artery*

**lienculus** /ləˈeŋkjʊləs/ noun a small secondary spleen sometimes found in the body (NOTE: The plural is **lienculi.**)

**lienorenal** /ˌlaɪənəʊˈriːn(ə)l/ adjective relating to or affecting both the spleen and the kidneys

**lientery** /ˈlaɪəntri/, **lienteric diarrhoea** /ˌlaɪənterɪk ˌdaɪəˈriːə/ noun a form of diarrhoea where the food passes through the intestine rapidly without being digested

**lie of fetus** /ˌlaɪ əv ˈfiːtəs/ noun the position of the fetus in the uterus ○ *Cause of rupture: abnormal lie of fetus.*

**life** /laɪf/ noun the quality that makes a person or thing alive and not dead or inorganic ○ *The surgeons saved the patient's life.* ○ *Her life is in danger because the drugs are not available.* ○ *The victim showed no sign of life.*

**life event** /ˈlaɪf ɪˌvent/ noun a significant event which alters a person's status as regards taxation, insurance or employment benefits, e.g. the birth of a child or the onset of a disability

**life expectancy** /laɪf ɪkˈspektənsi/ noun the number of years a person of a particular age is likely to live

**life-saving equipment** /ˌlaɪf ˌseɪvɪŋ ɪ ˈkwɪpmənt/ noun equipment kept ready in case of an emergency, e.g. boats, stretchers or first-aid kits

**life-support system** /laɪf səˈpɔːt ˌsɪstəm/ noun a machine that takes over one or more vital functions such as breathing when someone is unable to survive unaided because of a disease or injury

**life-threatening disease** /laɪf ˌθret(ə)nɪŋ dɪˈziːz/ noun a disease which may kill

**lift** /lɪft/ noun **1.** a particular way of carrying an injured or unconscious person ○ *a four-handed lift* ○ *a shoulder lift* **2.** a cosmetic operation to remove signs of age or to change a body feature ○ *a face lift*

**ligament** /ˈlɪgəmənt/ noun a thick band of fibrous tissue which connects the bones at a joint and forms the joint capsule

**ligate** /ˈlaɪgeɪt/ verb to tie something with a ligature, e.g. to tie a blood vessel to stop bleeding or to tie the Fallopian tubes as a sterilisation procedure (NOTE: **ligating – ligated**)

**ligation** /laɪˈgeɪʃ(ə)n/ noun a surgical operation to tie up a blood vessel

**ligature** /ˈlɪgətʃə/ noun a thread used to tie vessels or a lumen, e.g. to tie a blood vessel to stop bleeding ■ verb same as **ligate** (NOTE: **ligaturing – ligatured**)

**light** /laɪt/ adjective **1.** bright so that a person can see ○ *At six o'clock in the morning it was just getting light.* **2.** referring to hair or skin which is very pale ○ *She has a very light complexion.* ○ *He has light-coloured hair.* **3.** weighing a comparatively small amount ■ noun the energy that makes things bright and helps a person to see ○ *There's not enough light in here to take a photo.*

**light adaptation** /ˈlaɪt ædæpˌteɪʃ(ə)n/ noun changes in the eye to adapt to an unusually bright or dim light or to adapt to light after being in darkness

**lightening** /ˈlaɪtənɪŋ/ noun a late stage in pregnancy where the fetus goes down into the pelvic cavity

**lightning pains** /ˈlaɪtnɪŋ peɪnz/ plural noun sharp pains in the legs in someone who has tabes dorsalis

**light reflex** /ˈlaɪt ˌriːfleks/ noun same as **pupillary reaction**

**light therapy** /ˈlaɪt ˌθerəpi/, **light treatment** /ˈlaɪt ˌtriːtmənt/ noun the treatment of a disorder by exposing the person to light such as sunlight or infrared light

**light wave** /ˈlaɪt weɪv/ noun a wave travelling in all directions from a source of light which stimulates the retina and is visible

**lignocaine** /ˈlɪgnəkeɪn/ noun same as **lidocaine**

**limb** /lɪm/ noun one of the legs or arms

**limbi** /ˈlɪmbi/ plural of **limbus**

**limbic system** /ˈlɪmbɪk ˌsɪstəm/ noun a system of nerves in the brain, including the hippocampus, the amygdala and the hypothalamus, which are associated with emotions such as fear and anger

**limb lead** /ˈlɪm liːd/ noun an electrode attached to an arm or leg when taking an electrocardiogram

**limb lengthening** /ˈlɪm ˌleŋθənɪŋ/ noun a procedure in which an arm or a leg is made longer. Its bone is divided in two and new bone forms in the gap between the ends.

**limbless** /ˈlɪmləs/ adjective lacking one or more limbs

**limbus** /'lɪmbəs/ *noun* an edge, especially the edge of the cornea where it joins the sclera (NOTE: The plural is **limbi**.)

**liminal** /'lɪmɪn(ə)l/ *adjective* referring to a stimulus at the lowest level which can be sensed

**limp** /lɪmp/ *noun* a way of walking awkwardly because of pain, stiffness or malformation of a leg or foot ○ *She walks with a limp.* ■ *verb* to walk awkwardly because of pain, stiffness or malformation of a leg or foot ○ *He was still limping three weeks after the accident.*

**linctus** /'lɪŋktəs/ *noun* a sweet cough medicine

**line** /laɪn/ ♦ **catheter**

**linea** /'lɪnɪə/ *noun* a thin line (NOTE: The plural is **lineae**.)

**linea alba** /ˌlɪnɪə 'ælbə/ *noun* a tendon running from the breastbone to the pubic area, to which abdominal muscles are attached (NOTE: The plural is **lineae albae**.)

**linea nigra** /ˌlɪnɪə 'naɪɡrə/ *noun* a dark line on the skin from the navel to the pubis which appears during the later months of pregnancy (NOTE: The plural is **lineae nigrae**.)

**linear** /'lɪnɪə/ *adjective* **1.** long and narrow in shape **2.** able to be represented by a straight line

**lingual** /'lɪŋwəl/ *adjective* referring to the tongue

**lingual artery** /ˌlɪŋwəl 'ɑːtəri/ *noun* an artery which supplies blood to the tongue

**lingual tonsil** /ˌlɪŋwəl 'tɒns(ə)l/ *noun* a mass of lymphoid tissue on the top surface of the back of the tongue

**lingual vein** /ˌlɪŋwəl 'veɪn/ *noun* a vein which takes blood away from the tongue

**lingula** /'lɪŋɡjʊlə/ *noun* a long thin piece of bone or other tissue ○ *the lingula of the left lung* (NOTE: The plural is **lingulae**.)

**lingular** /'lɪŋɡjʊlə/ *adjective* relating to a lingula

**liniment** /'lɪnɪmənt/ *noun* an oily liquid rubbed on the skin to ease the pain or stiffness of a sprain or bruise by acting as a vasodilator or counterirritant. Also called **embrocation**

**lining** /'laɪnɪŋ/ *noun* a substance or tissue on the inside of an organ ○ *the thick lining of the aorta*

**link** /lɪŋk/ *verb* **1.** to join things together ○ *The ankle bone links the bones of the lower leg to the calcaneus.* **2.** to be related to or associated with something ○ *Health is linked to diet.*

**linkage** /'lɪŋkɪdʒ/ *noun* (*of genes*) the fact of being close together on a chromosome, and therefore likely to be inherited together

**linoleic acid** /ˌlɪnəʊliːɪk 'æsɪd/ *noun* one of the essential fatty acids, found in grains and seeds

**linolenic acid** /ˌlɪnəʊˌlenɪk 'æsɪd/ *noun* one of the essential fatty acids, found in linseed and other natural oils

**lint** /lɪnt/ *noun* thick flat cotton wadding, used as part of a surgical dressing

**liothyronine** /ˌlaɪəʊ'θaɪrəʊniːn/ *noun* a hormone produced by the thyroid gland which can be artificially synthesised for use as a rapid-acting treatment for hypothyroidism

**lip** /lɪp/ *noun* **1.** each of two fleshy muscular parts round the edge of the mouth ○ *Her lips were dry and cracked.* **2.** an edge of flesh round an opening **3.** same as **labium**

**lipaemia** /lɪ'piːmɪə/ *noun* an excessive amount of fat in the blood (NOTE: The US spelling is **lipemia**.)

**lipase** /'lɪpeɪz/ *noun* an enzyme which breaks down fats in the intestine. Also called **lipolytic enzyme**

**lipid** /'lɪpɪd/ *noun* an organic compound which is insoluble in water, e.g. a fat, oil or wax

COMMENT: Lipids are not water soluble. They float in the blood and can attach themselves to the walls of arteries causing atherosclerosis.

**lipid-lowering drug** /'lɪpɪd ˌləʊərɪŋ ˌdrʌg/ *noun* a drug which lowers serum triglycerides and low-density lipoprotein cholesterol and raises high-density lipoprotein cholesterol to reduce the progression of coronary artherosclerosis. Lipid-lowering drugs are used in people with, or at high risk of developing coronary heart disease. (NOTE: Lipid-lowering drugs have names ending in **-fibrate: bezafibrate**.)

**lipid metabolism** /ˌlɪpɪd mə'tæbəlɪz(ə)m/ *noun* the series of chemical changes by which lipids are broken down into fatty acids

**lipidosis** /ˌlɪpɪ'dəʊsɪs/ *noun* a disorder of lipid metabolism in which subcutaneous fat is not present in some parts of the body

**lipochondrodystrophy** /ˌlɪpəʊˌkɒndrəʊ'dɪstrəfi/ *noun* a congenital disorder affecting lipid metabolism, the bones and the main organs, causing learning difficulties and physical deformity

**lipodystrophy** /ˌlɪpəʊ'dɪstrəfi/ *noun* a disorder of lipid metabolism

**lipogenesis** /ˌlɪpəʊ'dʒenəsɪs/ *noun* the production or making of deposits of fat

**lipoid** /'lɪpɔɪd/ *noun* a compound lipid, or a fatty substance such as cholesterol which is like a lipid ■ *adjective* like a lipid

**lipoidosis** /ˌlɪpɔɪ'dəʊsɪs/ *noun* a group of diseases with reticuloendothelial hyperplasia and unusual deposits of lipoids in the cells

**lipolysis** /lɪ'pɒlɪsɪs/ *noun* the process of breaking down fat by lipase

**lipolytic enzyme** /ˌlɪpəlɪtɪk 'enzaɪm/ *noun* same as **lipase**

**lipoma** /lɪˈpəʊmə/ *noun* a benign tumour formed of fatty tissue (NOTE: The plural is **lipomas** or **lipomata**.)

**lipomatosis** /ˌlɪpəʊməˈtəʊsɪs/ *noun* an excessive deposit of fat in the tissues in tumour-like masses

**lipoprotein** /ˌlɪpəʊˈprəʊtiːn/ *noun* a protein which combines with lipids and carries them in the bloodstream and lymph system (NOTE: Lipoproteins are classified according to the percentage of protein which they carry.)

**liposarcoma** /ˌlɪpəʊsɑːˈkəʊmə/ *noun* a rare malignant tumour found in fatty tissue (NOTE: The plural is **liposarcomas** or **liposarcomata**.)

**liposuction** /ˈlɪpəʊˌsʌkʃ(ə)n/ *noun* the surgical removal of fatty tissue for cosmetic reasons

**lipotrophic** /ˌlɪpəʊˈtrɒfɪk/ *adjective* referring to a substance which increases the amount of fat present in the tissues

**Lippes loop** /ˌlɪpəz ˈluːp/ *noun* a type of intrauterine device

**lipping** /ˈlɪpɪŋ/ *noun* a condition in which bone tissue grows over other bones

**lip salve** /ˈlɪp sælv/ *noun* an ointment, usually sold as a soft stick, used to rub on lips to prevent them cracking

**lipuria** /lɪˈpjʊəriə/ *noun* the presence of fat or oily emulsion in the urine

**liquid diet** /ˌlɪkwɪd ˈdaɪət/ *noun* a diet consisting only of liquids ○ *The clear liquid diet is a temporary diet used in preparation for surgery.*

**liquid paraffin** /ˌlɪkwɪd ˈpærəfɪn/ *noun* an oil used as a laxative

**liquor** /ˈlɪkə/ *noun* (*in pharmacy*) a solution, usually aqueous, of a pure substance

**lisp** /lɪsp/ *noun* a speech condition in which someone replaces 's' sounds with 'th' ■ *verb* to talk with a lisp

**Listeria** /lɪˈstɪəriə/ *noun* a genus of bacteria found in domestic animals and in unpasteurised milk products which can cause uterine infection or meningitis

**listeriosis** /lɪˌstɪəriˈəʊsɪs/ *noun* an infectious disease transmitted from animals to humans by the bacterium *Listeria*

**listless** /ˈlɪstləs/ *adjective* weak and tired

**listlessness** /ˈlɪstləsnəs/ *noun* the fact of being generally weak and tired

**liter** /ˈliːtə/ *noun* US spelling of **litre**

**lith-** /lɪθ/ *prefix* same as **litho-** (*used before vowels*)

**lithaemia** /lɪˈθiːmiə/ *noun* an unusual amount of uric acid in the blood. Also called **uricacidaemia** (NOTE: The US spelling is **lithemia**.)

**lithagogue** /ˈlɪθəgɒg/ *noun* a drug which helps to remove stones from the urine

**lithiasis** /lɪˈθaɪəsɪs/ *noun* the formation of stones in an organ

**lithium** /ˈlɪθiəm/ *noun* a soft silver-white metallic element that forms compounds, used as a medical treatment for bipolar disorder

**litho-** *prefix* referring to a calculus

**litholapaxy** /lɪˈθɒləpæksi/ *noun* the evacuation of pieces of a stone in the bladder after crushing it with a lithotrite. Also called **lithotrity**

**lithonephrotomy** /ˌlɪθəʊnəˈfrɒtəmi/ *noun* a surgical operation to remove a stone in the kidney (NOTE: The plural is **lithonephrotomies**.)

**lithotomy** /lɪˈθɒtəmi/ *noun* a surgical operation to remove a stone from the bladder (NOTE: The plural is **lithotomies**.)

**lithotomy position** /lɪˈθɒtəmi pəˌzɪʃ(ə)n/ *noun* a position for some medical examinations in which the person lies on his or her back with the legs flexed and the thighs against the abdomen

**lithotripsy** /ˈlɪθətrɪpsi/ *noun* the process of breaking up kidney or gall bladder stones into small fragments that the body can eliminate them unaided

**lithotrite** /ˈlɪθətraɪt/ *noun* a surgical instrument which crushes a stone in the bladder

**lithotrity** /lɪˈθɒtrɪti/ *noun* same as **litholapaxy**

**lithuresis** /ˌlɪθjʊˈriːsɪs/ *noun* the passage of small stones from the bladder during urination

**lithuria** /lɪˈθjʊəriə/ *noun* the presence of excessive amounts of uric acid or urates in the urine

**litmus** /ˈlɪtməs/ *noun* a substance which turns red in acid and blue in alkali

**litmus paper** /ˈlɪtməs ˌpeɪpə/ *noun* a small piece of paper impregnated with litmus, used to test for acidity or alkalinity

**litre** /ˈliːtə/ *noun* a unit of measurement of liquids equal to 1.76 pints. Abbr **l**, **L** (NOTE: With figures, usually written **l** or **L**: *2.5l*, but it can be written in full to avoid confusion with the numeral **1**. The US spelling is **liter**.)

**little finger** /ˌlɪt(ə)l ˈfɪŋgə/ *noun* the smallest finger on the hand

**Little's area** /ˈlɪt(ə)lz ˌeəriə/ *noun* an area of blood vessels in the nasal septum

**Little's disease** /ˈlɪt(ə)lz dɪˌziːz/ *noun* same as **spastic diplegia** [Described 1843. After William John Little (1810–94), physician at the London Hospital, UK.]

**little toe** /ˌlɪt(ə)l ˈtəʊ/ *noun* the smallest toe on the foot ○ *Her little toe was crushed by the door.*

**live** *adjective* /laɪv/ **1.** living, not dead ○ *graft using live tissue* ◊ **birth 2.** carrying electricity ○ *He was killed when he touched a live wire.* ■ *verb* /lɪv/ to be alive ○ *She is very ill, and the doctor doesn't think she will live much longer.* (NOTE: **living – lived**)

**live birth** /ˌlaɪv ˈbɜːθ/ *noun* the birth of a baby which is alive ○ *The number of live births has remained steady.*

**livedo** /lɪˈviːdəʊ/ *noun* discoloured spots on the skin

**liver** /ˈlɪvə/ *noun* a large gland in the upper part of the abdomen. See illustration at DIGESTIVE SYSTEM in Supplement (NOTE: For other terms referring to the liver, see words beginning with **hepat-, hepato-**.)

COMMENT: The liver is situated in the top part of the abdomen on the right side of the body next to the stomach. It is the largest gland in the body, weighing almost 2 kg. Blood carrying nutrients from the intestines enters the liver by the hepatic portal vein; the nutrients are removed and the blood returned to the heart through the hepatic vein. The liver is the major detoxicating organ in the body; it destroys harmful organisms in the blood, produces clotting agents, secretes bile, stores glycogen and metabolises proteins, carbohydrates and fats. Diseases affecting the liver include hepatitis and cirrhosis; the symptom of liver disease is often jaundice.

**liver fluke** /ˈlɪvə fluːk/ *noun* a parasitic flatworm which can infest the liver

**liver spot** /ˈlɪvə spɒt/ *noun* a little brown patch on the skin of the backs of the hands, attributed to sun damage (NOTE: Liver spots are unconnected with any liver disorder.)

**liver transplant** /ˈlɪvə ˌtrænsplɑːnt/ *noun* a surgical operation to give a person the liver of another person who has died

**livid** /ˈlɪvɪd/ *adjective* referring to skin with a blue colour because of being bruised or because of asphyxiation

**living will** /ˌlɪvɪŋ ˈwɪl/ *noun* a document signed by a person while in good health to specify the decisions he or she wishes to be taken about medical treatment if he or she becomes incapable of making or communicating them

**LMC** *abbr* local medical committee

**loa loa** /ˌləʊə ˈləʊə/ *noun* a tropical disease of the eye caused when the threadworm *Loa loa* enters the eye or the skin around the eye

**Loa loa** /ˌləʊə ˈləʊə/ *noun* a tropical threadworm which digs under the skin, especially around and into the eye, causing loa loa and loiasis

**lobar** /ˈləʊbə/ *adjective* referring to a lobe

**lobar bronchi** /ˌləʊbə ˈbrɒŋkiː/ *plural noun* air passages supplying a lobe of a lung. Also called **secondary bronchi**

**lobar pneumonia** /ˌləʊbə njuːˈməʊniə/ *noun* pneumonia which affects one or more lobes of the lung

**lobe** /ləʊb/ *noun* 1. a rounded section of an organ such as the brain, lung or liver. See illustration at LUNGS in Supplement 2. the soft fleshy part at the bottom of the ear 3. a cusp on the crown of a tooth

**lobectomy** /ləʊˈbektəmi/ *noun* a surgical operation to remove one of the lobes of an organ such as the lung ○ *The plural is lobectomies.*

**lobotomy** /ləʊˈbɒtəmi/ *noun* a surgical operation formerly used to treat mental illness by cutting into a lobe of the brain to cut the nerve fibres (NOTE: The plural is **lobotomies**.)

**lobular** /ˈlɒbjʊlə/ *adjective* relating to a lobule ○ *lobular carcinoma*

**lobule** /ˈlɒbjuːl/ *noun* a small section of a lobe in the lung, formed of acini

**local** /ˈləʊk(ə)l/ *adjective* 1. referring to a separate place 2. confined to one part ■ *noun* same as **local anaesthetic**

**local anaesthesia** /ˌləʊk(ə)l ænəsˈθiːziə/ *noun* loss of feeling in a single part of the body

**local anaesthetic** /ˌləʊk(ə)l ænəsˈθetɪk/ *noun* an anaesthetic such as lignocaine which removes the feeling in a single part of the body only ○ *The surgeon removed the growth under local anaesthetic.*

**localise** /ˈləʊkəlaɪz/, **localize** *verb* 1. to restrict the spread of something to a specific area 2. to find where something is 3. to transfer power from a central authority to local organisations (NOTE: **localising – localised**)

**localised** /ˈləʊkəlaɪzd/, **localized** *adjective* referring to an infection which occurs in one part of the body only. Opposite **generalised**

**Local Medical Committee** /ˌləʊk(ə)l ˈmedɪk(ə)l kəˌmɪti/ *noun* a committee responsible for monitoring the interests of providers of primary care such as GPs, dentists and pharmacists in a district. Abbr **LMC**

**local supervising authority** /ˌləʊk(ə)l ˈsuːpəvaɪzɪŋ ɔːˌθɒrɪti/ *noun* an organisation which controls midwife services within its area

**lochia** /ˈlɒkiə/ *noun* a discharge from the vagina after childbirth or abortion

**lochial** /ˈləʊkiəl/ *adjective* referring to lochia

**lochiometra** /ˈlɒkiəmiːtrə/ *noun* a condition in which lochia remains in the uterus after a baby is born, making it swollen

**lock** /lɒk/ *verb* to fix something in a position

**locked-in syndrome** /ˌlɒkt ˈɪn ˌsɪndrəʊm/ *noun* a condition in which only the eyes and eyelids can move although the person is fully alert and conscious. It results from severe damage to the brain stem.

**locked knee** /ˌlɒkt ˈniː/ *noun* a condition in which a piece of the cartilage in the knee slips out of position. The symptom is a sharp pain, and the knee remains permanently bent.

**locking joint** /ˌlɒkɪŋ ˈdʒɔɪnt/ *noun* a joint which can be locked in an extended position, e.g. the knee or elbow

**lockjaw** /ˈlɒkjɔː/ *noun* same as **tetanus** (*dated informal*)

**locomotion** /ˌləʊkəˈməʊʃ(ə)n/ *noun* the fact of being able to move

**locomotor** /ˌləʊkəˈməʊtə/ *adjective* relating to locomotion

**locomotor ataxia** /ˌləʊkəˌməʊtər əˈtæksiə/ *noun* same as **tabes dorsalis**

**loculated** /ˈlɒkjʊleɪtɪd/ *adjective* referring to an organ or a growth which is divided into many compartments ○ *a loculated renal abscess*

**locule** /ˈlɒkjuːl/ *noun* same as **loculus**

**loculus** /ˈlɒkjʊləs/ *noun* a small space in an organ (NOTE: The plural is **loculi**.)

**locum** /ˈləʊkəm/ *noun* a healthcare professional such as a doctor or pharmacist who takes the place of another for a time. Also called **locum tenens**

**locum tenens** *noun* same as **locum** (NOTE: The plural is **locum tenentes**.)

**locus** /ˈləʊkəs/ *noun* **1.** an area or point where an infection or disease is to be found **2.** a position on a chromosome occupied by a gene (NOTE: The plural is **loci**.)

**lodge** /lɒdʒ/ *verb* to stay or stick somewhere, or to stick something somewhere ○ *The piece of bone lodged in her throat.* ○ *The larvae of the tapeworm lodge in the walls of the intestine.*

**lofepramine** /lɒˈfeprəmiːn/ *noun* an antidepressant drug

**log roll** /ˈlɒg rəʊl/ *noun* a method of turning people in bed onto their side by putting them into a straight position and pulling on the sheet under them

**logrolling** /ˈlɒgrəʊlɪŋ/ *noun* the process of moving a person who is lying down into another position using the log roll method

**-logy** /lədʒi/ *suffix* **1.** science or study ○ *psychology* ○ *embryology* **2.** speech or expression

**loiasis** /ləʊˈaɪəsɪs/ *noun* a tropical disease of the eye caused when the threadworm *Loa loa* enters the eye or the skin around the eye

**loin** /lɔɪn/ *noun* the lower back part of the body above the buttocks

**Lomotil** /ləʊˈməʊtɪl/ *a trade name for a preparation containing diphenoxalate*

**long-acting** /ˌlɒŋ ˈæktɪŋ/ *adjective* referring to a drug or treatment which has an effect that lasts a long time

**long bone** /ˈlɒŋ bəʊn/ *noun* any long limb bone that contains marrow and ends in a part that forms a joint with another bone

**longitudinal** /ˌlɒŋgɪˈtjuːdɪn(ə)l/ *adjective* **1.** positioned lengthwise **2.** in the direction of the long axis of the body

**longitudinal arch** /ˌlɒŋgɪtjuːdɪn(ə)l ˈɑːtʃ/ *noun* same as **plantar arch**

**longitudinal fissure** /ˌlɒŋgɪtjuːdɪn(ə)l ˈfɪʃə/ *noun* a groove separating the two cerebral hemispheres

**longitudinal lie** /ˌlɒŋgɪtjuːdɪn(ə)l ˈlaɪ/ *noun* the usual position of a fetus, lying along the axis of the mother's body

**longitudinal study** /ˌlɒŋgɪtjuːdɪn(ə)l ˈstʌdi/ *noun* a study of individuals or groups of people and of how some aspect such as their health or education changes over a long time

**longsighted** /ˌlɒŋˈsaɪtɪd/ *adjective* able to see clearly things which are far away but not things which are close

**longsightedness** /ˌlɒŋˈsaɪtɪdnəs/ *noun* the condition of being longsighted. Also called **hypermetropia**

**long-stay** /ˈlɒŋ steɪ/ *adjective* referring to staying a long time in hospital ○ *patients in long-stay units*

**long stay patient** /ˌlɒŋ steɪ ˈpeɪʃ(ə)nt/ *noun* a patient who will stay in hospital for a long time

**long stay ward** /ˌlɒŋ ˈsteɪ ˌwɔːd/ *noun* a ward for patients who will stay in hospital for a long time

**loo** /luː/ *noun* a toilet, or a room containing a toilet (*informal*) □ **to go to the loo** to urinate or defecate

**look after** /ˌlʊk ˈɑːftə/ *verb* to take care of a person and attend to his or her needs ○ *The nurses looked after him very well* or *He was very well looked after in hospital.* ○ *She is off work looking after her children who have mumps.*

**loop** /luːp/ *noun* **1.** a curve or bend in a line, especially one of the particular curves in a fingerprint **2.** a curved piece of wire placed in the uterus to prevent contraception

**loop of Henle** /ˌluːp əv ˈhenli/ *noun* a curved tube which forms the main part of a nephron in the kidney

**loperamide** /ləʊˈperəmaɪd/, **loperamide hydrochloride** /ləʊˌperəmaɪd ˌhaɪdrəʊˈklɔːraɪd/ *noun* a drug that relieves severe diarrhoea by slowing down the movements of the intestine

**loratidine** /lɒrˈætɪdiːn/ *noun* an antihistamine drug

**lorazepam** /lɔːˈræzɪpæm/ *noun* a mild tranquilliser that people often receive before surgery to lessen anxiety

**lordosis** /lɔːˈdəʊsɪs/ *noun* excessive forward curvature of the lower part of the spine. ◊ **kyphosis**

**lordotic** /lɔːˈdɒtɪk/ *adjective* referring to lordosis

**lotion** /ˈləʊʃ(ə)n/ *noun* a medicinal liquid used to rub on the skin ○ *a mild antiseptic lotion*

**louse** /laʊs/ *noun* a small insect of the *Pediculus* genus, which sucks blood and lives on the skin as a parasite on animals and humans (NOTE: The plural is **lice**.)

COMMENT: There are several forms of louse: the commonest are the body louse, the crab louse and the head louse. Some diseases can be transmitted by lice.

**low** /ləʊ/ *adjective* **1.** relatively little in height **2.** close to the bottom or base of something

**low blood pressure** /ˌləʊ ˈblʌd ˌpreʃə/ *noun* same as **hypotension**

**low-calorie diet** /ˌləʊ ˌkæləri ˈdaɪət/ *noun* a diet with few calories, to help a person to lose weight

**low-density lipoprotein** /ləʊ ˌdensɪti ˈlɪpəʊprəʊtiːn/ *noun* a lipoprotein with a large percentage of cholesterol which deposits fats in muscles and arteries. Abbr **LDL**

**lower** /ˈlaʊə/ *adjective* in a position below another thing

**lower jaw** /ˌləʊə ˈdʒɔː/ *noun* same as **mandible**

**lower limb** /ˌləʊə ˈlɪm/ *noun* a leg

**lower motor neurones** /ˌləʊə ˈməʊtə ˌnjʊərəʊnz/ *plural noun* linked neurones which carry motor impulses from the spinal cord to the muscles

**low-fat diet** /ˌləʊ ˌfæt ˈdaɪət/ *noun* a diet with little animal fat, which can help reduce the risk of heart disease and alleviate some skin conditions

**low-risk patient** /ˌləʊ rɪsk ˈpeɪʃ(ə)nt/ *noun* a person not likely to catch or develop a particular disease

**low-salt diet** /ˌləʊ ˌsɔːlt ˈdaɪət/ *noun* a diet with little salt, which has been shown to help reduce high blood pressure

**lozenge** /ˈlɒzɪndʒ/ *noun* a sweet medicinal tablet ○ *She was sucking a cough lozenge.*

**LPN** *abbr US* licensed practical nurse

**LRCP** *abbr* licentiate of the Royal College of Physicians

**LSA** *abbr* local supervising authority

**LSD** *abbr* lysergic acid diethylamide

**lubb-dupp** /lʌbˈdʌb/ *noun* two sounds made by the heart, which represent each cardiac cycle when heard through a stethoscope

**lubricant** /ˈluːbrɪkənt/ *noun* a fluid which lubricates

**lubricate** /ˈluːbrɪkeɪt/ *verb* to cover something with a fluid to reduce friction (NOTE: **lubricating – lubricated**)

**lubricating jelly** /ˈluːbrɪkeɪt ˌdʒeli/ *noun* a jelly used to make a surface slippery

**lucid** /ˈluːsɪd/ *adjective* with a clearly working mind ○ *In spite of the pain, he was still lucid.*

**lucid interval** /ˌluːsɪd ˈɪntəv(ə)l/ *noun* a period of clear thinking which occurs between two periods of unconsciousness or of mental illness

**Ludwig's angina** /ˌluːdvɪgz ænˈdʒaɪnə/ *noun* cellulitis of the mouth and some parts of the neck which causes the neck to swell and may obstruct the airway [Described 1836. After Wilhelm Friedrich von Ludwig (1790–1865), Professor of Surgery and Midwifery at Tübingen,

Germany, and Court Physician to King Frederick II.]

**lues** /ˈluːiːz/ *noun* a former name for syphilis or the plague

**lumbago** /lʌmˈbeɪgəʊ/ *noun* pain in the lower back (*informal*) ○ *She has been suffering from lumbago for years.* ○ *He has had an attack of lumbago.*

**lumbar** /ˈlʌmbə/ *adjective* referring to the lower part of the back

**lumbar artery** /ˈlʌmbə ˌɑːtəri/ *noun* one of four arteries which supply blood to the back muscles and skin

**lumbar cistern** /ˌlʌmbə ˈsɪstən/ *noun* a subarachnoid space in the spinal cord, where the dura mater ends, filled with cerebrospinal fluid

**lumbar enlargement** /ˌlʌmbə ɪn ˈlɑːdʒmənt/ *noun* the wider part of the spinal cord in the lower spine, where the nerves of the lower limbs are attached

**lumbar plexus** /ˌlʌmbə ˈpleksəs/ *noun* the point where several nerves which supply the thighs and abdomen join together, lying in the upper psoas muscle

**lumbar puncture** /ˌlʌmbə ˈpʌŋktʃə/ *noun* a surgical operation to remove a sample of cerebrospinal fluid by inserting a hollow needle into the lower part of the spinal canal. Also called **spinal puncture** (NOTE: The US term is usually **spinal tap**.)

**lumbar region** /ˈlʌmbə ˌriːdʒən/ *noun* the two parts of the abdomen on each side of the umbilical region

**lumbar vertebra** /ˌlʌmbə ˈvɜːtɪbrə/ *plural noun* each of the five vertebrae between the thoracic vertebrae and the sacrum

**lumbo-** /lʌmbəʊ/ *prefix* the lumbar region

**lumbosacral** /ˌlʌmbəʊˈseɪkrəl/ *adjective* referring to both the lumbar vertebrae and the sacrum

**lumbosacral joint** /ˌlʌmbəʊˈseɪkrəl dʒɔɪnt/ *noun* a joint at the bottom of the back between the lumbar vertebrae and the sacrum

**lumen** /ˈluːmɪn/ *noun* **1.** an SI unit of light emitted per second **2.** the inside width of a passage in the body or of an instrument such as an endoscope **3.** a hole at the end of an instrument such as an endoscope

**lump** /lʌmp/ *noun* a mass of hard tissue which rises on the surface or under the surface of the skin ○ *He has a lump where he hit his head on the low door.* ○ *She noticed a lump in her right breast and went to see the doctor.*

**lumpectomy** /lʌmˈpektəmi/ *noun* a surgical operation to remove a hard mass of tissue such as a breast tumour, leaving the surrounding tissue intact (NOTE: The plural is **lumpectomies**.)

**lunate** /ˈluːneɪt/, **lunate bone** /ˈluːneɪt bəʊn/ *noun* one of the eight small carpal bones in the wrist. See illustration at HAND in Supplement

**Lund and Browder chart** /ˌlʌnd ən ˈbraʊdə tʃɑːt/ *noun* a chart for calculating the surface area of a burn

**lung** /lʌŋ/ *noun* one of two organs of respiration in the body into which air is sucked when a person breathes (NOTE: For other terms referring to the lungs, see words beginning with **bronch-, broncho-, pneum-, pneumo-, pneumon-, pneumono-, pulmo-.**)

COMMENT: The two lungs are situated in the chest cavity, protected by the ribcage. The heart lies between the lungs. The right lung has three lobes, the left lung only two. Air goes down into the lungs through the trachea and bronchi. It passes to the alveoli where its oxygen is deposited in the blood in exchange for waste carbon dioxide which is exhaled (gas exchange). Lung cancer can be caused by smoking tobacco, and is commonest in people who are heavy smokers.

**lung cancer** /ˈlʌŋ ˌkænsə/ *noun* cancer in the lung

**lunula** /ˈluːnjʊlə/ *noun* a curved white mark at the base of a fingernail (NOTE: The plural is **lunulae.**)

**lupus** /ˈluːpəs/ *noun* a persistent skin disease, of which there are several unrelated types

**lupus erythematosus** /ˌluːpəs ˌerɪθiːməˈtəʊsəs/ *noun* an inflammatory disease of connective tissue of which the more serious, systemic, form affects the heart, joints and blood vessels. Abbr **LE**

**lupus vulgaris** /ˌluːpəs vʌlˈgeərɪs/ *noun* a form of tuberculosis of the skin in which red spots appear on the face and become infected

**lutein** /ˈluːtiːɪn/ *noun* a yellow pigment in the corpus luteum

**luteinising hormone** /ˈluːtiːɪnaɪzɪŋ ˌhɔːməʊn/, **luteinizing hormone** *noun* a hormone produced by the pituitary gland, which stimulates the formation of the corpus luteum in females and of testosterone in males. Abbr **LH.** Also called **interstitial cell stimulating hormone**

**luteo-** /ˈluːtiəʊ/ *prefix* **1.** yellow **2.** corpus luteum

**luxation** /lʌkˈseɪʃ(ə)n/ *noun* same as **dislocation**

**Lyme disease** /ˈlaɪm dɪˌziːz/ *noun* a viral disease caused by *Borrelia burgdorferi* transmitted by bites from deer ticks. It causes rashes, nervous pains, paralysis and, in extreme cases, death.

**lymph** /lɪmf/ *noun* a colourless liquid containing white blood cells which circulates in the lymph system from all body tissues, carrying waste matter away from tissues to the veins. Also called **lymph fluid**

COMMENT: Lymph drains from the tissues through capillaries into lymph vessels. It is formed of water, protein and white blood cells (lymphocytes). Waste matter such as infection in the lymph is filtered out and destroyed as it passes through the lymph nodes, which

then add further lymphocytes to the lymph before it continues in the system. It eventually drains into the brachiocephalic (innominate) veins, and joins the venous bloodstream. Lymph is not pumped round the body like blood but moves by muscle pressure on the lymph vessels and by the negative pressure of the large veins into which the vessels empty. Lymph is an essential part of the body's defence against infection.

**lymph-** /lɪmf/ *prefix meaning* same as **lympho-** (*used before vowels*)

**lymphaden-** /lɪmfædən/ *prefix* relating to the lymph nodes

**lymphadenectomy** /ˌlɪmfædəˈnektəmi/ *noun* the surgical removal of a lymph node (NOTE: The plural is **lymphadenectomies.**)

**lymphadenitis** /ˌlɪmfædəˈnaɪtɪs/ *noun* inflammation of the lymph nodes

**lymphadenoma** /ˌlɪmfædəˈnəʊmə/ *noun* same as **lymphoma**

**lymphadenopathy** /ˌlɪmfædəˈnɒpəθi/ *noun* any unusual condition of the lymph nodes (NOTE: The plural is **lymphadenopathies.**)

**lymphangi-** /lɪmfændʒi/ *prefix* lymphatic vessel

**lymphangiectasis** /ˌlɪmfændʒiˈektəsɪs/ *noun* swelling of the smaller lymph vessels as a result of obstructions in larger vessels

**lymphangiography** /ˌlɪmfændʒiˈɒɡrəfi/ *noun* an X-ray examination of the lymph vessels following introduction of radio-opaque material (NOTE: The plural is **lymphangiographies.**)

**lymphangioma** /ˌlɪmfændʒiˈəʊmə/ *noun* a benign tumour formed of lymph tissues (NOTE: The plural is **lymphangiomas** or **lymphangiomata.**)

**lymphangioplasty** /lɪmfˈændʒiəplæsti/ *noun* a surgical operation to make artificial lymph channels (NOTE: The plural is **lymphangioplasties.**)

**lymphangiosarcoma** /lɪmfˌændʒiəʊsɑːˈkəʊmə/ *noun* a malignant tumour of the endothelial cells lining the lymph vessels (NOTE: The plural is **lymphangiosarcomas** or **lymphangiosarcomata.**)

**lymphangitis** /ˌlɪmfænˈdʒaɪtɪs/ *noun* inflammation of the lymph vessels

**lymphatic** /lɪmˈfætɪk/ *adjective* referring to lymph

**lymphatic capillary** /lɪmˌfætɪk kəˈpɪləri/ *plural noun* any of the capillaries which lead from tissue and join lymphatic vessels

**lymphatic duct** /lɪmˈfætɪk dʌkt/ *noun* the main channel for carrying lymph

**lymphatic node** /lɪmˈfætɪk nəʊd/ *noun* same as **lymph gland**

**lymphatic nodule** /lɪmˌfætɪk ˈnɒdjuːl/ *noun* a small lymph node found in clusters in tissues

**lymphatic system** /lɪmˈfætɪk ˌsɪstəm/ *noun* a series of vessels which transport lymph from the tissues through the lymph nodes and into the bloodstream

**lymphatic vessel** /lɪmˈfætɪk ˌves(ə)l/ *noun* a tube which carries lymph round the body from the tissues to the veins

**lymph duct** /ˈlɪmf dʌkt/ *noun* any channel carrying lymph

**lymph fluid** /ˈlɪmf ˌfluːɪd/ *noun* same as **lymph**

**lymph gland** /ˈlɪmf glænd/, **lymph node** /ˈlɪmf nəʊd/ *noun* a mass of lymphoid tissue situated in various points of the lymphatic system, especially under the armpits and in the groin, through which lymph passes and in which lymphocytes are produced. Also called **lymphatic node**

**lympho-** /lɪmfəʊ/ *prefix meaning* lymph

**lymphoblast** /ˈlɪmfəʊblæst/ *noun* an unusual cell which forms in acute lymphoblastic leukaemia as a result of the change which takes place in a lymphocyte on contact with an antigen

**lymphoblastic** /ˌlɪmfəʊˈblæstɪk/ *adjective* referring to lymphoblasts, or forming lymphocytes

**lymphocele** /ˈlɪmfəsiːl/ *noun* a cyst containing lymph from injured or diseased lymph nodes or ducts

**lymphocyte** /ˈlɪmfəsaɪt/ *noun* a type of mature leucocyte or white blood cell formed by the lymph nodes and concerned with the production of antibodies

**lymphocytopenia** /ˌlɪmfəʊˌsaɪtəʊˈpiːniə/ *noun* same as **lymphopenia**

**lymphocytosis** /ˌlɪmfəʊsaɪˈtəʊsɪs/ *noun* an increased number of lymphocytes in the blood

**lymphoedema** /ˌlɪmfəʊɪˈdiːmə/ *noun* a swelling caused by obstruction of the lymph vessels or unusual development of lymph vessels (NOTE: The US spelling is **lymphedema**.)

**lymphogranuloma inguinale** /ˌlɪmfəʊ grænjʊˌləʊmə ˌɪŋgwɪˈneɪli/ *noun* same as **lymphogranuloma venereum**

**lymphogranuloma venereum** /ˌlɪmfəʊ ˌgrænjʊˌləʊmə vəˈnɪərəm/ *noun* a sexually transmitted bacterial infection that causes swelling of the genital lymph nodes and, especially in men, a genital ulcer. Abbr **l.g.v.**

**lymphography** /lɪmˈfɒgrəfi/ *noun* the making of images of the lymphatic system after having introduced a radio-opaque substance

**lymphoid** /ˈlɪmfɔɪd/ *adjective* referring to lymph, lymphatic tissue, or the lymphatic system

**lymphoid tissue** /ˈlɪmfɔɪd ˌtɪʃuː/ *noun* tissue in the lymph nodes, the tonsils and the spleen where masses of lymphocytes are supported by a network of reticular fibres and cells

**lymphokine** /ˈlɪmfəʊkaɪn/ *noun* a protein produced by lymphocytes that has an effect on other cells in the immune system. ◊ **cytokine**

**lymphoma** /lɪmˈfəʊmə/ *noun* a malignant tumour arising from lymphoid tissue. Also called **lymphadenoma** (NOTE: The plural is **lymphomas** or **lymphomata**.)

**lymphopenia** /ˌlɪmfəʊˈpiːniə/ *noun* a reduction in the number of lymphocytes in the blood. Also called **lymphocytopenia**

**lymphopoiesis** /ˌlɪmfəʊpɔɪˈiːsɪs/ *noun* the production of lymphocytes or lymphoid tissue

**lymphorrhagia** /ˌlɪmfəˈreɪdʒə/, **lymphorrhoea** /ˌlɪmfəˈriə/ *noun* escape of lymph from ruptured or severed lymphatic vessels

**lymphosarcoma** /ˌlɪmfəʊsɑːˈkəʊmə/ *noun* a malignant growth arising from lymphocytes and their cells of origin in the lymph nodes (NOTE: The plural is **lymphosarcomas** or **lymphosarcomata**.)

**lymphotropic** /ˌlɪmfəˈtrɒpɪk/ *adjective* affecting the lymphatic system

**lymphuria** /lɪmˈfjʊəriə/ *noun* the presence of lymph in the urine

**lymph vessel** /ˈlɪmf ˌves(ə)l/ *noun* one of the tubes which carry lymph round the body from the tissues to the veins

**lyophilisation** /laɪˌɒfɪlaɪˈzeɪʃ(ə)n/, **lyophilization** *noun* the act of preserving tissue, plasma or serum by freeze-drying it in a vacuum

**lyophilise** /laɪˈɒfɪlaɪz/, **lyophilize** *verb* to preserve tissue, plasma or serum by freeze-drying in a vacuum (NOTE: **lyophilising – lyophilised**)

**lysergic acid diethylamide** /laɪˈsɜːdʒɪk ˈæsɪd daɪˈeθɪləmaɪd/ *noun* a powerful hallucinogenic drug which can cause psychosis. Abbr **LSD**

**lysin** /ˈlaɪsɪn/ *noun* **1.** a protein in the blood which destroys the cell against which it is directed **2.** a toxin which causes the lysis of cells

**lysine** /ˈlaɪsiːn/ *noun* an essential amino acid

**lysis** /ˈlaɪsɪs/ *noun* **1.** the destruction of a cell by a lysin, in which the membrane of the cell is destroyed **2.** a reduction in a fever or disease slowly over a period of time. Opposite **crisis**

**-lysis** /lɪsɪs/ *suffix* referring to processes which involve breaking up or decaying, or to objects which are doing this ○ *haemolysis*

**lysol** /ˈlaɪsɒl/ *noun* a strong disinfectant, made of cresol and soap

**lysosome** /ˈlaɪsəsəʊm/ *noun* a particle in a cell which contains enzymes which break down substances such as bacteria which enter the cell

**lysozyme** /ˈlaɪsəzaɪm/ *noun* an enzyme found in the whites of eggs and in tears, which destroys specific bacteria

# M

**m** *symbol* **1.** metre **2.** milli-

**M** *symbol* mega-

**MAAG** *abbr* medical audit advisory group

**macerate** /'mæsəreɪt/ *verb* to make something soft by letting it lie in a liquid for a time (NOTE: **macerating – macerated**)

**maceration** /ˌmæsə'reɪʃ(ə)n/ *noun* the process of softening a solid by letting it lie in a liquid so that the soluble matter dissolves

**Mackenrodt's ligaments** /'mækənrəʊdz ˌlɪɡəmənts/ *plural noun* same as **cardinal ligaments**

**Macmillan nurse** /mək'mɪlən nɜːs/ *noun* a nurse who specialises in cancer care and is employed by the organisation Macmillan Cancer Relief

**macro-** /mækrəʊ/ *prefix* large. Opposite **micro-**

**macrobiotic** /ˌmækrəʊbaɪ'ɒtɪk/ *adjective* referring to food which has been produced naturally without artificial additives or preservatives

COMMENT: Macrobiotic diets are usually vegetarian and are prepared in a special way. They consist of beans, coarse flour, fruit and vegetables. They may not contain enough protein or trace elements, especially to satisfy the needs of children.

**macrocephaly** /ˌmækrəʊ'kefli/ *noun* the condition of having an unusually large head

**macrocheilia** /ˌmækrəʊ'kaɪliə/ *noun* the condition of having large lips

**macrocyte** /'mækrəʊsaɪt/ *noun* an unusually large red blood cell found in people who have pernicious anaemia

**macrocythaemia** /ˌmækrəʊsaɪ'θiːmiə/ *noun* same as **macrocytosis**

**macrocytic** /ˌmækrəʊ'sɪtɪk/ *adjective* referring to macrocytes

**macrocytic anaemia** /ˌmækrəʊsɪtɪk ə'niːmiə/ *noun* anaemia in which someone has unusually large red blood cells

**macrocytosis** /ˌmækrəʊsaɪ'təʊsɪs/ *noun* the condition of having macrocytes in the blood. Also called **macrocythaemia**

**macrodactyly** /ˌmækrəʊ'dæktɪli/ *noun* a condition in which a person has unusually large or long fingers or toes

**macrogenitosoma** /ˌmækrəʊˌdʒenɪtə'səʊmə/ *noun* premature development of the body with the genitals being of an unusually large size

**macroglobulin** /ˌmækrəʊ'ɡlɒbjʊlɪn/ *noun* a class of immunoglobulin, a globulin protein of high molecular weight, which serves as an antibody

**macroglossia** /ˌmækrəʊ'ɡlɒsiə/ *noun* the condition of having an unusually large tongue

**macrognathia** /ˌmækrəʊ'neɪθiə/ *noun* a condition in which the jaw is larger than usual

**macrolide drug** /'mækrəlaɪd drʌg/ *noun* a drug used in the treatment of bacterial infection, often in place of penicillin in people sensitive to penicillin (NOTE: Macrolide drugs have names ending in **-omycin: erythromycin.**)

**macromastia** /ˌmækrəʊ'mæstiə/ *noun* overdevelopment of the breasts

**macromelia** /ˌmækrəʊ'miːliə/ *noun* a condition in which a person has unusually large limbs

**macronutrient** /'mækrəʊˌnjuːtriənt/ *noun* a substance which an organism needs in large amounts for normal growth and development, e.g. nitrogen, carbon or potassium. Compare **micronutrient**

**macrophage** /'mækrəʊfeɪdʒ/ *noun* any of several large cells which destroy inflammatory tissue, found in connective tissue, wounds, lymph nodes and other parts

**macropsia** /mæ'krɒpsiə/ *noun* a condition in which a person sees objects larger than they really are, caused by an unusual development in the retina

**macroscopic** /ˌmækrəʊ'skɒpɪk/ *adjective* able to be seen with the naked eye

**macrosomia** /ˌmækrəʊ'səʊmiə/ *noun* a condition in which the body grows too much

**macrostomia** /ˌmækrəʊ'stəʊmiə/ *noun* a condition in which the mouth is too wide because the bones of the upper and lower jaw have not fused, either on one or on both sides

**macula** /'mækjʊlə/ *noun* **1.** same as **macule 2.** a small coloured area, e.g. a macula lutea **3.** an area of hair cells inside the utricle and saccule of the ear (NOTE: The plural is **maculae**.)

**macula lutea** /ˌmækjʊlə 'luːtiə/ *noun* a yellow spot on the retina, surrounding the fovea, the part of the eye which sees most clearly. Also called **yellow spot**

**macular** /'mækjʊlə/ *adjective* referring to a macula

**macular degeneration** /ˌmækjʊlə dɪˌdʒenəˈreɪʃ(ə)n/ *noun* an eye disorder in elderly people in which fluid leaks into the retina and destroys cones and rods, reducing central vision

**macular oedema** /ˌmækjʊlə ɪˈdiːmə/ *noun* a disorder of the eye in which fluid gathers in the fovea

**macule** /'mækjuːl/ *noun* a small flat coloured spot on the skin. Compare **papule**

**maculopapular** /ˌmækjʊləʊˈpæpjʊlə/ *adjective* made up of both macules and papules ○ *maculopapular rash*

**mad cow disease** *noun* same as **bovine spongiform encephalopathy** (*informal*)

**maduromycosis** /məˌdjʊərəʊmaɪˈkəʊsɪs/, **maduromycetoma** /məˌdjʊərəʊˌmaɪsə'təʊmə/, **Madura foot** /məˌdjʊərə 'fʊt/ *noun* a tropical fungus infection in the feet which can destroy tissue and infect bones

**Magendie's foramen** /məˌdʒendɪz fə 'reɪmen/ *noun* an opening in the fourth ventricle of the brain which allows cerebrospinal fluid to flow [Described 1828. After François Magendie (1783–1855), French physician and physiologist.]

**magna** /'mægnə/ ♦ **cisterna magna**

**magnesium** /mæg'niːziəm/ *noun* a chemical element found in green vegetables, which is essential especially for the correct functioning of muscles (NOTE: The chemical symbol is **Mg**.)

**magnesium sulphate** /mægˌniːziəm 'sʌlↄfeɪt/ *noun* a magnesium salt used as a laxative. Also called **Epsom salts**

**magnesium trisilicate** /mægˌniːziəm traɪ 'sɪlɪkət/ *noun* a magnesium compound used to treat peptic ulcers

**magnetic** /mæg'netɪk/ *adjective* able to attract objects, like a magnet

**magnetic field** /mægˌnetɪk 'fiːld/ *noun* an area round an object which is under the influence of the magnetic force exerted by the object

**magnetic resonance imaging** /mægˌnetɪk 'rezənəns ˌɪmɪdʒɪŋ/ *noun* a scanning technique which exposes the body to a strong magnetic field and uses the electromagnetic signals emitted by the body to form an image of soft tissue and cells. Abbr **MRI**

**magnum** /'mægnəm/ ♦ **foramen magnum**

**maim** /meɪm/ *verb* to incapacitate someone with a major injury

**main bronchi** /meɪn 'brɒŋkiː/ *plural noun* the two main air passages which branch from the trachea outside the lung. Also called **primary bronchi**

**major** /'meɪdʒə/ *adjective* **1.** important or serious **2.** more important or serious than others of the same type ○ *The operation was a major one.* ▶ opposite **minor**

**major surgery** /ˌmeɪdʒə 'sɜːdʒəri/ *noun* surgical operations involving important organs in the body. Compare **minor surgery**

**mal** /mæl/ *noun* an illness or disease

**mal-** /mæl/ *prefix* bad or unusual

**malabsorption** /ˌmæləbˈsɔːpʃən/ *noun* a situation where the intestines are unable to absorb the fluids and nutrients in food properly

**malabsorption syndrome** /ˌmæləb 'sɔːpʃən ˌsɪndrəʊm/ *noun* a group of symptoms and signs, including malnutrition, anaemia, oedema and dermatitis, which results from steatorrhoea and malabsorption of vitamins, protein, carbohydrates and water

**malacia** /məˈleɪʃə/ *noun* the pathological softening of an organ or tissue

**maladjusted** /ˌmæləˈdʒʌstɪd/ *adjective* referring to a person who has difficulty fitting into society or family

**maladjustment** /ˌmæləˈdʒʌstmənt/ *noun* difficulty experienced in fitting into society or family

**malaise** /məˈleɪz/ *noun* a feeling of discomfort

**malaligned** /ˌmælə'laɪnd/ *adjective* not in the correct position relative to other parts of the body

**malalignment** /ˌmælə'laɪnmənt/ *noun* a condition in which something is malaligned, especially in which a tooth is not in its correct position in the mouth

**malar** /'meɪlə/ *adjective* referring to the cheek

**malar bone** /'meɪlə bəʊn/ *noun* same as **cheekbone**

**malaria** /məˈleəriə/ *noun* a mainly tropical disease caused by a parasite *Plasmodium*, which enters the body after a bite from the female anopheles mosquito

COMMENT: Malaria is a recurrent disease. It produces headaches, shivering, vomiting, sweating and sometimes hallucinations which are caused by toxins coming from the waste of the parasite *Plasmodium* in the blood.

**malarial** /məˈleəriəl/ *adjective* referring to malaria

**malarial parasite** /məˌleəriəl 'pærəsaɪt/ *noun* a parasite transmitted into the human bloodstream by the bite of the female anopheles mosquito

**malarial therapy** /məˈleəriə ˌθerəpi/ *noun* a treatment in which a person is given a form of malaria in the belief that the high fevers they

**male menopause** **232**

experience can stimulate the immune system to fight off serious diseases such as syphilis and HIV

**male menopause** /meɪl ˈmenəpɔːz/ *noun* a period in middle age when a man may feel insecure and anxious about the fact that his physical powers are declining (*informal*)

**male sex hormone** /ˌmeɪl ˈseks ˌhɔːməʊn/ *noun* same as **testosterone**

**male sex organs** /ˌmeɪl ˈseks ˌɔːɡənz/ *plural noun* the testes, epididymis, vasa deferentia, seminal vesicles, ejaculatory ducts and penis

**malformation** /ˌmælfɔːˈmeɪʃ(ə)n/ *noun* an unusual variation in the shape, structure or development of something

**malformed** /mælˈfɔːmd/ *adjective* unusual in shape, structure or development

**malfunction** /mælˈfʌŋkʃən/ *noun* a situation in which a particular organ does not work in the usual way ○ *Her loss of consciousness was due to a malfunction of the kidneys* or *to a kidney malfunction.* ■ *verb* to fail to work correctly ○ *During the operation his heart began to malfunction.*

**malignancy** /məˈlɪɡnənsi/ *noun* **1.** the state of being malignant ○ *The tests confirmed the malignancy of the growth.* **2.** a cancerous growth (NOTE: The plural is **malignancies**.)

**malignant** /məˈlɪɡnənt/ *adjective* likely to cause death or serious disablement if not properly treated

**malignant hypertension** /məˌlɪɡnənt ˌhaɪpəˈtenʃən/ *noun* dangerously high blood pressure

**malignant melanoma** /məˌlɪɡnənt ˌmeləˈnəʊmə/ *noun* a dark tumour which develops on the skin from a mole, caused by exposure to strong sunlight

**malignant pustule** /məˌlɪɡnənt ˈpʌstjuːl/ *noun* a pus-filled swelling that results from infection of the skin with anthrax

**malignant tumour** /məˌlɪɡnənt ˈtjuːmə/ *noun* a tumour which is cancerous and can grow again or spread into other parts of the body, even if removed surgically. Opposite **benign tumour**

**malingerer** /məˈlɪŋɡərə/ *noun* a person who pretends to be ill

**malingering** /məˈlɪŋɡərɪŋ/ *adjective* the act of pretending to be ill

**malleolar** /məˈliːələ/ *adjective* referring to a malleolus

**malleolus** /məˈliːələs/ *noun* one of two bony prominences at each side of the ankle (NOTE: The plural is **malleoli**.)

**mallet finger** /ˌmælɪt ˈfɪŋɡə/ *noun* a finger which cannot be straightened because the tendon attaching the top joint has been torn

**malleus** /ˈmæliəs/ *noun* the largest of the three ossicles in the middle ear, shaped like a hammer. See illustration at EAR in Supplement

**Mallory bodies** /ˈmæləri ˌbɒdiz/ *plural noun* large irregular masses which occur in the cytoplasm of damaged liver cells, often a sign of an alcohol-related disease

**Mallory's stain** /ˈmæləriz steɪn/ *noun* trichrome stain, used in histology to distinguish collagen, cytoplasm and nuclei

**Mallory-Weiss syndrome** /ˌmæləri ˈvaɪs ˌsɪndrəʊm/, **Mallory-Weiss tear** /ˌmæləri ˈvaɪs ˌteə/ *noun* a condition in which there is a tearing in the mucous membrane where the stomach and oesophagus join, e.g. because of strain on them due to vomiting [Described 1929. After G. Kenneth Mallory (b. 1900), Professor of Pathology, Boston University, USA; Konrad Weiss (1898–1942) US physician.]

**malnourished** /mælˈnʌrɪʃt/ *adjective* not having enough to eat or having only poor-quality food, leading to ill-health

**malnutrition** /ˌmælnjuːˈtrɪʃ(ə)n/ *noun* **1.** a lack of food or of good-quality food, leading to ill-health **2.** the state of not having enough to eat

**malocclusion** /ˌmæləˈkluːʒ(ə)n/ *noun* a condition in which the teeth in the upper and lower jaws do not meet properly when the person's mouth is closed

**malodorous** /mælˈəʊdərəs/ *adjective* with a strong unpleasant smell

**Malpighian body** /mælˈpɪɡiən ˌbɒdi/, **Malpighian corpuscle** /mælˈpɪɡiən ˌkɔːpʌs(ə)l/ *noun* same as **renal corpuscle** [Described 1666. After Marcello Malpighi (1628–94), anatomist and physiologist in Rome and Bologna, Italy.]

**Malpighian glomerulus** /mælˌpɪɡiən ɡlɒˈmerʊləs/ *noun* same as **Bowman's capsule**

**Malpighian layer** /mælˈpɪɡiən ˌleɪə/ *noun* the deepest layer of the epidermis

**malposition** /ˌmælpəˈzɪʃ(ə)n/ *noun* an unusual or unexpected position of something such as a fetus in the uterus or fractured bones

**malpractice** /mælˈpræktɪs/ *noun* **1.** illegal, unethical, negligent or immoral behaviour by a professional person, especially a healthcare professional ○ *The surgeon was found guilty of malpractice.* **2.** wrong treatment of a patient for which a healthcare professional may be tried in court

**malpresentation** /ˌmælprez(ə)nˈteɪʃ(ə)n/ *noun* an unusual position of a fetus in the uterus just before it is ready to be born

**Malta fever** /ˈmɔːltə ˌfiːvə/ *noun* same as **brucellosis**

**maltase** /ˈmɔːlteɪz/ *noun* an enzyme in the small intestine which converts maltose into glucose

**maltose** /ˈmɔːltəʊs/ *noun* a sugar formed by digesting starch or glycogen

**malunion** /mælˈjuːnjən/ *noun* a bad join of the pieces of a broken bone

**mamilla** /məˈmɪlə/ *noun* another spelling of **mammilla**

**mamillary** /ˈmæmɪlri/ *adjective* another spelling of **mammillary**

**mamm-** *prefix* same as **mammo-** (*used before vowels*)

**mamma** /ˈmæmə/ *noun* same as **breast** (NOTE: The plural is **mammae**.)

**mammary** /ˈmæməri/ *adjective* referring to the breast

**mammary gland** /ˈmæməri ɡlænd/ *noun* a gland in female mammals which produces milk

**mammilla** /məˈmɪlə/, **mamilla** *noun* the protruding part in the centre of the breast, containing the milk ducts through which the milk flows. Also called **nipple**

**mammillary** /ˈmæmɪl(ə)ri/, **mamillary** *adjective* referring to the nipple

**mammillary body** /ˌmæmɪl(ə)ri ˈbɒdi/ *noun* one of two little projections on the base of the hypothalamus

**mammo-** *prefix* referring to breasts

**mammogram** /ˈmæməɡræm/ *noun* a picture of a breast made using a special X-ray technique

**mammography** /mæˈmɒɡrəfi/ *noun* examination of the breast using a special X-ray technique

'…mammography is the most effective technique available for the detection of occult (non-palpable) breast cancer. It has been estimated that mammography can detect a carcinoma two years before it becomes palpable.' [*Southern Medical Journal*]

**mammoplasty** /ˈmæməplæsti/ *noun* plastic surgery to alter the shape or size of the breasts

**mammothermography** /ˌmæməʊθɜːˈmɒɡrəfi/ *noun* thermography of a breast

**manage** /ˈmænɪdʒ/ *verb* **1.** to be in charge or control of something ○ *She manages the ward very efficiently.* ○ *Bleeding can usually be managed, but sometimes an operation may be necessary.* **2.** to be able to do something, or to succeed in doing something ○ *Did you manage to phone the doctor?* ○ *Can she manage to feed herself?* (NOTE: **managing – managed**)

**management** /ˈmænɪdʒmənt/ *noun* **1.** the organising or running of an organisation such as a hospital, clinic or health authority **2.** the organisation of a series of different treatments for a person

**manager** /ˈmænɪdʒə/ *noun* a person in charge of a department in the health service or in charge of a group of hospitals

**Manchester operation** /ˈmæntʃɪstər ɒpəˌreɪʃ(ə)n/ *noun* a surgical operation to correct downward movement of the uterus, involving removal of the cervix

**mandible** /ˈmændɪb(ə)l/ *noun* the lower bone in the jaw. Also called **lower jaw**

COMMENT: The jaw is formed of two bones, the mandible which is attached to the skull with a hinge joint and can move up and down, and the maxillae which are fixed parts of the skull.

**mandibular** /mænˈdɪbjʊlə/ *adjective* referring to the lower jaw

**mandibular fossae** /mænˌdɪbjʊlə ˈfɒsi/ *plural noun* sockets in the skull into which the ends of the lower jaw fit

**mandibular nerve** /mænˈdɪbjʊlə nɜːv/ *noun* a sensory nerve which supplies the teeth in the lower jaw, the temple, the floor of the mouth and the back part of the tongue

**mane** /ˈmeɪni/ *adverb* (*used on prescriptions*) during the daytime. Opposite **nocte**

'…he was diagnosed as having diabetes mellitus at age 14, and was successfully controlled on insulin 15 units mane and 10 units nocte' [*British Journal of Hospital Medicine*]

**manganese** /ˈmæŋɡəniːz/ *noun* a metallic trace element (NOTE: The chemical symbol is **Mn**.)

**mania** /ˈmeɪniə/ *noun* a state of bipolar disorder in which the person is excited, very sure of his or her own abilities and has increased energy

**-mania** /meɪniə/ *suffix* obsession with something

**maniac** /ˈmeɪniæk/ *noun* a person who behaves in an uncontrolled way or is considered to have an obsession (NOTE: This term is regarded as offensive.)

**manic** /ˈmænɪk/ *adjective* referring to mania

**manic depression** /ˌmænɪk dɪˈpreʃ(ə)n/ *noun* same as **bipolar disorder**

**manic-depressive** /ˌmænɪk dɪˈpresɪv/ *adjective* relating to bipolar disorder ■ *noun* a person with bipolar disorder

**manic-depressive illness** /ˌmænɪk dɪˈpresɪv ˌɪlnəs/, **manic-depressive psychosis** /ˌmænɪk dɪˌpresɪv saɪˈkəʊsɪs/ *noun* same as **bipolar disorder**

**manifestation** /ˌmænɪfeˈsteɪʃ(ə)n/ *noun* a sign, indication or symptom of a disease

'…the reason for this susceptibility is a profound abnormality of the immune system in children with sickle cell disease. The major manifestations of pneumococcal infection in SCD are septicaemia, meningitis and pneumonia.' [*Lancet*]

**manikin** /ˈmænɪkɪn/ *noun* an anatomical model of the human body, used in teaching anatomy

**manipulate** /məˈnɪpjʊˌleɪt/ *verb* to rub or move parts of the body with the hands to treat a joint, a slipped disc or a hernia (NOTE: **manipulating – manipulated**)

**manipulation** /məˌnɪpjʊˈleɪʃ(ə)n/ *noun* a form of treatment that involves moving or rubbing parts of the body with the hands, e.g. to treat a disorder of a joint

**manner** /ˈmænə/ *noun* a way of doing something or of behaving ○ *He was behaving in a strange manner.* ◊ **bedside manner**

**mannitol** /ˈmænɪtɒl/ *noun* a diuretic drug used in the treatment of oedema of the brain

**manometer** /məˈnɒmɪtə/ *noun* an instrument for comparing pressures

**manometry** /məˈnɒmɪtri/ *noun* the measurement of pressures within organs of the body which contain gases or liquids, e.g. the oesophagus or parts of the brain

**Mantoux test** /mæntuː test/ *noun* a test for tuberculosis, in which a person is given an intracutaneous injection of tuberculin. ◊ **Heaf test** [Described 1908. After Charles Mantoux (1877–1947), French physician.]

**manual** /ˈmænjuəl/ *adjective* done by hand

**manual examination** /ˌmænjuəl ɪɡˌzæmɪˈneɪʃ(ə)n/ *noun* an examination using the hands and fingers

**manubrium** /məˈnuːbriəm/ *noun* a handle-shaped anatomical part, e.g. part of the inner ear

**manubrium sterni** /məˌnuːbriəm ˈstɜːnaɪ/ *noun* the upper part of the sternum

**MAO** *abbr* monoamine oxidase

**MAOI** *abbr* monoamine oxidase inhibitor

**MAO inhibitor** /ˌem eɪ ˈəʊ ɪnˌhɪbɪtə/ *noun* same as **monoamine oxidase inhibitor**

**maple syrup urine disease** /ˌmeɪp(ə)l ˌsɪrəp ˈjʊərɪn dɪˌziːz/ *noun* an inherited condition caused by not having enough of a particular enzyme which helps the body to deal with amino acid. The urine smells like maple syrup. It can be fatal if not treated.

**marasmus** /məˈræzməs/ *noun* a wasting disease which affects small children who have difficulty in absorbing nutrients or who are malnourished. Also called **failure to thrive**

**marble bone disease** /ˌmɑːb(ə)l ˈbəʊn dɪˌziːz/ *noun* same as **osteopetrosis**

**Marburg disease** /ˈmɑːbɜːɡ dɪˌziːz/, **Marburg virus disease** /ˈmɑːbɜːɡ ˌvaɪrəs dɪˌziːz/ *noun* a severe viral infection causing high fever, bleeding from mucous membranes, vomiting and often death. Also called **green monkey disease**

COMMENT: The disease is transmitted to humans from green monkeys. Because the monkeys are used in laboratory experiments, the disease mainly affects laboratory workers.

**march fracture** /mɑːtʃ ˈfræktʃə/ *noun* a fracture of one of the metatarsal bones in the foot, caused by excessive exercise to which the body is not accustomed

**Marfan's syndrome** /ˈmɑːfɑːnz ˌsɪndrəʊm/, **Marfan syndrome** /ˈmɑːfɑːn ˌsɪndrəʊm/ *noun* a hereditary condition in which a person has extremely long fingers and toes, with disorders of the heart, aorta and eyes [Described 1896. After Bernard Jean Antonin Marfan (1858–1942), French paediatrician.]

**marijuana** /ˌmærɪˈwɑːnə/ *noun* same as **cannabis**

**mark** /mɑːk/ *noun* a spot or small area of a different colour ○ *There's a red mark where you hit your head.* ○ *The rash has left marks* on the chest and back. ■ *verb* to make a mark on something □ **the door is marked 'Supervisor'** the door has the word 'Supervisor' written on it

**marked** /mɑːkt/ *adjective* obvious or noticeable ○ *There has been a marked improvement in his condition.*

**marker** /ˈmɑːkə/ *noun* **1.** something which acts as an indicator of something else **2.** a substance introduced into the body to make internal structures clearer to X-rays

**marrow** /ˈmærəʊ/ *noun* soft tissue in cancellous bone. In young animals **red marrow** is concerned with blood formation while in adults it becomes progressively replaced with fat and is known as yellow marrow. Also called **bone marrow**. See illustration at BONE STRUCTURE in Supplement

**marsupialisation** /mɑːˌsuːpiəlaɪˈzeɪʃ(ə)n/, **marsupialization** *noun* a surgical procedure in which the inside of a cyst is opened up so that the cyst can be allowed to shrink gradually, because it cannot be cut out

**masculinisation** /ˌmæskjʊlɪnaɪˈzeɪʃ(ə)n/, **masculinization** *noun* the development of male characteristics such as body hair and a deep voice in a woman, caused by hormone deficiency or by treatment with male hormones

**mask** /mɑːsk/ *noun* **1.** a metal and rubber frame that fits over the nose and mouth and is used to administer an anaesthetic **2.** a piece of gauze which fits over the mouth and nose to prevent droplet infection **3.** a cover which fits over the face of a person who has suffered facial damage in an accident

**masked** /mɑːskt/ *adjective* used to describe diseases that are present but not observable

**Maslow's hierarchy of human needs** /ˌmæzləʊz ˌhaɪrɑːki əv ˌhjuːmən ˈniːdz/ *noun* a system which explains human behaviour by organising human needs in order of priority, from basic ones such as eating to complex ones such as finding self-fulfilment, a higher level of motivation not being activated until the lesser needs have been satisfied

**masochism** /ˈmæsəkɪz(ə)m/ *noun* a sexual condition in which a person takes pleasure in being hurt or badly treated

**masochist** /ˈmæsəkɪst/ *noun* a person suffering from masochism

**masochistic** /ˌmæsəˈkɪstɪk/ *adjective* referring to masochism

**mass** /mæs/ *noun* **1.** a large quantity, e.g. a large number of people ○ *The patient's back was covered with a mass of red spots.* **2.** a body of matter with no clear shape **3.** a mixture for making pills **4.** the main solid part of bone

**massage** /ˈmæsɑːʒ/ *noun* a treatment for muscular conditions which involves rubbing, stroking or pressing the body with the hands ■

*verb* to rub, stroke or press the body with the hands

**masseter** /mæˈsiːtə/, **masseter muscle** /mæˈsiːtə ˌmʌs(ə)l/ *noun* a muscle in the cheek which clenches the lower jaw making it move up, to allow chewing

**massive** /ˈmæsɪv/ *adjective* very large ○ *He was given a massive injection of penicillin.* ○ *She had a massive heart attack.*

**mass radiography** /ˌmæs ˌreɪdiˈɒɡrəfi/ *noun* the practice of taking X-ray photographs of large numbers of people to check for tuberculosis

**mass screening** /ˌmæs ˈskriːnɪŋ/ *noun* the practice of testing large numbers of people for the presence of a disease

**mast-** /mæst/ *prefix* same as **masto-** (*used before vowels*)

**mastalgia** /mæˈstældʒə/ *noun* pain in the mammary gland

**mastatrophy** /mæˈstætrəfi/ *noun* atrophy of the mammary gland

**mast cell** /ˈmæst sel/ *noun* a large cell in connective tissue, which carries histamine and reacts to allergens

**mastectomy** /mæˈstektəmi/ *noun* the surgical removal of a breast

**masticate** /ˈmæstɪkeɪt/ *verb* to chew food

**mastication** /ˌmæstɪˈkeɪʃ(ə)n/ *noun* the act of chewing food

**mastitis** /mæˈstaɪtɪs/ *noun* inflammation of the breast

**masto-** /mæstəʊ/ *prefix* referring to a breast

**mastoid** /ˈmæstɔɪd/ *adjective* 1. shaped like a nipple 2. belonging to the part of the temporal bone which protrudes at the side of the head behind the ear ■ *noun* same as **mastoid process**

**mastoid air cell** /ˌmæstɔɪd ˈeə sel/, **mastoid cell** /ˈmæstɔɪd sel/ *noun* an air cell in the mastoid process

**mastoid antrum** /ˌmæstɔɪd ˈæntrəm/ *noun* a cavity linking the air cells of the mastoid process with the middle ear

**mastoid bone** /ˈmæstɔɪd bəʊn/ *noun* same as **mastoid process**

**mastoidectomy** /ˌmæstɔɪˈdektəmi/ *noun* a surgical operation to remove part of the mastoid process, as a treatment for mastoiditis

**mastoiditis** /ˌmæstɔɪˈdaɪtɪs/ *noun* inflammation of the mastoid process and air cells. The symptoms are fever and pain in the ears.

COMMENT: The mastoid process can be infected by infection from the middle ear through the mastoid antrum. Mastoiditis can cause deafness and can affect the meninges if not treated.

**mastoidotomy** /ˌmæstɔɪˈdɒtəmi/ *noun* a surgical operation to make a cut into the mastoid process to treat infection

**mastoid process** /ˌmæstɔɪd ˈprəʊses/ *noun* part of the temporal bone which protrudes at the side of the head behind the ear

**masturbate** /ˈmæstəbeɪt/ *verb* to excite one's own genitals so as to produce an orgasm

**masturbation** /ˌmæstəˈbeɪʃ(ə)n/ *noun* stimulation of one's own genitals to produce an orgasm. Also called **onanism**

**match** /mætʃ/ *verb* 1. to examine two things to see if they are similar or fit together ○ *They are trying to match the donor to the recipient.* 2. to fit together in a specific way ○ *The two samples don't match.*

'…bone marrow from donors has to be carefully matched with the recipient or graft-versus-host disease will ensue' [*Hospital Update*]

**mater** /ˈmeɪtə/ ♦ **dura mater**

**material** /məˈtɪəriəl/ *noun* 1. matter which can be used to make something 2. cloth ○ *The wound should be covered with gauze or other light material.* 3. all that is necessary in surgery

**materia medica** /məˌtɪəriə ˈmedɪkə/ *noun* the study of drugs or dosages as used in treatment (NOTE: It comes from a Latin term meaning 'medical substance'.)

**maternal** /məˈtɜːn(ə)l/ *adjective* referring to a mother

**maternal death** /məˌtɜːn(ə)l ˈdeθ/ *noun* the death of a mother during pregnancy, childbirth or up to twelve months after childbirth

**maternal deprivation** /məˌtɜːn(ə)l ˌdeprɪˈveɪʃ(ə)n/ *noun* a psychological condition caused when a child does not have a proper relationship with a mother

**maternal dystocia** /məˌtɜːn(ə)l dɪsˈtəʊsiə/ *noun* difficult childbirth caused by a physical problem in the mother

**maternal instincts** /məˌtɜːn(ə)l ˈɪnstɪŋkts/ *plural noun* instinctive feelings in a woman to look after and protect her child

**maternity** /məˈtɜːnɪti/ *noun* childbirth, the fact of becoming a mother

**maternity case** /məˈtɜːnɪti keɪs/ *noun* a woman who is about to give birth

**maternity clinic** /məˈtɜːnɪti ˌklɪnɪk/ *noun* same as **antenatal clinic**

**maternity hospital** /məˈtɜːnɪti ˌhɒspɪt(ə)l/, **maternity ward** /məˈtɜːnɪti wɔːd/, **maternity unit** /məˈtɜːnɪti ˌjuːnɪt/ *noun* a hospital, ward or unit which deals only with women giving birth

**matrix** /ˈmeɪtrɪks/ *noun* an amorphous mass of cells forming the basis of connective tissue. Also called **ground substance**

**matron** /ˈmeɪtrən/ *noun* a title formerly given to a woman in charge of the nurses in a hospital. ◊ **modern matron**

**matter** /ˈmætə/ *noun* a substance

**mattress** /ˈmætrəs/ *noun* the thick soft part of a bed for lying on

**mattress suture** /'mætrəs ˌsuːtʃə/ *noun* a suture made with a loop on each side of the incision

**maturation** /ˌmætʃʊ'reɪʃ(ə)n/ *noun* the process of becoming mature or fully developed

**mature** /mə'tjʊə/ *adjective* fully developed

**mature follicle** /məˌtʃʊə 'fɒlɪk(ə)l/ *noun* a Graafian follicle just before ovulation

**maturing** /mə'tʃʊərɪŋ/ *adjective* becoming mature

**maturing egg** /məˌtʃʊərɪŋ 'eg/, **maturing ovum** /'əʊvəm/ *noun* an ovum contained by a Graafian follicle

**maturity** /mə'tʃʊərɪti/ *noun* **1.** being fully developed **2.** (*in psychology*) the state of being a responsible adult

**maxilla** /mæk'sɪlə/, **maxilla bone** /mæk'sɪlə bəʊn/ *noun* the upper jaw bone (NOTE: The plural is **maxillae**. It is more correct to refer to the upper jaw as the **maxillae**, as it is in fact formed of two bones which are fused together.)

**maxillary** /mæk'sɪləri/ *adjective* referring to the maxilla

**maxillary antrum** /mækˌsɪləri 'æntrəm/, **maxillary air sinus** /mækˌsɪləri 'eə ˌsaɪnəs/ *noun* one of two sinuses behind the cheekbones in the upper jaw. Also called **antrum of Highmore**

**maxillo-facial** /mækˌsɪləʊ'feɪʃ(ə)l/ *adjective* referring to the maxillary bone and the face ○ *maxillo-facial surgery*

**MB** *abbr* bachelor of medicine

**McBurney's point** /məkˌbɜːniz 'pɔɪnt/ *noun* a point which indicates the usual position of the appendix on the right side of the abdomen, between the hip bone and the navel, which is extremely painful if pressed when the person has appendicitis [Described 1899. After Charles McBurney (1845–1913), US surgeon.]

**McNaghten's Rules on Insanity at Law** /məkˌnɔːtənz ˌruːlz ɒn ɪnˌsænɪti ət 'lɔː/, **McNaghten's Rules** /məkˈnɔːtənz ˌruːlz/ *plural noun* a set of principles which explain how people can defend themselves in law by claiming that they committed a murder because they were mentally ill, and therefore not responsible for any of their actions. In 1957 it was adapted to include the idea of knowing that an action is wrong but being unable to stop yourself from committing it because of your mental condition.

**MCP joint** /ˌem siː 'piː ˌdʒɔɪnt/ *noun* same as **metacarpophalangeal joint**

**MCU, MCUG** *abbr* micturating cysto(-urethro)gram

**MD** *abbr* doctor of medicine

**ME** *abbr* myalgic encephalomyelitis

**meal** /miːl/ *noun* food eaten at a particular time

**measles** /'miːz(ə)lz/ *noun* an infectious disease of children, where the body is covered with a red rash ○ *She's in bed with measles.* ○ *He's got measles.* ○ *They caught measles from their friend at school.* ○ *Have you had the measles?* Also called **morbilli, rubeola** (NOTE: Takes a singular or plural verb.)

COMMENT: Measles can be a serious disease as it weakens the body's resistance to other diseases, especially bronchitis and ear infections. It can be prevented by immunisation. If caught by an adult it can be very serious.

**measure** /'meʒə/ *noun* a unit of size, quantity or degree ○ *A metre is a measure of length.* ■ *verb* **1.** to find out the size of something ○ *A thermometer measures temperature.* **2.** to be a particular size ○ *The room measures 3 metres by 2 metres.*

**measurement** /'meʒəmənt/ *noun* the size, length, etc. of something which has been measured

**meat** /miːt/ *noun* animal flesh which is eaten (NOTE: No plural: *some meat*, *a piece* or *a slice of meat*; *he refuses to eat meat.*)

**meat-** /mieɪt/ *prefix* relating to a meatus

**meatus** /mi'eɪtəs/ *noun* an opening leading to an internal passage in the body, e.g. the urethra or the nasal cavity (NOTE: The plural is **meatuses** or **meatus**.)

**mechanism** /'mekənɪz(ə)m/ *noun* **1.** a physical or chemical change by which a function is carried out **2.** a system in the body which carries out or controls a particular function ○ *The inner ear is the body's mechanism for the sense of balance.*

**mechanism of labour** /ˌmekənɪz(ə)m əv 'leɪbə/ *noun* all the forces and processes which combine to push a foetus out of the uterus during its birth, together with the ones which oppose it

**mechanotherapy** /ˌmekənəʊ'θerəpi/ *noun* the treatment of injuries through mechanical means, such as massage and exercise machines

**Meckel's diverticulum** /ˌmekəlz ˌdaɪvə'tɪkjʊləm/ *noun* a congenital formation of a diverticulum in the ileum [Described 1809. After Johann Friedrich Meckel II (1781–1833), German surgeon and anatomist.]

**meconism** /'mekəʊnɪz(ə)m/ *noun* poisoning by opium or morphine

**meconium** /mɪ'kəʊniəm/ *noun* the first dark green faeces produced by a newborn baby

**med.** *abbr* **1.** medical **2.** medicine

**media** /'miːdiə/ *noun* same as **tunica media**

**medial** /'miːdiəl/ *adjective* nearer to the central midline of the body or to the centre of an organ. Compare **lateral**

**medial arcuate ligament** /ˌmiːdiəl 'ɑːkjuɪt ˌlɪgəmənt/ *noun* a fibrous arch to which the diaphragm is attached

**medial epicondyle** /ˌmiːdiəl ˌepɪˈkɒndaɪl/ *noun* a medial projection on the condyle of the humerus

**medially** /ˈmiːdiəli/ *adverb* towards or on the sagittal plane of the body. See illustration at **ANATOMICAL TERMS** in Supplement

**medial malleolus** /ˌmiːdiəl məˈliːələs/ *noun* a bone at the end of the tibia which protrudes at the inside of the ankle

**medial rectus** /ˌmiːdiəl ˈrektəs/ *noun* a muscle inserted into the sclera of the eyeball

**median** /ˈmiːdiən/ *adjective* towards the central midline of the body, or placed in the middle

**median nerve** /ˈmiːdiən nɜːv/ *noun* one of the main nerves of the forearm and hand

**median plane** /ˈmiːdiən pleɪn/ *noun* an imaginary flat surface on the midline and at right angles to the coronal plane, which divides the body into right and left halves. See illustration at **ANATOMICAL TERMS** in Supplement

**mediastinal** /ˌmiːdiəˈstaɪn(ə)l/ *adjective* referring to the mediastinum ○ *the mediastinal surface of pleura* or *of the lungs*

**mediastinitis** /ˌmiːdiəstɪˈnaɪtɪs/ *noun* inflammation of the mediastinum

**mediastinoscopy** /ˌmiːdiəstɪˈnɒskəpi/ *noun* an operation in which a tube is put into the mediastinum so that its organs can be examined

**mediastinum** /ˌmiːdiəˈstaɪnəm/ *noun* the section of the chest between the lungs, where the heart, oesophagus and phrenic and vagus nerves are situated

**medic** /ˈmedɪk/ *noun* a doctor or medical student (*informal*)

**medical** /ˈmedɪk(ə)l/ *adjective* **1.** referring to the study of diseases ○ *a medical student* **2.** referring to treatment of disease which does not involve surgery ○ *Medical help was provided by the Red Cross.* **3.** referring to treatment given by a doctor, as opposed to a surgeon, in a hospital or in his or her surgery ■ *noun* an official examination of a person by a doctor ○ *He wanted to join the army, but failed his medical.* ○ *You will have to have a medical if you take out an insurance policy.*

**medical administration** /ˌmedɪk(ə)l ədˌmɪnɪˈstreɪʃ(ə)n/ *noun* the running of hospitals and other health services ○ *She started her career in medical administration.*

**medical aid** /ˈmedɪk(ə)l eɪd/ *noun* treatment of someone who is ill or injured, given by a doctor. ◊ **first aid**

**medical alert bracelet** /ˌmedɪk(ə)l əˈlɜːt ˌbreɪslət/ *noun* a band or chain worn around the wrist giving information about the wearer's medical needs, allergies or condition

**medical assistance** /ˌmedɪk(ə)l əˈsɪst(ə)ns/ *noun* help provided by a nurse, an ambulanceman or a member of an association

such as the Red Cross, to a person who is ill or injured

**medical assistant** /ˈmedɪk(ə)l əˌsɪst(ə)nt/ *noun* someone who performs routine administrative and clinical tasks to help in the offices and clinics of doctors and other medical practitioners

**medical audit** /ˌmedɪk(ə)l ˈɔːdɪt/ *noun* a systematic critical analysis of the quality of medical care provided to a person, which examines the procedures used for diagnosis and treatment, the use of resources and the resulting outcome and quality of life for the person

**medical audit advisory group** /ˌmedɪk(ə)l ˌɔːdɪt ədˈvaɪz(ə)ri gruːp/ *noun* a body with the responsibility of advising on medical audit in primary care. Abbr **MAAG**

**medical centre** /ˈmedɪk(ə)l ˌsentə/ *noun* a place where several different doctors and specialists practise

**medical certificate** /ˈmedɪk(ə)l səˌtɪfɪkət/ *noun* an official document signed by a doctor, giving someone permission to be away from work or not to do specific types of work

**medical committee** /ˈmedɪk(ə)l kəˌmɪti/ *noun* a committee of doctors in a hospital who advise the management on medical matters

**medical diathermy** /ˌmedɪk(ə)l ˌdaɪəˈθɜːmi/ *noun* the use of heat produced by electricity for treatment of muscle and joint disorders such as rheumatism

**medical doctor** /ˈmedɪk(ə)l ˌdɒktə/ *noun* a doctor who practises medicine, but is not usually a surgeon

**medical ethics** /ˌmedɪk(ə)l ˈeθɪks/ *plural noun* the moral and professional principles which govern how doctors and nurses should work, and, in particular, what type of relationship they should have with their patients

**medical examination** /ˌmedɪk(ə)l ɪgˌzæmɪˈneɪʃ(ə)n/ *noun* an examination of a person by a doctor

**medical history** /ˌmedɪk(ə)l ˈhɪst(ə)ri/ *noun* the details of a person's medical condition and treatment over a period of time

**medical intervention** /ˌmedɪk(ə)l ˌɪntəˈvenʃən/ *noun* the treatment of illness by drugs

**medicalisation** /ˌmedɪkəlaɪˈzeɪʃ(ə)n/, **medicalization** *noun* the act of looking at something as a medical issue or problem

**medical jurisprudence** /ˌmedɪk(ə)l dʒʊərɪsˈpruːd(ə)ns/ *noun* the use of the principles of law as they relate to the practice of medicine and the relationship of doctors with each other, their patients and society. ◊ **forensic medicine**

**Medical Officer of Health** /ˌmedɪk(ə)l ˌɒfɪsər əv ˈhelθ/ *noun* formerly, a local government official in charge of the health services in an area. Abbr **MOH**

**medical practitioner** /ˌmedɪk(ə)l ˈprækˈtɪʃ(ə)nə/ *noun* a person qualified in medicine, i.e. a doctor or surgeon

**medical profession** /ˈmedɪk(ə)l prəˌfeʃ(ə)n/ *noun* all doctors

**medical records** /ˈmedɪk(ə)l ˌrekɔːdz/ *plural noun* information about a person's medical history

**Medical Register** /ˌmedɪk(ə)l ˈredʒɪstə/ *noun* a list of doctors approved by the General Medical Council ○ *The committee ordered his name to be struck off the Medical Register.*

**Medical Research Council** /ˌmedɪk(ə)l rɪˈsɜːtʃ ˌkaʊnsəl/ *noun* a government body which organises and pays for medical research. Abbr **MRC**

**medical school** /ˈmedɪk(ə)l skuːl/ *noun* a section of a university which teaches medicine ○ *He is at medical school.*

**medical secretary** /ˌmedɪk(ə)l ˈsekrɪt(ə)ri/ *noun* a qualified secretary who specialises in medical documentation, either in a hospital or in a doctor's surgery

**medical social worker** /ˌmedɪk(ə)l ˈsəʊʃ(ə)l ˌwɜːkə/ *noun* someone who helps people with family problems or problems related to their work which may have an effect on their response to treatment

**medical ward** /ˈmedɪk(ə)l wɔːd/ *noun* a ward for people who do not have to undergo surgical operations

**Medicare** /ˈmedɪkeə/ *noun* a system of public health insurance in the US

**medicated** /ˈmedɪkeɪtɪd/ *adjective* containing a medicinal drug ○ *medicated cough sweet*

**medicated shampoo** /ˌmedɪkeɪtɪd ʃæmˈpuː/ *noun* a shampoo containing a chemical which is supposed to prevent dandruff

**medication** /ˌmedɪˈkeɪʃ(ə)n/ *noun* **1.** the treatment of illnesses by giving people drugs. ◊ **premedication 2.** a drug used to treat a particular illness ○ *What sort of medication has she been taking?* ○ *80% of elderly patients admitted to geriatric units are on medication.*

**medicinal** /məˈdɪsɪn(ə)l/ *adjective* which has healing properties or a beneficial effect on someone's health ○ *He has a drink of whisky before he goes to bed for medicinal purposes.*

**medicinal bath** /məˌdɪsɪn(ə)l ˈbɑːθ/ *noun* treatment in which someone lies in a bath of hot water containing particular chemicals, in hot mud or in other substances

**medicinal drug** /məˌdɪsɪn(ə)l ˈdrʌg/ *noun* a drug used to treat a disease as opposed to hallucinatory or addictive drugs

**medicinal leech** /məˌdɪsɪn(ə)l ˈliːtʃ/ *noun* a leech which is raised specially for use in medicine

**medicinally** /məˈdɪsɪn(ə)li/ *adverb* used as a medicine ○ *The herb can be used medicinally.*

**medicine** /ˈmed(ə)s(ə)n/ *noun* **1.** a preparation taken to treat a disease or condition, especially one in liquid form ○ *Take some cough medicine if your cough is bad.* ○ *You should take the medicine three times a day.* **2.** the study of diseases and how to cure or prevent them ○ *She is studying medicine because she wants to be a doctor.* **3.** the study and treatment of diseases which does not involve surgery

**medicine bottle** /ˈmed(ə)s(ə)n ˌbɒt(ə)l/ *noun* a special bottle which contains medicine

**medicine cabinet** /ˈmed(ə)s(ə)n ˌkæbɪnət/, **medicine chest** /ˈmed(ə)s(ə)n tʃest/ *noun* a cupboard where medicines, bandages, thermometers and other pieces of medical equipment can be left locked up, but ready for use in an emergency

**medico** /ˈmedɪkəʊ/ *noun* a doctor (*informal*) ○ *The medico said I was perfectly fit.*

**medico-** /medɪkəʊ/ *prefix* referring to medicine or to doctors

**medicochirurgical** /ˌmedɪkəʊkaɪˈrɜːdʒɪk(ə)l/ *adjective* referring to both medicine and surgery

**medicolegal** /ˌmedɪkəʊˈliːg(ə)l/ *adjective* referring to both medicine and the law

**medicosocial** /ˌmedɪkəʊ ˈsəʊʃ(ə)l/ *adjective* involving both medical and social factors

**medium** /ˈmiːdiəm/ *adjective* average, in the middle or at the halfway point ■ *noun* a substance through which something acts

**medroxyprogesterone** /məˌdrɒksɪprəʊˈdʒestərəʊn/ *noun* a synthetic hormone used to treat menstrual disorders, in oestrogen replacement therapy and as a contraceptive

**medulla** /meˈdʌlə/ *noun* **1.** the soft inner part of an organ, as opposed to the outer cortex. See illustration at **KIDNEY** in Supplement **2.** bone marrow **3.** any structure similar to bone marrow

**medulla oblongata** /meˌdʌlə ˌɒblɒŋˈgeɪtə/ *noun* a continuation of the spinal cord going through the foramen magnum into the brain

**medullary** /meˈdʌləri/ *adjective* **1.** similar to marrow **2.** referring to a medulla

**medullary cavity** /meˌdʌləri ˈkævɪti/ *noun* a hollow centre of a long bone, containing bone marrow. See illustration at **BONE STRUCTURE** in Supplement

**medullary cord** /meˈdʌləri kɔːd/ *noun* an epithelial fibre found near the hilum of the fetal ovary

**medullated nerve** /ˈmedəleɪtɪd nɜːv/ *noun* a nerve surrounded by a myelin sheath

**medulloblastoma** /meˌdʌləʊblæˈstəʊmə/ *noun* a tumour which develops in the medulla oblongata and the fourth ventricle of the brain in children

**mefenamic acid** /ˌmefənæmɪk ˈæsɪd/ *noun* a drug which reduces inflammation and pain,

used in the treatment of rheumatoid arthritis
and menstrual problems

**mefloquine** /'mefləkwiːn/, **mefloquine hydrochloride** /ˌmefləkwiːn ˌhaɪdrəʊ'klɔːraɪd/
*noun* a drug used in the prevention and treatment of malaria

**mega-** /megə/ *prefix* **1.** large. Opposite **micro-**
**2.** one million, or $10^6$

**megacolon** /ˌmegə'kəʊlən/ *noun* a condition in which the lower colon is very much
larger than normal, because part of the colon
above is constricted, making bowel movements impossible

**megajoule** /'megədʒuːl/ *noun* a unit of
measurement of energy equal to one million
joules. Symbol **Mj**

**megakaryocyte** /ˌmegə'kæriəsaɪt/ *noun* a
bone marrow cell which produces blood platelets

**megalo-** /megaləʊ/ *prefix* large

**megaloblast** /'megələʊblæst/ *noun* an unusually large blood cell found in the bone marrow of people who have some types of anaemia caused by Vitamin $B_{12}$ deficiency

**megaloblastic** /ˌmegələʊ'blæstɪk/ *adjective* referring to megaloblasts

**megaloblastic    anaemia**    /ˌmegələʊ
ˌblæstɪk ə'niːmiə/ *noun* anaemia caused by
Vitamin $B_{12}$ deficiency

**megalocephaly** /ˌmegələʊ'kefəli/ *noun* the
condition of having an unusually large head

**megalocyte** /'megələʊsaɪt/ *noun* an unusually large red blood cell, found in pernicious
anaemia

**megalomania** /ˌmegələʊ'meɪniə/ *noun* a
psychiatric disorder in which a person believes
they are very powerful and important

**megalomaniac** /ˌmegələʊ'meɪniæk/ *noun*
someone who has megalomania ■ *adjective*
having megalomania

**-megaly** /megəli/ *suffix* enlargement

**megaureter** /ˌmegəjʊ'riːtə/ *noun* a condition in which a part of the ureter becomes very
wide, above the site of a blockage

**meibomian cyst** /maɪˌbəʊmiən 'sɪst/ *noun*
the swelling of a sebaceous gland in the eyelid.
Also called **chalazion**

**meibomian gland** /maɪ'bəʊmiən ˌglænd/
*noun* a sebaceous gland on the edge of the eyelid which secretes a liquid to lubricate the eyelid. Also called **tarsal gland**

**meibomianitis** /maɪˌbəʊmiə'naɪtɪs/ *noun* a
condition in which the meibomian glands become swollen

**Meigs' syndrome** /'megz ˌsɪndrəʊm/ *noun*
a condition in which liquid collects in the chest
and abdominal cavities. It is associated with
pelvic tumours.

**meiosis** /maɪ'əʊsɪs/ *noun* the process of cell
division which results in two pairs of haploid
cells, i.e. cells with only one set of chromo-

somes. Compare **mitosis** (NOTE: The US spelling is **miosis**.)

**Meissner's       corpuscle**      /ˌmaɪsnəz
'kɔːpʌs(ə)l/ *noun* a receptor cell in the skin
which is thought to be sensitive to touch

**Meissner's plexus** /ˌmaɪsnəz 'pleksəs/
*noun* a network of nerve fibres in the wall of
the alimentary canal [Described 1853. After
Georg Meissner (1829–1905), German anatomist and physiologist.]

**melaena** /mə'liːnə/ *noun* black faeces where
the colour is caused by bleeding in the intestine

**melan-** /melən/ *prefix* same as **melano-** (*used
before vowels*)

**melancholia** /ˌmelən'kəʊliə/ *noun* **1.** a severe depressive illness occurring usually between the ages of 45 and 65 **2.** a clinical syndrome with a tendency to delusion, fixed personality and agitated movements

**melanin** /'melənɪn/ *noun* a dark pigment
which gives colour to skin and hair, also found
in the choroid of the eye and in some tumours

**melanism** /'melənɪz(ə)m/ *noun* **1.** the unexpected depositing of dark pigment **2.** the staining of all body tissue with melanin in a form of
carcinoma

**melano-** /melənəʊ/ *prefix* black or dark

**melanocyte** /'melənəʊsaɪt/ *noun* any cell
which carries pigment

**melanocyte-stimulating      hormone**      /
ˌmelənəʊsaɪt 'stɪmjʊleɪtɪŋ ˌhɔːməʊm/ *noun*
a hormone produced by the pituitary gland
which causes darkening in the colour of the
skin. Abbr **MSH**

**melanoderma** /ˌmelənəʊ'dɜːmə/ *noun* **1.** a
large amount of melanin in the skin **2.** discoloration of patches of the skin

**melanoma** /ˌmelə'nəʊmə/ *noun* a tumour
formed of dark pigmented cells

COMMENT: ABCD is the key to remember if you
want to know if there is a risk of developing a
melanoma: A = ASYMMETRY, ie. the two
sides are not quite the same, and the mole
does not have a perfect shape; B = BORDER,
the edge becomes irregular; C = COLOUR,
there may be a change in colour, with the
mole becoming darker; D = DIAMETER, any
change in diameter should be considered an
important factor. Among other features, pain
is rarely an important feature but itching could
be one.

**melanophore** /'melənəʊfɔː/ *noun* a cell
which contains melanin

**melanoplakia** /'melənəʊpleɪkiə/ *noun* areas
of pigment in the mucous membrane inside the
mouth

**melanosis** /ˌmelə'nəʊsɪs/ *noun* same as
**melanism**

**melanuria** /ˌmelə'njʊəriə/ *noun* **1.** the presence of dark colouring in the urine **2.** a condition in which the urine turns black after being

allowed to stand, e.g. in cases of malignant melanoma

**melasma** /mə'læzmə/ *noun* the presence of little brown, yellow or black spots on the skin

**melatonin** /ˌmelə'təʊnɪn/ *noun* a hormone produced by the pineal gland during the hours of darkness, which makes animals sleep during the winter months. It is thought to control the body's rhythms.

**melena** /mə'liːnə/ *noun* same as **melaena**

**mellitus** /'melɪtəs/ ♦ **diabetes mellitus**

**membrane** /'membreɪn/ *noun* a thin layer of tissue which lines or covers an organ

**membrane bone** /'membreɪn bəʊn/ *noun* a bone which develops from tissue and not from cartilage

**membranous** /'membrənəs/ *adjective* referring to membranes, or like a membrane

**membranous labyrinth** /ˌmembrənəs 'læbərɪnθ/ *noun* a series of ducts and canals formed of membrane inside the osseous labyrinth

**memory** /'mem(ə)ri/ *noun* the ability to remember ○ *He has a very good memory for dates.* ○ *He said the whole list from memory.*

**menarche** /mə'nɑːki/ *noun* the start of menstrual periods

**mend** /mend/ *verb* to repair something ○ *The surgeons are trying to mend the damaged heart valves.*

**Mendel's laws** /'mendəlz lɔːz/ *plural noun* the laws of heredity, that are the basis of the science of genetics [Described 1865. After Gregor Johann Mendel (1822–84), Austrian Augustinian monk and naturalist of Brno, whose work was rediscovered by de Vries in 1900.]

**Mendelson's syndrome** /'mendəlsənz ˌsɪndrəʊm/ *noun* a sometimes fatal condition in which acid fluid from the stomach is brought up into the windpipe and passes into the lungs, occurring mainly in obstetric patients [Described 1946. After Curtis L. Mendelson (b. 1913), US obstetrician and gynaecologist.]

**Ménière's disease** /meni'eəz dɪˌziːz/, **Ménière's syndrome** /'sɪndrəʊm/ *noun* a disease of the middle ear, in which someone becomes dizzy, hears ringing in the ears and may vomit, and becomes progressively deaf. The causes may include infections or allergies, which increase the fluid contents of the labyrinth in the middle ear. [Described 1861. After Prosper Ménière (1799–1862) and his son, Emile Antoine Ménière (1839–1905), French physicians.]

**mening-** /menɪndʒ/ *prefix* same as **meningo-** (used before vowels)

**meningeal** /me'nɪndʒiəl/ *adjective* referring to the meninges

**meningeal haemorrhage** /me,nɪndʒiəl 'hem(ə)rɪdʒ/ *noun* a haemorrhage from a meningeal artery

**meningeal sarcoma** /me,nɪndʒiəl sɑː 'kəʊmə/ *noun* a malignant tumour in the meninges

**meninges** /me'nɪndʒiːz/ *plural noun* the membranes which surround the brain and spinal cord (NOTE: The singular is **meninx**.)

COMMENT: The meninges are divided into three layers: the tough outer layer (dura mater) which protects the brain and spinal cord; the middle layer (arachnoid mater) and the delicate inner layer (pia mater) which contains the blood vessels. The cerebrospinal fluid flows in the space (subarachnoid space) between the arachnoid mater and pia mater.

**meningioma** /ˌmenɪndʒi'əʊmə/ *noun* a benign tumour in the meninges

**meningism** /me'nɪndʒɪz(ə)m/ *noun* a condition in which there are signs of meningeal irritation suggesting meningitis, but where there is no pathological change in the cerebrospinal fluid

**meningitis** /ˌmenɪn'dʒaɪtɪs/ *noun* inflammation of the meninges, causing someone to have violent headaches, fever, and stiff neck muscles, and sometimes to become delirious

COMMENT: Meningitis is a serious viral or bacterial disease which can cause brain damage and even death. The bacterial form can be treated with antibiotics. The most common forms of bacterial meningitis are Hib and meningococcal.

**meningo-** /mənɪŋgəʊ/ *prefix* referring to the meninges

**meningocele** /mə'nɪŋgəʊsiːl/ *noun* a condition in which the meninges protrude through the vertebral column or skull

**meningococcal** /mə,nɪŋgəʊ'kɒk(ə)l/ *adjective* referring to meningococci

**meningococcal disease** /mə,nɪŋgəʊ 'kɒk(ə)l dɪ,ziːz/ *noun* a disease caused by a meningococcus

**meningococcal meningitis** /mə,nɪŋgəʊ ,kɒk(ə)l ,menɪn'dʒaɪtɪs/ *noun* the commonest epidemic form of meningitis, caused by a bacterium *Neisseria meningitidis*, where the meninges become inflamed causing headaches and fever

**meningococcus** /mə,nɪŋgəʊ'kɒkəs/ *noun* the bacterium *Neisseria meningitidis* which causes meningococcal meningitis (NOTE: The plural is **meningococci**.)

**meningoencephalitis** /mə,nɪŋgəʊen,kefə 'laɪtɪs/ *noun* inflammation of the meninges and the brain

**meningoencephalocele** /mə,nɪŋgəʊen 'kefələʊsiːl/ *noun* a condition in which part of the meninges and the brain push through a gap in the skull

**meningomyelocele** /mə,nɪŋgəʊ'maɪələʊ siːl/ *noun* the pushing forward of part of the meninges and spinal cord through a gap in the spine. Also called **myelomeningocele, myelocele**

**meningovascular** /məˌnɪŋɡəʊˈvæskjʊlə/ *adjective* referring to the meningeal blood vessels

**meninx** /ˈmenɪŋks/ *noun* ♦ **meninges**

**meniscectomy** /ˌmenɪˈsektəmi/ *noun* the surgical removal of a cartilage from the knee

**meniscus** /məˈnɪskəs/ *noun* one of two pads of cartilage, the lateral meniscus and medial meniscus, between the femur and tibia in a knee joint. Also called **semilunar cartilage** (NOTE: The plural is **menisci**.)

**meno-** /menəʊ/ *prefix* referring to menstruation

**menopausal** /ˌmenəˈpɔːz(ə)l/ *adjective* referring to the menopause

**menopause** /ˈmenəpɔːz/ *noun* a period, usually between 45 and 55 years of age, when a woman stops menstruating and can no longer bear children. Also called **climacteric, change of life**

**menorrhagia** /ˌmenəˈreɪdʒiə/ *noun* very heavy bleeding during menstruation. Also called **flooding**

**menorrhoea** /ˌmenəˈriːə/ *noun* normal bleeding during menstruation

**menses** /ˈmensiːz/ *plural noun* same as **menstruation**

**menstrual** /ˈmenstruəl/ *adjective* referring to menstruation

**menstrual cramp** /ˌmenstruəl ˈkræmp/ *noun* a cramp in the muscles round the uterus during menstruation

**menstrual cycle** /ˈmenstruəl ˌsaɪk(ə)l/ *noun* a period, usually of 28 days, during which a woman ovulates, the walls of the uterus swell and bleeding takes place if the ovum has not been fertilised

**menstrual flow** /ˈmenstruəl fləʊ/ *noun* the discharge of blood from the uterus during menstruation

**menstruate** /ˈmenstrueɪt/ *verb* to bleed from the uterus during menstruation

**menstruation** /ˌmenstruˈeɪʃ(ə)n/ *noun* bleeding from the uterus which occurs in a woman each month when the lining of the uterus is shed because no fertilised egg is present

**menstruum** /ˈmenstruːəm/ *noun* a liquid used in the extract of active principles from an unrefined drug

**mental** /ˈment(ə)l/ *adjective* **1.** referring to the mind **2.** referring to the chin

**mental aberration** /ˌment(ə)l ˌæbəˈreɪʃ(ə)n/ *noun* slight forgetfulness or confusion (*often humorous*) ○ *I thought the meeting was at 11 – I must have had a mental aberration.*

**mental age** /ˌment(ə)l ˈeɪdʒ/ *noun* a measurement based on intelligence tests that shows a person's intellectual development, usually compared to standardised data for a chronological age □ **he's nine, but he has a mental age of five** although he is nine years old, his level of intellectual development is the same as that of an average child of five

**mental block** /ˌment(ə)l ˈblɒk/ *noun* a temporary inability to remember something, caused by the effect of nervous stress on the mental processes

**mental deficiency** /ˌment(ə)l dɪˈfɪʃ(ə)nsi/ *noun* a former term for learning disability (NOTE: This term is regarded as offensive.)

**mental development** /ˌment(ə)l dɪˈveləpmənt/ *noun* the development of the mind ○ *Her mental development is higher than usual for her age.*

**mental disorder** /ˌment(ə)l dɪsˈɔːdə/ *noun* a temporary or permanent change in a person's mental state which makes them function less effectively than they would usually, or than the average person would be expected to function

**mental faculties** /ˌment(ə)l ˈfæk(ə)ltiːz/ *plural noun* abilities such as thinking and decision-making ○ *There has been no impairment of the mental faculties.*

**mental handicap** /ˌment(ə)l ˈhændikæp/ *noun* a former term for learning disability (NOTE: This term is regarded as offensive.)

**mental health** /ˈment(ə)l helθ/ *noun* the condition of someone's mind

**Mental Health Acts** /ˌment(ə)l ˈhelθ ækts/ *plural noun* laws made by a parliament which lay down rules for the care of people with mental illness

**Mental Health Review Tribunal** /ˌment(ə)l helθ rɪˈvjuː traɪˌbjuːn(ə)l/ *noun* a committee which makes decisions about whether people who have been detained under the Mental Health Acts should be released. It consists of medical members, legal experts and lay members, who include people with experience in social services. Abbr **MHRT**

**mental hospital** /ˈment(ə)l ˌhɒspɪt(ə)l/ *noun* a psychiatric hospital (NOTE: This term is regarded as offensive.)

**mental illness** /ˌment(ə)l ˈɪlnəs/ *noun* any disorder which affects the mind

**mental impairment** /ˌment(ə)l ɪmˈpeəmənt/ *noun* a temporary or permanent condition which affects a person's mental state, making them function less effectively than they would usually, or than the average person would be expected to function

**mentalis muscle** /menˈteɪlɪs ˌmʌs(ə)l/ *noun* a muscle attached to the front of the lower jaw and the skin of the chin

**mentally** /ˈment(ə)li/ *adverb* in the mind ○ *Mentally, she is very advanced for her age.*

**mentally handicapped** /ˌment(ə)li ˈhændikæpt/ *adjective* a former term for someone with learning disability (NOTE: This term is usually regarded as offensive.)

**mentally ill** /ˌment(ə)li ˈɪl/ *adjective* experiencing mental illness

**mental nerve** /ˈment(ə)l nɜːv/ *noun* a nerve which supplies the chin

**mental patient** /ˈment(ə)l ˌpeɪʃ(ə)nt/ *noun* a former term of a patient who has mental illness (NOTE: This term is regarded as offensive.)

**mental retardation** /ˌment(ə)l ˌriːtɑːˈdeɪʃ(ə)n/ *noun* a former term for learning disability, a condition that results in someone finding it difficult to learn skills or information at the same rate as others of a similar age (NOTE: This term is regarded as offensive.)

**mental subnormality** /ˌment(ə)l ˌsʌbnɔːˈmælɪti/ *noun* a former term for mental impairment (NOTE: This term is usually regarded as offensive.)

**menthol** /ˈmenθɒl/ *noun* a strongly scented compound, produced from peppermint oil, used in cough medicines and in the treatment of neuralgia

**mentholated** /ˈmenθəleɪtɪd/ *adjective* impregnated with menthol

**mento-** /ˈmentəʊ/ *prefix* relating to the chin

**mentor** /ˈmentɔː/ *noun* somebody who advises and guides a younger, less experienced person ■ *verb* to act as a mentor to somebody

**mentum** /ˈmentəm/ *noun* the chin

**meralgia** /məˈrældʒə/, **meralgia paraesthetica** /məˌrældʒə ˌpæresˈθetɪkə/ *noun* pain in the top of the thigh caused by a pinched nerve

**mercurialism** /məˈkjʊəriəlɪz(ə)m/ *noun* mercury poisoning

**mercurochrome** /məˈkjʊərəʊkrəʊm/ *noun* a red antiseptic solution

**mercury** /ˈmɜːkjʊri/ *noun* a poisonous liquid metal, used in thermometers (NOTE: The chemical symbol is **Hg**.)

**mercury poisoning** /ˈmɜːkjʊri ˌpɔɪz(ə)nɪŋ/ *noun* poisoning by drinking mercury or mercury compounds or by inhaling mercury vapour

**mercy killing** /ˈmɜːsi ˌkɪlɪŋ/ *noun* same as **euthanasia**

**meridian** /məˈrɪdiən/ *noun* in acupuncture and Chinese medicine, one of the pathways in the body along which its energy is believed to flow

**Merkel's cells** /ˈmɜːkelz selz/, **Merkel's discs** /ˈmɜːkelz dɪsks/ *plural noun* epithelial cells in the deeper part of the dermis which form touch receptors [After Friedrich Siegmund Merkel (1845–1919), German anatomist]

**merocrine** /ˈmerəʊkraɪn/ *adjective* same as **eccrine**

**mes-** /mes/ *prefix* same as **meso-** (*used before vowels*)

**mesaortitis** /ˌmeseɪɔːˈtaɪtɪs/ *noun* inflammation of the media of the aorta

**mesarteritis** /mesˌɑːtəˈraɪtɪs/ *noun* inflammation of the media of an artery

**mesencephalon** /mesenˈkefəlɒn/ *noun* same as **midbrain**

**mesenteric** /ˌmesenˈterɪk/ *adjective* referring to the mesentery

**mesenterica** /mesenˈterɪkə/ ♦ **tabes mesenterica**

**mesenteric artery** /ˌmesenterɪk ˈɑːtəri/ *noun* one of two arteries, the superior and inferior mesenteric arteries, which supply the small intestine or the transverse colon and rectum

**mesenteric ganglion** /ˌmesenterɪk ˈɡæŋɡliən/ *noun* a plexus of sympathetic nerve fibres and ganglion cells around the superior mesenteric artery

**mesenteric vein** /ˌmesenterɪk ˈveɪn/ *noun* a vein in the portal system running from the intestine to the portal vein

**mesentery** /ˈmesent(ə)ri/ *noun* a double-layer peritoneum which attaches the small intestine and other abdominal organs to the abdominal wall

**mesial** /ˈmiːsiəl/ *adjective* **1.** in dentistry, relating to the middle of the front of the jaw, or occurring in a place near this **2.** relating to or located in the middle part of something

**meso-** /mesəʊ/ *prefix* middle

**mesoappendix** /ˌmesəʊəˈpendɪks/ *noun* a fold of peritoneum which links the appendix and the ileum

**mesocolon** /ˌmesəʊˈkəʊlən/ *noun* a fold of peritoneum which supports the colon. In an adult it supports the transverse and sigmoid sections only.

**mesoderm** /ˈmesəʊdɜːm/ *noun* the middle layer of an embryo, which develops into muscles, bones, blood, kidneys, cartilages, urinary ducts and the cardiovascular and lymphatic systems

**mesodermal** /ˌmesəʊˈdɜːm(ə)l/ *adjective* referring to the mesoderm

**mesometrium** /ˌmesəʊˈmiːtriəm/ *noun* a muscle layer of the uterus

**mesonephros** /ˌmesəʊˈnefrɒs/ *noun* kidney tissue which exists in a human embryo

**mesosalpinx** /ˌmesəʊˈsælpɪŋks/ *noun* the upper part of the broad ligament around the Fallopian tubes

**mesotendon** /ˌmesəʊˈtendən/ *noun* synovial membrane connecting the lining of the fibrous sheath to that of a tendon

**mesothelioma** /ˌmesəʊtiːliˈəʊmə/ *noun* a tumour of the serous membrane, which can be benign or malignant

**mesothelium** /ˌmesəʊˈθiːliəm/ *noun* a layer of cells lining a serous membrane. Compare **epithelium, endothelium**

**mesovarium** /ˌmesəʊˈveəriəm/ *noun* a fold of peritoneum around the ovaries

**messenger RNA** /ˌmes(ə)ndʒə ˌɑːr en 'eɪ/ noun a type of ribonucleic acid which transmits the genetic code from the DNA to the ribosomes which form the proteins coded on the DNA. Abbr **mRNA**

**mestranol** /'miːstrənɒl/ noun a synthetically produced oestrogen used in birth control pills

**meta-** /metə/ prefix referring to change

**meta analysis** /'metə əˌnæləsɪs/ noun a statistical procedure to combine the results from many studies to give a single estimate, giving weight to large studies

**metabolic** /ˌmetə'bɒlɪk/ adjective referring to metabolism

**metabolic acidosis** /ˌmetəbɒlɪk ˌæsɪ'dəʊsɪs/ noun acidosis caused by a malfunction of the body's metabolism

**metabolic alkalosis** /ˌmetəbɒlɪk ælkə'ləʊsɪs/ noun alkalosis caused by a malfunction of the body's metabolism

**metabolise** /mə'tæbəlaɪz/, **metabolize** verb to change the nature of something by metabolism ○ The liver metabolises proteins and carbohydrates.

**metabolism** /mə'tæbəlɪz(ə)m/ noun chemical processes which are continually taking place in the human body and which are essential to life, especially the processes that convert food into energy

COMMENT: Metabolism covers all changes which take place in the body: the building of tissue (anabolism); the breaking down of tissue (catabolism); the conversion of nutrients into tissue; the elimination of waste matter and the action of hormones.

**metabolite** /mə'tæbəlaɪt/ noun a substance produced by metabolism, or a substance taken into the body in food and then metabolised

**metacarpal bone** /ˌmetə'kɑːp(ə)l bəʊn/, **metacarpal** /ˌmetə'kɑːp(ə)l/ noun one of the five bones in the metacarpus

**metacarpophalangeal** /ˌmetəˌkɑːpəʊfə'lændʒiəl/ adjective relating to the part of the hand between the wrist and the fingers

**metacarpophalangeal joint** /ˌmetə ˌkɑːpəʊfə'lændʒiəl ˌdʒɔɪnt/ noun a joint between a metacarpal bone and a finger. Also called **MCP joint, MP joint**

'…replacement of the MCP joint is usually undertaken to relieve pain, deformity and immobility due to rheumatoid arthritis' [Nursing Times]

**metacarpus** /ˌmetə'kɑːpəs/ noun the five bones in the hand between the fingers and the wrist. See illustration at **HAND** in Supplement

**metal** /'met(ə)l/ noun material, either an element or a compound, which can carry heat and electricity. Some metals are essential for life.

**metallic** /me'tælɪk/ adjective like a metal, referring to a metal

**metallic element** /meˌtælɪk 'elɪmənt/ noun a chemical element which is a metal

**metamorphopsia** /ˌmetəmɔː'fɒpsiə/ noun a condition in which someone sees objects in distorted form, usually due to inflammation of the choroid

**metaphase** /'metəfeɪz/ noun one of the stages in mitosis or meiosis

**metaphysis** /me'tæfəsɪs/ noun the end of the central section of a long bone, where the bone grows and where it joins the epiphysis

**metaplasia** /metə'pleɪziə/ noun a change of one tissue to another

**metastasis** /me'tæstəsɪs/ noun the spreading of a malignant disease from one part of the body to another through the bloodstream and the lymph system. Also called **secondary growth** (NOTE: The plural is **metastases**.)

'…he suddenly developed problems with his balance and a solitary brain metastasis was diagnosed' [British Journal of Nursing]

**metastasise** /me'tæstəsaɪz/, **metastasize** verb to spread by metastasis

**metastatic** /ˌmetə'stætɪk/ adjective relating to, or produced by, metastasis ○ Metastatic growths developed in the liver.

**metatarsal** /ˌmetə'tɑːs(ə)l/ noun one of the five bones in the metatarsus ■ adjective relating to the metatarsus

**metatarsal arch** /ˌmetə'tɑːs(ə)l ɑːtʃ/ noun an arched part of the sole of the foot, running across the sole of the foot from side to side. Also called **transverse arch**

**metatarsalgia** /ˌmetətɑː'sældʒə/ noun pain in the heads of the metatarsal bones

**metatarsophalangeal joint** /metəˌtɑːsəʊ fə'lændʒiəl ˌdʒɔɪnt/ noun a joint between a metatarsal bone and a toe

**metatarsus** /ˌmetə'tɑːsəs/ noun the five long bones in the foot between the toes and the tarsus. See illustration at **FOOT** in Supplement (NOTE: The plural is **metatarsi**.)

**metatarsus adductus** /ˌmetətɑːsəs ə 'dʌktəs/ noun a condition found in newborn babies or young infants in which the front half of the foot is twisted inwards at an angle to the heel

**meteorism** /'miːtiərɪz(ə)m/ noun same as **tympanites**

**meter** /'miːtə/ noun US same as **metre**

**-meter** /miːtə, mɪtə/ suffix measuring instrument

**metformin** /met'fɔːmɪn/ noun a drug which reduces the level of the blood sugar levels, used to treat non-insulin dependent diabetes which does not respond to dietary measures

**methadone** /'meθədəʊn/ noun a synthetically produced narcotic drug, used to reduce pain and as a substitute for heroin in the treatment of addiction

**methaemoglobin** /metˌhiːməʊ'gləʊbɪn/ noun a dark brown substance formed from haemoglobin which develops during illness, following treatment with some drugs. Methaemoglobin cannot transport oxygen round the body, and so causes cyanosis.

**methaemoglobinaemia** /metˌhiːməʊˌɡləʊbɪˈniːmiə/ *noun* the presence of methaemoglobin in the blood

**methane** /ˈmiːθeɪn, ˈmeθeɪn/ *noun* a colourless flammable gas with no smell

**methanol** /ˈmeθənɒl/ *noun* a colourless poisonous liquid, used as a solvent and a fuel. It changes easily into a gas. Also called **methyl alcohol**

**methicillin** /ˌmeθɪˈsɪlɪn/ *noun* a synthetically produced antibiotic, used in the treatment of infections which are resistant to penicillin

**methicillin-resistant Staphylococcus aureus** /ˌmeθɪˌsɪlɪn rɪˌzɪstənt stæfɪləˌkɒkəs ˈɔːriəs/ *noun* a bacterium resistant to almost all antibiotics and which can cause life-threatening infection in people recovering from surgery. Abbr **MRSA**

**methionine** /meˈθaɪəniːn/ *noun* an essential amino acid

**method** /ˈmeθəd/ *noun* a way of doing something

**methotrexate** /ˌmeθəˈtrekseɪt/ *noun* a drug which helps to prevent cells reproducing, used in the treatment of cancer

**methyl alcohol** /ˌmiːθaɪl ˈælkəhɒl/ *noun* same as **methanol**

**methylated spirits** /ˌmeθəleɪtɪd ˈspɪrɪts/ *plural noun* almost pure alcohol, with wood alcohol and colouring added

**methylene blue** /ˌmeθɪliːn ˈbluː/ *noun* a blue dye, formerly used as a mild urinary antiseptic, now used to treat drug-induced methaemoglobinaemia

**methylenedioxymethamphetamine** /ˌmeθɪliːnˌdaɪɒksɪˌmeθæmˈfetəmiːn/ *noun* same as **ecstasy**

**methylphenidate** /ˌmiːθaɪlˈfenɪdeɪt/ *noun* a drug which stimulates the central nervous system, used in the treatment of narcolepsy and attention deficit disorder

**methylprednisolone** /ˌmiːθaɪlpredˈnɪsələʊn/ *noun* a corticosteroid drug which reduces inflammation, used in the treatment of arthritis, allergies and asthma

**metoclopramide** /ˌmetəʊˈkləʊprəmaɪd/ *noun* a drug used to treat nausea, vomiting and indigestion

**metoprolol** /mɪˈtɒprəlɒl/ *noun* a drug which controls the activity of the heart, used to treat angina and high blood pressure

**metr-** /metr/ *prefix* same as **metro-** (*used before vowels*)

**metra** /ˈmetrə/ *noun* the uterus

**metralgia** /meˈtrældʒə/ *noun* pain in the uterus

**metre** /ˈmiːtə/ *noun* an SI unit of length ○ *The room is four metres by three.* Symbol **m** (NOTE: The US spelling is **meter**.)

**metritis** /meˈtraɪtɪs/ *noun* same as **myometritis**

**metro-** /metrəʊ/ *prefix* referring to the uterus

**metrocolpocele** /ˌmetrəˈkɒlpəʊsiːl/ *noun* a condition in which the uterus protrudes into the vagina

**metronidazole** /ˌmetrəˈnɪdəzəʊl/ *noun* a yellow antibiotic compound, used especially in the treatment of vaginal infections

**metropathia haemorrhagica** /ˌmetrəpæθiə ˌheməˈreɪdʒɪkə/ *noun* an essential uterine haemorrhage, where the lining of the uterus swells and there is heavy menstrual bleeding

**metroptosis** /ˌmetrəˈtəʊsɪs/ *noun* a condition in which the uterus has moved downwards out of its usual position. Also called **prolapse of the uterus**

**metrorrhagia** /ˌmiːtrəʊˈreɪdʒiə/ *noun* unusual bleeding from the vagina between the menstrual periods

**metrostaxis** /ˌmiːtrəʊˈstæksɪs/ *noun* a continual light bleeding from the uterus

**-metry** /mətri/ *suffix* relating to the process of measuring, or to instruments which are used for measuring

**mg** *abbr* milligram

**MI** *abbr* **1.** mitral incompetence **2.** myocardial infarction

**micelle** /mɪˈsel/ *noun* a tiny particle formed by the digestion of fat in the small intestine

**Michel's clips** /mɪˌʃelz ˈklɪps/ *plural noun* metal clips used to suture a wound [After Gaston Michel (1874–1937), Professor of Clinical Surgery at Nancy, France]

**miconazole** /maɪˈkɒnəzəʊl/ *noun* a drug used to treat fungal infections of the skin and nails

**micro-** /maɪkrəʊ/ *prefix* **1.** very small. Opposite **macro-, mega-, megalo- 2.** one millionth ($10^{-6}$)

**microaneurysm** /ˌmaɪkrəʊˈænjərɪz(ə)m/ *noun* a tiny swelling in the wall of a capillary in the retina

**microangiopathy** /ˌmaɪkrəʊˌændʒiˈɒpəθi/ *noun* any disease of the capillaries

**microbe** /ˈmaɪkrəʊb/ *noun* a microorganism which may cause disease and which can only be seen with a microscope, e.g. a bacterium

**microbial** /maɪˈkrəʊbiəl/ *adjective* referring to microbes

**microbial disease** /maɪˌkrəʊbiəl dɪˈziːz/ *noun* a disease caused by a microbe

**microbiological** /ˌmaɪkrəʊˌbaɪəˈlɒdʒɪk(ə)l/ *adjective* referring to microbiology

**microbiologist** /ˌmaɪkrəʊbaɪˈɒlədʒɪst/ *noun* a scientist who specialises in the study of microorganisms

**microbiology** /ˌmaɪkrəʊbaɪˈɒlədʒi/ *noun* the scientific study of microorganisms

**microcephalic** /ˌmaɪkrəʊkeˈfælɪk/ *adjective* having microcephaly

**microcephaly** /ˌmaɪkrəʊˈkefəli/ *noun* a condition in which a person has an unusually small head, sometimes caused by the mother having had a rubella infection during pregnancy

**microcheilia** /ˌmaɪkrəʊˈkaɪliə/ *noun* the condition of having unusually small lips

**Micrococcus** /ˌmaɪkrəʊˈkɒkəs/ *noun* a genus of bacterium, some species of which cause arthritis, endocarditis and meningitis

**microcyte** /ˈmaɪkrəʊsaɪt/ *noun* an unusually small red blood cell

**microcythaemia** /ˌmaɪkrəʊsaɪˈθiːmiə/ *noun* same as **microcytosis**

**microcytic** /ˌmaɪkrəˈsɪtɪk/ *adjective* referring to microcytes

**microcytosis** /ˌmaɪkrəʊsaɪˈtəʊsɪs/ *noun* the presence of excess microcytes in the blood

**microdactylia** /ˌmaɪkrəʊdækˈtɪliə/, **microdactyly** /ˌmaɪkrəʊˈdæktɪli/ *noun* a condition in which a person has unusually small or short fingers or toes

**microdiscectomy** /ˌmaɪkrəʊdɪskˈektəmi/ *noun* a surgical operation to remove all or part of a disc in the spine which is pressing on a nerve

**microdontism** /ˌmaɪkrəʊˈdɒntɪz(ə)m/, **microdontia** /ˌmaɪkrəʊˈdɒntiə/ *noun* the condition of having unusually small teeth

**microglia** /maɪˈkrɒɡliə/ *noun* tissue in the central nervous system composed of tiny cells which destroy other cells

**microglossia** /ˌmaɪkrəʊˈɡlɒsiə/ *noun* a condition in which a person has an unusually small tongue

**micrognathia** /ˌmaɪkrəʊˈneɪθiə/ *noun* a condition in which one jaw is unusually smaller than the other

**microgram** /ˈmaɪkrəɡræm/ *noun* a unit of measurement of weight equal to one millionth of a gram

**micromastia** /ˌmaɪkrəʊˈmæstiə/ *noun* a condition in which a person has unusually small breasts

**micromelia** /ˌmaɪkrəʊˈmiːliə/ *noun* a condition in which a person has unusually small arms or legs

**micrometer** /maɪˈkrɒmɪtə/ *noun* **1.** an instrument for taking very small measurements, such as the width or thickness of very thin pieces of tissue **2.** *US* same as **micrometre**

**micrometre** /ˈmaɪkrəʊˌmiːtə/ *noun* a unit of measurement of thickness (= one millionth of a metre) (NOTE: With figures, usually written **μm**.)

**micromole** /ˈmaɪkrəʊˌməʊl/ *noun* a unit of measurement of the amount of substance equal to one millionth of a mole. Symbol **μ**

**micron** /ˈmaɪkrɒn/ *noun* same as **micrometre**

**micronutrient** /ˈmaɪkrəʊˌnjuːtriənt/ *noun* a substance which an organism needs for normal growth and development, but only in very small quantities, e.g. a vitamin or mineral. Compare **macronutrient**

**microorganism** /ˌmaɪkrəʊˈɔːɡənɪz(ə)m/ *noun* an organism which can only be seen under a microscope and which may cause disease. Viruses, bacteria and protozoa are microorganisms.

**microphthalmia** /ˌmaɪkrɒfˈθælmiə/ *noun* a condition in which the eyes are unusually small

**micropsia** /maɪˈkrɒpsiə/ *noun* a condition in which someone sees objects smaller than they really are, caused by an unusual development in the retina

**microscope** /ˈmaɪkrəskəʊp/ *noun* a scientific instrument with lenses, which makes very small objects appear larger ○ *The tissue was examined under the microscope.* ○ *Under the microscope it was possible to see the cancer cells.*

COMMENT: In an ordinary or light microscope the image is magnified by lenses. In an electron microscope the lenses are electromagnets and a beam of electrons is used instead of light, thereby achieving much greater magnifications.

**microscopic** /ˌmaɪkrəˈskɒpɪk/ *adjective* so small that it can only be seen through a microscope

**microscopy** /maɪˈkrɒskəpi/ *noun* the science of the use of microscopes

**microsecond** /ˈmaɪkrəʊˌsekənd/ *noun* a unit of measurement of time ( = one millionth of a second) (NOTE: With figures, usually written **μs**.)

**Microsporum** /ˈmaɪkrəʊspɔːrəm/ *noun* a type of fungus which causes ringworm of the hair, skin and sometimes nails

**microsurgery** /ˈmaɪkrəʊˌsɜːdʒəri/ *noun* surgery using tiny instruments and a microscope. Microsurgery is used in operations on eyes and ears, and also to connect severed nerves and blood vessels.

**microvillus** /ˌmaɪkrəʊˈvɪləs/ *noun* a very small process found on the surface of many cells, especially the epithelial cells in the intestine (NOTE: The plural is **microvilli**.)

**microwave therapy** /ˈmaɪkrəʊweɪv ˌθerəpi/ *noun* treatment using high-frequency radiation

**micturate** /ˈmɪktjʊreɪt/ *verb* same as **urinate**

**micturating cystogram** /ˌmɪktjʊreɪtɪŋ ˈsɪstəʊɡræm/, **micturating cysto-urethrogram** /ˌmɪktjʊreɪtɪŋ ˌsɪstəʊ jʊˈriːθrəɡræm/ *noun* an X-ray of the bladder and urethra taken while the bladder is being filled and then emptied. Abbr **MCU, MCUG**

**micturition** /ˌmɪktjʊˈrɪʃ(ə)n/ *noun* same as **urination**

**mid-** /mɪd/ *prefix* middle

**midazolam** /mɪˈdæzəlæm/ *noun* a drug used to produce sleepiness and to reduce anxiety before surgery or other procedures

**midbrain** /ˈmɪdbreɪn/ *noun* the small middle section of the brain stem above the pons and between the cerebrum and the hindbrain. Also called **mesencephalon**

**midcarpal** /mɪdˈkɑːp(ə)l/ *adjective* between the two rows of carpal bones

**middle** /ˈmɪd(ə)l/ *noun* **1.** the centre or central point of something **2.** the waist or stomach area (*informal*)

**middle-aged** /ˌmɪd(ə)l ˈeɪdʒd/ *adjective* not young and not old, in the middle years of life ○ *a disease which affects middle-aged women*

**middle colic** /ˌmɪd(ə)l ˈkɒlɪk/ *noun* an artery which leads from the superior mesenteric artery

**middle ear** /ˌmɪd(ə)l ˈɪə/ *noun* a section of the ear between the eardrum and the inner ear

COMMENT: The middle ear contains the three ossicles which receive vibrations from the eardrum and transmit them to the cochlea. The middle ear is connected to the throat by the Eustachian tube.

**middle ear infection** /ˌmɪd(ə)l ˈɪər ɪn ˌfekʃən/ *noun* same as **otitis media**

**middle finger** /ˌmɪd(ə)l ˈfɪŋgə/ *noun* the longest of the five fingers

**midgut** /ˈmɪdgʌt/ *noun* the middle part of the gut in an embryo, which develops into the small intestine

**mid-life crisis** /ˌmɪd laɪf ˈkraɪsɪs/ *noun* a period in early middle age when some people experience feelings of anxiety, insecurity and self-doubt

**midline** /ˈmɪdlaɪn/ *noun* an imaginary line drawn down the middle of the body from the head through the navel to the point between the feet

'…patients admitted with acute abdominal pains were referred for study. Abdominal puncture was carried out in the midline immediately above or below the umbilicus.' [*Lancet*]

**midriff** /ˈmɪdrɪf/ *noun* the diaphragm

**midstream specimen** /ˈmɪdstriːm ˌspesɪmɪn/, **midstream specimen of urine** /ˌmɪd striːm ˌspesɪmɪn əv ˈjʊərɪn/ *noun* a sample of urine collected in a sterile bottle in the middle of a flow of urine, because the first part of the flow may be contaminated with bacteria from the skin. Abbr **MSU**

**midtarsal** /mɪdˈtɑːs(ə)l/ *adjective* between the tarsal bones

**midwife** /ˈmɪdwaɪf/ *noun* a professional person who helps a woman give birth to a child, often at home

COMMENT: To become a Registered Midwife (RM), a Registered General Nurse has to follow a further 18 month course, or alternatively can follow a full 3 year course.

**midwifery** /mɪdˈwɪfəri/ *noun* **1.** the profession of a midwife **2.** the study of the practical aspects of obstetrics

**midwifery course** /mɪdˈwɪfəri kɔːs/ *noun* a training course to teach nurses the techniques of being a midwife

**migraine** /ˈmiːɡreɪn, ˈmaɪɡreɪn/, **migraine headache** /ˌmiːɡreɪn ˈhedeɪk/ *noun* a very severe throbbing headache which can be accompanied by nausea, vomiting, visual disturbance and vertigo. The cause is not known. Attacks may be preceded by an 'aura', where the patient sees flashing lights, or the eyesight becomes blurred. The pain is usually intense and affects one side of the head only.

**migrainous** /ˈmaɪɡreɪnəs/ *adjective* referring to someone who is subject to migraine attacks

**mild** /maɪld/ *adjective* not severe, not cold, gentle ○ *a mild throat infection*

**mildly** /ˈmaɪldli/ *adverb* slightly, not strongly ○ *a mildly infectious disease* ○ *a mildly antiseptic solution*

**milia** /ˈmɪliə/ plural of **milium**

**miliaria** /ˌmɪliˈeəriə/ *noun* itchy red spots which develop on the chest, under the armpits and between the thighs in hot countries, caused by blocked sweat glands. Also called **prickly heat, heat rash**

**miliary** /ˈmɪliəri/ *adjective* small in size, like a seed

**miliary tuberculosis** /ˌmɪliəri tjuːˌbɜːkjʊ ˈləʊsɪs/ *noun* a form of tuberculosis which occurs as little nodes in many parts of the body, including the meninges of the brain and spinal cord

**milium** /ˈmɪliəm/ *noun* **1.** a white pinhead-sized tumour on the face seen in adults **2.** a retention cyst in infants **3.** a cyst on the skin (NOTE: [all senses] The plural is **milia**.)

**milk** /mɪlk/ *noun* **1.** a white liquid produced by female mammals to feed their young. Cow's milk and other dairy products are important parts of most diets, especially children's. ○ *The patient can only drink warm milk.* (NOTE: No plural: *some milk, a bottle of milk* or *a glass of milk*.) **2.** the breast milk produced by a woman ○ *The milk will start to flow a few days after childbirth.* (NOTE: For other terms referring to milk, see words beginning with **galact-, galacto-, lact-, lacto-**.)

**milk dentition** /mɪlk denˈtɪʃ(ə)n/ *noun* same as **deciduous dentition**

**milk leg** /ˈmɪlk leg/ *noun* acute oedema of the leg, a condition which affects women after childbirth, where a leg becomes pale and inflamed as a result of lymphatic obstruction. Also called **white leg, phlegmasia alba dolens**

**milk rash** /ˈmɪlk ræʃ/ *noun* a temporary blotchiness of the skin seen in young babies

**milk sugar** /mɪlk 'ʃʊɡə/ *noun* same as **lactose**

**milk tooth** /'mɪlk tuːθ/ *noun* same as **primary tooth**

**milky** /'mɪlki/ *adjective* referring to liquid which is white like milk

**Miller-Abbott tube** /,mɪlər 'æbət tjuːb/ *noun* a tube with a balloon at the end, used to clear the small intestine. The balloon is inflated after the tip of the tube reaches an obstruction.

**milli-** /mɪlɪ/ *prefix* one thousandth (10⁻³). Symbol **m**

**milligram** /'mɪlɪɡræm/ *noun* a unit of measurement of weight equal to one thousandth of a gram. Symbol **mg**

**millilitre** /'mɪlɪ,liːtə/ *noun* a unit of measurement of liquid equal to one thousandth of a litre. Abbr **ml** (NOTE: The US spelling is **milliliter**.)

**millimetre** /'mɪlɪmiːtə/ *noun* a unit of measurement of length equal to one thousandth of a metre. Abbr **mm** (NOTE: The US spelling is **millimeter**.)

**millimole** /'mɪliməʊl/ *noun* a unit of measurement of the amount of a substance equal to one thousandth of a mole. Abbr **mmol**

**millisievert** /'mɪlisiːvət/ *noun* a unit of measurement of radiation □ **millisievert/year (mSv/year)** number of millisieverts per year

'…radiation limits for workers should be cut from 50 to 5 millisieverts, and those for members of the public from 5 to 0.25' [*Guardian*]

**Milroy's disease** /'mɪlrɔɪz dɪ,ziːz/ *noun* a hereditary condition where the lymph vessels are blocked and the legs swell [Described 1892. After William Forsyth Milroy (1855–1942), Professor of Clinical Medicine in Nebraska, USA.]

**Milwaukee brace** /mɪl,wɔːki 'breɪs/ *noun* a support for people with unusually curved spines, consisting of a leather or metal pelvic girdle with two bars at the back and one at the front, which connect into a neck ring

**mimesis** /mɪ'miːsɪs/ *noun* the appearance of the symptoms of a disease in someone who does not have the disease

**Minamata disease** /,mɪnə'mɑːtə dɪ,ziːz/ *noun* a form of mercury poisoning from eating polluted fish, found first in Japan

**mind** /maɪnd/ *noun* the part of the brain which controls memory, consciousness or reasoning □ **he's got something on his mind** he's worrying about something □ **let's try to take her mind off her exams** try to stop her worrying about them

**miner** /'maɪnə/ *noun* a person who works in a coal mine

**mineral** /'mɪn(ə)rəl/ *noun* an inorganic substance

COMMENT: The most important minerals required by the body are: calcium (found in cheese, milk and green vegetables) which helps the growth of bones and encourages blood clotting; iron (found in bread and liver) which helps produce red blood cells; phosphorus (found in bread and fish) which helps in the growth of bones and the metabolism of fats; iodine (found in fish) which is essential to the functioning of the thyroid gland.

**mineral water** /'mɪn(ə)rəl ,wɔːtə/ *noun* a drinking water containing dissolved mineral salts from the ground the water is piped from. It is bottled and sold.

**minim** /'mɪnɪm/ *noun* a liquid measure used in pharmacy (one sixtieth of a drachm)

**minimal** /'mɪnɪm(ə)l/ *adjective* very small

**minimally invasive surgery** /,mɪnɪm(ə)l ɪn,veɪsɪv 'sɜːdʒəri/ *noun* surgery which involves the least possible disturbance to the body. It often uses lasers and other high-tech devices.

**mini mental state examination** /,mɪni 'ment(ə)l ,steɪt ɪɡzæmɪ,neɪʃ(ə)n/ *noun* a test performed mainly by psychiatrists to determine someone's mental ability, used in the diagnosis of dementia

**minimum** /'mɪnɪməm/ *adjective* smallest possible ■ *noun* the smallest possible amount (NOTE: The plural is **minimums** or **minima**.)

**minimum lethal dose** /,mɪnɪməm ,liːθ(ə)l 'dəʊs/ *noun* the smallest amount of a substance required to kill someone or something. Abbr **MLD**

**ministroke** /'mɪnistrəʊk/ *noun* same as **transient ischaemic attack**

**minitracheostomy** /,mɪnitreɪki'ɒstəmi/ *noun* a temporary tracheostomy

**minor** /'maɪnə/ *adjective* **1.** not very serious or life-threatening **2.** less important or serious than others of the same type ▶ opposite **major**

'…practice nurses play a major role in the care of patients with chronic disease and they undertake many preventive procedures. They also deal with a substantial amount of minor trauma' [*Nursing Times*]

**minor illness** /,maɪnər 'ɪlnəs/ *noun* an illness which is not serious

**minor injuries unit** /,maɪnər 'ɪndʒəriz ,juːnɪt/ *noun* a hospital department which treats most accidents and emergencies. Abbr **MIU**

**minor surgery** /,maɪnə 'sɜːdʒəri/ *noun* surgery which can be undertaken even when there are no hospital facilities. Compare **major surgery**

**mio-** /maɪəʊ/ *prefix* less

**miosis** /maɪ'əʊsɪs/ *noun* **1.** the contraction of the pupil of the eye, as in bright light **2.** *US* same as **meiosis**

**miotic** /maɪ'ɒtɪk/ *noun* a drug which makes the pupil of the eye become smaller ■ *adjective* causing the pupil of the eye to become smaller

**mis-** /mɪs/ *prefix* wrong

**miscarriage** /'mɪskærɪdʒ/ *noun* a situation in which an unborn baby leaves the uterus before the end of the pregnancy, especially during the first seven months of pregnancy ○ *She had two miscarriages before having her first child.* Also called **spontaneous abortion**

**miscarry** /mɪsˈkæri/ *verb* to have a miscarriage ○ *The accident made her miscarry.* ○ *She miscarried after catching the infection.*

**misconduct** /mɪsˈkɒndʌkt/ *noun* action by a professional person such as a doctor which is considered wrong

**misdiagnose** /ˌmɪsˈdaɪəgˌnəʊz/ *verb* to make an incorrect diagnosis of a condition

**misdiagnosis** /ˌmɪsdaɪəgˈnəʊsɪs/ *noun* an incorrect diagnosis

**mismatch** /ˈmɪsmætʃ/ *verb* to match tissues wrongly

'...finding donors of correct histocompatible type is difficult but necessary because results using mismatched bone marrow are disappointing' [*Hospital Update*]

**miso-** /mɪsɒ/ *prefix* indicating hatred of something

**missed case** /ˌmɪst ˈkeɪs/ *noun* someone with an infection or disease which is not identified by a doctor

**mist.** /mɪst/, **mistura** /mɪsˈtjʊərə/ ♦ **re. mist.**

**misuse** *noun* /mɪsˈjuːs/ wrong use ○ *He was arrested for misuse of drugs.* ■ *verb* /mɪsˈjuːz/ to use something such as a drug wrongly

**Misuse of Drugs Act 1971** /mɪsˌjuːs əv ˈdrʌgz ækt/ *noun* a law relating to all aspects of the supply and possession of dangerous drugs such as morphine, anabolic steroids, LSD and cannabis. In 2002 many new benzodiazepines were added.

**mite** /maɪt/ *noun* a very small parasite, which causes dermatitis

**mitochondrial** /ˌmaɪtəˈkɒndriəl/ *adjective* referring to mitochondria

**mitochondrion** /ˌmaɪtəˈkɒndriən/ *noun* a tiny rod-shaped part of a cell's cytoplasm responsible for cell respiration (NOTE: The plural is **mitochondria**.)

**mitomycin C** /ˌmaɪtəʊmaɪsɪn ˈsiː/ *noun* an antibiotic which helps to prevent cancer cells from growing, used especially in the chemotherapy treatment of bladder and rectal cancers

**mitosis** /maɪˈtəʊsɪs/ *noun* the process of cell division, where the mother cell divides into two identical daughter cells. Compare **meiosis**

**mitral** /ˈmaɪtrəl/ *adjective* referring to the mitral valve

**mitral incompetence** /ˌmaɪtrəl ɪnˈkɒmpɪt(ə)ns/ *noun* Abbr **MI**. Now called **mitral regurgitation**

**mitral regurgitation** /ˌmaɪtrəl rɪˌgɜːdʒɪˈteɪʃ(ə)n/ *noun* a situation in which the mitral valve does not close completely so that blood goes back into the atrium

**mitral stenosis** /ˌmaɪtrəl steˈnəʊsɪs/ *noun* a condition in which the opening in the mitral valve becomes smaller because the cusps have

fused (NOTE: This condition is almost always the result of rheumatic endocarditis.)

**mitral valve** /ˈmaɪtrəl vælv/ *noun* a valve in the heart which allows blood to flow from the left atrium to the left ventricle but not in the opposite direction. Also called **bicuspid valve**

**mitral valvotomy** /ˌmaɪtrəl vælˈvɒtəmi/ *noun* a surgical operation to separate the cusps of the mitral valve in mitral stenosis

**mittelschmerz** /ˈmɪt(ə)lˌʃmeəts/ *noun* a pain felt by women in the lower abdomen at ovulation

**MIU** *abbr* minor injuries unit

**mix** /mɪks/ *verb* to put things together ○ *The pharmacist mixed the chemicals in a bottle.*

**mixture** /ˈmɪkstʃə/ *noun* chemical substances mixed together ○ *The doctor gave me an unpleasant mixture to drink.* ○ *Take one spoonful of the mixture every three hours.*

**ml** *abbr* millilitre

**MLD** *abbr* minimum lethal dose

**MLSO** *abbr* medical laboratory scientific officer

**mm** *abbr* millimetre

**mmol** *abbr* millimole

**MMR** /ˌem em ˈɑː/, **MMR vaccine** /ˌem em ˈɑː ˌvæksiːn/ *noun* a single vaccine given to small children to protect them against measles, mumps and rubella

**Mn** *symbol* manganese

**MND** *abbr* motor neurone disease

**MO** *abbr* medical officer

**mobile** /ˈməʊbaɪl/ *adjective* able to move about ○ *It is important for elderly patients to remain mobile.*

**mobilisation** /ˌməʊbɪlaɪˈzeɪʃ(ə)n/, **mobilization** *noun* the act of making something mobile

**mobility** /məʊˈbɪlɪti/ *noun* (*of patients*) the ability to move about

**mobility allowance** /məʊˈbɪlɪti əˌlaʊəns/ *noun* a government benefit to help disabled people pay for transport

**modality** /məʊˈdælɪti/ *noun* a method used in the treatment of a disorder, e.g. surgery or chemotherapy

**moderate** /ˈmɒd(ə)rət/ *adjective* not high or low

**moderately** /ˈmɒd(ə)rətli/ *adverb* not at one or other extreme ○ *The patient had a moderately comfortable night.*

**modern matron** /ˌmɒd(ə)n ˈmeɪtrən/ *noun* a nursing post which supports the ward sister in ensuring that basic care of patients, including cleanliness of the ward and infection control, is carried out to a high standard

**modiolus** /məʊˈdiːələs/ *noun* the central stalk in the cochlea

**MODS** *abbr* multiple organ dysfunction syndrome

**MOF** *abbr* **1.** male or female **2.** multi-organ failure

**Mogadon** /'mɒgədɒn/ a trade name for nitrazepam

**MOH** *abbr* Medical Officer of Health

**moist** /mɔɪst/ *adjective* slightly wet or damp ○ *The compress should be kept moist.*

**moisten** /'mɔɪs(ə)n/ *verb* to make something damp

**moist gangrene** /ˌmɔɪst 'gæŋgriːn/ *noun* a condition in which dead tissue decays and swells with fluid because of infection and the tissues have an unpleasant smell

**moisture** /'mɔɪstʃə/ *noun* water or other liquid

**moisture content** /'mɔɪstʃə ˌkɒntent/ *noun* the amount of water or other liquid which a substance contains

**mol** /məʊl/ *symbol* mole *noun* 2

**molar** /'məʊlə/ *adjective* **1.** referring to the large back teeth **2.** referring to the mole, the SI unit of amount of a substance ■ *noun* one of the large back teeth, used for grinding food. In milk teeth there are eight molars and in permanent teeth there are twelve. See illustration at TEETH in Supplement

**molarity** /məʊ'lærɪti/ *noun* the strength of a solution shown as the number of moles of a substance per litre of solution

**molasses** /mə'læsɪz/ *noun* a dark sweet substance made of sugar before it has been refined

**mole** /məʊl/ *noun* **1.** a dark raised spot on the skin ○ *She has a large mole on her chin.* ◊ melanoma **2.** an SI unit of measurement of the amount of a substance. Symbol **mol**

**molecular** /mə'lekjʊlə/ *adjective* referring to a molecule

**molecular biology** /məˌlekjʊlə baɪ'ɒlədʒi/ *noun* the study of the molecules of living matter

**molecular weight** /məˌlekjʊlə 'weɪt/ *noun* the weight of one molecule of a substance

**molecule** /'mɒlɪkjuːl/ *noun* the smallest independent mass of a substance

**molluscum** /mə'lʌskəm/ *noun* a soft round skin tumour

**molluscum contagiosum** /məˌlʌskəm kənˌteɪdʒi'əʊsəm/ *noun* a contagious viral skin infection which gives a small soft sore

**molluscum fibrosum** /məˌlʌskəm ˌfaɪ'brəʊsəm/ *noun* same as **neurofibromatosis**

**molluscum sebaceum** /məˌlʌskəm sɪ'beɪʃəm/ *noun* a benign skin tumour which disappears after a short time

**molybdenum** /mɒ'lɪbdənəm/ *noun* a metallic trace element (NOTE: The chemical symbol is **Mo**.)

**monaural** /mɒn'ɔːrəl/ *adjective* referring to the use of one ear only

**Mönckeberg's arteriosclerosis** /ˌmʌnkəbeəgz ˌɑːtiːriəʊskle'rəʊsɪs/ *noun* a condition of elderly people, where the media of the arteries in the legs harden, causing limping [Described 1903. After Johann Georg Mönckeberg (1877–1925), German physician and pathologist.]

**mongolism** /'mɒŋgəlɪz(ə)m/ *noun* a former name for Down's syndrome (NOTE: This term is regarded as offensive.)

**Monilia** /məʊ'nɪliə/ *noun* same as **Candida**

**moniliasis** /mɒni'laɪəsɪs/ *noun* same as **candidiasis**

**monitor** /'mɒnɪtə/ *noun* a screen on a computer ■ *verb* **1.** to check something **2.** to examine how someone is progressing

**monitoring** /'mɒnɪt(ə)rɪŋ/ *noun* the regular examination and recording of a person's temperature, weight, blood pressure and other essential indicators

**mono-** /mɒnəʊ/ *prefix* single or one

**monoamine oxidase** /ˌmɒnəʊˌæmiːn 'ɒksɪdeɪz/ *noun* an enzyme which breaks down the catecholamines to their inactive forms. Abbr **MAO**

**monoamine oxidase inhibitor** /ˌmɒnəʊˌæmiːn ˌɒksɪdeɪz ɪn'hɪbɪtə/ *noun* a drug which inhibits monoamine oxidase and is used to treat depression, e.g. phenelzine. Its use is limited, because of the potential for drug and dietary interactions and the necessity for slow withdrawal. It can also cause high blood pressure. Abbr **MAOI**. Also called **MAO inhibitor**

**monoblast** /'mɒnəʊblæst/ *noun* a cell which produces a monocyte

**monochromatism** /ˌmɒnəʊ'krəʊmətɪz(ə)m/ *noun* colour blindness in which all colours appear to be black, grey or white. Compare **dichromatism**, **trichromatism**

**monoclonal** /ˌmɒnəʊ'kləʊn(ə)l/ *adjective* referring to cells or products of cells which are formed or derived from a single clone

**monoclonal antibody** /ˌmɒnəʊkləʊn(ə)l 'æntɪbɒdi/ *noun* an antibody which can be easily made in the laboratory by a single clone of cells. It may be useful in the treatment of cancer.

**monocular** /mɒ'nɒkjʊlə/ *adjective* referring to one eye. Compare **binocular**

**monocular vision** /məˌnɒkjʊlə 'vɪʒ(ə)n/ *noun* the ability to see with one eye only, so that the sense of distance is impaired

**monocyte** /'mɒnəʊsaɪt/ *noun* a white blood cell with a nucleus shaped like a kidney, which destroys bacterial cells

**monocytosis** /ˌmɒnəʊsaɪ'təʊsɪs/ *noun* a condition in which there is an unusually high number of monocytes in the blood. Symptoms include sore throat, swelling of the lymph nodes and fever. It is probably caused by the Epstein–Barr virus. Also called **glandular fever**

**monodactylism** /ˌmɒnəʊˈdæktɪlɪz(ə)m/ noun a congenital condition in which only one finger or toe is present on the hand or foot

**monomania** /ˌmɒnəʊˈmeɪniə/ noun a state of mental disorder in which a person concentrates attention on one idea

**mononeuritis** /ˌmɒnəʊnjuˈraɪtɪs/ noun a neuritis which affects one nerve

**mononuclear** /ˌmɒnəʊˈnjuːkliə/ adjective referring to a cell such as a monocyte which has one nucleus

**mononucleosis** /ˌmɒnəʊˌnjuːkliˈəʊsɪs/ noun same as **monocytosis**

**monoplegia** /ˌmɒnəʊˈpliːdʒə/ noun the paralysis of one part of the body only, i.e. one muscle or one limb

**monorchism** /ˈmɒnɔːkɪz(ə)m/ noun a condition in which only one testis is visible

**monosaccharide** /ˌmɒnəʊˈsækraɪd/ noun a simple sugar which cannot be broken down any further, such as glucose or fructose

**monosodium glutamate** /ˌmɒnəʊˌsəʊdiəm ˈgluːtəmeɪt/ noun a sodium salt of glutamic acid, often used to make food taste better. ◊ **Chinese restaurant syndrome**

**monosomy** /ˈmɒnəʊsəʊmi/ noun a condition in which a person has a chromosome missing from one or more pairs

**monosynaptic** /ˌmɒnəʊsɪˈnæptɪk/ adjective referring to a nervous pathway with only one synapse

**monovalent** /ˌmɒnəʊˈveɪlənt/ adjective having a valency of one

**monoxide** /məˈnɒksaɪd/ ♦ **carbon**

**monozygotic twins** /ˌmɒnəʊzaɪˌgɒtɪk ˈtwɪnz/ plural noun same as **identical twins**

**mons** /mɒnz/ noun a fleshy body part which sticks out, especially the one formed by the pad of flesh where the pubic bones join (NOTE: The plural is **montes**.)

**mons pubis** /ˌmɒnz ˈpjuːbɪs/ noun a cushion of fat covering the pubis

**monster** /ˈmɒnstə/ noun a former term for a fetus or infant with severe developmental malformations, usually not able to live

**mons veneris** /ˌmɒnz vəˈnɪərɪs/ noun same as **mons pubis**

**Montezuma's revenge** /ˌmɒntɪzuːməz rɪˈvendʒ/ noun a diarrhoea which affects people travelling in foreign countries, often due to eating unwashed fruit or drinking water which has not been boiled (informal)

**Montgomery's glands** /məntˈgʌməriz glændz/ plural noun sebaceous glands around the nipple which become more marked in pregnancy [After William Fetherstone Montgomery (1797–1859), Dublin gynaecologist]

**mood** /muːd/ noun a person's mental state at a particular time ○ a mood of excitement □ **in a bad mood** feeling angry or irritable □ **in a good mood** feeling happy

**moon face** /ˈmuːn feɪs/ noun a condition in which someone has a round red face, occurring in Cushing's syndrome and when there are too many steroid hormones in the body

**Mooren's ulcer** /ˈmɔːrənz ˌʌlsə/ noun a persistent ulcer of the cornea, found in elderly people [After Albert Mooren (1828–99), ophthalmologist in Düsseldorf, Germany]

**morbid** /ˈmɔːbɪd/ adjective **1.** showing symptoms of being diseased ○ The X-ray showed a morbid condition of the kidneys. **2.** referring to disease **3.** referring to an unhealthy mental faculty

**morbid anatomy** /ˌmɔːbɪd əˈnætəmi/ noun same as **pathology**

**morbidity** /mɔːˈbɪdɪti/ noun the condition of being diseased or sick

'…apart from death, coronary heart disease causes considerable morbidity in the form of heart attack, angina and a number of related diseases' [Health Education Journal]

**morbidity rate** /mɔːˈbɪdɪti reɪt/ noun the number of cases of a disease per hundred thousand of population

**morbilli** /mɔːˈbɪli/ noun same as **measles**

**morbilliform** /mɔːˈbɪlifɔːm/ adjective referring to a rash which is similar to measles

**morbus** /ˈmɔːbəs/ noun disease

**moribund** /ˈmɒrɪbʌnd/ adjective dying ■ noun a dying person

**morning** /ˈmɔːnɪŋ/ noun the first part of the day before 12 o'clock noon

**morning-after feeling** /ˌmɔːnɪŋ ˈɑːftə ˌfiːlɪŋ/ noun ♦ **hangover** (informal)

**morning-after pill** /ˌmɔːnɪŋ ˈɑːftə pɪl/ noun a contraceptive pill taken after intercourse. Also called **next-day pill**

**morning sickness** /ˈmɔːnɪŋ ˌsɪknəs/ noun nausea and vomiting experienced by women in the early stages of pregnancy when they get up in the morning

**Moro reflex** /ˈmɔːrəʊ ˌriːfleks/ noun a reflex of a newborn baby when it hears a loud noise (NOTE: The baby is laid on a table and observed to see if it raises its arms when the table is struck.) [After Ernst Moro (1874–1951), paediatrician in Heidelberg, Germany]

**morphea** /mɔːˈfiə/ noun a form of scleroderma, a disease where the skin is replaced by thick connective tissue

**morphia** /ˈmɔːfiə/ same as **morphine**

**morphine** /ˈmɔːfiːn/ noun an analgesic derived from opium that is used to treat severe pain and may become addictive with prolonged use

**morpho-** /mɔːfəʊ/ prefix relating to form, shape or structure

**morphoea** /mɔːˈfiə/ noun same as **morphea**

**morphology** /mɔːˈfɒlədʒi/ noun the study of the structure and shape of living organisms

**-morphous** /mɔːfəs/ *suffix* relating to form or structure of a particular type

**mortality rate** /mɔːˈtælɪti reɪt/ *noun* the number of deaths per year, shown per hundred thousand of population

**mortification** /ˌmɔːtɪfɪˈkeɪʃ(ə)n/ *noun* ♦ necrosis

**mortis** /ˈmɔːtɪs/ ♦ rigor

**mortuary** /ˈmɔːtjuəri/ *noun* a room in a hospital where dead bodies are kept until removed by an undertaker for burial

**morula** /ˈmɒrʊlə/ *noun* an early stage in the development of an embryo, where the cleavage of the ovum creates a mass of cells

**mosquito** /mɒˈskiːtəʊ/ *noun* an insect which sucks human blood, some species of which can pass viruses or parasites into the bloodstream

COMMENT: In northern countries a mosquito bite merely produces an itchy spot. In tropical countries dengue, filariasis, malaria and yellow fever are transmitted by mosquitoes, and are major causes of morbidity and mortality. Mosquitoes breed in water and they spread rapidly in lakes or canals created by dams and other irrigation schemes as well as in containers of water stored for household use.

**mother** /ˈmʌðə/ *noun* a biological or adoptive female parent

**mother-fixation** /ˈmʌðə fɪkˌseɪʃ(ə)n/ *noun* a condition in which a person's development has been stopped at a stage where he or she remains like a child, dependent on his or her mother

**motile** /ˈməʊtaɪl/ *adjective* referring to a cell or microorganism which can move spontaneously ○ *Sperm cells are extremely motile.*

**motility** /məʊˈtɪlɪti/ *noun* **1.** (*of cells or microbes*) the fact of being able to move about **2.** (*of the gut*) the action of peristalsis

**motion** /ˈməʊʃ(ə)n/ *noun* **1.** movement **2.** same as **bowel movement**

**motionless** /ˈməʊʃ(ə)n(ə)ləs/ *adjective* not moving ○ *Catatonic patients can sit motionless for hours.*

**motion sickness** /ˌməʊʃ(ə)n ˈsɪknəs/ *noun* illness and nausea felt when travelling. It is caused by the movement of liquid inside the labyrinth of the middle ear and is particularly noticeable in vehicles which are closed, such as planes, coaches or hovercraft. (*informal*)

COMMENT: The movement of liquid inside the labyrinth of the middle ear causes motion sickness, which is particularly noticeable in vehicles which are closed, such as planes, coaches, hovercraft.

**motor** /ˈməʊtə/ *adjective* referring to movement, which produces movement

**motor area** /ˈməʊtər ˌeəriə/, **motor cortex** /ˌməʊtə ˈkɔːteks/ *noun* the part of the cortex in the brain which controls voluntary muscle movement by sending impulses to the motor nerves

**motor disorder** /ˈməʊtə dɪsˌɔːdə/ *noun* impairment of the nerves or neurons that cause muscles to contract to produce movement

**motor end plate** /ˌməʊtər ˈend pleɪt/ *noun* the end of a motor nerve where it joins muscle fibre

**motor nerve** /ˈməʊtə nɜːv/ *noun* a nerve which carries impulses from the brain and spinal cord to muscles and causes movements. Also called **efferent nerve**

**motor neurone** /ˌməʊtə ˈnjʊərəʊn/ *noun* a neurone which is part of a nerve pathway transmitting impulses from the brain to a muscle or gland

**motor neurone disease** /ˌməʊtə ˈnjʊərəʊn dɪˌziːz/ *noun* a disease of the nerve cells which control the movement of the muscles. Abbr **MND**

COMMENT: Motor neurone disease has three forms: progressive muscular atrophy (PMA), which affects movements of the hands, lateral sclerosis, and bulbar palsy, which affects the mouth and throat.

**motor pathway** /ˌməʊtə ˈpɑːθweɪ/ *noun* a series of motor neurones leading from the motor cortex to a muscle

**mottled** /ˈmɒt(ə)ld/ *adjective* with patches of different colours

**mountain fever** /ˈmaʊntɪn ˌfiːvə/ *noun* same as **brucellosis**

**mountain sickness** /ˈmaʊntɪn ˌsɪknəs/ *noun* same as **altitude sickness**

**mouth** /maʊθ/ *noun* an opening at the head of the alimentary canal, through which food and drink are taken in, and through which a person speaks and can breathe ○ *She was sleeping with her mouth open.* (NOTE: For other terms referring to the mouth, see **oral** and words beginning with **stomat-, stomato-**.)

**mouthful** /ˈmaʊθfʊl/ *noun* the amount which you can hold in your mouth

**mouth-to-mouth** /ˌmaʊθ tə ˈmaʊθ/, **mouth-to-mouth resuscitation** /ˌmaʊθ tə ˌmaʊθ rɪˌsʌsɪˈteɪʃ(ə)n/, **mouth-to-mouth ventilation** /ˌmaʊθ tə ˌmaʊθ ˌventɪˈleɪʃ(ə)n/ *noun* same as **cardiopulmonary resuscitation** (*informal*)

**mouth ulcer** /ˈmaʊθ ˌʌlsə/ *noun* a small white ulcer that appears in groups in the mouth and on the tongue

**mouthwash** /ˈmaʊθwɒʃ/ *noun* an antiseptic solution used to treat infection in the mouth

**move** /muːv/ *verb* to change from one place to another, or change something from one place to another ○ *Try to move your arm.* ○ *He found he was unable to move.*

**movement** /ˈmuːvmənt/ *noun* **1.** the act of changing position or the fact of not being still **2.** same as **bowel movement**

**moxybustion** /ˌmɒksɪˈbʌstʃ(ə)n/ *noun* a treatment used in the Far East, where dried herbs are placed on the skin and set on fire

**MP joint** /ˌem ˈpiː ˌdʒɔɪnt/ *noun* same as **metacarpophalangeal joint**

**MPS** *abbr* member of the pharmaceutical society

**MRC** *abbr* Medical Research Council

**MRCGP** *abbr* Member of the Royal College of General Practitioners

**MRCP** *abbr* Member of the Royal College of Physicians

**MRCS** *abbr* Member of the Royal College of Surgeons

**MRI** *abbr* magnetic resonance imaging

'…during an MRI scan, the patient lies within a strong magnetic field as selected sections of his body are stimulated with radio frequency waves. Resulting energy changes are measured and used by the MRI computer to generate images.' [*Nursing 87*]

**mRNA** *abbr* messenger RNA

**MRSA** *abbr* methicillin-resistant Staphylococcus aureus

**MS** *abbr* **1.** mitral stenosis **2.** multiple sclerosis

**MSH** *abbr* melanocyte-stimulating hormone

**MSU** *abbr* midstream specimen of urine

**mSv** *abbr* millisievert

**mucin** /ˈmjuːsɪn/ *noun* a compound of sugars and protein which is the main substance in mucus

**muco-** /mjuːkəʊ/ *prefix* referring to mucus

**mucocele** /ˈmjuːkəʊsiːl/ *noun* a cavity containing an accumulation of mucus

**mucociliary transport** /ˌmjuːkəʊˌsɪliəri ˈtrænspɔːt/ *noun* the process in which the cilia, the microscopic structures within the nose, move mucus towards the oesophagus, cleansing the nose of dust and bacteria

**mucocoele** /ˈmjuːkəʊsiːl/ *noun* **1.** a condition in which a cavity or organ becomes swollen because there is too much mucus in it **2.** the swelling produced by this condition

**mucocutaneous** /ˌmjuːkəʊkjuːˈteɪniəs/ *adjective* referring to both mucous membrane and the skin

**mucocutaneous leishmaniasis** /ˌmjuːkəʊkjuːˌteɪniəs ˌliːʃməˈnaɪəsɪs/ *noun* a disorder affecting the skin and mucous membrane

**mucoid** /ˈmjuːkɔɪd/ *adjective* similar to mucus

**mucolytic** /ˌmjuːkəʊˈlɪtɪk/ *noun* a substance which dissolves mucus

**mucomembranous colitis** /ˌmjuːkəʊ ˌmembrənəs kəˈlaɪtɪs/ *noun* same as **mucous colitis**

**mucoprotein** /ˌmjuːkəʊˈprəʊtiːn/ *noun* a form of protein found in blood plasma

**mucopurulent** /ˌmjuːkəʊˈpjʊərʊlənt/ *adjective* consisting of a mixture of mucus and pus

**mucopus** /ˌmjuːkəʊˈpʌs/ *noun* a mixture of mucus and pus

**mucormycosis** /ˌmjuːkɔːmaɪˈkəʊsɪs/ *noun* a disease of the ear and throat caused by the fungus *Mucor*

**mucosa** /mjuːˈkəʊzə/ *noun* same as **mucous membrane** (NOTE: The plural is **mucosae**.)

**mucosal** /mjuːˈkəʊz(ə)l/ *adjective* referring to a mucous membrane

**mucous** /ˈmjuːkəs/ *adjective* referring to mucus, covered in mucus

**mucous cell** /ˈmjuːkəs sel/ *noun* a cell which contains mucinogen which secretes mucin

**mucous colic** /ˌmjuːkəs ˈkɒlɪk/ *noun* an inflammation of the colon, with painful spasms in the muscles of the walls of the colon

**mucous colitis** /ˌmjuːkəs kəˈlaɪtɪs/ *noun* an inflammation of the mucous membrane in the intestine, in which the person experiences pain caused by spasms in the muscles of the walls of the colon, accompanied by constipation or diarrhoea or alternating attacks of both. Also called **irritable bowel syndrome**

**mucous membrane** /ˌmjuːkəs ˈmembreɪn/ *noun* a wet membrane which lines internal passages in the body, e.g. the nose, mouth, stomach and throat, and secretes mucus. Also called **mucosa**

**mucous plug** /ˈmjuːkəs plʌg/ *noun* a plug of mucus which blocks the cervical canal during pregnancy

**mucoviscidosis** /ˌmjuːkəʊvɪsɪˈdəʊsɪs/ *noun* same as **cystic fibrosis**

**mucus** /ˈmjuːkəs/ *noun* a slippery liquid secreted by mucous membranes inside the body, which protects those membranes (NOTE: For other terms referring to mucus, see words beginning with **blenno-**.)

**muddled** /ˈmʌd(ə)ld/ *adjective* referring to someone whose thought processes are confused

**Müllerian duct** /mʌˌlɪəriən ˈdʌkt/ *noun* same as **paramesonephric duct** [Described 1825. After Johannes Peter Müller (1801–58), Professor of Anatomy at Bonn, later Professor of Anatomy and Physiology at Berlin, Germany.]

**multi-** /mʌlti/ *prefix* many

**multicentric** /ˌmʌltiˈsentrɪk/ *adjective* in several centres

**multicentric trial** /ˌmʌltisentrɪk ˈtraɪəl/, **multicentric testing** /ˌmʌltisentrɪk ˈtestɪŋ/ *noun* trials carried out in several centres at the same time

**multidisciplinary** /ˌmʌltiˈdɪsɪplɪnəri/ *adjective* using or involving several specialised subjects or skills ○ *a multidisciplinary team*

**multifactorial** /ˌmʌltifækˈtɔːriəl/ *adjective* **1.** involving several different factors or elements **2.** referring to inheritance which depends on more than one gene. Height and weight are examples of characteristics determined by multifactorial inheritance.

**multifocal lens** /ˌmʌltiˌfəʊk(ə)l ˈlenz/ *noun* a lens in spectacles whose focus changes from top to bottom so that the person wearing the spectacles can see objects clearly at different distances

**multiforme** /ˈmʌltifɔːm/ ♦ **erythema multiforme**

**multigravida** /ˌmʌltiˈɡrævidə/ noun a pregnant woman who has been pregnant two or more times before

**multi-infarct dementia** /ˌmʌlti ˈɪnfɑːkt dɪ ˌmenʃə/ noun dementia caused by a number of small strokes, when the dementia is not progressive as in Alzheimer's disease but increases in steps as new strokes occur

**multilocular** /ˌmʌltiˈlɒkjʊlə/ adjective referring to a body part or growth which has a lot of separate compartments or locules

**multinucleated** /ˌmʌltiˈnjuːklieɪtɪd/ adjective referring to a cell with several nuclei, such as a megakaryocyte

**multi-organ failure** /ˌmʌlti ˈɔːɡən ˌfeɪljə/ noun an extremely serious condition in which several of the body's organs stop functioning at the same time. The person may survive, depending on how many organs fail and the length of time that the failure lasts. Abbr **MOF**

**multipara** /mʌlˈtɪpərə/ noun a woman who has given birth to two or more live children

**multiple** /ˈmʌltɪp(ə)l/ adjective occurring several times or in several places

**multiple birth** /ˌmʌltɪp(ə)l ˈbɜːθ/ noun a birth where more than one child is born at the same time

**multiple fracture** /ˌmʌltɪp(ə)l ˈfræktʃə/ noun a condition in which a bone is broken in several places

**multiple myeloma** /ˌmʌltɪp(ə)l ˌmaɪə ˈləʊmə/ noun a malignant tumour in bone marrow, most often affecting flat bones

**multiple organ dysfunction syndrome** /ˌmʌltɪp(ə)l ˌɔːɡən dɪsˈfʌŋkʃ(ə)n ˌsɪn drəʊm/ noun a state of continuous disturbances and abnormalities in organ systems, rather than true failure, e.g. following trauma and sepsis. It is often fatal. Abbr **MODS**

**multiple pregnancy** /ˌmʌltɪp(ə)l ˈpregnənsi/ noun a pregnancy where the mother is going to give birth to more than one child

**multiple sclerosis** /ˌmʌltɪp(ə)l sklə ˈrəʊsɪs/ noun a nervous disease which gets progressively worse, where patches of the fibres of the central nervous system lose their myelin, causing numbness in the limbs and progressive weakness and paralysis. Abbr **MS**. Also called **disseminated sclerosis**. ◊ arteriosclerosis, atherosclerosis

**multipolar neurone** /mʌltiˌpəʊlə ˈnjʊərəʊn/ noun a neurone with several processes. See illustration at NEURONE in Supplement. Compare **bipolar neurone, unipolar neurone**

**multiresistant** /ˌmʌltirɪˈzɪstənt/ adjective resistant to several types of antibiotic

**multivitamin** /ˈmʌltiˌvɪtəmɪn/ noun a preparation containing several vitamins and sometimes minerals, used as a dietary supplement ■ adjective referring to a preparation containing several vitamins, and sometimes minerals ○ multivitamin pills ○ multivitamin supplement

**mumps** /mʌmps/ noun an infectious disease of children, with fever and swellings in the salivary glands, caused by a paramyxovirus ○ He caught mumps from the children next door. Also called **infectious parotitis** (NOTE: Takes a singular or a plural verb.)

COMMENT: Mumps is a relatively mild disease in children. In adult males it can have serious complications and cause inflammation of the testicles (mumps orchitis).

**Münchausen's syndrome** /ˈmʌnt ʃaʊz(ə)nz ˌsɪndrəʊm/ noun a mental disorder in which someone tries to get hospital treatment by claiming symptoms of an illness which he or she does not have. Many people will undergo very painful procedures which they do not need. [Described by Richard Asher in 1951, and named after Baron von Münchhausen, a 16th century traveller and inveterate liar]

**Münchausen's syndrome by proxy** /ˌmʌntʃaʊz(ə)nz ˌsɪndrəʊm baɪ ˈprɒksi/ noun a mental disorder in which someone tries to get hospital treatment for someone else such as their child or an elderly relative. It is regarded as a form of child abuse, as the person may cause a child to be ill in order to receive attention.

**mural thrombus** /ˌmjʊərəl ˈθrɒmbəs/ noun a thrombus which forms on the wall of a vein or artery

**murder** /ˈmɜːdə/ noun the crime of killing someone intentionally ■ verb to kill someone intentionally

**murmur** /ˈmɜːmə/ noun a sound, usually the sound of the heart, heard through a stethoscope

**Murphy's sign** /ˈmɜːfiz saɪn/ noun a sign of an inflamed gall bladder, where the person will experience pain if the abdomen is pressed while he or she inhales [Described 1912. After John Benjamin Murphy (1857–1916), US surgeon.]

**muscae volitantes** /ˌmʌskaɪ ˌvɒli ˈtænteɪz/ plural noun pieces of cellular or blood debris present in the vitreous of the eye, common in old age but, if a sudden event, can be a symptom of retinal haemorrhage. Also called **floaters**

**muscarine** /ˈmʌskəriːn/ noun a poison found in fungi

**muscarinic** /ˌmʌskəˈrɪnɪk/ adjective referring to a neurone or receptor stimulated by acetylcholine and muscarine

**muscle** /ˈmʌs(ə)l/ noun 1. an organ in the body, which contracts to make part of the body move ○ *If you do a lot of exercises you develop strong muscles.* ○ *The muscles in his legs were still weak after he had spent two months in bed.* ○ *She had muscle cramp after going into the cold water.* See illustration at **EYE** in Supplement **2.** same as **muscle tissue**

COMMENT: There are two types of muscle: voluntary (striated) muscles, which are attached to bones and move parts of the body when made to do so by the brain, and involuntary (smooth) muscles which move essential organs such as the intestines and bladder automatically. The heart muscle also works automatically.

**muscle coat** /'mʌs(ə)l kəʊt/ *noun* one of two layers of muscle forming part of the lining of the intestine

**muscle fatigue** /'mʌs(ə)l fə,tiːg/, **muscular fatigue** /,mʌskjʊlə fə'tiːg/ *noun* tiredness in the muscles after strenuous exercise

**muscle fibre** /'mʌs(ə)l ,faɪbə/ *noun* a component fibre of muscles (NOTE: There are two types of fibre which form striated and smooth muscles.)

**muscle relaxant** /'mʌs(ə)l rɪ,læksənt/ *noun* a drug which reduces contractions in the muscles, e.g. baclofen

**muscle spasm** /'mʌs(ə)l ,spæz(ə)m/ *noun* a sudden contraction of a muscle

**muscle spindle** /'mʌs(ə)l ,spɪnd(ə)l/ *noun* one of the sensory receptors which lie along striated muscle fibres

**muscle tissue** /'mʌs(ə)l ,tɪʃuː/, **muscular tissue** /,mʌskjʊlə 'tɪʃuː/ *noun* the specialised type of tissue which forms the muscles and which can contract and expand

**muscle wasting** /'mʌs(ə)l ,weɪstɪŋ/ *noun* a condition in which the muscles lose weight and become thin

**muscular** /'mʌskjʊlə/ *adjective* referring to muscle

**muscular branch** /'mʌskjʊlə brɑːntʃ/ *noun* a branch of a nerve to a muscle carrying efferent impulses to produce contraction

**muscular defence** /,mʌskjʊlə dɪ'fens/ *noun* a rigidity of muscles associated with inflammation such as peritonitis

**muscular disorder** /'mʌskjʊlə dɪs,ɔːdə/ *noun* a disorder which affects the muscles, e.g. cramp or strain

**muscular dystrophy** /,mʌskjʊlə 'dɪstrəfi/ *noun* a type of muscle disease where some muscles become weak and are replaced with fatty tissue. ◊ **Duchenne muscular dystrophy**

**muscular fatigue** /,mʌskjʊlə fə'tiːg/ *noun* same as **muscle fatigue**

**muscularis** /,mʌskjʊ'leərɪs/ *noun* muscular layer of an internal organ

**muscular relaxant** /,mʌskjʊlə rɪ'læksənt/ *noun* a drug which relaxes the muscles

**muscular rheumatism** /,mʌskjʊlə 'ruːmə,tɪz(ə)m/ *noun* a disease giving pains in the

back or neck, usually caused by fibrositis or inflammation of the muscles

**muscular system** /'mʌskjʊlə ,sɪstəm/ *noun* the muscles in the body, usually applied only to striated muscles

**muscular tissue** /,mʌskjʊlə 'tɪʃuː/ *noun* same as **muscle tissue**

**musculo-** /mʌskjʊləʊ/ *prefix* relating to or affecting muscle

**musculocutaneous** /,mʌskjʊləʊkjuː'teɪniəs/ *adjective* referring to muscle and skin

**musculocutaneous nerve** /,mʌskjʊləʊ kjuː,teɪniəs 'nɜːv/ *noun* a nerve in the brachial plexus which supplies the muscles in the arm

**musculoskeletal** /,mʌskjʊləʊ'skelɪt(ə)l/ *adjective* referring to muscles and bone

**musculotendinous** /,mʌskjʊləʊ'tendɪnəs/ *adjective* referring to both muscular and tendinous tissue

**mutant** /'mjuːt(ə)nt/ *adjective* in which mutation has occurred ■ *noun* an organism carrying a mutant gene

**mutant gene** /,mjuːt(ə)nt 'dʒiːn/ *noun* a gene which has undergone mutation

**mutate** /mjuː'teɪt/ *verb* to undergo a genetic change ○ *Bacteria can mutate suddenly, and become increasingly able to infect.*

**mutation** /mjuː'teɪʃ(ə)n/ *noun* a change in DNA which changes the physiological effect of the DNA on the cell

COMMENT: A mutation in the gene for amyloid precursor protein (APP) in some families causes early-onset Alzheimer's disease, when unusual deposits of beta amyloid are formed and dementia occurs.

**mute** /mjuːt/ *adjective* **1.** unwilling or unable to speak **2.** felt or expressed without speech ■ *noun* somebody who is unable or unwilling to speak (NOTE: This term is sometimes considered offensive.)

**mutism** /'mjuːtɪz(ə)m/ *noun* the condition of being unable to speak. Also called **dumbness**

**my-** /maɪ/ *prefix* same as **myo-** (*used before vowels*)

**myalgia** /maɪ'ældʒə/ *noun* a muscle pain

**myalgic encephalomyelitis** /maɪ,ældʒɪk en,kefələʊmaɪə'laɪtɪs/ *noun* a long-term condition affecting the nervous system, in which someone feels tired and depressed and has pain and weakness in the muscles. Abbr **ME**. Also called **chronic fatigue syndrome, postviral fatigue syndrome**

**myasthenia** /,maɪəs'θiːniə/, **myasthenia gravis** /,maɪəs,θiːniə 'grɑːvɪs/ *noun* a general weakness and dysfunction of the muscles, caused by poor conduction at the motor end plates

**myc-** /maɪk, maɪs/ *prefix* same as **myco-** (*used before vowels*)

**mycelium** /maɪˈsiːliəm/ *noun* a mass of threads which forms the main part of a fungus

**mycetoma** /ˌmaɪsiˈtəʊmə/ *noun* same as **maduromycosis**

**myco-** /maɪkəʊ/ *prefix* referring to fungus

**Mycobacterium** /ˌmaɪkəʊbækˈtɪəriəm/ *noun* one of a group of bacteria including those which cause leprosy and tuberculosis

**mycology** /maɪˈkɒlədʒi/ *noun* the study of fungi

**Mycoplasma** /ˈmaɪkəʊˌplæzmə/ *noun* a type of microorganism, similar to a bacterium, associated with diseases such as pneumonia and urethritis

**mycosis** /maɪˈkəʊsɪs/ *noun* any disease caused by a fungus, e.g. athlete's foot

**mycosis fungoides** /maɪˌkəʊsɪs fʌŋˈɡɔɪdiz/ *noun* a form of skin cancer, with irritating nodules

**mydriasis** /maɪˈdraɪəsɪs/ *noun* an enlargement of the pupil of the eye

**mydriatic** /ˌmɪdriˈætɪk/ *noun* a drug which makes the pupil of the eye become larger

**myectomy** /maɪˈektəmi/ *noun* the surgical removal of part or all of a muscle

**myel-** /maɪəl/ *prefix* same as **myelo-** (*used before vowels*)

**myelin** /ˈmaɪəlɪn/ *noun* the substance of the cell membrane of Schwann cells that coils into a protective covering around nerve fibres called a myelin sheath

**myelinated** /ˈmaɪəlɪneɪtɪd/ *adjective* referring to nerve fibre covered by a myelin sheath

**myelination** /ˌmaɪəlɪˈneɪʃ(ə)n/ *noun* the process by which a myelin sheath forms around nerve fibres

**myelin sheath** /ˈmaɪəlɪn ʃiːθ/ *noun* a layer of myelin that insulates some nerve cells and speeds the conduction of nerve impulses. See illustration at NEURONE in Supplement

**myelitis** /ˌmaɪəˈlaɪtɪs/ *noun* 1. inflammation of the spinal cord 2. an inflammation of bone marrow

**myelo-** /maɪələʊ/ *prefix* 1. referring to bone marrow 2. referring to the spinal cord

**myeloblast** /ˈmaɪələblæst/ *noun* a precursor of a granulocyte

**myelocele** /ˈmaɪələsiːl/ *noun* same as **meningomyelocele**

**myelocyte** /ˈmaɪələsaɪt/ *noun* a cell in bone marrow which develops into a granulocyte

**myelofibrosis** /maɪələfaɪˈbrəʊsɪs/ *noun* fibrosis of bone marrow, associated with anaemia

**myelogram** /ˈmaɪələɡræm/ *noun* a record of the spinal cord taken by myelography

**myelography** /ˌmaɪəˈlɒɡrəfi/ *noun* an X-ray examination of the spinal cord and subarachnoid space after a radio-opaque substance has been injected

**myeloid** /ˈmaɪəlɔɪd/ *adjective* 1. referring to bone marrow, or produced by bone marrow 2. referring to the spinal cord

**myeloid leukaemia** /ˌmaɪəlɔɪd luːˈkiːmiə/ *noun* an acute form of leukaemia in adults

**myeloid tissue** /ˈmaɪəlɔɪd ˌtɪʃuː/ *noun* red bone marrow

**myeloma** /ˌmaɪəˈləʊmə/ *noun* a malignant tumour in bone marrow, at the ends of long bones or in the jaw

**myelomalacia** /ˌmaɪələʊməˈleɪʃə/ *noun* softening of tissue in the spinal cord

**myelomatosis** /ˌmaɪələʊməˈtəʊsɪs/ *noun* a disease where malignant tumours infiltrate the bone marrow

**myelomeningocele** /ˌmaɪələʊməˈnɪŋɡəʊsiːl/ *noun* same as **meningomyelocele**

**myelopathy** /ˌmaɪəˈlɒpəθi/ *noun* any disorder of the spinal cord or bone marrow

**myelosuppression** /ˌmaɪələʊsəˈpreʃ(ə)n/ *noun* a condition in which the bone marrow does not produce enough blood cells, often occurring after chemotherapy

**myenteron** /maɪˈentərɒn/ *noun* a layer of muscles in the small intestine, which produces peristalsis

**myiasis** /ˈmaɪəsɪs/ *noun* an infestation by larvae of flies

**mylohyoid** /ˌmaɪləˈhaɪɔɪd/ *noun, adjective* referring to the molar teeth in the lower jaw and the hyoid bone

**mylohyoid line** /ˌmaɪləˈhaɪɔɪd ˌlaɪn/ *noun* a line running along the outside of the lower jawbone, dividing the upper part of the bone which forms part of the mouth from the lower part which is part of the neck

**myo-** /maɪəʊ/ *prefix* referring to muscle

**myoblast** /ˈmaɪəblæst/ *noun* an embryonic cell which develops into muscle

**myoblastic** /ˌmaɪəʊˈblæstɪk/ *adjective* referring to myoblast

**myocardial** /ˌmaɪəʊˈkɑːdiəl/ *adjective* referring to the myocardium

**myocardial infarction** /ˌmaɪəʊˌkɑːdiəl ɪn ˈfɑːkʃən/ *noun* the death of part of the heart muscle after coronary thrombosis. Abbr **MI**

**myocarditis** /ˌmaɪəʊkɑːˈdaɪtɪs/ *noun* inflammation of the heart muscle

**myocardium** /ˌmaɪəʊˈkɑːdiəm/ *noun* the middle layer of the wall of the heart, formed of heart muscle. See illustration at HEART in Supplement

**myocele** /ˈmaɪəsiːl/ *noun* a condition in which a muscle pushes through a gap in the surrounding membrane

**myoclonic** /ˌmaɪəʊˈklɒnɪk/ *adjective* referring to myoclonus

**myoclonic epilepsy** /ˌmaɪəʊklɒnɪk ˈepɪ lepsi/ *noun* a form of epilepsy where the limbs jerk frequently

**myoclonus** /maɪˈɒklənəs/ *noun* a muscle spasm which makes a limb give an involuntary jerk

**myocyte** /ˈmaɪəʊsaɪt/ *noun* a muscle cell

**myodynia** /ˌmaɪəʊˈdɪniə/ *noun* a pain in the muscles

**myofibril** /ˌmaɪəʊˈfaɪbrɪl/ *noun* a long thread of striated muscle fibre

**myofibrosis** /ˌmaɪəʊfaɪˈbrəʊsɪs/ *noun* a condition in which muscle tissue is replaced by fibrous tissue

**myogenic** /ˌmaɪəʊˈdʒenɪk/ *adjective* referring to movement which comes from an involuntary muscle

**myoglobin** /ˌmaɪəʊˈɡləʊbɪn/ *noun* a muscle haemoglobin, which takes oxygen from blood and passes it to the muscle

**myoglobinuria** /ˌmaɪəʊˌɡləʊbɪˈnjʊəriə/ *noun* the presence of myoglobin in the urine

**myogram** /ˈmaɪəʊɡræm/ *noun* a record showing how a muscle is functioning

**myograph** /ˈmaɪəʊɡrɑːf/ *noun* an instrument which records the degree and strength of a muscle contraction

**myography** /maɪˈɒɡrəfi/ *noun* the process of recording the degree and strength of a muscle contraction with a myograph

**myokymia** /ˌmaɪəʊˈkɪmiə/ *noun* twitching of a particular muscle

**myology** /maɪˈɒlədʒi/ *noun* the study of muscles and associated structures and diseases

**myoma** /maɪˈəʊmə/ *noun* a benign tumour in a smooth muscle

**myomectomy** /ˌmaɪəʊˈmektəmi/ *noun* **1.** the surgical removal of a benign growth from a muscle, especially removal of a fibroid from the uterus **2.** same as **myectomy**

**myometritis** /ˌmaɪəʊməˈtraɪtɪs/ *noun* inflammation of the myometrium. Also called **metritis**

**myometrium** /ˌmaɪəʊˈmiːtriəm/ *noun* the muscular tissue in the uterus

**myoneural** /ˌmaɪəʊˈnjʊərəl/ *adjective* relating to or involving both the muscles and the nerves

**myoneural junction** /ˌmaɪəʊnjʊər(ə)l ˈdʒʌŋkʃ(ə)n/ *noun* same as **neuromuscular junction**

**myopathy** /maɪˈɒpəθi/ *noun* a disease of a muscle, especially one in which the muscle wastes away

**myopia** /maɪˈəʊpiə/ *noun* a condition in which someone can see clearly objects which are close, but not ones which are further away. Also called **shortsightedness**. Opposite **longsightedness**

**myopic** /maɪˈɒpɪk/ *adjective* able to see close objects clearly, but not objects which are further away. Also called **shortsighted**

**myoplasm** /ˈmaɪəʊplæz(ə)m/ *noun* same as **sarcoplasm**

**myoplasty** /ˈmaɪəʊplæsti/ *noun* a form of plastic surgery to repair a muscle

**myosarcoma** /ˌmaɪəʊsɑːˈkəʊmə/ *noun* **1.** a malignant tumour containing unstriated muscle **2.** combined myoma and sarcoma

**myosis** /maɪˈəʊsɪs/ *noun* another spelling of **miosis 1**

**myositis** /ˌmaɪəʊˈsaɪtɪs/ *noun* inflammation and degeneration of a muscle

**myotatic** /ˌmaɪəʊˈtætɪk/ *adjective* referring to the sense of touch in a muscle

**myotatic reflex** /ˌmaɪəʊtætɪk ˈriːfleks/ *noun* a reflex action in a muscle which contracts after being stretched

**myotic** /maɪˈɒtɪk/ *noun* a drug which causes the pupil of the eye to contract

**myotomy** /maɪˈɒtəmi/ *noun* a surgical operation to cut a muscle

**myotonia** /ˌmaɪəʊˈtəʊniə/ *noun* difficulty in relaxing a muscle after exercise

**myotonic** /ˌmaɪəʊˈtɒnɪk/ *adjective* referring to tone in a muscle

**myotonic dystrophy** /ˌmaɪəʊtɒnɪk ˈdɪstrəfi/ *noun* a hereditary disease with muscle stiffness leading to atrophy of the muscles of the face and neck

**myotonus** /maɪˈɒtənəs/ *noun* a muscle tone

**myringa** /mɪˈrɪŋɡə/ *noun* same as **eardrum**

**myringitis** /ˌmɪrɪnˈdʒaɪtɪs/ *noun* inflammation of the eardrum

**myringoplasty** /mɪˈrɪŋɡəʊplæsti/ *noun* the surgical repair of a perforated eardrum. Also called **tympanoplasty**

**myringotome** /mɪˈrɪŋɡəʊtəʊm/ *noun* a sharp knife used in myringotomy

**myringotomy** /ˌmɪrɪŋˈɡɒtəmi/ *noun* a surgical operation to make an opening in the eardrum to allow fluid to escape

**myx-** /mɪks/, **myxo-** /mɪksəʊ/ *prefix* referring to mucus

**myxoedema** /ˌmɪksəˈdiːmə/ *noun* a condition caused when the thyroid gland does not produce enough thyroid hormone. The person, often a middle-aged woman, becomes overweight, moves slowly and develops coarse skin. It can be treated with thyroxine. (NOTE: The US spelling is **myxedema**.)

**myxoedematous** /ˌmɪksəˈdemətəs/ *adjective* referring to myxoedema

**myxoid cyst** /ˌmɪksɔɪd ˈsɪst/ *noun* a cyst which develops at the base of a fingernail or toenail

**myxoma** /mɪkˈsəʊmə/ *noun* a benign tumour of mucous tissue, usually found in subcutaneous tissue of the limbs and neck

**myxosarcoma** /ˌmɪksəʊsɑːˈkəʊmə/ *noun* a malignant tumour of mucous tissue

**myxovirus** /ˌmɪksəʊˈvaɪrəs/ *noun* any virus which has an affinity for the mucoprotein receptors in red blood cells. One of these viruses causes influenza.

# N

**n** *symbol* nano-

**nabothian cyst** /nə,bəʊθiən 'sɪst/, **nabothian follicle** /nə,bəʊθiən 'fɒlɪk(ə)l/, **nabothian gland** /nə,bəʊθiən 'glænd/ *noun* a cyst which forms in the cervix of the uterus when the ducts in the cervical glands are blocked

**Naegele rule** /'neɪgələ ruːl/ *noun* a method used to determine when a pregnant woman is likely to go into labour, in which nine months and seven days are added to the date on which her last period started. If the woman does not have a 28-day menstrual cycle, an adjustment is made: e.g., if she has a 26-day cycle you would subtract 2 days from the Naegele's estimated due date.

**naevus** /'niːvəs/ *noun* same as **birthmark** (NOTE: The plural is **naevi**.)

**Naga sore** /'nɑːgə sɔː/ *noun* same as **tropical ulcer**

**nagging pain** /,nægɪŋ 'peɪn/ *noun* a dull, continuous throbbing pain

**NAI** *abbr* non-accidental injury

**nail** /neɪl/ *noun* a hard growth, made of keratin, which forms on the top surface at the end of each finger and toe. Also called **unguis** (NOTE: For terms referring to nail, see words beginning with **onych-, onycho-**.)

**nail avulsion** /'neɪl ə,vʌlʃən/ *noun* the act of pulling away an ingrowing toenail

**nail bed** /'neɪl bed/ *noun* the part of the finger which is just under the nail and on which the nail rests

**nail biting** /'neɪl ,baɪtɪŋ/ *noun* the obsessive chewing of the fingernails, usually a sign of stress

**nail matrix** /neɪl 'meɪtrɪks/ *noun* the internal structure of the nail, the part of the finger from which the nail grows

**naloxone** /nə'lɒksəʊn/ *noun* a drug resembling morphine, used in the diagnosis of narcotics addiction and to reverse the effects of narcotics poisoning

**named nurse** /,neɪmd 'nɜːs/ *noun* a nurse, midwife or health visitor who is responsible for communicating with a particular person and ensuring that his or her needs for care and information are met

**nandrolone** /'nændrələʊn/ *noun* an anabolic steroid which builds muscle. Its use is banned by the International Amateur Athletics Federation.

**nano-** /nænəʊ/ *prefix* one thousand millionth ($10^{-9}$). Symbol **n**

**nanometre** /'nænəʊmitə/ *noun* a unit of measurement of length equal to one thousand millionth of a metre. Symbol **nm**

**nanomole** /'nænəʊməʊl/ *noun* a unit of measurement of the amount of a substance equal to one thousand millionth of a mole. Symbol **nmol**

**nanosecond** /'nænəʊ,sekənd/ *noun* a unit of measurement of time equal to one thousand millionth of a second. Symbol **ns**

**nape** /neɪp/ *noun* the back of the neck. Also called **nucha**

**napkin** /'næpkɪn/ *noun* a soft cloth, used for wiping or absorbing

**nappy** /'næpi/ *noun* a cloth used to wrap round a baby's bottom and groin, to keep clothing clean and dry (NOTE: The US term is **diaper**.)

**nappy rash** /'næpi ræʃ/ *noun* sore red skin on a baby's buttocks and groin, caused by long contact with ammonia in a wet nappy (NOTE: The US term is **diaper rash**.)

**naproxen** /næ'prɒksen/ *noun* a drug which reduces inflammation and pain, used in the treatment of arthritis

**narcissism** /'nɑːsɪsɪz(ə)m/ *noun* in psychiatry, a personality disorder in which someone has a very confident opinion about their own appearance and abilities, and a great need to be admired by other people. It sometimes involves sexual interest in their own body.

**narco-** /nɑːkəʊ/ *prefix* referring to sleep or stupor

**narcoanalysis** /,nɑːkəʊə'næləsɪs/ *noun* the use of narcotics to induce a comatose state in someone about to undergo psychoanalysis which may be emotionally disturbing

**narcolepsy** /'nɑːkəlepsi/ *noun* a condition in which someone has an uncontrollable tendency to fall asleep at any time

**narcoleptic** /ˌnɑːkəˈleptɪk/ *adjective* **1.** causing narcolepsy **2.** having narcolepsy ■ *noun* **1.** a substance which causes narcolepsy **2.** someone who has narcolepsy

**narcosis** /nɑːˈkəʊsɪs/ *noun* a state of lowered consciousness induced by a drug

**narcotic** /nɑːˈkɒtɪk/ *noun* a pain-relieving drug which makes someone sleep or become unconscious ○ *The doctor put her to sleep with a powerful narcotic.* ■ *adjective* causing sleep or unconsciousness ○ *the narcotic side-effects of an antihistamine*

COMMENT: Although narcotics are used medicinally as painkillers, they are highly addictive. The main narcotics are barbiturates, cocaine and opium, and drugs derived from opium, such as morphine, codeine and heroin. Addictive narcotics are widely used for the relief of pain in terminally ill patients.

**nares** /ˈneəriːz/ *plural noun* the nostrils (NOTE: The singular is **naris**.)

**narrow** /ˈnærəʊ/ *adjective* not wide ○ *The blood vessel is a narrow channel which takes blood to the tissues.* ○ *The surgeon inserted a narrow tube into the vein.* ■ *verb* to make something narrow, or become narrow ○ *The bronchial tubes are narrowed causing asthma.*

**nasal** /ˈneɪz(ə)l/ *adjective* referring to the nose

**nasal apertures** /ˌneɪz(ə)l ˈæpətʃəs/ *plural noun* the two openings shaped like funnels leading from the nasal cavity to the pharynx. ◊ **choana**

**nasal bone** /ˈneɪz(ə)l bəʊn/ *noun* one of two small bones which form the bridge at the top of the nose

**nasal cartilage** /ˈneɪz(ə)l ˌkɑːtəlɪdʒ/ *noun* one of two cartilages in the nose. The upper is attached to the nasal bone and the front of the maxilla. The lower is thinner and curls round each nostril to the septum.

**nasal cavity** /ˌneɪz(ə)l ˈkævɪti/ *noun* the cavity behind the nose between the cribriform plates above and the hard palate below, divided in two by the nasal septum and leading to the nasopharynx

**nasal conchae** /ˌneɪz(ə)l ˈkɒŋkiː/ *plural noun* the three ridges of bone, called the superior, middle and inferior conchae, which project into the nasal cavity from the side walls. Also called **turbinate bones**

**nasal congestion** /ˌneɪz(ə)l kənˈdʒestʃ(ə)n/ *noun* the blocking of the nose by inflammation as a response to a cold or other infection

**nasal drops** /ˈneɪz(ə)l drɒps/ *plural noun* drops of liquid inserted into the nose

**nasal septum** /ˌneɪz(ə)l ˈseptəm/ *noun* a wall of cartilage between the two nostrils and the two parts of the nasal cavity

**nasal spray** /ˈneɪz(ə)l spreɪ/ *noun* a spray of liquid into the nose

**nascent** /ˈnæs(ə)nt, ˈneɪs(ə)nt/ *adjective* **1.** in the process of coming into existence and starting to develop **2.** referring to a substance, especially hydrogen, in the process of being created. At this stage it is often in a highly active form.

**Naseptin** /næˈseptɪn/ a trade name for a mixture containing chlorhexidine and neomycin, used to treat nasal infection by organisms such as staphylococci

**nasion** /ˈneɪzɪən/ *noun* the place at which the bridge of the nose meets the forehead

**naso-** /neɪzəʊ/ *prefix* referring to the nose

**nasogastric** /ˌneɪzəʊˈɡæstrɪk/ *adjective* referring to the nose and stomach

**nasogastrically** /ˌneɪzəʊˈɡæstrɪkli/ *adverb* referring to a method of feeding someone via a tube passed through the nose into the stomach

'…all patients requiring nutrition are fed enterally, whether nasogastrically or directly into the small intestine' [*British Journal of Nursing*]

**nasogastric tube** /ˌneɪzəʊˌɡæstrɪk ˈtjuːb/ *noun* a tube passed through the nose into the stomach

**nasolacrimal** /ˌneɪzəʊˈlækrɪm(ə)l/ *adjective* referring to the nose and the tear glands

**nasolacrimal duct** /ˌneɪzəʊˌlækrɪm(ə)l ˈdʌkt/ *noun* a duct which drains tears from the lacrimal sac into the nose

**nasopharyngeal** /ˌneɪzəʊˌfærɪnˈdʒiːəl/ *adjective* referring to the nasopharynx

**nasopharyngitis** /ˌneɪzəʊˌfærɪnˈdʒaɪtɪs/ *noun* inflammation of the mucous membrane of the nasal part of the pharynx

**nasopharynx** /ˌneɪzəʊˈfærɪŋks/ *noun* the top part of the pharynx which connects with the nose

**nasosinusitis** /ˌneɪzəʊˌsaɪnəˈsaɪtɪs/ *noun* a condition in which the nose and sinuses swell up

**nasty** /ˈnɑːsti/ *adjective* unpleasant ○ *This medicine has a nasty taste.* ○ *This new drug has some nasty side-effects.* (NOTE: **nastier – nastiest**)

**nates** /ˈneɪtiːz/ *noun* same as **buttock**

**National Boards** /ˌnæʃ(ə)nəl ˈbɔːrdz/ *plural noun* the National Boards for Nursing, Midwifery, and Health Visiting, which were formerly responsible for the education of professionals in these fields in England, Wales, Scotland and Northern Ireland

**National Council for Vocational Qualifications** /ˌnæʃ(ə)nəl ˌkaʊns(ə)l fə vəʊˌkeɪʃ(ə)nəl ˌkwɒlɪfɪˈkeɪʃ(ə)nz/ *noun* full form of **NCVQ**

**National Health Service** /ˌnæʃ(ə)nəl ˈhelθ ˌsɜːvɪs/ *noun* a government service in the UK which provides medical services free of charge at the point of delivery, or at reduced cost, to the whole population. The service is paid for out of tax revenue. Abbr **NHS** □ **on the NHS** paid for by the NHS ○ *He had his operation on* *the NHS.* ○ *She went to see a specialist on the NHS.* Compare **privately**

'…figures reveal that 5% more employees in the professional and technical category were working in the NHS compared with three years before' [*Nursing Times*]

**National Institute for Clinical Excellence** /ˌnæʃ(ə)n(ə)l ˌɪnstɪtjuːt fə ˌklɪnɪk(ə)l 'eksələns/ *noun* an organisation in the UK which produces recommendations for treatments based on clinical evidence and cost-effectiveness. Abbr **NICE**

**National Insurance** /ˌnæʃ(ə)nəl ɪn 'ʃʊərəns/ *noun* a weekly payment from a person's wages, with a supplement from the employer, which pays for state assistance and medical treatment, in the UK

**natriuretic** /ˌneɪtrijʊ'retɪk/ *noun* something which helps sodium to be excreted in the urine

**natural** /'nætʃ(ə)rəl/ *adjective* **1.** usual or expected in particular conditions ○ *It's natural for people to be anxious before an operation.* **2.** referring to something which comes from nature and is not made by humans ○ *natural products* **3.** relaxed and not consciously changed ○ *His behaviour seemed quite natural.*

**natural childbirth** /ˌnætʃ(ə)rəl 'tʃaɪldbɜːθ/ *noun* childbirth where the mother is not given any pain-killing drugs or anaesthetic but is encouraged to give birth after having prepared herself through relaxation and breathing exercises and a new psychological outlook

**natural immunity** /ˌnætʃ(ə)rəl ɪ'mjuːnɪti/ *noun* the immunity from disease which a newborn baby has from birth and which is inherited or acquired in the uterus or from the mother's milk

**natural killer cell** /ˌnætʃ(ə)rəl 'kɪlə sel/ *noun* a white blood cell which can recognise microorganisms and tumour cells as foreign without any previous exposure to them, and destroy them

**natural mother** /ˌnætʃ(ə)rəl 'mʌðə/, **natural parent** /ˌnætʃ(ə)rəl 'peərənt/ *noun* same as **birth mother, birth parent**

**nature** /'neɪtʃə/ *noun* **1.** the essential quality of something **2.** kind or sort **3.** the genetic make-up which affects personality, behaviour or risk of disease. ◊ **nurture 4.** plants and animals

**nature nurture debate** /ˌneɪtʃə 'nɜːtʃə dɪ ˌbeɪt/ *noun* the arguments put forward about whether human beings behave in the way they do because of their genetic make-up and instincts or because of the way they are educated and the influences they are exposed to when they are young

**naturopathy** /ˌneɪtʃə'rɒpəθi/ *noun* a method of treatment of diseases and disorders which does not use medical or surgical means, but

natural forces such as light, heat, massage, eating natural foods and using herbal remedies

**nausea** /'nɔːziə/ *noun* a feeling that you want to vomit ○ *She suffered from nausea in the morning.* ○ *He felt slight nausea after getting onto the boat.*

COMMENT: Nausea can be caused by eating habits, such as eating too much rich food or drinking too much alcohol. It can also be caused by sensations such as unpleasant smells or motion sickness. Other causes include stomach disorders, such as gastritis, ulcers and liver infections. Nausea is commonly experienced by women in the early stages of pregnancy, and is called morning sickness.

**nauseated** /'nɔːzieɪtɪd/ *adjective* feeling as if you are about to vomit ○ *The casualty may feel nauseated.* (NOTE: The US term is **nauseous**.)

**nauseous** /'nɔːziəs/ *adjective* having the feeling in the stomach that precedes the urge to vomit

**navel** /'neɪv(ə)l/ *noun* the scar with a depression in the middle of the abdomen where the umbilical cord was detached after birth. Also called **umbilicus** (NOTE: For other terms referring to the navel, see words beginning with **omphal-, omphalo-**.)

**navicular** /nə'vɪkjʊlə/ *adjective* relating to a navicular bone ■ *noun* same as **navicular bone**

**navicular bone** /nə'vɪkjʊlə bəʊn/ *noun* one of the tarsal bones in the foot. See illustration at FOOT in Supplement

**NCVQ** *noun* a government body in the UK responsible for setting standards of qualification for specific jobs. Full form **National Council for Vocational Qualifications**

**NDU** *abbr* Nursing Development Unit

**nearsighted** /nɪə'saɪtɪd/ *adjective* same as **myopic**

**nearsightedness** /ˌnɪə'saɪtɪdnəs/ *noun* same as **myopia**

**nebula** /'nebjʊlə/ *noun* **1.** a slightly cloudy spot on the cornea **2.** a spray of medicinal solution, applied to the nose or throat using a nebuliser

**nebuliser** /'nebjʊlaɪzə/, **nebulizer** *noun* same as **atomiser**

**Necator** /ne'keɪtə/ *noun* a genus of hookworm which infests the small intestine

**necatoriasis** /neˌkeɪtə'raɪəsɪs/ *noun* infestation of the small intestine by the parasite Necator

**neck** /nek/ *noun* **1.** the part of the body which joins the head to the body ○ *He is suffering from pains in the neck.* ○ *The front of the neck is swollen with goitre.* ○ *The jugular veins run down the side of the neck.* **2.** a narrow part of a bone or organ □ **neck of the femur, femoral neck** the narrow part between the head and the diaphysis of the femur □ **neck of a tooth** point where a tooth narrows slightly, between the crown and the root

# neck collar

COMMENT: The neck is formed of the seven cervical vertebrae, and is held vertical by strong muscles. Many organs pass through the neck, including the oesophagus, the larynx and the arteries and veins which connect the brain to the bloodstream. The front of the neck is usually referred to as the throat.

**neck collar** /'nek ˌkɒlə/ *noun* a strong high collar to support the head of a person with neck injuries or a condition such as cervical spondylosis

**necro-** /nekrəʊ/ *prefix* referring to death

**necrobiosis** /ˌnekrəʊbaɪ'əʊsɪs/ *noun* **1.** the death of cells surrounded by living tissue **2.** the gradual localised death of a part or tissue

**necrology** /ne'krɒlədʒi/ *noun* the scientific study of mortality statistics

**necrophilia** /ˌnekrəʊ'fɪliə/, **necrophilism** /ne'krɒfɪlɪz(ə)m/ *noun* **1.** unusual pleasure in corpses **2.** sexual attraction to dead bodies

**necropsy** /'nekrɒpsi/ *noun* same as **post mortem**

**necrosed** /'nekrəʊsd/ *adjective* referring to dead tissue or bone

**necrosis** /ne'krəʊsɪs/ *noun* the death of a part of the body such as a bone, tissue or an organ as a result of disease or injury ○ *Gangrene is a form of necrosis.*

**necrospermia** /ˌnekrəʊ'spɜːmiə/ *noun* a condition in which dead sperm exist in the semen

**necrotic** /ne'krɒtɪk/ *adjective* referring to, or affected with, necrosis ○ *necrotic tissue*

**necrotising enterocolitis** /ˌnekrətaɪzɪŋ ˌentərəʊkə'laɪtɪs/ *noun* a disorder in which patches of dead tissue are found in the small or large intestine as a result of severe bacterial infection. It occurs in babies, especially premature ones.

**necrotising fasciitis** /ˌnekrətaɪzɪŋ ˌfæʃi'aɪtɪs/ *noun* a severe bacterial infection that causes cell tissue to decay rapidly (NOTE: It is sometimes referred to in the media as the 'flesh-eating bug'.)

**necrotomy** /ne'krɒtəmi/ *noun* the dissection of a dead body (NOTE: The plural is **necrotomies.**)

**needle** /'niːd(ə)l/ *noun* **1.** a thin metal instrument with a sharp point at one end and a hole at the other for attaching a thread, used for sewing up surgical incisions **2.** the hollow pointed end of a hypodermic syringe, or the syringe itself

**needle myopathy** /ˌniːd(ə)l maɪ'ɒpəθi/ *noun* destruction of muscle tissue caused by using a large needle for intramuscular injections

**needlestick** /'niːd(ə)lstɪk/ *noun* an accidental pricking of your own skin by a needle, as by a nurse picking up a used syringe

**needlestick injury** /'niːd(ə)lstɪk ˌɪndʒəri/ *noun* the real or potential harm resulting from a prick with a needle previously used to take blood or give an injection. The main concern is the risk of HIV or hepatitis B infection.

**needling** /'niːdlɪŋ/ *noun* the puncture of a cataract with a needle

**needs assessment** /'niːdz əˌsesmənt/ *noun* the investigation of what a particular group of people need in terms of health and social care, so that services can be matched to their needs

**needs deprivation** /'niːdz deprɪˌveɪʃ(ə)n/ *noun* a state in which someone does not have the opportunity or capacity to fulfil his or her basic needs

**negative** /'negətɪv/ *adjective* **1.** meaning or showing 'no' □ **the answer is in the negative** the answer is 'no' **2.** indicating that something being tested for is not present ○ *The test results were negative.* Opposite **positive**

**negative feedback** /ˌnegətɪv 'fiːdbæk/ *noun* a situation in which the result of a process represses the process which caused it

**negativism** /'negətɪvɪz(ə)m/ *noun* the attitude of a person who opposes advice or instructions

COMMENT: There are two types of negativism: active, where someone does the opposite of what a doctor tells him or her, and passive, where someone does not do what he or she has been asked to do.

**negligence** /'neglɪdʒəns/ *noun* the act of causing injury or harm to another person or to property as the result of doing something wrongly or failing to provide a proper level of care

**Negri body** /'neɪgri ˌbɒdi/ *noun* a round or oval inclusion in the cytoplasm of nerve cells of people or animals who have rabies [Described 1903. After Adelchi Negri (1876–1912), Professor of Bacteriology at Pavia, Italy.]

**Neil Robertson stretcher** /ˌniːl 'rɒbətsən ˌstretʃə/ *noun* a stretcher to which a person can be strapped and moved about in an upright position

**Neisseria** /naɪ'sɪəriə/ *noun* a genus of bacteria which includes gonococcus, which causes gonorrhoea, and meningococcus, which causes meningitis

**nematode** /'nemətəʊd/ *noun* a type of parasitic roundworm, e.g. a hookworm, pinworm or roundworm

**neo-** /niːəʊ/ *prefix* new

**neoadjuvant chemotherapy** /ˌniːəʊ ˌædʒʊvənt ˌkiːməʊ'θerəpi/ *noun* chemotherapy given to people with tumours instead of immediate surgery or radiotherapy, in the hope of reducing the need for these later

**neocerebellum** /ˌniːəʊserə'beləm/ *noun* the middle part of the cerebellum (NOTE: The plural is **neocerebellums** or **neocerebella.**)

**neomycin** /ˌniːəʊ'maɪsɪn/ *noun* a drug used externally to treat bacterial infections

**neonatal** /ˌniːəʊ'neɪt(ə)l/ *adjective* referring to the first few weeks after birth

'…one of the most common routes of neonatal poisoning is percutaneous absorption following topical administration' [*Southern Medical Journal*]

**neonatal death rate** /ˌniːəʊneɪt(ə)l 'deθ ˌreɪt/ *noun* the number of babies who die soon after birth, shown per thousand babies born

**neonatal maceration** /ˌniːəʊneɪt(ə)l ˌmæsə'reɪʃ(ə)n/ *noun* softening or rotting of fetal tissue after the fetus has died in the uterus and has remained in the amniotic fluid

**neonatal screening** /ˌniːəʊˌneɪt(ə)l 'skriːnɪŋ/ *noun* a set of tests performed on babies soon after birth so that any problems can be treated immediately (NOTE: Tests for certain diseases such as hypothyroidism and phenylketonuria are a legal duty.)

**neonate** /'niːəʊneɪt/ *noun* a baby which is less than four weeks old

**neonatologist** /ˌniːənə'tɒlədʒɪst/ *noun* a specialist who looks after babies during the first few weeks of life, or premature babies and babies with some congenital disorders

**neonatology** /ˌniːəʊnə'tɒlədʒi/ *noun* the branch of medicine dealing with babies in the first few weeks of life

**neonatorum** /ˌniːəʊneɪ'tɔːrəm/ ♦ **asphyxia neonatorum**

**neoplasia** /ˌniːəʊ'pleɪziə/ *noun* the formation of tumours

**neoplasm** /'niːəʊplæz(ə)m/ *noun* any new and morbid formation of tissue

'…testicular cancer comprises only 1% of all malignant neoplasms in the male, but it is one of the most frequently occurring types of tumours in late adolescence' [*Journal of American College Health*]

**neoplastic** /ˌniːəʊ'plæstɪk/ *adjective* referring to neoplasms, neoplasty or neoplasia

**neoplasty** *noun* the surgical repair or replacement of damaged tissue

**neostigmine** /ˌniːəʊ'stɪgmiːn/ *noun* a white crystalline compound used in the treatment of muscle fatigue myasthenia and to reverse the effects of muscle relaxant drugs

**nephr-** /nefr/ *prefix* kidney

**nephralgia** /ne'frældʒə/ *noun* pain in the kidney

**nephralgic** /ne'frældʒɪk/ *adjective* relating to pain in the kidney

**nephrectomy** /ne'frektɒmi/ *noun* a surgical operation to remove the whole kidney (NOTE: The plural is **nephrectomies**.)

**nephric** /'nefrɪk/, **nephritic** /ne'frɪtɪk/ *adjective* referring to the kidneys

**nephritis** /ne'fraɪtɪs/ *noun* inflammation of the kidney

COMMENT: Acute nephritis can be caused by a streptococcal infection. Symptoms can include headaches, swollen ankles, and fever.

**nephroblastoma** /ˌnefrəʊblæ'stəʊmə/ *noun* a malignant tumour in the kidneys in young children, usually under the age of 10, leading to swelling of the abdomen. It is treated by removal of the affected kidney. Also called **Wilms' tumour** (NOTE: The plural is **nephroblastomas** or **nephrobrastomata**.)

**nephrocalcinosis** /ˌnefrəʊˌkælsɪ'nəʊsɪs/ *noun* a condition in which calcium deposits are found in the kidney

**nephrocapsulectomy** /ˌnefrəʊˌkæpsjʊ'lektəmi/ *noun* a surgical operation to remove the capsule round a kidney (NOTE: The plural is **nephrocapsulectomies**.)

**nephrogram** /'nefrəgræm/ *noun* a radiographic examination of the kidney

**nephrolith** /'nefrəlɪθ/ *noun* a stone in the kidney

**nephrolithiasis** /ˌnefrəʊlɪ'θaɪəsɪs/ *noun* a condition in which stones form in the kidney

**nephrolithotomy** /ˌnefrəʊlɪ'θɒtəmi/ *noun* a surgical operation to remove a stone in the kidney (NOTE: The plural is **nephrolithotomies**.)

**nephrologist** /ne'frɒlədʒɪst/ *noun* a doctor who specialises in the study of the kidney and its diseases

**nephrology** /ne'frɒlədʒi/ *noun* the study of the kidney and its diseases

**nephroma** /ne'frəʊmə/ *noun* a tumour in the kidney, or a tumour derived from renal substances (NOTE: The plural is **nephromas** or **nephromata**.)

**nephron** /'nefrɒn/ *noun* a tiny structure in the kidney through which fluid is filtered

COMMENT: A nephron is formed of a series of tubules, the loop of Henle, Bowman's capsule and a glomerulus. Blood enters the nephron from the renal artery, and waste materials are filtered out by the Bowman's capsule. Some substances return to the bloodstream by reabsorption in the tubules. Urine is collected in the ducts leading from the tubules to the ureters.

**nephropathy** /ne'frɒpəθi/ *noun* a disease or medical disorder of the kidney (NOTE: The plural is **nephropathies**.)

**nephropexy** /'nefrəʊpeksi/ *noun* a surgical operation to attach a mobile kidney (NOTE: The plural is **nephropexies**.)

**nephroptosis** /ˌnefrɒp'təʊsɪs/ *noun* a condition in which a kidney is mobile. Also called **floating kidney**

**nephrosclerosis** /ˌnefrəʊsklə'rəʊsɪs/ *noun* a kidney disease due to vascular change

**nephroscope** /'nefrəskəʊp/ *noun* a type of endoscope used to examine the kidneys

**nephrosis** /ne'frəʊsɪs/ *noun* degeneration of the tissue of a kidney

**nephrostomy** /ne'frɒstəmi/ *noun* a surgical operation to make a permanent opening into the pelvis of the kidney from the surface (NOTE: The plural is **nephrostomies**.)

**nephrotic** /ne'frɒtɪk/ *adjective* relating to or caused by nephrosis

**nephrotic syndrome** /neˌfrɒtɪk 'sɪn drəʊm/ *noun* increasing oedema, albuminuria and raised blood pressure resulting from nephrosis

**nephrotomy** /ne'frɒtəmi/ *noun* a surgical operation to cut into a kidney (NOTE: The plural is **nephrotomies**.)

**nephrotoxic** /ˌnefrəʊ'tɒksɪk/ *adjective* poisonous or damaging to kidney cells

**nephroureterectomy** /ˌnefrəʊˌjʊərɪtə 'rektəmi/ *noun* a surgical operation to remove all or part of a kidney and the ureter attached to it. Also called **ureteronephrectomy** (NOTE: The plural is **nephroureterectomies**.)

**nerve** /nɜːv/ *noun* **1.** a bundle of fibres that can transmit electrochemical impulses and that forms part of the network that connects the brain and spinal cord to the body's organs **2.** the sensitive tissue in the root of a tooth (NOTE: For other terms referring to nerves, see words beginning with **neur-, neuro-**.)

COMMENT: Nerves are the fibres along which impulses are carried. Motor nerves or efferent nerves take messages between the central nervous system and muscles, making the muscles move. Sensory nerves or afferent nerves transmit impulses such as sight or pain from the sense organs to the brain.

**nerve block** /'nɜːv blɒk/ *noun* the act of stopping the function of a nerve by injecting an anaesthetic

**nerve centre** /'nɜːv ˌsentə/ *noun* the point at which nerves come together

**nerve ending** /nɜːv 'endɪŋ/ *noun* same as **sensory receptor**

**nerve entrapment syndrome** /ˌnɜːv ɪn 'træpmənt ˌsɪndrəʊm/ *noun* pain caused by pressure on a nerve, especially where nerves occur in narrow passages such as the wrist (NOTE: The most common nerve entrapment syndrome in the body is carpal tunnel syndrome.)

**nerve fibre** /'nɜːv ˌfaɪbə/ *noun* a thin structure leading from a nerve cell and carrying nerve impulses, e.g. an axon

**nerve gas** /'nɜːv ɡæs/ *noun* a gas which attacks the nervous system

**nerve impulse** /nɜːv 'ɪmpʌls/ *noun* an electrochemical impulse which is transmitted by nerve cells

**nerve regeneration** /ˌnɜːv rɪdʒenə'reɪʃ(ə)n/ *noun* the growth of new nerve tissue after damage has occurred

**nerve root** /'nɜːv ruːt/ *noun* the first part of a nerve as it leaves or joins the spinal column (NOTE: The dorsal nerve root is the entry for a sensory nerve, and the ventral nerve root is the exit for a motor nerve.)

**nerve tissue** /'nɜːv ˌtɪʃuː/ *noun* tissue which forms nerves, and which is able to transmit nerve impulses

**nervosa** /nə'vəʊsə/ ♦ **anorexia nervosa**

**nervous** /'nɜːvəs/ *adjective* **1.** referring to nerves **2.** very easily worried ○ *Don't be nervous – the operation is a very simple one.*

**nervous breakdown** /ˌnɜːvəs 'breɪkdaʊn/ *noun* any sudden mental illness (*informal*)

**nervous complaint** /ˌnɜːvəs kəm'pleɪnt/, **nervous disorder** *noun* an emotional or mental illness (*informal*)

**nervousness** /'nɜːvəsnəs/ *noun* the state of being nervous

**nervous system** /'nɜːvəs ˌsɪstəm/ *noun* the nervous tissues of the body, including the peripheral nerves, spinal cord, ganglia and nerve centres

**nervy** /'nɜːvi/ *adjective* worried and nervous (*informal*)

**nether parts** /'neðə pɑːts/, **nether regions** /ˌneðə 'riːdʒ(ə)ns/ *plural noun* the lower part of the body, especially the buttocks or genital area (*informal*)

**nettle rash** /'net(ə)l ræʃ/ *noun* same as **urticaria**

**network** /'netwɜːk/ *noun* an interconnecting system of lines and spaces, like a net ○ *a network of fine blood vessels*

**Neuman's model** /'nɔɪmənz ˌmɒd(ə)l/ *noun* a modern model for nursing in which prevention is the primary nursing aim (NOTE: Prevention focuses on keeping both the things which cause stress and the patient's response to stress from having a damaging effect on the body.)

**neur-** /njʊər/ *prefix* same as **neuro-** (*used before vowels*)

**neural** /'njʊərəl/ *adjective* referring to a nerve or the nervous system

**neural arch** /ˌnjʊərəl 'ɑːtʃ/ *noun* a curved part of a vertebra, which forms the space through which the spinal cord passes

**neural crest** /'njʊərəl krest/ *noun* the ridge of cells in an embryo which forms nerve cells of the sensory and autonomic ganglia

**neuralgia** /njʊ'rældʒə/ *noun* a spasm of pain which runs along a nerve

**neural groove** /'njʊərəl gruːv/ *noun* a groove on the back of an embryo formed as the neural plate closes to form the neural tube

**neural plate** /'njʊərəl pleɪt/ *noun* a thickening of an embryonic disc which folds over to form the neural tube

**neural tube** /'njʊərəl tjuːb/ *noun* a tube lined with ectodermal cells running the length of an embryo, which develops into the brain and spinal cord

**neural tube defect** /ˌnjʊərəl 'tjuːb dɪ ˌfekt/ *noun* a congenital anomaly which occurs when the edges of the neural tube do not close up properly while the fetus develops in the uterus, e.g. spina bifida (NOTE: There is less risk of a neural tube defect if the mother takes folic acid during her pregnancy.)

**neurapraxia** /ˌnjʊərəˈpræksiə/ *noun* a lesion of a nerve which leads to paralysis for a very short time, giving a tingling feeling and loss of function

**neurasthenia** /ˌnjʊərəsˈθiːniə/ *noun* a type of neurosis in which a person is mentally and physically irritable and extremely fatigued

**neurasthenic** /ˌnjʊərəsˈθenɪk/ *noun* a person affected by neurasthenia

**neurectasis** /njʊˈrektəsɪs/ *noun* a surgical operation to stretch a peripheral nerve (NOTE: The plural is **neurectases**.)

**neurectomy** /njʊˈrektəmi/ *noun* a surgical operation to remove all or part of a nerve (NOTE: The plural is **neurectomies**.)

**neurilemma** /ˌnjʊərɪˈlemə/ *noun* the outer sheath, formed of Schwann cells, which covers the myelin sheath around a nerve fibre. Also called **neurolemma**. See illustration at NEURONE in Supplement

**neurilemmoma** /ˌnjʊərileˈməʊmə/, **neurinoma** /njʊəriˈnəʊmə/ *noun* a benign tumour of a nerve, formed from the neurilemma (NOTE: The plurals are **neurilemmomas** or **neurolemmomata** and **neurinomas** or **neurinomata**.)

**neuritis** /njʊˈraɪtɪs/ *noun* inflammation of a nerve, giving a constant pain

**neuro-** /njʊərəʊ/ *prefix* nerve or nervous system

**neuroanatomy** /ˌnjʊərəʊəˈnætəmi/ *noun* the scientific study of the structure of the nervous system

**neuroblast** /ˈnjʊərəʊblæst/ *noun* a cell in the embryonic spinal cord which forms a nerve cell

**neuroblastoma** /ˌnjʊərəʊblæˈstəʊmə/ *noun* a malignant tumour formed from the neural crest, found mainly in young children (NOTE: The plural is **neuroblastomas** or **neuroblastomata**.)

**neurocranium** /ˌnjʊərəʊˈkreɪniəm/ *noun* a part of the skull which encloses and protects the brain (NOTE: The plural is **neurocraniums** or **neurocrania**.)

**neurodegenerative** /ˌnjʊərəʊdɪˈdʒenərətɪv/ *adjective* referring to a disorder such as Alzheimer's disease or Parkinson's disease that causes damage to the nerves

**neurodermatitis** /ˌnjʊərəʊdɜːməˈtaɪtɪs/ *noun* inflammation of the skin caused by psychological factors

**neurodermatosis** /ˌnjʊərəʊdɜːməˈtəʊsɪs/ *noun* a nervous condition involving the skin

**neuroendocrine system** /ˌnjʊərəʊˈendəkrɪn ˌsɪstəm/ *noun* a system in which the central nervous system and hormonal systems interact to control the function of organs and tissues

**neuroepithelial** /ˌnjʊərəʊepɪˈθiːliəl/ *adjective* referring to the neuroepithelium

**neuroepithelioma** /ˌnjʊərəʊepɪθiːliˈəʊmə/ *noun* a malignant tumour in the retina (NOTE: The plural is **neuroepitheliomas** or **neuroepitheliomata**.)

**neuroepithelium** /ˌnjʊərəʊepɪˈθiːliəm/ *noun* the layer of epithelial cells forming part of the lining of the mucous membrane of the nose or the labyrinth of the middle ear

**neurofibril** /ˌnjʊərəʊˈfaɪbrɪl/ *noun* a fine thread in the cytoplasm of a neurone

**neurofibrilla** /ˌnjʊərəʊˈfɪbrɪlə/ *noun* same as **neurofibril**. see illustration at NEURONE in Supplement (NOTE: The plural is **neurofibrillae**.)

**neurofibroma** /ˌnjʊərəʊfaɪˈbrəʊmə/ *noun* a benign tumour of a nerve, formed from the neurilemma (NOTE: The plural is **neurofibromas** or **neurofibromata**.)

**neurofibromatosis** /ˌnjʊərəʊˌfaɪbrəʊməˈtəʊsɪs/ *noun* a hereditary condition in which a person has neurofibromata on the nerve trunks, limb plexuses or spinal roots, and pale brown spots appear on the skin. Abbr **NF**. Also called **molluscum fibrosum, von Recklinghausen's disease**

**neurogenesis** /ˌnjʊərəʊˈdʒenəsɪs/ *noun* the development and growth of nerves and nervous tissue

**neurogenic** /ˌnjʊərəʊˈdʒenɪk/ *adjective* **1.** coming from the nervous system **2.** referring to neurogenesis

**neurogenic bladder** /ˌnjʊərəʊdʒenɪk ˈblædə/ *noun* a disturbance of the bladder function caused by lesions in the nerve supply to the bladder

**neurogenic shock** /ˌnjʊərəʊˌdʒenɪk ˈʃɒk/ *noun* a state of shock caused by bad news or an unpleasant surprise

**neuroglandular junction** /ˌnjʊərəʊˌglændjʊlə ˈdʒʌŋkʃən/ *noun* the point where a nerve joins the gland which it controls

**neuroglia** /njʊˈrɒgliə/ *noun* same as **glia**

**neurohormone** /ˌnjʊərəʊˈhɔːməʊn/ *noun* a hormone produced in some nerve cells and secreted from the nerve endings

**neurohypophysis** /ˌnjʊərəʊhaɪˈpɒfəsɪs/ *noun* the lobe at the back of the pituitary gland, which secretes oxytocin and vasopressin (NOTE: The plural is **neurohypophyses**.)

**neurolemma** /ˌnjʊərəʊˈlemə/ *noun* same as **neurilemma**

**neuroleptic** /ˌnjʊərəʊˈleptɪk/ *noun* an antipsychotic drug which calms a person and stops him or her from worrying, e.g. chlorpromazine hydrochloride

**neurological** /ˌnjʊərəˈlɒdʒɪk(ə)l/ *adjective* referring to neurology

**neurological assessment** /ˌnjʊərəlɒdʒɪk(ə)l əˈsesmənt/ *noun* an evaluation of the health of a person with a disorder of the nervous system, using interviews, a physical examination, and specific diagnostic tests, sometimes with the help of a family member or close friend

**neurologist** /njʊˈrɒlədʒɪst/ *noun* a doctor who specialises in the study of the nervous system and the treatment of its diseases

**neurology** /njʊˈrɒlədʒi/ *noun* the scientific study of the nervous system and its diseases

**neuroma** /njʊˈrəʊmə/ *noun* a benign tumour formed of nerve cells and nerve fibres (NOTE: The plural is **neuromas** or **neuromata**.)

**neuromuscular** /ˌnjʊərəʊˈmʌskjʊlə/ *adjective* referring to both nerves and muscles

**neuromuscular junction** /ˌnjʊərəʊmʌskjʊlə ˈdʒʌŋkʃən/ *noun* the point where a motor nerve joins muscle fibre. Also called **myoneural junction**

**neuromyelitis optica** /ˌnjʊərəʊmaɪəlaɪtɪs ˈɒptɪkə/ *noun* a condition, similar to multiple sclerosis, in which a person has acute myelitis and the optic nerve is also affected. Also called **Devic's disease**

**neuron** /ˈnjʊərəʊn/, **neurone** /ˈnjʊərɒn/ *noun* a cell in the nervous system which transmits nerve impulses. Also called **nerve cell**

**neuropathic bladder** /ˌnjʊərəʊpæθik ˈblædə/ *noun* a condition in which the bladder does not function properly because its nerve supply is damaged, e.g. due to an injury to the spinal cord

**neuropathology** /ˌnjʊərəʊpəˈθɒlədʒi/ *noun* the study of diseases of the nervous system

**neuropathy** /njʊəˈrɒpəθi/ *noun* a disease involving destruction of the tissues of the nervous system (NOTE: The plural is **neuropathies**.)

**neurophysiology** /ˌnjʊərəʊfɪziˈɒlədʒi/ *noun* the study of the physiology of nerves

**neuroplasty** /ˈnjʊərəʊplæsti/ *noun* surgery to repair damaged nerves

**neuropsychiatric** /ˌnjʊərəʊsaɪkiˈætrik/ *adjective* referring to neuropsychiatry

**neuropsychiatrist** /ˌnjʊərəʊsaɪˈkaɪətrɪst/ *noun* a doctor who specialises in the study and treatment of mental and nervous disorders

**neuropsychiatry** /ˌnjʊərəʊsaɪˈkaɪətri/ *noun* the study of mental and nervous disorders

**neurorrhaphy** /njʊˈrɔːrəfi/ *noun* a surgical operation to join by suture a nerve which has been cut (NOTE: The plural is **neurorrhaphies**.)

**neurosarcoma** /ˌnjʊərəʊsɑːˈkəʊmə/ *noun* a malignant neuroma (NOTE: The plural is **neurosarcomas** or **neurosarcomata**.)

**neurosecretion** /ˌnjʊərəʊsɪˈkriːʃ(ə)n/ *noun* **1.** a substance secreted by a nerve cell **2.** the process of secretion of an active substance by nerve cells

**neurosis** /njʊˈrəʊsɪs/ *noun* a disorder of the personality in which a person experiences obsessive negative emotions towards someone or

something, e.g. fear of empty spaces or jealousy of a sibling. ◊ **psychoneurosis** (NOTE: The plural is **neuroses**.)

**neurosurgeon** /ˈnjʊərəʊˌsɜːdʒən/ *noun* a surgeon who operates on the nervous system, including the brain and spinal cord

**neurosurgery** /ˈnjʊərəʊˌsɜːdʒəri/ *noun* surgery on the nervous system, including the brain and spinal cord

**neurosyphilis** /ˌnjʊərəʊˈsɪfəlɪs/ *noun* syphilis which attacks the nervous system

**neurotic** /njʊˈrɒtɪk/ *adjective* relating to or having neurosis ■ *noun* a person who is worried about or obsessed with something (*informal*)

**neurotically** /njʊˈrɒtɪkli/ *adverb* in a neurotic way ○ *She is neurotically obsessed with keeping herself clean.*

**neurotmesis** /ˌnjʊərɒtˈmiːsɪs/ *noun* an act of cutting a nerve completely (NOTE: The plural is **neurotmeses**.)

**neurotomy** /njʊˈrɒtəmi/ *noun* a surgical operation to cut a nerve (NOTE: The plural is **neurotomies**.)

**neurotoxic** /ˌnjʊərəʊˈtɒksɪk/ *adjective* harmful or poisonous to nerve cells

**neurotransmitter** /ˌnjʊərəʊtrænsˈmɪtə/ *noun* a chemical substance which transmits nerve impulses from one neurone to another

COMMENT: The main neurotransmitters are the catecholamines (adrenaline, noradrenaline and 5-hydroxytryptamine) and acetylcholine. Other neurotransmitters such as gamma aminobutyric acid, glutamine and substance P are less common.

**neurotripsy** /ˈnjʊərəʊtrɪpsi/ *noun* surgical bruising or crushing of a nerve

**neurotrophic** /ˌnjʊərəʊˈtrəʊfɪk/ *adjective* relating to the nutrition and maintenance of tissue of the nervous system

**neurotropic** /ˌnjʊərəʊˈtrɒpɪk/ *adjective* referring to a bacterium which is attracted to and attacks nerves

**neuter** /ˈnjuːtə/ *adjective* neither male nor female

**neutral** /ˈnjuːtrəl/ *adjective* neither acid nor alkali ○ *A pH factor of 7 is neutral.*

**neutralise** /ˈnjuːtrəlaɪz/, **neutralize** *verb* **1.** to counteract the effect of something ○ *Alkali poisoning can be neutralised by applying acid solution.* (NOTE: **neutralising – neutralised**) **2.** to form a salt from an acid

**neutropenia** /ˌnjuːtrəˈpiːniə/ *noun* a condition in which there are fewer neutrophils than usual in the blood

**neutrophil** /ˈnjuːtrəfɪl/ *noun* a type of white blood cell with an irregular nucleus, which can attack and destroy bacteria. Also called **polymorph**

**newborn** /ˈnjuːbɔːn/ *adjective* born recently. ◊ **neonatal** ■ *noun* a recently born baby. ◊ **neonate**

**newton** /'nju:t(ə)n/ *noun* an SI unit of measurement of force. Symbol **N**

COMMENT: One newton is the force required to move one kilogram at the speed of one metre per second

**new variant CJD** /nju: ˌveəriənt ˌsi:dʒeɪ 'di:/ *noun* ♦ **variant CJD**

**next-day pill** /ˌnekst deɪ 'pɪl/ *noun* same as **morning-after pill**

**next of kin** /ˌnekst əv 'kɪn/ *noun* the person or persons who are most closely related to someone ○ *The hospital has notified the next of kin of the death of the accident victim.* (NOTE: Takes a singular or plural verb.)

**nexus** /'neksəs/ *noun* **1.** a link (NOTE: The plural is **nexus** or **nexuses**.) **2.** a point where two organs or tissues join

**NF** *abbr* neurofibromatosis

**NHS** *abbr* National Health Service

**NHS Direct** /ˌen eɪt ʃ es dɪ'rekt/ *noun* in the UK, a national telephone helpline run by nurses to provide information about health and health services for the public

**niacin** /'naɪəsɪn/ *noun* a vitamin of the vitamin B complex found in milk, meat, liver, kidney, yeast, beans, peas and bread, lack of which can cause mental disorders and pellagra. Also called **nicotinic acid**

**nicardipine** /nɪ'kɑːdɪpi:n/ *noun* a drug which slows down the movement of calcium ions into smooth muscle cells, used especially to treat angina

**NICE** /naɪs/ *abbr* National Institute for Clinical Excellence

**nick** /nɪk/ *noun* a little cut ○ *She had a nick in her ear lobe which bled.* ■ *verb* to make a little cut in something ○ *He nicked his chin while shaving.*

**niclosamide** /nɪ'kləʊsəmaɪd/ *noun* a drug used for removing tapeworms

**nicotine** /'nɪkəti:n/ *noun* the main alkaloid substance found in tobacco

**nicotine addiction** /'nɪkəti:n əˌdɪkʃən/ *noun* an addiction to nicotine, derived from smoking tobacco

**nicotine patch** /'nɪkəti:n pætʃ/ *noun* a patch containing nicotine which is released slowly into the bloodstream, applied to the skin as a method of curing nicotine addiction

**nicotine poisoning** /'nɪkəti:n ˌpɔɪz(ə)nɪŋ/ *noun* poisoning of the autonomic nervous system with large quantities of nicotine. Also called **nicotinism**

**nicotine receptor** /'nɪkəti:n rɪˌseptə/ *noun* a cholinergic receptor found at the neuromuscular junction on skeletal muscle and in the autonomic ganglia, which responds to nicotine and nicotine-like drugs. Also called **nicotinic receptor**

**nicotine replacement** /'nɪkəti:n rɪˌpleɪsmənt/ *noun* the use of nicotine patches or other products to help during an attempt to give up smoking

**nicotinic acid** /ˌnɪkətɪnɪk 'æsɪd/ same as **niacin**

**nicotinic receptor** /nɪkəˌtɪnɪk rɪ'septə/ *noun* same as **nicotine receptor**

**nicotinism** /'nɪkəti:nɪz(ə)m/ *noun* same as **nicotine poisoning**

**nictation** /nɪk'teɪʃ(ə)n/, **nictitation** /nɪktɪ'teɪʃ(ə)n/ *noun* the act of winking

**nidation** /naɪ'deɪʃ(ə)n/ *noun* **1.** the process of building the endometrial layers of the uterus between menstrual periods **2.** the point in the development of an embryo at which the fertilised ovum reaches the uterus and implants in the wall of the uterus. Also called **implantation**

**nidus** /'naɪdəs/ *noun* a site where bacteria can settle and breed, which becomes a centre of infection (NOTE: The plural is **niduses** or **nidi**.)

**Niemann-Pick disease** /ˌni:mən 'pɪk dɪ ˌzi:z/ *noun* a rare inherited disease of a group which affect metabolism. Signs in babies include feeding difficulties, a large abdomen within 3 to 6 months, and progressive loss of early motor skills.

**nifedipine** /nɪ'fedɪpi:n/ *noun* a drug which stops the heart muscles from taking up calcium, used in the treatment of high blood pressure and angina pectoris

**night duty** /'naɪt ˌdju:ti/ *noun* the situation of working at night ○ *Nurse Smith is on night duty this week.*

**Nightingale ward** *noun* an old-fashioned type of long ward with a row of beds along each wall and a centrally placed point for the nurse in charge to work from

**nightmare** /'naɪtmeə/ *noun* a dream which frightens the dreamer ○ *The child had a nightmare and woke up screaming.*

**night nurse** /'naɪt nɜːs/ *noun* a nurse who is on duty at night

**night sweat** /'naɪt swet/ *noun* heavy sweating when a person is asleep at night

**night terror** /'naɪt 'terə/ *noun* a period of disturbed sleep, which a child does not remember afterwards

**nigra** /'naɪgrə/ ♦ **linea nigra**

**nihilism** /'naɪhɪlɪz(ə)m/ *noun* the rejection of all the usual social conventions and beliefs, especially of morality and religion

**nihilistic** /ˌnaɪhɪ'lɪstɪk/ *adjective* relating to or showing a belief in nihilism

**ninety-nine** /ˌnaɪnti 'naɪn/ *number* a number which a doctor asks a person to say so that he or she can inspect the back of the throat ○ *The doctor told him to open his mouth wide and say ninety-nine.*

**nipple** /'nɪp(ə)l/ *noun* **1.** same as **mammilla 2.** *US* a rubber teat on a baby's feeding bottle

**Nissl granule** /'nɪs(ə)l ˌɡrænjuːl/, **Nissl body** /'nɪs(ə)l ˌbɒdi/ *noun* one of the coarse granules surrounding the nucleus in the cytoplasm of nerve cells. See illustration at NEURONE in Supplement [Described 1894. After Franz Nissl (1860–1919), German psychiatrist.]

**nit** /nɪt/ *noun* an egg or larva of a louse

**nitrate** /'naɪtreɪt/ *noun* **1.** a salt or an ester of nitric acid **2.** a drug such as glyceryl trinitrate which dilates the vessels leading to the heart muscle and lowers cardiac work by reducing venous return to the heart, for rapid relief of angina and in heart failure (NOTE: Patients can develop tolerance to these drugs.)

**-nitrate** /naɪtreɪt/ *suffix* used in names of nitrate drugs

**nitrazepam** /naɪ'træzɪpæm/ *noun* a tranquilliser used in some sleeping pills

**nitrofurantoin** /ˌnaɪtrəʊfjʊ'ræntəʊin/ *noun* a drug which helps to prevent the growth of bacteria, used in the treatment of urinary infections

**nitrogen** /'naɪtrədʒən/ *noun* a chemical element, which is a gas that is the main component of air and is an essential part of protein (NOTE: The chemical symbol is **N**.)

COMMENT: Nitrogen is taken into the body by digesting protein-rich foods; excess nitrogen is excreted in urine. When the intake of nitrogen and the excretion rate are equal, the body is in nitrogen balance or protein balance.

**nitrogen narcosis** /ˌnaɪtrədʒ(ə)n nɑː'kəʊsɪs/ *noun* loss of consciousness due to the formation of nitrogen in the tissues, caused by pressure change

**nitroglycerin** /ˌnaɪtrəʊ'ɡlɪsərɪn/ *noun* a drug which helps the veins and coronary arteries to become wider

**nitrous oxide** /ˌnaɪtrəs 'ɒksaɪd/ *noun* a colourless gas with a sweet smell, used in combination with other gases as an anaesthetic in dentistry and surgery. Also called **laughing gas**

**nm** *abbr* nanometre

**NMC** *abbr* Nursing and Midwifery Council

**nmol** *abbr* nanomole

**NMR** *abbr* nuclear magnetic resonance

**Nocardia** /nəʊ'kɑːdiə/ *noun* a genus of bacteria found in soil, some species of which cause nocardiosis and maduramycosis

**nocardiosis** /nəʊˌkɑːdi'əʊsɪs/, **nocardiasis** /ˌnəʊkɑː'daɪəsɪs/ *noun* a lung infection which may metastasise to other tissue, caused by *Nocardia*

**noci-** /nəʊsi/ *prefix* pain or injury

**nociassociation** /ˌnəʊsiəˌsəʊsi'eɪʃ(ə)n/ *noun* an unconscious release of nervous energy, e.g. as a result of shock

**nociceptive** /ˌnəʊsi'septɪv/ *adjective* referring to nerves which carry pain to the brain

**nociceptor** /'nəʊsiˌseptə/ *noun* a sensory nerve which carries pain to the brain

**noct-** /nɒkt/ *prefix* night

**noctambulation** /ˌnɒktæmbjuleɪʃ(ə)n/ *noun* same as **somnambulism**

**nocte** /'nɒkti/ *adverb* at night. Opposite **mane** (NOTE: used on prescriptions)

**nocturia** /nɒk'tjʊəriə/ *noun* the fact of passing an unusually large quantity of urine during the night

**nocturnal** /nɒk'tɜːn(ə)l/ *adjective* referring to or taking place at night

**nocturnal emission** /nɒkˌtɜːn(ə)l ɪ'mɪʃ(ə)n/ *noun* the production of semen from the penis while a man is asleep

**nocturnal enuresis** /nɒkˌtɜːn(ə)l enjʊ'riːsɪs/ *noun* the act of passing urine when asleep in bed at night. Also called **bedwetting**

**nodal** /'nəʊd(ə)l/ *adjective* referring to nodes

**nodal tachycardia** /ˌnəʊd(ə)l tæki'kɑːdiə/ *noun* a sudden attack of rapid heartbeats. Also called **paroxysmal tachycardia**

**node** /nəʊd/ *noun* **1.** a small mass of tissue **2.** a group of nerve cells

**node of Ranvier** /ˌnəʊd əv 'rænviə/ *noun* one of a series of gaps in the myelin sheath surrounding a nerve fibre. See illustration at NEURONE in Supplement

**nod off** *verb* to fall asleep (*informal*)

**nodosum** /nəʊ'dəʊsəm/ ♦ **erythema nodosum**

**nodular** /'nɒdjʊlə/ *adjective* formed of nodules

**nodule** /'nɒdjuːl/ *noun* **1.** a small node or group of cells. ◊ **Bohn's nodules 2.** the anterior part of the inferior vermis

**noma** /'nəʊmə/ *noun* same as **cancrum oris**

**nomen proprium** /ˌnəʊmən 'prəʊpriəm/ *noun* full form of **n.p.**

**non-** /nɒn/ *prefix* not

**non-A, non-B hepatitis** *noun* now called **hepatitis C**

**non-absorbable suture** /ˌnɒn əbˌzɔːbəb(ə)l 'suːtʃə/ *noun* a suture made of a substance which cannot be absorbed into the body and which eventually has to be removed

**non-accidental injury** /ˌnɒn æksɪˌdent(ə)l 'ɪndʒəri/ *noun* an injury which is not caused accidentally

**non-allergenic** /ˌnɒn ælə'dʒenɪk/ *adjective* not aggravating an allergy

**non-cancerous** /ˌnɒn 'kænsərəs/ *adjective* not malignant

**non-clinical** /ˌnɒn 'klɪnɪk(ə)l/ *adjective* referring to the wider non-medical aspects of patient care ○ *non-clinical services such as administration and catering* ○ *non-clinical guidelines including confidentiality protocols*

**non-compliance** /ˌnɒn kəm'plaɪəns/ *noun* the failure to take drugs at the correct times and in the dosages prescribed, or to take them at all

**non compos mentis** /ˌnɒn ˌkɒmpəs ˈmentɪs/ *adjective* referring to a person who is mentally incapable of managing his or her own affairs (NOTE: From a Latin phrase meaning 'not of sound mind'.)

**non-contagious** /ˌnɒn kənˈteɪdʒəs/ *adjective* not contagious

**non-drowsy** /ˌnɒn ˈdraʊzi/ *adjective* not causing drowsiness

**non-emergency surgery** /ˌnɒn ɪˈmɜːdʒənsi ˈsɜːdʒəri/ *noun* a surgical operation which does not need to be performed immediately because it is for a condition which is not life-threatening, e.g. joint replacement. Also called **non-urgent surgery**

**non-granular leucocyte** /ˌnɒn ˌgrænjʊlə ˈluːkəʊsaɪt/ *noun* a leucocyte which has no granules, e.g. a lymphocyte or monocyte

**non-Hodgkins lymphoma** /nɒn ˌhɒdʒkɪnz lɪmˈfəʊmə/ *noun* a cancer of the lymph nodes which differs from Hodgkin's disease by the absence of a particular type of cell with double nuclei

**non-insulin-dependent diabetes** /nɒn ˌɪnsjʊlɪn dɪˌpendənt ˌdaɪəˈbiːtiːz/ *noun* same as **Type II diabetes mellitus**

**non-invasive** /ˌnɒn ɪnˈveɪzɪv/ *adjective* referring to treatment which does not involve entering the body by making an incision

**non-maleficence** /nɒn məˈlefɪs(ə)ns/ *noun* the concept that professionals in the health service have a duty to protect the patient from harm (NOTE: Under this principle, professionals' obligations include keeping their knowledge and skills current, realising their own limitations and knowing when to refer a case to a specialist or other professional.)

**non-malignant** /ˌnɒn məˈlɪgnənt/ *adjective* not cancerous, or not life-threatening ○ *a non-malignant growth*

**non-medical** /ˌnɒn ˈmedɪk(ə)l/ *adjective* **1.** not relating to medicine ○ *non-medical genetics* **2.** not according to medical practice, or not as directed by a doctor ○ *non-medical use of stimulant drugs* **3.** not used in specialised medical speech ○ *'Nervous breakdown' is a non-medical term for a type of sudden mental illness.*

**non-nucleated** /ˌnɒn ˈnjuːkliːeɪtɪd/ *adjective* referring to a cell with no nucleus

**non-official drug** /ˌnɒn əˌfɪʃ(ə)l ˈdrʌg/ *noun* a drug that is not listed in the national pharmacopoiea

**non-palpable** /nɒn ˈpælpəb(ə)l/ *adjective* not able to be felt when touched

**non-paralytic poliomyelitis** /nɒn ˌpærəlɪtɪk ˌpəʊliəʊˌmaɪəˈlaɪtɪs/ *noun* a form of poliomyelitis similar to abortive poliomyelitis but which also affects the muscles to some degree

**non-secretor** /ˌnɒn sɪˈkriːtə/ *noun* a person who does not secrete substances indicating

ABO blood group into mucous fluids such as semen or saliva

**non-smoker** /nɒn ˈsməʊkə/ *noun* a person who does not smoke

**non-specific** /ˌnɒn spəˈsɪfɪk/ *adjective* not caused by any single identifiable cause

**non-specific urethritis** /ˌnɒn spəˌsɪfɪk ˌjʊərɪˈθraɪtɪs/ *noun* any sexually transmitted inflammation of the urethra not caused by gonorrhoea (*dated*) Abbr **NSU**

**non-sterile** /ˌnɒn ˈsterɪl/ *adjective* not sterile or sterilised

**non-steroidal** /ˌnɒn steˈrɔɪd(ə)l/ *adjective* not containing steroids

**non-steroidal anti-inflammatory drug** /ˌnɒnsteˌrɔɪd(ə)l ˌænti ɪnˈflæmət(ə)ri drʌg/ *noun* a drug used in the treatment of pain associated with inflammation, including rheumatic disease, post-operative analgesia and dysmenorrhoea, by inhibiting the release of prostaglandins. Abbr **NSAID** (NOTE: Non-steroidal anti-inflammatory drugs have names ending in **-fen: ibuprofen.**)

COMMENT: Serious gastro-intestinal side effects can occur, especially in the elderly. Asthma can worsen.

**non-union** /nɒn ˈjuːnjən/ *noun* a condition in which the two parts of a fractured bone do not join together and do not heal

**non-urgent surgery** /ˌnɒn ˌɜːdʒənt ˈsɜːdʒəri/ same as **non-emergency surgery**

**noradrenaline** /ˌnɔːrəˈdrenəlɪn/ *noun* a hormone secreted by the medulla of the adrenal glands which acts as a vasoconstrictor and is used to maintain blood pressure in shock, haemorrhage or hypotension (NOTE: The US term is **norepinephrine**.)

**norma** /ˈnɔːmə/ *noun* a view of the skull as seen from a particular angle (NOTE: The plural is **normae**.)

**normal** /ˈnɔːm(ə)l/ *adjective* usual, ordinary or conforming to a standard ○ *After he took the tablets, his blood pressure went back to normal.* ○ *Her temperature is two degrees above normal.* ○ *He had an above-normal pulse rate.* ○ *Is it normal for a person with myopia to suffer from headaches?*

**normally** /ˈnɔːm(ə)li/ *adverb* in an ordinary way, on most occasions or in most circumstances ○ *The patients are normally worried before the operation.* ○ *He was breathing normally.*

**normo-** /ˈnɔːməʊ/ *prefix* normal, usual or expected

**normoblast** /ˈnɔːməʊblæst/ *noun* an early form of a red blood cell, usually found only in bone marrow but occurring in the blood in some types of leukaemia and anaemia

**normocyte** /ˈnɔːməʊsaɪt/ *noun* a red blood cell

**normocytic** /ˌnɔːməʊˈsaɪtɪk/ *adjective* referring to a normocyte

**normocytosis** /ˌnɔːməʊsaɪˈtəʊsɪs/ *noun* the condition of having the standard number of red blood cells in the peripheral blood

**normotension** /ˌnɔːməʊˈtenʃən/ *noun* blood pressure at the usual level

**normotensive** /ˌnɔːməʊˈtensɪv/ *adjective* referring to blood pressure at the usual level

**Norton score** /ˈnɔːt(ə)n skɔː/ *noun* a scale for deciding how likely it is that pressure sores will develop, used mostly in assessing elderly patients

**nortriptyline** /nɔːˈtrɪptəliːn/ *noun* a drug used to reduce pain and as an antidepressant and tranquilliser

**nose** /nəʊz/ *noun* an organ through which a person breathes and smells □ **her nose is running** liquid mucus is dripping from her nose □ **he blew his nose** he blew air through his nose into a handkerchief to get rid of mucus in his nose □ **to speak through your nose** to speak as if your nose is blocked, so that you say 'b' instead of 'm' and 'd' instead of 'n'

COMMENT: The nose is formed of cartilage and small bones making the bridge at the top. It leads into two passages, the nostrils, which in turn lead to the nasal cavity, divided in two by the septum. The nasal passages connect with the sinuses, with the ears through the Eustachian tubes, and with the pharynx. The receptors which detect smell are in the top of the nasal passage.

**nosebleed** /ˈnəʊzbliːd/ *noun* an incident of bleeding from the nose, usually caused by a blow or by sneezing, by blowing the nose hard or by high blood pressure (*informal*) ○ *She had a headache, followed by a violent nosebleed.* Also called **epistaxis**

**noso-** /nɒsəʊ/ *prefix* disease

**nosocomial** /ˌnɒsəʊˈkəʊmiəl/ *adjective* referring to hospitals

**nosocomial infection** /ˌnɒsəʊˌkəʊmiəl ɪnˈfekʃən/ *noun* an infection which is passed on to a person being treated in a hospital

**nosology** /nɒˈsɒlədʒi/ *noun* the classification of diseases

**nostril** /ˈnɒstrɪl/ *noun* one of the two passages in the nose through which air is breathed in or out ○ *His right nostril is blocked.* (NOTE: The nostrils are also referred to as the **nares**.)

**notch** /nɒtʃ/ *noun* a depression on a surface, usually on a bone, but sometimes on an organ. ◊ **cardiac notch, occipital notch**

**notice** /ˈnəʊtɪs/ *noun* **1.** a piece of writing giving information, usually put in a place where everyone can see it **2.** a warning ○ *They had to leave with ten minutes' notice.* **3.** attention □ **to take notice (of something *or* someone)** to give attention (to something or someone) ○ *We need to take notice of this feedback.* ■ *verb* to see or be aware of something ○ *Nobody noticed that she was sweating.* ○ *Did you notice the development of any new symptoms?* (NOTE: **noticing – noticed**)

**noticeable** /ˈnəʊtɪsəb(ə)l/ *adjective* able to be noticed ○ *The disease has no easily noticeable symptoms.*

**noticeboard** /ˈnəʊtɪsbɔːd/ *noun* a flat piece of wood, or board fixed on a wall, on which notices can be pinned

**notifiable disease** /ˌnəʊtɪfaɪəb(ə)l dɪˈziːz/ *noun* a serious infectious disease which, in the UK, has to be reported by a doctor to the Department of Health so that steps can be taken to stop it spreading

COMMENT: The following are notifiable diseases: cholera, diphtheria, dysentery, encephalitis, food poisoning, jaundice, malaria, measles, meningitis, ophthalmia neonatorum, paratyphoid, plague, poliomyelitis, relapsing fever, scarlet fever, smallpox, tuberculosis, typhoid, typhus, whooping cough and yellow fever.

**notify** /ˈnəʊtɪfaɪ/ *verb* to inform a person or authority officially ○ *The local doctor notified the Health Service of the case of cholera.* (NOTE: **notifies – notifying – notified**. You notify a person **of** something.)

**nourish** /ˈnʌrɪʃ/ *verb* to give food or nutrients to a person

**nourishment** /ˈnʌrɪʃmənt/ *noun* **1.** the act of supplying nutrients to a person **2.** food and the nutrients in it, e.g. proteins, fats or vitamins

**noxious** /ˈnɒkʃəs/ *adjective* harmful ○ *a noxious gas*

**n.p.** *noun* the name of the drug written on the label of its container. Full form **nomen proprium**

**NPO** *abbreviation* used to refer to patients being kept without food ○ *The patient should be kept NPO for five hours before the operation.* Full form **ne per oris**

**NSAID** *abbr* non-steroidal anti-inflammatory drug

**NSU** *abbr* non-specific urethritis

**nucha** /ˈnjuːkə/ *noun* same as **nape** (NOTE: The plural is **nuchae**.)

**nuchal** /ˈnjuːk(ə)l/ *adjective* referring to the back of the neck

**nucle-** /njuːkli/ *prefix* same as **nucleo-** (*used before vowels*)

**nuclear** /ˈnjuːkliə/ *adjective* referring to nuclei, e.g. of a cell or an atom

**nuclear magnetic resonance** /ˌnjuːkliə mæɡˌnetɪk ˈrezənəns/ *noun* a scanning technique using magnetic fields and radio waves which reveals abnormalities in soft tissue and body fluids. ◊ **magnetic resonance imaging**. Abbr **NMR**

**nuclear medicine** /ˌnjuːkliə ˈmed(ə)s(ə)n/ *noun* the use of radioactive substances for detecting and treating disorders

**nuclease** /ˈnjuːklieɪz/ *noun* an enzyme which breaks down nucleic acids

**nucleic acid** /njuːˌkliːɪk ˈæsɪd/ *noun* an organic acid of a type found in all living cells, which consists of complex nucleotide chains which pass on genetic information, e.g. DNA or RNA

**nucleo-** /njuːkliəʊ/ *prefix* referring to a cell or atomic nucleus

**nucleolus** /njuˈkliːələs/ *noun* a structure inside a cell nucleus, containing RNA (NOTE: The plural is **nucleoli**.)

**nucleoprotein** /ˌnjuːkliəʊˈprəʊtiːn/ *noun* a compound of protein and nucleic acid, e.g. a chromosome or ribosome

**nucleus** /ˈnjuːkliəs/ *noun* **1.** a central part which has others grouped or built around it **2.** the central body in a cell, which contains DNA and RNA and controls the function and characteristics of the cell. See illustration at NEU-RONE in Supplement **3.** a group of nerve cells in the brain or spinal cord (NOTE: The plural is **nuclei**.)

**nucleus pulposus** /ˌnjuːkliəs pʊlˈpəʊsəs/ *noun* a soft central part of an intervertebral disc which disappears in old age (NOTE: The plural is **nuclei pulposi**)

**nullipara** /nʌˈlɪpərə/ *noun* a woman who has never had a child (NOTE: The plural is **nulliparas** or **nulliparae**.) ■ *adjective* referring to a woman who has never had a child

**numb** /nʌm/ *adjective* **1.** referring to a part of the body which has no feeling **2.** unable to feel emotion

**numbness** /ˈnʌmnəs/ *noun* a loss of feeling

**nurse** /nɜːs/ *noun* a person who looks after sick people in a hospital or helps a doctor in a local surgery. Some nurses may be trained to diagnose and treat patients. ○ *She works as a nurse in the local hospital.* ○ *He's training to be a nurse.* ◊ **nurse practitioner** ■ *verb* **1.** to look after a sick person, or to be employed as a nurse ○ *When he was ill his mother nursed him until he was better.* **2.** to behave so as not to aggravate a condition ○ *nursing a sprained ankle* (NOTE: **nurses – nursing – nursed**)

**nurse executive director** /nɜːs ɪg,zekjʊtɪv daɪˈrektə/ *noun* in the UK, a senior nurse who sits on the Board of an NHS Trust and has corporate as well as professional responsibilities in the organisation for nursing and sometimes other aspects such as quality or human resources

**nurse manager** /ˌnɜːs ˈmænɪdʒə/ *noun* a nurse who has administrative duties in a hospital or a health service

**nurse practitioner** /ˌnɜːs prækˈtɪʃ(ə)nə/ *noun* a nurse with additional clinical training at degree level who often works independently, assessing, diagnosing and treating patients, particularly in primary care

**nurse station** /ˈnɜːs ˌsteɪʃ(ə)n/, **nurses' station** /ˈnɜːsɪz ˌsteɪʃ(ə)n/ *noun* an area in or near a ward from which nurses work, keep records and control the activities of the ward

**nurse tutor** /ˌnɜːs ˈtjuːtə/ *noun* an experienced nurse who teaches student nurses

**nursing** /ˈnɜːsɪŋ/ *noun* **1.** the work or profession of being a nurse ○ *He has chosen nursing as his career.* **2.** care for sick people provided by a nurse ■ *adjective* providing care as a nurse

'…few would now dispute the need for clear, concise nursing plans to guide nursing practice, provide educational tools and give an accurate legal record' [*Nursing Times*]

'…all relevant sections of the nurses' care plan and nursing process records had been left blank' [*Nursing Times*]

**Nursing and Midwifery Council** /ˌnɜːsɪŋ ən ˌmɪdˈwɪfəri ˌkaʊnsəl/ *noun* in the UK, an organisation that sets standards for the education, practice and conduct of nurses, midwives and health visitors. Abbr **NMC**

**nursing audit** /ˈnɜːsɪŋ ˌɔːdɪt/ *noun* a formal detailed review of records or observation of nursing actions so that judgments can be made about the quality of nursing care being given (NOTE: The documented evidence is compared with accepted standards and criteria.)

**nursing development unit** /ˌnɜːsɪŋ dɪ ˈveləpmənt/ *noun* a nurse-led ward or unit that sets out to demonstrate by example innovative high-quality care, to reflect on practice and draw lessons from this experience, and to provide learning opportunities for other nurses. Abbr **NDU**

**nursing home** /ˈnɜːsɪŋ həʊm/ *noun* a house where convalescents or dependent elderly people can live under medical supervision by a qualified nurse

**nursing intervention** /ˌnɜːsɪŋ ɪntə ˈvenʃən/ *noun* the treatment of illness by nursing care, without surgery

**nursing model** /ˈnɜːsɪŋ ˌmɒd(ə)l/ *noun* a set of stated principles about nursing which gives professionals a way of formulating a plan of care, assessing its success and addressing any problems which arise from it

**nursing mother** /ˌnɜːsɪŋ ˈmʌðə/ *noun* a mother who breast-feeds her baby

**Nursing Officer** /ˈnɜːsɪŋ ˌɒfɪsə/ *noun* in the UK, a nurse employed by the Department of Health to assist the Chief Nursing Officer in providing professional advice to Ministers and policy-makers

**nursing practice** /ˈnɜːsɪŋ ˌpræktɪs/ *noun* treatment given by nurses

**nursing process** /ˌnɜːsɪŋ ˈprəʊses/ *noun* a standard method of treatment and documentation of treatment carried out by nurses

**nursing sister** /ˌnɜːsɪŋ ˈsɪstə/ *noun* a hospital sister who has administrative duties

**nursing standard** /ˈnɜːsɪŋ ˌstændəd/ *noun* an accepted level of achievement by which nursing care can be assessed or compared

**nurture** /'nɜːtʃə/ *noun* care given to a child while it is developing ■ *verb* to bring up and care for children (NOTE: **nurturing – nurtured**)

**nutans** /'njuːt(ə)ns/ ♦ **spasmus nutans**

**nutation** /njuː'teɪʃ(ə)n/ *noun* involuntary nodding of the head

**nutrient** /'njuːtriənt/ *noun* a substance in food which is necessary to provide energy or to help the body grow, e.g. protein, fat or a vitamin

**nutrition** /njuː'trɪʃ(ə)ⁿn/ *noun* **1.** the study of the supply of nutrients to the body from digesting food **2.** nourishment or food

**nutritional** /njuː'trɪʃ(ə)n(ə)l/ *adjective* referring to nutrition

**nutritional anaemia** /njuː,trɪʃ(ə)n(ə)l ə 'niːmiə/ *noun* anaemia caused by an imbalance in the diet

**nutritional disorder** /njuː'trɪʃ(ə)n(ə)l dɪs ,ɔːdə/ *noun* a disorder related to food and nutrients, e.g. obesity

**nutritionist** /njuː'trɪʃ(ə)nɪst/ *noun* a person who specialises in the study of nutrition and advises on diets. ◊ **dietitian**

**nyct-** /nɪkt/ *prefix* night or darkness

**nyctalopia** /,nɪktə'ləʊpiə/ *noun* the condition of being unable to see in bad light. Also called **night blindness**

**nyctophobia** /,nɪktə'fəʊbiə/ *noun* fear of the dark

**nymphae** /'nɪmfiː/ *plural noun* same as **labia minora**

**nympho-** /nɪmfəʊ/ *prefix* **1.** female sexuality **2.** nymphae

**nymphomania** /,nɪmfə'meɪniə/ *noun* an obsessive sexual urge in a woman (NOTE: A similar condition in a man is called **satyriasis**.)

**nymphomaniac** /,nɪmfə'meɪniæk/ *noun* a woman who has an unusually obsessive sexual urge (NOTE: This term is regarded as offensive.)

**nystagmus** /nɪ'stægməs/ *noun* a rapid, involuntary movement of the eyes up and down or from side to side

COMMENT: Nystagmus can be horizontal, vertical, torsional or rotary; it can be congenital, but is also a symptom of multiple sclerosis and Ménière's disease.

**nystatin** /naɪ'stætɪn/ *noun* an anti-microbial drug used in the treatment of fungal infections, especially thrush

# O

**oat cell carcinoma** /ˈəʊt sel kɑːsɪˌnəʊmə/ *noun* a type of cancer of the bronchi, with distinctive small cells

**OB** *abbr* obstetrics

**obese** /əʊˈbiːs/ *adjective* so overweight as to be at risk of several serious illnesses, including diabetes and heart disease

**obesity** /əʊˈbiːsɪti/ *noun* the condition of being seriously overweight

COMMENT: Obesity is caused by excess fat accumulating under the skin and around organs in the body. It is sometimes due to glandular disorders, but it is usually caused by eating or drinking too much. A tendency to obesity can be hereditary.

**obey** /əˈbeɪ/ *verb* to do what a person, authority or rule says you should do ○ *You ought to obey the doctor's instructions and go to bed.*

**objective** /əbˈdʒektɪv/ *noun* an aim or goal ■ *adjective* **1.** existing independently of any individual person's mind **2.** not influenced by any bias or prejudice caused by personal feelings **3.** referring to symptoms of illness which can be observed by somebody other than the person who is ill. Compare **subjective**

**obligate** /ˈɒblɪɡeɪt/ *adjective* referring to an organism which exists and develops in only one way, e.g. a virus which is a parasite only inside cells

**oblique** /əˈbliːk/ *adjective* lying at an angle ■ *noun* also called **oblique muscle**

'…there are four recti muscles and two oblique muscles in each eye, which coordinate the movement of the eyes and enable them to work as a pair' [*Nursing Times*]

**oblique fissure** /əˌbliːk ˈfɪʃə/ *noun* a groove between the superior and inferior lobes of a lung. See illustration at LUNGS in Supplement

**oblique fracture** /əˌbliːk ˈfræktʃə/ *noun* a fracture in which the bone is broken diagonally

**oblique muscle** /əˌbliːk ˈmʌs(ə)l/ *noun* **1.** each of two muscles in the wall of the abdomen **2.** each of two muscles which control the movement of the eyeball

**obliterate** /əˈblɪtəreɪt/ *verb* **1.** to destroy something completely **2.** to block a cavity completely (NOTE: **obliterating – obliterated**)

**obliteration** /əˌblɪtəˈreɪʃ(ə)n/ *noun* **1.** the complete destruction of something **2.** the complete blocking of something such as a cavity

**oblongata** /ˌɒblɒŋˈɡeɪtə/ ♦ **medulla oblongata**

**observable** /əbˈzɜːvəb(ə)l/ *noun* which can be seen or measured

**observation** /ˌɒbzəˈveɪʃ(ə)n/ *noun* the process of watching and examining a person or thing over a period of time ○ *She was admitted to hospital for observation.*

**observation register** /ˌɒbzəˈveɪʃ(ə)n ˌredʒɪstə/ *noun* a record of children who have had problems at birth, or soon after their birth, and so need particular follow-up care from a health visitor, general practitioner or social worker

**observe** /əbˈzɜːv/ *verb* **1.** to see something ○ *The nurses observed signs of improvement in the patient's condition.* ○ *The girl's mother observed symptoms of anorexia.* **2.** to watch a person or thing carefully in order to discover something ○ *Observe the way in which the patient is lying.* **3.** to take something into account ○ *You're expected to observe the rules of conduct.*

**obsessed** /əbˈsest/ *adjective* having an obsession ○ *He is obsessed with the idea that someone is trying to kill him.*

**obsession** /əbˈseʃ(ə)n/ *noun* a mental disorder in which a person has a fixed idea or emotion which he or she cannot get rid of, even if he or she knows it is wrong or unpleasant ○ *She has an obsession about cats.*

**obsessional** /əbˈseʃ(ə)n(ə)l/ *adjective* referring to or having an obsession ○ *He is suffering from an obsessional disorder.*

**obsessive** /əbˈsesɪv/ *adjective* having or showing an obsession ○ *He has an obsessive desire to steal little objects.*

**obsessive action** /əbˌsesɪv ˈækʃən/ *noun* an action such as washing which is repeated over and over again and indicates a mental disorder

**obsessive–compulsive disorder** /əbˌsel↓sɪv kəmˈpʌlʃɪv dɪsˌɔːdə/ *noun* a mental disorder characterised by the need to perform repeated ritual acts such as checking or cleaning, which can be treated with psychotherapy and antidepressants. Abbr **OCD**

**obstetric** /əb'stetrɪk(ə)l/, **obstetrical** /əb'stetrɪkəl/ *adjective* referring to obstetrics

**obstetrical forceps** /əb,stetrɪk(ə)l 'fɔːseps/ *plural noun* a type of large forceps used to hold a baby's head during childbirth

**obstetrician** /,ɒbstə'trɪʃ(ə)n/ *noun* a doctor who specialises in obstetrics

**obstetric patient** /əb'stetrɪk ,peɪʃ(ə)nt/ *noun* a woman who is being treated by an obstetrician

**obstetrics** /əb'stetrɪks/ *noun* a branch of medicine and surgery dealing with pregnancy, childbirth and the period immediately after childbirth. Abbr **OB**

**obstipation** /,ɒbstɪ'peɪʃ(ə)n/ *noun* severe constipation, often caused by a blockage in the intestines

**obstruct** /əb'strʌkt/ *verb* to block something ○ *The artery was obstructed by a blood clot.*

**obstruction** /əb'strʌkʃən/ *noun* **1.** something which blocks a passage or a blood vessel **2.** the blocking of a passage or blood vessel

**obstructive** /əb'strʌktɪv/ *adjective* caused by an obstruction

**obstructive jaundice** /əb,strʌktɪv 'dʒɔːndɪs/ *noun* jaundice caused by an obstruction of the bile ducts. Also called **posthepatic jaundice.** ◊ **acholuric jaundice, icterus gravis neonatorum**

**obstructive lung disease** /əb,strʌktɪv 'lʌŋ dɪ,ziːz/ *noun* bronchitis and emphysema

**obstructive sleep apnoea** /əb,strʌktɪv 'sliːp ,æpniə/ *noun* the stopping of breathing, or difficulty in breathing, during sleep, resulting in loud snoring

**obtain** /əb'teɪn/ *verb* to get something ○ *Some amino acids are obtained from food.* ○ *Where did he obtain the drugs?*

**obtrusive** /əb'truːsɪv/ *adjective* **1.** forcing your presence on others **2.** referring to a scar which is very noticeable

**obturation** /,ɒbtjʊ'reɪʃ(ə)n/ *noun* the act of obstructing a body passage, or the state of a body passage when it is obstructed, e.g. by hard faeces

**obturator** /'ɒbtjʊreɪtə/ *noun* **1.** one of two muscles in the pelvis which govern the movement of the hip and thigh **2.** a device which closes an opening, e.g. a dental prosthesis which covers a cleft palate **3.** a metal bulb which fits into a bronchoscope or sigmoidoscope

**obturator foramen** /,ɒbtjʊreɪtə fə'reɪmən/ *noun* an opening in the hip bone near the acetabulum. See illustration at PELVIS in Supplement (NOTE: The plural is **obturator foramina.**)

**obtusion** /əb'tjuːʒ(ə)n/ *noun* a condition in which perception and feelings become dulled

**OC** *abbr* oral contraceptive

**occipita** /ɒk'sɪpɪtə/ plural of **occiput**

**occipital** /ɒk'sɪpɪt(ə)l/ *adjective* referring to the back of the head ■ *noun* same as **occipital bone**

**occipital bone** /ɒk'sɪpɪt(ə)l bəʊn/ *noun* the bone at the back of the head. Also called **occipital**

**occipital condyle** /ɒk,sɪpɪt(ə)l 'kɒndaɪl/ *noun* a round part of the occipital bone which joins it to the atlas

**occipital lobe** /ɒk'sɪpɪt(ə)l ləʊb/ *noun* the lobe at the back of each cerebral hemisphere

**occipital notch** /ɒk'sɪpɪt(ə)l nɒtʃ/ *noun* a point on the lower edge of the cerebral hemisphere where the surface has a notch

**occipito-anterior** /ɒk,sɪpɪtəʊ æn'tɪəriə/ *adjective* referring to a position of a baby during birth, in which the baby faces the mother's back

**occipito-posterior** /ɒk,sɪpɪtəʊ pɒ'stɪəriə/ *adjective* referring to a position of a baby during birth in which the baby faces the front

**occiput** /'ɒksɪpʌt/ *noun* the lower part of the back of the head or skull (NOTE: The plural is **occiputs** or **occipita.**)

**occluded** /ə'kluːdɪd/ *adjective* closed or blocked

**occlusion** /ə'kluːʒ(ə)n/ *noun* **1.** a thing which blocks a passage or which closes an opening **2.** the way in which the teeth in the upper and lower jaws fit together when the jaws are closed (NOTE: A bad fit between the teeth is a **malocclusion.**)

**occlusive** /ə'kluːsɪv/ *adjective* referring to occlusion or blocking

**occlusive stroke** /ə,kluːsɪv 'strəʊk/ *noun* a stroke caused by a blood clot

**occlusive therapy** /ə,kluːsɪv 'θerəpi/ *noun* a treatment for a squint in which the good eye is covered up in order to encourage the squinting eye to become straight

**occult** /ə'kʌlt/ *adjective* **1.** not easy to see with the naked eye. Opposite **overt 2.** referring to a symptom or sign which is hidden

**occult blood** /ə,kʌlt 'blʌd/ *noun* very small quantities of blood in the faeces, which can only be detected by tests

**occupancy rate** /'ɒkjʊpənsi reɪt/ *noun* the number of beds occupied in a hospital, shown as a percentage of all the beds

**occupation** /,ɒkjʊ'peɪʃ(ə)n/ *noun* **1.** a job or work ○ *What is his occupation?* ○ *People in sedentary occupations are liable to digestive disorders.* **2.** the state or fact of occupying something or of being occupied

**occupational** /,ɒkjʊ'peɪʃ(ə)nəl/ *adjective* referring to work

**occupational asthma** /ˌɒkjʊpeɪʃ(ə)n(ə)l ˈæsmə/ noun asthma caused by materials with which people come into contact at work

**occupational dermatitis** /ˌɒkjʊpeɪʃ(ə)n(ə)l ˌdɜːməˈtaɪtɪs/ noun dermatitis caused by materials touched at work

**occupational disease** /ɒkjʊˈpeɪʃ(ə)nəl dɪˌziːz/ noun a disease which is caused by the type of work a person does or the conditions in which a person works, e.g. a disease caused by dust or chemicals in a factory

**occupational hazard** /ˌɒkjʊpeɪʃ(ə)n(ə)l ˈhæzəd/ noun a dangerous situation related to the working environment

**occupational health nurse** /ˌɒkjʊ peɪʃ(ə)n(ə)l ˈhelθ nɜːs/ noun a nurse who deals with health problems of people at work. Abbr **OH nurse**

**occupational medicine** /ˌɒkjʊ peɪʃ(ə)n(ə)l ˈmed(ə)sɪn/ noun the branch of medicine concerned with accidents and diseases connected with work

**occupational therapist** /ˌɒkjʊpeɪʃ(ə)n(ə)l ˈθerəpɪst/ noun a qualified health professional who offers patients occupational therapy

**occupational therapy** /ˌɒkjʊpeɪʃ(ə)n(ə)l ˈθerəpi/ noun light work or hobbies used as a means of treatment, especially for physically challenged or mentally ill people, to promote independence during the recovery period after an illness or operation

**occur** /əˈkɜː/ verb **1.** to take place ○ one of the most frequently occurring types of tumour ○ Thrombosis occurred in the artery. ○ a form of glaucoma which occurs in infants. **2.** to come into a person's mind ○ It occurred to her that she might be pregnant. (NOTE: **occurring – occurred**)

**occurrence** /əˈkʌrəns/ noun something that takes place ○ Neuralgia is a common occurrence after shingles.

**OCD** abbr obsessive-compulsive disorder

**ochronosis** /ˌɒkrəʊˈnəʊsɪs/ noun a condition in which cartilage, ligaments and other fibrous tissue become dark as a result of a metabolic disorder, and in which the urine turns black on exposure to air

**ocular** /ˈɒkjʊlə/ adjective referring to the eye ○ Opticians are trained to detect all kinds of ocular imbalance.

**ocular dominance** /ˌɒkjʊlə ˈdɒmɪnəns/ noun a condition in which a person uses one eye more than the other

**ocular prosthesis** /ˌɒkjʊlə prɒsˈθiːsɪs/ noun a false eye

**oculi** /ˈɒkjʊlaɪ/ ♦ orbicularis oculi

**oculist** /ˈɒkjʊlɪst/ noun a qualified physician or surgeon who specialises in the treatment of eye disorders

**oculo-** /ɒkjʊləʊ/ prefix eye

**oculogyric** /ˌɒkjʊləʊˈdʒaɪrɪk/ adjective causing eye movements

**oculomotor** /ˌɒkjʊləʊˈməʊtə/ adjective referring to movements of the eyeball

**oculomotor nerve** /ˌɒkjʊləʊˈməʊtə nɜːv/ noun the third cranial nerve which controls the eyeballs and eyelids

**oculonasal** /ˌɒkjʊləʊˈneɪz(ə)l/ adjective referring to both the eye and the nose

**oculoplethysmography** /ˌɒkjʊləʊˌpleθɪz ˈmɒɡrəfi/ noun measurement of the pressure inside the eyeball

**OD** abbr overdose

**o.d.** adverb (written on a prescription) every day. Full form **omni die**

**ODA** abbr operating department assistant

**odont-** /ɒdɒnt/ prefix same as **odonto-** (used before vowels)

**odontalgia** /ˌɒdɒnˈtældʒə/ noun same as **toothache**

**odontitis** /ˌɒdɒnˈtaɪtɪs/ noun inflammation of the pulpy interior of a tooth

**odonto-** /ɒdɒntəʊ/ prefix tooth

**odontoid** /ɒˈdɒntɔɪd/ adjective similar to a tooth, especially in shape

**odontoid process** /ɒˌdɒntɔɪd ˈprəʊses/ noun a projecting part of a vertebra, shaped like a tooth

**odontology** /ˌɒdɒnˈtɒlədʒi/ noun the study of teeth and associated structures, and their disorders

**odontoma** /ˌɒdɒnˈtəʊmə/, **odontome** /ˈɒdɒntəʊm/ noun **1.** a structure like a tooth which has an unusual arrangement of its component tissues **2.** a solid or cystic tumour derived from cells concerned with the development of a tooth (NOTE: The plural is **odontomas** or **odontomata**.)

**odourless** /ˈəʊdələs/ adjective with no smell

**odyn-** /ɒdɪn/ prefix same as **odyno-** (used before vowels)

**-odynia** /ədɪniə/ suffix pain

**odyno-** /ɒdɪnəʊ/ prefix pain

**odynophagia** /ɒˌdɪnəˈfeɪdʒə/ noun a condition in which pain occurs when food is swallowed

**oedema** /ɪˈdiːmə/ noun the swelling of part of the body caused by accumulation of fluid in the intercellular tissue spaces ○ Her main problem is oedema of the feet. Also called **dropsy**. ◊ **tumescence** (NOTE: The US spelling is **edema**.)

**oedematous** /ɪˈdemətəs/ adjective referring to oedema (NOTE: The US spelling is **edematous**.)

**Oedipus complex** /ˈiːdɪpəs ˌkɒmpleks/ noun (in Freudian psychology) a condition in which a boy feels sexually attracted to his mother and sees his father as an obstacle

**oesophag-** /iːsɒfədʒ/ prefix same as **oesophago-** (used before vowels)

**oesophageal** /iːˌsɒfəˈdʒiːəl/ *adjective* referring to the oesophagus (NOTE: The US spelling is **esophageal**.)

**oesophageal hiatus** /iːˌsɒfəˌdʒiːəl haɪˈeɪtəs/ *noun* the opening in the diaphragm through which the oesophagus passes

**oesophageal varices** /iːˌsɒfəˌdʒiːəl ˈværɪsiːz/ *plural noun* varicose veins in the oesophagus

**oesophagectomy** /iːˌsɒfəˈdʒektəmi/ *noun* a surgical operation to remove part of the oesophagus (NOTE: The plural is **oesophagectomies**.)

**oesophagi** /iːˈsɒfəgi/ plural of **oesophagus**

**oesophagitis** /iːˌsɒfəˈdʒaɪtɪs/ *noun* inflammation of the oesophagus, caused by acid juices from the stomach or by infection

**oesophago-** /iːsɒfəgəʊ/ *prefix* oesophagus (NOTE: The US spelling is **esophago-**.)

**oesophagocele** /iːˈsɒfəgəʊsiːl/ *noun* a condition in which the mucous membrane lining the oesophagus protrudes through the wall

**oesophagogastroduodenoscopy** /iːˌsɒfəgəʊˌgæstrəʊˌdjuːəʊdəˈnɒskəpi/ *noun* a surgical operation in which a tube is put down into the oesophagus so that the doctor can examine it, the stomach and the duodenum. Abbr **OGD** (NOTE: The plural is **oesophagogastroduodenoscopies**.)

**oesophagojejunostomy** /iːˌsɒfəgəʊdʒɪˌdʒuːˈnɒstəmi/ *noun* a surgical operation to create a junction between the jejunum and the oesophagus after the stomach has been removed (NOTE: The plural is **oesophagojejunostomies**.)

**oesophagoscope** /iːˈsɒfəgəʊskəʊp/ *noun* a thin tube with a light at the end, which is passed down the oesophagus to examine it

**oesophagoscopy** /iːˌsɒfəˈgɒskəpi/ *noun* an examination of the oesophagus with an oesophagoscope (NOTE: The plural is **oesophagoscopies**.)

**oesophagostomy** /iːˌsɒfəˈgɒstəmi/ *noun* a surgical operation to make an opening in the oesophagus to allow the person to be fed, usually after an operation on the pharynx (NOTE: The plural is **oesophagostomies**.)

**oesophagotomy** /iːˌsɒfəˈgɒtəmi/ *noun* a surgical operation to make an opening in the oesophagus to remove something which is blocking it (NOTE: The plural is **oesophagotomies**.)

**oesophagus** /iːˈsɒfəgəs/ *noun* a tube down which food passes from the pharynx to the stomach (NOTE: The plural is **oesophagi**. The US spellings are **esophagus** and **esophagi**.)

**oestradiol** /ˌiːstrəˈdaɪɒl/ *noun* a type of oestrogen secreted by an ovarian follicle, which stimulates the development of secondary sexual characteristics in females at puberty (NOTE: A synthetic form of oestradiol is given as treatment for oestrogen deficiency. The US spelling is **estradiol**.)

**oestriol** /ˈiːstrɪɒl/ *noun* a placental hormone with oestrogenic properties, found in the urine of pregnant women (NOTE: The US spelling is **estriol**.)

**oestrogen** /ˈiːstrədʒən/ *noun* any steroid hormone which stimulates the development of secondary sexual characteristics in females at puberty (NOTE: The US spelling is **estrogen**.)

COMMENT: Synthetic oestrogens form most oral contraceptives, and are also used in the treatment of menstrual and menopausal disorders.

**oestrogenic hormone** /ˌiːstrədʒenɪk ˈhɔːməʊn/ *noun* synthetic oestrogen used to treat conditions which develop during menopause (NOTE: The US spelling is **estrogenic hormone**.)

**oestrone** /ˈiːstrəʊn/ *noun* a type of oestrogen produced in the ovaries (NOTE: The US spelling is **estrone**.)

**official** /əˈfɪʃ(ə)l/ *adjective* **1.** accepted or permitted by an authority ○ *We need to undertake a review of the official procedures.* **2.** constituting an authority

**official drug** /əˌfɪʃ(ə)l ˈdrʌg/ *noun* any drug listed in the national pharmacopoeia

**officially** /əˈfɪʃ(ə)li/ *adverb* in a way that is approved by an authority ○ *officially listed as a dangerous drug*

**OGD** *abbr* oesophagogastroduodenoscopy

**OH nurse** /əʊ ˈeɪtʃ nɜːs/ *abbr* occupational health nurse

**-oid** /ɔɪd/ *suffix* like or related to

**oil** /ɔɪl/ *noun* a liquid which cannot be mixed with water (NOTE: There are three types of oil: fixed vegetable or animal oils, volatile oils and mineral oils.)

**oily** /ˈɔɪli/ *adjective* containing or resembling oil

**ointment** /ˈɔɪntmənt/ *noun* a smooth oily medicinal preparation which can be spread on the skin to soothe or to protect

**old age** /əʊld ˈeɪdʒ/ *noun* a period in a person's life, usually taken to be after the age of sixty-five

**oleaginous** /ˌəʊliˈædʒɪnəs/ *adjective* same as **oily**

**olecranon** /əʊˈlekrənɒn/, **olecranon process** /əʊˈlekrənɒn ˌprəʊsəs/ *noun* a curved projecting part at the end of the ulna at the elbow, which gives rise to a painful tingling sensation if hit by accident. Also called **funny bone**

**oleic** /əʊˈliːɪk/ *adjective* referring to oil

**oleic acid** /əʊˌliːɪk ˈæsɪd/ *noun* a fatty acid which is present in most oils

**oleo-** /əʊliəʊ/ *prefix* oil

**oleum** /ˈəʊliəm/ *noun* oil (*used in pharmacy*)

**olfaction** /ɒlˈfækʃən/ *noun* **1.** the sense of smell **2.** the way in which a person's sensory organs detect smells

**olfactory** /ɒlˈfækt(ə)ri/ *adjective* referring to the sense of smell

**olfactory area** /ɒlˌfækt(ə)ri ˈeəriə/ *noun* the part of the brain that registers smell

**olfactory bulb** /ɒlˈfækt(ə)ri bʌlb/ *noun* the end of the olfactory tract, where the processes of the sensory cells in the nose are linked to the fibres of the olfactory nerve

**olfactory cortex** /ɒlˌfækt(ə)ri ˈkɔːteks/ *noun* the parts of the cerebral cortex which receive information about smell

**olfactory nerve** /ɒlˈfækt(ə)ri nɜːv/ *noun* the first cranial nerve which controls the sense of smell

**olfactory tract** /ɒlˈfækt(ə)ri trækt/ *noun* a nerve tract which takes the olfactory nerve from the nose to the brain

**olig-** /ɒlɪg/ *prefix* same as **oligo-** (*used before vowels*)

**oligaemia** /ˌɒlɪˈɡiːmiə/ *noun* a condition in which a person has too little blood in his or her circulatory system (NOTE: The US spelling is **oligemia.**)

**oligo-** /ɒlɪɡəʊ/ *prefix* few or little

**oligodactylism** /ˌɒlɪɡəʊˈdæktɪlɪz(ə)m/ *noun* a congenital condition in which a baby is born without some fingers or toes

**oligodipsia** /ˌɒlɪɡəʊˈdɪpsiə/ *noun* a condition in which a person does not want to drink

**oligodontia** /ˌɒlɪɡəʊˈdɒnʃə/ *noun* a state in which most of the teeth are lacking

**oligohydramnios** /ˌɒlɪɡəʊhaɪˈdræmniəs/ *noun* a condition in which the amnion surrounding the fetus contains too little amniotic fluid

**oligomenorrhoea** /ˌɒlɪɡəʊmenəˈriːə/ *noun* a condition in which a person menstruates infrequently (NOTE: The US spelling is **oligomenorrhea.**)

**oligo-ovulation** /ˌɒlɪɡəʊ ˌɒvjʊˈleɪʃ(ə)n/ *noun* ovulation which does not occur as often as is usual

**oligospermia** /ɒlɪɡəʊˈspɜːmiə/ *noun* a condition in which there are too few spermatozoa in the semen

**oliguria** /ˌɒlɪˈɡjʊəriə/ *noun* a condition in which a person does not produce enough urine

**olive** /ˈɒlɪv/ *noun* **1.** the fruit of a tree, which gives an edible oil **2.** a swelling containing grey matter, on the side of the pyramid of the medulla oblongata

**-ology** /ɒlədʒi/ *suffix* area of study

**-olol** /əlɒl/ *suffix* beta blocker ○ *atenolol* ○ *propranolol hydrochloride*

**o.m.** *adverb* (*written on a prescription*) every morning. Full form **omni mane**

**-oma** /əʊmə/ *suffix* tumour

**Ombudsman** /ˈɒmbʊdzmən/ ♦ **Health Service Commissioner**

**oment-** /əʊment/ *prefix* omentum

**omenta** /əʊˈmentə/ plural of **omentum**

**omental** /əʊˈment(ə)l/ *adjective* referring to the omentum

**omentectomy** /ˌəʊmenˈtektəmi/ *noun* a surgical operation to remove part of the omentum (NOTE: The plural is **omentectomies.**)

**omentopexy** /əʊˈmentəpeksi/ *noun* a surgical operation to attach the omentum to the abdominal wall (NOTE: The plural is **omentopexies.**)

**omentum** /əʊˈmentəm/ *noun* a double fold of peritoneum hanging down over the intestines. Also called **epiploon** (NOTE: The plural is **omenta**. For other terms referring to the omentum see words beginning with **epiplo-**.)

COMMENT: The omentum is in two sections: the **greater omentum** which covers the intestines, and the **lesser omentum** which hangs between the liver and the stomach and the liver and the duodenum.

**omeprazole** /əʊˈmeprəzəʊl/ *noun* a drug which reduces the amount of acid released in the stomach, used in the treatment of ulcers and heartburn

**omphal-** /ɒmfəl/ *prefix* same as **omphalo-** (*used before vowels*)

**omphali** /ˈɒmfəli/ plural of **omphalus**

**omphalitis** /ˌɒmfəˈlaɪtɪs/ *noun* inflammation of the navel

**omphalo-** /ɒmfələʊ/ *prefix* navel

**omphalocele** /ˈɒmfələsiːl/ *noun* a hernia in which part of the intestine protrudes through the abdominal wall near the navel

**omphalus** /ˈɒmfələs/ *noun* a scar with a depression in the middle of the abdomen where the umbilical cord was detached after birth. Also called **navel, umbilicus** (NOTE: The plural is **omphali.**)

**-omycin** /əʊmaɪsɪn/ *suffix* macrolide drug ○ *erythromycin*

**o.n.** *adverb* (*written on a prescription*) every night. Full form **omni nocte**

**onanism** /ˈəʊnənɪz(ə)m/ *noun* same as **masturbation**

**Onchocerca** /ˌɒŋkəʊˈsɜːkə/ *noun* a genus of tropical parasitic threadworms

**onchocerciasis** /ˌɒŋkəʊsɜːˈkaɪəsɪs/ *noun* infestation with *Onchocerca* in which the larvae can move into the eye, causing river blindness

**onco-** /ɒŋkəʊ/ *prefix* tumour

**oncogene** /ˈɒŋkədʒiːn/ *noun* a part of the genetic system which causes malignant tumours to develop

'…all cancers may be reduced to fundamental mechanisms based on cancer risk genes or oncogenes within ourselves. An oncogene is a gene that encodes a protein that contributes to the malignant phenotype of the cell' [*British Medical Journal*]

**oncogenesis** /ˌɒŋkəˈdʒenəsɪs/ *noun* the origin and development of a tumour

**oncogenic** /ˌɒŋkəˈdʒenɪk/ *adjective* causing tumours to develop ○ *an oncogenic virus*

**oncologist** /ɒŋˈkɒlədʒɪst/ *noun* a doctor who specialises in oncology, especially cancer

**oncology** /ɒŋˈkɒlədʒi/ *noun* the scientific study of new growths, especially cancers

**oncolysis** /ɒŋˈkɒləsɪs/ *noun* the destruction of a tumour or of tumour cells

**oncometer** /ɒŋˈkɒmɪtə/ *noun* **1.** an instrument for measuring swelling in an arm or leg using changes in their blood pressure **2.** an instrument for measuring the variations in size of the kidney and other organs of the body

**oncotic** /ɒŋˈkɒtɪk/ *adjective* referring to a tumour

**ondansetron** /ɒnˈdænsɪtrɒn/ *noun* a drug which helps to prevent the production of serotonin, used to control nausea and vomiting caused by drug treatment and radiotherapy for cancer

**onset** /ˈɒnset/ *noun* the beginning of something ○ *The onset of the illness is marked by sudden high temperature.*

**ontogeny** /ɒnˈtɒdʒəni/ *noun* the origin and development of an individual organism

**onych-** /ɒnɪk/ *prefix* same as **onycho-** (*used before vowels*)

**onychauxis** /ˌɒnɪˈkɔːksɪs/ *noun* excessive growth of the nails of the fingers or toes

**onychia** /ɒˈnɪkiə/ *noun* an irregularity of the nails caused by inflammation of the matrix

**onycho-** /ɒnɪkəʊ/ *prefix* nails

**onychogryphosis** /ˌɒnɪkəʊɡrɪˈfəʊsɪs/ *noun* a condition in which the nails are bent or curved over the ends of the fingers or toes

**onycholysis** /ˌɒnɪˈkɒləsɪs/ *noun* a condition in which a nail becomes separated from its bed, without falling out

**onychomadesis** /ˌɒnɪkəʊməˈdiːsɪs/ *noun* a condition in which the nails fall out

**onychomycosis** /ˌɒnɪkəʊmaɪˈkəʊsɪs/ *noun* an infection of a nail with a fungus

**onychosis** /ˌɒnɪˈkəʊsɪs/ *noun* any disease of the nails (NOTE: The plural is **onychoses**.)

**o'nyong-nyong fever** /ˌəʊ ˈnjɒŋ ˌnjɒŋ ˌfiːvə/ *noun* an infectious virus disease prevalent in East Africa, spread by mosquitoes. The symptoms are high fever, inflammation of the lymph nodes and excruciating pains in the joints. Also called **joint-breaker fever**

**oo-** /əʊə/ *prefix* ovum or embryo

**oocyesis** /ˌəʊəsaɪˈiːsɪs/ *noun* a pregnancy which develops in the ovary (NOTE: The plural is **oocyeses**.)

**oocyte** /ˈəʊəsaɪt/ *noun* a cell which forms from an oogonium and becomes an ovum by meiosis

**oocyte donation** /ˌəʊəsaɪt dəʊˈneɪʃ(ə)n/ *noun* the transfer of oocytes from one woman

to another who cannot produce her own, so that she can have a baby. The oocytes are removed in a laparoscopy and fertilised in vitro.

**oogenesis** /ˌəʊəˈdʒenəsɪs/ *noun* the formation and development of ova

COMMENT: In oogenesis, an oogonium produces an oocyte, which develops through several stages to produce a mature ovum. Polar bodies are also formed which do not develop into ova.

**oogenetic** /ˌəʊədʒəˈnetɪk/ *adjective* referring to oogenesis

**oogonium** /ˌəʊəˈɡəʊniəm/ *noun* a cell produced at the beginning of the development of an ovum (NOTE: The plural is **oogonia**.)

**oophor-** /əʊəfəʊr/ *prefix* same as **oophoro-** (*used before vowels*)

**oophoralgia** /ˌəʊəfəˈrældʒə/ *noun* pain in the ovaries

**oophore** /ˈəʊəfɔː/ *noun* same as **ovary**

**oophorectomy** /ˌəʊəfəˈrektəmi/ *noun* a surgical operation to remove an ovary. Also called **ovariectomy** (NOTE: The plural is **oophorectomies**.)

**oophoritis** /ˌəʊəfəˈraɪtɪs/ *noun* inflammation in an ovary, which can be caused by mumps. Also called **ovaritis**

**oophoro-** /əʊɒfərəʊ/ *prefix* ovary

**oophorocystectomy** /əʊˌɒfərəʊsɪˈstektəmi/ *noun* a surgical operation to remove an ovarian cyst (NOTE: The plural is **oophorocystectomies**.)

**oophorocystosis** /əʊˌɒfərəʊsɪˈstəʊsɪs/ *noun* the development of one or more ovarian cysts

**oophoroma** /ˌəʊəfəˈrəʊmə/ *noun* a rare ovarian tumour, occurring in middle age (NOTE: The plural is **oophoromas** or **oophoromata**.)

**oophoron** /əʊˈɒfərɒn/ *noun* same as **ovary** (*technical*) (NOTE: The plural is **oophora**.)

**oophoropexy** /əʊˈɒfərəpeksi/ *noun* a surgical operation to attach an ovary (NOTE: The plural is **oophoropexies**.)

**oophorosalpingectomy** /əʊˌɒfərəˌsælpɪnˈdʒektəmi/ *noun* a surgical operation to remove an ovary and the Fallopian tube attached to it (NOTE: The plural is **oophorosalpingectomies**.)

**ooze** /uːz/ *verb* **1.** (*of pus, blood or other liquid*) to flow slowly **2.** to leak a substance such as pus or blood (NOTE: **oozing – oozed**)

**op** /ɒp/ *noun* an operation (*informal*)

**OP** *abbr* outpatient

**opacification** /əʊpæsɪfɪˈkeɪʃ(ə)n/ *noun* the fact of becoming opaque, as the lens does in a case of cataract

**opacity** /əʊˈpæsɪti/ *noun* **1.** the fact of not allowing light to pass through **2.** an area in the eye which is not clear (NOTE: The plural is **opacities**.)

**opaque** /əʊˈpeɪk/ *adjective* not allowing light to pass through. Opposite **transparent**

**open** /'əʊpən/ *adjective* not closed

**open-angle glaucoma** /ˌəʊpən ˌæŋg(ə)l glɔː'kəʊmə/ *noun* an unusually high pressure of fluid inside the eyeball caused by a blockage in the channel through which the aqueous humour drains. Also called **chronic glaucoma**

**open fracture** /ˌəʊpən 'fræktʃə/ *noun* same as **compound fracture**

**open-heart surgery** /ˌəʊpən 'hɑːt ˌsɜːdʒəri/ *noun* surgery to repair part of the heart or one of the coronary arteries performed while the heart has been bypassed and the blood is circulated by a pump

**opening** /'əʊp(ə)nɪŋ/ *noun* a place where something opens

**open visiting** /ˌəʊpən 'vɪzɪtɪŋ/ *noun* an arrangement in a hospital by which visitors can enter the wards at any time

**operable** /'ɒp(ə)rəb(ə)l/ *adjective* referring to a condition which can be treated by a surgical operation ○ *The cancer is still operable.*

**operant conditioning** /'ɒpərənt kənˌdɪʃ(ə)nɪŋ/ *noun* a form of learning which takes place when a piece of spontaneous behaviour is either reinforced by a reward or discouraged by punishment

**operate** /'ɒpəreɪt/ *verb* **1.** to function or work, or to make something function or work **2.** to treat a person for a condition by cutting open the body and removing a part which is diseased or repairing a part which is not functioning correctly ○ *The patient was operated on yesterday.* ○ *The surgeons decided to operate as the only way of saving the baby's life.* (NOTE: **operating – operated**)

**operating department** *noun* a hospital department specialising in surgical operations

**operating department assistant** /ˌɒpəreɪtɪŋ dɪˌpɑːtmənt ə'sɪstənt/ *noun* a person who works in an operating department. Abbr **ODA**

**operating microscope** /'ɒpəreɪtɪŋ ˌmaɪkrəskəʊp/ *noun* a special microscope with two eyepieces and a light, used in very delicate surgery

**operating room** *US* same as **operating theatre**. Abbr **OR**

**operating table** /'ɒpəreɪtɪŋ ˌteɪb(ə)l/ *noun* a special table on which the patient is placed to undergo a surgical operation

**operating theatre** /'ɒpəreɪtɪŋ ˌθɪətə/ *noun* a special room in a hospital, where surgical operations are carried out (NOTE: The US term is **operating room.**)

**operation** /ˌɒpə'reɪʃ(ə)n/ *noun* **1.** the way in which something operates **2.** a surgical procedure carried out to repair or remove a damaged body part ○ *She's had an operation on her foot.* ○ *The operation to remove the cataract was successful.* ○ *A team of surgeons performed the operation.* ○ *Heart operations are always difficult.* (NOTE: A surgeon **performs** or

**carries out** an operation **on** a patient.) **3.** the way in which a drug acts

**operative** /'ɒp(ə)rətɪv/ *adjective* taking place during a surgical operation. ◊ **peroperative, postoperative, preoperative**

**operator** /'ɒpəreɪtə/ *noun* **1.** someone whose job is to operate a machine or piece of equipment **2.** a surgeon who operates on people

**operculum** /ə'pɜːkjʊləm/ *noun* **1.** a part of the cerebral hemisphere which overlaps the insula **2.** a plug of mucus which can block the cervical canal during pregnancy (NOTE: The plural is **opercula** or **operculums.**)

**ophth-** /ɒfθ, ɒpθ/ *prefix* eye

**ophthalm-** /ɒfθælm, ɒpθælm/ *prefix* same as **ophthalmo-** (*used before vowels*)

**ophthalmectomy** /ˌɒfθæl'mektəmi/ *noun* a surgical operation to remove an eye (NOTE: The plural is **ophthalmectomies.**)

**ophthalmia** /ɒf'θælmiə/ *noun* inflammation of the eye

**ophthalmia neonatorum** /ɒfˌθælmiə niːəʊneɪ'tɔːrəm/ *noun* conjunctivitis of a newborn baby, beginning 21 days after birth, caused by infection in the birth canal

**ophthalmic** /ɒf'θælmɪk/ *adjective* referring to the eye

**ophthalmic nerve** /ɒf'θælmɪk nɜːv/ *noun* a branch of the trigeminal nerve, supplying the eyeball, the upper eyelid, the brow and one side of the scalp

**ophthalmic optician** /ɒfˌθælmɪk ɒp'tɪʃ(ə)n/, **ophthalmic practitioner** *noun* same as **optician**

**ophthalmic surgeon** /ɒfˌθælmɪk 'sɜːdʒən/ *noun* a surgeon who specialises in surgery to treat eye disorders

**ophthalmitis** /ˌɒfθæl'maɪtɪs/ *noun* inflammation of the eye

**ophthalmo-** /ɒfθælməʊ, ɒpθælməʊ/ *prefix* eye or eyeball

**ophthalmological** /ɒfˌθælmə'lɒdʒɪk(ə)l/ *adjective* referring to ophthalmology

**ophthalmologist** /ˌɒfθæl'mɒlədʒɪst/ *noun* a doctor who specialises in the study of the eye and its diseases. Also called **eye specialist**

**ophthalmology** /ˌɒfθæl'mɒlədʒi/ *noun* the study of the eye and its diseases

**ophthalmoplegia** /ˌɒfθælmə'pliːdʒə/ *noun* paralysis of the muscles of the eye

**ophthalmoscope** /ɒf'θælməskəʊp/ *noun* an instrument containing a bright light and small lenses, used by a doctor to examine the inside of an eye

**ophthalmoscopy** /ˌɒfθæl'mɒskəpi/ *noun* an examination of the inside of an eye using an ophthalmoscope (NOTE: The plural is **ophthalmoscopies.**)

**ophthalmotomy** /ˌɒfθæl'mɒtəmi/ *noun* a surgical operation to make a cut in the eyeball (NOTE: The plural is **ophthalmotomies.**)

**ophthalmotonometer** /ˌɒfθælmətəˈnɒmɪtə/ *noun* an instrument which measures pressure inside the eye

**-opia** /əʊpiə/ *suffix* eye condition

**opiate** /ˈəʊpiət/ *noun* a sedative which is pre- pared from opium, e.g. morphine or codeine

**opinion** /əˈpɪnjən/ *noun* what a person thinks about something ○ *What's the surgeon's opin- ion of the case?* ○ *The doctor asked the con- sultant for his opinion as to the best method of treatment.*

**opioid** /ˈəʊpiɔɪd/ *adjective* based on opium ○ *Codeine is an opioid analgesic.*

**opistho-** /ɒpɪsθəʊ/ *prefix* backbone

**opisthotonos** /ˌɒpɪsˈθɒtənəs/ *noun* a spasm of the body in which the spine is arched back- wards, occurring, e.g., in people with tetanus

**opium** /ˈəʊpiəm/ *noun* a substance made from poppies which is used in the preparation of codeine and heroin

**opponens** /əˈpəʊnənz/ *noun* one of a group of muscles which control the movements of the fingers, especially one which allows the thumb and little finger to come together

**opportunist** /ˌɒpəˈtjuːnɪst/, **opportunistic** /ˌɒpətjuːˈnɪstɪk/ *adjective* referring to a para- site or microorganism which takes advantage of the host's weakened state to cause infection

**opposition** /ˌɒpəˈzɪʃ(ə)n/ *noun* **1.** hostility towards something **2.** a movement of the hand muscles in which the tip of the thumb is made to touch the tip of another finger so as to hold something

**opsonic index** /ɒpˌsɒnɪk ˈɪndeks/ *noun* a number which gives the strength of a person's serum reaction to bacteria

**opsonin** /ˈɒpsənɪn/ *noun* a substance, usual- ly an antibody, in blood which sticks to the sur- face of bacteria and helps to destroy them

**optic** /ˈɒptɪk/ *adjective* referring to the eye or to sight

**optical** /ˈɒptɪk(ə)l/ *adjective* **1.** same as **optic 2.** relating to the visible light spectrum

**optical fibre** /ˌɒptɪk(ə)l ˈfaɪbə/ *noun* an arti- ficial fibre which can carry light or images

**optical illusion** /ˌɒptɪk(ə)l ɪˈluːʒ(ə)n/ *noun* something which is seen wrongly so that it ap- pears to be something else

**optic chiasma** /ˌɒptɪk kaɪˈæzmə/ *noun* a structure where some of the optic nerves from each eye partially cross each other in the hy- pothalamus

**optic disc** /ˈɒptɪk dɪsk/ *noun* the point on the retina where the optic nerve starts. Also called **optic papilla**

**optic fundus** /ˌɒptɪk ˈfʌndəs/ *noun* the back part of the inside of the eye, opposite the lens

**optician** /ɒpˈtɪʃ(ə)n/ *noun* a qualified person who specialises in making glasses and in test- ing eyes and prescribing lenses. Also called **ophthalmic optician** (NOTE: In US English, an

**optician** is a technician who makes lenses and fits glasses, but cannot test patient's eyesight.)

COMMENT: In the UK qualified opticians must be registered by the General Optical Council before they can practise.

**optic nerve** /ˈɒptɪk nɜːv/ *noun* the second cranial nerve which transmits the sensation of sight from the eye to the brain. See illustration at EYE in Supplement

**optic neuritis** /ˌɒptɪk njʊˈraɪtɪs/ *noun* same as **retrobulbar neuritis**

**optic papilla** /ˌɒptɪk pəˈpɪlə/ *noun* same as **optic disc**

**optic radiation** /ˌɒptɪk ˌreɪdiˈeɪʃ(ə)n/ *noun* a nerve tract which takes the optic impulses from the optic tract to the visual cortex

**optics** /ˈɒptɪks/ *noun* the study of the visible light spectrum and sight

**optic tract** /ˌɒptɪk ˈtrækt/ *noun* a nerve tract which takes the optic nerve from the optic ch- iasma to the optic radiation

**opto-** /ɒptəʊ/ *prefix* sight

**optometer** /ɒpˈtɒmɪtə/ *noun* same as **refrac- tometer**

**optometrist** /ɒpˈtɒmətrɪst/ *noun mainly US* a person who specialises in testing eyes and prescribing lenses

**optometry** /ɒpˈtɒmətri/ *noun* the testing of eyes and prescribing of lenses to correct sight

**-oquine** /əkwɪn/ *suffix* antimalarial drug ○ *chloroquine*

**OR** *abbr US* operating room

**ora** /ˈɔːrə/ *plural noun* plural of **os** *noun* 2

**oral** /ˈɔːrəl/ *adjective* **1.** referring to the mouth **2.** referring to medication that is swallowed ○ *an oral contraceptive* Compare **enteral, parenteral**

**oral cavity** /ˌɔːrəl ˈkævɪti/ *noun* the mouth

**oral contraceptive** /ˌɔːrəl ˌkɒntrəˈseptɪv/ *noun* a contraceptive pill which is swallowed

**oral hygiene** /ˌɔːrəl ˈhaɪdʒiːn/ *noun* the practice of keeping the mouth clean by gar- gling and mouthwashes

**orally** /ˈɔːrəli/ *adverb* by swallowing ○ *not to be taken orally*

**oral medication** /ˌɔːrəl ˌmedɪˈkeɪʃ(ə)n/ *noun* medication which is taken by swallowing

**oral rehydration solution** /ˌɔːrəl ˌriːhaɪ ˈdreɪʃ(ə)n səˌluːʃ(ə)n/ *noun* a liquid given as a drink to correct the water, mineral and nutri- tional deficiencies in a person who is affected by dehydration

**oral rehydration therapy** /ˌɔːrəl ˌriːhaɪ ˈdreɪʃ(ə)n ˌθerəpi/ *noun* the administration of a simple glucose and electrolyte solution to treat acute diarrhoea, particularly in children, which has greatly reduced the number of deaths from dehydration. Abbr **ORT**

**oral thermometer** /ˌɔːrəl θəˈmɒmɪtə/ *noun* a thermometer which is put into the mouth to take someone's temperature

**orbicularis** /ɔːˌbɪkjʊˈleərɪs/ *noun* a circular muscle in the face

**orbicularis oculi** /ɔːˌbɪkjʊˌleərɪs ˈɒkjʊlaɪ/ *noun* a muscle which opens and closes the eye

**orbicularis oris** /ɔːˌbɪkjʊˌleərɪs ˈɔːrɪs/ *noun* a muscle which closes the lips tight

**orbit** /ˈɔːbɪt/ *noun* the hollow bony depression in the front of the skull in which each eye and lacrimal gland are situated. Also called **eye socket**

**orbital** /ˈɔːbɪt(ə)l/ *adjective* referring to the orbit

**orchi-** /ɔːkɪ/ *prefix* testis

**orchidalgia** /ˌɔːkɪˈdældʒə/ *noun* a neuralgic-type pain in a testis

**orchidectomy** /ˌɔːkɪˈdektəmi/ *noun* a surgical operation to remove a testis (NOTE: The plural is **orchidectomies**.)

**orchidopexy** /ˈɔːkɪdəʊˌpeksi/ *noun* a surgical operation to place an undescended testis in the scrotum. Also called **orchiopexy** (NOTE: The plural is **orchidopexies**.)

**orchidotomy** /ˌɔːkɪˈdɒtəmi/ *noun* a surgical operation to make a cut into a testis (NOTE: The plural is **orchidotomies**.)

**orchiepididymitis** /ˌɔːkiˌepɪdɪdɪˈmaɪtɪs/ *noun* a condition in which a testicle and its epididymis become swollen

**orchiopexy** /ˈɔːkiəʊˌpeksi/ *noun* same as **orchidopexy** (NOTE: The plural is **orchiopexies**.)

**orchis** /ˈɔːkɪs/ *noun* a testis

**orchitis** /ɔːˈkaɪtɪs/ *noun* inflammation of the testes, characterised by hypertrophy, pain and a sensation of weight

**orderly** /ˈɔːdəli/ *noun* a person who does general work in a hospital (NOTE: The plural is **orderlies**.)

**Orem's model** /ˈɔːrəmz ˌmɒd(ə)l/ *noun* a modern model for nursing which focuses on a person's ability to perform self-care, defined as activities which individuals initiate and perform on their own behalf to maintain life, health and well-being

**organ** /ˈɔːgən/ *noun* a part of the body which is distinct from other parts and has a particular function, e.g. the liver, an eye or ovaries

**organic** /ɔːˈgænɪk/ *adjective* **1.** referring to organs in the body **2.** coming from an animal, plant or other organism **3.** referring to food which has been cultivated naturally, without certain fertilisers or pesticides

**organically** /ɔːˈgænɪkli/ *adverb* in a natural or apparently natural way

**organic disease** /ɔːˌgænɪk dɪˈziːz/, **organic disorder** /ɔːˌgænɪk dɪsˈɔːdə/ *noun* a disease or disorder associated with physical changes in one or more organs of the body

**organisation** /ˌɔːgənaɪˈzeɪʃ(ə)n/, **organization** *noun* **1.** a group of people set up for a particular purpose **2.** the planning or arranging of something ○ *the organisation of the rota* **3.** the

way in which the component parts of something are arranged

**organism** /ˈɔːgənɪz(ə)m/ *noun* any single plant, animal, bacterium, fungus or other living thing

**organo-** /ɔːgənəʊ, ɔːgænəʊ/ *prefix* organ

**organ of Corti** /ˌɔːgən əv ˈkɔːti/ *noun* a membrane in the cochlea which takes sounds and converts them into impulses sent to the brain along the auditory nerve. Also called **spiral organ** [Described 1851. After Marquis Alfonso Corti (1822–88), Italian anatomist and histologist.]

**organotherapy** /ˌɔːgənəʊˈθerəpi/ *noun* the treatment of a disease by using an extract from the organ of an animal, e.g. using liver extract to treat anaemia

**organ transplant** /ˈɔːgən ˌtrænsplɑːnt/ *noun* a surgical operation to transplant an organ from one person to another

**orgasm** /ˈɔːgæz(ə)m/ *noun* the climax of the sexual act, when a person experiences a moment of great excitement

**oriental sore** /ˌɔːrient(ə)l ˈsɔː/ *noun* a skin disease of tropical countries caused by the parasite *Leishmania*. ◊ **leishmaniasis**

**orifice** /ˈɒrɪfɪs/ *noun* an opening in the body, e.g. the mouth or anus

**origin** /ˈɒrɪdʒɪn/ *noun* **1.** the source or beginning of something **2.** a place where a muscle is attached, or where the branch of a nerve or blood vessel begins

**original** /əˈrɪdʒən(ə)l/ *adjective* as before a change was made ○ *The surgeon was able to move the organ back to its original position.*

**originate** /əˈrɪdʒɪneɪt/ *verb* to start in a place, or make something start ○ *drugs which originated in the tropics* ○ *The treatment originated in China.* (NOTE: **originating – originated**)

**oris** /ˈɔːrɪs/ *noun* ◆ **cancrum oris, orbicularis oris**

**ornithine** /ˈɔːnɪθaɪn/ *noun* an amino acid produced by the liver

**ornithosis** /ˌɔːnɪˈθəʊsɪs/ *noun* a disease of birds which can be passed to humans as a form of pneumonia

**oro-** /ɔːrəʊ/ *prefix* mouth

**orogenital** /ˌɔːrəʊˈdʒenɪt(ə)l/ *adjective* relating to both the mouth and the genitals

**oropharynx** /ˌɔːrəʊˈfærɪŋks/ *noun* a part of the pharynx below the soft palate at the back of the mouth (NOTE: The plural is **oropharynxes** or **oropharynges**.)

**ORT** *abbr* oral rehydration therapy

**ortho-** /ɔːθəʊ/ *prefix* correct or straight

**orthodiagraph** /ˌɔːθəʊˈdaɪəgrɑːf/ *noun* an X-ray photograph of an organ taken using only a thin stream of X-rays which allows accurate measurements of the organ to be made

**orthodontia** /ˌɔːθəˈdɒnʃə/ *noun US* same as **orthodontics**

**orthodontic** /ˌɔːθəʊˈdɒntɪk/ adjective correcting badly formed or placed teeth ○ He had to undergo a course of orthodontic treatment.

**orthodontics** /ˌɔːθəʊˈdɒntɪks/ noun a branch of dentistry which deals with correcting badly placed teeth (NOTE: The US term is **orthodontia**.)

**orthodontist** /ˌɔːθəʊˈdɒntɪst/ noun a dental surgeon who specialises in correcting badly placed teeth

**orthopaedic** /ˌɔːθəˈpiːdɪk/ adjective 1. referring to treatment which corrects badly formed bones or joints 2. referring to or used in orthopaedics (NOTE: The US spelling is **orthopedic**.)

**orthopaedic collar** /ˌɔːθəˈpiːdɪk ˈkɒlə/ noun a special strong collar to support the head of a person with neck injuries or a condition such as cervical spondylosis

**orthopaedic hospital** /ˌɔːθəpiːdɪk ˈhɒspɪt(ə)l/ noun a hospital which specialises in operations to correct badly formed joints or bones

**orthopaedics** /ˌɔːθəˈpiːdɪks/ noun a branch of surgery dealing with irregularities, diseases and injuries of the locomotor system (NOTE: The US spelling is **orthopedics**.)

**orthopaedic surgeon** /ˌɔːθəpiːdɪk ˈsɜːdʒən/ noun a surgeon who specialises in orthopaedics

**orthopaedist** /ˌɔːθəˈpiːdɪst/ noun a surgeon who specialises in orthopaedics (NOTE: The US spelling is **orthopedist**.)

**orthopnoea** /ˌɔːθəpˈniːə/ noun a condition in which a person has great difficulty in breathing while lying down. ◊ **dyspnoea** (NOTE: The US spelling is **orthopnea**.)

**orthopnoeic** /ˌɔːθəpˈniːɪk/ adjective referring to orthopnoea (NOTE: The US spelling is **orthopneic**.)

**orthopsychiatry** /ˌɔːθəʊsaɪˈkaɪətri/ noun the science and treatment of behavioural and personality disorders

**orthoptics** /ɔːˈθɒptɪks/ noun the study of methods used to treat squints

**orthoptist** /ɔːˈθɒptɪst/ noun an eye specialist, working in an eye hospital, who treats squints and other disorders of eye movement

**orthoptoscope** /ɔːˈθɒptəskəʊp/ noun same as **amblyoscope**

**orthosis** /ɔːˈθəʊsɪs/ noun a device which is fitted to the outside of the body to support a weakness or correct a malformation, e.g. a surgical collar or leg brace (NOTE: The plural is **orthoses**.)

**orthostatic** /ˌɔːθəˈstætɪk/ adjective referring to the position of the body when standing up straight

**orthostatic hypotension** /ˌɔːθəstætɪk haɪpəʊˈtenʃən/ noun a common condition where the blood pressure drops when a person stands up suddenly, causing dizziness

**orthotics** /ɔːˈθɒtɪks/ plural noun the branch of medical engineering which deals with the design and fitting of devices such as braces in the treatment of orthopaedic disorders

**orthotist** /ˈɔːθətɪst/ noun a qualified person who fits orthoses

**Ortolani's sign** /ˌɔːtəˈlɑːniz saɪn/, **Ortolani manoeuvre** /ˌɔːtəˈlɑːni məˌnuːvə/, **Ortolani's test** /ˌɔːtəˈlɑːniz test/ noun a test for congenital dislocation of the hip in babies aged 6–12, in which the hip makes sharp sounds if the joint is rotated [Described 1937. After Marius Ortolani, Italian orthopaedic surgeon.]

**os** /ɒs/ noun (technical) 1. a bone (NOTE: The plural is **ossa**.) 2. the mouth (NOTE: The plural is **ora**.)

**OSA** abbr obstructive sleep apnoea

**oscillation** /ˌɒsɪˈleɪʃ(ə)n/ noun 1. the action of moving backwards and forwards between two points at a regular speed 2. a single movement between two points

**oscilloscope** /ɒˈsɪləskəʊp/ noun a device which produces a visual record of an electrical current on a screen using a cathode ray tube. It is used in the testing of electronic equipment and in measuring electrical impulses of the heart or the brain.

**osculum** /ˈɒskjʊləm/ noun a small opening or pore (NOTE: The plural is **oscula**.)

**-osis** /əʊsɪs/ suffix disease

**Osler's nodes** /ˈɒsləz nəʊdz/ plural noun tender swellings at the ends of fingers and toes in people who have subacute bacterial endocarditis [Described 1885. After Sir William Osler (1849–1919), Professor of Medicine in Montreal, Philadelphia, Baltimore and then Oxford.]

**osm-** /ɒzm/ prefix 1. smell 2. osmosis

**osmoreceptor** /ˌɒzməʊrɪˈseptə/ noun a cell in the hypothalamus which checks the level of osmotic pressure in the blood by altering the secretion of ADH and regulates the amount of water in the blood

**osmosis** /ɒzˈməʊsɪs/ noun the movement of a solvent from one part of the body through a semipermeable membrane to another part where there is a higher concentration of molecules

**osmotic pressure** /ɒzˌmɒtɪk ˈpreʃə/ noun the pressure required to stop the flow of a solvent through a membrane

**ossa** /ˈɒsə/ plural of **os** noun 1

**osseous** /ˈɒsɪəs/ adjective referring to or resembling bone

**osseous labyrinth** /ˌɒsɪəs ˈlæbərɪnθ/ noun same as **bony labyrinth**

**ossicle** /ˈɒsɪk(ə)l/ noun a small bone

COMMENT: The auditory ossicles pick up the vibrations from the eardrum and transmit them through the oval window to the cochlea in the inner ear. The three bones are articulated together; the stapes is attached to the membrane of the oval window, the malleus to the eardrum, and the incus lies between the other two.

**ossification** /ˌɒsɪfɪˈkeɪʃ(ə)n/ *noun* the formation of bone. Also called **osteogenesis**

**ossium** /ˈɒsɪəm/ ♦ fragilitas ossium

**ost-** /ɒst/ *prefix* same as **osteo-** (used before vowels)

**ostectomy** /ɒˈstektəmi/ *noun* a surgical operation in which a bone, or a piece of bone, is removed (NOTE: The plural is **ostectomies**.)

**osteitis** /ˌɒstiˈaɪtɪs/ *noun* inflammation of a bone due to injury or infection

**osteitis deformans** /ˌɒstiˌaɪtɪs diː ˈfɔːmənz/ *noun* a disease which gradually softens bones in the spine, legs and skull, so that they become curved. Also called **Paget's disease**

**osteitis fibrosis cystica** /ˌɒstiaɪtɪs faɪ ˌbrəʊsɪs ˈsɪstɪkə/ *noun* a generalised weakness of bones, caused by excessive activity of the thyroid gland and associated with formation of cysts, in which bone tissue is replaced by fibrous tissue. Also called **von Recklinghausen's disease** (NOTE: The localised form is **osteitis fibrosis localista**.)

**osteo-** /ɒstiəʊ/ *prefix* bone

**osteoarthritis** /ˌɒstiəʊɑːˈθraɪtɪs/ *noun* a degenerative disease of middle-aged and elderly people characterised by inflamed joints which become stiff and painful. Also called **osteoarthrosis**

**osteoarthropathy** /ˌɒstiəʊɑːˈθrɒpəθi/ *noun* a disease of the bone and cartilage at a joint, particularly the ankles, knees or wrists, associated with carcinoma of the bronchi

**osteoarthrosis** /ˌɒstiəʊɑːˈθrəʊsɪs/ *noun* same as **osteoarthritis**

**osteoarthrotomy** /ˌɒstiəʊɑːˈθrɒtəmi/ *noun* a surgical operation to remove the articular end of a bone (NOTE: The plural is **osteoarthrotomies**.)

**osteoblast** /ˈɒstiəʊblæst/ *noun* a cell in an embryo which forms bone

**osteochondritis** /ˌɒstiəʊkɒnˈdraɪtɪs/ *noun* degeneration of the epiphyses

**osteochondritis dissecans** /ˌɒstiəʊkɒn ˌdraɪtɪs ˈdɪsəkænz/ *noun* a painful condition where pieces of articular cartilage become detached from the joint surface

**osteochondroma** /ˌɒstiəʊkənˈdrəʊmə/ *noun* a tumour containing both bony and cartilaginous cells (NOTE: The plural is **osteochondromas** or **osteochondromata**.)

**osteochondrosis** /ˌɒstiəʊkɒnˈdrəʊsɪs/ *noun* a disorder of cartilage and bone formation which affects the joints in children, causing pain and a limp, probably due to circulation disturbances to that part of the bone

**osteoclasia** /ˌɒstiəʊˈkleɪziə/, **osteoclasis** /ˌɒstiˈɒkləsɪs/ *noun* 1. destruction of bone tissue by osteoclasts 2. a surgical operation to

fracture or refracture bone to correct a deformity

**osteoclast** /ˈɒstiəʊklæst/ *noun* 1. a cell which destroys bone 2. a surgical instrument for breaking bones

**osteoclastoma** /ˌɒstiəʊklæˈstəʊmə/ *noun* a usually benign tumour occurring at the ends of long bones (NOTE: The plural is **osteoclastomas** or **osteoclastomata**.)

**osteocyte** /ˈɒstiəʊsaɪt/ *noun* a bone cell

**osteodystrophia** /ˌɒstiəʊdɪˈstrəʊfiə/, **osteodystrophy** /ˌɒstiəʊˈdɪstrəfi/ *noun* a bone disease, especially one caused by disorder of the metabolism

**osteogenesis** /ˌɒstiəʊˈdʒenəsɪs/ *noun* same as **ossification**

**osteogenesis imperfecta** /ˌɒstiəʊ ˌdʒenəsɪs ɪmpəˈfektə/ *noun* a congenital condition in which bones are brittle and break easily due to unusual bone formation. Also called **brittle bone disease**

**osteogenic** /ˌɒstiəʊˈdʒenɪk/ *adjective* made of or originating in bone tissue

**osteology** /ˌɒstiˈɒlədʒi/ *noun* the study of bones and their structure

**osteolysis** /ˌɒstiˈɒləsɪs/ *noun* 1. destruction of bone tissue by osteoclasts 2. loss of bone calcium

**osteolytic** /ˌɒstiəʊˈlɪtɪk/ *adjective* referring to osteolysis

**osteoma** /ˌɒstiˈəʊmə/ *noun* a benign tumour in a bone (NOTE: The plural is **osteomas** or **osteomata**.)

**osteomalacia** /ˌɒstiəʊməˈleɪʃə/ *noun* a condition in adults in which the bones become soft because of lack of calcium and Vitamin D, or limited exposure to sunlight

**osteomyelitis** /ˌɒstiəʊmaɪəˈlaɪtɪs/ *noun* inflammation of the interior of bone, especially the marrow spaces

**osteon** /ˈɒstiɒn/ *noun* same as **Haversian system**

**osteopath** /ˈɒstiəʊˌpæθ/ *noun* a person who practises osteopathy

**osteopathy** /ˌɒstiˈɒpəθi/ *noun* 1. the treatment of disorders by massage and manipulation of joints 2. any disease of bone (NOTE: The plural is **osteopathies**.)

**osteopetrosis** /ˌɒstiəʊpəˈtrəʊsɪs/ *noun* a disease of a group in which bones increase in density. Also called **marble bone disease**

**osteophony** /ˌɒstiˈɒfəni/ *noun* the conduction of sound by bone, as occurs in the ear. Also called **bone conduction**

**osteophyte** /ˈɒstiəʊfaɪt/ *noun* a bony growth

**osteoplastic necrotomy** /ˌɒstiəʊplæstɪk nekˈrɒtəmi/ *noun* a surgical operation to remove a piece of dead bone tissue

**osteoplasty** /ˈɒstiəʊplæsti/ *noun* plastic surgery on bones

**osteoporosis** /ˌɒstiəʊpɔːˈrəʊsɪs/ *noun* a condition in which the bones become thin, porous and brittle, due to low levels of oestrogen, lack of calcium and lack of physical exercise. Also called **brittle bone disease**

COMMENT: Osteoporosis mainly affects postmenopausal women, increasing the risk of fractures. Hormone replacement therapy is the most effective method of preventing osteoporosis though there are other risks to health from long-term use.

**osteosarcoma** /ˌɒstiəʊsɑːˈkəʊmə/ *noun* a malignant tumour of bone cells (NOTE: The plural is **osteosarcomas** or **osteosarcomata**.)

**osteosclerosis** /ˌɒstiəʊskləˈrəʊsɪs/ *noun* a condition in which the bony spaces become hardened as a result of persistent inflammation

**osteotome** /ˈɒstiəʊtəʊm/ *noun* a type of chisel used by surgeons to cut bone

**osteotomy** /ˌɒstiˈɒtəmi/ *noun* a surgical operation to cut a bone, especially to relieve pain in a joint (NOTE: The plural is **osteotomies**.)

**ostia** /ˈɒstiə/ plural of **ostium**

**ostium** /ˈɒstiəm/ *noun* an opening into a passage (NOTE: The plural is **ostia**.)

**ostomy** /ˈɒstəmi/ *noun* a colostomy or ileostomy (*informal*) (NOTE: The plural is **ostomies**.)

**-ostomy** /ɒstəmi/ *suffix* operation to make an opening

**OT** *abbr* occupational therapist

**ot-** /əʊt/ *prefix* same as **oto-** (*used before vowels*)

**otalgia** /əʊˈtældʒə/ *noun* same as **earache**

**OTC** *abbreviation* referring to medication which can be bought freely at a chemist's shop, and does not need a prescription. Full form **over the counter**

**OTC drug** /ˌəʊ tiː ˈsiː drʌg/ *noun* same as **over-the-counter drug**

**otic** /ˈəʊtɪk/ *adjective* referring to the ear

**otic ganglion** /ˌəʊtɪk ˈgæŋgliən/ *noun* a ganglion associated with the mandibular nerve where it leaves the skull

**otitis** /əʊˈtaɪtɪs/ *noun* inflammation of the ear

**otitis externa** /əʊˌtaɪtɪs ɪkˈstɜːnə/ *noun* inflammation of the external auditory meatus to the eardrum

**otitis interna** /əʊˌtaɪtɪs ɪnˈtɜːnə/ *noun* inflammation of the inner ear. Also called **labyrinthitis**

**otitis media** /əʊˌtaɪtɪs ˈmiːdiə/ *noun* an infection of the middle ear, usually accompanied by headaches and fever. Also called **middle ear infection, tympanitis**

**oto-** /əʊtəʊ/ *prefix* ear

**otolaryngologist** /ˌəʊtəʊlærɪŋˈgɒlədʒɪst/ *noun* a doctor who specialises in treatment of diseases of the ear and throat

**otolaryngology** /ˌəʊtəʊlærɪŋˈgɒlədʒi/ *noun* the study of diseases of the ear and throat

**otolith** /ˈəʊtəlɪθ/ *noun* a tiny piece of calcium carbonate attached to the hair cells in the saccule and utricle of the inner ear

**otolith organ** /ˌəʊtəlɪθ ˈɔːgən/ *noun* one of two pairs of sensory organs in the inner ear, the saccule and the utricle, which pass information to the brain about the position of the head

**otologist** /əʊˈtɒlədʒɪst/ *noun* a doctor who specialises in the study of the ear

**otology** /əʊˈtɒlədʒi/ *noun* the scientific study of the ear and its diseases

**-otomy** /ɒtəmi/ *suffix* an act of cutting into an organ or part of the body in a surgical operation

**otomycosis** /ˌəʊtəmaɪˈkəʊsɪs/ *noun* an infection of the external auditory meatus by a fungus

**otoplasty** /ˈəʊtəplæsti/ *noun* plastic surgery of the external ear to repair damage or deformity

**otorhinolaryngologist** /ˌəʊtəʊˌraɪnəʊˌlærɪŋˈgɒlədʒɪst/ *noun* a doctor who specialises in the study of the ear, nose and throat

**otorhinolaryngology** /ˌəʊtəʊˌraɪnəʊˌlærɪŋˈgɒlədʒi/ *noun* the study of the ear, nose and throat. Also called **ENT**

**otorrhagia** /ˌəʊtəˈreɪdʒə/ *noun* bleeding from the external ear

**otorrhoea** /ˌəʊtəˈriːə/ *noun* the discharge of pus from the ear (NOTE: The US spelling is **otorrhea**.)

**otosclerosis** /ˌəʊtəʊskləˈrəʊsɪs/ *noun* a condition in which the ossicles in the middle ear become thicker and the stapes becomes fixed to the oval window leading to deafness

**otoscope** /ˈəʊtəskəʊp/ *noun* same as **auriscope**

**otospongiosis** /ˌəʊtəˌspʌndʒiˈəʊsɪs/ *noun* the formation of spongy bone in the labyrinth of the ear which occurs in otosclerosis

**Otosporin** /ˈəʊtəspɔːrɪn/ *noun* a trade name for ear drops containing hydrocortisone, neomycin and polymyxin

**ototoxic** /ˌəʊtəˈtɒksɪk/ *adjective* referring to a drug or an effect which is damaging to organs or nerves involved in hearing or balance

**outbreak** /ˈaʊtbreɪk/ *noun* a series of cases of a disease which starts suddenly ○ *There was an outbreak of typhoid fever* or *a typhoid outbreak.*

**outcome** /ˈaʊtkʌm/ *noun* **1.** what happens as the result of something **2.** a measure of the result of an intervention or treatment, e.g. the mortality rate following different methods of surgery ○ *medical outcomes*

**outer** /ˈaʊtə/ *adjective* outside or external

**outer ear** /ˌaʊtər ˈɪə/ *noun* the part of the ear which is on the outside of the head, together with the passage leading to the eardrum. Also called **external ear**

**outer pleura** /ˌaʊtə ˈplʊərə/ *noun* same as **parietal pleura**

**outlet** /ˈaʊtlet/ *noun* an opening or channel through which something can go out

**out-of-body experience** /ˌaʊt əv ˈbɒdi ɪk ˌspɪəriəns/ *noun* an occasion when a person feels as though they have left their body and, often, travelled along a tunnel towards a bright light (NOTE: It may happen after anaesthesia, perhaps caused by the brain not having enough oxygen.)

**outpatient** /ˈaʊtpeɪʃ(ə)nt/ *noun* someone who comes to a hospital for treatment but does not stay overnight ○ *She goes for treatment as an outpatient.* Abbr **OP**. Compare **inpatient**

**outpatient department** /ˈaʊtpeɪʃ(ə)nt dɪ ˌpɑːtmənt/, **outpatients' department** /ˈaʊt peɪʃ(ə)nts dɪˌpɑːtmənt/, **outpatients' clinic** /ˈaʊtpeɪʃ(ə)nts ˌklɪnɪk/ *noun* a department of a hospital which deals with outpatients

**outreach** /ˈaʊtriːtʃ/ *noun* services provided for patients or the public in general, outside a hospital or clinic

**ova** /ˈəʊvə/ plural of **ovum**

**oval window** /ˈəʊv(ə)l ˌwɪndəʊ/ *noun* an oval opening between the middle ear and the inner ear. Also called **fenestra ovalis**. See illustration at **EAR** in Supplement

**ovar-** /ˈəʊvər/ *prefix* same as **ovari-** (*used before vowels*)

**ovaralgia** /ˌəʊvəˈrældʒə/ *noun* pain in the ovaries. Also called **ovarialgia**

**ovari-** /ˈəʊvəri/ *prefix* ovaries

**ovarialgia** /ˌəʊveəriˈældʒə/ *noun* same as **ovaralgia**

**ovarian** /əʊˈveəriən/ *adjective* referring to the ovaries

**ovarian cancer** /əʊˌveəriən ˈkænsə/ *noun* a malignant tumour of the ovary, which occurs especially after the menopause

**ovarian cycle** /əʊˌveəriən ˈsaɪk(ə)l/ *noun* the regular changes in the ovary during a woman's reproductive life

**ovarian cyst** /əʊˌveəriən ˈsɪst/ *noun* a cyst which develops in the ovaries

**ovarian follicle** /əʊˌveəriən ˈfɒlɪk(ə)l/ *noun* a cell which contains an ovum. Also called **Graafian follicle**

**ovariectomy** /ˌəʊvəriˈektəmi/ *noun* same as **oophorectomy** (NOTE: The plural is **ovariectomies**.)

**ovariocele** /əʊˈveəriəʊsiːl/ *noun* a hernia of an ovary

**ovariotomy** /ˌəʊvəriˈɒtəmi/ *noun* a surgical operation to remove an ovary or a tumour in an ovary (NOTE: The plural is **ovariotomies**.)

**ovaritis** /ˌəʊvəˈraɪtɪs/ *noun* same as **oophoritis**

**ovary** /ˈəʊv(ə)ri/ *noun* one of two organs in a woman which produce ova or egg cells and secrete the female hormone oestrogen. Also

called **oophoron**. See illustration at **UROGENITAL SYSTEM (FEMALE)** in Supplement (NOTE: The plural is **ovaries**. For other terms referring to ovaries, see words beginning with **oophor-, oophoro-**.)

**over-** /ˈəʊvə/ *prefix* too much

**overbite** /ˈəʊvəbaɪt/ *noun* the usual formation of the teeth, in which the top incisors come down over and in front of the bottom incisors when the jaws are closed

**overcome** /ˌəʊvəˈkʌm/ *verb* 1. to fight something and win 2. to make a person lose consciousness ○ *Two people were overcome by smoke in the fire.* (NOTE: **overcoming – overcame – overcome**)

**overcompensate** /ˌəʊvəˈkɒmpənseɪt/ *verb* to try too hard to cover the effects of a condition or quality (NOTE: **overcompensating – overcompensated**)

**overcompensation** /ˌəʊvəkɒmpən ˈseɪʃ(ə)n/ *noun* an attempt by a person to re-duce the bad effects of a mistake or a fault in their character in which they make too much effort, and so cause some other problem

**overdo** /ˌəʊvəˈduː/ *verb* □ **to overdo it** *or* **to overdo things** to work too hard or to do too much exercise (*informal*) ○ *She overdid it, working until 9 o'clock every evening.* ○ *He has been overdoing things and has to rest.*

**overdose** /ˈəʊvədəʊs/ *noun* a dose of a drug which is larger than the recommended or usual dose

**overeating** /ˌəʊvərˈiːtɪŋ/ *noun* eating too much food

**overexertion** /ˌəʊvərɪgˈzɜːʃ(ə)n/ *noun* doing too much physical work or taking too much exercise

**overflow incontinence** /ˌəʊvəfləʊ ɪnˈkɒn tɪnəns/ *noun* a leakage of urine because the bladder is too full

**overgrow** /ˌəʊvəˈgrəʊ/ *verb* (*of a tissue*) to grow over another tissue (NOTE: **overgrew – overgrown**)

**overgrowth** /ˈəʊvəgrəʊθ/ *noun* a growth of tissue over another tissue

**overjet** /ˈəʊvədʒet/ *noun* a space which separates the top incisors from the bottom incisors when the jaws are closed

**overlap** /ˌəʊvəˈlæp/ *verb* (*of bandages, etc.*) to lie partly on top of another (NOTE: **overlapping – overlapped**)

**overprescribe** /ˌəʊvəprɪˈskraɪb/ *verb* to issue too many prescriptions for something ○ *Some doctors seriously overprescribe tranquillisers.* (NOTE: **overprescribing – overprescribed**)

**overproduction** /ˌəʊvəprəˈdʌkʃən/ *noun* the act of producing too much of something ○ *The condition is caused by overproduction of thyroxine by the thyroid gland.*

**oversew** /ˈəʊvəsəʊ/ verb to sew a patch of tissue over a perforation (NOTE: **oversewing – oversewed – oversewn**)

**overt** /əʊˈvɜːt/ adjective easily seen with the naked eye. Opposite **occult**

**over-the-counter drug** /ˌəʊvə ðə ˈkaʊntə drʌg/ noun a drug which you can buy from a pharmacy without a doctor's prescription. Also called **OTC drug**

**overweight** /ˌəʊvəˈweɪt/ adjective fatter and heavier than is medically advisable ○ He is several kilos overweight for his age and height.

**overwork** /ˌəʊvəˈwɜːk/ noun too much work ○ He collapsed from overwork. ■ verb to work too much, or make something work too much ○ He has been overworking his heart.

**overwrought** /ˌəʊvəˈrɔːt/ adjective very tense and nervous

**ovi-** /əʊvi/ prefix eggs or ova

**oviduct** /ˈəʊvidʌkt/ noun same as **Fallopian tube**

**ovulate** /ˈɒvjuleɪt/ verb to release a mature ovum into a Fallopian tube (NOTE: **ovulating – ovulated**)

**ovulation** /ˌɒvjuˈleɪʃ(ə)n/ noun the release of an ovum from the mature ovarian follicle into the Fallopian tube

**ovum** /ˈəʊvəm/ noun a female egg cell which, when fertilised by a spermatozoon, begins to develop into an embryo (NOTE: The plural is **ova**. For other terms referring to ova, see words beginning with **oo-**.)

**-oxacin** /ɒksəsɪn/ suffix quinolone drug ○ ciprofloxacin

**oxidase** /ˈɒksɪdeɪz/ noun an enzyme which encourages oxidation by removing hydrogen. ◊ **monoamine oxidase**

**oxidation** /ˌɒksɪˈdeɪʃ(ə)n/ noun the action of making oxides by combining with oxygen or removing hydrogen

COMMENT: Carbon compounds form oxides when metabolised with oxygen in the body, producing carbon dioxide.

**oxide** /ˈɒksaɪd/ noun a compound formed with oxygen

**oximeter** /ɒkˈsɪmɪtə/ noun an instrument which measures the amount of oxygen in something, especially in blood

**oxybutynin** /ˌɒksiˈbjuːtənɪn/, **oxybutinin** noun a drug which reduces the need to pass urine

**oxycephalic** /ˌɒksikəˈfælɪk/ adjective referring to oxycephaly

**oxycephaly** /ˌɒksiˈkefəli/ noun a condition in which the skull is shaped into a point, with exophthalmos and poor sight. Also called **turricephaly**

**oxygen** /ˈɒksɪdʒən/ noun a chemical element that is a common colourless gas which is present in the air and essential to human life (NOTE: The chemical symbol is **O**.)

COMMENT: Oxygen is absorbed into the bloodstream through the lungs and is carried to the tissues along the arteries. It is essential to healthy metabolism and given to patients with breathing difficulties.

**oxygenate** /ˈɒksɪdʒəneɪt/ verb to combine blood with oxygen (NOTE: **oxygenating – oxygenated**)

**oxygenated blood** /ˌɒksɪdʒəneɪtɪd ˈblʌd/ noun blood which has received oxygen in the lungs and is being carried to the tissues along the arteries. Also called **arterial blood**. Compare **deoxygenated blood** (NOTE: Oxygenated blood is brighter red than venous deoxygenated blood.)

**oxygenation** /ˌɒksɪdʒəˈneɪʃ(ə)n/ noun the fact of becoming combined or filled with oxygen ○ Blood is carried along the pulmonary artery to the lungs for oxygenation.

**oxygenator** /ˈɒksɪdʒə,neɪtə/ noun a machine which puts oxygen into the blood, used as an artificial lung in surgery

**oxygen cylinder** /ˈɒksɪdʒən ,sɪlɪndə/ noun a heavy metal tube which contains oxygen and is connected to a patient's oxygen mask

**oxygen mask** /ˈɒksɪdʒən mɑːsk/ noun a mask connected to a supply of oxygen, which can be put over the face to help someone with breathing difficulties

**oxygen tent** /ˈɒksɪdʒən tent/ noun a type of cover put over a person so that he or she can breathe in oxygen

**oxygen therapy** /ˈɒksɪdʒən θerəpi/ noun any treatment involving the administering of oxygen, e.g. in an oxygen tent or in emergency treatment for heart failure

**oxyhaemoglobin** /ˌɒksi,hiːməˈgləʊbɪn/ noun a compound of haemoglobin and oxygen, which is the way oxygen is carried in arterial blood from the lungs to the tissues. ◊ **haemoglobin** (NOTE: The US spelling is **oxyhemoglobin**.)

**oxyntic** /ɒkˈsɪntɪk/ adjective referring to glands and cells in the stomach which produce acid

**oxyntic cell** /ɒkˈsɪntɪk sel/ noun a cell in the gastric gland which secretes hydrochloric acid. Also called **parietal cell**

**oxytetracycline** /ˌɒksi,tetrəˈsaɪkliːn/ noun an antibiotic which is effective against a wide range of organisms

**oxytocic** /ˌɒksiˈtəʊsɪk/ noun a drug which helps to start the process of childbirth, or speeds it up ■ adjective starting or speeding up childbirth by causing contractions in the muscles of the uterus

**oxytocin** /ˌɒksiˈtəʊsɪn/ noun a hormone secreted by the posterior pituitary gland, which controls the contractions of the uterus and encourages the flow of milk

COMMENT: An extract of oxytocin is used as an injection to start contractions of the uterus and to assist in the third stage of labour.

**oxyuriasis** /ˌɒksɪjʊˈraɪəsɪs/ *noun* same as **enterobiasis**

**Oxyuris** /ˌɒksɪˈjʊərɪs/ *noun* same as **Enterobius**

**ozaena** /əʊˈziːnə/ *noun* **1.** a disease of the nose in which the nasal passage is blocked and mucus forms, giving off an unpleasant smell **2.** any unpleasant discharge from the nose (NOTE: The US spelling is **ozena**.)

**ozone** /ˈəʊzəʊn/ *noun* a gas present in the atmosphere in small quantities, which is harmful at high levels of concentration

COMMENT: The maximum amount of ozone which is considered safe for humans to breathe is 80 parts per billion. Even in lower concentrations it irritates the throat, makes people cough and gives headaches and asthma attacks similar to hay fever. The ozone layer in the stratosphere acts as a protection against the harmful effects of the sun's radiation, and the destruction or reduction of the layer has the effect of allowing more radiation to pass through the atmosphere with harmful effects such as skin cancer on humans.

**ozone sickness** /ˈəʊzəʊn ˌsɪknəs/ *noun* a condition experienced by jet travellers, due to levels of ozone in aircraft

# P

**P** ♦ substance P

**Pa** *abbr* pascal

**pacemaker** /ˈpeɪsmeɪkə/ *noun* **1.** a node in the heart which regulates the heartbeat. Also called **sinoatrial node, SA node 2.** ♦ **cardiac pacemaker, epicardial pacemaker**

COMMENT: An electrode is usually attached to the epicardium and linked to the device which can be implanted in various positions in the chest.

**pachy-** /pæki/ *prefix* thickening

**pachydactyly** /ˌpæki'dæktɪli/ *noun* a condition in which the fingers and toes become thicker than usual

**pachydermia** /ˌpæki'dɜːmiə/, **pachyderma** /ˌpæki'dɜːmə/ *noun* a condition in which the skin becomes thicker than normal

**pachymeningitis** /ˌpæki,menɪn'dʒaɪtɪs/ *noun* inflammation of the dura mater

**pachymeninx** /ˌpæki'miːnɪŋks/ *noun* same as **dura mater**

**pachyonychia** /ˌpækiə'nɪkiə/ *noun* unusual thickness of the nails

**pachysomia** /ˌpæki'səʊmiə/ *noun* a condition in which soft tissues of the body become unusually thick

**pacifier** /ˈpæsɪfaɪə/ *noun US* a child's dummy

**pacing** /ˈpeɪsɪŋ/ *noun* a surgical operation to implant or attach a cardiac pacemaker

**Pacinian corpuscle** /pə,sɪniən 'kɔːpʌs(ə)l/ *noun* a sensory nerve ending in the skin which is sensitive to touch and vibrations

**pack** /pæk/ *noun* **1.** a tampon of gauze or cotton wool, used to fill an orifice such as the nose or vagina **2.** a piece of wet material folded tightly, used to press on the body **3.** a treatment in which a blanket or sheet is used to wrap round the body **4.** a box or bag of goods for sale ○ *a pack of sticking plaster* ○ *The cough tablets are sold in packs of fifty.* ■ *verb* **1.** to fill an orifice with a tampon ○ *The ear was packed with cotton wool to absorb the discharge.* **2.** to put things in cases or boxes ○ *The transplant organ arrived at the hospital packed in ice.*

**packed cell volume** /ˌpækt 'sel ,vɒljuːm/ *noun* the volume of red blood cells in a person's blood shown against the total volume of blood. Also called **haematocrit**

**packing** /ˈpækɪŋ/ *noun* absorbent material put into a wound or part of the body to absorb fluids

**pack up** /ˌpæk 'ʌp/ *verb* to stop working (*informal*) ○ *His heart simply packed up under the strain.*

**PACT** *abbr* prescribing analyses and cost

**pad** /pæd/ *noun* **1.** a piece or mass of soft absorbent material, placed on part of the body to protect it ○ *She wrapped a pad of soft cotton wool round the sore.* **2.** a thickening of part of the skin

**paed-** /piːd/ *prefix* same as **paedo-** (*used before vowels*) (NOTE: The US spelling is **ped-**.)

**paediatric** /ˌpiːdi'ætrɪk/ *adjective* referring to the treatment of the diseases of children ○ *A new paediatric hospital has been opened.* ○ *Parents can visit children in the paediatric wards at any time.*

'Paediatric day surgery minimizes the length of hospital stay and therefore is less traumatic for both child and parents' [*British Journal of Nursing*]

**paediatrician** /ˌpiːdiə'trɪʃ(ə)n/ *noun* a doctor who specialises in the treatment of diseases of children

**paediatrics** /ˌpiːdi'ætrɪks/ *noun* the study of children, their development and diseases. Compare **geriatrics**

**paedo-** /piːdəʊ/ *prefix* referring to children

**paedodontia** *noun* another spelling of **pedodontia**

**Paget's disease** /ˈpædʒəts dɪ,ziːz/ *noun* **1.** same as **osteitis deformans 2.** a form of breast cancer which starts as an itchy rash round the nipple [Described 1877. After Sir James Paget (1814–99), British surgeon.]

**pain** /peɪn/ *noun* the feeling of severe discomfort which a person has when hurt ○ *The doctor gave him an injection to relieve the pain.* ○ *She is suffering from back pain.* (NOTE: Pain can be used in the plural to show that it recurs: **She has pains in her left leg.**) □ **to be in great**

**pain** to have very sharp pains which are difficult to bear

COMMENT: Pain is carried by the sensory nerves to the central nervous system. From the site it travels up the spinal column to the medulla and through a series of neurones which use Substance P as the neurotransmitter to the sensory cortex. Pain is the method by which a person knows that part of the body is damaged or infected, though the pain is not always felt in the affected part. See synalgia.

**pain clinic** /'peɪn ˌklɪnɪk/ *noun* a centre which looks after people with severe persistent pain and whose staff include professionals from many specialist areas of medicine

**painful** /'peɪnf(ə)l/ *adjective* causing pain ○ *She has a painful skin disease.* ○ *His foot is so painful he can hardly walk.* ○ *Your eye looks very red – is it very painful?*

**painkiller** /'peɪnkɪlə/ *noun* a drug that reduces pain

**painless** /'peɪnləs/ *adjective* not causing pain ○ *a painless method of removing warts*

**pain pathway** /'peɪn ˌpɑːθweɪ/ *noun* a series of linking nerve fibres and neurones which carry impulses of pain from the site to the sensory cortex

**pain receptor** /'peɪn rɪˌseptə/ *noun* a nerve ending which is sensitive to pain

**pain relief** /'peɪn rɪˌliːf/ *noun* the act of easing pain by using analgesics

**paint** /peɪnt/ *noun* a coloured antiseptic, analgesic or astringent liquid which is put on the surface of the body ■ *verb* to cover a wound with an antiseptic, analgesic or astringent liquid or lotion ○ *She painted the rash with calamine.*

**painter's colic** /ˌpeɪntəz 'kɒlɪk/ *noun* a form of lead poisoning caused, especially formerly, by working with paint

**pain threshold** /'peɪn ˌθreʃhəʊld/ *noun* the point at which a person finds it impossible to bear pain without crying

**palatal** /'pælət(ə)l/ *adjective* referring to the palate

**palate** /'pælət/ *noun* the roof of the mouth and floor of the nasal cavity, formed of the hard and soft palates

**palate bone** /'pælət bəʊn/ *noun* one of two bones which form part of the hard palate, the orbits of the eyes and the cavity behind the nose. Also called **palatine bone**

**palatine** /'pælətaɪn/ *adjective* referring to the palate

**palatine arch** /'pælətaɪn ɑːtʃ/ *noun* a fold of tissue between the soft palate and the pharynx

**palatine bone** /'pælətaɪn bəʊn/ *noun* same as **palate bone**

**palatine tonsil** /ˌpælətaɪn 'tɒns(ə)l/ *noun* same as **tonsil**

**palato-** /'pælətəʊ/ *prefix* the palate

**palatoglossal arch** /ˌpælətəʊˌglɒs(ə)l 'ɑːtʃ/ *noun* a fold between the soft palate and the tongue, anterior to the tonsil

**palatopharyngeal arch** /ˌpælətəʊfærɪnˌdʒɪəl 'ɑːtʃ/ *noun* a fold between the soft palate and the pharynx, posterior to the tonsil

**palatoplasty** /'pælətəplæsti/ *noun* plastic surgery of the roof of the mouth, e.g. to repair a cleft palate

**palatoplegia** /ˌpælətə'pliːdʒə/ *noun* paralysis of the soft palate

**palatorrhaphy** /ˌpælə'tɔːrəfi/ *noun* a surgical operation to suture and close a cleft palate. Also called **staphylorrhaphy, uraniscorrhaphy**

**pale** /peɪl/ *adjective* light coloured or white ○ *After her illness she looked pale and tired.* □ **to turn pale** to become white in the face, because the flow of blood is reduced ○ *Some people turn pale at the sight of blood.*

**paleness** /'peɪlnəs/ *noun* the fact of being pale

**pali-** /'pæli/ *prefix* same as **palin-**

**palilalia** /ˌpæli'leɪliə/ *noun* a speech disorder in which the person repeats words

**palin-** /'pælɪn/ *prefix* repeating

**palindromic** /ˌpælɪn'drəʊmɪk/ *adjective* recurring ○ *a palindromic disease*

**palliative** /'pæliətɪv/ *noun* a treatment or drug which relieves symptoms but does nothing to cure the disease which causes the symptoms. For example, a painkiller can reduce the pain in a tooth, but will not cure the caries which causes the pain. ■ *adjective* providing relief

'…coronary artery bypass grafting is a palliative procedure aimed at the relief of persistent angina pectoris' [*British Journal of Hospital Medicine*]

**palliative care** /ˌpæliətɪv 'keə/, **palliative treatment** /ˌpæliətɪv 'triːtmənt/ *noun* treatment which helps to reduce the symptoms of a disease, especially a terminal or chronic condition, but does not cure it

COMMENT: Palliative care may involve giving antibiotics, transfusions, pain-killing drugs, low-dose chemotherapy and psychological and social support to help the person and their family adjust to the illness. The treatment is often provided in a hospice.

**pallidotomy** /ˌpæli'dɒtəmi/ *noun* an operation on the brain which can reduce many of the symptoms of Parkinson's disease, such as tremor, bradykinesia and bent posture

**pallium** /'pæliəm/ *noun* the layer of grey matter on the surface of the cerebral cortex

**pallor** /'pælə/ *noun* the condition of being pale

**palm** /pɑːm/ *noun* the inner surface of the hand, extending from the bases of the fingers to the wrist

**palmar** /'pælmə/ *adjective* referring to the palm of the hand

**palmar arch** /ˈpælmər ɑːtʃ/ *noun* one of two arches or joins within the palm formed by two arteries which link together

**palmar fascia** /ˌpælmə ˈfeɪʃə/ *noun* the tendons in the palm of the hand

**palmar interosseus** /ˌpælmər ˌɪntər ˈɒsiəs/ *noun* a deep muscle between the bones in the hand

**palmar region** /ˈpælmə ˌriːdʒ(ə)n/ *noun* an area of skin around the palm

**palpable** /ˈpælpəb(ə)l/ *adjective* **1.** able to be felt when touched **2.** able to be examined with the hand

'…mammography is the most effective technique available for the detection of occult (non-palpable) breast cancer. It has been estimated that mammography can detect a carcinoma two years before it becomes palpable' [*Southern Medical Journal*]

**palpate** /pælˈpeɪt/ *verb* to examine part of the body by feeling it with the hand

**palpation** /pælˈpeɪʃ(ə)n/ *noun* an examination of part of the body by feeling it with the hand

**palpebra** /ˈpælpɪbrə/ *noun* same as **eyelid** (NOTE: The plural is **palpebrae**.)

**palpebral** /ˈpælpɪbrəl/ *adjective* referring to the eyelids

**palpitate** /ˈpælpɪteɪt/ *verb* to beat rapidly or irregularly

**palpitation** /pælpɪˈteɪʃ(ə)n/ *noun* awareness that the heart is beating rapidly or irregularly, possibly caused by stress or by a disease

**pan-** /pæn/ *prefix* referring to everything

**panacea** /ˌpænəˈsiːə/ *noun* a medicine which is supposed to cure everything

**Panadol** /ˈpænədɒl/ a trade name for paracetamol

**panarthritis** /ˌpænɑːˈθraɪtɪs/ *noun* inflammation of all the tissues of a joint or of all the joints in the body

**pancarditis** /ˌpænkɑːˈdaɪtɪs/ *noun* inflammation of all the tissues in the heart, i.e. the heart muscle, the endocardium and the pericardium

**pancreas** /ˈpæŋkriəs/ *noun* a gland which lies across the back of the body between the kidneys. See illustration at **DIGESTIVE SYSTEM** in Supplement

COMMENT: The pancreas has two functions: the first is to secrete the pancreatic juice which goes into the duodenum and digests proteins and carbohydrates; the second function is to produce the hormone insulin which regulates the use of sugar by the body. This hormone is secreted into the bloodstream by the islets of Langerhans which are in the pancreas.

**pancreatectomy** /ˌpæŋkriəˈtektəmi/ *noun* the surgical removal of all or part of the pancreas

**pancreatic** /ˌpæŋkriˈætɪk/ *adjective* referring to the pancreas

**pancreatic duct** /ˌpæŋkriˈætɪk dʌkt/ *noun* a duct leading through the pancreas to the duodenum

**pancreatic juice** /ˌpæŋkriˈætɪk dʒuːs/, **pancreatic secretion** /ˌpæŋkriˌætɪk sɪˈkriːʃ(ə)n/ *noun* a digestive juice, formed of enzymes produced by the pancreas, which digests fats and carbohydrates

**pancreatin** /ˈpæŋkriətɪn/ *noun* a substance made from enzymes secreted by the pancreas, used to treat someone whose pancreas does not produce pancreatic enzymes

**pancreatitis** /ˌpæŋkriəˈtaɪtɪs/ *noun* inflammation of the pancreas

**pancreatomy** /ˌpæŋkriˈætəmi/, **pancreatotomy** /ˌpæŋkriəˈtɒtəmi/ *noun* a surgical operation to open the pancreatic duct

**pancytopenia** /ˌpænsaɪtəˈpiːniə/ *noun* a condition in which there are too few red and white blood cells and blood platelets

**pandemic** /pænˈdemɪk/ *noun* an epidemic disease which affects many parts of the world. Compare **endemic, epidemic** ■ *adjective* widespread

**pang** /pæŋ/ *noun* a sudden sharp pain, especially in the intestine ○ *After not eating for a day, she suffered pangs of hunger.*

**panhysterectomy** /ˌpænhɪstəˈrektmi/ *noun* the surgical removal of all the uterus and the cervix

**panic** /ˈpænɪk/ *noun* a feeling of great fear which cannot be stopped and which sometimes results in irrational behaviour ○ *He was in a panic as he sat in the consultant's waiting room.* ■ *verb* to be suddenly afraid ○ *She panicked when the surgeon told her she might need to have an operation.*

**panic attack** /ˈpænɪk əˌtæk/ *noun* a sudden onset of panic

**panic disorder** /ˈpænɪk dɪsˌɔːdə/ *noun* a condition in which somebody has frequent panic attacks

**panniculitis** /pəˌnɪkjʊˈlaɪtɪs/ *noun* inflammation of the panniculus adiposus, producing tender swellings on the thighs and breasts

**panniculus** /pəˈnɪkjʊləs/ *noun* a layer of membranous tissue

**panniculus adiposus** /pəˌnɪkjʊləs ˌædɪˈpəʊsəs/ *noun* a layer of fat underneath the skin

**pannus** /ˈpænəs/ *noun* a growth on the cornea containing tiny blood vessels

**panophthalmia** /ˌpænɒfˈθælmiə/, **panophthalmitis** /ˌpænɒfθælˈmaɪtɪs/ *noun* inflammation of the whole of the eye

**panosteitis** /ˌpænɒstiˈaɪtɪs/, **panostitis** /pænɒˈstaɪtɪs/ *noun* inflammation of the whole of a bone

**panotitis** /ˌpænəʊˈtaɪtɪs/ *noun* inflammation affecting all of the ear, but especially the middle ear

**panproctocolectomy** /ˌpænprɒktəkəˈlektəmi/ *noun* the surgical removal of the whole of the rectum and the colon

**pant** /pænt/ *verb* to take short breaths because of too much exercise, to gasp for breath ○ *He was panting when he reached the top of the stairs.*

**pant-** /pænt/ *prefix* same as **pan-**

**panto-** /pæntəʊ/ *prefix* same as **pan-**

**pantothenic acid** /ˌpæntəˌθenɪk ˈæsɪd/ *noun* a vitamin of the vitamin B complex, found in liver, yeast and eggs

**pantotropic** /ˌpæntəˈtrɒpɪk/, **pantropic** /pænˈtrɒpɪk/ *adjective* referring to a virus which attacks many different parts of the body

**Papanicolaou test** /ˌpæpənɪkəˈleɪu: test/ *noun* a method of staining samples from various body secretions to test for malignancy, e.g. testing a cervical smear sample to see if cancer is present. Also called **Pap test** [Described 1933. After George Nicholas Papanicolaou (1883–1962), Greek anatomist and physician who worked in the USA.]

**papaveretum** /pəˌpævəˈriːtəm/ *noun* a preparation of opium used to reduce pain

**papilla** /pəˈpɪlə/ *noun* a small swelling which sticks up above the usual surface level ○ *The upper surface of the tongue is covered with papillae.* (NOTE: The plural is **papillae**.)

**papillary** /pəˈpɪləri/ *adjective* referring to papillae

**papillitis** /ˌpæpɪˈlaɪtɪs/ *noun* inflammation of the optic disc at the back of the eye

**papilloedema** /ˌpæpɪləʊˈdiːmə/ *noun* an accumulation of fluid in the optic disc at the back of the eye

**papilloma** /ˌpæpɪˈləʊmə/ *noun* a benign tumour on the skin or mucous membrane (NOTE: The plural is **papillomas** or **papillomata**.)

**papillomatosis** /ˌpæpɪləʊməˈtəʊsɪs/ *noun* **1.** being affected with papillomata **2.** the formation of papillomata

**papillotomy** /ˌpæpɪˈlɒtəmi/ *noun* the operation of cutting into the body at the point where the common bile duct and pancreatic duct meet to go into the duodenum, in order to improve bile drainage and allow any stones to pass out

**papovavirus** /pəˈpəʊvəvaɪrəs/ *noun* a family of viruses which start tumours, some of which are malignant, and some of which, such as warts, are benign

**Pap test** /ˈpæp test/, **Pap smear** /ˈpæp smɪə/ *noun* same as **Papanicolaou test**

**papular** /ˈpæpjʊlə/ *adjective* referring to papule

**papule** /ˈpæpjuːl/ *noun* a small coloured spot raised above the surface of the skin as part of a rash (NOTE: A flat spot is a **macule**.)

**papulo-** /pæpjʊləʊ/ *prefix* relating to a papule

**papulopustular** /ˌpæpjʊləʊˈpʌstjʊlə/ *adjective* referring to a rash with both papules and pustules

**papulosquamous** /ˌpæpjʊləʊˈskweɪməs/ *adjective* referring to a rash with papules and a scaly skin

**para-** /pærə/ *prefix* **1.** similar to or near **2.** changed or beyond

**parabiosis** /ˌpærəbaɪˈəʊsɪs/ *noun* a condition in which two individuals are joined, e.g. conjoined twins

**paracentesis** /ˌpærəsenˈtiːsɪs/ *noun* the procedure of draining fluid from a cavity inside the body using a hollow needle, either for diagnostic purposes or because the fluid is harmful. Also called **tapping**

**paracetamol** /ˌpærəˈsiːtəmɒl/ *noun* a common drug used to relieve mild to moderate pain and reduce fever (NOTE: The US name is **acetaminophen**.)

**paracolpitis** /ˌpærəkɒlˈpaɪtɪs/ same as **pericolpitis**

**paracusis** /ˌpærəˈkjuːsɪs/, **paracousia** /ˌpærəˈkuːsiə/ *noun* a disorder of hearing

**paradoxical breathing** /ˌpærədɒksɪk(ə)l ˈbriːðɪŋ/, **paradoxical respiration** /ˌpærədɒksɪk(ə)l ˌrespɪˈreɪʃ(ə)n/ *noun* a condition affecting someone with broken ribs, where the chest appears to move in when he or she breathes in, and appears to move out when he or she breathes out

**paradoxical sleep** /ˌpærədɒksɪk(ə)l ˈsliːp/ *noun* same as **REM sleep**

**paradoxus** /ˌpærəˈdɒksəs/ ♦ **pulsus paradoxus**

**paraesthesia** /ˌpæriːsˈθiːziə/ *noun* an unexplained tingling sensation. ◊ **pins and needles** (NOTE: The plural is **paraesthesiae**.)

'…the sensory symptoms are paraesthesiae which may spread up the arm over the course of about 20 minutes' [*British Journal of Hospital Medicine*]

**paraffin** /ˈpærəfɪn/ *noun* an oil produced from petroleum, forming the base of some ointments, and also used for heating and light

**paraffin gauze** /ˈpærəfɪn gɔːz/ *noun* gauze covered with solid paraffin, used as a dressing

**parageusia** /ˌpærəˈgjuːsiə/ *noun* **1.** a disorder of the sense of taste **2.** an unpleasant taste in the mouth

**paragonimiasis** /ˌpærəgɒnəˈmaɪəsɪs/ *noun* a tropical disease in which the lungs are infested with the fluke of the genus Paragonimus and the person has bronchitis and coughs up blood. Also called **endemic haemoptysis**

**paragraphia** /ˌpærəˈgræfiə/ *noun* the writing of different words or letters from the ones intended, as a result of a stroke or disease

**paraguard stretcher** /ˈpærəgɑːd ˌstretʃə/ *noun* a type of strong stretcher to which the injured person is attached securely, so that he or she can be carried upright. It is used for rescu-

# para-influenza virus

ing people from mountains or from tall buildings.

**para-influenza virus** /ˌpærə ˌɪnfluˈenzə ˌvaɪrəs/ *noun* a virus which causes upper respiratory tract infection. In its structure it is identical to paramyxoviruses and the measles virus.

**paralyse** /ˈpærəlaɪz/ *verb* to make a part of the body unable to carry out voluntary movements by weakening or damaging muscles or nerves so that they cannot function, or by using a drug ○ *His arm was paralysed after the stroke.* ○ *She is paralysed from the waist down.* (NOTE: The US spelling is **paralyze**.)

**paralysis** /pəˈrælɪsɪs/ *noun* a condition in which part of the body cannot be moved because the motor nerves have been damaged or the muscles have been weakened ○ *The condition causes paralysis of the lower limbs.* ○ *He suffered temporary paralysis of the right arm.*
   COMMENT: Paralysis can have many causes: the commonest are injuries to or diseases of the brain or the spinal column.

**paralysis agitans** /pəˌrælɪsɪs ˈædʒɪtəns/ *noun* same as **Parkinsonism**

**paralytic** /ˌpærəˈlɪtɪk/ *adjective* **1.** referring to paralysis **2.** referring to a person who is paralysed

**paralytica** /ˌpærəˈlɪtɪkə/ ♦ **dementia paralytica**

**paralytic ileus** /ˌpærəlɪtɪk ˈɪliəs/ *noun* an obstruction in the ileum caused by paralysis of the muscles of the intestine. Also called **adynamic ileus**

**paralytic poliomyelitis** /ˌpærəlɪtɪk ˌpəʊliəʊˌmaɪəˈlaɪtɪs/ *noun* poliomyelitis which affects the muscles

**paramedian** /ˌpærəˈmiːdiən/ *adjective* near the midline of the body

**paramedian plane** /ˌpærəˈmiːdiən pleɪn/ *noun* a plane near the midline of the body, parallel to the sagittal plane and at right angles to the coronal plane. See illustration at ANATOMICAL TERMS in Supplement

**paramedic** /ˌpærəˈmedɪk/ *noun* a person whose work involves the restoration of health and normal functioning (NOTE: **Paramedic** is used to refer to all types of services and staff, from therapists and hygienists, to ambulance drivers and radiographers, but does not include doctors, nurses or midwives.)

**paramedical** /ˌpærəˈmedɪk(ə)l/ *adjective* referring to services linked to those given by nurses, doctors and surgeons

**paramesonephric duct** /ˌpærəmesəˈnefrɪk ˌdʌkt/ *noun* one of the two ducts in an embryo which develop into the uterus and Fallopian tubes. Also called **Müllerian duct**

**parameter** /pəˈræmɪtə/ *noun* a measurement of something such as blood pressure which may be an important consideration in treating the condition which the person has

**parametritis** /ˌpærəmɪˈtraɪtɪs/ *noun* inflammation of the parametrium

**parametrium** /ˌpærəˈmiːtriəm/ *noun* the connective tissue around the uterus

**paramnesia** /ˌpæræmˈniːziə/ *noun* a disorder of the memory in which someone remembers events which have not happened

**paramyxovirus** /ˌpærəmɪksəʊˈvaɪrəs/ *noun* one of a group of viruses, which cause mumps, measles and other infectious diseases

**paranasal** /ˌpærəˈneɪz(ə)l/ *adjective* by the side of the nose

**paranasal sinus** /ˌpærəneɪz(ə)l ˈsaɪnəs/, **paranasal air sinus** /ˌpærəneɪz(ə)l ˈeə ˌsaɪnəs/ *noun* one of the four pairs of sinuses in the skull near the nose, which open into the nasal cavity and are lined with sticky mucus (NOTE: They are the frontal, maxillary, ethmoidal and sphenoidal sinuses.)

**paranoia** /ˌpærəˈnɔɪə/ *noun* a behaviour characterised by mistaken ideas or delusions of persecution or self-importance

**paranoiac** /ˌpærəˈnɔɪæk/ *noun* a person affected by paranoia

**paranoid** /ˈpærənɔɪd/ *adjective* having a fixed delusion

**paranoid disorder** /ˌpærənɔɪd dɪsˈɔːdə/ *noun* a mental disorder which causes someone experiencing it to believe strongly that something is not right with them, with someone else or with the world generally and to maintain the belief even when given evidence against it (NOTE: The preferred term is delusional disorder.)

**paranoid schizophrenia** /ˌpærənɔɪd ˌskɪtsəʊˈfriːniə/ *noun* a form of schizophrenia in which the person believes he or she is being persecuted

**paraparesis** /ˌpærəpəˈriːsɪs/ *noun* incomplete paralysis of the legs

**paraphasia** /ˌpærəˈfeɪziə/ *noun* a speech disorder in which the person uses a wrong sound in the place of the correct word or phrase

**paraphimosis** /ˌpærəfaɪˈməʊsɪs/ *noun* a condition in which the foreskin around the penis is tight and may have to be removed by circumcision

**paraphrenia** /ˌpærəˈfriːniə/ *noun* a dated term for a mental disorder involving delusions without severe personality deterioration

**paraplegia** /ˌpærəˈpliːdʒə/ *noun* paralysis which affects the lower part of the body and the legs, usually caused by an injury to the spinal cord

**paraplegic** /ˌpærəˈpliːdʒɪk/ *noun* someone who has paraplegia ■ *adjective* paralysed in the lower part of the body and legs

**paraprofessional** /ˌpærəprəˈfeʃ(ə)n(ə)l/ *noun* somebody with training who acts as an assistant to a professional person

**parapsoriasis** /ˌpærəsəˈraɪəsɪs/ *noun* a group of skin diseases with scales, similar to psoriasis

**parapsychology** /ˌpærəsaɪˈkɒlədʒi/ *noun* the study of effects of the mind which appear not to be explained by known psychological or scientific principles, e.g. extrasensory perception and telepathy

**Paraquat** /ˈpærəkwɒt/ *noun* a trade name for dimethyl dupyridilium used as a weedkiller

**parasagittal** /ˌpærəˈsædʒɪt(ə)l/ *adjective* near the midline of the body

**parasagittal plane** /ˌpærəˈsædʒɪt(ə)l pleɪn/ *noun* a plane near the midline of the body, parallel to the sagittal plane and at right angles to the coronal plane. Also called **paramedian plane**. See illustration at ANATOMICAL TERMS in Supplement

**parasitaemia** /ˌpærəsɪˈtiːmiə/ *noun* the presence of parasites in the blood

**parasite** /ˈpærəsaɪt/ *noun* a plant or animal which lives on or inside another organism and draws nourishment from that organism

COMMENT: The commonest parasites affecting humans are lice on the skin, and various types of worms in the intestines. Many diseases such as malaria and amoebic dysentery are caused by infestation with parasites.

**parasitic** /ˌpærəˈsɪtɪk/ *adjective* referring to parasites

**parasitic cyst** /ˌpærəsɪtɪk ˈsɪst/ *noun* a cyst caused by the growing larvae of a parasite in the body

**parasiticide** /ˌpærəˈsaɪtɪsaɪd/ *noun* a substance which kills parasites ■ *adjective* killing parasites

**parasitology** /ˌpærəsaɪˈtɒlədʒi/ *noun* the scientific study of parasites

**parasuicide** /ˌpærəˈsuːɪsaɪd/ *noun* an act where someone tries to kill himself or herself, but without really intending to do so, rather as a way of drawing attention to his or her psychological condition

**parasympathetic** /ˌpærəsɪmpəˈθetɪk/ *adjective* referring to the parasympathetic nervous system

**parasympathetic nervous system** /ˌpærəsɪmpəˌθetɪk ˈnɜːvəs ˌsɪstəm/, **parasympathetic system** /ˌpærəsɪmpəˈθetɪk ˌsɪstəm/ *noun* one of two parts of the autonomic nervous system. Its messages reach the organs of the body through the cranial and sacral nerves to the eyes, the gastrointestinal system and other organs. ◊ **sympathetic nervous system**

COMMENT: The parasympathetic nervous system acts in opposition to the sympathetic nervous system, slowing down the action of the heart, reducing blood pressure and increasing the rate of digestion.

**parasympatholytic** /ˌpærəsɪmˌpæθəˈlɪtɪk/ *noun* a drug which reduces the effects of the parasympathetic nervous system by relaxing smooth muscle, reducing the amount of sweat and saliva produced and widening the pupil of the eye. An example is atropine. ■ *adjective* relating to a parasympatholytic drug

**parasympathomimetic** /ˌpærəsɪmˌpæθəʊmɪˈmetɪk/ *noun* a drug which stimulates the parasympathetic nervous system by making smooth muscle more tense, widening the blood vessels, slowing the heart rate, increasing the amount of sweat and saliva produced and contracting the pupil of the eye ■ *adjective* producing effects similar to those of a parasympathomimetic drug

**parathormone** /ˌpærəˈθɔːməʊn/ *noun* the hormone secreted by the parathyroid glands which regulates the level of calcium in blood plasma. Also called **parathyroid hormone**

**parathyroid** /ˌpærəˈθaɪrɔɪd/ *noun* same as **parathyroid gland** ■ *adjective* **1.** relating to a parathyroid gland **2.** located close to the thyroid gland

**parathyroidectomy** /ˌpærəˌθaɪrɔɪˈdektəmi/ *noun* the surgical removal of a parathyroid gland

**parathyroid gland** /ˌpærəˈθaɪrɔɪd glænd/ *noun* one of four small glands which are situated in or near the wall of the thyroid gland and secrete a hormone which controls the way in which calcium and phosphorus are deposited in bones

**parathyroid hormone** /ˌpærəˈθaɪrɔɪd ˌhɔːməʊn/ *noun* same as **parathormone**

**paratyphoid** /ˌpærəˈtaɪfɔɪd/, **paratyphoid fever** /ˌpærəˈtaɪfɔɪd ˌfiːvə/ *noun* an infectious disease which has similar symptoms to typhoid and is caused by bacteria transmitted by humans or animals

COMMENT: There are three forms of paratyphoid fever, known by the letters A, B, and C, caused by three types of bacterium, *Salmonella paratyphi* A, B, and C. TAB injections give immunity against paratyphoid A and B, but not against C.

**paravertebral** /ˌpærəˈvɜːtɪbrəl/ *adjective* near the vertebrae, beside the spinal column

**paravertebral injection** /ˌpærəˌvɜːtɪbrəl ɪnˈdʒekʃən/ *noun* an injection of local anaesthetic into the back near the vertebrae

**parenchyma** /pəˈreŋkɪmə/ *noun* tissues which contain the working cells of an organ

**parenchymal** /pəˈreŋkɪməl/ *adjective* relating to parenchyma

**parent** /ˈpeərənt/ *noun* a biological or adoptive mother or father ■ *verb* to carry out the role of a parent

'...in most paediatric wards today open visiting is the norm, with parent care much in evidence. Parents who are resident in the hospital also need time spent with them' [*Nursing Times*]

**parent cell** /ˈpeərənt sel/ *noun* an original cell which divides into daughter cells by mitosis

**parenteral** /pæˈrentərəl/ *adjective* referring to medication which is not given by mouth but in the form of injections or suppositories. Compare **enteral, oral**

**parenteral nutrition** /pæˌrentərəl njuːˈtrɪʃ(ə)n/, **parenteral feeding** /pæˌrentərəl ˈfiːdɪŋ/ *noun* the process of feeding someone by means other than the digestive tract, especially by giving injections of glucose to someone critically ill

**parenthood** /ˈpeərənthʊd/ *noun* the state of being a parent

**parenting** /ˈpeərəntɪŋ/ *noun* the activities involved in bringing up children □ **parenting skills** the abilities and experience that make someone a good parent

**paresis** /pəˈriːsɪs/ *noun* partial paralysis

**paresthesia** /ˌpæriːsˈθiːziə/ *noun US* same as **paraesthesia**

**paries** /ˈpeəriːz/ *noun* 1. a superficial part of a structure of an organ 2. the wall of a cavity (NOTE: [all senses] The plural is **parietes**.)

**parietal** /pəˈraɪət(ə)l/ *adjective* referring to the wall of a cavity or any organ

**parietal bone** /pəˈraɪət(ə)l bəʊn/, **parietal** /pəˈraɪət(ə)l/ *noun* one of two bones which form the sides of the skull

**parietal cell** /pəˈraɪət(ə)l sel/ *noun* same as **oxyntic cell**

**parietal lobe** /pəˈraɪət(ə)l ləʊb/ *noun* the middle lobe of the cerebral hemisphere, which is associated with language and other mental processes, and also contains the postcentral gyrus

**parietal pericardium** /pəˌraɪət(ə)l ˌperiˈkɑːdiəm/ *noun* the outer layer of the serous pericardium, not in direct contact with the heart muscle, which lies inside and is attached to the fibrous pericardium

**parietal peritoneum** /pəˌraɪət(ə)l ˌperitəˈniːəm/ *noun* part of the peritoneum which lines the abdominal cavity and covers the abdominal viscera

**parietal pleura** /pəˌraɪət(ə)l ˈplʊərə/ *noun* a membrane attached to the diaphragm and covering the chest cavity. Also called **outer pleura**. See illustration at LUNGS in Supplement

**-parin** /pərɪn/ *suffix* used for anticoagulants ○ *heparin*

**Paris** /ˈpærɪs/ ♦ **plaster of Paris**

**parity** /ˈpærɪti/ *noun* 1. equality of status or position, especially in terms of pay or rank 2. the number of children that a woman has given birth to

**parkinsonian** /ˌpɑːkɪnˈsəʊniən/ *adjective* referring to Parkinson's disease ○ *parkinsonian tremor*

**Parkinsonism** /ˈpɑːkɪnsənɪz(ə)m/ *noun* a progressive nervous disorder, which may be an effect of some drugs, repeated head injuries or brain tumours. The main symptoms are trem-

bling hands and a slow shuffling walk. Also called **paralysis agitans**

**Parkinson's disease** /ˈpɑːkɪnsənz dɪˌziːz/ *noun* a progressive nervous disorder without a known cause which is a type of Parkinsonism, the main symptoms of which are trembling hands, a slow shuffling walk and difficulty in speaking [Described 1817. After James Parkinson (1755–1824), English physician.]

COMMENT: Parkinson's disease affects the basal ganglia of the brain which control movement, due to the destruction of dopaminergic neurones. Some cases can be improved by treatment with levodopa, which is the precursor of the missing neurotransmitter dopamine, or by drugs which inhibit the breakdown of dopamine.

**paronychia** /ˌpærəˈnɪkiə/ *noun* inflammation near the nail which forms pus, caused by an infection in the fleshy part of the tip of a finger. ◊ **whitlow**

**parosmia** /pəˈrɒzmiə/ *noun* a disorder of the sense of smell

**parotid** /pəˈrɒtɪd/ *adjective* near the ear

**parotid gland** /pəˈrɒtɪd glænd/, **parotid** /pəˈrɒtɪd/ *noun* one of the glands which produces saliva, situated in the neck behind the joint of the jaw and ear

**parotitis** /ˌpærəˈtaɪtɪs/ *noun* inflammation of the parotid glands

COMMENT: Mumps is the commonest form of parotitis, where the parotid gland becomes swollen and the sides of the face appear fat.

**parous** /ˈpeərəs/ *adjective* referring to a woman who has given birth to one or more children

**paroxetine** /pəˈrɒksɪtiːn/ *noun* an antidepressant drug which prolongs the effects of serotonin in the brain

**paroxysm** /ˈpærəksɪz(ə)m/ *noun* 1. a sudden movement of the muscles ○ *She suffered paroxysms of coughing during the night.* 2. the sudden re-appearance of symptoms of the disease 3. a sudden attack of coughing or sneezing

**paroxysmal** /ˌpærəkˈsɪzm(ə)l/ *adjective* referring to a paroxysm, or similar to a paroxysm

**paroxysmal dyspnoea** /pærəkˌsɪzm(ə)l dɪspˈniːə/ *noun* an attack of breathlessness at night, usually caused by congestive heart failure

**paroxysmal tachycardia** /pærəkˌsɪzm(ə)l tæki'kɑːdiə/ *noun* same as **nodal tachycardia**

**parrot disease** /ˈpærət dɪˌziːz/ *noun* same as **psittacosis**

**pars** /pɑːz/ *noun* the Latin word for part

**part** /pɑːt/ *noun* a piece, one of the sections which make up a whole organ or body

**partial** /ˈpɑːʃ(ə)l/ *adjective* not complete, affecting only part of something ○ *He only made a partial recovery.*

**partial amnesia** /ˌpɑːʃ(ə)l æmˈniːziə/ *noun* an inability to remember specific facts, such as names of people

**partial deafness** /ˌpɑːʃ(ə)l ˈdefnəs/ *noun* the condition of being able to hear some sounds but not all

**partial denture** /ˌpɑːʃ(ə)l ˈdentʃə/ *noun* part of a set of false teeth, replacing only a few teeth

**partial gastrectomy** /ˌpɑːʃ(ə)l gæˈstrektəmi/ *noun* an operation to remove part of the stomach

**partially** /ˈpɑːʃ(ə)li/ *adverb* not completely ○ *He is partially paralysed in his right side.* □ **partially deaf** able to hear some sounds but not all □ **partially sighted** having only partial vision ○ *Large print books are available for people who are partially sighted.*

**partially sighted register** /ˌpɑːʃ(ə)li ˈsaɪtɪd ˌredʒɪstə/ *noun* a list of people who have poor sight but are not blind, and may require some special services

**partial mastectomy** /ˌpɑːʃ(ə)l mæˈstektəmi/ *noun* an operation to remove part of a breast

**partial pancreatectomy** /ˌpɑːʃ(ə)l ˌpæŋkriəˈtektəmi/ *noun* an operation to remove part of the pancreas

**partial thickness burn** /ˌpɑːʃ(ə)l ˈθɪknəs bɜːn/ *noun* a burn which leaves enough tissue for the skin to grow again. Also called **superficial thickness burn**

**partial vision** /ˌpɑːʃ(ə)l ˈvɪʒ(ə)n/ *noun* the ability to see only a part of the total field of vision, or not being able to see anything very clearly

**particle** /ˈpɑːtɪk(ə)l/ *noun* a very small piece of matter

**particulate** /pɑːˈtɪkjʊlət/ *adjective* **1.** referring to or composed of particles **2.** made up of separate particles

**particulate matter** /pɑːˈtɪkjʊlət ˌmætə/ *noun* particles of less than a specified size, usually of carbon, which are used as a measure of air pollution and can affect asthma

**partly** /ˈpɑːtli/ *adverb* not completely ○ *She is partly paralysed.*

**parturient** /pɑːˈtjʊəriənt/ *adjective* referring to childbirth ■ *noun* a woman who is in labour

**parturifacient** /pɑːˌtjʊəriˈfeɪʃənt/ *adjective* starting off birth or making it easier to give birth ■ *noun* a drug that starts off birth or makes it easier to give birth

**parturition** /ˌpɑːtjʊˈrɪʃ(ə)n/ *noun* same as **childbirth**

**parulis** /pəˈruːlɪs/ same as **gumboil**

**Paschen bodies** /ˈpæʃken ˌbɒdiz/ *plural noun* particles which occur in the skin lesions of people who have smallpox [After Enrique Paschen (1860–1936), German pathologist]

**pass** /pɑːs/ *verb* to allow faeces, urine or any other body product to come out of the body ○ *Have you passed anything this morning?* ○ *He passed a small stone in his urine.* □ **to pass blood** to produce faeces or urine that contain blood □ **to pass water** to urinate (*informal*)

**passage** /ˈpæsɪdʒ/ *noun* **1.** a long narrow channel inside the body **2.** the process of moving from one place to another **3.** evacuation of the bowels **4.** the introduction of an instrument into a cavity □ **air passage** a tube which takes air to the lungs

**pass away** /ˌpɑːs əˈweɪ/ *verb* used to avoid saying 'die' (*informal*) ○ *Mother passed away during the night.*

**passive** /ˈpæsɪv/ *adjective* receiving rather than initiating an action

**passive immunity** /ˌpæsɪv ɪˈmjuːnɪti/ *noun* immunity which is acquired by a baby in the uterus or by a person through an injection with an antitoxin

**passive movement** /ˌpæsɪv ˈmuːvmənt/ *noun* movement of a limb or other body part by a doctor or therapist, not by the person

**passive smoking** /ˌpæsɪv ˈsməʊkɪŋ/ *noun* the act of breathing in smoke from other people's cigarettes when you do not smoke yourself

**pass on** /ˌpɑːs ˈɒn/ *verb* **1.** to give a disease to someone ○ *Haemophilia is passed on by a woman to her sons.* ○ *The disease was quickly passed on by carriers to the rest of the population.* **2.** used to avoid saying 'die' ○ *My father passed on two years ago.*

**pass out** /ˌpɑːs ˈaʊt/ *verb* to faint (*informal*) ○ *When we told her that her father was ill, she passed out.*

**past** /pɑːst/ *adjective* referring to time which has passed

**paste** /peɪst/ *noun* a medicinal ointment which is very thick and is spread or rubbed onto the skin

**Pasteurella** /ˌpæstəˈrelə/ *noun* a genus of parasitic bacteria, one of which causes the plague

**pasteurisation** /ˌpɑːstʃəraɪˈzeɪʃ(ə)n/, **pasteurization** *noun* the process of heating food or food products to destroy bacteria [After Louis Pasteur (1822–95), French chemist and bacteriologist]

COMMENT: Pasteurisation is carried out by heating food for a short time at a lower temperature than that used for sterilisation: the two methods used are heating to 72°C for fifteen seconds (the high-temperature short-time method) or to 65°C for half an hour, and then cooling rapidly. This will kill tuberculosis bacteria that may be present in milk, for example.

**pasteurise** /ˈpɑːstʃəraɪz/, **pasteurize** *verb* to kill bacteria in food by heating it ○ *The government is telling people to drink only pasteurised milk.*

**past history** /ˌpɑːst ˈhɪst(ə)ri/ *noun* records of earlier illnesses ○ *He has no past history of renal disease.*

**pastille** /ˈpæst(ə)l/ *noun* **1.** a sweet jelly with medication in it, which can be sucked to relieve a sore throat **2.** a small paper disc covered with barium platinocyanide, which changes colour when exposed to radiation

**pat** /pæt/ *verb* to hit someone or something lightly and gently with the palm of the hand or some other flat surface ○ *She patted the baby on the back to make it burp.*

**patch** /pætʃ/ *noun* a piece of sticking plaster with a substance on it, which is stuck to the skin so that the substance to be gradually absorbed into the system through the skin, e.g. in HRT

COMMENT: Patches are available on prescription for various treatments, especially for administering hormone replacement therapy. They are also used for treating nicotine addiction and can be bought without a prescription.

**patch test** /ˈpætʃ test/ *noun* a test for allergies or tuberculosis, where a piece of sticking plaster containing an allergic substance or tuberculin is stuck to the skin to see if there is a reaction

**patella** /pəˈtelə/ *noun* the small bone in front of the knee joint. Also called **kneecap**

**patellar** /pəˈtelə/ *adjective* referring to the kneecap

**patellar reflex** /pəˌtelə ˈriːfleks/ *noun* the jerk made as a reflex action by the knee, when the legs are crossed and the patellar tendon is tapped sharply. Also called **knee jerk**

**patellar tendon** /pəˌtelə ˈtendən/ *noun* a tendon just below the kneecap

**patellectomy** /ˌpætəˈlektəmi/ *noun* a surgical operation to remove the kneecap

**patency** /ˈpeɪtənsi/ *noun* the condition of being wide open ○ *A salpingostomy was performed to restore the patency of the Fallopian tube.*

**patent** /ˈpeɪtənt, ˈpætənt/ *adjective* open, exposed ○ *The presence of a pulse shows that the main blood vessels from the heart to the site of the pulse are patent.*

**patent ductus arteriosus** /ˌpeɪtənt ˌdʌktəs ɑːˌtɪəriˈəʊsəs/ *noun* a congenital condition in which the ductus arteriosus does not close, allowing blood into the circulation without having passed through the lungs

**patent medicine** /ˌpeɪtənt ˈmed(ə)sɪn/ *noun* a medicinal preparation which is made and sold under a trade name and is protected by law from being copied or sold by other manufacturers for a certain length of time after its invention. ◊ **proprietary medicine**

**paternity** /pəˈtɜːnɪti/ *noun* **1.** the fact of being or becoming a father ○ *paternity leave* Compare **maternity 2.** the identity of a father

**paternity test** /pəˈtɜːnɪti test/ *noun* a test such as blood grouping which makes it possible to determine the identity of the father of a child

COMMENT: DNA fingerprinting may be required in order to identify a man who might be the father according to his blood group and that of the child, but is not in fact the father.

**path-** /pæθ/, **patho-** /ˈpæθəʊ/ *prefix* referring to disease

**pathogen** /ˈpæθədʒən/ *noun* a microorganism which causes a disease

**pathogenesis** /ˌpæθəˈdʒenəsɪs/ *noun* the origin, production and development of a morbid or diseased condition

**pathogenetic** /ˌpæθədʒəˈnetɪk/ *adjective* referring to pathogenesis

**pathogenic** /pæθəˈdʒenɪk/ *adjective* causing or producing a disease

**pathogenicity** /ˌpæθədʒəˈnɪsɪti/ *noun* the ability of a pathogen to cause a disease

**pathognomonic** /ˌpæθəɡnəʊˈmɒnɪk/ *adjective* referring to a symptom which is typical and characteristic, and which indicates that someone has a particular disease

**pathological** /ˌpæθəˈlɒdʒɪk(ə)l/, **pathologic** /ˌpæθəˈlɒdʒɪk/ *adjective* **1.** referring to a disease, or caused by a disease **2.** indicating a disease

**pathological depression** /ˌpæθə ˌlɒdʒɪk(ə)l dɪˈpreʃ(ə)n/ *noun* an unusually severe state of depression, possibly leading to suicide

**pathological dislocation** /ˌpæθəlɒdʒɪk(ə)l ˌdɪsləˈkeɪʃ(ə)n/ *noun* the dislocation of a diseased joint

**pathological fracture** /ˌpæθəˌlɒdʒɪk(ə)l ˈfræktʃə/ *noun* a fracture of a diseased bone

**pathologist** /pəˈθɒlədʒɪst/ *noun* **1.** a doctor who specialises in the study of diseases and the changes in the body caused by disease, examining tissue specimens from patients and reporting on the presence or absence of disease in them **2.** a doctor who examines dead bodies in order to find out the cause of death

**pathology** /pəˈθɒlədʒi/ *noun* the study of diseases and the changes in structure and function which diseases cause in the body. Also called **morbid anatomy**

**pathology report** /pəˈθɒlədʒi rɪˌpɔːt/ *noun* a report on tests carried out to find the cause of a disease

**pathophysiology** /ˌpæθəʊfɪziˈɒlədʒi/ *noun* the study of unusual or diseased organs

**pathway** /ˈpɑːθweɪ/ *noun* a series of linked neurones along which nerve impulses travel

**-pathy** /pəθi/ *suffix* **1.** disease **2.** treatment of a disease

**patient** /ˈpeɪʃ(ə)nt/ *adjective* being able to wait a long time without becoming annoyed ○ *You will have to be patient if you are waiting for treatment – the doctor is late with his ap-*

**pointments.** ■ *noun* a person who is in hospital or who is being treated by a doctor ○ *The patients are all asleep in their beds.* ○ *The doctor is taking the patient's temperature.*

**patient allocation** /ˌpeɪʃ(ə)nt ˌælə'keɪʃ(ə)n/ *noun* a system of assigning each patient to a particular nurse for all their care needs

**patient identifier** /ˌpeɪʃ(ə)nt aɪ'dentɪfaɪə/ *noun* a code of letters and numbers attached to the patient's medical records by which all information concerning the patient can be tracked, e.g. cause of death

**patulous** /'pætjʊləs/ *adjective* stretched open, patent

**Paul–Bunnell reaction** /ˌpɔːl 'bʌn(ə)l rɪ ˌækʃən/, **Paul–Bunnell test** /ˌpɔːl 'bʌn(ə)l ˌtest/ *noun* a blood test to see if someone has glandular fever, where the person's blood is tested against a solution containing glandular fever bacilli [Described 1932. After John Rodman Paul (b. 1893), US physician; Walls Willard Bunnell (1902–66), US physician.]

**Paul's tube** /'pɔːlz tjuːb/ *noun* a glass tube used to remove the contents of the bowel after an opening has been made between the intestine and the abdominal wall [Described 1891. After Frank Thomas Paul (1851–1941), British surgeon.]

**pavement epithelium** /'peɪvmənt epɪ ˌθiːliəm/ *noun* same as **squamous epithelium**

**Pavlov's method** /'pævlɒvz ˌmeθəd/ *noun* a set of procedures for the study or production of conditioned reflexes

**PBI test** /ˌpi: bi: 'aɪ test/ *noun* same as **protein-bound iodine test**

**p.c.** /ˌpi: 'si:/ *adverb* (*used on prescriptions*) after food. Full form **post cibum**

**PCC** *abbr* Professional Conduct Committee

**PCG** *abbr* primary care group

**PCOD** *abbr* polycystic ovary disease

**PCOS** *abbr* polycystic ovary syndrome

**PCP** *abbr* pneumocystis carinii pneumonia

**PCR** *abbr* polymerase chain reaction

**PCT** *abbr* primary care trust

**p.d.¹** *adverb* (*used on prescriptions*) per day. Full form **per diem**

**p.d.²** *abbr* per diem

**PE** *abbr* pulmonary embolism

**peak** /pi:k/ *noun* the highest point

**peak expiratory flow rate** /ˌpi:k ɪk ˌspaɪərət(ə)ri 'fləʊ ˌreɪt/ *noun* the rate at which someone can expel air from their lungs when they are full and with no time limit. Abbr **PEFR**

**peak period** /'pi:k ˌpɪəriəd/ *noun* the time of the day, days of the month or months of the year, during which something such as a fever, tiredness, infectious disease or cold reaches its highest point or occurs most frequently in a population

**peaky** /'pi:ki/ *adjective* thin, pale, and sickly in appearance (*informal*)

**pearl** /pɜːl/ ♦ **Bohn's nodules**

**Pearson bed** /'pɪəs(ə)n bed/ *noun* a type of bed with a Balkan frame, a rectangular frame attached to and overhanging the bed, used mainly for people with splints

**peau d'orange** /ˌpəʊ dɒ'rɑːnʒ/ *noun* thickened skin with many little depressions caused by lymphoedema which forms over a breast tumour or in elephantiasis (NOTE: From the French phrase meaning 'orange peel'.)

**pecten** /'pektən/ *noun* **1.** the middle section of the wall of the anal passage **2.** a hard ridge on the pubis

**pectineal** /pek'tɪniəl/ *adjective* **1.** referring to the pecten of the pubis **2.** referring to a structure with ridges like a comb

**pectoral** /'pekt(ə)rəl/ *noun* **1.** a therapeutic substance which has a good effect on respiratory disease **2.** same as **pectoral muscle** ■ *adjective* referring to the chest

**pectoral girdle** /ˌpekt(ə)rəl 'gɜːd(ə)l/ *noun* the shoulder bones, the scapulae and clavicles, to which the upper arm bones are attached. Also called **shoulder girdle**

**pectoralis** /ˌpektə'reɪlɪs/ *noun* a chest muscle

**pectoralis major** /pektəˌreɪlɪs 'meɪdʒə/ *noun* a large chest muscle which pulls the arm forward or rotates it

**pectoralis minor** /pektəˌreɪlɪs 'maɪnə/ *noun* a small chest muscle which allows the shoulder to be depressed

**pectoral muscle** /'pekt(ə)rəl ˌmʌs(ə)l/ *noun* one of two muscles which lie across the chest and control movements of the shoulder and arm. Also called **chest muscle**

**pectus** /'pektəs/ *noun* the anterior part of the chest

**pectus carinatum** /ˌpektəs ˌkærɪ'nɑːtəm/ *noun* a condition in which the sternum is unusually prominent. Also called **pigeon breast**

**pectus excavatum** /ˌpektəs ˌekskə'veɪtəm/ *noun* a congenital condition, in which the chest is depressed in the centre because the lower part of the breastbone is curved backwards. Also called **funnel chest**

**pedes** /'pi:di:z/ plural of **pes**

**pediatrics** /ˌpi:di'ætrɪks/ *noun* US same as **paediatrics**

**pedicle** /'pedɪk(ə)l/ *noun* **1.** a long thin piece of skin which attaches a skin graft to the place where it was growing originally **2.** a piece of tissue which connects a tumour to healthy tissue **3.** a bridge which connects the lamina of a vertebra to the body

**pediculicide** /pɪ'dɪkjʊlɪsaɪd/ *noun* a chemical substance that kills lice

**pediculosis** /pɪˌdɪkjʊ'ləʊsɪs/ *noun* a skin disease caused by being infested with lice

**Pediculus** /pɪˈdɪkjʊləs/ *noun* same as **louse** (NOTE: The plural is **Pediculi**.)

**Pediculus capitis** /pɪˌdɪkjʊləs kəˈpaɪtɪs/ *noun* same as **head louse**

**pedo-** /piːd/ *prefix* same as **paedo-**

**pedodontia** /ˌpiːdəˈdɒnʃə/ *noun* the study of children's teeth

**pedodontist** /ˌpiːdəˈdɒntɪst/ *noun* a dentist who specialises in the treatment of children's teeth

**peduncle** /pɪˈdʌŋkəl/ *noun* a stem or stalk

**pedunculate** /pɪˈdʌŋkjʊleɪt/ *adjective* having a stem or stalk. Opposite **sessile**

**pee** /piː/ *verb* same as **urinate** (*informal*)

**peel** /piːl/ *verb* 1. to take the skin off a fruit or vegetable 2. (*of skin*) to come off in pieces ○ *After getting sunburnt, his skin began to peel.*

**PEEP** *abbr* positive end-expiratory pressure

**peer review** /ˈpɪə rɪˌvjuː/ *noun* an assessment of a piece of someone's work by people who are experts on the subject

**PEFR** *abbr* peak expiratory flow rate

**Pel–Ebstein fever** /ˌpel ˈebstaɪn ˌfiːvə/ *noun* a fever associated with Hodgkin's disease which recurs regularly [Described 1885. After Pieter Klaases Pel (1852–1919), Professor of Medicine in Amsterdam, Netherlands; Wilhelm Ebstein (1836–1912), Professor of Medicine at Göttingen, Germany.]

**pellagra** /pəˈlægrə/ *noun* a disease caused by a deficiency of nicotinic acid, riboflavine and pyridoxine from the vitamin B complex, where patches of skin become inflamed, and the person has anorexia, nausea and diarrhoea

COMMENT: In some cases of pellagra the patient's mental faculties can be affected, with depression, headaches and numbness of the extremities. Treatment is by improving the patient's diet.

**Pellegrini–Stieda's disease** /peləˌgriːni ˈstiːdəz dɪˌziːz/ *noun* a disease where an injury to the knee causes the ligament to become calcified [Described 1905. After Augusto Pellegrini, surgeon in Florence, Italy; Alfred Stieda (1869–1945), Professor of Surgery at Königsberg, Germany.]

**pellet** /ˈpelɪt/ *noun* 1. a small rod- or oval-shaped pill of steroid hormone, usually either oestrogen or testosterone, that is implanted under the skin for slow absorption 2. solid sediment at the base of a container after centrifuging

**pellicle** /ˈpelɪk(ə)l/ *noun* a thin layer of skin tissue

**pellucida** /pɪˈluːsɪdə/ ♦ **zona pellucida**

**pelves** /ˈpelviːz/ plural of **pelvis**

**pelvic** /ˈpelvɪk/ *adjective* referring to the pelvis

**pelvic brim** /ˌpelvɪk ˈbrɪm/ *noun* a line on the ilium which separates the false pelvis from the true pelvis

**pelvic cavity** /ˌpelvɪk ˈkævɪti/ *noun* a space below the abdominal cavity, above the pelvis

**pelvic colon** /ˌpelvɪk ˈkəʊlɒn/ *noun* same as **sigmoid colon**

**pelvic diaphragm** /ˌpelvɪk ˈdaɪəfræm/ *noun* a sheet of muscle between the pelvic cavity and the peritoneum

**pelvic floor** /ˌpelvɪk ˈflɔː/ *noun* the lower part of the space beneath the pelvic girdle, formed of muscle

**pelvic fracture** /ˌpelvɪk ˈfræktʃə/ *noun* a fracture of the pelvis

**pelvic girdle** /ˌpelvɪk ˈgɜːd(ə)l/ *noun* the ring formed by the two hip bones to which the thigh bones are attached. Also called **hip girdle**

**pelvic inflammatory disease** /ˌpelvɪk ɪnˈflæmət(ə)ri dɪˌziːz/ *noun* an inflammation of a woman's reproductive organs in the pelvic area, which can cause infertility

**pelvic outlet** /ˌpelvɪk ˈaʊtlet/ *noun* an opening at the base of the pelvis

**pelvic version** /ˌpelvɪk ˈvɜːʃ(ə)n/ *noun* turning a fetus around in the uterus by moving the buttocks of the fetus

**pelvimeter** /pelˈvɪmɪtə/ *noun* an instrument to measure the diameter and capacity of the pelvis

**pelvimetry** /pelˈvɪmɪtri/ *noun* the act of measuring the pelvis, especially to see if the internal ring is wide enough for a baby to pass through in childbirth

**pelvis** /ˈpelvɪs/ *noun* 1. the strong basin-shaped ring of bone near the bottom of the spine, formed of the hip bones at the front and sides and the sacrum and coccyx at the back 2. the internal space inside the pelvic girdle (NOTE: [all senses] The plural is **pelvises** or **pelves**.)

COMMENT: The hip bones are each in three sections: the ilium, the ischium and the pubis and are linked in front by the pubic symphysis. The pelvic girdle is shaped in a different way in men and women, the internal space being wider in women. The top part of the pelvis, which does not form a complete ring, is called the 'false pelvis'; the lower part is the 'true pelvis'.

**pelvis of the kidney** /ˌpelvɪs əv ðə ˈkɪdni/ *noun* same as **renal pelvis**. See illustration at KIDNEY in Supplement (NOTE: For other terms referring to the pelvis of the kidney, see words beginning with **pyel-, pyelo-**.)

**pemphigoid** /ˈpemfɪgɔɪd/ *noun* a skin disease which is similar to pemphigus ■ *adjective* referring to a skin disease similar to pemphigus

**pemphigus** /ˈpemfɪgəs/ *noun* a rare disease where large blisters form inside the skin

**pendulous** /ˈpendjʊləs/ *adjective* referring to an object or body part which hangs loosely or swings freely

**penes** /ˈpiːniz/ plural of **penis**

**penetrate** /ˈpenɪtreɪt/ *verb* to go through or into something ○ *The end of the broken bone has penetrated the liver.* ○ *The ulcer burst, penetrating the wall of the duodenum.*

**penetration** /ˌpenɪˈtreɪʃ(ə)n/ *noun* the act of penetrating ○ *the penetration of the vagina by the penis* ○ *penetration of an ovum by a spermatozoon*

**-penia** /piːniə/ *suffix* meaning a deficiency or not enough of something

**penicillamine** /ˌpenɪˈsɪləmiːn/ *noun* a chelating agent which is used to help the body get rid of toxic metals

**penicillin** /ˌpenɪˈsɪlɪn/ *noun* a common antibiotic originally produced from a fungus (NOTE: Penicillin drugs have names ending in -cillin: amoxicillin.)

COMMENT: Penicillin is effective against many microbial diseases, but some people can be allergic to it, and this fact should be noted on medical record cards.

**penicillinase** /ˌpenɪˈsɪlɪneɪz/ *noun* an enzyme produced by some bacteria that inactivates penicillin, used to treat adverse reactions to penicillin

**penicillin resistance** /ˌpenɪsɪlɪn rɪˈzɪstəns/ *noun* the ability of bacteria to resist penicillin

**Penicillium** /ˌpenɪˈsɪliəm/ *noun* the fungus from which penicillin is derived

**penile** /ˈpiːnaɪl/ *adjective* referring to the penis

**penile urethra** /ˌpiːnaɪl jʊˈriːθrə/ *noun* a tube in the penis through which urine and semen pass

**penis** /ˈpiːnɪs/ *noun* the male genital organ, which also passes urine. See illustration at UROGENITAL SYSTEM (MALE) in Supplement. ◊ **kraurosis penis**

COMMENT: The penis is a mass of tissue containing the urethra. When stimulated the tissue of the penis fills with blood and becomes erect.

**pentamidine** /penˈtæmɪdiːn/ *noun* an antibiotic used in the treatment of African sleeping sickness and of pneumonia in people with AIDS

**pentazocine** /penˈtæzəsiːn/ *noun* an artificially produced narcotic drug used to reduce pain

**pentose** /ˈpentəʊz/ *noun* a sugar containing five carbon atoms

**pentosuria** /ˌpentəˈsjʊəriə/ *noun* a condition in which pentose is present in the urine

**Pentothal** /ˈpentəθæl/ a trade name for thiopentone

**Peplau's model** /ˈpeplaʊ ˌmɒd(ə)l/ *noun* a model for nursing which describes the individual as a system with physiological, psychological and social components. The nurse and patient work together to define the patient's problems and to understand their reactions to

one another, and the nurse takes on different roles in each phase of the relationship, such as a teacher, counsellor, leader, and technical expert, until the patient no longer needs their care.

**pepsin** /ˈpepsɪn/ *noun* an enzyme in the stomach which breaks down the proteins in food into peptones

**pepsinogen** /pepˈsɪnədʒən/ *noun* a secretion from the gastric gland which is the inactive form of pepsin

**peptic** /ˈpeptɪk/ *adjective* referring to digestion or to the digestive system

**peptic ulcer** /ˌpeptɪk ˈʌlsə/ *noun* a benign ulcer in the duodenum or in the stomach

**peptidase** /ˈpeptɪdeɪz/ *noun* an enzyme which breaks down proteins in the intestine into amino acids

**peptide** /ˈpeptaɪd/ *noun* a compound formed of two or more amino acids

**peptone** /ˈpeptəʊn/ *noun* a substance produced by the action of pepsins on proteins in food

**peptonuria** /ˌpeptəˈnjʊəriə/ *noun* a condition in which peptones are present in the urine

**per** /pɜː, pə/ *preposition* **1.** out of each ○ *ten per thousand* **2.** by or through ○ *per rectum*

**per cent** /pə ˈsent/ *noun, adjective, adverb* in or for every hundred ○ *Fifty per cent (50%) of the tests were positive.* ○ *Seventy-five per cent (75%) of hospital cases remain in hospital for less than four days.* □ **there has been a five per cent increase in applications** the number of applications has gone up by five in every hundred □ **new cases have decreased twenty per cent this year** the number of new cases has gone down by twenty in every hundred

**percentage** /pəˈsentɪdʒ/ *noun* the proportion rate in every hundred or for every hundred ○ *What is the percentage of long-stay patients in the hospital?*

**perception** /pəˈsepʃən/ *noun* an impression formed in the brain as a result of information about the outside world which is passed back by the senses

**perceptive deafness** /peˌseptɪv ˈdefnəs/ *noun* same as **sensorineural deafness**

**percussion** /pəˈkʌʃ(ə)n/ *noun* a test, usually on the heart and lungs, in which the doctor taps part of the person's body and listens to the sound produced

**percutaneous** /ˌpɜːkjuːˈteɪniəs/ *adjective* through the skin

**percutaneous absorption** /ˌpɜːkjuːˌteɪniəs əbˈzɔːpʃən/ *noun* the process of absorbing a substance through the skin

**percutaneous angioplasty** /ˌpɜːkjuːˌteɪniəs ˈændʒiəplæsti/ *noun* the repair of a narrowed artery by passing a balloon into the artery through a catheter and then inflating it. Also called **balloon angioplasty**

**percutaneous epididymal sperm aspiration** /ˌpɜːkjuːˈteɪniəs ˌepɪdɪdɪm(ə)l ˈspɜːm ˌæspɪreɪʃ(ə)n/ *noun* the removal of sperm from the epididymis by withdrawing it through the skin, usually as part of fertility treatment. Abbr **PESA**

**per diem** /pɜː ˈdiːem/ *adverb* (*written on prescriptions*) per day

**perennial** /pəˈreniəl/ *adjective* which continues all the time, for a period of years ○ *She has perennial bronchial asthma.*

**perforate** /ˈpɜːfəreɪt/ *verb* to make a hole through something ○ *The ulcer perforated the duodenum.*

**perforated eardrum** /ˌpɜːfəreɪtɪd ˈɪədrʌm/ *noun* an eardrum with a hole in it

**perforated ulcer** /ˌpɜːfəreɪtɪd ˈʌlsə/ *noun* an ulcer which has made a hole in the wall of the intestine

**perforation** /ˌpɜːfəˈreɪʃ(ə)n/ *noun* a hole through the whole thickness of a tissue or membrane such as the intestine or eardrum

**perform** /pəˈfɔːm/ *verb* **1.** to do an operation ○ *A team of three surgeons performed the heart transplant operation.* **2.** to work ○ *The new heart has performed very well.* ○ *The kidneys are not performing as well as they should.*

**performance** /pəˈfɔːməns/ *noun* a way in which something works ○ *The doctors are not satisfied with the performance of the transplanted heart.*

**performance indicators** /pəˈfɔːməns ˌɪndɪkeɪtəz/ *plural noun* statistical information needed for analysis of how effectively health organisations are meeting their objectives, produced by health authorities and sent to the government. Abbr **PIs**

**perfuse** /pəˈfjuːz/ *verb* to introduce a liquid into tissue or an organ, especially by circulating it through blood vessels

**perfusion** /pəˈfjuːʒ(ə)n/ *noun* the process of passing a liquid through vessels, an organ or tissue, e.g. the flow of blood into lung tissue

**perfusion scan** /pəˈfjuːʒ(ə)n skæn/ *noun* a procedure in which radioactive or radiopaque substances are introduced into the body so that the blood supply of an organ can be traced

**peri-** /peri/ *prefix* near, around or enclosing

**periadenitis** /ˌperiədɪˈnaɪtɪs/ *noun* inflammation of tissue around a gland

**perianal** /ˌperiˈeɪn(ə)l/ *adjective* around the anus

**perianal haematoma** /ˌperieɪn(ə)l ˌhiːməˈtəʊmə/ *noun* a small painful swelling outside the anus caused by forcing a bowel movement

**periarteritis** /ˌperiɑːtəˈraɪtɪs/ *noun* inflammation of the outer coat of an artery and the tissue round it

**periarteritis nodosa** /ˌperiɑːtəˌraɪtɪs nəʊˈdəʊsə/ *noun* same as **polyarteritis nodosa**

**periarthritis** /ˌperiɑːˈθraɪtɪs/ *noun* inflammation of the tissue round a joint

**pericard-** /perikɑːd/ *prefix* referring to the pericardium

**pericardectomy** /ˌperikɑːˈdektəmi/ *noun* the surgical removal of the pericardium

**pericardial** /ˌperiˈkɑːdiəl/ *adjective* referring to the pericardium

**pericardial effusion** /ˌperikɑːdiəl ɪˈfjuːʒ(ə)n/ *noun* an excess of fluid which forms in the pericardial sac

**pericardial friction** /ˌperikɑːdiəl ˈfrɪkʃ(ə)n/ *noun* the rubbing together of the two parts of the pericardium in pericarditis

**pericardial sac** /ˌperikɑːdiəl ˈsæk/ *noun* the inner part of the pericardium forming a bag-like structure or sac which contains fluid to prevent the two parts of the pericardium rubbing together

**pericardiectomy** /perikɑːdiˈektəmi/ *noun* same as **pericardectomy**

**pericardiocentesis** /ˌperiˌkɑːdiəʊsenˈtiːsɪs/ *noun* the puncture of the pericardium to remove fluid

**pericardiorrhaphy** /ˌperikɑːdiˈɔːrəfi/ *noun* a surgical operation to repair a wound in the pericardium

**pericardiostomy** /ˌperikɑːdiˈɒstəmi/ *noun* a surgical operation to open the pericardium through the thoracic wall to drain off fluid

**pericardiotomy** /ˌperikɑːdiˈɒtəmi/ *noun* same as **pericardotomy**

**pericarditis** /ˌperikɑːˈdaɪtɪs/ *noun* inflammation of the pericardium □ **acute pericarditis** a sudden attack of fever and pains in the chest, caused by the two parts of the pericardium rubbing together

**pericardium** /ˌperiˈkɑːdiəm/ *noun* a membrane which surrounds and supports the heart

**pericardotomy** /ˌperikɑːˈdɒtəmi/ *noun* a surgical operation to open the pericardium

**perichondritis** /ˌperikɒnˈdraɪtɪs/ *noun* inflammation of cartilage, especially in the outer ear

**perichondrium** /ˌperiˈkɒndriəm/ *noun* the fibrous connective tissue which covers cartilage

**pericolpitis** /ˌperikɒlˈpaɪtɪs/ *noun* inflammation of the connective tissue round the vagina. Also called **paracolpitis**

**pericranium** /ˌperiˈkreɪniəm/ *noun* connective tissue which covers the surface of the skull

**pericystitis** /ˌperisɪˈstaɪtɪs/ *noun* inflammation of the structures round the bladder, usually caused by infection in the uterus

**perifolliculitis** /ˌperiˌfɒlɪkjuˈlaɪtɪs/ *noun* inflammation of the skin round hair follicles

**perihepatitis** /ˌperihepəˈtaɪtɪs/ *noun* inflammation of the membrane round the liver

**perilymph** /ˈperilɪmf/ *noun* a fluid found in the labyrinth of the inner ear

**perimenopause** /ˌperiˈmenəpɔːz/ *noun* the few years before the menopause, in which oestrogen levels start to fall

**perimeter** /pəˈrɪmɪtə/ *noun* **1.** an instrument to measure the field of vision **2.** the length of the outside line around an enclosed area

**perimetritis** /ˌperɪməˈtraɪtɪs/ *noun* inflammation of the perimetrium

**perimetrium** /ˌperiˈmiːtriəm/ *noun* a membrane round the uterus

**perimetry** /pəˈrɪmɪtri/ *noun* a measurement of the field of vision

**perimysium** /ˌperiˈmaɪsiəm/ *noun* a sheath which surrounds a bundle of muscle fibres

**perinatal** /ˌperɪˈneɪt(ə)l/ *adjective* referring to the period just before and after childbirth

**perinatal mortality rate** /ˌperineɪt(ə)l mɔːˈtælɪti reɪt/ *noun* the number of babies born dead or who die during the period immediately after childbirth, shown per thousand babies born

**perinatal period** /ˌperiˈneɪt(ə)l ˌpɪəriəd/ *noun* the period of time before and after childbirth, from the 28th week after conception to the first week after delivery

**perinatologist** /ˌperinəˈtɒlədʒɪst/ *noun* an obstetrician who is a specialist in perinatology

**perinatology** /ˌperinəˈtɒlədʒi/ *noun* a branch of medicine which studies and treats physiological and pathological conditions affecting the mother and/or infant just before and just after the birth of a baby

**perineal** /ˌperɪˈniːəl/ *adjective* referring to the perineum

**perineal body** /ˌperɪniːəl ˈbɒdi/ *noun* the mass of muscle and fibres between the anus and the vagina or prostate

**perineal muscle** /ˌperɪniːəl ˈmʌs(ə)l/ *noun* one of the muscles which lie in the perineum

**perineoplasty** /ˌperiˈniːəplæsti/ *noun* a surgical operation to repair the perineum by grafting tissue

**perineorrhaphy** /ˌperiniˈɔːrəfi/ *noun* a surgical operation to stitch up a perineum which has torn during childbirth

**perinephric** /ˌperiˈnefrɪk/ *adjective* around the kidney

**perinephritis** /ˌperinɪˈfraɪtɪs/ *noun* inflammation of tissue round the kidney, which spreads from an infected kidney

**perinephrium** /ˌperiˈnefriəm/ *noun* the fatty tissue that is around a kidney

**perineum** /ˌperɪˈniːəm/ *noun* the skin and tissue between the opening of the urethra and the anus

**perineurium** /ˌperiˈnjʊəriəm/ *noun* connective tissue which surrounds bundles of nerve fibres

**periocular** /ˌperiˈɒkjʊlə/ *adjective* around the eyeball

**period** /ˈpɪəriəd/ *noun* **1.** a length of time ○ *The patient regained consciousness after a short period of time.* ○ *She is allowed out of bed for two periods each day.* **2.** menstruation or the menses, bleeding from the uterus which occurs in a woman each month when the lining of the uterus is shed because no fertilised egg is present ○ *She always has heavy periods.* ○ *Some women experience abdominal pain during their periods.* ○ *She has bleeding between periods.*

**periodic** /ˌpɪəriˈɒdɪk/ *adjective* occurring from time to time ○ *He has periodic attacks of migraine.* ○ *She has to go to the clinic for periodic checkups.*

**periodic fever** /ˌpɪəriɒdɪk ˈfiːvə/ *noun* a disease of the kidneys, common in Mediterranean countries

**periodicity** /ˌpɪəriəˈdɪsɪti/ *noun* the timing of recurrent attacks of a disease

**periodic paralysis** /ˌpɪəriɒdɪk pəˈræləsɪs/ *noun* recurrent attacks of weakness where the level of potassium in the blood is low

**periodontal** /ˌperiəʊˈdɒnt(ə)l/, **periodontic** /ˌperiəʊˈdɒntɪk/ *adjective* referring to the area around the teeth

**periodontal membrane** /ˌperiəʊˌdɒnt(ə)l ˈmembreɪn/, **periodontal ligament** /ˌperiəʊ ˌdɒnt(ə)l ˈlɪgəmənt/ *noun* a ligament which attaches a tooth to the bone of the jaw

**periodontics** /ˌperiəʊˈdɒntɪks/, **periodontia** /ˌperiəʊˈdɒnʃə/ *noun* the study of diseases of the periodontal membrane

**periodontist** /ˌperiəʊˈdɒntɪst/ *noun* a dentist who specialises in the treatment of gum diseases

**periodontitis** /ˌperiəʊdɒnˈtaɪtɪs/ *noun* an infection of the periodontal membrane leading to pyorrhoea, and resulting in the teeth falling out if untreated

**periodontium** /ˌperiəʊˈdɒnʃiəm/ *noun* **1.** the gums, bone and periodontal membrane around a tooth **2.** same as **periodontal membrane**

**perionychia** /ˌperiəʊˈnɪkiə/, **perionyxis** /ˌperiəʊˈnɪksɪs/ *noun* a painful swelling round a fingernail

**perionychium** /ˌperiəʊˈnɪkiəm/ *noun* the skin that is round a fingernail or toenail

**perioperative** /ˌperiˈɒp(ə)rətɪv/ *adjective* before and after a surgical operation

'During the perioperative period little attention is given to thermoregulation.' [*British Journal of Nursing*]

**periorbital** /ˌperiəʊˈɔːbɪt(ə)l/ *adjective* around the eye socket

**periosteal** /ˌperiˈɒstiəl/ *adjective* referring to, or attached to, the periosteum

**periosteotome** /periˈɒstiəʊtəʊm/ *noun* a surgical instrument used to cut the periosteum

**periosteum** /ˌperiˈɒstiəm/ *noun* a dense layer of connective tissue around a bone. See illustration at **BONE STRUCTURE** in Supplement

**periosteum elevator** /ˌperiˌɒstiəm ˈeləveɪtə/ *noun* a surgical instrument used to remove the periosteum from a bone

**periostitis** /ˌperiəˈstaɪtɪs/ *noun* inflammation of the periosteum

**periotic** /ˌperiˈɒtɪk/ *adjective* referring to the area around the ear, especially the bones around the inner ear

**peripheral** /pəˈrɪf(ə)rⁿəl/ *adjective* at the edge

**peripheral nerves** /pəˈrɪf(ə)rəl nɜːvz/ *plural noun* the parts of motor and sensory nerves which branch from the brain and spinal cord

**peripheral nervous system** /pəˌrɪf(ə)rəl ˈnɜːvəs ˌsɪstəm/ *noun* all the nerves in different parts of the body which are linked and governed by the central nervous system. Abbr **PNS**

**peripheral resistance** /pəˌrɪf(ə)rəl rɪˈzɪstəns/ *noun* the ability of the peripheral blood vessels to slow down the flow of blood inside them

**peripheral vascular disease** /pəˌrɪf(ə)rəl ˈvæskjʊlə dɪˌziːz/ *noun* a disease affecting the blood vessels which supply the arms and legs

**peripheral vasodilator** /pəˌrɪf(ə)rəl ˌveɪzəʊdaɪˈleɪtə/ *noun* a chemical substance which acts to widen the blood vessels in the arms and legs and so improves bad circulation

**periphery** /pəˈrɪf(ə)ri/ *noun* **1.** the regions of the body where the nerves end, such as the sense organs or the muscles **2.** the surface of something

**periphlebitis** /ˌperɪfləˈbaɪtɪs/ *noun* **1.** inflammation of the outer coat of a vein **2.** an inflammation of the connective tissue round a vein

**periproctitis** /ˌperiprɒkˈtaɪtɪs/ *noun* swelling of the tissues around the rectum

**perisalpingitis** /ˌperisælpɪnˈdʒaɪtɪs/ *noun* inflammation of the peritoneum and other parts round a Fallopian tube

**perisplenitis** /ˌperispləˈnaɪtɪs/ *noun* inflammation of the peritoneum and other parts round the spleen

**peristalsis** /ˌperiˈstælsɪs/ *noun* the movement, like waves, produced by alternate contraction and relaxation of muscles along an organ such as the intestine or oesophagus, which pushes the contents of the organ along it. Compare **antiperistalsis**

**peristaltic** /ˌperiˈstæltɪk/ *adjective* occurring in waves, as in peristalsis

**peritendinitis** /peritendiˈnaɪtɪs/ *noun* same as **tenosynovitis**

**peritomy** /pəˈrɪtəmi/ *noun* **1.** a surgical operation on the eye, where the conjunctiva is cut in a circle round the cornea **2.** circumcision

**peritoneal** /ˌperitəˈniːəl/ *adjective* referring to, or belonging to, the peritoneum

**peritoneal cavity** /ˌperitəˌniːəl ˈkævɪti/ *noun* a space between the layers of the peritoneum, containing the major organs of the abdomen

**peritoneal dialysis** /ˌperitəˌniːəl daɪˈæləsɪs/ *noun* removing waste matter from someone's blood by introducing fluid into the peritoneum which then acts as a filter, as opposed to haemodialysis

**peritoneoscope** /ˌperiˈtəʊniəskəʊp/ *noun* same as **laparoscope**

**peritoneoscopy** /ˌperitəʊniˈɒskəpi/ *noun* same as **laparoscopy**

**peritoneum** /ˌperitəˈniːəm/ *noun* a membrane which lines the abdominal cavity and covers the organs in it

**peritonitis** /ˌperitəˈnaɪtɪs/ *noun* inflammation of the peritoneum as a result of bacterial infection

> COMMENT: Peritonitis is a serious condition and can have many causes. One of its effects is to stop the peristalsis of the intestine so making it impossible for a person to eat and digest.

**peritonsillar** /ˌperiˈtɒnsɪlə/ *adjective* around the tonsils

**peritonsillar abscess** /ˌperiˌtɒnsɪlə ˈæbses/ *noun* same as **quinsy**

**peritrichous** /pəˈrɪtrɪkəs/ *adjective* referring to bacteria where the surface of the cell is covered with flagella

**perityphlitis** /ˌperitɪˈflaɪtɪs/ *noun* swelling of the tissues around the caecum

**periumbilical** /ˌperiʌmˈbɪlɪk(ə)l/ *adjective* around the navel

**periureteritis** /ˌperijʊəritəˈraɪtɪs/ *noun* inflammation of the tissue round a ureter, usually caused by inflammation of the ureter itself

**periurethral** /ˌperijʊəˈriːθrəl/ *adjective* around the urethra

**PERLA** *abbreviation* Pupils Equal and Reactive to Light and Accommodation

**perle** /pɜːl/ *noun* a soft capsule of medicine

**perleche** /pɜːˈleʃ/ *noun* **1.** inflammation, with small cracks, at the corners of the mouth, caused by infection, poor diet, or producing too much saliva **2.** candidiasis

**permanent** /ˈpɜːmənənt/ *adjective* always existing ○ *The accident left him with a permanent disability.*

**permanently** /ˈpɜːmənəntli/ *adverb* always, forever ○ *He was permanently disabled by the accident.*

**permanent teeth** /ˈpɜːmənənt tiːθ/ *noun* the teeth in an adult, which replace the child's milk teeth during childhood

COMMENT: The permanent teeth consist of eight incisors, four canines, eight premolars and twelve molars, the last four molars (one on each side of the upper and lower jaw) being called the wisdom teeth.

**permeability** /ˌpɜːmiəˈbɪlɪti/ *noun* (*of a membrane*) the ability to allow some substances to pass through

**permeable membrane** /ˌpɜːmiəb(ə)l ˈmembreɪn/ *noun* a membrane which allows some substances to pass through it

**pernicious** /pəˈnɪʃəs/ *adjective* harmful or dangerous, or unusually severe and likely to end in death

**pernicious anaemia** /pəˌnɪʃəs əˈniːmiə/ *noun* a disease where an inability to absorb vitamin B₁₂ prevents the production of red blood cells and damages the spinal cord. Also called **Addison's anaemia**

**perniosis** /ˌpɜːniˈəʊsɪs/ *noun* any condition caused by cold which affects blood vessels in the skin

**pero-** /perəʊ/ *prefix* malformed or impaired

**peromelia** /ˌperəʊˈmiːliə/ *noun* a congenital condition in which the limbs have developed unusually

**peroneal** /ˌperəʊˈniːəl/ *adjective* referring to the outside of the leg

**peroneal muscle** /ˌperəʊˈniːəl ˌmʌs(ə)l/, **peroneus** /ˌperəʊˈniːəs/ *noun* one of three muscles, the peroneus brevis, longus and tertius, on the outside of the lower leg which make the leg turn outwards

**peroperative** /pəˈrɒp(ə)rətɪv/ *adjective* taking place during a surgical operation

**peroral** /pəˈrɔːrəl/ *adjective* through the mouth

**per os** /pər ˈɒs/ *adverb* referring to a drug or other substance to be taken through the mouth

**persecute** /ˈpɜːsɪkjuːt/ *verb* to make someone suffer all the time ○ *In paranoia, the patient feels he is being persecuted.*

**persecution** /ˌpɜːsɪˈkjuːʃ(ə)n/ *noun* the act of being made to suffer

**perseveration** /ˌpɜːsevəˈreɪʃ(ə)n/ *noun* the act of repeating actions or words without any stimulus

**persist** /pəˈsɪst/ *verb* to continue for some time ○ *The weakness in the right arm persisted for two weeks.*

**persistent** /pəˈsɪstənt/ *adjective* continuing for some time ○ *treatment aimed at the relief of persistent angina* ○ *She had a persistent cough.*

**persistent vegetative state** /pəˌsɪstənt ˈvedʒɪtətɪv steɪt/ *noun* a condition in which someone is alive and breathes, but shows no brain activity, and will never recover consciousness. Abbr **PVS**

**person** /ˈpɜːs(ə)n/ *noun* a man or woman

**personal** /ˈpɜːs(ə)n(ə)l/ *adjective* referring or belonging to a person ○ *Only certain senior members of staff can consult the personal records of the patients.*

**personal care** /ˈpɜːs(ə)nəl keə/ *noun* the act of washing, toileting and dressing someone who cannot do these things for themselves

**personal hygiene** /ˌpɜːs(ə)n(ə)l ˈhaɪdʒiːn/ *noun* the standards someone has of looking after parts of their body such as hair, skin, teeth and breath, hands and nails, and keeping them clean

**personality** /ˌpɜːsəˈnælɪti/ *noun* all the characteristics which are typical of one particular person and the way he or she thinks and behaves, and which make him or her different from other people

'Alzheimer's disease is a progressive disorder which sees a gradual decline in intellectual functioning and deterioration of personality and physical coordination and activity' [*Nursing Times*]

**personality disorder** /ˌpɜːsəˈnælɪti dɪsˌɔːdə/ *noun* a disorder which affects the way a person behaves, especially in relation to other people

**personnel** /ˌpɜːsəˈnel/ *noun* members of staff ○ *All hospital personnel must be immunised against hepatitis.* ○ *Only senior personnel can inspect the patients' medical records.* (NOTE: **Personnel** is singular.)

**perspiration** /ˌpɜːspəˈreɪʃ(ə)n/ *noun* sweat or the action of sweating ○ *Perspiration broke out on her forehead.*

COMMENT: Perspiration is formed in the sweat glands under the epidermis and cools the body as the moisture evaporates from the skin. Sweat contains salt, and in hot countries it may be necessary to take salt tablets to replace the salt lost through perspiration.

**perspire** /pəˈspaɪə/ *verb* to produce moisture through the sweat glands

**Perthes' disease** /ˈpɜːtiːz dɪˌziːz/, **Perthes' hip** /ˌpɜːtiːz ˈhɪp/ *noun* a disease found in young boys, in which the upper end of the femur degenerates and does not develop as expected, sometimes resulting in a permanent limp

**pertussis** /pəˈtʌsɪs/ *noun* same as **whooping cough**

**perversion** /pəˈvɜːʃ(ə)n/ *noun* a form of behaviour which is thought to be unnatural, dangerous or disgusting ○ *He is suffering from a form of sexual perversion.*

**pes** /pes/ *noun* a foot

**PESA** *abbr* percutaneous epididymal sperm aspiration

**pes cavus** /pes ˈkeɪvəs/ *noun* same as **claw foot**

**pes planus** /pes ˈpleɪnəs/ *noun* same as **flat foot**

**pessary** /ˈpesəri/ *noun* **1.** a drug in soluble material which is pushed into the vagina and absorbed into the blood there. Also called **vaginal suppository 2.** a contraceptive device worn inside the vagina to prevent spermatozoa entering **3.** a device like a ring, which is put into the vagina as treatment for prolapse of the uterus

**pest** /pest/ *noun* an animal which carries disease, attacks plants and animals and harms or kills them ○ *a spray to remove insect pests*

**pesticide** /'pestɪsaɪd/ *noun* a substance which kills pests

**PET** *abbr* positron-emission tomography

**petechia** /pe'tiːkiə/ *noun* a small red spot which does not go white when pressed, caused by bleeding under the skin (NOTE: The plural is **petechiae**.)

**pethidine** /'peθɪdiːn/ *noun* a synthetically produced narcotic drug, used to reduce pain and as a sedative

**petit mal** /,peti 'mæl/ *noun* a less severe form of epilepsy, where loss of consciousness attacks last only a few seconds and the person appears simply to be thinking deeply. Compare **grand mal**

**Petri dish** /'piːtri dɪʃ/ *noun* a small glass or plastic dish with a lid, in which a culture is grown

**petrissage** /,petrɪ'sɑːʒ/ *noun* an action used in massaging the muscles

**petrosal** /pə'trəʊs(ə)l/ *adjective* referring to the petrous part of the temporal bone

**petrositis** /,petrəʊ'saɪtɪs/ *noun* inflammation of the petrous part of the temporal bone

**petrous** /'petrəs/ *adjective* **1.** like stone **2.** petrosal

**petrous bone** /'petrəs bəʊn/ *noun* the part of the temporal bone which forms the base of the skull and the inner and middle ears

**PET scan** /'pet skæn/ *noun* an image of a cross-section, usually of the brain, that shows metabolic processes

**-pexy** /peksi/ *suffix* referring to fixation of an organ by surgery

**Peyer's patches** /,paɪəz 'pætʃɪz/ *plural noun* patches of lymphoid tissue on the mucous membrane of the small intestine [Described 1677. After Johann Conrad Peyer (1653–1712), Swiss anatomist.]

**Peyronie's disease** /'perəniːz dɪ,ziːz/ *noun* a condition associated with Dupuytren's contracture in which hard fibre develops in the penis which becomes painful when erect [Described 1743. After François de la Peyronie (1678–1747), Surgeon to Louis XV in Paris, France.]

**PGEA** *abbr* postgraduate education allowance

**pH** /,pi: 'eɪtʃ/ *noun* the concentration of hydrogen ions in a solution, which determines its acidity

COMMENT: The pH factor is shown as a number: pH 7 is neutral, pH 8 and above show that the solution is alkaline and pH 6 and below show that the solution is acid.

**phaco-** /fækəʊ/ *prefix* referring to the lens of the eye

**phacoemulsification** /,fækəʊɪ,mʌlsɪfɪ'keɪʃ(ə)n/ *noun* an ultrasonic technique which turns a cataract in the eye into liquid. It is then removed by suction and a plastic lens is put into the eye.

**phaeochromocytoma** /,fiːəʊ,krəʊməʊsaɪ'təʊmə/ *noun* a tumour of the adrenal glands which affects the secretion of hormones such as adrenaline, which in turn results in hypertension and hyperglycaemia

**phag-** /fæg/ *prefix* same as **phago-** (*used before vowels*)

**phage** /feɪdʒ/ *noun* same as **bacteriophage**

**-phage** /feɪdʒ/ *suffix* referring to something which eats

**phagedaena** /,fædʒə'diːnə/ *noun* an ulcer that spreads rapidly

**-phagia** /feɪdʒə/ *suffix* referring to eating

**phago-** /fægəʊ/ *prefix* referring to eating

**phagocyte** /'fægəʊ,saɪt/ *noun* a cell, especially a white blood cell, which can surround and destroy other cells such as bacteria cells

**phagocytic** /,fægə'sɪtɪk/ *adjective* **1.** referring to phagocytes ○ *Monocytes become phagocytic during infection.* **2.** destroying cells

**phagocytosis** /,fægəʊsaɪ'təʊsɪs/ *noun* destruction of bacteria cells and foreign bodies by phagocytes

**phakic** /'fækɪk/ *adjective* referring to an eye which has its natural lens

**phako-** /fækəʊ/ *prefix* same as **phaco-**

**phalangeal** /fə'lændʒiəl/ *adjective* referring to the phalanges

**phalanges** /fə'lændʒiːz/ *plural of* **phalanx**

**phalangitis** /,fælən'dʒaɪtɪs/ *noun* inflammation of the fingers or toes caused by infection of tissue

**phalanx** /'fælæŋks/ *noun* a bone in a finger or toe. See illustration at HAND in Supplement, FOOT in Supplement

COMMENT: The fingers and toes have three phalanges each, except the thumb and big toe, which have only two.

**phalloplasty** /'fæləʊplæsti/ *noun* a surgical operation to repair a damaged or deformed penis

**phantom** /'fæntəm/ *noun* **1.** a model of the whole body or part of the body, used to practise or demonstrate surgical operations **2.** an image not brought about by actual stimuli, something which is not there but seems to be there

**phantom limb** /,fæntəm 'lɪm/ *noun* a condition in which someone seems to feel sensations in a limb which has been amputated

**phantom pregnancy** /,fæntəm 'pregnənsi/ *noun* same as **pseudocyesis**

**phantom tumour** /,fæntəm 'tjuːmə/ *noun* a condition in which a swelling occurs which imitates a swelling caused by a tumour

**Pharm.** *abbr* **1.** pharmacopoeia **2.** pharmacy **3.** pharmaceutical

**pharmaceutical** /ˌfɑːməˈsjuːtɪk(ə)l/ *adjective* referring to pharmacy or drugs

**pharmaceutical products** /ˌfɑːmə ˌsjuːtɪk(ə)l ˈprɒdʌkts/ *plural noun* medicines, pills, lozenges or creams which are sold in chemists' shops

**pharmaceuticals** /ˌfɑːməˈsjuːtɪk(ə)lz/ *plural noun* drugs prescribed as medicines

**Pharmaceutical Society** /ˌfɑːmə ˈsjuːtɪk(ə)l səˌsaɪəti/ *noun* a professional association for pharmacists

**pharmaceutics** /ˌfɑːməˈsjuːtɪks/ *noun* the science of the preparation and dispensing of prescribed drugs ■ *plural noun* drugs prescribed as medicines

**pharmacist** /ˈfɑːməsɪst/ *noun* a trained person who is qualified to prepare medicines according to the instructions on a doctor's prescription

COMMENT: In the UK, qualified pharmacists must be registered by the Royal Pharmaceutical Society of Great Britain before they can practise.

**pharmaco-** /ˈfɑːməkəʊ/ *prefix* referring to drugs

**pharmacodynamic** /ˌfɑːməkəʊdaɪ ˈnæmɪk/ *adjective* referring to a property of a drug which affects the part where it is applied

**pharmacodynamics** /ˌfɑːməkəʊdaɪ ˈnæmɪks/ *plural noun* the study of the effects of drugs on living organisms, and especially of how much the body's response changes when you increase the dose of a drug. Compare **pharmacokinetics** (NOTE: Takes a singular verb.)

**pharmacogenomics** /ˌfɑːməkəʊdʒi ˈnɒmɪks/ *plural noun* the study of the relationship between a person's genetic makeup and response to drug treatments (NOTE: Takes a singular verb.)

**pharmacokinetic** /ˌfɑːməkəʊkaɪˈnetɪk/ *adjective* referring to a property of a drug which has an effect over a period of time

**pharmacokinetics** /ˌfɑːməkəʊkaɪˈnetɪks/ *plural noun* **1.** the study of how the body reacts to drugs over a period of time. Compare **pharmacodynamics** (NOTE: Takes a singular verb.) **2.** the way in which a drug interacts with the body

**pharmacological** /ˌfɑːməkəˈlɒdʒɪk(ə)l/ *adjective* referring to pharmacology

**pharmacologist** /ˌfɑːməˈkɒlədʒɪst/ *noun* a scientist who specialises in the study of drugs

**pharmacology** /ˌfɑːməˈkɒlədʒi/ *noun* the study of drugs or medicines, and their actions, properties and characteristics

**pharmacopoeia** /ˌfɑːməkəˈpiːə/ *noun* an official list of drugs, their methods of preparation, dosages and the ways in which they should be used

COMMENT: The British Pharmacopoeia is the official list of drugs used in the UK The drugs listed in it have the letters BP after their name. In the US the official list is the United States Pharmacopeia or USP.

**pharmacotherapy** /ˌfɑːməkəʊˈθerəpi/ *noun* the use of drugs to treat conditions, especially psychiatric disorders

**pharmacy** /ˈfɑːməsi/ *noun* **1.** the study of the making and dispensing of drugs ○ *He has a qualification in pharmacy.* **2.** a shop or department in a hospital where drugs are prepared

**Pharmacy Act** /ˈfɑːməsi ækt/ *noun* in the UK, one of several Acts of Parliament which regulate the making, prescribing and selling of drugs, e.g. the Pharmacy and Poisons Act 1933, the Misuse of Drugs Act 1971 and the Poisons Act 1972

**pharyng-** /færɪndʒ/ *prefix* same as **pharyngo-** (used before vowels)

**pharyngeal** /ˌfærɪnˈdʒiːəl/ *adjective* referring to the pharynx

**pharyngeal pouch** /ˌfærɪndʒiːəl ˈpaʊtʃ/ *noun* one of the pouches on each side of the throat of an embryo. Also called **visceral pouch**

**pharyngeal tonsils** /ˌfærɪndʒiːəl ˈtɒns(ə)lz/ *plural noun* same as **adenoids**

**pharyngectomy** /ˌfærɪnˈdʒektəmi/ *noun* the surgical removal of part of the pharynx, especially in cases of cancer of the pharynx

**pharynges** /fəˈrɪndʒiːz/ *plural of* **pharynx**

**pharyngismus** /ˌfærɪnˈdʒɪzməs/, **pharyngism** /ˈfærɪndʒɪz(ə)m/ *noun* a spasm which contracts the muscles of the pharynx

**pharyngitis** /ˌfærɪnˈdʒaɪtɪs/ *noun* inflammation of the pharynx

**pharyngo-** /fərɪŋgəʊ/ *prefix* referring to the pharynx

**pharyngocele** /fəˈrɪŋgəʊsiːl/ *noun* **1.** a cyst which opens off the pharynx **2.** a hernia of part of the pharynx

**pharyngolaryngeal** /fəˌrɪŋgəʊləˈrɪndʒiəl/ *adjective* referring to the pharynx and the larynx

**pharyngology** /ˌfærɪnˈgɒlədʒi/ *noun* the specialty in medicine that deals with the throat, its diseases and their treatment

**pharyngoscope** /fəˈrɪŋgəʊskəʊp/ *noun* an instrument with a light attached, used by a doctor to examine the pharynx

**pharyngotympanic tube** /fəˌrɪŋgəʊtɪm ˌpænɪk ˈtjuːb/ *noun* one of two tubes which connect the back of the throat to the middle ear. Also called **Eustachian tube**

**pharynx** /ˈfærɪŋks/ *noun* a muscular passage leading from the back of the mouth to the oesophagus (NOTE: The plural is **pharynges** or **pharynxes**.)

COMMENT: The nasal cavity (or nasopharynx) leads to the back of the mouth (or oropharynx) and then into the pharynx itself, which in turn becomes the oesophagus when it reaches the sixth cervical vertebra. The pharynx is the channel both for air and food; the trachea (or windpipe) leads off it before it joins the oesophagus. The upper part of the pharynx (the nasopharynx) connects with the middle ear through the Eustachian tubes. When air pressure in the middle ear is not equal to that outside, as when going up or down in an aeroplane, the tube becomes blocked and pressure can be reduced by swallowing.

**phase** /feɪz/ *noun* a stage or period of development ○ *If the cancer is diagnosed in its early phase, the chances of complete cure are much greater.*

**phenazopyridine** /fə,næzəʊˈpɪrɪdiːn/ *noun* a drug used to reduce pain in conditions of the urinary tract, such as cystitis

**phenobarbitone** /,fiːnəʊˈbɑːbɪtəʊn/ *noun* a barbiturate drug which is used as a sedative, a hypnotic and an anticonvulsant

**phenol** /ˈfiːnɒl/ *noun* a strong disinfectant used for external use. Also called **carbolic acid**

**phenomenon** /fəˈnɒmɪnən/ *noun* **1.** a fact or situation which can be observed **2.** someone or something that is considered to be extraordinary and marvellous

**phenotype** /ˈfiːnəʊtaɪp/ *noun* the particular characteristics of an organism. Compare **genotype**

'...all cancers may be reduced to fundamental mechanisms based on cancer risk genes or oncogenes within ourselves. An oncogene is a gene that encodes a protein that contributes to the malignant phenotype of the cell.' [*British Medical Journal*]

**phenylalanine** /,fiːnaɪlˈæləniːn/ *noun* an essential amino acid

**phenylketonuria** /,fiːnaɪl,kiːtəʊˈnjʊəriə/ *noun* a hereditary condition which affects the way in which the body breaks down phenylalanine, which in turn concentrates toxic metabolites in the nervous system causing brain damage

COMMENT: To have phenylketonuria, a child has to inherit the gene from both parents. The condition can be treated by giving the child a special diet but early diagnosis is essential to avoid brain damage.

**phenytoin** /ˈfenɪtɔɪn/ *noun* a drug which helps to prevent convulsions, used in the treatment of epilepsy

**pH factor** /,piː ˈeɪtʃ ,fæktə/ *noun* a factor which indicates acidity or alkalinity

**phial** /ˈfaɪəl/ *noun* a small medicine bottle

**-philia** /fɪliə/ *suffix* attraction to or liking for something

**philtrum** /ˈfɪltrəm/ *noun* **1.** a groove in the centre of the top lip **2.** a drug believed to stimulate sexual desire

**phimosis** /faɪˈməʊsɪs/ *noun* a condition in which the foreskin is tight and has to be removed by circumcision

**phleb-** /fleb/ *prefix* same as **phlebo-** (*used before vowels*)

**phlebectomy** /flɪˈbektəmi/ *noun* the surgical removal of a vein or part of a vein

**phlebitis** /flɪˈbaɪtɪs/ *noun* inflammation of a vein

**phlebo-** /flebəʊ/ *prefix* referring to a vein

**phlebogram** /ˈflebəgræm/ *noun* an X-ray picture of a vein or system of veins. Also called **venogram**

**phlebography** /flɪˈbɒɡrəfi/ *noun* an X-ray examination of a vein using a radio-opaque dye so that the vein will show up on the film. Also called **venography**

**phlebolith** /ˈflebəlɪθ/ *noun* a stone which forms in a vein as a result of an old thrombus becoming calcified

**phlebothrombosis** /,flebəʊθrɒmˈbəʊsɪs/ *noun* a blood clot in a deep vein in the legs or pelvis, which can easily detach and form an embolus in a lung

**phlebotomise** /flɪˈbɒtəmaɪz/, **phlebotomize** *verb* to make a cut in a person's vein to take blood for testing

**phlebotomy** /flɪˈbɒtəmi/ *noun* an operation where a vein or an artery is cut so that blood can be removed, as when taking blood from a donor

**phlegm** /flem/ *noun* same as **sputum** ○ *She was coughing up phlegm into her handkerchief.*

**phlegmasia alba dolens** /fleg,meɪziə ,ælbə ˈdəʊləns/ *noun* same as **milk leg**

**phlyctena** /flɪkˈtiːnə/, **phlycten** /ˈflɪktən/ *noun* **1.** a small blister caused by a burn **2.** a small vesicle on the conjunctiva

**phlyctenule** /flɪkˈtenjuːl/ *noun* **1.** a tiny blister on the cornea or conjunctiva **2.** any small blister

**phobia** /ˈfəʊbiə/ *noun* an unusually strong and irrational fear ○ *She has a phobia about of dogs.* ○ *Fear of snakes is one of the commonest phobias.*

**-phobia** /fəʊbiə/ *suffix* neurotic fear of something ○ *agoraphobia* ○ *claustrophobia*

**phobic** /ˈfəʊbɪk/ *adjective* referring to a phobia

**-phobic** /fəʊbɪk/ *suffix* a person who has a phobia of something

**phobic anxiety** /,fəʊbɪk æŋˈzaɪəti/ *noun* state of worry caused by a phobia

**phocomelia** /,fəʊkəˈmiːliə/, **phocomely** /fəʊˈkɒməli/ *noun* **1.** a congenital condition in which the upper parts of the limbs are missing or poorly developed, leaving the hands or feet directly attached to the body **2.** a congenital condition in which the legs develop as usual, but the arms are absent or underdeveloped

**phon-** /fəʊn/ *prefix* same as **phono-** (*used before vowels*)

**phonation** /fəʊˈneɪʃ(ə)n/ *noun* the production of vocal sounds, especially speech

**phoniatrics** /ˌfəʊniˈætrɪks/ *noun* the study of speech and disorders related to it

**phono-** /ˈfəʊnəʊ/ *prefix* referring to sound or voice

**phonocardiogram** /ˌfəʊnəʊˈkɑːdɪəgræm/ *noun* a chart of the sounds made by the heart

**phonocardiograph** /ˌfəʊnəʊˈkɑːdɪəgræf/ *noun* an instrument that amplifies heart sounds and converts them into a visual display

**phonocardiography** /ˌfəʊnəʊˌkɑːdiˈɒgrəfi/ *noun* the process of recording the sounds made by the heart

**phonology** /fəˈnɒlədʒi/ *noun* the study of the system of speech sounds used in a particular language or in human speech generally

**phonosurgery** /ˈfəʊnəʊˌsɜːdʒəri/ *noun* surgery performed to alter the quality of the voice

**phosphataemia** /ˌfɒsfəˈtiːmiə/ *noun* the presence of excess phosphates in the blood

**phosphatase** /ˈfɒsfəteɪz/ *noun* a group of enzymes which are important in the cycle of muscle contraction and in the calcification of bones

**phosphate** /ˈfɒsfeɪt/ *noun* a salt of phosphoric acid

**phosphaturia** /ˌfɒsfəˈtjʊəriə/ *noun* the presence of excess phosphates in the urine

COMMENT: In phosphaturia the urine becomes cloudy, which can indicate stones in the bladder or kidney.

**phospholipid** /ˌfɒsfəʊˈlɪpɪd/ *noun* a compound with fatty acids, which is one of the main components of membranous tissue

**phosphonecrosis** /ˌfɒsfəʊneˈkrəʊsɪs/ *noun* a necrotic condition affecting the kidneys, liver and bones, usually seen in people who work with phosphorus

**phosphorescent** /ˌfɒsfəˈres(ə)nt/ *adjective* shining without producing heat

**phosphoric acid** /fɒsˌfɒrɪk ˈæsɪd/ *noun* an acid which is very soluble in water and gives rise to acid, neutral and alkali salts

**phosphorus** /ˈfɒsf(ə)rəs/ *noun* a toxic chemical element which is present in very small quantities in bones and nerve tissue. It causes burns if it touches the skin, and can poison if swallowed. (NOTE: The chemical symbol is **P.**)

**phosphorylase** /fɒsˈfɒrɪleɪz/ *noun* an enzyme that aids the process of carbohydrate metabolism

**phossy jaw** /ˈfɒsi ˌdʒɔː/ *noun* a type of phosphonecrosis, caused by inhaling phosphorus fumes, which results in disintegration of the bones of the lower jaw. The disease was once common among workers in match factories.

**phot-** /fɒt, fəʊt/ *prefix* same as **photo-** (*used before vowels*)

**photalgia** /fəʊˈtældʒə/ *noun* **1.** pain in the eye caused by bright light **2.** severe photophobia

**photo-** /ˈfəʊtəʊ/ *prefix* referring to light

**photoablation** /ˌfəʊtəʊəˈbleɪʃ(ə)n/ *noun* the removal of tissue using lasers

**photocoagulation** /ˌfəʊtəʊkəʊæɡjuˈleɪʃ(ə)n/ *noun* the process in which tissue coagulates from the heat caused by light, used to treat a detached retina

**photodermatosis** /ˌfəʊtəʊˌdɜːməˈtəʊsɪs/ *noun* a lesion of the skin after exposure to bright light

**photogenic** /ˌfəʊtəˈdʒenɪk/ *adjective* **1.** produced by the action of light **2.** producing light

**photograph** /ˈfəʊtəɡrɑːf/ *noun* a picture taken with a camera, which uses the chemical action of light on sensitive film ■ *verb* to take a picture of something with a camera

**photography** /fəˈtɒɡrəfi/ *noun* the act of taking pictures with a camera ○ *The development of X-ray photography has meant that internal disorders can be more easily diagnosed.*

**photophobia** /ˌfəʊtəʊˈfəʊbiə/ *noun* **1.** a condition in which the eyes become sensitive to light and conjunctivitis may be caused (NOTE: It can be associated with measles and some other infectious diseases.) **2.** a morbid fear of light

**photophobic** /ˌfəʊtəʊˈfəʊbɪk/ *adjective* having an unusual fear of light

**photophthalmia** /ˌfəʊtɒfˈθælmiə/ *noun* inflammation of the eye caused by bright light, as in snow blindness

**photopic vision** /fəʊˌtɒpɪk ˈvɪʒ(ə)n/ *noun* vision which is adapted to bright light such as daylight, using the cones in the retina instead of the rods, which are used in scotopic vision. ◊ **light adaptation**

**photopsia** /fəʊˈtɒpsiə/ *noun* a condition of the eye in which someone sees flashes of light

**photoreceptor neurone** /ˌfəʊtəʊrɪˌseptə ˈnjʊərəʊn/ *noun* a rod or cone in the retina, which is sensitive to light or colour

**photoretinitis** /ˌfəʊtəʊretiˈnaɪtɪs/ *noun* damage to a retina caused by looking directly at the sun. Also called **sun blindness**

**photosensitive** /ˌfəʊtəʊˈsensɪtɪv/ *adjective* sensitive to light, or stimulated by light

**photosensitivity** /ˌfəʊtəʊsensəˈtɪvəti/ *noun* the fact of being sensitive to light

**phototherapy** /ˌfəʊtəʊˈθerəpi/ *noun* a treatment for jaundice and vitamin D deficiency, which involves exposing the person to ultraviolet rays

**phototoxic** /ˌfəʊtəʊˈtɒksɪk/ *adjective* making the skin unusually sensitive to damage by light, as in sunburn

**phototoxicity** /ˌfəʊtəʊtɒkˈsɪsɪti/ *noun* a cause of damage to the retina of the eye due to exposure to too much ultraviolet light or radiation ○ *Children's retinas are more likely to experience damage as a result of phototoxicity from excess ultraviolet light than those of adults.* ◊ **retinopathy**

**photuria** /fəʊˈtjʊəriə/ *noun* phosphorescent urine

**phren-** /fren/ *prefix* same as **phreno-** (used before vowels)

**phrenemphraxis** /ˌfrenemˈfræksɪs/ *noun* a surgical operation to crush the phrenic nerve in order to paralyse the diaphragm

**-phrenia** /friːniə/ *suffix* disorder of the mind

**phrenic** /ˈfrenɪk/ *adjective* **1.** referring to the diaphragm **2.** referring to the mind or intellect

**phrenic avulsion** /ˌfrenɪk əˈvʌlʃ(ə)n/ *noun* the surgical removal of part of the phrenic nerve in order to paralyse the diaphragm

**phrenicectomy** /ˌfrenɪˈsektəmi/ *noun* the surgical removal of all or part of the phrenic nerve

**phreniclasia** /ˌfrenɪˈkleɪziə/ *noun* an operation to clamp the phrenic nerve

**phrenic nerve** /ˈfrenɪk nɜːv/ *noun* a pair of nerves which controls the muscles in the diaphragm

**phrenicotomy** /ˌfrenɪˈkɒtəmi/ *noun* an operation to divide the phrenic nerve

**phreno-** /frenəʊ/ *prefix* **1.** referring to the brain **2.** referring to the phrenic nerve

**pH test** /ˌpiː ˈeɪtʃ test/ *noun* a test to see how acid or alkaline a solution is

**phthiriasis** /θɪˈraɪəsɪs/ *noun* infestation with the crab louse

**Phthirius pubis** /ˌθaɪəriəs ˈpjuːbɪs/ *noun* a louse which infests the pubic region. Also called **pubic louse, crab**

**phthisis** /ˈθaɪsɪs/ *noun* an old term for tuberculosis

**phycomycosis** /ˌfaɪkəʊmaɪˈkəʊsɪs/ *noun* an acute infection of the lungs, central nervous system and other organs by a fungus

**physi-** /fɪzi/ *prefix* same as **physio-** (used before vowels)

**physical** /ˈfɪzɪk(ə)l/ *adjective* referring to the body, as opposed to the mind ■ *noun* a physical examination ○ *He has to pass a physical before being accepted by the police force.*

**physical dependence** /ˌfɪzɪk(ə)l dɪ ˈpendəns/, **physical drug dependence** /ˌfɪzɪk(ə)l ˈdrʌg dɪˌpendəns/ *noun* a state where a person is addicted to a drug such as heroin and suffers physical effects if he or she stops taking the drug

**physical education** /ˌfɪzɪk(ə)l ˌedjʊ ˈkeɪʃ(ə)n/ *noun* the teaching of sports and exercises in school

**physical examination** /ˌfɪzɪk(ə)l ɪgˌzæmɪ ˈneɪʃ(ə)n/ *noun* an examination of someone's body to see if he or she is healthy

**physical genetic trait** /ˌfɪzɪk(ə)l dʒəˈnetɪk treɪt/ *noun* a characteristic of the body of a

person, e.g. red hair or big feet, which is inherited

**physically** /ˈfɪzɪkli/ *adverb* referring to the body ○ *Physically he is very weak, but his mind is still alert.*

**physically challenged** /ˌfɪzɪkli ˈtʃælɪndʒd/ *adjective* describing someone whose condition makes it difficult to perform some or all of the basic activities of daily life

**physical medicine** /ˌfɪzɪk(ə)l ˈmed(ə)sɪn/ *noun* a branch of medicine which deals with physical disabilities or with treatment of disorders after they have been diagnosed

**physical sign** /ˌfɪzɪk(ə)l ˈsaɪn/ *noun* a symptom which can be seen on someone's body or which can be produced by percussion and palpitation

**physical therapy** /ˌfɪzɪk(ə)l ˈθerəpi/ *noun* the treatment of disorders by heat, by massage, by exercise and other physical means

**physician** /fɪˈzɪʃ(ə)n/ *noun* a registered doctor who is not a surgeon (NOTE: In British English, physician refers to a specialist doctor, though not usually a surgeon, while in US English it is used for any qualified doctor.)

**physio** /ˈfɪziəʊ/ *noun* (*informal*) **1.** a session of physiotherapy treatment **2.** a physiotherapist

**physio-** /fɪziəʊ/ *prefix* **1.** referring to physiology **2.** physical

**physiological** /ˌfɪziəˈlɒdʒɪk(ə)l/ *adjective* referring to physiology and the regular functions of the body

**physiological saline** /ˌfɪziəlɒdʒɪk(ə)l ˈseɪ laɪn/, **physiological solution** /ˌfɪziəlɒdʒɪk(ə)l səˈluːʃ(ə)n/ *noun* any solution used to keep cells or tissue alive

**physiological tremor** /ˌfɪziəˌlɒdʒɪk(ə)l ˈtremə/ *noun* a small movement of the limbs which takes place when a person tries to remain still

**physiologist** /ˌfɪziˈɒlədʒɪst/ *noun* a scientist who specialises in the study of the functions of living organisms

**physiology** /ˌfɪziˈɒlədʒi/ *noun* the study of regular body functions

**physiotherapist** /ˌfɪziəʊˈθerəpɪst/ *noun* a trained specialist who gives physiotherapy

**physiotherapy** /ˌfɪziəʊˈθerəpi/ *noun* the treatment of a disorder or condition by exercise, massage, heat treatment, infrared lamps or other external means, e.g. to restore strength or function after a disease or injury

**physiotherapy clinic** /ˌfɪziəʊˈθerəpi ˌklɪnɪk/ *noun* a clinic where people can have physiotherapy

**physique** /fɪˈziːk/ *noun* the shape and size of a person's body

**physo-** /faɪsəʊ/ *prefix* **1.** tending to swell **2.** relating to air or gas

**physostigmine** /ˌfaɪsəʊˈstɪgmiːn/ *noun* an extract of the dried leaves of the vine that produces Calabar bean, which is toxic but may be used in the treatment of glaucoma and to counter the effects of anticholinergic drugs on the central nervous system

**phyt-** /faɪt/, **phyto-** /faɪtəʊ/ *prefix* referring to plants or coming from plants

**phytooestrogen** /ˌfaɪtəʊˈiːstrədʒən/ *noun* a substance obtained from cereals, legumes and seeds which has a similar effect on the body as oestrogen, used increasingly as an alternative to hormone replacement therapy

**phyto-photo dermatitis** /ˌfaɪtəʊ ˌfəʊtəʊ ˌdɜːməˈtaɪtɪs/ *noun* an acute skin reaction due to the combination of plant irritation and sunlight

**PI** *abbr* pressure index

**pia** /ˈpaɪə/, **pia mater** /ˌpaɪə ˈmeɪtə/ *noun* the delicate innermost membrane of the three which cover the brain. ◊ **arachnoid, dura mater**

**pian** /piːˈɑːn/ *noun* same as **yaws**

**pica** /ˈpaɪkə/ *noun* a desire to eat things which are not food, e.g. wood or paper, often found in pregnant women and small children

**pick** /pɪk/ *verb* to take away small pieces of something with the fingers or with a tool ○ *She picked the pieces of glass out of the wound with tweezers.*

**Pick's disease** /ˈpɪks dɪˌziːz/ *noun* a rare form of presenile dementia, in which a disorder of the lipoid metabolism causes mental impairment, anaemia, loss of weight and swelling of the spleen and liver

**pick up** /ˌpɪk ˈʌp/ *verb* (*informal*) **1.** to catch a disease ○ *She must have picked up the disease when she was travelling in Africa.* **2.** to get stronger or better ○ *He was ill for months, but he's picking up now.*

**pico-** /piːkəʊ/ *prefix* one million millionth (10⁻¹²). Symbol **p**

**picomole** /ˈpiːkəʊməʊl/ *noun* a unit of measurement of the amount of substance equal to one million millionth of a mole. Symbol **pmol**

**picornavirus** /piːˈkɔːnəˌvaɪrəs/ *noun* a virus containing RNA, e.g. enteroa viruses and rhinoa viruses

**PID** *abbr* prolapsed intervertebral disc

**PIDS** *abbr* primary immune deficiency syndrome

**Pierre Robin syndrome** /ˌpjeə rɒˈbæn ˌsɪndrəʊm/ *noun* a combination of facial features including a small lower jaw and a cleft palate that exist at birth, causing breathing and feeding problems early in a child's life

**pigeon breast** /ˈpɪdʒɪn brest/, **pigeon chest** /ˈpɪdʒɪn tʃest/ *noun* same as **pectus carinatum**

**pigeon toes** /ˈpɪdʒɪn təʊz/ *plural noun* a condition in which the feet turn towards the inside when a person is standing upright

**pigment** /ˈpɪgmənt/ *noun* **1.** a substance which gives colour to part of the body such as blood, the skin or hair **2.** (*in pharmacy*) a paint

COMMENT: The body contains several substances which control colour: melanin gives dark colour to the skin and hair; bilirubin gives yellow colour to bile and urine; haemoglobin in the blood gives the skin a pink colour; carotene can give a reddish-yellow colour to the skin if the patient eats too many tomatoes or carrots. Some pigment cells can carry oxygen and are called 'respiratory pigments'.

**pigmentation** /ˌpɪgmənˈteɪʃ(ə)n/ *noun* the colouring of the body, especially that produced by deposits of pigment

**pigmented** /ˈpɪgmentɪd/ *adjective* **1.** coloured **2.** showing an unusual colour

**pigmented epithelium** /ˌpɪgməntɪd ˌepɪˈθiːliəm/, **pigmented layer** /ˌpɪgməntɪd ˈleɪə/ *noun* coloured tissue at the back of the retina

**PIH** *abbr* pregnancy-induced hypertension

**Pilates** /pɪˈlɑːtiz/ *noun* a holistic form of exercise and postural therapy that develops the deep abdominal muscles to control body movement and protect the back

**piles** /paɪlz/ *plural noun* same as **haemorrhoids**

**pili** /ˈpaɪlaɪ/ ♦ **arrector pili**

**pill** /pɪl/ *noun* a small hard round ball of medication that is taken by swallowing ○ *He has to take the pills twice a day.* □ **the pill** an oral contraceptive. ◊ **morning-after pill** □ **on the pill** taking a regular course of contraceptive pills

**pillar** /ˈpɪlə/ *noun* a part that is long and thin

**pillow** /ˈpɪləʊ/ *noun* a soft cushion on a bed which the head lies on when the person is lying down ○ *The nurse gave her an extra pillow to keep her head raised.*

**pill-rolling** /ˈpɪl ˌrəʊlɪŋ/ *noun* nervous action of the fingers, in which the person seems to be rolling a very small object, associated with Parkinson's disease

**pilo-** /paɪləʊ/ *prefix* referring to hair

**pilocarpine** /ˌpaɪləʊˈkɑːpiːn/ *noun* an organic compound of plant origin which is used in eye drops to treat glaucoma

**pilomotor** /ˌpaɪləʊˈməʊtə/ *adjective* referring to something that moves the hairs of the skin

**pilomotor nerve** /ˌpaɪləʊˈməʊtə nɜːv/ *noun* a nerve which supplies the arrector pili muscles attached to hair follicles

**pilomotor reflex** /ˌpaɪləʊˈməʊtə ˌriːfleks/ *noun* a reaction of the dermal papillae of the skin to cold and fear which causes the hairs on the skin to become erect

**pilonidal** /ˌpaɪləˈnaɪd(ə)l/ *adjective* relating to a cyst or cavity which has a growth of hair

**pilonidal cyst** /ˌpaɪləˌnaɪd(ə)l ˈsɪst/ *noun* a cyst containing hair, usually found at the bottom of the spine near the buttocks

**pilonidal sinus** /ˌpaɪləˌnaɪd(ə)l ˈsaɪnəs/ noun a small depression with hairs at the base of the spine

**pilosebaceous** /ˌpaɪləʊsəˈbeɪʃəs/ adjective referring to the hair follicles and the glands attached to them

**pilosis** /paɪˈləʊsɪs/, **pilosism** /ˈpaɪləsɪz(ə)m/ noun a condition in which someone has an unusual amount of hair or where hair is present in an unusual place

**pilot study** /ˈpaɪlət ˌstʌdi/ noun a small version of a project which is carried out first, in order to discover how well it works and to solve any problems, before going ahead with the full version

**pilus** /ˈpaɪləs/ noun 1. one hair (NOTE: The plural is **pili**.) 2. hair-like process on the surface of a bacterium

**pimple** /ˈpɪmpəl/ noun a small swelling on the skin, containing pus ○ He had pimples on his neck.

**pimply** /ˈpɪmpli/ adjective covered with pimples

**pin** /pɪn/ noun 1. a small sharp piece of metal for attaching things together ○ The nurse fastened the bandage with a pin. 2. a metal nail used to attach broken bones ○ He has had a pin inserted in his hip. ■ verb to attach something with a pin ○ She pinned the bandages carefully to stop them slipping. ○ The bone had fractured in several places and needed pinning.

**pinch** /pɪntʃ/ noun 1. an act of squeezing the thumb and first finger together 2. a quantity of something which can be held between the thumb and first finger ○ She put a pinch of salt into the water. ■ verb 1. to squeeze something tightly between the thumb and first finger 2. to squeeze something ○ She developed a sore on her ankle where her shoe pinched.

**pineal** /ˈpɪniəl/ adjective relating to or released by the pineal gland

**pineal body** /ˈpɪniəl ˌbɒdi/, **pineal gland** /ˈpɪniəl glænd/ noun a small cone-shaped gland situated below the corpus callosum in the brain, which produces melatonin and is believed to be associated with the circadian rhythm. See illustration at BRAIN in Supplement

**pinguecula** /pɪŋˈgwekjʊlə/, **pinguicula** /pɪŋˈgwɪkjʊlə/ noun a condition affecting elderly people, in which the conjunctiva in the eyes has small yellow growths near the edge of the cornea, usually on the nasal side

**pink disease** /ˈpɪŋk dɪˌziːz/ noun same as **acrodynia**

**pinna** /ˈpɪnə/ noun the outer ear, the part of the ear which is outside the head, connected by a passage to the eardrum. See illustration at EAR in Supplement

**pinnaplasty** /ˈpɪnəplæsti/ noun a cosmetic surgical procedure to correct the shape of the ear

**pinocytosis** /ˌpiːnəʊsaɪˈtəʊsɪs/ noun the process by which a cell surrounds and takes in fluid

**pins and needles** /ˌpɪnz ən ˈniːd(ə)lz/ noun an unpleasant tingling sensation, usually occurring after a temporarily restricted blood supply returns to an arm or leg (informal) ◊ **paraesthesia**

**pint** /paɪnt/ noun a unit of measurement of liquids ( = about 0.56 of a litre) ○ He lost two pints of blood during the operation.

**pinta** /ˈpɪntə/ noun a skin disease of the tropical regions of America, in which the skin on the hands and feet swells and loses colour, caused by a spirochaete Treponema

**pinworm** /ˈpɪnwɜːm/ noun US same as **threadworm**

**PIP** abbr proximal interphalangeal joint

**pipette** /pɪˈpet/ noun a thin glass tube used in the laboratory for taking or measuring samples of liquid

**piriform fossae** /ˌpɪrifɔːm ˈfɒsiː/ plural noun the two hollows at the sides of the upper end of the larynx

**Piriton** /ˈpɪrɪtɒn/ a trade name for chlorpheniramine

**piroxicam** /pɪˈrɒksɪkæm/ noun a non-steroidal anti-inflammatory drug used in the treatment of rheumatoid arthritis and osteoarthritis

**PIs** abbr performance indicators

**pisiform** /ˈpɪsifɔːm/, **pisiform bone** /ˈpɪsiˌfɔːm bəʊn/ noun one of the eight small carpal bones in the wrist. See illustration at HAND in Supplement

**pit** /pɪt/ noun a hollow place on a surface □ **the pit of the stomach** the epigastrium, the part of the upper abdomen between the ribcage above the navel. ◊ **armpit**

**pithiatism** /pɪˈθaɪətɪz(ə)m/ noun a way of influencing someone's mind by persuading him or her of something, as when a doctor treats a condition by telling the person that he or she is in fact well

**pitted** /ˈpɪtɪd/ adjective covered with small hollows ○ His skin was pitted by acne.

**pitting** /ˈpɪtɪŋ/ noun the formation of hollows in the skin

**pituitary** /pɪˈtjuːɪt(ə)ri/ adjective 1. relating to or produced by the pituitary gland 2. caused by a disturbance of the pituitary gland ■ noun same as **pituitary gland**

**pituitary body** /pɪˈtjuːɪt(ə)ri ˌbɒdi/ noun same as **pituitary gland**

**pituitary fossa** /pɪˌtjuːɪt(ə)ri ˈfɒsə/ noun same as **sella turcica**

**pituitary gland** /pɪˈtjuːɪt(ə)ri ˌglænd/ noun the main endocrine gland in the body which secretes hormones that stimulate other glands.

Also called **pituitary body, hypophysis cerebri**. See illustration at BRAIN in Supplement

COMMENT: The pituitary gland is about the size of a pea and hangs down from the base of the brain, inside the sphenoid bone, on a stalk which attaches it to the hypothalamus. The front lobe of the gland (the adenohypophysis) secretes several hormones (TSH, ACTH) which stimulate the adrenal and thyroid glands, or which stimulate the production of sex hormones, melanin and milk. The posterior lobe of the pituitary gland (the neurohypophysis) secretes the antidiuretic hormone (ADH) and oxytocin.

**pituitrin** /pɪˈtjuːɪtrɪn/ *noun* a hormone secreted by the pituitary gland

**pityriasis** /ˌpɪtɪˈraɪəsɪs/ *noun* any skin disease in which the skin develops thin scales

**pityriasis alba** /pɪtɪˌraɪəsɪs ˈælbə/ *noun* a disease affecting children which results in flat white patches on the cheeks that usually heal naturally

**pityriasis capitis** /pɪtɪˌraɪəsɪs kəˈpaɪtɪs/ *noun* ♦ dandruff

**pityriasis rosea** /pɪtɪˌraɪəsɪs ˈrəʊziə/ *noun* a mild irritating rash affecting young people, which appears especially in the early part of the year and has no known cause

**pityriasis rubra** /pɪtɪˌraɪəsɪs ˈruːbrə/ *noun* a serious, sometimes fatal, skin disease, a type of exfoliative dermatitis in which the skin turns dark red and is covered with white scales

**pivot** /ˈpɪvət/ *noun* a stem used to attach an artificial crown to the root of a tooth ■ *verb* to rest and turn on a point ○ *The atlas bone pivots on the second vertebra.*

**pivot joint** /ˈpɪvət dʒɔɪnt/ *noun* same as **trochoid joint**

**PKD** *abbr* polycystic kidney disease

**PKU** *abbr* phenylketonuria

**placebo** /pləˈsiːbəʊ/ *noun* a tablet which appears to be a drug, but has no medicinal substance in it

COMMENT: Placebos may be given to patients who have imaginary illnesses. Placebos can also help in treating real disorders by stimulating the patient's psychological will to be cured. Placebos are also used on control groups in tests of new drugs (a placebo-controlled study).

**placebo effect** /pləˈsiːbəʊ ɪˌfekt/ *noun* the apparently beneficial effect of telling someone that he or she is having a treatment, even if this is not true, caused by the hope that the treatment will be effective

**placenta** /pləˈsentə/ *noun* the tissue which grows inside the uterus during pregnancy and links the baby to the mother

COMMENT: The vascular system of the fetus is not directly connected to that of the mother. The placenta allows an exchange of oxygen and nutrients to be passed from the mother to the fetus to which she is linked by the umbilical cord. It stops functioning when the baby breathes for the first time and is then passed out of the uterus as the afterbirth.

**placental** /pləˈsent(ə)l/ *adjective* referring to the placenta

**placental barrier** /plə,sent(ə)l ˈbæriə/ *noun* a barrier which prevents the blood of a fetus and that of the mother from mixing, but allows water, oxygen and hormones to pass from mother to fetus

**placental insufficiency** /plə,sent(ə)l ˌɪnsəˈfɪʃ(ə)nsi/ *noun* a condition in which the placenta does not provide the fetus with the necessary oxygen and nutrients

**placenta praevia** /plə,sentə ˈpriːviə/ *noun* a condition in which the fertilised egg becomes implanted in the lower part of the uterus, which means that the placenta lies across the cervix and may become detached during childbirth and cause brain damage to the baby

**placentography** /ˌplæsənˈtɒɡrəfi/ *noun* an X-ray examination of the placenta of a pregnant woman after a radiopaque dye has been injected

**Placido's disc** /pləˈsaɪdəʊz dɪsk/ *noun* same as **keratoscope** [After A. Placido, Portuguese oculist.]

**plagiocephaly** /ˌpleɪdʒiəˈkefəli/ *noun* a condition in which a person has a distorted head shape, from irregular closure of the cranial sutures

**plague** /pleɪɡ/ *noun* an infectious disease which occurs in epidemics where many people are killed

COMMENT: Bubonic plague was the Black Death of the Middle Ages; its symptoms are fever, delirium, prostration, rigor and swellings on the lymph nodes.

**plan** /plæn/ *noun* arrangement of how something should be done ■ *verb* to arrange how something is going to be done □ **they are planning to have a family** they expect to have children and so are not taking contraceptives

'…one issue has arisen – the amount of time and effort which nurses need to put into the writing of detailed care plans. Few would now dispute the need for clear, concise nursing plans to guide nursing practice, provide educational tools and give an accurate legal record' [*Nursing Times*]

**plane** /pleɪn/ *noun* a flat surface, especially that of the body seen from a specific angle

**planned parenthood** /ˌplænd ˈpeərənthʊd/ *noun* a situation in which two people plan to have a specific number of children, and take contraceptives to control the number of children in the family

**planning** /ˈplænɪŋ/ *noun* the work of deciding and arranging how something should be done

**planta** /ˈplæntə/ *noun* the sole of the foot

**plantar** /ˈplæntə/ *adjective* referring to the sole of the foot

**plantar arch** /ˌplæntər ˈɑːtʃ/ *noun* the curved part of the sole of the foot running along the length of the foot. Also called **longitudinal arch**

**plantar flexion** /ˌplæntə 'flekʃən/ *noun* the bending of the toes downwards

**plantar reflex** /ˌplæntə 'riːfleks/, **plantar response** /ˌplæntə rɪ'spɒns/ *noun* the usual downward movement of the toes when the sole of the foot is stroked in the Babinski test

**plantar region** /ˈplæntə ˌriːdʒən/ *noun* the sole of the foot

**plantar surface** /ˈplæntə ˌsɜːfɪs/ *noun* the skin of the sole of the foot

**plantar wart** /ˈplæntə wɔːt/ *noun* a wart on the sole of the foot

**planus** /ˈpleɪnəs/ ✦ **lichen planus**

**plaque** /plæk, plɑːk/ *noun* **1.** a flat area **2.** a film of saliva, mucus, bacteria and food residues that builds up on the surface of teeth and can cause gum damage

**-plasia** /pleɪzɪə/ *suffix* referring to something which develops or grows

**plasm-** /plæz(ə)m/ *prefix* same as **plasmo-** (*used before vowels*)

**plasma** /ˈplæzmə/ *noun* **1.** a yellow watery liquid which makes up the main part of blood **2.** lymph with no corpuscles **3.** cytoplasm

COMMENT: If blood does not clot it separates into blood corpuscles and plasma, which is formed of water and proteins, including the clotting agent fibrinogen. If blood clots, the corpuscles separate from serum, which is a watery liquid similar to plasma, but not containing fibrinogen. Dried plasma can be kept for a long time, and is used, after water has been added, for transfusions.

**plasma cell** /ˈplæzmə sel/ *noun* a lymphocyte which produces a particular type of antibody

**plasmacytoma** /ˌplæzməsaɪ'təumə/ *noun* a malignant tumour of plasma cells, usually found in lymph nodes or bone marrow

**plasmapheresis** /ˌplæzməfə'riːsɪs/ *noun* an operation to take blood from someone, then to separate the red blood cells from the plasma, and to return the red blood cells suspended in a saline solution to the patient through a transfusion

**plasma protein** /ˈplæzmə ˌprəutiːn/ *noun* a protein in plasma, e.g. albumin, gamma globulin or fibrinogen

**plasmin** /ˈplæzmɪn/ *noun* same as **fibrinolysin**

**plasminogen** /plæz'mɪnədʒən/ *noun* a substance in blood plasma which becomes activated and forms plasmin

**plasmo-** /plæzməu/ *prefix* referring to blood plasma

**Plasmodium** /plæz'məudiəm/ *noun* a type of parasite which infests red blood cells and causes malaria

**plasmolysis** /plæz'mɒlɪsɪs/ *noun* the contraction of a cell protoplasm by dehydration,

where the surrounding cell wall becomes smaller

**plaster** /ˈplɑːstə/ *noun* a white powder which is mixed with water and used to make a solid support to cover a broken limb ○ *After his accident he had his leg in plaster for two months.*

**plaster cast** /ˈplɑːstə kɑːst/ *noun* a hard support made of bandage soaked in liquid plaster of Paris, which is allowed to harden after being wrapped round a broken limb and which prevents the limb moving while the bone heals

**plaster of Paris** /ˌplɑːstər əv 'pærɪs/ *noun* a fine white plaster used to make plaster casts

**plastic** /ˈplæstɪk/ *noun* an artificial material made from petroleum, and used to make many objects, including replacement organs ■ *adjective* able to change shape or develop in different shapes

**plastic lymph** /ˈplæstɪk lɪmf/ *noun* a yellow liquid produced by an inflamed wound which helps the healing process

**plastic surgeon** /ˌplæstɪk 'sɜːdʒən/ *noun* a surgeon who specialises in plastic surgery

**plastic surgery** /ˌplæstɪk 'sɜːdʒəri/ *noun* surgery to repair damaged or malformed parts of the body (*informal*) ◊ **reconstructive surgery**

COMMENT: Plastic surgery is especially important in treating accident victims or people who have suffered burns. It is also used to correct congenital disorders such as a cleft palate. When the aim is simply to improve the patient's appearance, it is usually referred to as 'cosmetic surgery'.

**plastin** /ˈplæstɪn/ *noun* same as **fibrinolysin**

**-plasty** /plæsti/ *suffix* referring to plastic surgery

**plate** /pleɪt/ *noun* **1.** a flat sheet of metal or bone ○ *The surgeon inserted a plate in her skull.* **2.** a flat piece of metal attached to a fractured bone to hold the broken parts together

**platelet** /ˈpleɪtlət/ *noun* a small blood cell which releases thromboplastin and which multiplies rapidly after an injury, encouraging the coagulation of blood. Also called **thrombocyte**

**platelet count** /ˈpleɪt(ə)lət kaunt/ *noun* a test to count the number of platelets in a specific quantity of blood

**platy-** /plæti/ *prefix* flat

**platysma** /plə'tɪzmə/ *noun* a flat muscle running from the collarbone to the lower jaw

**pledget** /ˈpledʒɪt/ *noun* a small piece of gauze or cotton wool used to protect or apply medication to a small enclosed space, such as the ear passage

**-plegia** /pliːdʒə/ *suffix* paralysis

**pleio-** /plaɪəu/ *prefix* same as **pleo-**

**pleo-** /pliːəu/ *prefix* too many

**pleocytosis** /ˌpliːəʊsaɪˈtəʊsɪs/ *noun* a condition in which there are an unusual number of leucocytes in the cerebrospinal fluid

**pleoptics** /pliːˈɒptɪks/ *noun* treatment to help the partially sighted

**plessor** /ˈplesə/ *noun* a little hammer with a rubber tip, used by doctors to tap tendons to test for reflexes or for percussion of the chest. Also called **plexor**

**plethora** /ˈpleθərə/ *noun* too much blood in a part of the body

**plethoric** /pleˈθɒrɪk/ *adjective* referring to an appearance that is due to dilatation of superficial blood vessels, e.g. a red complexion

**plethysmography** /ˌpleθɪzˈmɒɡrəfi/ *noun* a method of recording the changes in the volume of organs, mainly used to measure blood flow in the limbs

**pleur-** /plʊər/ *prefix* same as **pleuro-** (*used before vowels*)

**pleura** /ˈplʊərə/ *noun* one of two membranes lining the chest cavity and covering each lung (NOTE: The plural is **pleuras** or **pleurae**.)

**pleuracentesis** /ˌplʊərəsenˈtiːsɪs/ *noun* same as **pleurocentesis**

**pleural** /ˈplʊərəl/ *adjective* referring to the pleura

**pleural cavity** /ˌplʊərəl ˈkævɪti/ *noun* a space between the inner and outer pleura of the chest. See illustration at LUNGS in Supplement

**pleural effusion** /ˌplʊərəl ɪˈfjuːʒ(ə)n/ *noun* an excess of fluid formed in the pleural sac

**pleural fluid** /ˌplʊərəl ˈfluːɪd/ *noun* a fluid which forms between the layers of the pleura in pleurisy

**pleural membrane** /ˌplʊərəl ˈmembreɪn/ *noun* same as **pleura**

**pleural mesothelioma** /ˌplʊərəl ˌmesəʊθeliˈəʊmə/ *noun* a tumour of the pleura, caused by inhaling asbestos dust

**pleurectomy** /plʊəˈrektəmi/ *noun* the surgical removal of part of the pleura which has been thickened or made stiff by chronic empyema

**pleurisy** /ˈplʊərɪsi/ *noun* inflammation of the pleura, usually caused by pneumonia

COMMENT: The symptoms of pleurisy are coughing, fever, and sharp pains when breathing, caused by the two layers of pleura rubbing together.

**pleuritis** /plʊəˈraɪtɪs/ *noun* same as **pleurisy**

**pleuro-** /plʊərəʊ/ *prefix* referring to the pleura

**pleurocele** /ˈplʊərəʊsiːl/ *noun* 1. a condition in which part of the lung or pleura is herniated 2. fluid in the pleural cavity

**pleurocentesis** /ˌplʊərəʊsenˈtiːsɪs/ *noun* an operation in which a hollow needle is put into the pleura to drain liquid. Also called **pleuracentesis**

**pleurodesis** /ˌplʊərəʊˈdiːsɪs/ *noun* treatment for a collapsed lung, in which the inner and outer pleura are stuck together

**pleurodynia** /ˌplʊərəʊˈdɪniə/ *noun* pain in the muscles between the ribs, due to rheumatic inflammation

**pleuron** /ˈplʊərɒn/ *noun* a membrane that encases the lung

**pleuropneumonia** /ˌplʊərəʊnjuːˈməʊniə/ *noun* acute lobar pneumonia, the classic type of pneumonia

**plexor** /ˈpleksə/ *noun* same as **plessor**

**plexus** /ˈpleksəs/ *noun* a network of nerves, blood vessels or lymphatics

**pliable** /ˈplaɪəb(ə)l/ *adjective* able to be bent easily

**plica** /ˈplaɪkə/ *noun* a fold

**plicate** /ˈplaɪkeɪt/ *adjective* folded

**plication** /plaɪˈkeɪʃ(ə)n/ *noun* 1. a surgical operation to reduce the size of a tissue or a hollow organ by making folds in its walls and attaching them 2. the action of folding 3. a fold

**ploidy** /ˈplɔɪdi/ *noun* the number of sets of chromosomes within a cell

**plombage** /plɒmˈbɑːʒ/ *noun* 1. the act of packing bone cavities with antiseptic material 2. the act of packing of the lung or pleural cavities with inert material

**PLSS** *abbr* portable life-support system

**plumbing** /ˈplʌmɪŋ/ *noun* any system of tubes or vessels in the body, but especially the urinary system (*informal humorous*)

**plumbism** /ˈplʌmbɪz(ə)m/ *noun* same as **lead poisoning**

**Plummer–Vinson syndrome** /ˌplʌmə ˈvɪnsən ˌsɪndrəʊm/ *noun* a type of iron-deficiency anaemia, in which the tongue and mouth become inflamed and the person cannot swallow [Described 1912 by Plummer, 1919 by Vinson (also described in 1919 by Patterson and Brown Kelly, whose names are frequently associated with the syndrome). Henry Stanley Plummer (1874–1937), US physician; Porter Paisley Vinson (1890–1959), physician at the Mayo Clinic, Minnesota, USA.]

**plunger** /ˈplʌndʒə/ *noun* the part of a hypodermic syringe which slides up and down inside the tube, either sucking liquid into the syringe or forcing the contents out

**pluri-** /plʊəri/ *prefix* indicating more than one of something

**PM** *abbr* 1. particulate matter 2. post mortem

**PMA** *abbr* progressive muscular atrophy

**pmol** *symbol* picomole

**PMR** *abbr* polymyalgia rheumatica

**PMS** *abbr* premenstrual syndrome

**PMT** *abbr* premenstrual tension

**-pnea** /pniːə/ *suffix* same as **-pnoea**

**pneo-** /niːəʊ/ *prefix* relating to breathing

**pneum-** /njuːm/ *prefix* same as **pneumo-** (used before vowels)

**pneumat-** /njuːmət/ *prefix* same as **pneumato-** (used before vowels)

**pneumato-** /njuːmətəʊ/ *prefix* relating to air, gas or breath

**pneumatocele** /njuːˈmætəʊsiːl/ *noun* 1. a sac or tumour filled with gas 2. herniation of the lung

**pneumatonometer** /ˌnjuːmətəˈnɒmɪtə/ *noun* an instrument which measures the air pressure in the eye, used in testing for glaucoma. It blows a puff of air onto the cornea.

**pneumatosis** /ˌnjuːməˈtəʊsɪs/ *noun* the occurrence of gas in an unusual place in the body

**pneumaturia** /ˌnjuːməˈtjʊəriə/ *noun* the act of passing air or gas in the urine

**pneumo-** /njuːməʊ/ *prefix* referring to air, to the lungs or to breathing

**pneumocephalus** /ˌnjuːməʊˈkefələs/ *noun* the presence of air or gas in the brain

**pneumococcal** /ˌnjuːməʊˈkɒk(ə)l/ *adjective* referring to pneumococci

**pneumococcus** /ˌnjuːməʊˈkɒkəs/ *noun* a bacterium which causes respiratory tract infections including pneumonia (NOTE: The plural is **pneumococci.**)

**pneumoconiosis** /ˌnjuːməʊkəʊniˈəʊsɪs/ *noun* a lung disease in which fibrous tissue forms in the lungs because the person has inhaled particles of stone or dust over a long period of time

**pneumocystis carinii pneumonia** /ˌnjuːməʊsɪstɪs kəˌriːniː njuːˈməʊniə/ *noun* a form of pneumonia found in people with impaired immune systems after radiotherapy or with AIDS. Abbr **PCP**

**pneumocyte** /ˈnjuːməʊsaɪt/ *noun* a cell of the walls between the air sacs in the lung

**pneumoencephalography** /ˌnjuːməʊenˌkefəˈlɒɡrəfi/ *noun* same as **encephalogram**

**pneumogastric** /ˌnjuːməʊˈɡæstrɪk/ *adjective* referring to the lungs and the stomach

**pneumograph** /ˈnjuːməɡrɑːf/ *noun* an instrument which records chest movements during breathing

**pneumohaemothorax** /ˌnjuːməʊˌhiːməʊˈθɔːræks/ *noun* blood or air in the pleural cavity. Also called **haemopneumothorax**

**pneumomycosis** /ˌnjuːməʊmaɪˈkəʊsɪs/ *noun* an infection of the lungs caused by a fungus

**pneumon-** /njuːmən/ *prefix* same as **pneumono-** (used before vowels)

**pneumonectomy** /ˌnjuːməˈnektəmi/ *noun* the surgical removal of all or part of a lung. Also called **pulmonectomy**

**pneumonia** /njuːˈməʊniə/ *noun* inflammation of a lung, where the tiny alveoli of the lung become filled with fluid ○ *He developed pneumonia and had to be hospitalised.* ○ *She died of pneumonia.*

COMMENT: The symptoms of pneumonia are shivering, pains in the chest, high temperature and sputum brought up by coughing.

**pneumonic** /njuːˈmɒnɪk/ *adjective* 1. referring to the lungs 2. referring to pneumonia

**pneumonic plague** /njuːˌmɒnɪk ˈpleɪɡ/ *noun* a form of bubonic plague which mainly affects the lungs

**pneumonitis** /ˌnjuːməʊˈnaɪtɪs/ *noun* inflammation of the lungs

**pneumono-** /njuːmənəʊ/ *prefix* referring to the lungs

**pneumoperitoneum** /ˌnjuːməʊperɪtəˈniːəm/ *noun* air in the peritoneal cavity

**pneumoradiography** /ˌnjuːməʊˌreɪdiˈɒɡrəfi/ *noun* an X-ray examination of part of the body after air or a gas has been inserted to make the organs show more clearly

**pneumothorax** /ˌnjuːməʊˈθɔːræks/ *noun* a condition in which air or gas is in the thorax. Also called **collapsed lung**

**-pnoea** /pniːə/ *suffix* referring to breathing

**PNS** *abbr* peripheral nervous system

**pock** /pɒk/ *noun* a localised lesion on the skin, due to smallpox or chickenpox

**pocket** /ˈpɒkɪt/ *noun* a cavity in the body □ **pocket of infection** place where an infection remains

**pockmark** /ˈpɒkmɑːk/ *noun* a scar left by a pustule, as in smallpox

**pockmarked** /ˈpɒkmɑːkt/ *adjective* referring to a face with scars from smallpox

**pod-** /pɒd/ *prefix* referring to the foot

**podagra** /pɒˈdæɡrə/ same as **gout**

**podalic** /pəʊˈdælɪk/ *adjective* relating to the feet

**podalic version** /pəʊˌdælɪk ˈvɜːʃ(ə)n/ *noun* the procedure of turning a fetus in the uterus by its feet

**podarthritis** /ˌpəʊdɑːˈθraɪtɪs/ *noun* the swelling of one or more joints of the foot

**podiatrist** /pəʊˈdaɪətrɪst/ *noun* US a person who specialises in the care of the foot and its diseases

**podiatry** /pəʊˈdaɪətri/ *noun* US the study of minor diseases and disorders of the feet

**-poiesis** /pɔɪˈsɪs/ *suffix* referring to something which forms

**poikilo-** /pɔɪkɪləʊ/ *prefix* irregular or varied

**poikilocyte** /ˈpɔɪkɪləʊsaɪt/ *noun* an unusually large red blood cell with an irregular shape

**poikilocytosis** /ˌpɔɪkɪləʊsaɪˈtəʊsɪs/ *noun* a condition in which poikilocytes exist in the blood

**point** /pɔɪnt/ *noun* 1. a sharp end ○ *Surgical needles have to have very sharp points.* 2. the dot used to show the division between whole numbers and parts of numbers (NOTE: **3.256:** say 'three point two five six'; **his temperature**

**was 38.7:** say 'thirty-eight point seven'.) **3.** a mark in a series of numbers ○ *the freezing point of water*

**pointed** /'pɔɪntɪd/ *adjective* with a sharp point

**poison** /'pɔɪz(ə)n/ *noun* a substance which can kill or harm body tissues if eaten or drunk ■ *verb* to harm or kill someone with a poison

COMMENT: The commonest poisons, of which even a small amount can kill, are arsenic, cyanide and strychnine. Many common foods and drugs can be poisonous if taken in large doses. Common household materials such as bleach, glue and insecticides can also be poisonous. Some types of poisoning, such as Salmonella, can be passed to other people through lack of hygienic conditions.

**poisoning** /'pɔɪz(ə)nɪŋ/ *noun* a condition in which a person is made ill or is killed by a poisonous substance

**poison ivy** /ˌpɔɪz(ə)n 'aɪvi/, **poison oak** /ˌpɔɪz(ə)n 'əʊk/ *noun* American plants whose leaves can cause a painful rash if touched

**poisonous** /'pɔɪz(ə)nəs/ *adjective* referring to a substance which is full of poison or which can kill or harm

**poisonous gas** /ˌpɔɪz(ə)nəs 'gæs/ *noun* a gas which can kill or can make someone ill

**Poisons Act** /'pɔɪz(ə)nz ækt/ *noun* in the UK, one of several Acts of Parliament which regulate the making, prescribing and selling of drugs, e.g. the Pharmacy and Poisons Act 1933, Misuse of Drugs Act 1971, or Poisons Act 1972

**polar** /'pəʊlə/ *adjective* with a pole

**polar body** /ˌpəʊlə 'bɒdi/ *noun* a small cell which is produced from an oocyte but does not develop into an ovum

**pole** /pəʊl/ *noun* **1.** the end of an axis **2.** the end of a rounded organ, e.g. the end of a lobe in the cerebral hemisphere

**pole and canvas stretcher** /ˌpəʊl ən 'kænvəs ˌstretʃə/ *noun* a simple stretcher made of a piece of canvas and two poles which slide into tubes at the side of the canvas

**poli-** /pɒli/ *prefix* same as **polio-** (*used before vowels*)

**polio** /'pəʊliəʊ/ *noun* same as **poliomyelitis** (*informal*)

**polio-** /pəʊliəʊ/ *prefix* grey matter in the nervous system

**polioencephalitis** /ˌpəʊliəʊenˌkefə'laɪtɪs/ *noun* a type of viral encephalitis, an inflammation of the grey matter in the brain caused by the same virus as poliomyelitis

**polioencephalomyelitis** /ˌpəʊliəʊenˌkefələʊˌmaɪə'laɪtɪs/ *noun* polioencephalitis which also affects the spinal cord

**poliomyelitis** /ˌpəʊliəʊˌmaɪə'laɪtɪs/ *noun* an infection of the anterior horn cells of the spinal cord caused by a virus which attacks the motor neurones and can lead to paralysis. Also called **polio, infantile paralysis**

COMMENT: Symptoms of poliomyelitis are paralysis of the limbs, fever and stiffness in the neck. The bulbar form may start with difficulty in swallowing. Poliomyelitis can be prevented by immunisation and two vaccines are used: Sabin vaccine is formed of live polio virus and is taken orally on a piece of sugar; Salk vaccine is given as an injection of dead virus.

**poliovirus** /'pəʊliəʊˌvaɪrəs/ *noun* a virus which causes poliomyelitis

**Politzer bag** /'pɒlɪtsə bæg/ *noun* a rubber bag which is used to blow air into the middle ear to unblock a Eustachian tube [Described 1863. After Adam Politzer (1835–1920), Professor of Otology in Vienna, Austria.]

**pollen** /'pɒlən/ *noun* a powdery substance consisting of male gametes from plants, produced by the flower stamens, which floats in the air in spring and summer, and which causes hay fever

**pollen count** /'pɒlən kaʊnt/ *noun* a figure which shows the amount of pollen in a sample of air

**pollex** /'pɒleks/ *noun* the thumb (*technical*) (NOTE: The plural is **pollices**.)

**pollutant** /pə'luːt(ə)nt/ *noun* a substance which causes pollution

**pollute** /pə'luːt/ *verb* to make e.g. the air, a river or the sea dirty, especially with industrial waste (NOTE: **polluting – polluted**)

**pollution** /pə'luːʃ(ə)n/ *noun* the act of making dirty, or substances which make e.g. air or water impure

**poly-** /pɒli/ *prefix* **1.** many or much **2.** touching many organs

**polyarteritis** /ˌpɒliɑːtə'raɪtɪs/ *noun* a condition in which a lot of arteries swell up at the same time

**polyarteritis nodosa** /ˌpɒliɑːtəˌraɪtɪs nə'dəʊsə/ *noun* a collagen disease in which the walls of the arteries in various parts of the body become inflamed, leading to asthma, high blood pressure and kidney failure. Also called **periarteritis nodosa**

**polyarthritis** /ˌpɒliɑː'θraɪtɪs/ *noun* inflammation of several joints, as in rheumatoid arthritis

**polycystic** /ˌpɒli'sɪstɪk/ *adjective* referring to an organ which has developed more than one cyst, or to a disease caused by the development of cysts

**polycystic kidney disease** /ˌpɒlisɪstɪk 'kɪdni dɪˌziːz/ *noun* a condition in which there are multiple cysts on each kidney which grow and multiply over time. Abbr **PKD**

COMMENT: The diseased kidney finally shuts down in over 60% of cases, and dialysis and transplantation are the only forms of treatment.

**polycystic ovary disease** /ˌpɒlɪsɪstɪk ˈəʊvəri dɪˌziːz/ *noun* same as **polycystic ovary syndrome**. Abbr **PCOD**

**polycystic ovary syndrome** /ˌpɒlɪsɪstɪk ˈəʊvəri ˌsɪndrəʊm/, **polycystic ovarian syndrome** /ˌpɒlɪsɪstɪk əʊˈveəriən ˌsɪndrəʊm/ *noun* a hormonal disorder in which a woman's ovaries are enlarged and contain many small painless cysts, hair growth is excessive, acne develops and infertility may occur. Also called **Stein Leventhal syndrome**. Abbr **PCOS**

**polycystitis** /ˌpɒlɪsɪˈstaɪtɪs/ *noun* a congenital disease in which several cysts form in the kidney at the same time

**polycythaemia** /ˌpɒlɪsaɪˈθiːmiə/ *noun* a condition in which the number of red blood cells increases (NOTE: The US spelling is **polycythemia**.)

**polycythaemia vera** /ˌpɒlɪsaɪθiːmiə ˈvɪərə/ *noun* a blood disease in which the number of red blood cells increases, together with an increase in the number of white blood cells, making the blood thicker and slowing its flow. Also called **erythraemia, Vaquez-Osler disease**

**polydactyl** /ˌpɒliˈdæktɪl/ *adjective* having more than the usual number of fingers or toes

**polydactylism** /ˌpɒliˈdæktɪlɪz(ə)m/ *noun* same as **hyperdactylism**

**polydipsia** /ˌpɒliˈdɪpsiə/ *noun* a condition, often caused by diabetes insipidus, in which a person is unusually thirsty

**polygraph** /ˈpɒligrɑːf/ *noun* an instrument which records the pulse in several parts of the body at the same time

**polymenorrhoea** /ˌpɒlimenəˈriːə/ *noun* unusually frequent menstruations (NOTE: The US spelling is **polymenorrhea**.)

**polymerase chain reaction** /ˌpɒliməreɪz ˌtʃeɪn riˈækʃ(ə)n/ *noun* the technique used to amplify genetic material in order to analyse it for genetic disorders, e.g. material from a single cell in an embryo. Abbr **PCR**

**polymorph** /ˈpɒlimɔːf/ *noun* same as **neutrophil**

**polymyalgia rheumatica** /ˌpɒlimaɪˌældʒə ruːˈmætɪkə/ *noun* a disease of elderly people characterised by pain and stiffness in the shoulder and hip muscles making them weak and sensitive

**polymyositis** /ˌpɒlimaɪəʊˈsaɪtɪs/ *noun* a condition in which a lot of muscles swell up at the same time, especially the ones in the trunk of the body, causing weakness. It is treated with steroid drugs or immunosuppressants, and also exercise.

**polyneuritis** /ˌpɒlinjʊˈraɪtɪs/ *noun* inflammation of many nerves

**polyneuropathy** /ˌpɒlinjʊˈrɒpəθi/ *noun* any disease which affects several nerves (NOTE: The plural is **polyneuropathies**.)

**polyopia** /ˌpɒliˈəʊpiə/, **polyopsia** /ˌpɒliˈɒpsiə/, **polyopy** /ˈpɒliəʊpi/ *noun* a condition in which a person sees several images of one object at the same time. Compare **diplopia**

**polyp** /ˈpɒlɪp/ *noun* a tumour growing on a stalk in mucous membrane, which can be cauterised. Polyps are often found in the nose, mouth or throat. Also called **polypus**

**polypectomy** /ˌpɒlɪˈpektəmi/ *noun* a surgical operation to remove a polyp (NOTE: The plural is **polypectomies**.)

**polypeptide** /ˌpɒliˈpeptaɪd/ *noun* a type of protein formed of linked amino acids

**polyphagia** /ˌpɒliˈfeɪdʒə/ *noun* **1.** a condition in which a person eats too much **2.** a compulsive desire for every kind of food

**polypharmacy** /ˌpɒliˈfɑːməsi/ *noun* the practice of prescribing several drugs to be taken at the same time

**polyploid** /ˈpɒlɪplɔɪd/ *adjective* referring to a cell where there are more than two copies of each chromosome, which is not viable in humans

**polypoid** /ˈpɒlɪpɔɪd/ *adjective* looking like a polyp

**polyposis** /ˌpɒlɪˈpəʊsɪs/ *noun* a condition in which many polyps form in the mucous membrane of the colon. ◊ **familial adenomatous polyposis**

**polypus** /ˈpɒlɪpəs/ *noun* same as **polyp** (NOTE: The plural is **polypi**.)

**polyradiculitis** /ˌpɒliræˌdɪkjuˈlaɪtɪs/ *noun* a disease of the nervous system which affects the roots of the nerves

**polysaccharide** /ˌpɒliˈsækəraɪd/ *noun* a type of carbohydrate made up of a lot of monosaccharides joined together in chains. They include starch and cellulose, are insoluble in water and do not form crystals.

**polyserositis** /ˌpɒlisɪərəʊˈsaɪtɪs/ *noun* inflammation of the membranes lining the abdomen, chest and joints and exudation of serous fluid

**polysomnograph** /ˌpɒliˈsɒmnəgrɑːf/ *noun* a record of bodily activity during sleep to identify possible causes of sleep disorders

**polyspermia** /ˌpɒliˈspɜːmiə/, **polyspermism** /ˌpɒliˈspɜːmɪz(ə)m/, **polyspermy** /ˌpɒliˈspɜːmi/ *noun* **1.** excessive seminal secretion **2.** fertilisation of one ovum by several spermatozoa

**polyunsaturated fat** /ˌpɒliʌnsætʃəreɪtɪd ˈfæt/ *noun* a fatty acid capable of absorbing more hydrogen than most others, typical of vegetable and fish oils

**polyuria** /ˌpɒliˈjʊəriə/ *noun* a condition in which a person passes a large quantity of urine, usually as a result of diabetes insipidus

**polyvalent** /ˌpɒliˈveɪlənt/ *adjective* having more than one valency

**POM** *abbr* prescription-only medicine

**pompholyx** /'pɒmfɒlɪks/ *noun* **1.** a type of eczema with many irritating little blisters on the hands and feet **2.** a skin condition with bulbous swellings

**pons** /pɒnz/ *noun* a bridge of tissue joining parts of an organ. See illustration at BRAIN in Supplement (NOTE: The plural is **pontes**.)

**pons Varolii** /,pɒnz və'rəʊliaɪ/ *noun* part of the hindbrain, formed of fibres which continue the medulla oblongata. See illustration at BRAIN in Supplement (NOTE: The plural is **pontes Varolii**.) [After Constanzo Varolius (1543–75), Italian physician and anatomist, doctor to Pope Gregory XIII]

**pontes** /'pɒntiz/ plural of **pons**

**pontine** /'pɒntaɪn/ *adjective* referring to a pons

**pontine cistern** /,pɒntaɪn 'sɪstən/ *noun* a subarachnoid space in front of the pons, containing the basilar artery

**poor** /pɔː/ *adjective* not very good ○ *He's in poor health.* ○ *She's always had poor circulation.*

**poorly** /'pɔːli/ *adjective* not very well (*informal*) ○ *Her mother has been quite poorly recently.* ○ *He felt poorly and stayed in bed.*

**POP** *abbr* progesterone only pill

**popeyes** /'pɒpaɪz/ *plural noun* US protruding eyes

**popliteal** /,pɒplɪ'tiːəl/ *adjective* referring to the back of the knee

**popliteal artery** /,pɒplɪtiːəl 'ɑːtəri/ *noun* an artery which branches from the femoral artery behind the knee and leads into the tibial arteries

**popliteal fossa** /,pɒplɪtiːəl 'fɒsə/ *noun* a space behind the knee between the hamstring and the calf muscle. Also called **popliteal space**

**popliteal muscle** /,pɒplɪ'tiːəl ,mʌs(ə)l/ *noun* same as **popliteus**

**popliteal space** /,pɒplɪtiːəl 'speɪs/ *noun* same as **popliteal fossa**

**popliteus** /pɒ'plɪtiəs/ *noun* a muscle at the back of the knee. Also called **popliteal muscle**

**population** /,pɒpjʊ'leɪʃ(ə)n/ *noun* **1.** the number of people living in a country or town ○ *Population statistics show that the birth rate is slowing down.* ○ *The government has decided to screen the whole population of the area.* **2.** the number of patients in hospital ○ *The hospital population in the area has fallen below 10,000.*

**pore** /pɔː/ *noun* **1.** a tiny hole in the skin through which the sweat passes **2.** a small communicating passage between cavities

**porencephaly** /,pɔːren'kefəli/, **porencephalia** /,pɔːrenkə'feɪliə/, **porencephalus** /,pɔːren'kefələs/ *noun* a condition in which there are cysts in the cerebral cortex, as a result of unusual development

**porous** /'pɔːrəs/ *adjective* **1.** containing pores ○ *Porous bone surrounds the Eustachian tubes.* **2.** referring to tissue which allows fluid to pass through it

**porphyria** /pɔː'fɪriə/ *noun* a hereditary disease affecting the metabolism of porphyrin pigments

COMMENT: Porphyria causes abdominal pains and attacks of mental confusion. The skin becomes sensitive to light and the urine becomes coloured and turns dark brown when exposed to the light.

**porphyrin** /'pɔːfərɪn/ *noun* a member of a family of metal-containing biological pigments, the commonest of which is protoporphyrin IX

**porphyrinuria** /,pɔːfɪri'njʊəriə/ *noun* the presence of excess porphyrins in the urine, a sign of porphyria or of metal poisoning

**porta** /'pɔːtə/ *noun* an opening which allows blood vessels to pass into an organ (NOTE: The plural is **portae**.)

**portable** /'pɔːtəb(ə)l/ *adjective* referring to something which can be carried ○ *He keeps a portable first aid kit in his car.* ○ *The ambulance team carried a portable blood testing unit.*

**Portacath** /'pɔːtəkæθ/ *noun* a type of catheter put in place under a person's skin to make it easier to have chemotherapy, transfusions and blood tests. It is accessed by the use of a special needle and flushed regularly with sterile saline.

**portacaval** /,pɔːtə'keɪv(ə)l/ *adjective* another spelling of **portocaval**

**portae** /'pɔːti/ plural of **porta**

**porta hepatis** /,pɔːtə 'hepətɪs/ *noun* an opening in the liver through which the hepatic artery, hepatic duct and portal vein pass (NOTE: The plural is **portae hepatitis**.)

**portal** /'pɔːt(ə)l/ *adjective* referring to a porta, especially the portal system or the portal vein

**portal hypertension** /,pɔːt(ə)l ,haɪpə'tenʃən/ *noun* high pressure in the portal vein, caused by cirrhosis of the liver or a clot in the vein and causing internal bleeding

**portal pyaemia** /,pɔːt(ə)l paɪ'iːmiə/ *noun* an infection of the portal vein in the liver, giving abscesses

**portal system** /'pɔːt(ə)l ,sɪstəm/ *noun* a group of veins which have capillaries at both ends and do not go to the heart

**portal vein** /'pɔːt(ə)l veɪn/ *noun* a vein which takes blood from the stomach, pancreas, gall bladder, intestines and spleen to the liver (NOTE: For other terms referring to the portal vein, see words beginning with **pyl-, pyle-**.)

**porter** /'pɔːtə/ *noun* a hospital worker who does general work such as wheeling a patient's trolley into the operating theatre or moving heavy equipment

**portocaval** /ˌpɔːtəʊˈkeɪv(ə)l/ *adjective* linking the portal vein to the inferior vena cava

**portocaval anastomosis** /ˌpɔːtəʊˌkeɪv(ə)l ənæstəˈməʊsɪs/ *noun* a surgical operation to join the portal vein to the inferior vena cava and divert blood past the liver

**portocaval shunt** /ˌpɔːtəʊˌkeɪv(ə)l ˈʃʌnt/ *noun* an artificial passage made between the portal vein and the inferior vena cava to relieve portal hypertension

**porto-systemic encephalopathy** /ˌpɔːtəʊ sɪsˌtiːmɪk ˌenkefəˈlɒpəθi/ *noun* a mental disorder and coma caused by liver disorder due to portal hypertension

**port wine stain** /pɔːt ˈwaɪn steɪn/ *noun* a purple birthmark

**position** /pəˈzɪʃ(ə)n/ *noun* **1.** the place where something is ○ *The exact position of the tumour is located by an X-ray.* **2.** the way a person's body is arranged ○ *in a sitting position* ○ *The accident victim had been placed in the recovery position.* ■ *verb* to place something in a particular position ○ *The fetus is correctly positioned in the uterus.*

**positive** /ˈpɒzɪtɪv/ *adjective* **1.** indicating the answer 'yes' **2.** indicating the presence of something being tested for ○ *Her cervical smear was positive.* Opposite **negative**

**positive end-expiratory pressure** /ˌpɒzɪtɪv ˌend ɪkˌspɪrət(ə)ri ˈpreʃə/ *noun* the procedure of forcing a person to breathe through a mask in cases where fluid has collected in the lungs. Abbr **PEEP**

**positive feedback** /ˌpɒzɪtɪv ˈfiːdbæk/ *noun* a situation in which the result of a process stimulates the process which caused it

**positively** /ˈpɒzɪtɪvli/ *adverb* in a positive way ○ *She reacted positively to the test.*

**positive pressure respirator** /ˌpɒzɪtɪv ˈpreʃə ˌrespɪreɪtə/ *noun* a machine which forces air into the lungs through a tube inserted in the mouth

**positive pressure ventilation** /ˌpɒzɪtɪv ˈpreʃə ventɪˌleɪʃ(ə)n/ *noun* the act of forcing air into the lungs to encourage them to expand. Abbr **PPV**

**positron-emission tomography** /ˌpɒzɪtrɒn ɪˈmɪʃ(ə)n təˌmɒgrəfi/ *noun* a method of scanning the tissues of the brain, chest and abdomen for unusual metabolic activity after injecting a radioactive substance into the body. Abbr **PET**

**posology** /pəˈsɒlədʒi/ *noun* the study of doses of medicine

**posseting** /ˈpɒsɪtɪŋ/ *noun* (*in babies*) the act of bringing up small quantities of curdled milk into the mouth after feeding

**Possum** /ˈpɒsəm/ *noun* a device using electronic switches which helps a person who is severely paralysed to work a machine such as a telephone (NOTE: The name is derived from the first letters of **patient-operated selector mechanism**.)

**post-** /pəʊst/ *prefix* after or later

**postcentral gyrus** /pəʊstˌsentr(ə)l ˈdʒaɪrəs/ *noun* a sensory area of the cerebral cortex which receives impulses from receptor cells and registers sensations such as pain, heat and touch

**post-cibal** /pəʊst ˈsaɪb(ə)l/ *adjective* after having eaten food

**post cibum** *adverb* full form of **p.c.**

**post-coital** /pəʊst ˈkɔɪt(ə)l/ *adjective* taking place after sexual intercourse

**postconcussional syndrome** /ˌpəʊstkən ˈkʌʃ(ə)n(ə)l ˌsɪndrəʊm/ *noun* a set of symptoms which sometimes follow a head injury in which a person lost consciousness, including headache, loss of concentration, memory loss, depression and irritability

**post-epileptic** /ˌpəʊst epɪˈleptɪk/ *adjective* taking place after an epileptic fit

**posterior** /pɒˈstɪəriə/ *adjective* at the back. Opposite **anterior** □ **posterior to** behind ○ *The cerebellum is posterior to the medulla oblongata.* ■ *noun* same as **buttock** (*informal*)

**posterior approach** /pɒˈstɪəriər əˌprəʊtʃ/ *noun* an operation carried out from the back

**posterior aspect** /pɒˈstɪəriər ˌæspekt/ *noun* a view of the back of the body, or of the back of part of the body. See illustration at ANATOMICAL TERMS in Supplement

**posterior chamber** /pɒˌstɪəriə ˈtʃeɪmbə/ *noun* a part of the aqueous chamber which is behind the iris. Compare **anterior chamber**

**posterior fontanelle** /pɒˌstɪəriə fɒntəˈnel/ *noun* a cartilage at the back of the head where the parietal bones join the occipital. ◊ **bregma**

**posterior lobe** *noun* same as **caudate lobe**

**posteriorly** /pɒˈstɪəriəli/ *adverb* in or from a position behind ○ *An artery leads to a posteriorly placed organ.* ○ *Rectal biopsy specimens are best taken posteriorly.*

**posterior nares** /pɒˌstɪəriə ˈneəriːz/ *plural noun* same as **internal nares**

**posterior synechia** /pɒˌstɪəriə sɪˈnekiə/ *noun* a condition of the eye in which the iris sticks to the anterior surface of the lens

**postero-** /pɒstərəʊ/ *prefix* back or behind

**posteroanterior** /ˌpɒstərəʊænˈtɪəriə/ *adjective* lying from the back to the front

**post-exposure prophylaxis** /ˌpəʊst ɪk ˌspəʊʒə ˌprɒfəˈlæksɪs/ *noun* a treatment given to a person who has been exposed to a harmful agent, in an effort to prevent or reduce injury or infection

**postganglionic** /ˌpəʊstgæŋliˈɒnɪk/ *adjective* placed after a ganglion

**postganglionic fibre** /ˌpəʊstgæŋliˌɒnɪk ˈfaɪbə/ *noun* an axon of a nerve cell which starts in a ganglion and extends beyond the ganglion

COMMENT: Postganglionic fibres go to the nose, palate, pharynx and lacrimal glands.

**postganglionic neurone** /ˌpəʊstɡæŋgli ˌɒnɪk ˈnjʊərəʊn/ *noun* a neurone which starts in a ganglion and ends in a gland or unstriated muscle

**postgastrectomy syndrome** /ˌpəʊst gæ ˈstrektəmi ˌsɪndrəʊm/ *noun* a group of symptoms which can occur after eating in people who have had stomach operations. It is caused by a lot of food passing into the small intestine too fast and can cause dizziness, nausea, sweating and weakness. Also called **dumping syndrome**

**postgraduate education allowance** /ˈpəʊstˈɡrædjʊət edjʊˈkeɪʃ(ə)n əˈlaʊəns/ *noun* a payment made to GPs to reward continued education. Abbr **PGEA**

**posthepatic** /ˌpəʊsthɪˈpætɪk/ *adjective* positioned behind or coming into effect after the liver

**posthepatic bilirubin** /ˌpəʊsthɪˌpætɪk ˌbɪli ˈruːbɪn/ *noun* bilirubin which enters the plasma after being treated by the liver

**posthepatic jaundice** /ˌpəʊsthɪˌpætɪk ˈdʒɔːndɪs/ *noun* same as **obstructive jaundice**

**post herpetic neuralgia** /ˌpəʊst həˌpetɪk njʊˈrældʒə/ *noun* pains felt after an attack of shingles

**posthitis** /pɒsˈθaɪtɪs/ *noun* inflammation of the foreskin

**posthumous** /ˈpɒstjʊməs/ *adjective* occurring after death ◇ **posthumous birth 1.** the birth of a baby after the death of the father **2.** the birth of a baby by caesarean section after the mother has died

**post-irradiation** /ˌpəʊst ɪˌreɪdiˈeɪʃ(ə)n/ *adjective* referring to pain or disorder caused by X-rays

**post-irradiation enteritis** /ˌpəʊst ɪˌreɪdi eɪʃ(ə)n ˌentəˈraɪtɪs/ *noun* enteritis caused by X-rays

**postmature** /ˌpəʊstməˈtʃʊə/ *adjective* referring to a baby born after the usual gestation period of 42 weeks

**postmaturity** /ˌpəʊstməˈtʃʊərɪti/ *noun* a pregnancy which lasts longer than the usual gestation period of 42 weeks

**postmenopausal** /ˌpəʊstmenəʊˈpɔːz(ə)l/ *adjective* happening or existing after the menopause ○ *She experienced some postmenopausal bleeding.*

**post mortem** /pəʊst ˈmɔːtəm/, **post mortem examination** /pəʊst ˈmɔːtəm ɪɡˌzæmɪ ˌneɪʃ(ə)n/ *noun* an examination of a dead body by a pathologist to find out the cause of death ○ *The post mortem showed that he had been poisoned.* Abbr **PM**. Also called **autopsy**

**postnasal** /pəʊstˈneɪz(ə)l/ *adjective* situated or happening behind the nose

**postnasal drip** /pəʊstˌneɪz(ə)l ˈdrɪp/ *noun* a condition in which mucus from the nose runs down into the throat and is swallowed

**postnatal** /ˌpəʊstˈneɪt(ə)l/ *adjective* referring to the period after the birth of a child

**postnatal care** /pəʊstˌneɪt(ə)l ˈkeə/ *noun* the care given to a woman after the birth of her child

**postnatal depression** /pəʊstˌneɪt(ə)l dɪ ˈpreʃ(ə)n/ *noun* depression which sometimes affects a woman after childbirth

**postnecrotic cirrhosis** /ˌpəʊstnekrɒtɪk sɪ ˈrəʊsɪs/ *noun* cirrhosis of the liver caused by viral hepatitis

**post-op** /pəʊst ˈɒp/ (*informal*) *adjective* same as **postoperative** ■ *adverb* same as **postoperatively**

**postoperative** /ˌpəʊstˈɒp(ə)rətɪv/ *adjective* referring to the period after a surgical operation ○ *The patient has suffered postoperative nausea and vomiting.* ○ *Occlusion may appear as postoperative angina pectoris.*

'...the nurse will help ensure that the parent is physically fit to cope with the postoperative child' [*British Journal of Nursing*]

**postoperatively** /ˌpəʊstˈɒp(ə)rətɪvli/ *adverb* after a surgical operation

**postoperative pain** /pəʊstˌɒp(ə)rətɪv ˈpeɪn/ *noun* pain felt after a surgical operation

**postorbital** /ˌpəʊstˈɔːbɪt(ə)l/ *adjective* situated behind the eye or the eye socket

**postpartum** /ˌpəʊstˈpɑːtəm/ *adjective* referring to the period after the birth of a child

**postpartum fever** /pəʊstˌpɑːtəm ˈfiːvə/ *noun* same as **puerperal infection**

**postpartum haemorrhage** /pəʊstˌpɑːtəm ˈhem(ə)rɪdʒ/ *noun* heavy bleeding after childbirth. Abbr **PPH**

**post-primary tuberculosis** /ˌpəʊst ˌpraɪməri tjuːˌbɜːkjʊˈləʊsɪs/ *noun* the reappearance of tuberculosis in a person who has been infected with it before

**post-registration education and practice** /ˌpəʊst redʒɪˌstreɪʃ(ə)n edjʊˌkeɪʃ(ə)n ənd ˈpræktɪs/ *noun* in the UK, the requirement for all registered nurses and midwives to undertake educational activities and keep up with contemporary practice, and also for their employers to address the learning needs of staff. It was started by the UKCC in 1993. Abbr **PREP**

**postsynaptic** /ˌpəʊstsɪˈnæptɪk/ *adjective* situated behind a synapse

**postsynaptic axon** /ˌpəʊstsɪnæptɪk ˈæksɒn/ *noun* an axon of the nerves on either side of a synapse

**post-traumatic** /ˌpəʊst trɔːˈmætɪk/ *adjective* appearing after a trauma, e.g. after an accident, rape or fire

**post-traumatic amnesia** /ˌpəʊst trɔː ˌmætɪk æmˈniːziə/ *noun* amnesia which follows a trauma

**post-traumatic stress disorder** /ˌpəʊst trɔːˌmætɪk ˈstres dɪsˌɔːdə/ noun a psychological condition affecting people who have suffered severe emotional trauma, e.g. occasioned by war or natural disaster. Its symptoms include chest pain, dizziness, sleep disturbances, flashbacks, anxiety, tiredness, and depression. Abbr **PTSD**

**postural** /ˈpɒstʃərəl/ adjective referring to posture ○ a study of postural disorders

**postural drainage** /ˌpɒstʃərəl ˈdreɪnɪdʒ/ noun a procedure for removing matter from infected lungs by making the person lie down with the head lower than the feet, so that he or she can cough more easily

**postural hypotension** /ˌpɒstʃərəl haɪpəʊˈtenʃən/ noun low blood pressure when standing up suddenly, causing dizziness

**posture** /ˈpɒstʃə/ noun the position in which a body is arranged, or the way a person usually holds his or her body when standing ○ Bad posture can cause pain in the back. ○ She has to do exercises to correct her bad posture.

**postviral** /pəʊstˈvaɪrəl/ adjective occurring after a viral infection

**postviral fatigue syndrome** /pəʊstˌvaɪrəl fəˈtiːɡ ˌsɪndrəʊm/ noun same as **myalgic encephalomyelitis**

**potassium** /pəˈtæsiəm/ noun a metallic element (NOTE: The chemical symbol is **K**.)

**potassium permanganate** /pəˌtæsiəm pəˈmæŋɡənət/ noun a purple-coloured poisonous salt, used as a disinfectant

**potentiate** /pəˈtenʃieɪt/ verb to improve the effectiveness of a drug or treatment, especially by adding another drug or agent (NOTE: **potentiating – potentiated**)

**Pott's disease** /ˈpɒts dɪˌziːz/, **Pott's caries** /ˈpɒts ˌkeəriːz/ noun tuberculosis of the spine, causing paralysis [Described 1779. After Sir Percivall Pott (1714–88), London surgeon.]

**Pott's fracture** /ˈpɒts ˌfræktʃə/ noun a fracture of the lower end of the fibula together with displacement of the ankle and foot outwards [Described 1765. After Sir Percivall Pott (1714–88), London surgeon.]

**pouch** /paʊtʃ/ noun a small sac or pocket attached to an organ

**poultice** /ˈpəʊltɪs/ noun a compress made of hot water and flour paste or other substances which is pressed onto an infected part to draw out pus, to relieve pain or to encourage the circulation. Also called **fomentation**

**pound** /paʊnd/ noun a measure of weight equal to about 450 grams ○ The baby weighed only four pounds at birth. Abbr **lb** (NOTE: With figures, usually written **lb: The baby weighs 6lb**.)

**Poupart's ligament** /ˈpuːpɑːts ˌlɪɡəmənt/ noun same as **inguinal ligament** [Described

1705. After François Poupart (1616–1708), French surgeon and anatomist.]

**powder** /ˈpaʊdə/ noun a medicine in the form of a fine dry dust made from particles of drugs ○ He took a powder to help his indigestion or He took an indigestion powder.

**powdered** /ˈpaʊdəd/ adjective crushed so that it forms a fine dry dust ○ The medicine is available in tablets or in powdered form.

**pox** /pɒks/ noun **1.** a disease with eruption of vesicles or pustules **2.** same as **syphilis** (old)

**poxvirus** /ˈpɒksˌvaɪrəs/ noun any of a group of viruses which cause cowpox, smallpox and related diseases

'Molluscum contagiosum is a harmless skin infection caused by a poxvirus that affects mainly children and young adults' [British Medical Journal]

**p.p.** abbreviation after a meal. Full form **post prandium**. Compare **a.p.**

**PPD** abbr purified protein derivative

**PPH** abbr postpartum haemorrhage

**PPV** abbr positive pressure ventilation

**PQRST complex** noun the set of deflections on an electrocardiogram, labelled P to T, which show ventricular contraction

**p.r.** adverb (of an examination) by the rectum. Full form **per rectum**

**practice** /ˈpræktɪs/ noun **1.** the business, or the premises occupied by, a doctor, dentist, or a group of doctors or dentists working together ○ After qualifying she joined her father's practice. □ **in practice** doing the work of a doctor or dentist ○ He has been in practice for six years. **2.** the fact of doing something, as opposed to thinking or talking about it ○ theory and practice **3.** a usual way of doing something ○ Such practices are now regarded as unsafe.

**practice nurse** /ˈpræktɪs nɜːs/ noun a nurse employed by a GP or primary care trust to work in a GP's practice providing treatment, health promotion, screening and other services to patients of the practice

'…practice nurses play a major role in the care of patients with chronic disease and they undertake many preventive procedures' [Nursing Times]

**practise** /ˈpræktɪs/ verb **1.** to work as a doctor ○ He practises in North London. ○ She practises homeopathy. **2.** to work in a particular branch of medicine (NOTE: **practising – practised**. The US spelling is **practice**.)

**practitioner** /prækˈtɪʃ(ə)nə/ noun a qualified person who works in the medical profession ◇ **nurse practitioner** US **1.** a nurse employed by a clinic or doctor's practice who can give advice to patients **2.** a trained nurse who has not been licensed

**praecox** /ˈpriːkɒks/ noun ♦ **ejaculatio praecox**

**praevia** /ˈpriːviə/ noun ♦ **placenta praevia**

**pravastatin** /ˌprævəˈstætɪn/ *noun* a drug used to reduce unusually high levels of blood cholesterol

**prazosin** /ˈpræzəsɪn/ *noun* a drug which relaxes or widens the blood vessels, used to treat hypertension

**pre-** /priː/ *prefix* before or in front of

**preadmission information** /ˌpriːəd ˈmɪʃ(ə)n ɪnfəˌmeɪʃ(ə)n/ *noun* information given to a person before he or she is admitted to hospital

**pre-anaesthetic round** /ˌpriːænəsˈθetɪk raʊnd/ *noun* an examination of patients by the surgeon before they are anaesthetised

**precancer** /priːˈkænsə/ *noun* a growth or cell which is not malignant but which may become cancerous

**precancerous** /priːˈkænsərəs/ *adjective* referring to a growth which is not malignant now, but which can become cancerous later

**precaution** /prɪˈkɔːʃ(ə)n/ *noun* an action taken before something happens ○ *She took the tablets as a precaution against seasickness.*

**precede** /prɪˈsiːd/ *verb* to happen before or earlier than something ○ *The attack was preceded by a sudden rise in body temperature.* (NOTE: **preceding – preceded**)

**precentral gyrus** /priːˌsentr(ə)l ˈdʒaɪrəs/ *noun* a motor area of the cerebral cortex

**preceptor** /prɪˈseptə/ *noun* a specialist who gives practical training to a student

**preceptorship** /prɪˈseptəʃɪp/ *noun* a period of time during which a recently trained nurse, midwife or health visitor can gain practical experience working with a specialist who advises and guides them

**precipitate** /prɪˈsɪpɪtət/ *noun* a substance which is precipitated during a chemical reaction ■ *verb* **1.** to make a substance separate from a chemical compound and fall to the bottom of a liquid during a chemical reaction ○ *Casein is precipitated when milk comes into contact with an acid.* **2.** to make something start suddenly (NOTE: [all verb senses] **precipitating – precipitated**)

'...it has been established that myocardial infarction and sudden coronary death are precipitated in the majority of patients by thrombus formation in the coronary arteries' [*British Journal of Hospital Medicine*]

**precipitate labour** /prɪˌsɪpɪtət ˈleɪbə/ *noun* unusually fast labour, lasting two hours or less. It can be dangerous both to the mother and to the child.

**precipitation** /prɪˌsɪpɪˈteɪʃ(ə)n/ *noun* the action of forming a precipitate

**precipitin** /prɪˈsɪpɪtɪn/ *noun* an antibody which reacts to an antigen and forms a precipitate, used in many diagnostic tests

**precise** /prɪˈsaɪs/ *adjective* very exact or correct ○ *The instrument can give precise measurements of changes in heartbeat.*

**preclinical** /priːˈklɪnɪk(ə)l/ *adjective* **1.** taking place before diagnosis ○ *the preclinical stage of an infection* **2.** referring to the first part of a medical course, before the students are allowed to examine real patients

**precocious** /prɪˈkəʊʃəs/ *adjective* more physically or mentally developed than is usual for a specific age

**precocious puberty** /prɪˌkəʊʃəs ˈpjuːbəti/ *noun* the development of signs of puberty in girls before the age of seven, and in boys before the age of nine. If untreated, affected boys typically grow no taller than 1.6 metres and girls rarely reach 1.5 metres.

**precocity** /prɪˈkɒsɪti/ *noun* the state or fact of being precocious

**precordia** /priːˈkɔːdiə/ *plural noun* plural of **precordium**

**precordial** /priːˈkɔːdiəl/ *adjective* referring to the precordium

**precordium** /priːˈkɔːdiəm/ *noun* the part of the thorax over the heart (NOTE: The plural is **precordia**.)

**precursor** /prɪˈkɜːsə/ *noun* a substance or cell from which another substance or cell is developed, e.g. dopa, the precursor for dopamine, which is converted to dopamine by the enzyme dopa decarboxylase

**predict** /prɪˈdɪkt/ *verb* to say what will happen in the future ○ *Doctors are predicting a rise in cases of whooping cough.*

**prediction** /prɪˈdɪkʃən/ *noun* an act of saying what you expect will happen in the future, or what is said ○ *the Health Ministry's prediction of a rise in cases of hepatitis B*

**predictive** /prɪˈdɪktɪv/ *adjective* referring to prediction ○ *The predictive value of the test is high.*

**predigest** /ˌpriːdaɪˈdʒest/ *verb* to treat food with chemicals or enzymes so that it is more easily digested by people with digestion problems

**predigested food** /ˌpriːdaɪdʒestɪd ˈfuːd/ *noun* food which has undergone predigestion

**predigestion** /ˌpriːdaɪˈdʒestʃ(ə)n/ *noun* the artificial starting of the digestive process before food is eaten

**predisposed to** /ˌpriːdɪˈspəʊzd tʊ/ *adjective* having a tendency or susceptibility to a condition ○ *All the members of the family are predisposed to vascular diseases.*

**predisposing factor** /ˌpriːdɪspəʊzɪŋ ˈfæktə/ *noun* a factor which will increase the risk of disease

**predisposition** /ˌpriːdɪspəˈzɪʃ(ə)n/ *noun* a tendency or susceptibility ○ *She has a predisposition to obesity.*

**prednisolone** /predˈnɪsələʊn/ *noun* a synthetically produced steroid hormone, similar to cortisone, used especially to control inflammatory diseases such as rheumatoid arthritis

**prednisone** /predˈnɪsəʊn/ *noun* a synthetically produced steroid hormone produced from cortisone, used to treat allergies and rheumatoid arthritis

**predominant** /prɪˈdɒmɪnənt/ *adjective* more powerful than others

**pre-eclampsia** /ˌpriː ɪˈklæmpsiə/ *noun* a condition in pregnant women towards the end of the pregnancy which may lead to eclampsia. Symptoms are high blood pressure, oedema and protein in the urine. Also called **pregnancy-induced hypertension**

**preemie** /ˈpriːmi/ *noun US* a premature baby (*informal*)

**prefrontal** /priːˈfrʌnt(ə)l/ *adjective* situated in or affecting the front part of the frontal lobe

**prefrontal leucotomy** /priːˌfrʌnt(ə)l luːˈkɒtəmi/ *noun* a surgical operation to divide some of the white matter in the prefrontal lobe, formerly used as a treatment for schizophrenia

**prefrontal lobe** /priːˈfrʌnt(ə)l ləʊb/ *noun* an area of the brain in the front part of each hemisphere, in front of the frontal lobe, which is concerned with memory and learning

**preganglionic** /ˌpriːɡæŋɡlɪˈɒnɪk/ *adjective* near to and in front of a ganglion

**preganglionic fibre** /ˌpriːɡæŋɡlɪɒnɪk ˈfaɪbə/ *noun* a nerve fibre which ends in a ganglion where it is linked in a synapse to a postganglionic fibre

**preganglionic neurone** /ˌpriːɡæŋɡlɪˌɒnɪk ˈnjʊərəʊn/ *noun* a neurone which ends in a ganglion

**pregnancy** /ˈpreɡnənsi/ *noun* **1.** same as **gestation period 2.** the condition of being pregnant. Also called **cyesis**

**pregnancy-associated hypertension** /ˌpreɡnənsi əˌsəʊsieɪtɪd ˌhaɪpəˈtenʃən/ *noun* high blood pressure which is associated with pregnancy

**pregnancy-induced hypertension** /ˌpreɡnənsi ɪnˈdjuːsd ˌhaɪpəˈtenʃən/ *noun* Abbr **PIH**. same as **pre-eclampsia**

**pregnancy test** /ˈpreɡnənsi test/ *noun* a test to see if a woman is pregnant or not

**pregnant** /ˈpreɡnənt/ *adjective* with an unborn child in the uterus ○ *She is six months pregnant.*

**prehepatic** /priːhɪˈpætɪk/ *adjective* in front of or before the liver

**prehepatic bilirubin** /priːhɪˌpætɪk bɪliˈruːbɪn/ *noun* bilirubin in plasma before it passes through the liver

**prehepatic jaundice** /ˌpriːhɪˌpætɪk ˈdʒɔːndɪs/ *noun* same as **haemolytic jaundice**

**prem** /prem/ (*informal*) *adjective* same as **premature** ■ *noun* a premature baby

**premature** /ˈpremətʃə/ *adjective* before the expected or desirable time ○ *The baby was five weeks premature.*

COMMENT: Babies can survive even if born several weeks premature. Even babies weighing less than one kilo at birth can survive in an incubator, and develop healthily.

**premature baby** /ˌpremətʃə ˈbeɪbi/ *noun* a baby born earlier than 37 weeks from conception, or weighing less than 2.5 kg, but capable of independent life

**premature birth** /ˌpremətʃə ˈbɜːθ/ *noun* the birth of a baby earlier than 37 weeks from conception

**premature ejaculation** /ˌpremətʃə ɪˌdʒækjʊˈleɪʃ(ə)n/ *noun* a situation in which a man ejaculates too early during sexual intercourse

**premature labour** /ˌpremətʃə ˈleɪbə/ *noun* the condition of starting to give birth earlier than 37 weeks from conception ○ *After the accident she went into premature labour.*

**prematurely** /ˈpremətʃʊəli/ *adverb* before the expected or desirable time ○ *The baby was born two weeks prematurely.* ○ *A large number of people die prematurely from ischaemic heart disease.*

**prematurity** /ˌpreməˈtʃʊərɪti/ *noun* a situation in which something occurs before the expected or desirable time

**premed** /ˈpriːmed/ *noun* a stage of being given premedication (*informal*) ○ *The patient is in premed.*

**premedical** /priːˈmedɪk(ə)l/ *adjective* referring to the studies that a person must complete before entering medical school

**premedication** /ˌpriːmedɪˈkeɪʃ(ə)n/, **premedicant drug** /priːˈmedɪkənt ˈdrʌɡ/ *noun* a drug given before an operation in order to block the parasympathetic nervous system and prevent vomiting during the operation, e.g. a sedative

**premenopausal** /ˌpriːmenəˈpɔːz(ə)l/ *adjective* referring to the stage in a woman's life just before the start of the menopause

**premenstrual** /priːˈmenstruəl/ *adjective* happening before menstruation

**premenstrual syndrome** /priːˌmenstruəl ˈsɪndrəʊm/, **premenstrual tension** /priːˌmenstruəl ˈtenʃən/ *noun* nervous stress experienced by a woman for one or two weeks before a menstrual period starts. Abbr **PMS, PMT**

**premolar** /priːˈməʊlə/ *noun* a tooth with two points, situated between the canines and the first proper molar. See illustration at TEETH in Supplement

**prenatal** /priːˈneɪt(ə)l/ *adjective* during the period between conception and childbirth

**prenatal diagnosis** /priːˌneɪt(ə)l ˌdaɪəɡˈnəʊsɪs/ *noun* same as **antenatal diagnosis**

**pre-op** /ˌpriː ˈɒp/ *adjective* same as **preoperative** (*informal*)

**preoperative** /priːˈɒp(ə)rətɪv/ *adjective* during the period before a surgical operation

**preoperatively** /priːˈɒp(ə)rətɪvli/ *adverb* before a surgical operation

**preoperative medication** /priːˌɒp(ə)rətɪv ˌmedɪˈkeɪʃən/ *noun* a drug given before an operation, e.g. a sedative

**preovulatory** /priːˈɒvjələt(ə)ri/ *adjective* referring to the 6 to 13 days in the menstrual cycle between menstruation and ovulation

**prep** /prep/ (*informal*) *noun* same as **preparation** ○ *The prep is finished, so the patient can be taken to the operating theatre.* ■ *verb* same as **prepare** ○ *Has the patient been prepped?* (NOTE: **prepping – prepped**)

**PREP** *abbr* post-registration education and practice

**preparation** /ˌprepəˈreɪʃ(ə)n/ *noun* **1.** the act of getting a person ready for a surgical operation. Also called **prep 2.** a medicine or liquid containing a drug ○ *He was given a preparation containing an antihistamine.*

**prepare** /prɪˈpeə/ *verb* **1.** to get something or someone ready ○ *Six rooms in the hospital were prepared for the accident victims.* ○ *The nurses were preparing him for the operation.* **2.** to make something ○ *He prepared a soothing linctus.*

**prepatellar bursitis** /ˌpriːpəˌtelə bɜːˈsaɪtɪs/ *noun* a condition in which the fluid sac at the knee becomes inflamed, caused by kneeling on hard surfaces. Also called **housemaid's knee**

**prepubertal** /priːˈpjuːbət(ə)l/ *adjective* referring to the period before puberty

**prepuberty** /priːˈpjuːbəti/ *noun* the period before puberty

**prepubescent** /ˌpriːpjuːˈbesənt/ *adjective* referring to a person at the stage of life just before puberty

**prepuce** /ˈpriːpjuːs/ *noun* same as **foreskin**

**presby-** /ˈprezbi/ *prefix* same as **presbyo-** (used before vowels)

**presbyacusis** /ˌprezbiˈkuːsɪs/ *noun* a condition in which an elderly person's hearing fails gradually, through to degeneration of the internal ear

**presbyo-** /prezbiəʊ/ *prefix* referring to the last stages of the natural life span

**presbyopia** /ˌprezbiˈəʊpiə/ *noun* a condition in which an elderly person's sight fails gradually, through hardening of the lens

**prescribe** /prɪˈskraɪb/ *verb* to give instructions for a person to get a specific dosage of a drug or a specific form of therapeutic treatment ○ *The doctor prescribed a course of antibiotics.* (NOTE: **prescribing – prescribed**)

**prescribed disease** /prɪˌskraɪbd dɪˈziːz/ *noun* an illness caused by the type of work a person does which is on an annually reviewed official list, entitling the person to claim bene-

fit. Examples are deafness, pneumoconiosis and RSI.

**prescribed illness** /prɪˌskraɪbd ˈɪlnəs/ *noun* an illness developing in the workplace from exposure to chemicals, e.g. mercury poisoning, or to dangerous activities, e.g. decompression sickness

**prescribing analyses and cost** /prɪ ˌskraɪbɪŋ əˌnælɪsiːz ənd ˈkɒst/ *plural noun* data on the prescribing of drugs in primary care. Abbr **PACT**

**prescription** /prɪˈskrɪpʃən/ *noun* an order written by a doctor to a pharmacist asking for a drug to be prepared and given or sold to a person

**prescription drug** /prɪˈskrɪpʃən drʌg/ *noun* a drug which can only be obtained by having a legally valid prescription

**presence** /ˈprez(ə)ns/ *noun* the act or fact of being there ○ *Tests showed the presence of sugar in the urine.*

**presenile** /priːˈsiːnaɪl/ *adjective* **1.** prematurely showing the effects of advanced age **2.** referring to a condition which affects people of early or middle age but has characteristics of a more advanced age

**presenile dementia** /priːˌsiːnaɪl dɪˈmenʃə/ *noun* mental degeneration affecting adults of around 40–60 years of age (*dated*)

COMMENT: Patients used to be diagnosed with presenile dementia if they showed symptoms of dementia and were under the age of 65, and senile dementia if over 65. However, the terms are no longer often used and instead the type of dementia is used for diagnostic purposes, e.g. Alzheimer's disease, multi-infarct or vascular

**presenility** /ˌpriːsəˈnɪlɪti/ *noun* the ageing of the body or brain before the expected time, with a person showing symptoms which are usually associated with people of very advanced years

**present** *verb* /prɪˈzent/ **1.** (*of a patient*) to show particular symptoms ○ *The patient presented with severe chest pains.* **2.** (*of a symptom*) to be present ○ *The doctors' first task is to relieve the presenting symptoms.* ○ *The condition may also present in a baby.* **3.** (*of a baby*) to appear in the vaginal channel ■ *adjective* /ˈprez(ə)nt/ currently existing in a place ○ *All the symptoms of the disease are present.*

'…chlamydia in the male commonly presents a urethritis characterized by dysuria' [*Journal of American College Health*]

'26 patients were selected from the outpatient department on grounds of disabling breathlessness present for at least five years' [*Lancet*]

'…sickle cell chest syndrome is a common complication of sickle cell disease, presenting with chest pain, fever and leucocytosis' [*British Medical Journal*]

'…a 24 year-old woman presents with an influenza-like illness of five days' duration' [*British Journal of Hospital Medicine*]

'…the presenting symptoms of Crohn's disease may be extremely variable' [New Zealand Medical Journal]

**presentation** /ˌprez(ə)nˈteɪʃ(ə)n/ noun the way in which a baby will be born, in respect of the part of the baby's body which will appear first in the vaginal channel

**presenting part** /prɪˈzentɪŋ pɑːt/ noun the part of a baby which appears first during birth

**preservation** /ˌprezəˈveɪʃ(ə)n/ noun the keeping of a tissue sample or donor organ in good condition

**preserve** /prɪˈzɜːv/ verb to keep something from rotting (NOTE: **preserving – preserved**)

**press** /pres/ verb to push or squeeze something ○ The tumour is pressing against a nerve.

**pressor** /ˈpresə/ adjective **1.** referring to a nerve which increases the action of part of the body **2.** raising blood pressure

**pressure** /ˈpreʃə/ noun **1.** the action of squeezing or forcing something **2.** the force of something on its surroundings **3.** mental or physical stress caused by external events

**pressure area** /ˈpreʃər ˌeəriə/ noun an area of the body where a bone is near the surface of the skin, so that if the skin is pressed the circulation will be cut off

**pressure bandage** /ˈpreʃə ˌbændɪdʒ/ noun a bandage which presses on a part of the body

**pressure index** /ˈpreʃər ˌɪndeks/ noun a method for determining the extent of obstruction to the artery in the leg by measuring the blood pressure in the arms and legs and then dividing the systolic pressure in the leg by that in the arm. Abbr **PI**

**pressure point** /ˈpreʃə pɔɪnt/ noun a place where an artery crosses over a bone, so that the blood can be cut off by pressing with the finger

**presynaptic** /ˌpriːsɪˈnæptɪk/ adjective situated in front of a synapse

**presynaptic axon** /ˌprisɪnæptɪk ˈnɜːv/ noun a nerve leading to one side of a synapse

**presystole** /priːˈsɪstəli/ noun the period before systole in the cycle of heartbeats

**preterm birth** /ˌpriːˈtɜːm bɜːθ/ noun the birth of a baby before 37 completed weeks of pregnancy, which presents a greater risk of serious health problems (NOTE: About 12 per cent of births in the UK are preterm births.)

**prevalence** /ˈprevələns/ noun the number of cases of a disease in a specific place at a specific time ○ the prevalence of malaria in some tropical countries ○ the prevalence of cases of malnutrition in large towns ○ a high prevalence of renal disease

**prevalent** /ˈprevələnt/ adjective common in comparison to something else ○ The disease is prevalent in some African countries. ○ The condition is more prevalent in the cold winter months.

**prevent** /prɪˈvent/ verb to stop something from happening, or a person from doing something ○ The treatment is given to prevent the patient's condition from getting worse. ○ Doctors are trying to prevent the spread of the outbreak of Legionnaires' disease.

**preventative** /prɪˈventətɪv/ adjective same as **preventive**

**prevention** /prɪˈvenʃən/ noun action to stop something happening

**preventive** /prɪˈventɪv/ adjective referring to an action taken to stop something happening, especially to stop a disease or infection from spreading ○ preventive treatment ○ preventive action

**preventive measure** /prɪˌventɪv ˈmeʒə/ noun an action taken to prevent a disease from occurring or spreading

COMMENT: Preventive measures include immunisation, vaccination, sterilisation, quarantine and improving standards of housing and sanitation. Health education also has an important role to play in the prevention of disease.

**preventive medicine** /prɪˌventɪv ˈmed(ə)s(ə)n/ noun action carried out to stop disease from occurring, e.g. by education in health-related issues, immunisation and screening for known diseases

**prevertebral** /priːˈvɜːtɪbr(ə)l/ adjective situated in front of the spinal column or a vertebra

**Priadel** /ˈpraɪədel/ a trade name for lithium

**priapism** /ˈpraɪəpɪz(ə)m/ noun an erection of the penis without sexual stimulus, caused by a blood clot in the tissue of the penis, injury to the spinal cord or stone in the urinary bladder

**prick** /prɪk/ verb to make a small hole in something with a sharp point ○ The nurse pricked the patient's finger to take a blood sample.

**prickle cell** /ˈprɪk(ə)l sel/ noun a cell with many processes connecting it to other cells, found in the inner layer of the epidermis

**prickly heat** /ˈprɪkli hiːt/ noun same as **miliaria**

**-pril** /prɪl/ suffix used for ACE inhibitors ○ Captopril

**prilocaine** /ˈpraɪləkeɪn/ noun a local anaesthetic used especially in dentistry

**primaquine** /ˈpraɪməkwiːn/ noun a synthetically produced drug used in the treatment of malaria

**primary** /ˈpraɪməri/ adjective **1.** happening first, and leading to something else **2.** most important **3.** referring to a condition which comes first and is followed by another. Compare **secondary**

**primary amenorrhoea** /ˌpraɪməri ˌeɪmenəˈriːə/ noun a condition in which a woman has never had menstrual periods

**primary biliary cirrhosis** /ˌpraɪməri ˌbɪliəri sɪˈrəʊsɪs/ *noun* cirrhosis of the liver caused by autoimmune disease

**primary bronchi** /ˌpraɪməri ˈbrɒŋkiː/ *plural noun* same as **main bronchi**

**primary care** /ˌpraɪməri ˈkeə/ *noun* in the UK, health services offered directly to individuals by GPs, dentists, opticians and other health professionals who may also refer a patient on to specialists for further treatment. Also called **primary health care, primary medical care**. Compare **secondary care, tertiary care**

'…primary care is largely concerned with clinical management of individual patients, while community medicine tends to view the whole population as its patient'  [*Journal of the Royal College of General Practitioners*]

**primary care group** /ˌpraɪməri ˈkeə gruːp/ *noun* an organisation responsible for overseeing the provision of primary healthcare and the commissioning of secondary care in a district. Key members include GPs, community nurses, social services and lay members. Abbr **PCG**

**primary care team** /ˌpraɪməri ˈkeə tiːm/ *noun* same as **primary health care team**

**primary care trust** /ˌpraɪməri ˈkeə trʌst/ *noun* in the UK, the top level of the primary care group with extra responsibilities such as direct employment of community staff. Abbr **PCT**

**primary cartilaginous joint** /ˌpraɪməri ˌkɑːtəˈlædʒɪnəs dʒɔɪnt/ *noun* a temporary joint where the intervening cartilage is converted into adult bone

**primary complex** /ˌpraɪməri ˈkɒmpleks/ *noun* the first lymph node to be infected by tuberculosis

**primary dysmenorrhoea** /ˌpraɪməri ˌdɪsmenəˈriːə/ *noun* dysmenorrhoea which occurs at the first menstrual period. Also called **essential dysmenorrhoea**

**primary haemorrhage** /ˌpraɪməri ˈhem(ə)rɪdʒ/ *noun* bleeding which occurs immediately after an injury has taken place

**primary health care** /ˌpraɪməri ˈhelθ keə/ *noun* same as **primary care**

'…among primary health care services, 1.5% of all GP consultations are due to coronary heart disease' [*Health Services Journal*]

**primary health care team** /ˌpraɪməri ˈhelθ keə ˌtiːm/ *noun* a group of professional medical workers who have first contact with someone needing medical attention and are responsible for delivering a range of health care services. Abbr **PHCT**

**primary medical care** /ˌpraɪməri ˈmedɪk(ə)l keə/ *noun* same as **primary care**

**primary nurse** /ˌpraɪməri ˈnɜːs/ *noun* a nurse who is responsible for planning a person's nursing care in consultation with that person and his or her family. In the absence of the primary nurse, associate nurses provide care based on the plan designed by the primary nurse.

**primary nursing** /ˌpraɪməri ˈnɜːsɪŋ/ *noun* a model of nursing that involves the delivery of comprehensive, continuous, co-ordinated and individualised patient care through a primary nurse, who has autonomy, accountability and authority in relation to his or her patient's care

**primary peritonitis** /ˌpraɪməri ˌperɪtəˈnaɪtɪs/ *noun* peritonitis caused by direct infection from the blood or the lymph

**primary tooth** /ˈpraɪməri tuːθ/ *noun* any one of the first twenty teeth which develop in children between about six months and two-and-a-half years of age, and are replaced by the permanent teeth at around the age of six. Also called **milk tooth, deciduous tooth**

**primary tubercle** /ˌpraɪməri ˈtjuːbək(ə)l/ *noun* the first infected spot where tuberculosis starts to infect a lung

**primary tuberculosis** /ˌpraɪməri tjuːˌbɜːkjʊˈləʊsɪs/ *noun* a person's first infection with tuberculosis

**primary tumour** /ˌpraɪməri ˈtjuːmə/ *noun* a site of the original malignant growth from which cancer spreads

**prime** /praɪm/ *adjective* **1.** of the greatest importance or the highest rank **2.** of the highest quality ■ *noun* the best state or period of something, especially the most active and enjoyable period in adult life ■ *verb* to make something ready for use, or to become ready for use (NOTE: **priming – primed**)

**prime mover** /praɪm ˈmuːvə/ *noun* **1.** same as **agonist 2.** somebody or something which has the most influence over the starting of a process or activity

**primigravida** /ˌpraɪmɪˈɡrævɪdə/, **primigravid patient** /ˌpraɪmɪˈɡrævɪd ˈpeɪʃ(ə)nt/ *noun* a woman who is pregnant for the first time (NOTE: The plural is **primigravidas** or **primigravidae**.)

**primipara** /praɪˈmɪpərə/ *noun* a woman who has given birth to one child. Also called **unipara** (NOTE: The plural is **primiparas** or **primiparae**.)

**primordial** /praɪˈmɔːdiəl/ *adjective* in the very first stage of development

**primordial follicle** /praɪˌmɔːdiəl ˈfɒlɪk(ə)l/ *noun* the first stage of development of an ovarian follicle

**principle** /ˈprɪnsɪp(ə)l/ *noun* **1.** a rule or theory **2.** a standard of ethical behaviour

**P-R interval** /ˌpiː ˈɑːr ˌɪntəv(ə)l/ *noun* the time recorded on an electrocardiogram between the start of atrial activity and ventricular activity

**prion** /ˈpriːɒn/ *noun* a particle of protein which contains no nucleic acid, does not trigger an immune response and is not destroyed by extreme heat or cold. Prions are considered to be the agents responsible for scrapie, BSE, and Creutzfeldt-Jakob disease.

**priority despatch** /praɪˈɒrəti dɪˌspætʃ/ noun the process of talking to people who need medical help on the telephone in order to make sure that ambulances are sent to the most urgent cases first

**priority matrix** /praɪˈɒrəti ˌmeɪtrɪks/ noun a way of trying to make sure that each community has a fair number of services for its particular health needs

**private** /ˈpraɪvət/ adjective not supported by government or paid for by the National Health Service ○ He runs a private clinic for alcoholics.

**private hospital** /ˌpraɪvət ˈhɒspɪt(ə)l/ noun a hospital which takes only paying patients

**privately** /ˈpraɪvətli/ adverb by a private practitioner or company, not by the National Health Service ○ She decided to have the operation done privately.

**private parts** /ˈpraɪvət pɑːts/ plural noun the genital area (informal) Also called **privates**

**private patient** /ˌpraɪvət ˈpeɪʃ(ə)nt/ noun a patient who is paying for treatment and who is not being treated under the National Health Service

**private practice** /ˌpraɪvət ˈpræktɪs/ noun the services of a doctor, surgeon or dentist which are paid for by the patients themselves or by a medical insurance company, but not by the National Health Service

**privates** /ˈpraɪvəts/ plural noun same as **private parts** (informal)

**p.r.n.** adverb (written on a prescription) as and when required. Full form **pro re nata**

**pro-** /prəʊ/ prefix before or in front of

**probang** /ˈprəʊbæŋ/ noun a surgical instrument like a long rod with a brush at one end, formerly used to test and find strictures in the oesophagus and to push foreign bodies into the stomach

**probe** /prəʊb/ noun 1. an instrument used to explore inside a cavity or wound 2. a device inserted into a medium to obtain information ■ verb to investigate the inside of something ○ The surgeon probed the wound with a scalpel. (NOTE: **probing – probed**)

**problem** /ˈprɒbləm/ noun 1. something which is difficult to find an answer to ○ Scientists are trying to find a solution to the problem of drug-related disease. 2. a medical disorder ○ heart problems 3. an addiction to something ○ has a drug problem

**problem child** /ˈprɒbləm tʃaɪld/ noun a child who is difficult to control

**problem drinking** /ˌprɒbləm ˈdrɪŋkɪŋ/ noun alcoholism or heavy drinking which has a bad effect on a person's behaviour or work

**problem-oriented record** /ˌprɒbləm ˌɔːrien tɪd ˈrekɔːd/ noun a record of patient care which links patients' clinical data with their problems, so that all aspects of the care process are focused on resolving those problems

**problem-solving approach** /ˈprɒbləm ˌsɒlvɪŋ əˌprəʊtʃ/ noun the provision of nursing care based on assessment, problem identification (nursing diagnosis), planning implementation (nursing intervention) and evaluation

**procedure** /prəˈsiːdʒə/ noun 1. a standard way of doing something 2. a type of treatment ○ The hospital has developed some new procedures for treating Parkinson's disease. 3. a treatment given at one time ○ We are hoping to increase the number of procedures carried out per day.

'…disposable items now available for medical and nursing procedures range from cheap syringes to expensive cardiac pacemakers' [Nursing Times]

'…the electromyograms and CT scans were done as outpatient procedures' [Southern Medical Journal]

**process** /ˈprəʊses/ noun 1. a technical or scientific action ○ A new process for testing serum samples has been developed in the research laboratory. 2. a projecting part of the body ■ verb 1. to deal with a person or thing according to a standard procedure 2. to examine or test samples ○ The blood samples are being processed by the laboratory.

'…the nursing process serves to divide overall patient care into that part performed by nurses and that performed by the other professions' [Nursing Times]

**prochlorperazine** /ˌprəʊklɔːˈperəziːn/ noun a drug used to control nausea and vomiting, and to reduce the symptoms of Ménière's disease, migraine and anxiety

**procidentia** /ˌprəʊsɪˈdenʃə/ noun movement of an organ downwards

**proct-** /prɒkt/ prefix same as **procto-** (used before vowels)

**proctalgia** /prɒkˈtældʒə/ noun pain in the lower rectum or anus, caused by neuralgia

**proctalgia fugax** /prɒkˌtældʒə ˈfjuːgæks/ noun a condition in which a person has sudden pains in the rectum during the night, usually relieved by eating or drinking

**proctatresia** /ˌprɒktəˈtriːziə/ noun a condition in which the anus does not have an opening. Also called **imperforate anus**

**proctectasia** /ˌprɒktekˈteɪziə/ noun a condition in which the rectum or anus is dilated because of continued constipation

**proctectomy** /prɒkˈtektəmi/ noun a surgical operation to remove the rectum (NOTE: The plural is **proctectomies**.)

**proctitis** /prɒkˈtaɪtɪs/ noun inflammation of the rectum

**procto-** /prɒktəʊ/ prefix the anus or rectum

**proctocele** /ˈprɒktəsiːl/ noun same as **rectocele**

**proctoclysis** /ˌprɒkˈtɒkləsɪs/ *noun* the introduction of a lot of fluid into the rectum slowly

**proctocolectomy** /ˌprɒktəʊkɒˈlektəmi/ *noun* a surgical operation to remove the rectum and the colon (NOTE: The plural is **proctocolectomies.**)

**proctocolitis** /ˌprɒktəkəˈlaɪtɪs/ *noun* inflammation of the rectum and part of the colon

**proctodynia** /ˌprɒktəˈdɪniə/ *noun* a sensation of pain in the anus

**proctogram** /ˈprɒktəgræm/ *noun* an X-ray photograph of the rectum taken after a contrast agent is introduced

**proctologist** /prɒkˈtɒlədʒɪst/ *noun* a specialist in proctology

**proctology** /prɒkˈtɒlədʒi/ *noun* the scientific study of the rectum and anus and their associated diseases

**proctorrhaphy** /prɒkˈtɔːrəfi/ *noun* a surgical operation to stitch up a tear in the rectum or anus (NOTE: The plural is **proctorrhaphies.**)

**proctoscope** /ˈprɒktəskəʊp/ *noun* a surgical instrument consisting of a long tube with a light in the end, used to examine the rectum

**proctoscopy** /prɒkˈtɒskəpi/ *noun* an examination of the rectum using a proctoscope (NOTE: The plural is **proctoscopies.**)

**proctosigmoiditis** /ˌprɒktəʊˌsɪgmɔɪˈdaɪtɪs/ *noun* inflammation of the rectum and the sigmoid colon

**proctotomy** /prɒkˈtɒtəmi/ *noun* **1.** a surgical operation to divide a structure of the rectum or anus **2.** an opening of an imperforate anus (NOTE: [all senses] The plural is **proctotomies.**)

**prodromal** /prəʊˈdrəʊml/ *adjective* occurring between the appearance of the first symptoms of a disease and the major effect, e.g. a fever or rash

**prodromal rash** /prəʊˌdrəʊmˈ(ə)l ˈræʃ/ *noun* a rash which appears as a symptom of a disease before the major rash

**prodrome** /ˈprəʊdrəʊm/, **prodroma** /prəʊˈdrəʊmə/ *noun* an early symptom of an attack of a disease

'…in classic migraine a prodrome is followed by an aura, then a headache, and finally a recovery phase. The prodrome may not be recognised' [*British Journal of Hospital Medicine*]

**produce** /prəˈdjuːs/ *verb* to make or cause something ○ *The drug produces a sensation of dizziness.* ○ *Doctors are worried by the side-effects produced by the new painkiller.* (NOTE: **producing – produced**)

**product** /ˈprɒdʌkt/ *noun* **1.** something which is produced **2.** a result or effect of a process

**productive cough** /prəˌdʌktɪv ˈkɒf/ *noun* a cough where phlegm is produced

**proenzyme** /prəʊˈenzaɪm/ *noun* the first mature form of an enzyme, before it develops into an active enzyme. Also called **zymogen**

**profession** /prəˈfeʃ(ə)n/ *noun* **1.** a type of job for which special training is needed **2.** all people working in a specialised type of employment for which they have been trained ○ *They are both doctors by profession.*

**professional** /prəˈfeʃ(ə)n(ə)l/ *adjective* referring to a profession

**professional body** /prəˌfeʃ(ə)n(ə)l ˈbɒdi/ *noun* an organisation which acts for all the members of a profession

**Professional Conduct Committee** /prəˌfeʃ(ə)n(ə)l ˈkɒndʌkt kəˌmɪti/ *noun* a committee of the General Medical Council which decides on cases of professional misconduct. Abbr **PCC**

**professional misconduct** /prəˌfeʃ(ə)n(ə)l mɪsˈkɒndʌkt/ *noun* actions which are considered to be wrong by the body which regulates a profession, e.g. an action by a doctor which is considered wrong by the Professional Conduct Committee of the General Medical Council

**profile** /ˈprəʊfaɪl/ *noun* **1.** a brief description of the characteristics of a person or thing **2.** a set of data, usually in graph or table form, which indicates to what extent something has the same characteristics as a group tested or considered standard **3.** the amount that other people notice somebody or something ■ *verb* to give a short description or assessment of somebody or something (NOTE: **profiling – profiled**)

**profound** /prəˈfaʊnd/ *adjective* very great or serious ○ *a profound impairment of the immune system*

**profunda** /prəˈfʌndə/ *adjective* referring to blood vessels which lie deep in tissues

**profundaplasty** /prəˈfʌndəplæsti/ *noun* a surgical operation to widen a junction of the femoral artery, in order to relieve narrowing by atherosclerosis (NOTE: The plural is **profundaplasties.**)

**profuse** /prəˈfjuːs/ *adjective* existing in very large quantities ○ *fever accompanied by profuse sweating* ○ *pains with profuse internal bleeding*

**progeny** /ˈprɒdʒəni/ *noun* a person's child or children (NOTE: Takes a singular or plural verb.)

**progeria** /prəʊˈdʒɪəriə/ *noun* a condition of premature ageing. Also called **Hutchinson-Gilford syndrome**

**progestational** /prəʊˌdʒesˈteɪʃ(ə)nəl/ *adjective* referring to the stage of the menstrual cycle after ovulation when progesterone is produced

**progesterone** /prəʊˈdʒestərəʊn/ *noun* a hormone which is produced in the second part of the menstrual cycle by the corpus luteum and which stimulates the formation of the placenta if an ovum is fertilised (NOTE: Progesterone is also produced by the placenta itself.)

**progestogen** /prəˈdʒestədʒən/ *noun* any substance which has the same effect as progesterone

COMMENT: Because natural progesterones prevent ovulation during pregnancy, synthetically produced progestogens are used to make contraceptive pills.

**prognathic jaw** /prɒɡˌnæθɪk ˈdʒɔː/ *noun* a jaw which protrudes further than the other

**prognathism** /ˈprɒɡnəθɪz(ə)m/ *noun* a condition in which one jaw, especially the lower jaw, or both jaws protrude

**prognosis** /prɒɡˈnəʊsɪs/ *noun* an opinion of how a disease or disorder will develop ○ *This cancer has a prognosis of about two years.* ○ *The prognosis is not good.* (NOTE: The plural is **prognoses**.)

**prognostic** /prɒɡˈnɒstɪk/ *adjective* referring to a prognosis

**prognostic test** /prɒɡˌnɒstɪk ˈtest/ *noun* a test to suggest how a disease will develop or how long a person will survive after an operation

**programme** /ˈprəʊɡræm/ *noun* a series of medical treatments given in a set way at set times ○ *The doctor prescribed a programme of injections.* ○ *She took a programme of steroid treatment.* (NOTE: The US spelling is **program**.)

**progress** *noun* /ˈprəʊɡres/ **1.** development and improvement ○ *Progress has been made in cutting waiting times.* **2.** the way in which a person is becoming well ○ *The doctors seem pleased that she has made such good progress since her operation.* ■ *verb* /prəʊˈɡres/ **1.** to develop and improve, or to continue to do well ○ *The patient is progressing well.* **2.** to move to a more advanced stage ○ *As the disease progressed, he spent more and more time sleeping.*

**progression** /prəʊˈɡreʃ(ə)n/ *noun* development ○ *The progression of the disease was swift.*

**progressive** /prəˈɡresɪv/ *adjective* developing all the time ○ *Alzheimer's disease is a progressive disorder which sees a gradual decline in intellectual functioning.*

**progressive deafness** /prəˌɡresɪv ˈdefnəs/ *noun* a condition, common in people as they get older, in which a person gradually becomes more and more deaf

**progressively** /prəʊˈɡresɪvli/ *adverb* more and more ○ *He became progressively more disabled.*

**progressive muscular atrophy** /prəˌɡresɪv ˌmʌskjʊlə ˈætrəfi/ *noun* muscular dystrophy, with progressive weakening of the muscles, particularly in the pelvic and shoulder girdles

**proguanil** /prəʊˈɡwænɪl/ *noun* a drug used in the prevention and treatment of malaria

**proinsulin** /prəʊˈɪnsʊlɪn/ *noun* a substance produced by the pancreas, then converted to insulin

**project** /prəˈdʒekt/ *verb* to protrude or stick out

**projection** /prəˈdʒekʃən/ *noun* **1.** a part of the body which sticks out or stands out. Also called **prominence**. Compare **promontory 2.** (*in psychology*) mental action in which a person blames another person for his or her own faults

**projection tract** /prəˈdʒekʃ(ə)n trækt/ *noun* fibres connecting the cerebral cortex with the lower parts of the brain and spinal cord

**prolactin** /prəʊˈlæktɪn/ *noun* a hormone secreted by the pituitary gland which stimulates the production of milk. Also called **lactogenic hormone**

**prolapse** /ˈprəʊlæps/ *noun* a condition in which an organ has moved downwards out of its usual position ■ *verb* to move downwards out of the usual position (NOTE: **prolapsing – prolapsed**)

**prolapsed intervertebral disc** /prəʊˌlæpsd ɪntəˌvɜːtəbrəl ˈdɪsk/ *noun* a condition in which an intervertebral disc becomes displaced or where the soft centre of a disc passes through the hard cartilage of the exterior and presses onto a nerve. Abbr **PID**. Also called **slipped disc**

**prolapse of the rectum** /ˌprəʊlæps əv ðə ˈrektəm/ *noun* a condition in which mucous membrane of the rectum moves downwards and passes through the anus

**prolapse of the uterus** /ˌprəʊlæps əv ðə ˈjuːtərəs/, **prolapse of the womb** /ˌprəʊlæps əv ðə ˈwuːm/ *noun* a movement of the uterus downwards due to weakening of the structures of the pelvic floor, e.g. because of age or a difficult childbirth. Also called **metroptosis, prolapsed uterus, uterine prolapse**

**proliferate** /prəˈlɪfəreɪt/ *verb* to produce many similar cells or parts, and so grow (NOTE: **proliferating – proliferated**)

**proliferation** /prəˌlɪfəˈreɪʃ(ə)n/ *noun* the process of proliferating

**proliferative** /prəˈlɪfərətɪv/ *adjective* multiplying

**proliferative phase** /prəˈlɪfərətɪv feɪz/ *noun* a period when a disease is spreading fast

**proline** /ˈprəʊlɪn/ *noun* an amino acid found in proteins, especially in collagen

**prolong** /prəˈlɒŋ/ *verb* to make something last longer ○ *The treatment prolonged her life by three years.*

**prolonged** /prəˈlɒŋd/ *adjective* very long ○ *She had to undergo a prolonged course of radiation treatment.*

**promethazine** /prəʊˈmeθəziːn/ *noun* an antihistamine drug used in the treatment of allergies and motion sickness

**prominence** /ˈprɒmɪnəns/ *noun* a part of the body which sticks out or stands out. Also called **projection**. Compare **promontory**

**prominent** /ˈprɒmɪnənt/ *adjective* standing out, very visible ○ *She had a prominent scar* *on her neck which she wanted to have removed.*

**promontory** /ˈprɒmənt(ə)ri/ *noun* a section of an organ, especially the middle ear and sacrum which stands out above the rest. Compare **projection, prominence**

**promote** /prəˈməʊt/ *verb* **1.** to help something to take place ○ *The drug is used to promote blood clotting.* **2.** to raise a person to a more senior job or a higher position (NOTE: **promoting – promoted**)

**pronate** /ˈprəʊneɪt/ *verb* **1.** to lie face downwards **2.** to turn the hand so that palm faces downwards (NOTE: **pronating – pronated**)

**pronation** /prəʊˈneɪʃ(ə)n/ *noun* the act of turning the hand round so that the palm faces downwards. Opposite **supination**. See illustration at ANATOMICAL TERMS in Supplement

**pronator** /prəʊˈneɪtə/ *noun* a muscle which makes the hand turn face downwards

**prone** /prəʊn/ *adjective* **1.** lying face downwards. Opposite **supine 2.** referring to the arm with the palm facing downwards

**pronounced** /prəˈnaʊnst/ *adjective* very obvious or marked ○ *She has a pronounced limp.*

**propagate** /ˈprɒpəgeɪt/ *verb* to multiply something, or cause something to multiply (NOTE: **propagating – propagated**)

**propagation** /ˌprɒpəˈgeɪʃ(ə)n/ *noun* an act of causing something to spread or multiply

**properdin** /ˈprəʊpədɪn/ *noun* protein in blood plasma which can destroy Gram-negative bacteria and neutralise viruses when acting together with magnesium

**prophase** /ˈprəʊfeɪz/ *noun* the first stage of mitosis when the chromosomes are visible as long thin double threads

**prophylactic** /ˌprɒfəˈlæktɪk/ *noun* a substance which helps to prevent the development of a disease ■ *adjective* preventive

**prophylaxis** /ˌprɒfəˈlæksɪs/ *noun* **1.** the prevention of disease **2.** a preventive treatment (NOTE: [all senses] The plural is **prophylaxes**.)

**proportion** /prəˈpɔːʃ(ə)n/ *noun* a quantity of something, especially as compared to the whole ○ *A high proportion of cancers can be treated by surgery.* ○ *The proportion of outpatients to inpatients is increasing.*

'…the target cells for adult myeloid leukaemia are located in the bone marrow, and there is now evidence that a substantial proportion of childhood leukaemias also arise in the bone marrow' [*British Medical Journal*]

**propranolol** /prəʊˈpænəlɒl/ *noun* a drug that slows heart rate and heart output, used in the treatment of angina pectoris, irregular heart rhythms, migraine and high blood pressure

**proprietary** /prəˈpraɪət(ə)ri/ *adjective* belonging to a commercial company

**proprietary medicine** /prəˌpraɪət(ə)ri ˈmed(ə)s(ə)n/, **proprietary drug** /prə

ˌpraɪət(ə)ri ˈdrʌg/ *noun* a drug which is sold under a trade name. ◊ **patent medicine**

**proprietary name** /prəˌpraɪət(ə)ri ˈneɪm/ *noun* a trade name for a drug

**proprioception** /ˌprəʊprɪəˈsepʃən/ *noun* the reaction of nerves to body movements and the relaying of information about movements to the brain

**proprioceptive** /ˌprəʊprɪəˈseptɪv/ *adjective* referring to sensory impulses from the joints, muscles and tendons, which relay information about body movements to the brain

**proprioceptor** /ˌprəʊprɪəˈseptə/ *noun* the end of a sensory nerve which reacts to stimuli from muscles and tendons as they move

**proptosis** /prɒpˈtəʊsɪs/ *noun* forward displacement of the eyeball

**prop up** /ˌprɒp ˈʌp/ *verb* to support a person, e.g. with pillows (NOTE: **propping up – propped up**)

**prospective** /prəˈspektɪv/ *adjective* **1.** applying to the future. ◊ **retrospective 2.** following what happens to selected patients

**prostaglandin** /ˌprɒstəˈglændɪn/ *noun* any of a class of unsaturated fatty acids found in all mammals which control smooth muscle contraction, inflammation and body temperature, are associated with the sensation of pain and have an effect on the nervous system, blood pressure and in particular the uterus at menstruation

**prostate** /ˈprɒsteɪt/ *noun* same as **prostate gland** (NOTE: Do not confuse with **prostrate**.) □ **prostate trouble** inflammation or enlargement of the prostate gland (*informal*)

**prostate cancer** /ˈprɒsteɪt ˌkænsə/ *noun* a malignant tumour of the prostate gland, found especially in men over 55

**prostatectomy** /ˌprɒstəˈtektəmi/ *noun* a surgical operation to remove all or part of the prostate gland (NOTE: The plural is **prostatectomies**.)

**prostate gland** /ˈprɒsteɪt glænd/ *noun* an O-shaped gland in males which surrounds the urethra below the bladder and secretes a fluid containing enzymes into the sperm. See illustration at UROGENITAL SYSTEM (MALE) in Supplement. Also called **prostate**

COMMENT: As a man grows older, the prostate gland tends to enlarge and constrict the point at which the urethra leaves the bladder, making it difficult to pass urine.

**prostatic** /prɒˈstætɪk/ *adjective* referring to or belonging to the prostate gland

**prostatic hypertrophy** /prɒˌstætɪk haɪ ˈpɜːtrəfi/ *noun* an enlargement of the prostate gland

**prostatic massage** /prɒˌstætɪk ˈmæsɑːʒ/ *noun* the removal of fluid from the prostate gland through the rectum

**prostatic urethra** /prɒˌstætɪk juːˈriːθrə/ *noun* a section of the urethra which passes through the prostate gland

**prostatic utricle** /prɒˌstætɪk ˈjuːtrɪk(ə)l/ *noun* a sac branching off the urethra as it passes through the prostate gland

**prostatism** /ˈprɒsteɪtɪz(ə)m/ *noun* a disorder of the prostate gland, especially enlargement that blocks or inhibits urine flow

**prostatitis** /ˌprɒstəˈtaɪtɪs/ *noun* inflammation of the prostate gland

**prostatocystitis** /ˌprɒstætəʊsɪˈstaɪtɪs/ *noun* inflammation of the prostatic urethra and the bladder

**prostatorrhoea** /ˌprɒstətəˈriːə/ *noun* discharge of fluid from the prostate gland (NOTE: The US spelling is **prostatorrhea**.)

**prosthesis** /prɒsˈθiːsɪs/ *noun* a device which is attached to the body to take the place of a part which is missing, e.g. an artificial leg or glass eye (NOTE: The plural is **prostheses**.)
'The average life span of a joint prosthesis is 10–15 years' [*British Journal of Nursing*]

**prosthetic** /prɒsˈθetɪk/ *adjective* replacing a part of the body which has been amputated or removed ○ *He was fitted with a prosthetic hand.*

**prosthetic dentistry** /prɒsˌθetɪk ˈdentɪstri/ *noun* the branch of dentistry which deals with replacing missing teeth parts of the jaw, and fitting dentures, bridges and crowns. Also called **prosthodontics**

**prosthetics** /prɒsˈθetɪks/ *noun* the study and making of prostheses

**prosthetist** /ˈprɒsθətɪst/ *noun* a qualified person who fits prostheses

**prosthodontics** /ˌprɒsθəˈdɒntɪks/ *noun* same as **prosthetic dentistry** (NOTE: Takes a singular verb.)

**prostrate** /ˈprɒstreɪt/ *adjective* lying face down (NOTE: Do not confuse with **prostate**.)

**prostration** /prɒˈstreɪʃ(ə)n/ *noun* extreme tiredness of body or mind

**protamine** /ˈprəʊtəmiːn/ *noun* a simple protein found in fish, used with insulin to slow down the insulin absorption rate

**protanopia** /ˌprəʊtəˈnəʊpiə/ *noun* same as **Daltonism**

**protease** /ˈprəʊtieɪz/ *noun* a digestive enzyme which breaks down protein in food by splitting the peptide link. Also called **proteolytic enzyme**

**protect** /prəˈtekt/ *verb* to keep a person or thing safe from harm ○ *The population must be protected against the spread of the virus.*

**protection** /prəˈtekʃən/ *noun* **1.** the act of keeping a person or thing safe from harm **2.** something which protects ○ *Children are vaccinated as a protection against disease.*

**Protection of Children Act 1999** /prəˌtekʃən əv ˈtʃɪldrən ækt/ *noun* in the UK, an Act of Parliament to protect children by restricting the employment of certain nurses, teachers or other workers whose jobs bring them into contact with children, on grounds such as misconduct or health

**protective** /prəˈtektɪv/ *adjective* providing protection

**protective isolation** /prəˌtektɪv ˌaɪsəˈleɪʃ(ə)n/ *noun* a set of procedures used to protect people who have impaired resistance to infectious disease, e.g. those with leukaemia and lymphoma, Aids and graft patients. Also called **reverse isolation**

**protein** /ˈprəʊtiːn/ *noun* a nitrogen compound which is present in and is an essential part of all living cells in the body, formed by the linking of amino acids
COMMENT: Proteins are necessary for growth and repair of the body's tissue. They are mainly formed of carbon, nitrogen and oxygen in various combinations as amino acids. Foods such as beans, meat, eggs, fish and milk are rich in protein.

**protein balance** /ˈprəʊtiːn ˌbæləns/ *noun* a situation when the nitrogen intake in protein is equal to the excretion rate in the urine

**protein-bound iodine** /ˌprəʊtiːn baʊnd ˈaɪədiːn/ *noun* a compound of thyroxine and iodine

**protein-bound iodine test** /ˌprəʊtiːn baʊnd ˈaɪədiːn test/ *noun* a test to measure if the thyroid gland is producing adequate quantities of thyroxine. Abbr **PBI test**

**protein deficiency** /ˈprəʊtiːn dɪˌfɪʃ(ə)nsi/ *noun* a lack of enough proteins in the diet

**proteinuria** /ˌprəʊtɪˈnjʊəriə/ *noun* a condition in which there are proteins in the urine

**proteolysis** /ˌprəʊtiˈɒləsɪs/ *noun* the breaking down of proteins in food into amino acids by enzymes

**proteolytic** /ˌprəʊtiəʊˈlɪtɪk/ *adjective* referring to proteolysis

**proteolytic enzyme** /ˌprəʊtiəʊlɪtɪk ˈenzaɪm/ *noun* same as **protease**

**proteose** /ˈprəʊtiəʊs/ *noun* a water-soluble compound formed during hydrolytic processes such as digestion

**Proteus** /ˈprəʊtiəs/ *noun* a genus of bacteria commonly found in the intestines

**prothrombin** /prəʊˈθrɒmbɪn/ *noun* a protein in blood which helps blood to coagulate and which needs Vitamin K to be effective. Also called **Factor II**

**prothrombin time** /prəʊˈθrɒmbɪn taɪm/ *noun* the time taken in Quick test for clotting to take place

**proto-** /prəʊtəʊ/ *prefix* first or at the beginning

**protocol** /ˈprəʊtəkɒl/ *noun* the set of instructions for the clinical management of a particular condition, including tests, surgery and drug treatments

**proton pump** /ˈprəʊtɒn pʌmp/ *noun* an enzyme system within the gastric mucosa that secretes gastric acids ○ *The drug acts on the proton pump mechanism.*

**proton-pump inhibitor** /ˈprəʊtɒn pʌmp ɪnˌhɪbɪtə/ *noun* a drug which suppresses the final stage of gastric acid secretion by the proton pump in the gastric mucosa

**protopathic** /ˌprəʊtəʊˈpæθɪk/ *adjective* **1.** referring to nerves which are able to sense only strong sensations **2.** referring to a first symptom or lesion **3.** referring to the first sign of partially restored function in an injured nerve ▶ compare **epicritic**

**protoplasm** /ˈprəʊtəʊˌplæz(ə)m/ *noun* a substance like a jelly which makes up the largest part of each cell

**protoplasmic** /ˌprəʊtəʊˈplæzmɪk/ *adjective* referring to protoplasm

**protoporphyrin IX** /ˌprəʊtəʊˌpɔːfərɪn ˈnaɪn/ *noun* the commonest form of porphyrin, found in haemoglobin and chlorophyll

**protozoa** /ˌprəʊtəˈzəʊə/ plural of **protozoon**

**protozoan** /ˌprəʊtəˈzəʊən/ *adjective* referring to protozoa

**protozoon** *noun* a tiny simple organism with a single cell (NOTE: The plural is **protozoa** or **protozoons**.)

COMMENT: Parasitic protozoa can cause several diseases, including amoebiasis, malaria and other tropical diseases.

**protract** /prəʊˈtrækt/ *verb* **1.** to make something last a long time **2.** to extend or lengthen a body part

**protractor** /prəˈtræktə/ *noun* a muscle with the function of extending a body part

**protrude** /prəˈtruːd/ *verb* to stick out ○ *She wears a brace to correct her protruding teeth.* ○ *Protruding eyes are associated with some forms of goitre.* (NOTE: **protruding – protruded**)

**protuberance** /prəˈtjuːb(ə)rəns/ *noun* a rounded part of the body which projects above the rest

**proud flesh** /ˌpraʊd ˈfleʃ/ *noun* new vessels and young fibrous tissue which form when a wound, incision or lesion is healing

**provide** /prəˈvaɪd/ *verb* to supply something ○ *A balanced diet should provide the necessary proteins required by the body.* ○ *The hospital provides an ambulance service to the whole area.* (NOTE: **providing – provided**)

**provider** /prəˈvaɪdə/ *noun* a hospital which provides secondary care which is paid for by another body such as a PCG or social services. ◊ **purchaser**

**provision** /prəˈvɪʒ(ə)n/ *noun* **1.** the act of providing something ○ *the provision of aftercare facilities for patients recently discharged from hospital* **2.** something provided

**provisional** /prəˈvɪʒ(ə)n(ə)l/ *adjective* temporary and which may be changed ○ *The hos-pital has given me a provisional date for the operation.* ○ *The paramedical team attached sticks to the broken leg to act as provisional splints.*

**provisionally** /prəˈvɪʒ(ə)nəli/ *adverb* in a temporary way, not certainly ○ *She has provisionally accepted the offer of a bed in the hospital.*

**provitamin** /prəʊˈvɪtəmɪn/ *noun* a chemical compound which is converted to a vitamin during usual biochemical processes, e.g. the amino acid tryptophan, which is converted to niacin, and beta carotene, which is converted into vitamin A

**provoke** /prəˈvəʊk/ *verb* **1.** to make a person angry **2.** to make something happen ○ *The medication provoked a sudden rise in body temperature.* ○ *The fit was provoked by the shock of the accident.* **3.** to make something be felt ○ *His lack of visitors provoked the nurses' sympathy.* (NOTE: **provokes – provoking – provoked**)

**proximal** /ˈprɒksɪm(ə)l/ *adjective* near the midline, the central part of the body

**proximal convoluted tubule** /ˌprɒksɪm(ə)l ˌkɒnvəluːtɪd ˈtjuːbjuːl/ *noun* a part of the kidney filtering system between the loop of Henle and the glomerulus

**proximal interphalangeal joint** /ˌprɒksɪm(ə)l ɪntəfəˈlændʒiəl dʒɔɪnt/ *noun* a joint nearest the point of attachment of a finger or toe. Abbr **PIP**

**proximally** /ˈprɒksɪmli/ *adverb* further towards the centre or point of attachment. Opposite **distally**. See illustration at ANATOMICAL TERMS in Supplement

**Prozac** /ˈprəʊzæk/ a trade name for fluoxetine

**prurigo** /pruəˈraɪgəʊ/ *noun* an itchy eruption of papules

**pruritus** /pruəˈraɪtəs/ *noun* an irritation of the skin which makes a person want to scratch. Also called **itching**

**pruritus ani** /pruəˌraɪtɪs ˈeɪnaɪ/ *noun* itching round the anal orifice

**pruritus vulvae** /pruəˌraɪtɪs ˈvʌlviː/ *noun* itching round the vulva

**prussic acid** /ˌprʌsɪk ˈæsɪd/ *noun* same as **cyanide**

**PSA test** /ˌpiː es ˈeɪ test/ *noun* a blood test for prostate cancer which detects a protein produced by prostate cells. Full form **prostatic specific antigen test**

**pseud-** /sjuːd/ *prefix* same as **pseudo-** (used before vowels)

**pseudarthrosis** /sjuːdɑːˈθrəʊsɪs/ *noun* a false joint, as when the two broken ends of a fractured bone do not bind together but heal separately (NOTE: The plural is **pseudarthroses**.)

**pseudo-** /ˈsjuːdəʊ/ prefix similar to something but not the same

**pseudoangina** /ˌsjuːdəʊænˈdʒaɪnə/ noun pain in the chest, caused by worry but not indicating heart disease

**pseudocoxalgia** /ˌsjuːdəʊkɒkˈsældʒə/ noun the degeneration of the upper end of the femur in young boys which prevents the femur from growing properly and can result in a permanent limp. Also called **Legg-Calvé-Perthes disease**

**pseudocrisis** /ˈsjuːdəʊˌkraɪsɪs/ noun a sudden fall in the temperature of a person with fever which does not mark the end of the fever

**pseudocroup** /ˌsjuːdəʊˈkruːp/ noun **1.** same as **laryngismus 2.** a form of asthma in which contractions take place in the larynx

**pseudocyesis** /ˌsjuːdəʊsaɪˈiːsɪs/ noun a condition in which a woman has the physical symptoms of pregnancy but is not pregnant. Also called **phantom pregnancy, pseudopregnancy**

**pseudocyst** /ˈsjuːdəʊsɪst/ noun a space which fills with fluid in an organ but without the walls which would form a cyst, as a result of softening or necrosis of the tissue

**pseudodementia** /ˌsjuːdəʊdɪˈmenʃə/ noun a condition of extreme apathy found in hysterical people in which their behaviour corresponds to what they imagine to be insanity, though they show no signs of true dementia

**pseudogynaecomastia** /ˌsjuːdəʊ ˌgaɪnɪkəʊˈmæstiə/ noun enlargement of the male breast because of extra fatty tissue (NOTE: The US spelling is **pseudogynecomastia**.)

**pseudohermaphroditism** /ˌsjuːdəʊhɜː ˈmæfrədaɪtɪz(ə)m/ noun a condition in which a person has either ovaries or testes but external genitalia that are not clearly of either sex

**pseudohypertrophic muscular dystrophy** /ˌsjuːdəʊhaɪpəˌtrɒfɪk ˌmʌskjʊlə ˈdɪstrəfi/ noun a hereditary disease affecting the muscles, which swell and become weak, beginning in early childhood. Also called **Duchenne muscular dystrophy**

**pseudohypertrophy** /ˌsjuːdəʊhaɪ ˈpɜːtrəfi/ noun an overgrowth of fatty or fibrous tissue in a part or organ, which results in the part or organ being enlarged

**pseudomonad** /ˌsjuːdəʊˈməʊnəd/ noun a rod-shaped bacterium which lives in soil or decomposing organic material and can cause disease in plants and sometimes in humans

**pseudomyxoma** /ˌsjuːdəʊmɪkˈsəʊmə/ noun a tumour rich in mucus (NOTE: The plural is **pseudomyxomas** or **pseudomyxomata**.)

**pseudo-obstruction** /ˌsjuːdəʊ əbˈstrʌkʃən/ noun a condition in which symptoms such as stomach cramps, nausea and bloating indicate a blockage in the intestines although no blockage exists

**pseudoplegia** /ˌsjuːdəʊˈpliːdʒə/, **pseudoparalysis** /ˌsjuːdəʊpəˈræləsɪs/ noun **1.** loss of muscular power in the limbs without true paralysis **2.** paralysis caused by hysteria

**pseudopolyposis** /ˌsjuːdəʊpɒliˈpəʊsɪs/ noun a condition in which polyps are found in many places in the intestine, usually resulting from an earlier infection

**pseudopregnancy** /ˌsjuːdəʊˈpregnənsi/ noun also called **pseudocyesis**

**psilosis** /saɪˈləʊsɪs/ noun a disease of the small intestine which prevents a person from absorbing food properly. Also called **sprue**

COMMENT: The condition is often found in the tropics, and results in diarrhoea and loss of weight.

**psittacosis** /ˌsɪtəˈkəʊsɪs/ noun a disease of parrots which can be transmitted to humans. It is similar to typhoid fever, but atypical pneumonia is present. Symptoms include fever, diarrhoea and distension of the abdomen. Also called **parrot disease**

**psoas** /ˈsəʊəs/ noun either of two pairs of muscles in the groin, psoas major and psoas minor, which help to move the hip joint

**psoas major** /ˌsəʊəs ˈmeɪdʒə/ noun a muscle in the groin which flexes the hip

**psoas minor** /ˌsəʊəs ˈmaɪnə/ noun a small muscle similar to the psoas major but not always present

**psoriasis** /səˈraɪəsɪs/ noun a common inflammatory skin disease where red patches of skin are covered with white scales

**psoriatic** /ˌsɔːriˈætɪk/ adjective referring to psoriasis

**psoriatic arthritis** /ˌsɔːriætɪk ɑːˈθraɪtɪs/ noun a form of psoriasis which is associated with arthritis

**psych-** /saɪk/ prefix same as **psycho-** (used before vowels)

**psychasthenia** /ˌsaɪkæsˈθiːniə/ noun **1.** any psychoneurosis other than hysteria **2.** psychoneurosis characterised by fears and phobias

**psyche** /ˈsaɪki/ noun the mind

**psychedelic** /ˌsaɪkəˈdelɪk/ adjective referring to drugs such as LSD which expand a person's consciousness

**psychiatric** /ˌsaɪkiˈætrɪk/ adjective referring to psychiatry ○ He is undergoing psychiatric treatment.

**psychiatric hospital** /ˌsaɪkiˈætrɪk ˌhɒs pɪt(ə)l/ noun a hospital which specialises in the treatment of patients with mental disorders

**psychiatrist** /saɪˈkaɪətrɪst/ noun a doctor who specialises in the diagnosis and treatment of mental and behavioural disorders

**psychiatry** /saɪˈkaɪətri/ noun a branch of medicine concerned with the diagnosis and treatment of mental and behavioural disorders

**psychic** /'saɪkɪk/, **psychical** /'saɪkɪk(ə)l/ *adjective* **1.** referring to a person who is supposedly able to guess thoughts which people have not expressed, or to foresee the future **2.** relating to or originating in the human mind

**psycho-** /saɪkəʊ/ *prefix* referring to the mind

**psychoanalysis** /,saɪkəʊə'næləsɪs/ *noun* a form of treatment for mental disorders in which a specialist and patient talk and together analyse the patient's condition and past events which may have contributed to it

**psychoanalyst** /,saɪkəʊ'æn(ə)lɪst/ *noun* a person who is trained in psychoanalysis

**psychodrama** /'saɪkəʊ,drɑːmə/ *noun* a type of psychotherapy in which patients act out roles in dramas illustrating their emotional problems, in front of other patients

**psychodynamics** /,saɪkəʊdaɪ'næmɪks/ *noun* the study of how the forces which affect human behaviour and mental states work, especially on a subconscious level

**psychogenic** /,saɪkə'dʒenɪk/, **psychogenetic** /,saɪkəʊdʒə'netɪk/, **psychogenous** /saɪ'kɒdʒənəs/ *adjective* referring to an illness which starts in the mind, rather than in a physical state

**psychogeriatrics** /,saɪkəʊdʒeri'ætrɪks/ *noun* the study of the mental disorders of the late stages of the natural life span

**psychological** /,saɪkə'lɒdʒɪk(ə)l/ *adjective* referring to psychology, or caused by a mental state

**psychological dependence** /,saɪkə,lɒdʒɪk(ə)l dɪ'pendəns/, **psychological drug dependence** /,saɪkə,lɒdʒɪk(ə)l 'drʌg dɪ,pendəns/ *noun* a state in which a person is addicted to a drug such as cannabis or alcohol but does not suffer physical effects if he or she stops taking it

**psychologically** /,saɪkə'lɒdʒɪkli/ *adverb* in a way which is caused by a mental state ○ *He is psychologically addicted to tobacco.*

**psychologist** /saɪ'kɒlədʒɪst/ *noun* a person who specialises in the study of the mind and mental processes

**psychology** /saɪ'kɒlədʒi/ *noun* the study of the mind and mental processes

**psychometrics** /,saɪkə'metrɪks/ *noun* a way of measuring intelligence and personality in which the result is shown as a number on a scale

**psychomotor** /,saɪkə'məʊtə/ *adjective* referring to muscle movements caused by mental activity

**psychomotor disturbance** /,saɪkəməʊtə dɪ'stɜːbəns/ *noun* muscle movements caused by a mental disorder, e.g. twitching

**psychomotor epilepsy** /,saɪkəməʊtə 'epɪlepsi/ *noun* epilepsy in which fits are characterised by blurring of consciousness and ac-

companied by coordinated but wrong movements

**psychomotor retardation** /,saɪkəməʊtə ,riːtɑː'deɪʃ(ə)n/ *noun* the slowing of movement and speech, caused by depression

**psychoneuroimmunology** /,saɪkəʊ ,njʊərəʊ,ɪmjʊ'nɒlədʒi/ *noun* a branch of medicine which deals with how emotions affect the immune system

**psychoneurosis** /,saɪkəʊnjʊ'rəʊsɪs/ *noun* any of a group of mental disorders in which a person has a faulty response to the stresses of life. ◊ **neurosis** (NOTE: The plural is **psychoneuroses**.)

**psychopath** /'saɪkəpæθ/ *noun* a person with a long-term mental disorder characterised by antisocial and often violent behaviour

**psychopathic** /,saɪkə'pæθɪk/ *adjective* referring to psychopaths or psychopathy

**psychopathological** /,saɪkəʊpæθə 'lɒdʒɪk(ə)l/ *adjective* referring to psychopathology

**psychopathology** /,saɪkəpə'θɒlədʒi/ *noun* a branch of medicine concerned with the pathology of mental disorders and diseases

**psychopathy** /saɪ'kɒpəθi/ *noun* any disease of the mind (NOTE: The plural is **psychopathies**.)

**psychopharmacology** /,saɪkəʊ,fɑːmə 'kɒlədʒi/ *noun* the study of the actions and applications of drugs which have a powerful effect on the mind and behaviour

**psychophysiological** /,saɪkəʊ,fɪziə 'lɒdʒɪk(ə)l/ *adjective* referring to psychophysiology

**psychophysiology** /,saɪkəʊ,fɪzi'ɒlədʒi/ *noun* the physiology of the mind and its functions

**psychoses** /saɪ'kəʊsiːz/ plural of **psychosis**

**psychosexual** /,saɪkəʊ'sekʃuəl/ *adjective* relating to the mental and emotional aspects of sexuality and sexual development

**psychosexual development** /,saɪkəʊ ,sekʃuəl dɪ'veləpmənt/ *noun* the development of human personality in stages based upon the ability to experience sexual pleasure, and the way in which sexuality plays a role in a person's life

**psychosis** /saɪ'kəʊsɪs/ *noun* any serious mental disorder in which a person has a distorted perception of reality (NOTE: The plural is **psychoses**.)

**psychosocial** /,saɪkəʊ'səʊʃ(ə)l/ *adjective* relating to the interaction of psychological and social factors

'...recent efforts to redefine nursing have moved away from the traditional medically dominated approach towards psychosocial care and forming relationships with patients' [*British Journal of Nursing*]

**psychosomatic** /ˌsaɪkəʊsə'mætɪk/ adjective referring to the relationship between body and mind

COMMENT: Many physical disorders, including duodenal ulcers and high blood pressure, can be caused by mental conditions like worry or stress, and are then termed psychosomatic in order to distinguish them from the same conditions having physical or hereditary causes.

**psychosurgery** /ˌsaɪkəʊ'sɜːdʒəri/ noun brain surgery, used as a treatment for psychological disorders

**psychosurgical** /ˌsaɪkəʊ'sɜːdʒɪk(ə)l/ adjective referring to psychosurgery

**psychotherapeutic** /ˌsaɪkəʊθerə'pjuːtɪk/ adjective referring to psychotherapy

**psychotherapist** /ˌsaɪkəʊ'θerəpɪst/ noun a person trained to give psychotherapy

**psychotherapy** /ˌsaɪkəʊ'θerəpi/ noun the treatment of mental disorders by psychological methods, as when a psychotherapist encourages a person to talk about his or her problems. ◊ **therapy**

**psychotic** /saɪ'kɒtɪk/ adjective **1.** referring to psychosis **2.** characterised by mental disorder

**psychotropic** /ˌsaɪkə'trɒpɪk/ adjective referring to a drug such as a stimulant or sedative which affects a person's mood

**pt** abbr pint

**pterion** /'tɪəriɒn/ noun the point on the side of the skull where the frontal, temporal parietal and sphenoid bones meet

**pteroylglutamic acid** /ˌterəʊaɪlgluːˌtæmɪk 'æsɪd/ noun same as **folic acid**

**pterygium** /tə'rɪdʒiəm/ noun a degenerative condition in which a triangular growth of conjunctiva covers part of the cornea, with its apex towards the pupil

**pterygo-** /terɪgəʊ/ suffix the pterygoid process

**pterygoid plate** /ˌterɪgɔɪd 'pleɪt/ noun a small flat bony projection on the pterygoid process

**pterygoid plexus** /ˌterɪgɔɪd 'pleksəs/ noun a group of veins and sinuses which join together behind the cheek

**pterygoid process** /'terɪgɔɪd ˌprəʊses/ noun one of two projecting parts on the sphenoid bone

**pterygomandibular** /ˌterɪgəʊmæn'dɪbjʊlə/ adjective referring to the pterygoid process and the mandible

**pterygopalatine fossa** /ˌterɪgəʊpælətaɪn 'fɒsə/ noun the space between the pterygoid process and the upper jaw

**pterygopalatine ganglion** /ˌterɪgəʊ pælətaɪn 'gæŋliən/ noun a ganglion in the pterygopalatine fossa associated with the maxillary nerve. Also called **sphenopalatine ganglion**

**ptomaine** /'təʊmeɪn/ noun a group of nitrogenous substances produced in rotting food, which gives the food a special smell (NOTE: **Ptomaine poisoning** was the term formerly used to refer to any form of food poisoning.)

**ptosis** /'təʊsɪs/ noun **1.** prolapse of an organ **2.** drooping of the upper eyelid, which makes the eye stay half closed

**-ptosis** /təʊsɪs/ suffix prolapse

**PTSD** abbr post-traumatic stress disorder

**ptyal-** /taɪəl/ prefix same as **ptyalo-** (used before vowels)

**ptyalin** /'taɪəlɪn/ noun an enzyme in saliva which cleanses the mouth and converts starch into sugar

**ptyalism** /'taɪəlɪz(ə)m/ noun the production of an excessive amount of saliva

**ptyalith** /'taɪəlɪθ/ noun same as **sialolith**

**ptyalo-** /taɪələʊ/ prefix referring to saliva

**ptyalography** /ˌtaɪə'lɒgrəfi/ noun same as **sialography**

**pubertal** /'pjuːbət(ə)l/, **puberal** /'pjuːbərəl/ adjective referring to puberty

**puberty** /'pjuːbəti/ noun **1.** the physical and psychological changes which take place when childhood ends and adolescence and sexual maturity begin and the sex glands become active **2.** the time when these changes take place

COMMENT: Puberty starts at about the age of 10 in girls, and slightly later in boys.

**pubes¹** /'pjuːbiːz/ noun the part of the body just above the groin, where the pubic bones are found

**pubes²** /'pjuːbiːz/ plural of **pubis**

**pubescent** /pjuː'besənt/ adjective reaching or having reached puberty

**pubic** /'pjuːbɪk/ adjective referring to the area near the genitals

**pubic bone** /ˌpjuːbɪk 'bəʊn/ noun the bone in front of the pelvis. Also called **pubis**. See illustration at **UROGENITAL SYSTEM (MALE)** in Supplement

**pubic hair** /ˌpjuːbɪk 'heə/ noun tough hair growing in the genital region

**pubic louse** /ˌpjuːbɪk 'laʊs/ noun also called **Pediculus pubis**

**pubic symphysis** /ˌpjuːbɪk 'sɪmfəsɪs/ noun a piece of cartilage which joins the two sections of the pubic bone. Also called **symphysis pubis**

COMMENT: In a pregnant woman, the pubic symphysis stretches to allow the pelvic girdle to expand so that there is room for the baby to pass through.

**pubiotomy** /ˌpjuːbi'ɒtəmi/ noun a surgical operation to divide the pubic bone during labour, in order to make the pelvis wide enough for the child to be born safely (NOTE: The plural is **pubiotomies**.)

**pubis** /'pjuːbɪs/ noun a bone forming the front part of the pelvis. See illustration at **PELVIS** in Supplement (NOTE: The plural is **pubes**.)

**public health** /ˌpʌblɪk 'helθ/ *noun* the study of illness, health and disease in the community

**public health laboratory service** /ˌpʌblɪk ˌhelθ ləˈbɒrət(ə)ri ˌsɜːvɪs/ *noun* in the UK, a former service of the NHS which detected, diagnosed and monitored suspected cases of infectious disease in a countrywide network of laboratories. Abbr **PHLS**

**public health medicine** /ˌpʌblɪk ˌhelθ 'med(ə)s(ə)n/ *noun* the branch of medicine concerned with health and disease in populations, with the responsibilities of monitoring health, identification of health needs, development of policies which promote health and evaluation of health services

**public health nurse** /ˌpʌblɪk ˌhelθ 'nɜːs/ *noun* a nurse such as a school nurse, health visitor or other community nurse who monitors health and works to prevent illness in community situations

**public health physician** /ˌpʌblɪk ˌhelθ fɪ 'zɪʃ(ə)n/ *noun* a consultant who has special training in public health medicine

**pudenda** /pjuːˈdendə/ plural of **pudendum**

**pudendal** /pjuːˈdend(ə)l/ *adjective* referring to the pudendum

**pudendal block** /pjuːˌdend(ə)l 'blɒk/ *noun* an operation to anaesthetise the pudendum during childbirth

**pudendum** /pjuːˈdendəm/ *noun* an external genital organ of a woman (NOTE: The plural is **pudenda**.)

**puerpera** /pjuːˈɜːp(ə)rə/ *noun* a woman who has recently given birth, or is giving birth, and whose uterus is still distended (NOTE: The plural is **puerperae**.)

**puerperal** /pjuːˈɜːp(ə)rəl/ *adjective* **1.** referring to the puerperium **2.** referring to childbirth **3.** occurring after childbirth

**puerperal infection** /pjuːˌɜːp(ə)rəl ɪn 'fekʃən/, **puerperal fever** /pjuːˌɜːp(ə)rəl 'fiːvə/ *noun* an infection of the uterus and genital tract after the birth of a baby, which is more common in women who have had a caesarean section. It causes a high fever, and occasionally sepsis, which can be fatal and was commonly so in the past. Also called **postpartum fever**

**puerperalism** /pjuːˈɜːp(ə)rəlɪz(ə)m/ *noun* an illness of a baby or its mother resulting from or associated with childbirth

**puerperal psychosis** /pjuːˌɜːp(ə)rəl saɪ 'kəʊsɪs/ *noun* a psychiatric disorder that some women may experience in the first two weeks after giving birth

**puerperal sepsis** /pjuːˌɜːp(ə)rəl 'sepsɪs/ *noun* blood poisoning following childbirth, caused by infection of the placental site

**puerperium** /ˌpjuːɪəˈpɪəriəm/ *noun* a period of about six weeks which follows immediately after the birth of a child, during which the mother's sexual organs recover from childbirth

**puerperous** /pjuːˈɜːprəs/ *adjective* same as **puerperal**

**puke** /pjuːk/ *verb* same as **vomit** (*informal*)

**Pulex** /'pjuːleks/ *noun* a genus of human fleas

**pull** /pʊl/ *verb* to make a muscle move in a wrong direction ○ *He pulled a muscle in his back.* □ **to pull the plug** to switch off life support (*informal*) ■ □ **to pull yourself together** to become calmer ○ *Although he was very angry he soon pulled himself together.*

**pulley** /'pʊli/ *noun* a device with rings through which wires or cords pass, used in traction to make wires tense

**pull through** /ˌpʊl 'θruː/ *verb* to recover from a serious illness (*informal*) ○ *The doctor says she is strong and should pull through.*

**pulmo-** /'pʌlməʊ/, **pulmon-** /'pʌlmən/ *prefix* referring to the lungs

**pulmonale** /ˌpʌlməˈneɪli/ ♦ **cor pulmonale**

**pulmonary** /'pʌlmən(ə)ri/ *adjective* referring to the lungs

**pulmonary artery** /ˌpʌlmən(ə)ri 'ɑːtəri/ *noun* one of the two arteries which take deoxygenated blood from the heart to the lungs for oxygenation. See illustration at HEART in Supplement

**pulmonary circulation** /ˌpʌlmən(ə)ri ˌsɜːkjʊ'leɪʃ(ə)n/ *noun* the circulation of blood from the heart through the pulmonary arteries to the lungs for oxygenation and back to the heart through the pulmonary veins. Also called **lesser circulation**

**pulmonary embolism** /ˌpʌlmən(ə)ri 'embəlɪz(ə)m/ *noun* a blockage of a pulmonary artery by a blood clot. Abbr **PE**

**pulmonary hypertension** /ˌpʌlmən(ə)ri ˌhaɪpə'tenʃən/ *noun* high blood pressure in the blood vessels supplying blood to the lungs

**pulmonary insufficiency** /ˌpʌlmən(ə)ri ˌɪnsə'fɪʃ(ə)nsi/, **pulmonary incompetence** /ˌpʌlmən(ə)ri ɪn'kɒmpɪt(ə)ns/ *noun* a condition characterised by dilatation of the main pulmonary artery and stretching of the valve ring, due to pulmonary hypertension

**pulmonary oedema** /ˌpʌlmən(ə)ri ɪ 'diːmə/ *noun* the collection of fluid in the lungs, as occurs in left-sided heart failure

**pulmonary stenosis** /ˌpʌlmən(ə)ri ste 'nəʊsɪs/ *noun* a condition in which the opening to the pulmonary artery in the right ventricle becomes narrow

**pulmonary tuberculosis** /ˌpʌlmən(ə)ri tjuːˌbɜːkjuː'ləʊsɪs/ *noun* tuberculosis in the lungs, which makes the person lose weight, cough blood and have a fever

**pulmonary valve** /'pʌlmən(ə)ri vælv/ *noun* a valve at the opening of the pulmonary artery

**pulmonary vein** /'pʌlmən(ə)ri veɪn/ *noun* one of the four veins which carry oxygenated blood from the lungs back to the left atrium of the heart. See illustration at HEART in Supplement (NOTE: The pulmonary veins are the only veins which carry oxygenated blood.)

**pulmonectomy** /ˌpʌlmə'nektəmi/ noun same as **pneumonectomy** (NOTE: The plural is **pulmonectomies**.)

**pulmonology** /ˌpʌlmən'ɒlədʒi/ noun the branch of medicine that deals with the structure, physiology and diseases of the lungs

**pulp** /pʌlp/ noun soft tissue, especially when surrounded by hard tissue as in the inside of a tooth

**pulp cavity** /'pʌlp ˌkævɪti/ noun the central part of a tooth containing soft tissue

**pulpy** /'pʌlpi/ adjective made of pulp ○ the pulpy tissue inside a tooth

**puisate** /pʌl'seɪt/ verb to expand and contract with a strong regular beat (NOTE: **pulsating – pulsated**)

**pulsation** /pʌl'seɪʃ(ə)n/ noun the action of beating regularly, e.g. the visible pulse which can be seen under the skin in some parts of the body

**pulse** /pʌls/ noun the regular expansion and contraction of an artery caused by the heart pumping blood through the body, which can be felt with the fingers especially where an artery is near the surface of the body, as in the wrist or neck ○ Her pulse is very irregular. □ **to take** or **feel a person's pulse** to measure a person's pulse rate by pressing on the skin above an artery with the fingers ○ Has the patient's pulse been taken?

COMMENT: The standard adult pulse is about 72 beats per minute, but it is higher in children. The pulse is usually taken by placing the fingers on the patient's wrist, at the point where the radial artery passes through the depression just below the thumb.

**pulseless** /'pʌlsləs/ adjective referring to a person who has no pulse because the heart is beating very weakly

**pulse oximetry** /ˌpʌls ɒk'sɪmətri/ noun a method of measuring the oxygen content of arterial blood

**pulse point** /'pʌls pɔɪnt/ noun a place on the body where the pulse can be taken

**pulse pressure** /'pʌls ˌpreʃə/ noun the difference between the diastolic and systolic pressure. ◊ **Corrigan's pulse**

**pulse rate** /'pʌls reɪt/ noun the number of times the pulse beats per minute

**pulsus** /'pʌlsəs/ noun same as **pulse**

**pulsus alternans** /ˌpʌlsəs 'ɔːltənænz/ noun a pulse with a beat which is alternately strong and weak

**pulsus bigeminus** /ˌpʌlsəs baɪ'gemɪnəs/ noun a double pulse, with an extra ectopic beat

**pulsus paradoxus** /ˌpʌlsəs pærə'dɒksəs/ noun a condition in which there is a sharp fall in the pulse when the person breathes in

**pulvis** /'pʌlvɪs/ noun powder

**pump** /pʌmp/ noun a machine which forces liquids or air into or out of something ■ verb to force liquid or air along a tube ○ The heart pumps blood round the body. ○ The nurses tried to pump the poison out of the stomach.

**pumping chamber** /'pʌmpɪŋ ˌtʃeɪmbə/ noun one of the sections of the heart where blood is pumped

**punch drunk syndrome** /pʌntʃ 'drʌŋk ˌsɪndrəʊm/ noun a condition affecting a person, usually a boxer, who has been hit on the head many times and develops impaired mental faculties, trembling limbs and speech disorders

**puncta** /'pʌŋktə/ plural of **punctum**

**puncta lacrimalia** /ˌpʌŋktə lækrɪ'meɪliə/ plural noun small openings at the corners of the eyes through which tears drain into the nose

**punctate** /'pʌŋkteɪt/ adjective referring to tissue or a surface which has tiny spots, holes or dents in it

**punctum** /'pʌŋktəm/ noun a point (NOTE: The plural is **puncta**.)

**puncture** /'pʌŋktʃə/ noun **1.** a neat hole made by a sharp instrument **2.** the making of a hole in an organ or swelling to take a sample of the contents or to remove fluid ■ verb to make a hole in tissue with a sharp instrument (NOTE: **puncturing – punctured**)

**puncture wound** /'pʌŋktʃə wuːnd/ noun a wound made by a sharp instrument which makes a hole in the tissue

**pupil** /'pjuːp(ə)l/ noun the central opening in the iris of the eye, through which light enters the eye. See illustration at EYE in Supplement

**pupillary** /'pjuːpɪləri/ adjective referring to the pupil

**pupillary reaction** /ˌpjuːpɪləri ri'ækʃən/ noun a reflex of the pupil of the eye which contracts when exposed to bright light. Also called **light reflex**

**purchaser** /'pɜːtʃɪsə/ noun a body, usually a PCG, which commissions health care and manages the budget to pay for the service. ◊ **provider**

**pure** /pjʊə/ adjective **1.** not mixed with other substances **2.** very clean

**pure alcohol** /ˌpjʊə 'ælkəhɒl/ noun alcohol BP, alcohol with 5% water

**purgation** /pɜː'geɪʃ(ə)n/ noun the use of a drug to cause a bowel movement

**purgative** /'pɜːgətɪv/ noun a drug used to empty the bowels. ◊ **laxative**

**purge** /pɜːdʒ/ verb to induce evacuation of the bowels (NOTE: **purging – purged**)

**purified protein derivative** /ˌpjʊərɪfaɪd 'prəʊtiːn dɪˌrɪvətɪv/ noun a pure form of tuberculin, used in tuberculin tests. Abbr **PPD**

**purify** /'pjʊərɪfaɪ/ verb to make something pure (NOTE: **purifies – purifying – purified**)

**purine** /ˈpjʊəriːn/ *noun* **1.** a nitrogen-containing substance derived from uric acid which is the parent compound of several biologically important substances **2.** a derivative of purine, especially either of the bases adenine and guanine, which are found in RNA and DNA

**Purkinje cells** /pəˈkɪndʒi selz/ *plural noun* neurones in the cerebellar cortex [Described 1837. After Johannes Evangelista Purkinje (1787–1869), Professor of Physiology at Breslau, now in Poland, and then Prague, Czech Republic.]

**Purkinje fibres** /pəˈkɪndʒi ˌfaɪbəz/ *plural noun* a bundle of fibres which form the atrioventricular bundle and pass from the atrioventricular node to the septum [Described 1839. After Johannes Evangelista Purkinje (1787–1869), Professor of Physiology at Breslau, now in Poland, and then Prague, Czech Republic.]

**Purkinje shift** /pəˈkɪndʒi ʃɪft/ *noun* the change in colour sensitivity which takes place in the eye in low light when the eye starts using the rods in the retina because the light is too weak to stimulate the cones

**purpura** /ˈpɜːpjʊrə/ *noun* a purple colouring on the skin, similar to a bruise, caused by blood disease and not by trauma

**pursestring operation** /ˌpɜːsstrɪŋ ˌɒpəˈreɪʃ(ə)n/ same as **Shirodkar's operation**

**pursestring stitch** /ˈpɜːsstrɪŋ stɪtʃ/ *noun* same as **Shirodkar suture**

**purulent** /ˈpjʊərʊlənt/ *adjective* containing or producing pus

**pus** /pʌs/ *noun* a yellow liquid composed of blood serum, pieces of dead tissue, white blood cells and the remains of bacteria, formed by the body in reaction to infection (NOTE: For other terms referring to pus, see words beginning with **py-** or **pyo-**.)

**pustular** /ˈpʌstjʊlə/ *adjective* **1.** covered with or composed of pustules **2.** referring to pustules

**pustulate** /ˈpʌstjʊleɪt/ *verb* to become covered with pustules, or cause pustules to appear on the skin (NOTE: **pustulating – pustulated**) ■ *adjective* covered with pustules

**pustule** /ˈpʌstjuːl/ *noun* a small pimple filled with pus

**putrefaction** /ˌpjuːtrɪˈfækʃən/ *noun* the decomposition of organic substances by bacteria, making an unpleasant smell

**putrefy** /ˈpjuːtrɪfaɪ/ *verb* to rot or decompose (NOTE: **putrefies – putrefying – putrefied**)

**put up** /ˌpʊt ˈʌp/ *verb* to arrange something such as a drip (NOTE: **putting up – put up**)

**p.v.** *adverb* by way of the vagina. Full form **per vaginam**

**PVS** *abbr* persistent vegetative state

**PWA** /ˌpiː dʌbljuː ˈeɪ/ *noun* a person with Aids

**py-** /paɪ/, **pyo-** /paɪəʊ/ *prefix* same as **pyo-** (*used before vowels*)

**pyaemia** /paɪˈiːmiə/ *noun* invasion of blood with bacteria which then multiply and form many little abscesses in various parts of the body (NOTE: The US spelling is **pyemia**.)

**pyarthrosis** /ˌpaɪɑːˈθrəʊsɪs/ *noun* a condition in which a joint becomes infected with pyogenic organisms and fills with pus. Also called **acute suppurative arthritis**

**pyel-** /paɪəl/ *prefix* same as **pyelo-** (*used before vowels*)

**pyelitis** /ˌpaɪəˈlaɪtɪs/ *noun* inflammation of the central part of the kidney

**pyelo-** /paɪələʊ/ *prefix* referring to the pelvis of the kidney

**pyelocystitis** /ˌpaɪələʊsɪˈstaɪtɪs/ *noun* inflammation of the pelvis of the kidney and the urinary bladder

**pyelogram** /ˈpaɪələgræm/ *noun* an X-ray photograph of a kidney and the urinary tract

**pyelography** /ˌpaɪəˈlɒgrəfi/ *noun* X-ray examination of a kidney after introduction of a contrast medium

**pyelolithotomy** /ˌpaɪələʊlɪˈθɒtəmi/ *noun* a surgical operation to remove a stone from the pelvis of the kidney (NOTE: The plural is **pyelolithotomies**.)

**pyelonephritis** /ˌpaɪələʊnɪˈfraɪtɪs/ *noun* inflammation of the kidney and the pelvis of the kidney

**pyeloplasty** /ˈpaɪələplæsti/ *noun* any surgical operation on the pelvis of the kidney (NOTE: The plural is **pyeloplasties**.)

**pyelotomy** /ˌpaɪəˈlɒtəmi/ *noun* a surgical operation to make an opening in the pelvis of the kidney (NOTE: The plural is **pyelotomies**.)

**pyemia** /paɪˈiːmiə/ *noun US* same as **pyaemia**

**pykno-** /pɪknəʊ/ *prefix* indicating thickness or density

**pyknolepsy** /ˈpɪknəˌlepsi/ *noun* a former name for a type of frequent attack of petit mal epilepsy affecting children

**pyl-** /paɪl/, **pyle-** /ˈpaɪli/ *prefix* referring to the portal vein

**pylephlebitis** /ˌpaɪlɪfləˈbaɪtɪs/ *noun* thrombosis of the portal vein

**pylethrombosis** /ˌpaɪliθrɒmˈbəʊsɪs/ *noun* a condition in which blood clots are present in the portal vein or any of its branches

**pylor-** /paɪˈlɔːr/ *prefix* same as **pyloro-** (*used before vowels*)

**pylorectomy** /ˌpaɪləˈrektəmi/ *noun* a surgical operation to remove the pylorus and the antrum of the stomach (NOTE: The plural is **pylorectomies**.)

**pylori** /paɪˈlɔːri/ *plural of* **pylorus**

**pyloric** /paɪˈlɒrɪk/ *adjective* referring to the pylorus

**pyloric antrum** /paɪˌlɒrɪk ˈæntrəm/ *noun* a space at the bottom of the stomach, before the pyloric sphincter

**pyloric orifice** /paɪˌlɒrɪk ˈɒrɪfɪs/ *noun* an opening where the stomach joins the duodenum

**pyloric sphincter** /paɪˌlɒrɪk ˈsfɪŋktə/ *noun* a muscle which surrounds the pylorus, makes it contract and separates it from the duodenum

**pyloric stenosis** /paɪˌlɒrɪk steˈnəʊsɪs/ *noun* a blockage of the pylorus, which prevents food from passing from the stomach into the duodenum

**pyloro-** /paɪˈlɔːrəʊ/ *prefix* the pylorus

**pyloroplasty** /paɪˈlɔːrəplæsti/ *noun* a surgical operation to make the pylorus larger, sometimes combined with treatment for peptic ulcers (NOTE: The plural is **pyloroplasties**.)

**pylorospasm** /paɪˈlɔːrəspæz(ə)m/ *noun* a muscle spasm which closes the pylorus so that food cannot pass through into the duodenum

**pylorotomy** /ˌpaɪləˈrɒtəmi/ *noun* a surgical operation to cut into the muscle surrounding the pylorus to relieve pyloric stenosis. Also called **Ramstedt's operation** (NOTE: The plural is **pylorotomies**.)

**pylorus** /paɪˈlɔːrəs/ *noun* an opening at the bottom of the stomach leading into the duodenum (NOTE: The plural is **pylori**.)

**pyo-** /paɪəʊ/ *prefix* referring to pus

**pyocele** /ˈpaɪəsiːl/ *noun* an enlargement of a tube or cavity due to accumulation of pus

**pyocolpos** /ˌpaɪəˈkɒlpəs/ *noun* an accumulation of pus in the vagina

**pyoderma** /ˌpaɪəˈdɜːmə/ *noun* an eruption of pus in the skin

**pyoderma gangrenosum** /ˌpaɪədɜːmə ˌɡæŋɡrɪˈnəʊsəm/ *noun* a serious ulcerating disease of the skin, especially the legs, usually treated with steroid drugs

**pyogenesis** /ˌpaɪəˈdʒenɪsɪs/ *noun* the production or formation of pus

**pyogenic** /ˌpaɪəˈdʒenɪk/ *adjective* producing or forming pus

**pyometra** /ˌpaɪəˈmiːtrə/ *noun* an accumulation of pus in the uterus

**pyomyositis** /ˌpaɪəʊmaɪəˈsaɪtɪs/ *noun* inflammation of a muscle caused by staphylococci or streptococci

**pyonephrosis** /ˌpaɪəʊnɪˈfrəʊsɪs/ *noun* the distension of the kidney with pus

**pyopericarditis** /ˌpaɪəʊperikɑːˈdaɪtɪs/ *noun* an inflammation of the pericardium due to infection with staphylococci, streptococci or pneumococci

**pyopneumothorax** /ˌpaɪəʊˌnjuːməʊˈθɔːræks/ *noun* an accumulation of pus and gas or air in the pleural cavity

**pyorrhoea** /ˌpaɪəˈriə/ *noun* discharge of pus (NOTE: The US spelling is **pyorrhea**.)

**pyorrhoea alveolaris** /ˌpaɪəriə ˌælviəʊˈlɑːrɪs/ *noun* suppuration from the supporting tissues round the teeth

**pyosalpinx** /ˌpaɪəˈsælpɪŋks/ *noun* inflammation and formation of pus in a Fallopian tube

**pyothorax** /ˌpaɪəˈθɔːræks/ *noun* same as **empyema**

**pyr-** /paɪr/ *prefix* same as **pyro-** (used before vowels)

**pyramid** /ˈpɪrəmɪd/ *noun* a cone-shaped part of the body, especially a cone-shaped projection on the surface of the medulla oblongata or in the medulla of the kidney. See illustration at **KIDNEY** in Supplement

**pyramidal** /pɪˈræmɪd(ə)l/ *adjective* referring to a pyramid

**pyramidal cell** /pɪˈræmɪd(ə)l sel/ *noun* a cone-shaped cell in the cerebral cortex

**pyramidal system** /pɪˈræmɪd(ə)l ˈsɪstəm/, **pyramidal tract** /pɪˈræmɪd(ə)l trækt/ *noun* a group of nerve fibres within the pyramid of the medulla oblongata in the brain. It is thought to be vital in controlling movement and speech.

**pyretic** /paɪˈretɪk/ *adjective* referring to fever ■ *noun* an agent that causes fever

**pyrexia** /paɪˈreksiə/ *noun* same as **fever**

**pyrexic** /paɪˈreksɪk/ *adjective* having fever

**pyridostigmine** /ˌpɪrɪdəʊˈstɪɡmiːn/ *noun* a drug which stops or delays the action of the enzyme cholinesterase, used to treat myasthenia gravis

**pyridoxine** /ˌpɪrɪˈdɒksɪn/ *noun* same as **Vitamin B₆**

**pyrimidine** /pɪˈrɪmɪdiːn/ *noun* 1. a strong-smelling nitrogenous based compound with a six-sided ring structure that is the parent compound of several biologically important substances 2. a derivative of pyrimidine, especially any of the bases cytosine, thymine, and uracil which are found in RNA and DNA

**pyro-** /paɪrəʊ/ *prefix* burning or fever

**pyrogen** /ˈpaɪrədʒen/ *noun* a substance which causes a fever

**pyrogenic** /ˌpaɪrəˈdʒenɪk/ *adjective* causing a fever

**pyromania** /ˌpaɪrəʊˈmeɪniə/ *noun* an uncontrollable desire to start fires

**pyrophobia** /ˌpaɪrəʊˈfəʊbiə/ *noun* an unusual fear of fire

**pyruvic acid** /paɪˌruːvɪk ˈæsɪd/ *noun* a substance formed from glycogen in the muscles when it is broken down to release energy

**pyuria** /paɪˈjʊəriə/ *noun* pus in the urine

# Q

**q.d.s.** *adverb* (*written on prescriptions*) to be taken four times a day. Full form **quater in die sumendus**

**Q fever** /'kjuː ˌfiːvə/ *noun* an infectious rickettsial disease of sheep and cows caused by *Coxiella burnetti* transmitted to humans

COMMENT: Q fever mainly affects farm workers and workers in the meat industry. The symptoms are fever, cough and headaches.

**q.i.d.** *adverb* (*written on prescriptions*) four times a day. Full form **quater in die**

**q.l.** *adverb* (*written on prescriptions*) as much as you like. Full form **quantum libet**

**q.m.** *adverb* (*written on prescriptions*) every morning. Full form **quaque mane**

**q.n.** *adverb* (*written on prescriptions*) every night. Full form **quaque nocte**

**QRS complex** /ˌkjuː ɑːr 'es ˌkɒmpleks/ *noun* the deflections on an electrocardiogram, labelled Q, R, and S, which show ventricular contraction. ◊ **PQRST complex**

**q.s.** *adverb* (*written on prescriptions*) as much as necessary. Full form **quantum sufficiat**

**Q-T interval** /ˌkjuː 'tiː ˌɪntəv(ə)l/, **Q-S2 interval** /ˌkjuː es 'tuː ˌɪntəv(ə)l/ *noun* the length of the QRS complex in an electrocardiogram. ◊ **PQRST complex**

**quad** /kwɒd/ *noun* same as **quadruplet** (*informal*)

**quadrant** /'kwɒdrənt/ *noun* one of four sectors of the body thought of as being divided by the sagittal plane and the intertubercular plane ○ *tenderness in the right lower quadrant*

**quadrantanopia** /ˌkwɒdræntə'nəʊpiə/ *noun* blindness in a quarter of the field of vision

**quadrate lobe** /'kwɒdreɪt ləʊb/ *noun* a lobe on the lower side of the liver

**quadratus** /kwɒ'dreɪtəs/ *noun* any muscle with four sides

**quadratus femoris** /kwɒˌdreɪtəs 'femərɪs/ *noun* a muscle at the top of the femur which rotates the thigh

**quadri-** /kwɒdri/ *prefix* four

**quadriceps** /'kwɒdrɪseps/, **quadriceps femoris** /ˌkwɒdrɪseps 'femrɪs/ *noun* a large muscle in the front of the thigh, which extends to the leg

COMMENT: The quadriceps femoris is divided into four parts: the rectus femoris, vastus lateralis, vastus medialis and vastus intermedius. It is the sensory receptors in the quadriceps which react to give a knee jerk when the patellar tendon is tapped.

**quadriplegia** /ˌkwɒdrɪ'pliːdʒə/ *noun* paralysis of all four limbs, both arms and both legs

**quadriplegic** /ˌkwɒdrɪ'pliːdʒɪk/ *adjective* paralysed in both arms and both legs ■ *noun* a person paralysed in both arms and both legs

**quadruple** /'kwɒdrʊp(ə)l/ *adjective* **1.** consisting of four times as much **2.** having four parts

**quadruplet** /'kwɒdrʊplət/ *noun* one of four babies born to a mother at the same time. Also called **quad**

**quadruple vaccine** /ˌkwɒdrʊp(ə)l 'væksiːn/ *noun* a vaccine which immunises against four diseases, diphtheria, whooping cough, poliomyelitis and tetanus

**quadrupod** /'kwɒdrʊpɒd/ *noun* a walking stick which ends in four little legs

**qualification** /ˌkwɒlɪfɪ'keɪʃ(ə)n/ *noun* **1.** a quality which makes a person suitable to do something **2.** an official recognition of a standard of achievement, e.g. a degree or diploma ○ *She has a qualification in pharmacy.* ○ *Are his qualifications recognised in Great Britain?*

**qualify** /'kwɒlɪfaɪ/ *verb* **1.** to make a person suitable to do something **2.** to pass a course of study and be accepted as being able to practise ○ *He qualified as a doctor two years ago.* (NOTE: [all senses] **qualifies – qualifying – qualified**)

**qualitative** /'kwɒlɪtətɪv/ *adjective* referring to a study in which descriptive information is collected. Compare **quantitative**

**quality** /'kwɒlɪti/ *noun* **1.** a characteristic of somebody or something **2.** the general standard or grade of something **3.** the highest or finest standard

**quality assurance** /'kwɒlɪti əˌʃʊərəns/ *noun* a set of criteria which are designed to check that people in an organisation maintain a high standard in the products or services they supply

**quality circle** /ˈkwɒləti ˌsɜːk(ə)l/ *noun* a group of employees from different levels of an organisation who meet regularly to discuss ways of improving the quality of its products or services

**Qualpacs** /ˈkwɒlpæks/, **Quality Patient Care Scale** /ˌkwɒliti ˌpeɪʃ(ə)nt ˈkeə skeɪl/ *noun* a method which guides nurses to evaluate their activity in terms of efficiency of cost, time, use of skill level and workload

**quantitative** /ˈkwɒntɪtətɪv/ *adjective* referring to a study in which numerical information is collected. Compare **qualitative**

**quantitative digital radiography** /ˌkwɒntɪtətɪv ˌdɪdʒɪt(ə)l reɪdiˈɒgrəfi/ *noun* the use of digital X-ray scans to find out whether a person has a bone disease such as osteoporosis. The levels of calcium in the bones are measured, usually in the spine and hip.

**quarantine** /ˈkwɒrəntiːn/ *noun* **1.** the situation in which a person, animal or ship just arrived in a country is kept isolated in case it carries a serious disease, to allow the disease time to develop and be detected **2.** the period of such isolation to prevent the spread of disease ○ *six months' quarantine* ■ *verb* to put a person or animal in quarantine (NOTE: **quarantining – quarantined**)

COMMENT: People who are suspected of having an infectious disease can be kept in quarantine for a period which varies according to the incubation period of the disease. The main diseases concerned are cholera, yellow fever and typhus.

**quartan** /ˈkwɔːt(ə)n/ *adjective* referring to a fever which occurs every fourth day, e.g. in some types of malaria

**quartan fever** /ˈkwɔːt(ə)n ˌfiːvə/ *noun* a form of malaria caused by *Plasmodium malariae* in which the fever returns every four days. ◊ **tertian fever**

**queasiness** /ˈkwiːzɪnəs/ *noun* the feeling of being about to vomit

**queasy** /ˈkwiːzi/ *adjective* feeling as though about to vomit

**Queckenstedt test** /ˈkwekənsted test/ *noun* a test done during a lumbar puncture in which pressure is applied to the jugular veins to see if the cerebrospinal fluid is flowing correctly [Described 1916. After Hans Heinrich George Queckenstedt (1876–1918), German physician.]

**quickening** /ˈkwɪknɪŋ/ *noun* the first sign of life in an unborn baby, usually after about four months of pregnancy, when the mother can feel it moving in her uterus

**Quick test** /ˈkwɪk test/, **Quick's test** *noun* a test to identify the clotting factors in a blood sample [Described 1932. After Armand James Quick (1894–1978), Professor of Biochemistry, Marquette University, USA.]

**quiescent** /kwiˈes(ə)nt/ *adjective* referring to a disease with symptoms reduced either by treatment or in the usual course of the disease

**quin** /kwɪn/ *noun* same as **quintuplet** (*informal*) (NOTE: The US term is **quint**.)

**quinine** /kwɪˈniːn/ *noun* an alkaloid drug made from the bark of cinchona, a South American tree

COMMENT: Quinine was formerly used to treat the fever symptoms of malaria, but is not often used now because of its side-effects. Small amounts of quinine have a tonic effect and are used in tonic water.

**quinine poisoning** /kwɪˈniːn ˌpɔɪz(ə)nɪŋ/, **quininism** /ˈkwɪniːnɪz(ə)m/, **quinism** /ˈkwɪnɪz(ə)m/ *noun* an illness caused by taking too much quinine, leading to dizziness and noises in the head

**quinolone** /kwɪnəˈləʊn/ *noun* a drug used to treat Gram-negative and Gram-positive bacterial infections of the respiratory and urinary tracts and of the gastro-intestinal system (NOTE: Quinolone drugs have names ending in -**oxacin: ciprofloxacin**)

COMMENT: Contraindications include use in pregnancy, renal disease and for use in children.

**quinsy** /ˈkwɪnzi/ *noun* acute throat inflammation with an abscess round a tonsil. Also called **peritonsillar abscess**

**quint** /kwɪnt/ *noun US* same as **quintuplet**

**quintan** /ˈkwɪntən/ *adjective* referring to a fever that occurs every fifth day

**quintuplet** /ˈkwɪntjʊplət/ *noun* one of five babies born to a mother at the same time. Also called **quin, quint**

**quotidian** /kwəʊˈtɪdiən/ *adjective* recurring daily

**quotidian fever** /kwəʊˌtɪdiən ˈfiːvə/ *noun* a violent form of malaria in which the fever returns at daily or even shorter intervals

**quotient** /ˈkwəʊʃ(ə)nt/ *noun* the result when one number is divided by another

**Q wave** /ˈkjuː weɪv/ *noun* a negative deflection at the start of the QRS complex on an electrocardiogram, going downwards

# R

**R** *symbol* roentgen

**R/** *abbreviation* prescription. Full form **recipe**

**rabbit fever** /'ræbɪt ,fiːvə/ *noun* same as **tularaemia**

**rabid** /'ræbɪd/ *adjective* referring to rabies, or affected by rabies ○ *She was bitten by a rabid dog.*

**rabid encephalitis** /,ræbɪd en,kefə'laɪtɪs/ *noun* a fatal form of encephalitis resulting from the bite of a rabid animal

**rabies** /'reɪbiːz/ *noun* a frequently fatal viral disease transmitted to humans by infected animals ○ *The hospital ordered a batch of rabies vaccine.* Also called **hydrophobia**

COMMENT: Rabies affects the mental balance, and the symptoms include difficulty in breathing or swallowing and an intense fear of water (hydrophobia) to the point of causing convulsions at the sight of water.

**racemose** /'ræsɪməʊs/ *adjective* referring to glands which look like a bunch of grapes

**rachi-** /reɪki/ *prefix* same as **rachio-** (*used before vowels*)

**rachianaesthesia** /,reɪkiænəs'θiːziə/ same as **spinal anaesthesia** (NOTE: The US spelling is **rachianesthesia.**)

**rachio-** /reɪkiəʊ/ *prefix* referring to the spine

**rachiotomy** /,reɪki'ɒtəmi/ *noun* same as **laminectomy** (NOTE: The plural is **rachiotomies.**)

**rachis** /'reɪkɪs/ *noun* same as **backbone** (NOTE: The plural is **rachises** or **rachides.**)

**rachischisis** /reɪ'kɪskɪsɪs/ *noun* same as **spina bifida**

**rachitic** /rə'kɪtɪk/ *adjective* referring to rickets

**rachitis** /rə'kaɪtɪs/ *noun* same as **rickets**

**rad** /ræd/ *noun* a unit of measurement of absorbed radiation dose. ◊ **becquerel, gray** (NOTE: **Gray** is now used to mean one hundred rads.)

**radial** /'reɪdɪəl/ *adjective* **1.** referring to something which branches **2.** referring to the radius bone in the arm

**radial artery** /'reɪdɪəl ɑːtəri/ *noun* an artery which branches from the brachial artery, running near the radius, from the elbow to the palm of the hand

**radial nerve** /'reɪdɪəl nɜːv/ *noun* the main motor nerve in the arm, running down the back of the upper arm and the outer side of the forearm

**radial pulse** /'reɪdɪəl pʌls/ *noun* the main pulse in the wrist, taken near the outer edge of the forearm just above the wrist

**radial recurrent** /,reɪdɪəl rɪ'kʌrənt/ *noun* an artery in the arm which forms a loop beside the brachial artery

**radial reflex** /,reɪdɪəl 'riːfleks/ *noun* a jerk made by the forearm when the insertion in the radius of one of the muscles, the brachioradialis, is hit

**radiate** /'reɪdɪeɪt/ *verb* **1.** to spread out in all directions from a central point ○ *The pain radiates from the site of the infection.* **2.** to send out rays ○ *Heat radiates from the body.* (NOTE: **radiating – radiated**)

**radiation** /,reɪdi'eɪʃ(ə)n/ *noun* waves of energy which are given off by some substances, especially radioactive substances

COMMENT: Prolonged exposure to many types of radiation can be harmful. Nuclear radiation is the most obvious, but exposure to X-rays, either as a patient being treated or as a radiographer, can cause radiation sickness. First symptoms of the sickness are diarrhoea and vomiting, but radiation exposure can also be followed by skin burns and loss of hair. Massive exposure to radiation can kill quickly, and any person exposed to radiation is more likely to develop certain types of cancer than other members of the population.

**radiation burn** /,reɪdi'eɪʃ(ə)n bɜːn/ *noun* a burn on the skin caused by exposure to large amounts of radiation

**radiation enteritis** /,reɪdieɪʃ(ə)n ,entə'raɪtɪs/ *noun* enteritis caused by X-rays

**radiation sickness** /,reɪdi'eɪʃ(ə)n ,sɪknəs/ *noun* an illness caused by exposure to radiation from radioactive substances

**radiation treatment** /,reɪdi'eɪʃ(ə)n ,triːtmənt/ *noun* same as **radiotherapy**

**radical** /'rædɪk(ə)l/ *adjective* **1.** aiming to deal with the root of a problem, taking thorough action to remove the source of a disease rather than treat its symptoms **2.** referring to an operation which removes the whole of a part or of an organ, together with its lymph system and other tissue

**radical mastectomy** /ˌrædɪk(ə)l mæ ˈstektəmi/ *noun* a surgical operation to remove a breast and the lymph nodes and muscles associated with it

**radical mastoidectomy** /ˌrædɪk(ə)l mæstɔɪˈdektəmi/ *noun* a surgical operation to remove all of the mastoid process

**radical treatment** /ˌrædɪk(ə)l ˈtriːtmənt/ *noun* treatment which aims at complete eradication of a disease

**radicle** /ˈrædɪk(ə)l/ *noun* **1.** a small root or vein **2.** a tiny fibre which forms the root of a nerve

**radicular** /rəˈdɪkjʊlə/ *adjective* referring to a radicle

**radiculitis** /rəˌdɪkjʊˈlaɪtɪs/ *noun* inflammation of a radicle of a cranial or spinal nerve

**radio-** /ˈreɪdiəʊ/ *prefix* **1.** referring to radiation **2.** referring to radioactive substances **3.** referring to the radius in the arm

**radioactive** /ˌreɪdiəʊˈæktɪv/ *adjective* with a nucleus which disintegrates and gives off energy in the form of radiation which can pass through other substances

COMMENT: The commonest naturally radioactive substances are radium and uranium. Other substances can be made radioactive for medical purposes by making their nuclei unstable, so forming radioactive isotopes. Radioactive iodine is used to treat conditions such as thyrotoxicosis. Radioactive isotopes of various chemicals are used to check the functioning of, or disease in, internal organs.

**radioactive isotope** /ˌreɪdiəʊæktɪv ˈaɪsətəʊp/ *noun* an isotope which sends out radiation, used in radiotherapy and scanning

**radioactivity** /ˌreɪdiəʊækˈtɪvɪti/ *noun* energy in the form of radiation emitted by a radioactive substance

**radiobiologist** /ˌreɪdiəʊbaɪˈɒlədʒɪst/ *noun* a doctor who specialises in radiobiology

**radiobiology** /ˌreɪdiəʊbaɪˈɒlədʒi/ *noun* the scientific study of radiation and its effects on living things

**radiocarpal joint** /reɪdiəʊˈkɑːp(ə)l dʒɔɪnt/ *noun* the joint where the radius articulates with the scaphoid, one of the carpal bones. Also called **wrist joint**

**radiodermatitis** /ˌreɪdiəʊˌdɜːməˈtaɪtɪs/ *noun* inflammation of the skin caused by exposure to radiation

**radiodiagnosis** /ˌreɪdiəʊdaɪəgˈnəʊsɪs/ *noun* an X-ray diagnosis

**radiograph** /ˈreɪdiəɡrɑːf/ *noun* an image produced on film or another sensitive surface when radiation such as X-rays or gamma rays passes through an object ■ *verb* to make a radiograph of something, especially a part of the body

**radiographer** /ˌreɪdiˈɒɡrəfə/ *noun* **1.** a person specially trained to operate a machine to take X-ray photographs or radiographs. Also called **diagnostic radiographer 2.** a person specially trained to use X-rays or radioactive isotopes in the treatment of patients. Also called **therapeutic radiographer**

**radiography** /ˌreɪdiˈɒɡrəfi/ *noun* the work of examining the internal parts of the body by taking X-ray photographs

**radioimmunoassay** /ˌreɪdiəʊˌɪmjʊnəʊ ˈæseɪ/ *noun* the use of radioactive tracers to investigate the presence of antibodies in blood samples, in order to measure the antibodies themselves or the amount of particular substances, such as hormones, in the blood

**radioisotope** /ˌreɪdiəʊˈaɪsətəʊp/ *noun* an isotope of a chemical element which is radioactive

COMMENT: Radioisotopes are used in medicine to provide radiation for radiation treatment. Radioactive isotopes of various chemicals are used to check the way organs function or if they are diseased: for example, radioisotopes of iodine are used to investigate thyroid activity.

**radiologist** /ˌreɪdiˈɒlədʒɪst/ *noun* a doctor who specialises in radiology

**radiology** /ˌreɪdiˈɒlədʒi/ *noun* the use of radiation to diagnose disorders, e.g. through the use of X-rays or radioactive tracers, or to treat diseases such as cancer

**radiomimetic** /ˌreɪdiəʊmɪˈmetɪk/ *adjective* referring to a drug or chemical which produces similar effects to those of radiation, e.g. the nitrogen mustard group of chemicals used in chemotherapy

**radionuclide** /ˌreɪdiəʊˈnjuːklaɪd/ *noun* an element which gives out radiation

**radionuclide scan** /ˌreɪdiəʊˈnjuːklaɪd ˌskæn/ *noun* a scan, especially of the brain, where radionuclides are put in compounds which are concentrated in particular parts of the body

**radio-opaque** /ˌreɪdiəʊ əʊˈpeɪk/ *adjective* absorbing and blocking radiant energy, e.g. X-rays

COMMENT: Radio-opaque substances appear light or white on X-rays and are used to make it easier to have clear radiographs of certain organs.

**radio-opaque dye** /ˌreɪdiəʊ əʊˌpeɪk ˈdaɪ/ *noun* a liquid which appears on an X-ray, and which is introduced into soft organs such as the kidney so that they show up clearly on an X-ray photograph

**radiopaque** /ˌreɪdiəʊˈpeɪk/ *adjective* same as **radio-opaque**

**radiopharmaceutical** /ˌreɪdiəʊˌfɑːmə ˈsuːtɪk(ə)l/ *noun* a radioisotope used in medical diagnosis or treatment

**radio pill** /ˈreɪdiəʊ pɪl/ *noun* a tablet with a tiny radio transmitter

COMMENT: The person swallows the pill and as it passes through the body it gives off information about the digestive system.

**radioscopy** /ˌreɪdiˈɒskəpi/ *noun* an examination of an X-ray photograph on a fluorescent screen

**radiosensitive** /ˌreɪdiəʊˈsensɪtɪv/ *adjective* referring to a cancer cell which is sensitive to radiation and can be treated by radiotherapy

**radiosensitivity** /ˌreɪdiəʊsensəˈtɪvɪti/ *noun* sensitivity of a cell to radiation

**radiotherapist** /ˌreɪdiəʊˈθerəpɪst/ *noun* a doctor who specialises in radiotherapy

**radiotherapy** /ˌreɪdiəʊˈθerəpi/ *noun* the treatment of diseases by exposing the affected part to radioactive rays such as X-rays or gamma rays

COMMENT: Many forms of cancer can be treated by directing radiation at the diseased part of the body.

**radium** /ˈreɪdiəm/ *noun* a radioactive metallic element (NOTE: The chemical symbol is **Ra**.)

**radius** /ˈreɪdiəs/ *noun* the shorter and outer of the two bones in the forearm between the elbow and the wrist. See illustration at HAND in Supplement (NOTE: The plural is **radii**. The other bone in the forearm is the **ulna**.)

**radix** /ˈreɪdɪks/ *noun* same as **root** (NOTE: The plural is **radices** or **radixes**.)

**radon** /ˈreɪdɒn/ *noun* a radioactive gas, formed from the radioactive decay of radium, and used in capsules called radon seeds to treat cancers inside the body (NOTE: The chemical symbol is **Rn**.)

COMMENT: Radon occurs naturally in soil, in construction materials and even in ground water. It can seep into houses and causes radiation sickness.

**raise** /reɪz/ *verb* 1. to lift something ○ *Lie with your legs raised above the level of your head.* 2. to increase something ○ *Anaemia causes a raised level of white blood cells in the body.*

**rale** /rɑːl/ *noun* same as **crepitation**

**rally** /ˈræli/ *verb* to recover after a period of illness ■ *noun* a sudden recovery after a period of illness

**Ramstedt's operation** /ˈrɑːmstets ɒpəˌreɪʃ(ə)n/ *noun* same as **pylorotomy** [Described 1912. After Wilhelm Conrad Ramstedt (1867–1963), German surgeon.]

**ramus** /ˈreɪməs/ *noun* 1. a branch of a nerve, artery or vein 2. the ascending part on each side of the mandible (NOTE: The plural is **rami**.)

**R & D** /ˌɑːr ən ˈdiː/ *abbr* research and development

**randomised** /ˈrændəmaɪzd/, **randomized** *adjective* involving subjects which have been selected without a prearranged plan and in no particular pattern or order

**range** /reɪndʒ/ *noun* 1. a series of different but similar things ○ *The drug offers protection against a wide range of diseases.* ○ *Doctors*

*have a range of drugs which can be used to treat arthritis.* 2. the difference between lowest and highest values in a series of data

**ranitidine** /ræˈnɪtɪdiːn/ *noun* a drug which reduces the amount of acid released by the stomach. It is used to treat peptic ulcers and gastritis.

**ranula** /ˈrænjʊlə/ *noun* a small cyst under the tongue, on the floor of the mouth, which forms when a salivary duct is blocked

**Ranvier** /ˈrɑːnvɪˌeɪ/ ♦ **node of Ranvier**

**rape** /reɪp/ *noun* the crime of forcing somebody to have sexual intercourse ■ *verb* to force somebody to have sexual intercourse

**raphe** /ˈreɪfi/ *noun* a long thin fold which looks like a seam, along a midline such as on the dorsal face of the tongue

**rapid** /ˈræpɪd/ *adjective* fast

**rapid-acting** /ˌræpɪd ˈæktɪŋ/ *adjective* referring to a drug or treatment which has an effect very quickly

**rapid eye movement sleep** /ˌræpɪd aɪ ˈmuːvmənt sliːp/ *noun* same as **REM sleep**

**rapport** /ræˈpɔː/ *noun* an emotional bond or friendly relationship between people ○ *a psychiatrist who quickly establishes a rapport with his patients*

**rare** /reə/ *adjective* referring to something such as a disease of which there are very few cases ○ *He is suffering from a rare blood disorder.*

**rarefaction** /ˌreərɪˈfækʃən/ *noun* a condition in which bone tissue becomes more porous and less dense because of a lack of calcium

**rarefy** /ˈreərɪfaɪ/ *verb* 1. (*of bones*) to become less dense 2. to make something less dense

**rash** /ræʃ/ *noun* a mass of small spots which stays on the skin for a period of time, and then disappears □ **to break out in a rash** to have a rash which starts suddenly ○ *She had a high temperature and then broke out in a rash.*

COMMENT: Many common diseases such as chickenpox and measles have a characteristic rash as their main symptom. Rashes can be very irritating, but the itching can be relieved by applying calamine lotion.

**raspatory** /ˈræspət(ə)ri/ *noun* a surgical instrument like a file, which is used to scrape the surface of a bone

**ratbite fever** /ˈrætbaɪt ˌfiːvə/, **ratbite disease** /ˈrætbaɪt dɪˌziːz/ *noun* fever caused by either of two bacteria *Spirillum minor* or *Streptobacillus moniliformis* and transmitted to humans by rats

**rate** /reɪt/ *noun* 1. the amount or proportion of something compared with something else 2. the number of times something happens in a set time ○ *The heart was beating at a rate of only 59 per minute.*

**ratio** /ˈreɪʃiəʊ/ *noun* a number which shows a proportion or which is the result of one number divided by another ○ *An IQ is the ratio* *of the person's mental age to his or her chronological age.*

**rattle** /'ræt(ə)l/ *noun* a harsh noise made in the throat, caused by a blockage to breathing and heard especially near death

**Rauwolfia** /rɔː'wʊlfiə/ *noun* a tranquillising drug extracted from the plant *Rauwolfia serpentine*, sometimes used to treat high blood pressure

**raw** /rɔː/ *adjective* **1.** not cooked **2.** sensitive ○ *The scab came off leaving the raw wound exposed to the air.* **3.** referring to skin scraped or partly removed

**ray** /reɪ/ *noun* a line of light, radiation or heat

**Raynaud's disease** /'reɪnəʊ dɪˌziːz/, **Raynaud's phenomenon** /'reɪnəʊ fɪˌnɒmɪnən/ *noun* a condition with various possible causes in which the blood supply to the fingers and toes is restricted and they become cold, white and numb. Also called **dead man's fingers, vasospasm** [Described 1862. After Maurice Raynaud (1834–81), French physician.]

**RBC** *abbr* red blood cell

**RCGP** *abbr* Royal College of General Practitioners

**RCN** *abbr* Royal College of Nursing

**RCOG** *abbr* Royal College of Obstetricians and Gynaecologists

**RCP** *abbr* Royal College of Physicians

**RCPsych** /ˌɑː siː 'saɪk/ *abbr* Royal College of Psychiatrists

**RCS** *abbr* Royal College of Surgeons

**RCT** *abbr* randomised controlled trial

**reabsorb** /ˌriːəb'zɔːb/ *verb* to absorb or take up something again ○ *Glucose is reabsorbed by the tubules in the kidney.*

**reabsorption** /ˌriːəb'zɔːpʃ(ə)n/ *noun* the process of being reabsorbed ○ *Some substances which are filtered into the tubules of the kidney, then pass into the bloodstream by tubular reabsorption.*

**reach** /riːtʃ/ *noun* **1.** the distance which one can stretch to get hold of or touch something ○ *Medicines should be kept out of the reach of children.* **2.** the distance which one can travel easily ○ *The hospital is in easy reach of the railway station.* ■ *verb* to arrive at a point ○ *The infection has reached the lungs.*

**react** /ri'ækt/ *verb* **1.** □ **to react to something** to act because of something else, to act in response to something ○ *The tissues reacted to the cortisone injection.* ○ *The patient reacted badly to the penicillin.* ○ *She reacted positively to the Widal test.* **2.** □ **to react with something** (*of a chemical substance*) to change because of the presence of another substance

**reaction** /ri'ækʃən/ *noun* **1.** an action which takes place as a direct result of something which has happened earlier ○ *A rash appeared as a reaction to the penicillin injection.* **2.** an effect produced by a stimulus ○ *The patient*

*experienced an allergic reaction to oranges.* **3.** the particular response of someone to a test

**reactionary** /ri'ækʃən(ə)ri/ *adjective* same as **reactive**

**reactionary haemorrhage** /riˌækʃən(ə)ri 'hem(ə)rɪdʒ/ *noun* bleeding which follows an operation

**reactivate** /ri'æktɪveɪt/ *verb* to make something active again ○ *His general physical weakness has reactivated the dormant virus.*

**reactive** /ri'æktɪv/ *adjective* taking place as a reaction to something else

**reactive arthritis** /riˌæktɪv ɑː'θraɪtɪs/ *noun* arthritis caused by a reaction to something

**reactive hyperaemia** /riˌæktɪv ˌhaɪpər 'iːmiə/ *noun* congestion of blood vessels after an occlusion has been removed

**reading** /'riːdɪŋ/ *noun* a note taken of figures, especially of degrees on a scale ○ *The sphygmomanometer gave a diastolic reading of 70.*

**reagent** /ri'eɪdʒənt/ *noun* a chemical substance which reacts with another substance, especially one which is used to detect the presence of the second substance

**reagin** /'riədʒɪn/ *noun* an antibody which reacts against an allergen

**real-time imaging** /ˌrɪəl taɪm 'ɪmɪdʒɪŋ/ *noun* the use of ultrasound information to produce a series of images of a process or changing object almost instantly

**reappear** /ˌriːə'pɪə/ *verb* to appear again

**rear** /rɪə/, **rear end** /rɪə end/ *noun* same as **buttock** (*informal*)

**reason** /'riːz(ə)n/ *noun* **1.** something which explains why something happens ○ *What was the reason for the sudden drop in the patient's pulse rate?* **2.** the fact of being mentally stable ○ *Her reason was beginning to fail.*

**reassurance** /ˌriːə'ʃʊərəns/ *noun* an act of reassuring

**reassure** /ˌriːə'ʃʊə/ *verb* to calm someone who is worried and give them hope ○ *The doctor reassured her that the drug had no unpleasant side-effects.* ○ *He reassured the old lady that she should be able to walk again in a few weeks.*

**Reaven's Syndrome** /'riːvənz ˌsɪndrəʊm/ *noun* a clinical syndrome characterised by Type 2 diabetes, abdominal obesity, hypertension and dyslipidaemia. Insulin resistance may be a key factor. [Described 1988. After Gerald Reaven, US physician.]

**rebore** /'riːbɔː/ *noun* same as **endarterectomy** (*informal*)

**rebuild** /riː'bɪld/ *verb* to make good again a damaged structure or part of the body ○ *After the accident, she had several operations to rebuild her pelvis.*

**recalcitrant** /rɪ'kælsɪtrənt/ *adjective* not responding to treatment ○ *a recalcitrant condition*

**recall** /rɪˈkɔːl/ *noun* the act of remembering something from the past ■ *verb* to remember something which happened in the past

**recanalisation** /riːˌkænəlaɪˈzeɪʃ(ə)n/, **recanalization** *noun* surgery to unblock a vessel within the body or reconnect a tube or duct

**receive** /rɪˈsiːv/ *verb* to get something, especially a transplanted organ ○ *She received six pints of blood in a transfusion.* ○ *He received a new kidney from his brother.*

**receptaculum** /riːsepˈtækjʊləm/ *noun* part of a tube which is expanded to form a sac

**receptor** /rɪˈseptə/, **receptor cell** /rɪˈseptə sel/ *noun* a nerve ending or cell which senses a change such as cold or heat in the surrounding environment or in the body and reacts to it by sending an impulse to the central nervous system

**recess** /rɪˈses/ *noun* a hollow part in an organ

**recessive** /rɪˈsesɪv/ *adjective* (*of an allele*) having the characteristic that leads to the trait which it controls being suppressed by the presence of the corresponding dominant allele. Compare **dominant**

COMMENT: Since each physical characteristic is governed by two genes, if one is dominant and the other recessive, the resulting trait will be that of the dominant gene. Traits governed by recessive genes will appear if both genes are recessive.

**recipient** /rɪˈsɪpiənt/ *noun* a person who receives something such as a transplant or a blood transfusion from a donor

'…bone marrow from donors has to be carefully matched with the recipient or graft-versus-host disease will ensue' [*Hospital Update*]

**recognise** /ˈrekəgnaɪz/, **recognize** *verb* **1.** to see or sense something or someone and remember it from an earlier occasion ○ *She did not recognise her mother.* **2.** to approve of something officially ○ *The diploma is recognised by the Department of Health.*

**recombinant DNA** /rɪˌkɒmbɪnənt diː en ˈeɪ/ *noun* DNA extracted from two or more different sources and joined together to form a single molecule or fragment. This technology is used to produce molecules and organisms with new properties.

**recommend** /ˌrekəˈmend/ *verb* to suggest that it would be a good thing if someone did something ○ *The doctor recommended that she should stay in bed.* ○ *I would recommend following a diet to try to lose some weight.*

**reconstruct** /ˌriːkənˈstrʌkt/ *verb* to repair and rebuild a damaged part of the body

**reconstruction** /ˌriːkənˈstrʌkʃən/ *noun* the process of repairing and rebuilding a damaged part of the body

**reconstructive surgery** /ˌriːkənstrʌktɪv ˈsɜːdʒəri/ *noun* surgery which rebuilds a damaged part of the body. ◊ **plastic surgery**

**record** /ˈrekɔːd/ *verb* /rɪˈkɔːd/ to note information ○ *The chart records the variations in the patient's blood pressure.* ○ *You must take the patient's temperature every hour and record it in this book.* ■ *noun* a piece of information about something

COMMENT: Patients now have a legal right to have access to their medical records.

**recover** /rɪˈkʌvə/ *verb* **1.** to get better after an illness, operation or accident ○ *She recovered from her concussion in a few days.* ○ *It will take him weeks to recover from the accident.* (NOTE: You recover **from** an illness.) **2.** to get back something which has been lost ○ *Will he ever recover the use of his legs?* ○ *She recovered her eyesight even though the doctors had thought she would be permanently blind.*

**recovery** /rɪˈkʌv(ə)ri/ *noun* the process of returning to health after being ill or injured □ **he is well on the way to recovery** he is getting better □ **she made only a partial recovery** she is better, but is not completely well □ **she has made a complete** or **splendid recovery** she is completely well

**recovery position** /rɪˈkʌvəri pəˌzɪʃ(ə)n/ *noun* a position in which someone is lying face downwards, with one knee and one arm bent forwards and the face turned to one side

COMMENT: It is called the recovery position because it is recommended for accident victims or for people who are suddenly ill, while waiting for an ambulance to arrive. The position prevents the person from swallowing and choking on blood or vomit.

**recovery room** /rɪˈkʌv(ə)ri ruːm/ *noun* a room in a hospital where patients are cared for after they have had a surgical operation and are recovering from the effects of the anaesthetic. Abbr **RR**

**recreational drug** /ˌrekriˈeɪʃ(ə)n(ə)l drʌg/ *noun* a drug that is taken for pleasure rather than because of medical need

**recrudescence** /ˌriːkruːˈdes(ə)ns/ *noun* the reappearance of symptoms of a disease which seemed to have got better

**recrudescent** /ˌriːkruːˈdes(ə)nt/ *adjective* referring to a symptom which has reappeared

**recruit** /rɪˈkruːt/ *verb* to get people to join the staff or a group ○ *We are trying to recruit more nursing staff.*

'…patients presenting with symptoms of urinary tract infection were recruited in a general practice surgery' [*Journal of the Royal College of General Practitioners*]

**rect-** /rekt/ *prefix* same as **recto-** (used before vowels)

**recta** /ˈrektə/ plural of **rectum**

**rectal** /ˈrekt(ə)l/ *adjective* referring to the rectum

**rectal fissure** /ˌrekt(ə)l ˈfɪʃə/ *noun* a crack in the wall of the anal canal

**rectally** /ˈrekt(ə)li/ *adverb* through the rectum ○ *The temperature was taken rectally.*

**rectal prolapse** /ˌrekt(ə)l ˈprəʊlæps/ *noun* a condition in which part of the rectum moves downwards and passes through the anus

**rectal temperature** /ˌrekt(ə)l ˈtemprɪtʃə/ *noun* the temperature in the rectum, taken with a rectal thermometer

**rectal thermometer** /ˌrekt(ə)l θəˈmɒmɪtə/ *noun* a thermometer which is inserted into the rectum to take the person's temperature

**rectal triangle** /ˌrekt(ə)l ˈtraɪæŋg(ə)l/ *noun* same as **anal triangle**

**recti** /ˈrekti/ plural of **rectus**

**recto-** /rektəʊ/ *prefix* referring to the rectum

**rectocele** /ˈrektəʊsiːl/ *noun* a condition associated with prolapse of the uterus, in which the rectum protrudes into the vagina. Also called **proctocele**

**rectopexy** /ˈrektəʊpeksi/ *noun* a surgical operation to attach a rectum which has prolapsed

**rectoscope** /ˈrektəskəʊp/ *noun* an instrument for looking into the rectum

**rectosigmoid** /ˌrektəʊˈsɪgmɔɪd/ *noun* the part of the large intestine where the sigmoid colon joins the rectum

**rectosigmoidectomy** /ˌrektəʊˌsɪgmɔɪˈdektəmi/ *noun* the surgical removal of the sigmoid colon and the rectum

**rectovaginal** /ˌrektəʊvəˈdʒaɪn(ə)l/ *adjective* relating to both the rectum and the vagina

**rectovaginal examination** /ˌrektəʊvəˌdʒaɪn(ə)l ɪgˌzæmɪˈneɪʃ(ə)n/ *noun* an examination of the rectum and vagina

**rectovesical** /ˌrektəʊˈvesɪk(ə)l/ *adjective* referring to the rectum and the bladder

**rectum** /ˈrektəm/ *noun* the end part of the large intestine leading from the sigmoid colon to the anus. See illustration at DIGESTIVE SYSTEM in Supplement, UROGENITAL SYSTEM (MALE) in Supplement (NOTE: For other terms referring to the rectum, see words beginning with **proct-**, **procto-**.)

**rectus** /ˈrektəs/ *noun* a straight muscle (NOTE: The plural is **recti**.)

    '...there are four recti muscles and two oblique muscles in each eye, which coordinate the movement of the eyes and enable them to work as a pair' [*Nursing Times*]

**rectus abdominis** /ˌrektəs æbˈdɒmɪnɪs/ *noun* a long straight muscle which runs down the front of the abdomen

**rectus femoris** /ˌrektəs ˈfemərɪs/ *noun* a flexor muscle in the front of the thigh, one of the four parts of the quadriceps femoris. ◊ **medial**

**recumbent** /rɪˈkʌmbənt/ *adjective* lying down

**recuperate** /rɪˈkuːpəreɪt/ *verb* to recover, to get better after an illness or accident ○ *He is recuperating after an attack of flu.* ○ *She is going to stay with her mother while she recuperates.*

**recuperation** /rɪˌkuːpəˈreɪʃ(ə)n/ *noun* the process of getting better after an illness ○ *His recuperation will take several months.*

**recur** /rɪˈkɜː/ *verb* to return ○ *The headaches recurred frequently, but usually after the patient had eaten chocolate.*

**recurrence** /rɪˈkʌrəns/ *noun* an act of returning ○ *He had a recurrence of a fever which he had caught in the tropics.*

**recurrent** /rɪˈkʌrənt/ *adjective* **1.** occurring in the same way many times **2.** referring to a vein, artery or nerve which forms a loop

**recurrent abortion** /rɪˌkʌrənt əˈbɔːʃ(ə)n/ *noun* a condition in which a woman has abortions with one pregnancy after another

**recurrent fever** /rɪˌkʌrənt ˈfiːvə/ *noun* a fever like malaria which returns at regular intervals

**red** /red/ *adjective* **1.** of a similar colour to blood ○ *Blood in an artery is bright red, but venous blood is darker.* **2.** (of an area of skin) with an increased blood flow because of heat or infection ■ *noun* a colour similar to that of blood

**red blood cell** /red blʌd sel/ *noun* a blood cell which contains haemoglobin and carries oxygen to the tissues and takes carbon dioxide from them. Abbr **RBC**. Also called **erythrocyte**

**red corpuscle** /ˌred ˈkɔːpʌs(ə)l/ *noun* same as **red blood cell**

**Red Crescent** /red ˈkrez(ə)nt/ *noun* in Islamic countries, an international organisation dedicated to the medical care of the sick and wounded in wars and natural disasters (NOTE: It is known as the Red Cross elsewhere.)

**Red Cross** /red ˈkrɒs/ *noun* an international organisation dedicated to the medical care of the sick and wounded in wars and natural disasters (NOTE: It is known as the Red Crescent in Islamic countries.)

**red–green colourblindness** /ˌred griːn ˈkʌləˌblaɪndnəs/ *noun* same as **deuteranopia**

**Redivac drain** /ˈredɪvæk dreɪn/, **Redivac drainage tube** /ˌredɪvæk ˈdreɪnɪdʒ tjuːb/ *trademark* a tube which drains fluid away from the inside of a wound into a bottle, used mainly after operations on the abdomen

**red marrow** /ˌred ˈmærəʊ/ *noun* the type of bone marrow where red blood cells and some white blood cells are formed

**redness** /ˈrednəs/ *noun* **1.** an area of skin to which the blood flow is increased because of heat or infection ○ *The redness showed where the skin had reacted to the injection.* **2.** a red colour

**reduce** /rɪˈdjuːs/ *verb* **1.** to make something smaller or lower ○ *They used ice packs to try to reduce the patient's temperature.* **2.** to put something such as a dislocated or fractured bone, a displaced organ or part or a hernia back into its proper position so that it can heal

'...blood pressure control reduces the incidence of first stroke and aspirin appears to reduce the risk of stroke after transient ischaemic attacks by some 15%' [*British Journal of Hospital Medicine*]

**reducible** /rɪ'djuːsɪb(ə)l/ *adjective* capable of being reduced

**reducible hernia** /rɪˌdjuːsɪb(ə)l 'hɜːniə/ *noun* a hernia where the organ can be pushed back into place without an operation

**reduction** /rɪ'dʌkʃən/ *noun* **1.** the lessening of something, the process of becoming less ○ *They noted a reduction in body temperature.* **2.** the action of putting a hernia, a dislocated joint or a broken bone back into the correct position

**reduction division** /rɪ'dʌkʃən dɪˌvɪʒ(ə)n/ *noun* same as **meiosis**

**re-emerge** /ˌriː ɪ'mɜːdʒ/ *verb* to come out again

**re-emergence** /ˌriː ɪ'mɜːdʒəns/ *noun* an act of coming out again

**refer** /rɪ'fɜː/ *verb* **1.** to mention or to talk about something ○ *The doctor referred to the patient's history of sinus problems.* **2.** to suggest that someone should consult something ○ *For method of use, please refer to the manufacturer's instructions.* ○ *The user is referred to the page giving the results of the tests.* **3.** to pass on information about a patient to someone else ○ *They referred her case to a gynaecologist.* **4.** to send someone to another doctor, usually a specialist, for advice or treatment ○ *She was referred to a cardiologist.* □ **the GP referred the patient to a consultant** he or she passed details about the patient's case to the consultant so that the consultant could examine them

'27 adult patients admitted to hospital with acute abdominal pains were referred for study because their attending clinicians were uncertain whether to advise an urgent laparotomy' [*Lancet*]

'...many patients from outside districts were referred to London hospitals by their GPs' [*Nursing Times*]

**referral** /rɪ'fɜːrəl/ *noun* the act of sending someone to a specialist ○ *She asked for a referral to a gynaecologist.*

'...he subsequently developed colicky abdominal pain and tenderness which caused his referral' [*British Journal of Hospital Medicine*]

**referred pain** /rɪˌfɜːd 'peɪn/ *noun* same as **synalgia**

**reflection** /rɪ'flekʃən/ *noun* **1.** the image of somebody or something which is seen in a mirror or still water **2.** the process of reflecting something, especially light, sound or heat **3.** careful thought **4.** a situation in which an anatomical structure bends back upon itself

**reflective practice** /rɪˌflektɪv 'præktɪs/ *noun* the process of improving professional skills by monitoring your own actions while they are being carried out, and by then later evaluating them by talking or writing about

them and asking other professionals to give their assessments of you

**reflex** /'riːfleks/, **reflex action** /'riːfleks ˌækʃən/ *noun* a physiological reaction without any conscious thought involved, e.g. a knee jerk or a sneeze, which happens in response to a particular stimulus □ **light reflex**, **pupillary reflex to light** reaction of the pupil of the eye which changes size according to the amount of light going into the eye

**reflex arc** /'riːfleks ˌɑːk/ *noun* the basic system of a reflex action, where a receptor is linked to a motor neurone which in turn is linked to an effector muscle

**reflexologist** /ˌriːflək'sɒlədʒɪst/ *noun* a person specialising in reflexology

**reflexology** /ˌriːflek'sɒlədʒi/ *noun* a treatment to relieve tension by massaging the soles of the feet and thereby stimulating the nerves and increasing the blood supply

**reflux** /'riːflʌks/ *noun* a situation where a fluid flows in the opposite direction to its usual flow ○ *The valves in the veins prevent blood reflux.* ◊ **vesicoureteric reflux**

**reflux oesophagitis** /ˌriːflʌks iːˌsɒfə'dʒaɪtɪs/ *noun* inflammation of the oesophagus caused by regurgitation of acid juices from the stomach

**refract** /rɪ'frækt/ *verb* to make light rays change direction as they go from one medium such as air to another such as water at an angle ○ *The refracting media in the eye are the cornea, the aqueous humour, the vitreous humour and the lens.*

**refraction** /rɪ'frækʃən/ *noun* **1.** a change of direction of light rays as they enter a medium such as the eye **2.** the measurement of the angle at which the light rays bend, as a test to see if someone needs to wear glasses

**refractive** /rɪ'fræktɪv/ *adjective* referring to refraction

**refractometer** /ˌriːfræk'tɒmɪtə/ *noun* an instrument which measures the refraction of the eye. Also called **optometer**

**refractory** /rɪ'frækt(ə)ri/ *adjective* difficult or impossible to treat, or not responding to treatment

**refractory period** /rɪˌfrækt(ə)ri 'pɪəriəd/ *noun* a short space of time after the ventricles of the heart have contracted, when they cannot contract again

**refrigerate** /rɪ'frɪdʒəreɪt/ *verb* to make something cold ○ *The serum should be kept refrigerated.*

**refrigeration** /rɪˌfrɪdʒə'reɪʃ(ə)n/ *noun* **1.** the process of making something cold **2.** the process of making part of the body very cold, to give the effect of an anaesthetic

**refrigerator** /rɪ'frɪdʒəreɪtə/ *noun* a machine which cools and keeps things cold

**regain** /rɪ'geɪn/ *verb* to get back something which was lost ○ *He has regained the use of his left arm.* ○ *She went into a coma and never regained consciousness.*

**regenerate** /rɪ'dʒenəreɪt/ *verb* to grow again, or grow something again

**regeneration** /rɪ,dʒenə'reɪʃ(ə)n/ *noun* the process where tissue that has been destroyed grows again

**regenerative medicine** /rɪ,dʒenərətɪv 'med(ə)s(ə)n/ *noun* the branch of medicine that deals with the repair or replacement of tissues and organs by using advanced materials and methods such as cloning

**regimen** /'redʒɪmən/ *noun* a fixed course of treatment, e.g. a course of drugs or a special diet

**region** /'riːdʒən/ *noun* an area or part which is around something ○ *She experienced itching in the anal region.* ○ *The rash started in the region of the upper thigh.* ○ *The plantar region is very sensitive.*

**regional** /'riːdʒ(ə)nəl/ *adjective* in a particular region, referring to a particular region

**regional enteritis** /,riːdʒ(ə)nəl ,entə 'raɪtɪs/ *noun* same as **Crohn's disease**

**Regional Health Authority** /,riːdʒ(ə)nəl 'helθ ɔː,θɒrɪti/ *noun* an administrative unit in the National Health Service which is responsible for planning the health service in a region. Abbr **RHA**

**regional ileitis** /,riːdʒ(ə)nəl ,ɪli'aɪtɪs/ *noun* compare **ulcerative colitis**. same as **Crohn's disease**

**register** /'redʒɪstə/ *noun* an official list ■ *verb* to write a name on an official list, especially the official list of patients treated by a GP or dentist, or the list of people with a particular disease ○ *He is a registered heroin addict.* ○ *They went to register the birth with the Registrar of Births, Marriages and Deaths.* □ **to register with someone** to put your name on someone's official list, especially the list of patients treated by a GP or dentist ○ *Before registering with the GP, she asked if she could visit him.* ○ *All practising doctors are registered with the General Medical Council.*

**registered midwife** /,redʒɪstəd 'mɪdwaɪf/ *noun* a qualified midwife who is registered to practise

**Registered Nurse** /'redʒɪstəd 'nɜːs/, **Registered General Nurse** /,redʒɪstəd 'dʒen(ə)rəl nɜːs/, **Registered Theatre Nurse** /,redʒɪstəd 'θɪətə nɜːs/ *noun* a nurse who has been registered by the UKCC. Abbr **RN, RGN, RTN**

**registrar** /,redʒɪ'strɑː/ *noun* **1.** a qualified doctor or surgeon in a hospital who supervises house officers **2.** a person who registers something officially

**Registrar of Births, Marriages and Deaths** /,redʒɪstrɑː əv ,bɜːθs ,mærɪdʒɪz ən 'deθs/ *noun* an official who keeps the records of people who have been born, married or who have died in a particular area

**registration** /,redʒɪ'streɪʃ(ə)n/ *noun* the act of registering ○ *A doctor cannot practise without registration by the General Medical Council.*

**regress** /rɪ'gres/ *verb* to return to an earlier stage or condition

**regression** /rɪ'greʃ(ə)n/ *noun* **1.** a stage where symptoms of a disease are disappearing and the person is getting better **2.** (*in psychiatry*) the process of returning to a mental state which existed when the person was younger

**regular** /'regjʊlə/ *adjective* **1.** taking place again and again after the same period of time ○ *He was advised to make regular visits to the dentist.* ○ *She had her regular six-monthly checkup.* **2.** happening at the same time each day

**regularly** /'regjʊləli/ *adverb* happening repeatedly after the same period of time ○ *The tablets must be taken regularly every evening.* ○ *You should go to the dentist regularly.*

**regulate** /'regjʊleɪt/ *verb* to make something work in a regular way ○ *The heartbeat is regulated by the sinoatrial node.*

**regulation** /,regjʊ'leɪʃ(ə)n/ *noun* the act of regulating ○ *the regulation of the body's temperature*

**regurgitate** /rɪ'gɜːdʒɪteɪt/ *verb* to bring into the mouth food which has been partly digested in the stomach

**regurgitation** /rɪ,gɜːdʒɪ'teɪʃ(ə)n/ *noun* the process of flowing back in the opposite direction to the usual flow, especially of bringing up partly digested food from the stomach into the mouth

**rehabilitate** /,riːə'bɪlɪteɪt/ *verb* to make someone fit to work or to lead their usual life

**rehabilitation** /,riːəbɪlɪ'teɪʃ(ə)n/ *noun* the process of making someone fit to work or to lead an ordinary life again

**rehydrate** /,riːhaɪ'dreɪt/ *verb* to restore body fluids to a healthy level, or cause this to occur

**rehydration** /,riːhaɪ'dreɪʃ(ə)n/ *noun* the act of giving water or liquid to someone who has dehydration

**reinfect** /,riːɪn'fekt/ *verb* to infect someone or something again

**reinfection** /,riːɪn'fekʃ(ə)n/ *noun* infection of an area for another time after recovery, especially with the same microorganism

**Reiter's syndrome** /'raɪtəz ,sɪndrəʊm/, **Reiter's disease** /'raɪtəz dɪ'ziːz/ *noun* an illness which may be sexually transmitted and affects mainly men, causing arthritis, urethritis and conjunctivitis at the same time [Described 1916. After Hans Conrad Reiter (1881–1969), German bacteriologist and hygienist.]

**reject** /rɪ'dʒekt/ *verb* **1.** to refuse to accept something **2.** to be unable to tolerate tissue or an organ transplanted from another body because it is immunologically incompatible ○ *The new heart was rejected by the body.* ○ *They gave the patient drugs to prevent the transplant being rejected.* **3.** to be unable to keep food down and vomit it up again

**rejection** /rɪ'dʒekʃən/ *noun* the act of rejecting tissue ○ *The patient was given drugs to reduce the possibility of tissue rejection.*

**relapse** /'riːlæps, rɪ'læps/ *noun* a situation in which someone gets worse after seeming to be getting better, or where a disease appears again after seeming to be cured ■ *verb* to return to an earlier and worse state, especially to get ill again after getting better ○ *She relapsed into a coma.*

**relapsing fever** /rɪ'læpsɪŋ ˌfiːvə/ *noun* a disease caused by a bacterium, where attacks of fever recur from time to time

**relapsing pancreatitis** /rɪˌlæpsɪŋ ˌpæŋkriə'taɪtɪs/ *noun* a form of pancreatitis where the symptoms recur, but in a less painful form

**relate** /rɪ'leɪt/ *verb* to connect something to something else ○ *The disease is related to the weakness of the heart muscles.*

**-related** /rɪleɪtɪd/ *suffix* connected to ○ *drug-related diseases*

**relationship** /rɪ'leɪʃ(ə)nʃɪp/ *noun* a way in which someone or something is connected to another ○ *The incidence of the disease has a close relationship to the environment.* ○ *He became withdrawn and broke off all relationships with his family.*

**relative density** /ˌrelətɪv 'densɪti/ *noun* the ratio of the density of a substance to the density of a standard substance at the same temperature and pressure. For liquids and solids the standard substance is usually water, and for gases, it is air.

**relative risk** /ˌrelətɪv 'rɪsk/ *noun* a measure of the likelihood of developing a disease for people who are exposed to a particular risk, relative to people who are not exposed to the same risk. For example, the relative risk of myocardial infarction for oral contraceptive users is 1.6 times that of non-users. Abbr **RR**

**relax** /rɪ'læks/ *verb* to become less tense, or cause someone or something to become less tense ○ *He was given a drug to relax the muscles.* ○ *The muscle should be fully relaxed.*

**relaxant** /rɪ'læksənt/ *noun* a substance which relieves strain ■ *adjective* relieving strain

**relaxation** /ˌriːlæk'seɪʃ(ə)n/ *noun* **1.** the process of reducing strain in a muscle **2.** the reduction of stress in a person

**relaxation therapy** /ˌriːlæk'seɪʃ(ə)n ˌθerəpi/ *noun* a treatment in which people are encouraged to relax their muscles to reduce stress

**relaxative** /rɪ'læksətɪv/ *noun US* a drug which reduces stress

**relaxin** /rɪ'læksɪn/ *noun* a hormone which is secreted by the placenta to make the cervix relax and open fully in the final stages of pregnancy before childbirth

**release** /rɪ'liːs/ *noun* the process of allowing something to go out ○ *the slow release of the drug into the bloodstream* ■ *verb* to let something out ○ *Hormones are released into the body by glands.*

**releasing factor** /rɪ'liːsɪŋ ˌfæktə/ *noun* a substance produced in the hypothalamus which encourages the release of hormones

**releasing hormone** /rɪ'liːsɪŋ ˌhɔːməʊn/ *noun* a hormone secreted by the hypothalamus which makes the pituitary gland release particular hormones. Also called **hypothalamic hormone**

**relief** /rɪ'liːf/ *noun* the process of making something better or easier ○ *The drug provides rapid relief for patients with bronchial spasms.*

'…complete relief of angina is experienced by 85% of patients subjected to coronary artery bypass surgery' [*British Journal of Hospital Medicine*]

**relieve** /rɪ'liːv/ *verb* to make something better or easier ○ *Nasal congestion can be relieved by antihistamines.* ○ *The patient was given an injection of morphine to relieve the pain.* ○ *The condition is relieved by applying cold compresses.*

'…replacement of the metacarpophalangeal joint is mainly undertaken to relieve pain, deformity and immobility due to rheumatoid arthritis' [*Nursing Times*]

**rem** /rem/ *noun* a unit for measuring amounts of radiation, equal to the effect that one roentgen of X-rays or gamma-rays would produce in a human being. It is used in radiation protection and monitoring.

**REM** /rem/ *abbr* rapid eye movement. ♦ **REM sleep**

**remedial** /rɪ'miːdiəl/ *adjective* acting as a cure

**remedy** /'remədi/ *noun* a cure, a drug which will cure ○ *Honey and glycerine is an old remedy for sore throats.*

**remember** /rɪ'membə/ *verb* to bring back into the mind something which has been seen or heard before ○ *He remembers nothing* or *he can't remember anything about the accident.*

**remission** /rɪ'mɪʃ(ə)n/ *noun* a period when an illness or fever is less severe

**re. mist.** /ˌriː 'mɪst/ *adverb* (*on a prescription*) repeat the same mixture. Full form **repetatur mistura**

**remittent** /rɪ'mɪtənt/ *adjective* lessening and then intensifying again at intervals

**remittent fever** /rɪˌmɪtənt 'fiːvə/ *noun* fever which goes down for a period each day, like typhoid fever

**removal** /rɪ'muːv(ə)l/ *noun* the action of removing something ○ *An appendicectomy is the surgical removal of an appendix.*

**remove** /rɪ'muːv/ *verb* to take something away ○ *He will have an operation to remove an ingrowing toenail.*

**REM sleep** /'rem sliːp/ *noun* a stage of sleep which happens several times each night and is characterised by dreaming, rapid eye movement and increased pulse rate and brain activity. Also called **rapid eye movement sleep**

> COMMENT: During REM sleep, a person dreams, breathes lightly and has a raised blood pressure and an increased rate of heartbeat. The eyes may be half-open, and the sleeper may make facial movements.

**ren-** /riːn/ *prefix* same as **reno-** (*used before vowels*)

**renal** /'riːn(ə)l/ *adjective* referring to the kidneys

**renal artery** /ˌriːn(ə)l 'ɑːtəri/ *noun* one of two arteries running from the abdominal aorta to the kidneys

**renal calculus** /ˌriːn(ə)l 'kælkjʊləs/ *noun* a small hard mineral mass called a stone in the kidney

**renal capsule** /ˌriːn(ə)l 'kæpsjuːl/ *noun* same as **fibrous capsule**

**renal clearance** /'riːn(ə)l ˌklɪərəns/ *noun* the measurement of the rate at which kidneys filter impurities from blood

**renal colic** /ˌriːn(ə)l 'kɒlɪk/ *noun* a sudden pain caused by a kidney stone or stones in the ureter

**renal corpuscle** /ˌriːn(ə)l 'kɔːpʌs(ə)l/ *noun* part of a nephron in the cortex of a kidney. Also called **Malpighian body**

**renal cortex** /ˌriːn(ə)l 'kɔːteks/ *noun* the outer covering of the kidney, immediately beneath the capsule. See illustration at **KIDNEY** in Supplement

**renal dialysis** /ˌriːn(ə)l daɪ'æləsɪs/ *noun* a method of artificially maintaining the chemical balance of the blood when the kidneys have failed, or the process of using this method. Also called **dialysis**

**renal hypertension** /ˌriːn(ə)l ˌhaɪpə'tenʃən/ *noun* high blood pressure linked to kidney disease

**renal medulla** /ˌriːn(ə)l me'dʌlə/ *noun* the inner part of a kidney containing no glomeruli. See illustration at **KIDNEY** in Supplement

**renal pelvis** /ˌriːn(ə)l 'pelvɪs/ *noun* the upper and wider part of the ureter leading from the kidney where urine is collected before passing down the ureter into the bladder. Also called **pelvis of the kidney**. See illustration at **KIDNEY** in Supplement

**renal rickets** /ˌriːn(ə)l 'rɪkɪts/ *noun* a form of rickets caused by kidneys which do not function properly

**renal sinus** /ˌriːn(ə)l 'saɪnəs/ *noun* a cavity in which the renal pelvis and other tubes leading into the kidney fit

**renal transplant** /ˌriːn(ə)l 'trænsplɑːnt/ *noun* a kidney transplant

**renal tubule** /ˌriːn(ə)l 'tjuːbjuːl/ *noun* a tiny tube which is part of a nephron. Also called **uriniferous tubule**

**renew** /rɪ'njuː/ *verb* □ **to renew a prescription** to get a new prescription for the same drug as before

**reni-** /riːni/ *prefix* referring to the kidneys

**renin** /'riːnɪn/ *noun* an enzyme secreted by the kidney to prevent loss of sodium, and which also affects blood pressure

**rennin** /'renɪn/ *noun* an enzyme which makes milk coagulate in the stomach, so as to slow down the passage of the milk through the digestive system

**reno-** /riːnəʊ/ *prefix* referring to the kidneys

**renogram** /'riːnəʊgræm/ *noun* **1.** an X-ray image of a kidney **2.** a visual record of kidney function that shows how quickly a radioactive substance introduced into the bloodstream is removed by the kidneys

**renography** /riː'nɒɡrəfi/ *noun* an examination of a kidney after injection of a radioactive substance, using a gamma camera

**renovascular** /ˌriːnəʊ'væskjʊlə/ *adjective* relating to the blood vessels of the kidneys

**renovascular system** /ˌriːnəʊ'væskjʊlə ˌsɪstəm/ *noun* the blood vessels associated with the kidney

**reorganisation** /riːˌɔːɡənaɪ'zeɪʃ(ə)n/, **reorganization** *noun* **1.** a change in the way something is organised or done **2.** the process of changing the way something is organised or done **3.** an occasion when a business or organisation is given a completely new structure

**reovirus** /'riːəʊˌvaɪrəs/ *noun* a virus which affects both the intestine and the respiratory system, but does not cause serious illness. Compare **echovirus**

**rep** /rep/ *adverb* (*written on a prescription*) repeat. Full form **repetatur**

**repair** /rɪ'peə/ *verb* to make something that is damaged good again ○ *Surgeons operated to repair a hernia.*

**repeat** /rɪ'piːt/ *verb* to say or do something again ○ *The course of treatment was repeated after two months.*

**repeat prescription** /rɪˌpiːt prɪ'skrɪpʃən/ *noun* a prescription which is exactly the same as the previous one, and is often given without examination of the person by the doctor and may sometimes be requested by telephone

**repel** /rɪ'pel/ *verb* to make something go away ○ *If you spread this cream on your skin it will repel insects.*

**repetitive strain injury** /rɪˌpetɪtɪv 'streɪn ˌɪndʒəri/, **repetitive stress injury** /rɪˌpetɪtɪv 'stres ˌɪndʒəri/ *noun* pain, usually in a limb, felt by someone who performs the same movement many times over a period, e.g. when operating a computer terminal or playing a musical instrument. Abbr **RSI**

**replace** /rɪ'pleɪs/ *verb* **1.** to put something back ○ *an operation to replace a prolapsed uterus* **2.** to exchange one part for another ○ *The surgeons replaced the diseased hip with a metal one.*

**replacement** /rɪ'pleɪsmənt/ *noun* an operation to replace part of the body with an artificial part

**replacement transfusion** /rɪˌpleɪsmənt ˌtrænsˈfjuːʒ(ə)n/ *noun* an exchange transfusion, a treatment for leukaemia or erythroblastosis where almost all the unhealthy blood is removed from the body and replaced by healthy blood

**replant** /riː'plɑːnt/ *verb* to reattach or reinsert a body part such as a limb or tooth that has become detached

**replantation** /ˌriːplɑːn'teɪʃ(ə)n/ *noun* a surgical technique which reattaches parts of the body which have been accidentally cut or torn off

**replicate** /'replɪkeɪt/ *verb* (*of a cell*) to make a copy of itself

**replication** /ˌreplɪ'keɪʃ(ə)n/ *noun* the process in the division of a cell, where the DNA makes copies of itself

**repolarisation** /riːˌpəʊləraɪ'zeɪʃ(ə)n/, **repolarization** *noun* the restoration of the usual electrical polarity of a nerve or muscle cell membrane after reversal of its polarity while a nerve impulse or muscle contraction travelled along it

**report** /rɪ'pɔːt/ *noun* an official note stating what action has been taken, what treatment given or what results have come from a test ○ *The patient's report card has to be filled in by the nurse.* ○ *The inspector's report on the hospital kitchens is good.* ■ *verb* to make an official report about something ○ *The patient reported her doctor for misconduct.* ○ *Occupational diseases or serious accidents at work must be reported to the local officials.*

**reportable diseases** /rɪˌpɔːtəb(ə)l dɪ 'ziːzɪz/ *plural noun* diseases such as asbestosis, hepatitis or anthrax which may be caused by working conditions or may infect other workers and must be reported to the District Health Authority

**repositor** /rɪ'pɒzɪtə/ *noun* a surgical instrument used to push a prolapsed organ back into its usual position

**repress** /rɪ'pres/ *verb* to decide to ignore or forget feelings or thoughts which may be unpleasant or painful

**repression** /rɪ'preʃ(ə)n/ *noun* (*in psychiatry*) the act of ignoring or forgetting feelings or thoughts which might be unpleasant

**reproduce** /ˌriːprə'djuːs/ *verb* **1.** to produce children **2.** (*of microorganisms*) to produce new cells **3.** to do a test again in exactly the same way

**reproduction** /ˌriːprə'dʌkʃən/ *noun* the process of making new living beings by existing ones, e.g. producing children or derived other descendants

**reproductive** /ˌriːprə'dʌktɪv/ *adjective* referring to reproduction

**reproductive organs** /ˌriːprə'dʌktɪv ˌɔːgənz/ *plural noun* parts of the bodies of men and women which are involved in the conception and development of a fetus

**reproductive system** /ˌriːprə'dʌktɪv ˌsɪstəm/ *noun* the arrangement of organs and ducts in the bodies of men and women which produce spermatozoa or ova

COMMENT: In the human male, the testes produce the spermatozoa which pass through the vasa efferentia and the vasa deferentia where they receive liquid from the seminal vesicles, then out of the body through the urethra and penis on ejaculation. In the female, an ovum, produced by one of the two ovaries, passes through the Fallopian tube where it is fertilised by a spermatozoon from the male. The fertilised ovum moves down into the uterus where it develops into an embryo.

**reproductive tract** /ˌriːprə'dʌktɪv trækt/ *noun* the series of tubes and ducts which carry spermatozoa or ova from one part of the body to another

**require** /rɪ'kwaɪə/ *verb* to need something ○ *His condition may require surgery.* ○ *Is it a condition which requires immediate treatment?* □ **required effect** effect which a drug is expected to have ○ *If the drug does not produce the required effect, the dose should be increased.*

**requirement** /rɪ'kwaɪəmənt/ *noun* something which is necessary ○ *One of the requirements of the position is a qualification in pharmacy.*

**RES** *abbr* reticuloendothelial system

**research** /rɪ'sɜːtʃ/ *noun* a scientific study which investigates something new ○ *He is the director of a medical research unit.* ○ *She is doing research into finding a cure for leprosy.* ○ *Research workers or Research teams are trying to find a vaccine against AIDS.* ■ *verb* to carry out scientific study ○ *He is researching the origins of cancer.*

**research and development** /rɪˌsɜːtʃ ən dɪ 'veləpmənt/ *noun* the process by which pharmaceutical companies find new drugs and test their suitability. Abbr **R & D**

**resect** /rɪ'sekt/ *verb* to remove any part of the body by surgery

**resection** /rɪ'sekʃən/ *noun* the surgical removal of any part of the body

**resection of the prostate** /rɪˌsekʃən əv ðə ˈprɒsteɪt/ *noun* same as **transurethral prostatectomy**

**resectoscope** /rɪˈsektəskəʊp/ *noun* a surgical instrument used to carry out a transurethral resection

**reservoir** /ˈrezəvwɑː/ *noun* **1.** a cavity in an organ or group of tissues in which fluids collect and are stored **2.** an organism in which a parasite lives and develops without damaging it, but from which the parasite then passes to another species which is damaged by it **3.** a part of a machine or piece of equipment where liquid is stored for it to use

**reset** /riːˈset/ *verb* to break a badly set bone and set it again correctly ○ *His arm had to be reset.*

**residency** /ˈrezɪd(ə)nsi/ *noun US* a period when a doctor is receiving specialist training in a hospital

**resident** /ˈrezɪd(ə)nt/ *noun* **1.** someone who lives in a place ○ *All the residents of the old people's home were tested for food poisoning.* **2.** *US* a qualified doctor who is employed by a hospital and sometimes lives in the hospital. Compare **intern** ■ *adjective* living in a place

**resident doctor** /ˌrezɪd(ə)nt ˈdɒktə/ *noun* a doctor who lives in a building such as an old people's home

**residential** /ˌrezɪˈdenʃəl/ *adjective* **1.** living in a hospital **2.** living at home

**residential care** /ˌrezɪˈdenʃəl keə/ *noun* the care of patients either in a hospital or at home, but not as outpatients

**residual** /rɪˈzɪdjuəl/ *adjective* remaining, which is left behind

**residual air** /rɪˌzɪdjuəl ˈeə/, **residual volume** /rɪˌzɪdjuəl ˈvɒljuːm/ *noun* air left in the lungs after a person has breathed out as much air as possible

**residual urine** /rɪˌzɪdjuəl ˈjʊərɪn/ *noun* urine left in the bladder after a person has passed as much urine as possible

**resin** /ˈrezɪn/ *noun* a sticky sap or liquid which comes from some types of tree

**resist** /rɪˈzɪst/ *verb* to be strong enough to avoid being killed or attacked by a disease ○ *A healthy body can resist some infections.*

**resistance** /rɪˈzɪstəns/ *noun* **1.** the ability of a person not to get a disease **2.** the ability of bacteria or a virus to remain unaffected by a drug ○ *The bacteria have developed a resistance to certain antibiotics.* **3.** opposition to a force

**resistant** /rɪˈzɪst(ə)nt/ *adjective* able not to be affected by something ○ *The bacteria are resistant to some antibiotics.*

**resistant strain** /rɪˌzɪst(ə)nt ˈstreɪn/ *noun* a strain of bacterium which is not affected by antibiotics

**resolution** /ˌrezəˈluːʃ(ə)n/ *noun* **1.** the amount of detail which can be seen in a microscope or on a computer monitor **2.** a point in the development of a disease where the inflammation begins to disappear

**resolve** /rɪˈzɒlv/ *verb* (*of inflammation*) to begin to disappear

'…valve fluttering disappears as the pneumothorax resolves. Always confirm resolution with a physical examination and X-ray' [*American Journal of Nursing*]

**resolvent** /rɪˈzɒlvənt/ *adjective* able to reduce inflammation or swelling

**resonance** /ˈrez(ə)nəns/ *noun* a sound made by a hollow part of the body when hit. ◊ **magnetic**

**resorption** /rɪˈsɔːpʃən/ *noun* the process of absorbing a substance produced by the body back into the body

**respiration** /ˌrespəˈreɪʃ(ə)n/ *noun* the act of taking air into the lungs and blowing it out again through the mouth or nose. Also called **breathing**

COMMENT: Respiration includes two stages: breathing in (inhalation) and breathing out (exhalation). Air is taken into the respiratory system through the nose or mouth, and goes down into the lungs through the pharynx, larynx and windpipe. In the lungs, the bronchi take the air to the alveoli (air sacs) where oxygen in the air is passed to the bloodstream in exchange for waste carbon dioxide which is then breathed out.

**respiration rate** /ˌrespəˈreɪʃ(ə)n reɪt/ *noun* the number of times a person breathes per minute

**respirator** /ˈrespəreɪtə/ *noun* **1.** same as **ventilator** □ **the patient was put on a respirator** the patient was attached to a machine which forced him to breathe **2.** a mask worn to prevent someone breathing harmful gas or fumes

**respiratory** /rɪˈspɪrət(ə)ri/ *adjective* referring to breathing

**respiratory allergy** /rɪˌspɪrət(ə)ri ˈælədʒi/ *noun* an allergy caused by a substance which is inhaled. ◊ **alveolitis, food allergy**

**respiratory bronchiole** /rɪˌspɪrət(ə)ri ˈbrɒŋkiəʊl/ *noun* the end part of a bronchiole in the lung, which joins the alveoli

**respiratory centre** /rɪˌspɪrət(ə)ri ˈsentə/ *noun* a nerve centre in the brain which regulates the breathing

**respiratory distress syndrome** /rɪˌspɪrət(ə)ri dɪˈstres ˌsɪndrəʊm/ *noun* a condition of newborn babies, and especially common in premature babies, in which the lungs do not expand properly, due to lack of surfactant. Also called **hyaline membrane disease**

**respiratory failure** /rɪˌspɪrət(ə)ri ˈfeɪljə/ *noun* failure of the lungs to oxygenate the blood correctly

**respiratory illness** /rɪˌspɪrət(ə)ri ˈɪlnəs/ *noun* an illness which affects someone's breathing

**respiratory pigment** /rɪˌspɪrət(ə)ri ˈpɪgmənt/ *noun* blood pigment which can carry oxygen collected in the lungs and release it in tissues

**respiratory quotient** /rɪˌspɪrət(ə)ri ˈkwəʊʃ(ə)nt/ *noun* the ratio of the amount of carbon dioxide taken into the alveoli of the lungs from the blood to the amount of oxygen which the alveoli take from the air. Abbr **RQ**

**respiratory syncytial virus** /rɪˌspɪrət(ə)ri sɪnˈsɪtiəl ˌvaɪrəs/ *noun* a virus which causes infections of the nose and throat in adults, but serious bronchiolitis in children. Abbr **RSV**

**respiratory system** /rɪˈspɪrət(ə)ri ˈsɪstəm/, **respiratory tract** /rɪˈspɪrət(ə)ri trækt/ *noun* the series of organs and passages which take air into the lungs, and exchange oxygen for carbon dioxide

**respite care** /ˈrespaɪt keə/ *noun* temporary care provided to people with disabilities, serious conditions or terminal illness, so that their families can have a rest from the daily routine

**respond** /rɪˈspɒnd/ *verb* **1.** to react to something ○ *The cancer is not responding to drugs.* **2.** to begin to get better because of a treatment ○ *She is responding to treatment.*

'...many severely confused patients, particularly those in advanced stages of Alzheimer's disease, do not respond to verbal communication' [*Nursing Times*]

**response** /rɪˈspɒns/ *noun* a reaction by an organ, tissue or a person to an external stimulus ◇ **immune response 1.** reaction of a body to an antigen **2.** reaction of a body which rejects a transplant

'...anaemia may be due to insufficient erythrocyte production, in which case the reticulocyte count will be low, or to haemolysis or haemorrhage, in which cases there should be a reticulocyte response' [*Southern Medical Journal*]

**responsibility** /rɪˌspɒnsɪˈbɪlɪti/ *noun* **1.** somebody or something which a person or organisation has a duty to take care of ○ *Checking the drip is your responsibility.* **2.** the blame for something bad which has happened ○ *She has taken full responsibility for the mix-up.* **3.** the position of having to explain to somebody why something was done ○ *Whose responsibility is it to talk to the family?*

**responsible** /rɪˈspɒnsɪb(ə)l/ *adjective* referring to something which is the cause of something else ○ *the allergen which is responsible for the patient's reaction* ○ *This is one of several factors which can be responsible for high blood pressure.*

**responsive** /rɪˈspɒnsɪv/ *adjective* reacting positively to medical treatment

**responsiveness** /rɪˈspɒnsɪvnəs/ *noun* the ability to respond to other people or to sensations

**rest** /rest/ *noun* a period of time spent relaxing or sleeping ○ *What you need is a good night's rest.* ■ *verb* **1.** to spend time relaxing or sleeping **2.** to use a body part less for a period of time ○ *Rest your arm for a week.*

**restenosis** /ˌriːstəˈnəʊsɪs/ *noun* an occasion when something becomes narrow again, e.g. a coronary artery which has previously been widened by balloon angioplasty (NOTE: The plural is **restenoses**.)

**restless** /ˈrestləs/ *adjective* not able to relax or be still ○ *restless sleep* ○ *She had a restless night.*

**restless leg syndrome** /ˌrestləs ˈleg ˌsɪndrəʊm/ *noun* painful discomfort in the legs when not active that can lead to interrupted sleep and fatigue

**restore** /rɪˈstɔː/ *verb* to give something back ○ *She needs vitamins to restore her strength.* ○ *The physiotherapy should restore the strength of the muscles.* ○ *A salpingostomy was performed to restore the patency of the Fallopian tube.*

**restrict** /rɪˈstrɪkt/ *verb* **1.** to make something less or smaller ○ *The blood supply is restricted by the tight bandage.* **2.** to set limits to something ○ *The doctor suggested she should restrict her intake of alcohol.*

**restrictive** /rɪˈstrɪktɪv/ *adjective* restricting, making something smaller

**result** /rɪˈzʌlt/ *noun* figures at the end of a calculation, at the end of a test ○ *What was the result of the test?* ○ *The doctor told the patient the result of the pregnancy test.* ○ *The result of the operation will not be known for some weeks.*

**resuscitate** /rɪˈsʌsɪteɪt/ *verb* to make someone who appears to be dead start breathing again, and to restart the circulation of blood

**resuscitation** /rɪˌsʌsɪˈteɪʃ(ə)n/ *noun* the act of reviving someone who seems to be dead, by making him or her breathe again and restarting the heart

COMMENT: The commonest methods of resuscitation are artificial respiration and cardiac massage.

**retain** /rɪˈteɪn/ *verb* to keep or hold something ○ *He was incontinent and unable to retain urine in his bladder.* ◊ **retention**

**retard** /rɪˈtɑːd/ *verb* to make something slower, e.g. to slow down the action of a drug ○ *The drug will retard the onset of the fever.* ○ *The injections retard the effect of the anaesthetic.*

**retardation** /ˌriːtɑːˈdeɪʃ(ə)n/ *noun* the process of making something slower

**retch** /retʃ/ *verb* to try to vomit without bringing any food up from the stomach

**retching** /ˈretʃɪŋ/ *noun* the fact of attempting to vomit without being able to do so

**rete** /ˈriːtiː/ *noun* a network of veins, arteries or nerve fibres in the body. ◊ **reticular** (NOTE: The plural is **retia**.)

**retention** /rɪ'tenʃən/ *noun* the act of not letting out something, especially a fluid, which is usually released from the body, e.g. holding back urine in the bladder

**retention cyst** /rɪ'tenʃən sɪst/ *noun* a cyst which is formed when a duct from a gland is blocked

**retention of urine** /rɪ,tenʃən əv 'jʊərɪn/ *noun* a condition in which passing urine is difficult or impossible because the urethra is blocked or because the prostate gland is enlarged

**rete testis** /,riːtiː 'testɪs/ *noun* a network of channels in the testis which take the sperm to the epididymis. ◊ **reticular**

**retia** /'riːʃiə/ plural of **rete**

**reticular** /rɪ'tɪkjʊlə/ *adjective* relating to or in the form of a network

**reticular fibres** /rɪ,tɪkjʊlə 'faɪbəs/ *plural noun* fibres in connective tissue which support, e.g., organs or blood vessels

**reticular tissue** /rɪ,tɪkjʊlə 'tɪʃuː/ *noun* same as **reticular fibres**

**reticulin** /rɪ'tɪkjʊliːn/ *noun* a fibrous protein which is one of the most important components of reticular fibres

**reticulocyte** /rɪ'tɪkjʊləʊsaɪt/ *noun* a red blood cell which has not yet fully developed

**reticulocytosis** /rɪ,tɪkjʊləʊsaɪ'təʊsɪs/ *noun* a condition in which the number of reticulocytes in the blood increases unusually

**reticuloendothelial cell** /rɪ,tɪkjʊləʊ ,endəʊ'θiːliəl sel/ *noun* a phagocytic cell in the reticuloendolethial system

**reticuloendothelial system** /rɪ,tɪkjʊləʊ ,endəʊ'θiːliəl ,sɪstəm/ *noun* a series of phagocytic cells in the body, found especially in bone marrow, lymph nodes, liver and spleen, which attack and destroy bacteria and form antibodies. Abbr **RES**

**reticuloendotheliosis** /rɪ,tɪkjʊləʊ,endəʊ θiːli'əʊsɪs/ *noun* a condition in which cells in the RES grow large and form swellings in bone marrow or destroy bones

**reticulosis** /rɪ,tɪkjʊ'ləʊsɪs/ *noun* any of several conditions where cells in the reticuloendothelial system grow large and form usually malignant tumours

**reticulum** /rɪ'tɪkjʊləm/ *noun* a series of small fibres or tubes forming a network

**retin-** /retɪn/ *prefix* same as **retino-** (*used before vowels*)

**retina** /'retɪnə/ *noun* the inside layer of the eye which is sensitive to light. ◊ **detached retina**. See illustration at **EYE** in Supplement
(NOTE: The plural is **retinae**.)

COMMENT: Light enters the eye through the pupil and strikes the retina. Light-sensitive cells in the retina (cones and rods) convert the light to nervous impulses. The optic nerve sends these impulses to the brain which interprets them as images. The point where the optic nerve joins the retina has no light-sensitive cells, and is known as the blind spot.

**retinaculum** /,retɪ'nækjʊləm/ *noun* a band of tissue which holds a structure in place, as found in the wrist and ankle over the flexor tendons

**retinae** /'retɪni/ plural of **retina**

**retinal** /'retɪn(ə)l/ *adjective* referring to the retina

**retinal artery** /'retɪn(ə)l ,ɑːtəri/ *noun* the only artery of the retina, which accompanies the optic nerve

**retinal detachment** /,retɪn(ə)l dɪ'tætʃmənt/ *noun* a condition in which the retina is partly detached from the choroid

**retinitis** /,retɪ'naɪtɪs/ *noun* inflammation of the retina

**retinitis pigmentosa** /,retɪ,naɪtɪs ,pɪgmen 'təʊsə/ *noun* a hereditary condition in which inflammation of the retina can result in blindness

**retino-** /retɪnəʊ/ *prefix* referring to the retina

**retinoblastoma** /,retɪnəʊblæ'stəʊmə/ *noun* a rare tumour in the retina, affecting infants

**retinol** /'retɪnɒl/ *noun* a vitamin found in liver, vegetables, eggs and cod liver oil which is essential for good vision. Also called **Vitamin A**

**retinopathy** /,retɪ'nɒpəθi/ *noun* any disease of the retina

**retinoscope** /'retɪnəskəʊp/ *noun* an instrument with various lenses, used to measure the refraction of the eye

**retinoscopy** /,retɪ'nɒskəpi/ *noun* a method of measuring refractive errors in the eye using a retinoscope

**retire** /rɪ'taɪə/ *verb* to stop work at a particular age ○ *Most men retire at 65, but women only go on working until they are 60.* ○ *Although she has retired, she still does voluntary work at the clinic.*

**retirement** /rɪ'taɪəmənt/ *noun* **1.** the act of retiring ○ *The retirement age for men is 65.* **2.** the act of being retired

**retraction** /rɪ'trækʃən/ *noun* the fact of moving backwards or becoming shorter ○ *There is retraction of the overlying skin.*

**retraction ring** /rɪ'trækʃən rɪŋ/ *noun* a groove round the uterus, separating its upper and lower parts, which, in obstructed labour, prevents the baby from moving forward as expected into the cervical canal. Also called **Bandl's ring**

**retractor** /rɪ'træktə/ *noun* a surgical instrument which pulls and holds back the edge of the incision in an operation

**retro-** /retrəʊ/ *prefix* at the back, behind

**retrobulbar** /,retrəʊ'bʌlbə/ *adjective* behind the eyeball

**retrobulbar neuritis** /,retrəʊ,bʌlbə njuː 'raɪtɪs/ *noun* inflammation of the optic nerve which makes objects appear blurred. Also called **optic neuritis**

**retroflexion** /ˌretrəʊˈflekʃ(ə)n/ *noun* the fact of being bent backwards □ **retroflexion of the uterus** a condition in which the uterus bends backwards away from its usual position

**retrograde** /ˈretrəʊɡreɪd/ *adjective* going backwards or deteriorating, getting worse

**retrograde pyelography** /ˌretrəʊɡreɪd ˌpaɪəˈlɒɡrəfi/ *noun* an X-ray examination of the kidney where a catheter is passed into the kidney and an opaque liquid is injected directly into it

**retrogression** /ˌretrəʊˈɡreʃ(ə)n/ *noun* returning to an earlier state

**retrolental fibroplasia** /ˌretrəʊˌlent(ə)l ˌfaɪbrəʊˈpleɪziə/ *noun* a condition in which fibrous tissue develops behind the lens of the eye, resulting in blindness

COMMENT: Retrolental fibroplasia can occur in premature babies if they are treated with large amounts of oxygen immediately after birth.

**retro-ocular** /ˌretrəʊ ˈɒkjʊlə/ *adjective* at the back of the eye

**retroperitoneal** /ˌretrəʊˌperɪtəˈniːəl/ *adjective* at the back of the peritoneum

**retroperitoneal space** /ˌretrəʊˌperɪtəʊniːəl ˈspeɪs/ *noun* the area between the posterior parietal peritoneum and the posterior abdominal wall, containing the kidneys, adrenal glands, duodenum, ureters and pancreas

**retropharyngeal** /ˌretrəʊˌfærɪnˈdʒiːəl/ *adjective* at the back of the pharynx

**retropubic** /ˌretrəʊˈpjuːbɪk/ *adjective* at the back of the pubis

**retropubic prostatectomy** /ˌretrəʊpjuːbɪk ˌprɒstəˈtektəmi/ *noun* removal of the prostate gland which is carried out by a suprapubic incision and by cutting the membrane which surrounds the gland

**retrospection** /ˌretrəˈspekʃən/ *noun* the act of recalling what happened in the past

**retrospective** /ˌretrəˈspektɪv/ *adjective* applying to the past, tracing what has happened already to selected people

**retroversion** /ˌretrəʊˈvɜːʃ(ə)n/ *noun* the fact of sloping backwards □ **retroversion of the uterus** Same as **retroverted uterus**

**retroverted uterus** /ˌretrəʊvɜːtɪd ˈjuːtərəs/ *noun* a condition in which the uterus slopes backwards away from its usual position. Also called **retroversion of the uterus, tipped womb**

**retrovirus** /ˈretrəʊvaɪrəs/ *noun* a virus whose genetic material contains RNA from which DNA is synthesised (NOTE: The AIDS virus and many carcinogenic viruses are retroviruses.)

**revascularisation** /riːˌvæskjʊləraɪˈzeɪʃ(ə)n/, **revascularization** *noun* **1.** the act of restoring an adequate blood supply to an organ or tissue, especially in a surgical operation using a blood vessel graft **2.** the condition of having an adequate blood supply restored

**reveal** /rɪˈviːl/ *verb* to show something ○ *Digital palpation revealed a growth in the breast.*

**reversal** /rɪˈvɜːs(ə)l/ *noun* the procedure to change something back ○ *reversal of sterilisation*

**reverse isolation** /rɪˌvɜːs ˌaɪsəˈleɪʃ(ə)n/ *noun* same as **protective isolation**

**revision** /rɪˈvɪʒ(ə)n/ *noun* an examination of a surgical operation after it has been carried out ○ *a revision of a radical mastoidectomy*

**revive** /rɪˈvaɪv/ *verb* to bring someone back to life or to consciousness ○ *They tried to revive him with artificial respiration.* ○ *She collapsed on the floor and had to be revived by the nurse.*

**Reye's syndrome** /ˈraɪz ˌsɪndrəʊm/ *noun* a form of brain disease affecting young children, which is possibly due to viral infection and has a suspected link with aspirin

**RGN** *abbr* Registered General Nurse

**Rh** *abbr* rhesus

**RHA** *abbr* Regional Health Authority

**rhabdomyosarcoma** /ˌræbdəʊˌmaɪəʊsɑːˈkəʊmə/ *noun* a malignant tumour of striated muscle tissue. It occurs mostly in children.

**rhabdovirus** /ˈræbdəʊvaɪrəs/ *noun* any of a group of viruses containing RNA, one of which causes rabies

**rhachio-** /ˈreɪkiəʊ/ *prefix* referring to the spine

**rhagades** /ˈræɡədiːz/ *plural noun* long thin scars in the skin round the nose, mouth or anus, seen in syphilis. ◊ **fissure**

**Rh disease** /ɑːr ˈeɪtʃ dɪˌziːz/ *noun* same as **rhesus factor disease**

**rheo-** /riːəʊ/ *prefix* **1.** relating to the flow of liquids **2.** relating to the flow of electrical current

**rheometer** /riˈɒmɪtə/ *noun* a device that measures the flow of thick liquids such as blood

**rhesus baby** /ˈriːsəs ˌbeɪbi/ *noun* a baby with erythroblastosis fetalis

**rhesus factor** /ˈriːsəs ˌfæktə/ *noun* an antigen in red blood cells, which is an element in blood grouping. Also called **Rh factor**

COMMENT: The rhesus factor is important in blood grouping, because, although most people are Rh-positive, an Rh-negative patient should not receive an Rh-positive blood transfusion as this will cause the formation of permanent antibodies. If an Rh-negative mother has a child by an Rh-positive father, the baby will inherit Rh-positive blood, which may then pass into the mother's circulation at childbirth and cause antibodies to form. This can be prevented by an injection of anti D immunoglobulin immediately after the birth of the first Rh-positive child and any subsequent Rh-positive children. If an Rh-negative mother has formed antibodies to Rh-positive blood in the past, these antibodies will affect the blood of the fetus and may cause erythroblastosis fetalis.

**rhesus factor disease** /ˈriːsəs ˌfæktə dɪ ˌziːz/ *noun* a disease which occurs when the blood of a fetus has a different rhesus factor from that of the mother. Also called **Rh disease**

**rheumatic** /ruːˈmætɪk/ *adjective* referring to rheumatism

**rheumatic fever** /ruːˌmætɪk ˈfiːvə/ *noun* a collagen disease of young people and children, caused by haemolytic streptococci, where the joints and also the valves and lining of the heart become inflamed. Also called **acute rheumatism**

COMMENT: Rheumatic fever often follows another streptococcal infection such as a strep throat or tonsillitis. Symptoms are high fever, pains in the joints, which become red, formation of nodules on the ends of bones and difficulty in breathing. Although recovery can be complete, rheumatic fever can recur and damage the heart permanently.

**rheumatism** /ˈruːmətɪz(ə)m/ *noun* pains and stiffness in the joints and muscles (*informal*) ○ *She has rheumatism in her hips.* ○ *He complained of rheumatism in the knees.*

**rheumatoid** /ˈruːmətɔɪd/ *adjective* relating to rheumatism

**rheumatoid arthritis** /ˌruːmətɔɪd ɑːˈθraɪtɪs/ *noun* a general painful disabling collagen disease affecting any joint, but especially the hands, feet and hips, making them swollen and inflamed. ◊ **osteoarthritis**

'...rheumatoid arthritis is a chronic inflammatory disease which can affect many systems of the body, but mainly the joints. 70% of sufferers develop the condition in the metacarpophalangeal joints' [*Nursing Times*]

**rheumatoid erosion** /ˌruːmətɔɪd ɪ ˈrəʊʒ(ə)n/ *noun* erosion of bone and cartilage in the joints caused by rheumatoid arthritis

**rheumatoid factor** /ˈruːmətɔɪd ˌfæktə/ *noun* an antibody found in the blood serum of many people who have rheumatoid arthritis

**rheumatologist** /ˌruːməˈtɒlədʒɪst/ *noun* a doctor who specialises in rheumatology

**rheumatology** /ˌruːməˈtɒlədʒi/ *noun* a branch of medicine dealing with rheumatic disease of muscles and joints

**Rh factor** /ˌɑːr ˈeɪtʃ ˌfæktə/ *noun* same as **rhesus factor**

**rhin-** /raɪn/ *prefix* same as **rhino-** (*used before vowels*)

**rhinal** /ˈraɪn(ə)l/ *adjective* referring to the nose

**rhinencephalon** /ˌraɪnenˈkefəlɒn/ *noun* the area of the forebrain that controls the sense of smell

**rhinitis** /raɪˈnaɪtɪs/ *noun* inflammation of the mucous membrane in the nose, which makes the nose run, caused, e.g., by a virus infection or an allergic reaction to dust or flowers

**rhino-** /raɪnəʊ/ *prefix* referring to the nose

**rhinology** /raɪˈnɒlədʒi/ *noun* a branch of medicine dealing with diseases of the nose and the nasal passages

**rhinomycosis** /ˌraɪnəʊmaɪˈkəʊsɪs/ *noun* an infection of the nasal passages by a fungus

**rhinopharyngitis** /ˌraɪnəʊfærɪnˈdʒaɪtɪs/ *noun* inflammation of the mucous membranes in the nose and pharynx

**rhinophyma** /ˌraɪnəʊˈfaɪmə/ *noun* a condition caused by rosacea, in which the nose becomes permanently red and swollen

**rhinoplasty** /ˈraɪnəʊplæsti/ *noun* plastic surgery to correct the appearance of the nose

**rhinorrhoea** /ˌraɪnəʊˈrɪə/ *noun* a watery discharge from the nose

**rhinoscope** /ˈraɪnəskəʊp/ *noun* an instrument for examining the inside of the nose

**rhinoscopy** /raɪˈnɒskəpi/ *noun* an examination of the inside of the nose

**rhinosinusitis** /ˌraɪnəʊˌsaɪnəˈsaɪtɪs/ *noun* swelling of the lining of the nose and paranasal sinuses, as a result of either a viral infection or allergic rhinitis. It is usually treated with antibiotics, antihistamines or steroids.

**rhinosporidiosis** /ˌraɪnəʊˌspɒrɪdiˈəʊsɪs/ *noun* an infection of the nose, eyes, larynx and genital organs by the fungus *Rhinosporidium seeberi*

**rhinovirus** /ˈraɪnəʊˌvaɪrəs/ *noun* a group of viruses containing RNA, which cause infection of the nose and include the virus which causes the common cold

**rhiz-** /raɪz/, **rhizo-** /ˈraɪzəʊ/ *prefix* referring to a root

**rhizotomy** /raɪˈzɒtəmi/ *noun* a surgical operation to cut or divide the roots of a nerve to relieve severe pain

**Rh-negative** /ˌɑː eɪtʃ ˈnegətɪv/ *adjective* who does not have the rhesus factor in his or her blood

**rhodopsin** /rəʊˈdɒpsɪn/ *noun* a light-sensitive purple pigment in the rods of the retina, which makes it possible to see in dim light. Also called **visual purple**

**rhombencephalon** /ˌrɒmbenˈkefəlɒn/ *noun* the hindbrain, the part of the brain which contains the cerebellum, the medulla oblongata and the pons

**rhomboid** /ˈrɒmbɔɪd/ *noun* one of two muscles in the top part of the back which move the shoulder blades

**rhonchus** /ˈrɒŋkəs/ *noun* an unusual sound in the chest, heard through a stethoscope, caused by a partial blockage in the bronchi (NOTE: The plural is **rhonchi**.)

**Rh-positive** /ˌɑː eɪtʃ ˈpɒzɪtɪv/ *adjective* who has the rhesus factor in his or her blood

**rhythm** /ˈrɪð(ə)m/ *noun* a regular movement or beat

**rhythmic** /ˈrɪðmɪk/ *adjective* regular, with a repeated rhythm

**rhythm method** /ˈrɪð(ə)m ˌmeθəd/ *noun* a method of birth control where sexual intercourse should take place only during the safe periods when conception is least likely to occur, i.e. at the beginning and at the end of the menstrual cycle

COMMENT: This method is not as safe or reliable as other methods of contraception because the time when ovulation takes place cannot be accurately calculated if a woman does not have regular periods.

**rib** /rɪb/ *noun* one of twenty-four curved bones which protect the chest (NOTE: For other terms referring to the ribs, see words beginning with cost-, costo-.)

**ribavirin** /ˈraɪbəˌvaɪrɪn/ *noun* a synthetic drug which helps to prevent the synthesis of viral DNA and RNA, used in the treatment of viral diseases

**rib cage** /ˈrɪb keɪdʒ/ *noun* the ribs and the space enclosed by them

COMMENT: The rib cage is formed of twelve pairs of curved bones. The top seven pairs, the true ribs, are joined to the breastbone in front by costal cartilage. The other five pairs of ribs, the false ribs, are not attached to the breastbone, though the 8th, 9th and 10th pairs are each attached to the rib above. The bottom two pairs, which are not attached to the breastbone at all, are called the floating ribs.

**riboflavine** /ˌraɪbəʊˈfleɪvɪn/ same as **Vitamin B₂** (NOTE: The US spelling is **riboflavin**.)

**ribonuclease** /ˌraɪbəʊˈnjuːklieɪz/ *noun* an enzyme which breaks down RNA

**ribonucleic acid** /ˌraɪbəʊnjuːˌkliːɪk ˈæsɪd/ *noun* one of the nucleic acids in the nucleus of all living cells, which takes coded information from DNA and translates it into specific enzymes and proteins. ◊ **DNA**. Abbr **RNA**

**ribose** /ˈraɪbəʊs/ *noun* a type of sugar found in RNA

**ribosomal** /ˌraɪbəˈsəʊm(ə)l/ *adjective* referring to ribosomes

**ribosome** /ˈraɪbəsəʊm/ *noun* a tiny particle in a cell, containing RNA and protein, where protein is synthesised

**ricewater stools** /ˈraɪswɔːtə stuːlz/ *plural noun* watery faeces that are typically passed by people who have cholera

**rich** /rɪtʃ/ *adjective* **1.** well supplied **2.** referring to food which has a high calorific value

'...the sublingual region has a rich blood supply derived from the carotid artery' [*Nursing Times*]

**ricin** /ˈraɪsɪn/ *noun* a highly toxic albumin found in the seeds of the castor oil plant

**rick** /rɪk/ *noun* a slight injury to a joint caused by wrenching or spraining it ■ *verb* to wrench or sprain a joint of the body slightly

**rickets** /ˈrɪkɪts/ *noun* a disease of children, where the bones are soft and do not develop

properly due to lack of Vitamin D. Also called **rachitis**

COMMENT: Initial treatment for rickets in children is a vitamin-rich diet, together with exposure to sunshine which causes vitamin D to form in the skin.

**Rickettsia** /rɪˈketsiə/ *noun* a genus of microorganisms which causes several diseases including Q fever and typhus

**rickettsial** /rɪˈketsiəl/ *adjective* referring to Rickettsia

**rickettsial pox** /rɪˈketsiəl pɒks/ *noun* a disease found in North America, caused by *Rickettsia akari* passed to humans by bites from mites which live on mice

**rid** /rɪd/ *verb* □ **to get rid of something** to make something go away ○ *He can't get rid of his cold – he's had it for weeks.* □ **to be rid of something** not to have something unpleasant any more ○ *I'm very glad to be rid of my flu.*

**ridge** /rɪdʒ/ *noun* a long raised part on the surface of a bone or organ

**rifampicin** /rɪfˈæmpɪsɪn/ *noun* an antibiotic which works by interfering with RNA synthesis in the infecting bacteria, used in the treatment of tuberculosis, leprosy and other bacterial infections

**right** /raɪt/ *noun* the fact of being legally entitled to do or to have something ○ *You always have the right to ask for a second opinion.*

**right colic** /ˌraɪt ˈkɒlɪk/ *noun* an artery which leads from the superior mesenteric artery

**right-handed** /ˌraɪt ˈhændɪd/ *adjective* using the right hand more often than the left ○ *He's right-handed.* ○ *Most people are right-handed.*

**right-left shunt** /ˌraɪt left ˈʃʌnt/ *noun* a malformation in the heart, allowing blood to flow from the pulmonary artery to the aorta

**right lymphatic duct** /ˌraɪt lɪmˌfætɪk ˈdʌkt/ *noun* one of the main terminal channels for carrying lymph, draining the right side of the head and neck and entering the junction of the right subclavian and internal jugular veins. It is the smaller of the two main discharge points of the lymphatic system into the venous system, the larger being the thoracic duct.

**rigid** /ˈrɪdʒɪd/ *adjective* stiff, not moving

**rigidity** /rɪˈdʒɪdɪti/ *noun* the fact of being rigid, bent or not able to be moved. ◊ **spasticity**

**rigor** /ˈrɪgə/ *noun* an attack of shivering, often with fever

**rigor mortis** /ˌrɪgə ˈmɔːtɪs/ *noun* a condition in which the muscles of a dead body become stiff after death and then become relaxed again

COMMENT: Rigor mortis starts about eight hours after death, and begins to disappear several hours later. Environment and temperature play a large part in the timing.

**rima** /ˈraɪmə/ *noun* a narrow crack or cleft

**rima glottidis** /ˌriːmə ˈglɒtɪdɪs/ *noun* a space between the vocal cords

**ring** /rɪŋ/ noun a circle of tissue, or tissue or muscle shaped like a circle

**ring block** /'rɪŋ blɒk/ noun the process of inserting local anaesthetic all the way round a digit, e.g. a finger, in order to perform a procedure distal to the block.

**Ringer's solution** /'rɪŋəz səˌluːʃ(ə)n/ noun a solution of inorganic salts which is used both to treat burns and cuts and to keep cells, tissues or organs alive outside the body

**ring finger** /'rɪŋ ˌfɪŋgə/ noun the third finger, the finger between the little finger and the middle finger

**ringing in the ear** /ˌrɪŋɪŋ ɪn ðɪ 'ɪə/ ♦ tinnitus

**ringworm** /'rɪŋwɜːm/ noun any of various infections of the skin by a fungus, in which the infection spreads out in a circle from a central point. It is very contagious and difficult to get rid of. Also called **tinea**

**Rinne's test** /'rɪniz test/ noun a hearing test in which a tuning fork is hit and its handle placed near the ear, to test for air conduction, and then on the mastoid process, to test for bone conduction. It is then possible to determine the type of lesion which exists by finding if the sound is heard for a longer period by air or by bone conduction. [Described 1855. After Friedrich Heinrich Rinne (1819–68), otologist at Göttingen, Germany.]

**rinse out** /ˌrɪns 'aʊt/ verb to lightly wash the inside of something to make it clean, e.g. to get rid of soap ○ *She rinsed out the measuring jar.* ○ *Rinse your mouth out with mouthwash.*

**ripple bed** /'rɪp(ə)l bed/ noun a type of bed with an air-filled mattress divided into sections, in which the pressure is continuously being changed so that the body can be massaged and bedsores can be avoided

**rise** /raɪz/ verb to go up ○ *His temperature rose sharply.* (NOTE: **rising – rose – risen**)

**risk** /rɪsk/ noun the possibility of something harmful happening ○ *There is a risk of a cholera epidemic.* ○ *There is no risk of the disease spreading to other members of the family.* □ **at risk** in danger of being harmed ○ *Businessmen are particularly at risk of having a heart attack.* □ **children at risk** children who are more likely to be harmed or to catch a disease ■ verb to do something which may possibly cause harm or have bad results ○ *If the patient is not moved to an isolation ward, all the patients and staff in the hospital risk catching the disease.*

'…adenomatous polyps are a risk factor for carcinoma of the stomach' [*Nursing Times*]

'…three quarters of patients aged 35–64 on GPs' lists have at least one major risk factor: high cholesterol, high blood pressure or addiction to tobacco' [*Health Services Journal*]

**risk factor** /'rɪsk ˌfæktə/ noun a characteristic that increases a person's likelihood of getting a particular disease ○ *Smoking is a risk factor for lung cancer.* ○ *Obesity is a risk factor for diabetes.*

**risus sardonicus** /ˌraɪsəs sɑː'dɒnɪkəs/ noun a twisted smile which is a symptom of tetanus

**rite of passage** /ˌraɪt əv 'pæsɪdʒ/ noun a ceremony which shows that somebody is moving from one stage of their life to another, e.g. from childhood to puberty or from unmarried to married life

**river blindness** /'rɪvə ˌblaɪndnəs/ noun blindness caused by larvae getting into the eye in cases of onchocerciasis

**RM** abbr Registered Midwife

**RMN** abbr Registered Mental Nurse

**RN** abbr Registered Nurse

**RNA** abbr ribonucleic acid

**RNMH** abbr Registered Nurse for the Mentally Handicapped

**Rocky Mountain spotted fever** /ˌrɒki ˌmaʊntɪn ˌspɒtɪd 'fiːvə/ noun a type of typhus caused by *Rickettsia rickettsii,* transmitted to humans by ticks

**rod** /rɒd/ noun **1.** a stick shape with rounded ends ○ *Some bacteria are shaped like rods* or *are rod-shaped.* **2.** one of two types of light-sensitive cell in the retina of the eye. Rods are sensitive to dim light, but not to colour. ♦ **cone**

COMMENT: Rod cells in the eye are sensitive to poor light. They contain rhodopsin or visual purple, which produces the nervous impulse which the rod transmits to the optic nerve.

**rodent ulcer** /ˌrəʊd(ə)nt 'ʌlsə/ noun a malignant tumour on the face

COMMENT: Rodent ulcers are different from some other types of cancer in that they do not spread to other parts of the body and do not metastasise, but remain on the face, usually near the mouth or eyes. Rodent ulcer is rare before middle age.

**roentgen** /'rɒntgən/ noun a unit of radiation used to measure the exposure of someone or something to X-rays or gamma rays. Symbol **R** [After Wilhelm Konrad von Röntgen (1845–1923), physicist at Strasbourg, Geissen, Würzburg and Munich, and then Director of the physics laboratory at Würzburg where he discovered X-rays in 1895. Nobel prize for Physics 1901.]

**roentgenogram** /'rɒntgənəgræm/ noun an X-ray photograph

**roentgenology** /ˌrɒntgə'nɒlədʒi/ noun the study of X-rays and their use in medicine

**roentgen ray** /'rɒntgən reɪ/ noun an X-ray or gamma ray which can pass through tissue and leave an image on a photographic film

**role** /rəʊl/ noun **1.** the usual or expected function of somebody or something in a particular process or event ○ *the role of haemoglobin in blood clotting* **2.** the characteristic or expected pattern of behaviour of a particular member of a social group ○ *the eldest child's role in the family*

**role playing** /ˈrəʊl ˌpleɪɪŋ/ *noun* the act of pretending to be somebody else in a situation, so that you have to imagine how that person feels and thinks. It usually involves several people. It is used in many training exercises and psychiatric evaluations.

**rolled bandage** /ˌrəʊld ˈbændɪdʒ/, **roller bandage** /ˌrəʊlə ˈbændɪdʒ/ *noun* a bandage in the form of a long strip of cloth which is rolled up from one or both ends

**Romberg's sign** /ˈrɒmbɜːgz saɪn/ *noun* a swaying of the body or falling when standing with the feet close together and the eyes closed, the result of loss of the joint position sense [Described 1846. After Moritz Heinrich Romberg (1795–1873), German physician and pioneer neurologist.]

COMMENT: If a patient cannot stand upright when his or her eyes are closed, this shows that nerves in the lower limbs which transmit joint position sense to the brain are damaged.

**rongeur** /rɒŋˈɡɜː/ *noun* a strong surgical instrument like a pair of pliers, used for cutting bone

**roof** /ruːf/ *noun* the top part of a cavity □ **roof of the mouth** Same as **palate**

**root** /ruːt/ *noun* **1.** a point from which a part of the body grows ○ *root of hair* or *hair root* ○ *root of nerve* or *nerve root* **2.** part of a tooth which is connected to a socket in the jaw ▶ also called **radix**

**root canal** /ˈruːt kəˌnæl/ *noun* a canal in the root of a tooth through which the nerves and blood vessels pass

**rooting reflex** /ˈruːtɪŋ ˌriːfleks/ *noun* the instinct in new babies to turn their heads towards a touch on the cheek or mouth, which is important for breastfeeding

**Roper, Logan and Tierney model** /ˌrəʊpə ˌləʊɡən ən ˈtɪəni ˌmɒd(ə)l/ *noun* an important model of nursing developed in the UK in 1980. Various factors such as necessary daily tasks, lifespan and health status are used to assess the relative independence of an individual, which the nurse will help them to increase.

**Rorschach test** /ˈrɔːʃɑːk test/ *noun* the ink blot test, used in psychological diagnosis, where someone is shown a series of blots of ink on paper and is asked to say what each blot reminds him or her of. The answers give information about the person's psychological state. [Described 1921. After Hermann Rorschach (1884–1922), German-born psychiatrist who worked in Bern, Switzerland.]

**rosacea** /rəʊˈzeɪʃə/ *noun* a common skin disease seen from middle age affecting the face, and especially the nose, which becomes red because of enlarged blood vessels. The cause is not known. Also called **acne rosacea** (NOTE: Despite its alternative name, rosacea is not a type of acne.)

**rosea** /ˈrəʊzɪə/ ♦ **pityriasis**

**roseola infantum** /rəʊˌziːələ ɪnˈfæntəm/ *noun* a sudden infection of small children, with fever, swelling of the lymph glands and a rash. It is caused by herpesvirus 6. Also called **exanthem subitum**

**rostral** /ˈrɒstr(ə)l/ *adjective* like the beak of a bird

**rostrum** /ˈrɒstrəm/ *noun* a projecting part of a bone or structure shaped like a beak (NOTE: The plural is **rostra**.)

**rot** /rɒt/ *verb* to decay, to become putrefied ○ *The flesh was rotting round the wound as gangrene set in.* ○ *The fingers can rot away in leprosy.*

**rotate** /rəʊˈteɪt/ *verb* to move in a circle, or make something move in a circle

**rotation** /rəʊˈteɪʃ(ə)n/ *noun* the act of moving in a circle. See illustration at ANATOMICAL TERMS in Supplement □ **lateral and medial rotation** turning part of the body to the side, towards the midline

**rotator** /rəʊˈteɪtə/ *noun* a muscle which makes a limb rotate

**rotavirus** /ˈrəʊtəvaɪrəs/ *noun* any of a group of viruses associated with gastroenteritis in children

'…rotavirus is now widely accepted as an important cause of childhood diarrhoea in many different parts of the world' [*East African Medical Journal*]

**Rothera's test** /ˈrɒðərəz test/ *noun* a test to see if acetone is present in urine, a sign of ketosis which is a complication of diabetes mellitus [After Arthur Cecil Hamel Rothera (1880–1915), biochemist in Melbourne, Australia]

**Roth spot** /ˈrəʊt spɒt/ *noun* a pale spot which sometimes occurs on the retina of a person who has leukaemia or some other diseases [After Moritz Roth (1839–1915), Swiss pathologist and physician]

**rotunda** /rəʊˈtʌndə/ ♦ **fenestra**

**rough** /rʌf/ *adjective* not smooth ○ *rough skin*

**roughage** /ˈrʌfɪdʒ/ *noun* same as **dietary fibre**

COMMENT: Roughage is found in cereals, nuts, fruit and vegetables. It is believed to be necessary to help digestion and avoid developing constipation and obesity.

**rouleau** /ruːˈləʊ/ *noun* a roll of red blood cells which have stuck together like a column of coins (NOTE: The plural is **rouleaux**.)

**round** /raʊnd/ *adjective* shaped like a circle ■ *noun* a regular visit □ **to do the rounds of the wards** to visit various wards in a hospital and talk to the nurses and check on patients' progress or condition □ **a health visitor's rounds** regular series of visits made by a health visitor

**round ligament** /raʊnd ˈlɪɡəmənt/ *noun* a band of muscle which stretches from the uterus to the labia

**round window** /raʊnd ˈwɪndəʊ/ *noun* a round opening between the middle ear and the cochlea, and closed by a membrane. Also called **fenestra rotunda**. See illustration at EAR in Supplement

**roundworm** /'raʊndwɜːm/ *noun* any of several common types of parasitic worms with round bodies, such as hookworms. Compare **flatworm**

**Rovsing's sign** /'rɒvsɪŋz saɪn/ *noun* pain in the right iliac fossa when the left iliac fossa is pressed, which is a sign of acute appendicitis [Described 1907. After Nils Thorkild Rovsing (1862–1927), Professor of Surgery at Copenhagen, Denmark.]

**Royal College of General Practitioners** /ˌrɔɪəl ˌkɒlɪdʒ əv 'dʒen(ə)rəl/ *noun* a professional association which represents family doctors. Abbr **RCGP**

**Royal College of Nursing** /ˌrɔɪəl ˌkɒlɪdʒ əv 'nɜːsɪŋ/ *noun* a professional association which represents nurses. Abbr **RCN**

**Roy's model** /'rɔɪz ˌmɒd(ə)l/ *noun* a model for nursing developed in the US in the 1970s. It describes a person's health as being a state of successful positive adaptation to all those stimuli from the environment which could interfere with their basic need satisfaction. Illness results from an inability to adapt to such stimuli, so nurses should help patients to overcome this.

**RQ** *abbr* respiratory quotient

**RR** *abbr* **1.** recovery room **2.** relative risk

**-rrhage** /rɪdʒ/, **-rrhagia** /'reɪdʒə/ *suffix* referring to an unusual flow or discharge of blood

**-rrhaphy** /rəfi/ *suffix* referring to surgical sewing or suturing

**-rrhexis** /reksɪs/ *suffix* referring to splitting or rupture

**-rrhoea** /rɪə/ *suffix* referring to an unusual flow or discharge of fluid from an organ

**RSCN** *abbr* Registered Sick Children's Nurse

**RSI** *abbr* repetitive strain injury

**RSV** *abbr* respiratory syncytial virus

**RTN** *abbr* Registered Theatre Nurse

**rub** /rʌb/ *noun* a lotion used to rub on the skin ○ *The ointment is used as a rub.* ■ *verb* **1.** to move something, especially the hands, backwards and forwards over a surface ○ *She rubbed her leg after she knocked it against the table.* ○ *He rubbed his hands to make the circulation return.* **2.** □ **to rub into** to make an ointment go into the skin by rubbing ○ *Rub the liniment gently into the skin.*

**rubber** /'rʌbə/ *noun* **1.** a material which can be stretched and compressed, made from the thick white liquid called latex, from a tropical tree **2.** a condom (*informal*)

**rubber sheet** /ˌrʌbə 'ʃiːt/ *noun* a waterproof sheet put on hospital beds or on the bed of a child who is prone to bedwetting, to protect the mattress

**rubbing alcohol** /'rʌbɪŋ ˌælkəhɒl/ *noun* US same as **surgical spirit**

**rubefacient** /ˌruːbɪ'feɪʃ(ə)nt/ *noun* a substance which makes the skin warm, and pink or red ■ *adjective* causing the skin to become red

**rubella** /ruː'belə/ *noun* a common infectious viral disease of children with mild fever, swollen lymph nodes and rash. Also called **German measles**

COMMENT: Rubella can cause stillbirth or malformation of an unborn baby if the mother catches the disease while pregnant. One component of the MMR vaccine immunises against rubella.

**rubeola** /ruː'biːələ/ *noun* same as **measles**

**Rubin's test** /'ruːbɪnz test/ *noun* a test to see if the Fallopian tubes are free from obstruction [After Isador Clinton Rubin (b. 1883), US gynaecologist]

**rubor** /'ruːbə/ *noun* redness of the skin or tissue

**rudimentary** /ˌruːdɪ'ment(ə)ri/ *adjective* existing in a small form, or not developed fully ○ *The child was born with rudimentary arms.*

**Ruffini corpuscles** /ruː'fiːni ˌkɔːpʌs(ə)lz/, **Ruffini nerve endings** /ruːˌfiːni 'nɜːv ˌendɪŋz/ *plural noun* branching nerve endings in the skin, which are thought to be sensitive to heat

**ruga** /'ruːgə/ *noun* a fold or ridge, especially in a mucous membrane such as the lining of the stomach (NOTE: The plural is **rugae**.)

**rule out** /ˌruːl 'aʊt/ *verb* to state that someone does not have a specific disease ○ *We can rule out shingles.*

**rumbling** /'rʌmblɪŋ/ *noun* borborygmus, noise in the abdomen, caused by gas in the intestine

**rumination** /ˌruːmɪ'neɪʃ(ə)n/ *noun* **1.** a condition in which someone has constant irrational thoughts which they cannot control **2.** the regurgitation of food from the stomach which is then swallowed again

**run** /rʌn/ *verb* (*of the nose*) to drip with liquid secreted from the mucous membrane in the nasal passage ○ *His nose is running.* ○ *If your nose is running, blow it on a handkerchief.* ○ *One of the symptoms of a cold is a running nose.*

**run-down** /ˌrʌn 'daʊn/ *adjective* exhausted and unwell

**running** /'rʌnɪŋ/ *adjective* from which liquid is flowing ○ *running eyes*

**running sore** /ˌrʌnɪŋ 'sɔː/ *noun* a sore which is discharging pus

**runny nose** /ˌrʌni 'nəʊz/ *noun* a nose which is dripping with liquid from the mucous membrane

**runs** /rʌnz/ *noun* **the runs** same as **diarrhoea** (*informal*) ○ *I've got the runs again.* (NOTE: Takes a singular or plural verb.)

**rupture** /'rʌptʃə/ *noun* **1.** the breaking or tearing of an organ such as the appendix **2.** same as **hernia** ■ *verb* to break or tear something

**ruptured spleen** /ˌrʌptʃəd 'spliːn/ *noun* a spleen which has been torn by piercing or by a blow

**Russell traction** /'rʌs(ə)l ˌtrækʃ(ə)n/ *noun* a type of traction with weights and slings used to straighten a femur which has been fractured

[Described 1924. After R. Hamilton Russell (1860–1933), Australian surgeon.]

**Ryle's tube** /'raɪlz ˌtjuːb/ *noun* a thin tube which is passed into the stomach through either the nose or mouth, used to pump out the contents of the stomach or to introduce a barium meal in the stomach [Described 1921. After John Alfred Ryle (1882–1950), physician at London, Cambridge and Oxford, UK.]

# S

**Sabin vaccine** /'seɪbɪn ˌvæksiːn/ *noun* an oral vaccine against poliomyelitis, consisting of weak live polio virus. Compare **Salk vaccine** (NOTE: This is the vaccine used in the UK) [Developed 1955. After Albert Bruce Sabin (1906–93), Russian-born New York bacteriologist.]

**sac** /sæk/ *noun* a part of the body shaped like a bag

**saccades** /sæ'keɪdz/ *plural noun* controlled rapid movements of the eyes made when a person is changing the direction in which they are focusing, e.g. when they are reading

**sacchar-** /sækə/ *prefix* same as **saccharo-** (*used before vowels*)

**saccharide** /'sækəraɪd/ *noun* a form of carbohydrate

**saccharin** /'sækərɪn/ *noun* a white crystalline substance, used in place of sugar because, although it is nearly 500 times sweeter than sugar, it contains no carbohydrates

**saccharine** /'sækəraɪn/ *adjective* relating to, resembling or containing sugar

**saccharo-** /sækərəʊ/ *prefix* referring to sugar

**saccule** /'sækjuːl/, **sacculus** /'sækjʊləs/ *noun* the smaller of two sacs in the vestibule of the inner ear which is part of the mechanism which relates information about the position of the head in space

**sacra** /'seɪkrə/ plural of **sacrum**

**sacral** /'seɪkrəl/ *adjective* referring to the sacrum

**sacral foramen** /ˌseɪkrəl fə'reɪmən/ *noun* one of the openings in the sacrum through which the sacral nerves pass. See illustration at PELVIS in Supplement (NOTE: The plural is **sacral foramina**.)

**sacralisation** /ˌsækrəlaɪ'zeɪʃ(ə)n/, **sacralization** *noun* a condition in which the lowest lumbar vertebra fuses with the sacrum

**sacral nerve** /'sækrəl ˌnɜːv/ *noun* one of the nerves which branch from the spinal cord in the sacrum and govern the legs, the arms and the genital area

**sacral plexus** /ˌseɪkrəl 'pleksəs/ *noun* a group of nerves inside the pelvis near the sacrum which lead to nerves in the buttocks, back of the thigh and lower leg and foot

**sacral vertebrae** /ˌseɪkrəl 'vɜːtɪbriː/ *plural noun* the five vertebrae in the lower part of the spine which are fused together to form the sacrum

**sacro-** /seɪkrəʊ/ *prefix* referring to the sacrum

**sacrococcygeal** /ˌseɪkrəʊkɒk'siːdʒiəl/ *adjective* referring to the sacrum and the coccyx

**sacroiliac** /ˌseɪkrəʊ'ɪliæk/ *adjective* referring to the sacrum and the ilium

**sacroiliac joint** /ˌseɪkrəʊ'ɪliæk dʒɔɪnt/ *noun* a joint where the sacrum joins the ilium

**sacroiliitis** /ˌseɪkrəʊɪli'aɪtɪs/ *noun* inflammation of the sacroiliac joint

**sacrotuberous ligament** /ˌseɪkrəʊˌtjuːbərəs 'lɪgəmənt/ *noun* the large ligament between the iliac spine, the sacrum, the coccyx and the ischial tuberosity

**sacro-uterine ligament** /ˌseɪkrəʊˌjuːtəraɪn 'lɪgəmənt/ *noun* a ligament which goes from the neck of the uterus to the sacrum, passing on each side of the rectum

**sacrum** /'seɪkrəm/ *noun* a flat triangular bone, formed of five sacral vertebrae fused together, located between the lumbar vertebrae and the coccyx. It articulates with the coccyx and also with the hip bones. See illustration at PELVIS in Supplement (NOTE: The plural is **sacra**.)

**SAD** *abbr* seasonal affective disorder

**saddle joint** /'sæd(ə)l dʒɔɪnt/ *noun* a synovial joint where one element is concave and the other convex, like the joint between the thumb and the wrist

**saddle-nose** /'sæd(ə)l nəʊz/ *noun* a deep bridge of the nose, usually a sign of injury but sometimes a sign of tertiary syphilis

**sadism** /'seɪdɪz(ə)m/ *noun* a sexual condition in which a person finds sexual pleasure in hurting others

**sadist** /'seɪdɪst/ *noun* a person whose sexual urge is linked to sadism

**sadistic** /sə'dɪstɪk/ *adjective* referring to sadism. Compare **masochism**

**SADS** *abbr* seasonal affective disorder syndrome

**safe** /seɪf/ *adjective* **1.** not likely to cause harm ○ *Is it safe to use this drug on someone who is diabetic?* **2.** in a protected place or situation and not likely to be harmed or lost ○ *Keep the drugs in a safe place.* ○ *He's safe in hospital being looked after by the doctors and nurses.* (NOTE: **safer – safest**)

'…a good collateral blood supply makes occlusion of a single branch of the coeliac axis safe' [*British Medical Journal*]

**safe dose** /seɪf 'dəʊs/ *noun* the amount of a drug which can be given without being harmful

**safely** /ˈseɪfli/ *adverb* without danger, without being hurt ○ *You can safely take six tablets a day without any risk of side-effects.*

**safe period** /seɪf ˌpɪəriəd/ *noun* the time during the menstrual cycle, when conception is not likely to occur, and sexual intercourse can take place, used as a method of contraception. ◊ **rhythm method**

**safe sex** /seɪf 'seks/ *noun* the use of measures such as a contraceptive sheath and having only one sexual partner to reduce the possibility of catching a sexually transmitted disease

**safety** /ˈseɪfti/ *noun* the fact of being safe □ **to take safety precautions** to do things which make your actions or condition safe

**safety pin** /ˈseɪfti pɪn/ *noun* a special type of bent pin with a guard which protects the point, used for attaching nappies or bandages

**sagittal** /ˈsædʒɪt(ə)l/ *adjective* going from the front of the body to the back, dividing it into right and left

**sagittal plane** /ˌsædʒɪt(ə)l 'pleɪn/ *noun* the division of the body along the midline, at right angles to the coronal plane, dividing the body into right and left parts. Also called **median plane**. See illustration at ANATOMICAL TERMS in Supplement

**sagittal section** /ˌsædʒɪt(ə)l 'sekʃən/ *noun* any section or cut through the body, going from the front to the back along the length of the body

**sagittal suture** /ˌsædʒɪt(ə)l 'suːtʃə/ *noun* a joint along the top of the head where the two parietal bones are fused

**StHA** *abbr* Strategic Health Authority

**St John Ambulance Association and Brigade** /sənt ˌdʒɒn 'æmbjʊləns əˌsəʊsieɪʃ(ə)n ən brɪ'geɪd/ *noun* a voluntary organisation which gives training in first aid and whose members provide first aid at public events such as football matches and demonstrations

**St Louis encephalitis** /seɪnt ˌluːɪs enˌkefə'laɪtɪs/ *noun* a sometimes fatal form of encephalitis, transmitted by the ordinary house mosquito, *Culex pipiens* [After St Louis, Missouri, USA, where it was first diagnosed]

**St Vitus's dance** /sənt 'vaɪtəsɪz dɑːns/ *noun* a former name for Sydenham's chorea

**salbutamol** /sæl'bjuːtəmɒl/ *noun* a drug which relaxes and dilates the bronchi, used in the relief of asthma, emphysema and chronic bronchitis

**salicylate** /sə'lɪsɪleɪt/ *noun* one of various pain-killing substances derived from salicylic acid, e.g. aspirin

**salicylic acid** /ˌsælɪˌsɪlɪk 'æsɪd/ *noun* a white antiseptic substance which destroys bacteria and fungi and which is used in ointments to treat corns, warts and other skin disorders

**salicylism** /ˈsælɪsɪlɪz(ə)m/ *noun* the effects of poisoning due to too much salicylic acid. Symptoms include headache, tinnitus, faintness and vomiting.

**saline** /ˈseɪlaɪn/ *adjective* referring to or containing salt ○ *The patient was given a saline transfusion.* ■ *noun* same as saline solution

**saline drip** /ˌseɪlaɪn 'drɪp/ *noun* a drip containing a saline solution

**saline solution** /ˈseɪlaɪn səˌluːʃ(ə)n/ *noun* a solution made of distilled water and sodium chloride, which is introduced into the body intravenously through a drip

**saliva** /sə'laɪvə/ *noun* a fluid in the mouth, secreted by the salivary glands, which starts the process of digesting food (NOTE: For terms referring to saliva, see words beginning with **ptyal-**, **ptyalo-** or **sial-, sialo-**.)

COMMENT: Saliva is a mixture of a large quantity of water and a small amount of mucus, secreted by the salivary glands. Saliva acts to keep the mouth and throat moist, allowing food to be swallowed easily. It also contains the enzyme ptyalin, which begins the digestive process of converting starch into sugar while food is still in the mouth. Because of this association with food, the salivary glands produce saliva automatically when food is seen, smelt or even simply talked about.

**salivary** /sə'laɪv(ə)ri/ *adjective* referring to saliva

**salivary calculus** /səˌlaɪv(ə)ri 'kælkjʊləs/ *noun* a stone which forms in a salivary gland

**salivary gland** /sə'laɪv(ə)ri ɡlænd/ *noun* a gland which secretes saliva, situated under the tongue (the **sublingual gland**), beneath the lower jaw (the **submandibular gland**) and in the neck at the back of the lower jaw joint (the **parotid gland**)

**salivate** /ˈsælɪveɪt/ *verb* to produce saliva

**salivation** /ˌsælɪ'veɪʃ(ə)n/ *noun* the production of saliva

**Salk vaccine** /ˈsɔːk ˌvæksiːn/ *noun* an injected vaccine against poliomyelitis, consisting of inactivated polio virus. Compare **Sabin vaccine** [Developed 1954. After Jonas Edward Salk (1914–95), virologist in Pittsburgh, USA.]

**salmeterol** /sæl'metərɒl/ *noun* a drug which relaxes and widens the airways, used to treat severe asthma

**Salmonella** /ˌsælməˈnelə/ *noun* a genus of pathogenic bacteria which live in the intestines and are usually acquired by eating contaminated food, responsible for many cases of gastroenteritis and for typhoid or paratyphoid fever (NOTE: The plural is **Salmonellae**.)

**Salmonella poisoning** /ˌsælməˈnelə ˌpɔɪz(ə)nɪŋ/ *noun* poisoning caused by Salmonellae which develop in the intestines ○ *Five people were taken to hospital with Salmonella poisoning.*

**salmonellosis** /ˌsælməneˈləʊsɪs/ *noun* food poisoning caused by *Salmonella* in the digestive system

**salping-** /sælpɪndʒ/ *prefix* same as **salpingo-** (used before vowels)

**salpingectomy** /ˌsælpɪnˈdʒektəmi/ *noun* a surgical operation to remove or cut a Fallopian tube, used as a method of contraception

**salpingitis** /ˌsælpɪnˈdʒaɪtɪs/ *noun* inflammation, usually of a Fallopian tube

**salpingo-** /sælpɪŋgəʊ/ *prefix* **1.** referring to the Fallopian tubes **2.** referring to the auditory meatus

**salpingography** /ˌsælpɪŋˈgɒgrəfi/ *noun* an X-ray examination of the Fallopian tubes

**salpingolysis** /ˌsælpɪŋˈgɒlɪsɪs/ *noun* a surgical operation to open up blocked Fallopian tubes by removing any adhesions near the ovaries

**salpingo-oophorectomy** /sælˌpɪŋgəʊ ˌəʊəfəˈrektəmi/ *noun* a surgical operation to remove a Fallopian tube and ovary

**salpingo-oophoritis** /sælˌpɪŋgəʊ ˌəʊəfə ˈraɪtɪs/, **salpingo-oothecitis** /sælˌpɪŋgəʊ ˌəʊəθɪˈsaɪtɪs/ *noun* inflammation of a Fallopian tube and the ovary connected to it

**salpingo-oophorocele** /sælˌpɪŋgəʊ əʊ ˈnfərəʊsiːl/, **salpingo-oothecocele** /sæl ˌpɪŋgəʊ əʊəˈθiːkəʊsiːl/ *noun* a hernia where a Fallopian tube and its ovary pass through a weak point in the surrounding tissue

**salpingostomy** /ˌsælpɪŋˈgɒstəmi/ *noun* a surgical operation to open up a blocked Fallopian tube

**salpinx** /ˈsælpɪŋks/ *noun* same as **Fallopian tube** (NOTE: The plural is **salpinges**.)

**salt** /sɔːlt/ *noun* **1.** small white crystals mainly of sodium chloride used to flavour and preserve food **2.** a crystalline compound, usually containing a metal, formed when an acid is neutralised by an alkali

COMMENT: Salt forms a necessary part of diet, as it replaces salt lost in sweating and helps to control the water balance in the body. It also improves the working of the muscles and nerves. Most diets contain more salt than each person actually needs, and although it has not been proved to be harmful, it is generally wise to cut down on salt consumption. Salt is one of the four tastes, the others being sweet, sour and bitter.

**salt depletion** /ˈsɔːlt dɪˌpliːʃ(ə)n/ *noun* loss of salt from the body, by sweating or vomiting, which causes cramp

**salt-free diet** /ˌsɔːlt friː ˈdaɪət/ *noun* a diet in which no salt is allowed

**salve** /sælv/ *noun* an ointment

**sample** /ˈsɑːmpəl/ *noun* a small quantity of something used for testing ○ *Blood samples were taken from all the staff in the hospital.* ○ *The doctor asked her to provide a urine sample.*

**sanatorium** /ˌsænəˈtɔːriəm/ *noun* an institution, similar to a hospital, which treats particular types of disorder such as tuberculosis, or offers special treatment such as hot baths or massage (NOTE: The plural is **sanatoria** or **sanatoriums**.)

**sandflea** /ˈsændfliː/ *noun* the jigger, a tropical insect which enters the skin between the toes and digs under the skin, causing intense irritation

**sandfly fever** /ˈsændflaɪ ˌfiːvə/ *noun* a virus infection like influenza, which is transmitted by the bite of the sandfly *Phlebotomus papatasii* and is common in the Middle East

**sandwich therapy** /ˈsænwɪdʃ ˌθerəpi/ *noun* a system in which one type of treatment is used between exposures to a different treatment, e.g., chemotherapy given before and after radiation, or radiation given before and after surgery

**sangui-** /sæŋgwi/ *prefix* relating to blood

**sanguineous** /sæŋˈgwɪniəs/ *adjective* referring to blood, containing blood

**sanies** /ˈseɪniːz/ *noun* a discharge from a sore or wound which has an unpleasant smell

**sanitary** /ˈsænɪt(ə)ri/ *adjective* **1.** clean **2.** referring to hygiene or to health

**sanitary towel** /ˈsænɪt(ə)ri ˌtaʊəl/ *noun* a disposable pad of absorbent material worn by women to absorb the blood flow during menstruation

**sanitation** /ˌsænɪˈteɪʃ(ə)n/ *noun* the practice of being hygienic, especially referring to public hygiene ○ *Poor sanitation in crowded conditions can result in the spread of disease.*

**SA node** /ˌes ˈeɪ nəʊd/, **S-A node** *noun* same as **sinoatrial node**

**saphena** /səˈfiːnə/ *noun* same as **saphenous vein** (NOTE: The plural is **saphenae**.)

**saphenous** /səˈfiːnəs/ *adjective* relating to the saphenous veins

**saphenous nerve** /səˈfiːnəs nɜːv/ *noun* a branch of the femoral nerve which connects with the sensory nerves in the skin of the lower leg

**saphenous opening** /səˌfiːnəs ˈəʊp(ə)nɪŋ/ *noun* a hole in the fascia of the thigh through which the saphenous vein passes

# 363

scald

**saphenous vein** /sə'fiːnəs veɪn/ *noun* one of two veins which take blood from the foot up the leg. Also called **saphena**

COMMENT: The long (internal) saphenous vein, the longest vein in the body, runs from the foot up the inside of the leg and joins the femoral vein. The short (posterior) saphenous vein runs up the back of the lower leg and joins the popliteal vein.

**sapphism** /'sæfɪz(ə)m/ *noun* same as **lesbianism**

**sapraemia** /sæ'priːmiə/ *noun* blood poisoning by saprophytes

**saprophyte** /'sæprəfaɪt/ *noun* a microorganism which lives on dead or decaying tissue

**saprophytic** /sæprəʊ'fɪtɪk/ *adjective* referring to an organism which lives on dead or decaying tissue

**sarc-** /saːk/, **sarco-** /saːkəʊ/ *prefix* 1. referring to flesh 2. referring to muscle

**sarcoid** /'saːkɔɪd/ *noun* a tumour which is like a sarcoma ■ *adjective* like a sarcoma

**sarcoidosis** /saːkɔɪ'dəʊsɪs/ *noun* a disease causing enlargement of the lymph nodes, where small nodules or granulomas form in certain tissues, especially in the lungs or liver and other parts of the body. Also called **Boeck's disease, Boeck's sarcoid** (NOTE: The Kveim test confirms the presence of sarcoidosis.)

**sarcolemma** /saːkəʊ'lemə/ *noun* a membrane surrounding a muscle fibre

**sarcoma** /saː'kəʊmə/ *noun* a cancer of connective tissue such as bone, muscle or cartilage

**sarcomatosis** /saːkəʊmə'təʊsɪs/ *noun* a condition in which a sarcoma has spread through the bloodstream to many parts of the body

**sarcomatous** /saː'kɒmətəs/ *adjective* referring to a sarcoma

**sarcomere** /'saːkəmɪə/ *noun* a filament in myofibril

**sarcoplasm** /'saːkəplæz(ə)m/ *noun* semiliquid cytoplasm in muscle membrane. Also called **myoplasm**

**sarcoplasmic** /saːkəʊ'plæzmɪk/ *adjective* referring to sarcoplasm

**sarcoplasmic reticulum** /saːkəʊ plæzmɪk rɪ'tɪkjʊləm/ *noun* a network in the cytoplasm of striated muscle fibres

**sarcoptes** /saː'kɒptiːz/ *noun* a type of mite which causes scabies

**sardonicus** /saː'dɒnɪkəs/ ♦ **risus sardonicus**

**SARS** /saːz/ *noun* a serious, sometimes fatal, infection affecting the respiratory system, first seen in China. Suspected cases of SARS must be isolated with full barrier nursing precautions. Full form **severe acute respiratory syndrome**

**sartorius** /saː'tɔːriəs/ *noun* a very long muscle, the longest muscle in the body, which runs from the anterior iliac spine, across the thigh down to the tibia

**saturated fat** /sætʃəreɪtɪd 'fæt/ *noun* a fat which has the largest amount of hydrogen possible

COMMENT: Animal fats such as butter and fat meat are saturated fatty acids. It is thought that increasing the amount of unsaturated and polyunsaturated fats, mainly vegetable fats and oils, and fish oil, and reducing saturated fats in the food intake helps reduce the level of cholesterol in the blood, and so lessens the risk of atherosclerosis.

**saturnism** /'sætənɪz(ə)m/ *noun* lead poisoning

**satyriasis** /sætə'raɪəsɪs/ *noun* an obsessive sexual urge in a man (NOTE: A similar condition in a woman is called **nymphomania**.)

**saucerisation** /sɔːsəraɪ'zeɪʃ(ə)n/, **saucerization** *noun* 1. a surgical operation in which tissue is cut out in the form of a saucer-like depression, usually in order to help material drain away from infected areas of bone 2. the shallow saucer-like appearance of the upper surface of a vertebra after a compression fracture

**save** /seɪv/ *verb* 1. to stop someone from being hurt or killed ○ *The doctors saved the little boy from dying of cancer.* □ **the surgeons saved her life** they stopped the patient from dying 2. to stop something from being damaged ○ *The surgeons were unable to save the sight of their patient.*

**saw** /sɔː/ *noun* a tool with a long metal blade with teeth along its edge, used for cutting ■ *verb* to cut something with a saw (NOTE: **sawing – sawed – sawn**)

**Sayre's jacket** /'seɪəz ˌdʒækɪt/ *noun* a plaster cast which supports the spine when vertebrae have been deformed by tuberculosis or spinal disease [After Lewis Albert Sayre (1820–1901), US surgeon]

**s.c.** *abbr* subcutaneous

**scab** /skæb/ *noun* a crust of dry blood which forms over a wound and protects it

**scabicide** /'skeɪbəsaɪd/ *noun* a solution which kills mites ■ *adjective* killing mites

**scabies** /'skeɪbiːz/ *noun* a very irritating infection of the skin caused by a mite which lives under the skin

**scala** /'skaːlə/ *noun* a spiral canal in the cochlea

COMMENT: The cochlea is formed of three spiral canals: the **scala vestibuli** which is filled with perilymph and connects with the oval window; the **scala media** which is filled with endolymph and transmits vibrations from the scala vestibuli through the basilar membrane to the **scala tympani**, which in turn transmits the sound vibrations to the round window.

**scald** /skɔːld/ *noun* an injury to the skin caused by touching a very hot liquid or steam. Also called **wet burn** ■ *verb* to injure the skin with a very hot liquid or steam

**scalding** /ˈskɔːldɪŋ/ *adjective* **1.** referring to a liquid which is very hot **2.** referring to urine which gives a burning sensation when passed

**scale** /skeɪl/ *noun* **1.** a thin flat piece of something such as dead skin **2.** same as **tartar 3.** a system of measurement or valuation based on a series of marks or levels with regular intervals between them ○ *a pay scale* **4.** same as **scales** ◼ *verb* to remove the calcium deposits from teeth

**scalenus** /skeɪˈliːnəs/, **scalene** /ˈskeɪliːn/ *noun* one of a group of muscles in the neck which bend the neck forwards and sideways, and also help expand the lungs in deep breathing

**scalenus syndrome** /skeɪˈliːnəs ˌsɪnↆdrəʊm/ *noun* a pain in an arm, caused by the scalenus anterior muscle pressing the subclavian artery and the brachial plexus against the vertebrae. Also called **thoracic outlet syndrome**

**scale off** /ˌskeɪl ˈɒf/ *verb* to fall off in scales

**scaler** /ˈskeɪlə/ *noun* a surgical instrument for scaling teeth

**scales** /skeɪlz/ *noun* a machine for weighing ○ *The nurses weighed the baby on the scales.*

**scalp** /skælp/ *noun* the thick skin and muscle, with the hair, which covers the skull

**scalpel** /ˈskælpəl/ *noun* a small sharp-pointed knife used in surgery

**scaly** /ˈskeɪli/ *adjective* covered in scales ○ *The pustules harden and become scaly.*

**scan** /skæn/ *noun* **1.** an examination of part of the body using computer-interpreted X-rays to create a picture of the part on a screen **2.** a picture of part of the body created on a screen using computer-interpreted X-rays ◼ *verb* to examine part of the body using computer-interpreted X-rays to create a picture of the part on a screen

**scanner** /ˈskænə/ *noun* **1.** a machine which scans a part of the body **2.** a person who examines a test slide **3.** a person who operates a scanning machine

**scanning** /ˈskænɪŋ/ *noun* **1.** the act of examining an area with the eyes **2.** the act of examining internal organs of the body with a piece of electronic equipment

**scanning speech** /ˈskænɪŋ spiːtʃ/ *noun* a disorder in speaking, where each sound is spoken separately and given equal stress

**scaphocephalic** /ˌskæfəʊsəˈfælɪk/ *adjective* having a long narrow skull

**scaphocephaly** /ˌskæfəʊˈkefəli, ˌskæfəʊˈsefəli/ *noun* a condition in which the skull is unusually long and narrow

**scaphoid** /ˈskæfɔɪd/, **scaphoid bone** /ˈskæfɔɪd bəʊn/ *noun* one of the carpal bones in the wrist. See illustration at **HAND** in Supplement

**scapula** /ˈskæpjʊlə/ *noun* one of two large flat bones covering the top part of the back. Also called **shoulder blade** (NOTE: The plural is **scapulae**.)

**scapular** /ˈskæpjʊlə/ *adjective* referring to the shoulder blade

**scapulo-** /ˈskæpjʊləʊ/ *prefix* relating to the scapula

**scapulohumeral** /ˌskæpjʊləʊˈhjuːmərəl/ *adjective* referring to the scapula and humerus

**scar** /skɑː/ *noun* the mark left on the skin after a wound or surgical incision has healed ○ *He still has the scar of his appendicectomy.* Also called **cicatrix** ◼ *verb* to leave a scar on the skin ○ *The burns have scarred him for life.* ○ *Plastic surgeons have tried to repair the scarred arm.* ○ *Patients were given special clothes to reduce hypertrophic scarring.*

**scarification** /ˌskærɪfɪˈkeɪʃ(ə)n/ *noun* scratching, making minute cuts on the surface of the skin, e.g. for a smallpox vaccination

**scarificator** /ˈskærɪfəkeɪtə/ *noun* an instrument used for scarification

**scarlatina** /ˌskɑːləˈtiːnə/, **scarlet fever** /ˌskɑːlət ˈfiːvə/ *noun* an infectious disease with a fever, sore throat and a red rash. It is caused by a haemolytic streptococcus and can sometimes have serious complications if the kidneys are infected.

**Scarpa's triangle** /ˌskɑːpɑːz ˈtraɪæŋgəl/ *noun* same as **femoral triangle** [After Antonio Scarpa (1747–1832), Italian anatomist and surgeon]

**scar tissue** /ˈskɑː ˌtɪʃuː/ *noun* fibrous tissue which forms a scar

**scat-** /skæt/, **scato-** /ˈskætəʊ/ *prefix* referring to the faeces

**scatole** /ˈskætəʊl/ *noun* a substance in faeces, formed in the intestine, which causes a strong smell (NOTE: Also spelled **skatole**.)

**SCC** *abbr* squamous cell carcinoma

**scent** /sent/ *noun* **1.** a pleasant smell ○ *The scent of flowers makes me sneeze.* **2.** a cosmetic substance which has a pleasant smell **3.** a smell given off by a substance which stimulates the sense of smell

**scented** /ˈsentɪd/ *adjective* with a strong pleasant smell ○ *He is allergic to scented soap.*

**schema** /ˈskiːmə/ *noun* same as **body image**

**Scheuermann's disease** /ˈʃɔɪəmənz dɪˌziːz/ *noun* inflammation of the bones and cartilage in the spine, usually affecting adolescents [Described 1920. After Holger Werfel Scheuermann (1877–1960), Danish orthopaedic surgeon and radiologist.]

**Schick test** /ˈʃɪk test/ *noun* a test to see if a person is immune to diphtheria [Described 1908. After Bela Schick (1877–1967), paediatrician in Vienna, Austria, and New York, USA.]

COMMENT: In the Schick test, a small amount of diphtheria toxin is injected, and if the point of injection becomes inflamed it shows the person is not immune to the disease (a positive reaction).

**Schilling test** /ˈʃɪlɪŋ test/ *noun* a test to see if someone can absorb Vitamin B$_{12}$ through the intestines, to determine cases of pernicious anaemia [After Robert Frederick Schilling (b. 1919), US physician]

**-schisis** /skaɪsɪs/ *suffix* referring to a fissure or split

**schisto-** /ʃɪstəʊ/ *prefix* referring to something which is split

**Schistosoma** /ˌʃɪstəˈsəʊmə/, **schistosome** /ˈʃɪstəsəʊm/ same as **bilharzia**

**schistosomiasis** /ˌʃɪstəsəʊˈmaɪəsɪs/ *noun* same as **bilharziasis**

**schiz-** /skɪts/, **schizo-** /skɪtsəʊ/ *prefix* referring to something which is split

**schizoid** /ˈskɪtsɔɪd/ *adjective* referring to schizophrenia ■ *noun* a person who has a less severe form of schizophrenia

**schizoid personality** /ˌskɪtsɔɪd ˌpɜːsəˈnælɪti/ *noun* a disorder in which someone is cold towards other people, thinks mainly about himself or herself and behaves in an odd way. Also called **split personality**

**schizophrenia** /ˌskɪtsəʊˈfriːniə/ *noun* a mental disorder in which someone withdraws from contact with other people, has delusions and seems to lose contact with the real world

**schizophrenic** /ˌskɪtsəʊˈfrenɪk/ *noun* someone who has schizophrenia ■ *adjective* having schizophrenia

**schizotypal personality disorder** /ˌskɪtsəʊtaɪpəl ˌpɜːsəˈnælɪti dɪsˌɔːdə/ *noun* a schizoid personality type disorder

**Schlatter's disease** /ˈʃlætəz dɪˌziːz/ *noun* inflammation in the bones and cartilage at the top of the tibia [Described 1903. After Carl Schlatter (1864–1934), Professor of Surgery at Zürich, Switzerland.]

**Schlemm's canal** /ˈʃlemz kəˌnæl/ *noun* a circular canal in the sclera of the eye, which drains the aqueous humour [Described 1830. After Friedrich Schlemm (1795–1858), Professor of Anatomy in Berlin, Germany.]

**Schönlein–Henoch purpura** /ˌʃɜːnlaɪn ˈhenɒk ˌpɜːpjʊrə/, **Schönlein's purpura** /ˈʃɜːnlaɪnz ˌpɜːpjʊrə/ *noun* a blood disorder of children, in which the skin becomes purple on the buttocks and lower legs, the joints are swollen and painful and there are gastrointestinal problems

**school** /skuːl/ *noun* 1. a place where children are taught 2. a specialised section of a university

**school health service** /skuːl ˈhelθ ˌsɜːvɪs/ *noun* a special service, part of the local health authority, which looks after the health of children in school

**school nurse** /skuːl ˈnɜːs/ *noun* a nurse who works in a school, treating health problems and promoting health and safety

**Schwann cells** /ˈʃvɒn selz/ *plural noun* the cells which form the myelin sheath around a nerve fibre. See illustration at **NEURONE** in Supplement [Described 1839. After Friedrich Theodor Schwann (1810–82), German anatomist.]

**schwannoma** /ʃvɒˈnəʊmə/ *noun* a neurofibroma, a benign tumour of a peripheral nerve

**Schwartze's operation** /ˈʃvɔːtsɪz ˌɒpəreɪʃ(ə)n/ *noun* the original surgical operation to drain fluid and remove infected tissue from the mastoid process [After Hermann Schwartze (1837–1910), German otologist]

**sciatic** /saɪˈætɪk/ *adjective* 1. referring to the hip 2. referring to the sciatic nerve

**sciatica** /saɪˈætɪkə/ *noun* pain along the sciatic nerve, usually at the back of the thighs and legs

COMMENT: Sciatica can be caused by a slipped disc which presses on a spinal nerve, or can simply be caused by straining a muscle in the back.

**sciatic nerve** /saɪˈætɪk nɜːv/ *noun* one of two main nerves which run from the sacral plexus into each of the thighs, dividing into a series of nerves in the lower legs and feet. They are the largest nerves in the body.

**SCID** *abbr* severe combined immunodeficiency

**science** /ˈsaɪəns/ *noun* a study based on looking at and recording facts, especially facts arranged into a system

**scientific** /ˌsaɪənˈtɪfɪk/ *adjective* referring to science ○ *He carried out scientific experiments.*

**scientist** /ˈsaɪəntɪst/ *noun* a person who specialises in scientific studies

**scintigram** /ˈsɪntɪɡræm/ *noun* an image recording radiation from radioactive isotopes injected into the body

**scintillascope** /sɪnˈtɪləskəʊp/ *noun* an instrument which produces a scintigram

**scintillator** /ˈsɪntɪleɪtə/ *noun* a substance which produces a flash of light when struck by radiation

**scintiscan** /ˈsɪntɪskæn/ *noun* a scintigram which shows the variations in radiation from one part of the body to another

**scirrhous** /ˈsɪrəs/ *adjective* hard ○ *a scirrhous tumour*

**scirrhus** /ˈsɪrəs/ *noun* a hard malignant tumour, especially in the breast

**scissor leg** /ˈsɪzə leg/ *noun* a condition in which someone walks with one leg crossing over the other, usually as a result of spasticity of the leg's adductor muscles

**scissor legs** /ˈsɪzə legz/ *plural noun* malformed legs, where one leg is permanently crossed over in front of the other

**scissors** /'sɪzəz/ *plural noun* an instrument for cutting, made of two blades and two handles fastened together

**scissura** /sɪ'ʃʊrə/ *noun* an opening in something or a splitting of something

**scler-** /sklɪə/ *prefix* same as **sclero-** (*used before vowels*)

**sclera** /'sklɪərə/ *noun* the hard white outer covering of the eyeball. See illustration at **EYE** in Supplement. Also called **sclerotic, sclerotic coat, albuginea oculi**

COMMENT: The front part of the sclera is the transparent cornea, through which the light enters the eye. The conjunctiva, or inner skin of the eyelids, connects with the sclera and covers the front of the eyeball.

**scleral** /'sklɪərəl/ *adjective* referring to the sclera

**scleral lens** /'sklɪərəl lenz/ *noun* a large contact lens which covers most of the front of the eye

**scleritis** /sklə'raɪtɪs/ *noun* inflammation of the sclera

**sclero-** /sklɪərəʊ/ *prefix* 1. hard, thick 2. referring to the sclera

**scleroderma** /ˌsklɪərə'dɜːmə/ *noun* a collagen disease which thickens connective tissue and produces a hard thick skin

**scleroma** /sklə'rəʊmə/ *noun* a patch of hard skin or hard mucous membrane

**scleromalacia** /ˌsklɪərəʊmə,leɪʃiə pə'fɔːrəns/, **scleromalacia perforans** /ˌsklɪərəʊmə'leɪʃiə/ *noun* a condition of the sclera in which holes appear in it

**sclerosant agent** /sklə'rəʊs(ə)nt ,eɪdʒənt/ *noun* an irritating liquid injected into tissue to harden it

**sclerosing** /sklə'rəʊsɪŋ/ *adjective* becoming hard, or making tissue hard

**sclerosing agent** /sklə'rəʊsɪŋ ,eɪdʒ(ə)nt/, **sclerosing solution** /sklə'rəʊsɪŋ sə,luːʃ(ə)n/ *noun* same as **sclerosant agent**

**sclerosis** /sklə'rəʊsɪs/ *noun* a condition in which tissue becomes hard

**sclerotherapy** /ˌsklɪərəʊ'θerəpi/ *noun* the treatment of a varicose vein by injecting a sclerosant agent into the vein, and so encouraging the blood in the vein to clot

**sclerotic** /sklə'rɒtɪk/ *adjective* referring to sclerosis, or having sclerosis ■ *noun* same as **sclera**

**sclerotic coat** /sklə,rɒtɪk 'kəʊt/ *noun* same as **sclera**

**sclerotome** /'sklɪərətəʊm/ *noun* a sharp knife used in sclerotomy

**sclerotomy** /sklə'rɒtəmi/ *noun* a surgical operation to cut into the sclera

**scolex** /'skəʊleks/ *noun* the head of a tapeworm, with hooks which attach it to the wall of the intestine (NOTE: The plural is **scolices** or **scolexes**.)

**scoliosis** /ˌskəʊli'əʊsɪs/ *noun* a condition in which the spine curves sideways

**scoliotic** /ˌskəʊli'ɒtɪk/ *adjective* referring to a spine which curves sideways

**scoop stretcher** /'skuːp ,stretʃə/ *noun* a type of stretcher formed of two jointed sections which can slide under someone and lock together

**-scope** /skəʊp/ *suffix* referring to an instrument for examining by sight

**scopolamine** /skə'pɒləmiːn/ *noun* a colourless thick liquid poisonous alkaloid found in some plants of the nightshade family. It is used especially to prevent motion sickness and as a sedative.

**scorbutic** /skɔː'bjuːtɪk/ *adjective* referring to scurvy

**scorbutus** /skɔː'bjuːtəs/ *noun* same as **scurvy**

**scoto-** /skəʊtə/ *prefix* dark

**scotoma** /skɒ'təʊmə/ *noun* a small area in the field of vision where someone cannot see

**scotometer** /skəʊ'tɒmɪtə/ *noun* an instrument used to measure areas of impaired vision

**scotopia** /skəʊ'təʊpiə/ *noun* the power of the eye to adapt to poor lighting conditions and darkness

**scotopic** /skəʊ'tɒpɪk/ *adjective* referring to scotopia

**scotopic vision** /skəʊ,tɒpɪk 'vɪʒ(ə)n/ *noun* vision in the dark and in dim light, where the rods of the retina are used instead of the cones, which are used for photopic vision. ♦ **dark adaptation**

**scrape** /skreɪp/ *verb* to remove the surface of something by moving a sharp knife across it

**scratch** /skrætʃ/ *noun* a slight wound on the skin made when a sharp point is pulled across it ○ *She had scratches on her legs and arms.* ○ *Wash the dirt out of that scratch in case it gets infected.* ■ *verb* to harm the skin by moving a sharp point across it ○ *The cat scratched the girl's face.* ○ *Be careful not to scratch yourself on the wire.*

**scratch test** /'skrætʃ test/ *noun* a test for allergy, in which a small amount of a substance is placed on a lightly scratched area of skin to see if a reaction occurs

**scream** /skriːm/ *noun* a loud sharp cry ■ *verb* to make a loud sharp cry

**screen** /skriːn/ *noun* 1. a light wall, sometimes with a curtain, which can be moved about and put round a bed to shield a person 2. same as **screening** ■ *verb* to examine large numbers of people to test them for a disease ○ *The population of the village was screened for meningitis.*

'…in the UK the main screen is carried out by health visitors at 6–10 months. With adequately staffed and trained community services, this method of screening can be extremely effective' [*Lancet*]

**screening** /'skri:nɪŋ/ *noun* the process of testing large numbers of people to see if any of them have a particular type of disease. ◊ **genetic screening**

'GPs are increasingly requesting blood screening for patients concerned about HIV' [*Journal of the Royal College of General Practitioners*]

**screening test** /'skri:nɪŋ test/ *noun* a test for a particular disease which is given to people who have no symptoms in order to identify how many of them have that disease or are showing early signs of it

**scrip** /skrɪp/ *noun* a doctor's prescription (*informal*)

**scrofula** /'skrɒfjʊlə/ *noun* a form of tuberculosis in the lymph nodes in the neck, formerly caused by unpasteurised milk but now rare

**scrofuloderma** /ˌskrɒfjʊləʊ'dɜːmə/ *noun* a form of tuberculosis of the skin, forming ulcers, and secondary to tuberculous infection of an underlying lymph gland or structure

**scrota** /'skrəʊtə/ *plural of* **scrotum**

**scrotal** /'skrəʊt(ə)l/ *adjective* referring to the scrotum

**scrototomy** /skrəʊ'tɒtəmi/ *noun* a surgical operation to open up and examine the scrotum (NOTE: The plural is **scrototomies**.)

**scrotum** /'skrəʊtəm/ *noun* a bag of skin hanging from behind the penis, containing the testes, epididymides and part of the spermatic cord. See illustration at UROGENITAL SYSTEM (MALE) in Supplement (NOTE: The plural is **scrotums** or **scrota**.)

**scrub nurse** /'skrʌb ˌnɜːs/ *noun* a nurse who cleans the operation site on someone's body before an operation

**scrub typhus** /'skrʌb ˌtaɪfəs/ *noun* same as **tsutsugamushi disease**

**scrub up** /ˌskrʌb 'ʌp/ *verb* (*of a surgeon or theatre nurse*) to clean the hands and arms thoroughly before performing surgery (NOTE: **scrubbing up – scrubbed up**)

**scrumpox** /'skrʌmpɒks/ *noun* a form of herpes simplex found especially in male sports players, passed on easily due to the presence of small cuts in the skin combined with the abrasive effects of facial stubble

**scurf** /skɜːf/ *noun* same as **dandruff**

**scurvy** /'skɜːvi/ *noun* a disease caused by lack of vitamin C or ascorbic acid which is found in fruit and vegetables. Also called **scorbutus**

COMMENT: Scurvy causes general weakness and anaemia, with bleeding from the gums and joints, and under the skin. In severe cases, the teeth drop out. Treatment consists of vitamin C tablets and a change of diet to include more fruit and vegetables.

**scybalum** /'sɪbələm/ *noun* very hard faeces

**seasick** /'siːsɪk/ *adjective* feeling sick because of the movement of a ship ○ *As soon as the ferry started to move she felt seasick.*

**seasickness** /'siːsɪknəs/ *noun* illness, with nausea, vomiting and sometimes headache, caused by the movement of a ship ○ *Take some seasickness tablets if you are going on a long journey.*

**seasonal affective disorder** /ˌsiːz(ə)nl ə'fektɪv dɪsˌɔːdə/, **seasonal affective disorder syndrome** /ˌsiːz(ə)nl ə'fektɪv dɪs ˌɔːdə ˌsɪndrəʊm/ *noun* a condition in which a person becomes depressed and anxious during the winter when there are fewer hours of daylight. Its precise cause is not known, but it is thought that the shortage of daylight may provoke a reaction between various hormones and neurotransmitters in the brain. Abbr **SAD, SADS**

**seat-belt syndrome** /'siːt belt ˌsɪndrəʊm/ *noun* a group of injuries between the neck and the abdomen which occur in a car accident when a person is using either a lap belt or a shoulder belt incorrectly, not over the strongest part of the chest

**sebaceous** /sə'beɪʃəs/ *adjective* **1.** referring to sebum **2.** producing sebum

**sebaceous cyst** /səˌbeɪʃəs 'sɪst/ *noun* a cyst which forms when a sebaceous gland is blocked. ◊ **steatoma**

**sebaceous gland** /səˌbeɪʃəs 'glænd/ *noun* a gland in the skin which secretes sebum at the base of each hair follicle

**seborrhoea** /ˌsebə'riːə/ *noun* an excessive secretion of sebum by the sebaceous glands, common in young people at puberty, and sometimes linked to seborrhoeic dermatitis (NOTE: The US spelling is **seborrhea**.)

**seborrhoeic** /ˌsebə'riːɪk/ *adjective* **1.** caused by seborrhoea **2.** having an oily secretion (NOTE: [all senses] The US spelling is **seborrheic**.)

**seborrhoeic dermatitis** /ˌsebəriːɪk ˌdɜːmə 'taɪtɪs/, **seborrhoeic eczema** /ˌsebəriːɪk 'ekˌsɪmə/ *noun* a type of eczema where scales form on the skin

**seborrhoeic rash** /ˌsebəriːɪk 'ræʃ/ *noun* ◊ **seborrhoeic dermatitis**

**sebum** /'siːbəm/ *noun* an oily substance secreted by a sebaceous gland, which makes the skin smooth. It also protects the skin against bacteria and the body against rapid evaporation of water.

**second** /'sekənd/ *noun* a unit of time equal to 1/60 of a minute ■ *adjective* coming after the first

**secondary** /'sekənd(ə)ri/ *adjective* **1.** occurring after the first stage **2.** less important than something else **3.** referring to a condition which develops from another condition ■ *noun* a malignant tumour which has developed and spread from another malignant tumour. ◊ **primary** (NOTE: The plural is **secondaries**.)

**secondary amenorrhoea** /ˌsekənd(ə)ri eɪmenə'riːə/ *noun* a situation in which a premenopausal woman's menstrual periods have stopped

**secondary biliary cirrhosis** /ˌsekənd(ə)ri ˌbɪliəri səˈrəʊsɪs/ *noun* cirrhosis of the liver caused by an obstruction of the bile ducts

**secondary bronchi** /ˌsekənd(ə)ri ˈbrɒŋkiː/ *plural noun* same as **lobar bronchi**

**secondary care** /ˌsekənd(ə)ri ˈkeə/ *noun* treatment provided by the professional team in a hospital, rather than by a GP or other primary care provider and the primary health care team. Compare **primary care, tertiary care**. Also called **secondary health care**

**secondary cartilaginous joint** /ˌsekənd(ə)ri kɑːtəˈlædʒɪnəs ˌdʒɔɪnt/ *noun* a joint where the surfaces of the two bones are connected by a piece of cartilage so that they cannot move, e.g. the pubic symphysis

**secondary dysmenorrhoea** /ˌsekənd(ə)ri dɪsˌmenəˈriːə/ *noun* dysmenorrhoea which starts at some time after the first menstruation

**secondary growth** /ˌsekənd(ə)ri ˈɡrəʊθ/ *noun* same as **metastasis**

**secondary haemorrhage** /ˌsekənd(ə)ri ˈhem(ə)rɪdʒ/ *noun* a haemorrhage which occurs some time after an injury, usually due to infection of the wound

**secondary health care** /ˌsekənd(ə)ri ˈhelθ keə/ *noun* same as secondary care

**secondary infection** /ˌsekənd(ə)ri ɪnˈfekʃən/ *noun* an infection which affects a person while he or she is weakened through having another infection

**secondary medical care** /ˌsekənd(ə)ri ˈmedɪk(ə)l keə/ *noun* specialised treatment provided by a hospital

**secondary peritonitis** /ˌsekənd(ə)ri ˌperɪtəˈnaɪtɪs/ *noun* peritonitis caused by infection from an adjoining tissue, e.g. from the rupturing of the appendix

**secondary prevention** /ˌsekənd(ə)ri prɪˈvenʃən/ *noun* the use of methods such as screening tests which avoid a serious disease by detecting it early

**secondary sexual characteristic** /ˌsekənd(ə)ri ˌsekʃuəl kærɪktəˈrɪstɪk/ *noun* a sexual characteristic which develops after puberty, e.g. pubic hair or breasts

**second-degree burn** /ˌsekənd dɪˌɡriː ˈbɜːn/ *noun* a burn where the skin becomes very red and blisters

**second-degree haemorrhoids** /ˌsekənd dɪˌɡriː ˈhemərɔɪds/ *plural noun* haemorrhoids which protrude into the anus but return into the rectum automatically

**second intention** /ˌsekənd ɪnˈtenʃ(ə)n/ *noun* healing of an infected wound or ulcer, which takes place slowly and leaves a prominent scar

**second-level nurse** /ˌsekənd ˌlev(ə)l ˈnɜːs/, **second-level registered nurse** /ˌsekənd ˌlev(ə)l ˌredʒɪstəd ˈnɜːs/ *noun* a trained person who delivers nursing care under the direction and supervision of a first-level nurse. Compare **first-level nurse**

**second molar** /ˌsekənd ˈməʊlə/ *noun* any of the molars at the back of the jaw, before the wisdom teeth, erupting at about 12 years of age

**second opinion** /ˌsekənd əˈpɪnjən/ *noun* a diagnosis or opinion on treatment from a second doctor, often a hospital specialist

**secrete** /sɪˈkriːt/ *verb* (*of a gland*) to produce a substance such as hormone, oil or enzyme (NOTE: **secreting – secreted**)

**secretin** /sɪˈkriːtɪn/ *noun* a hormone secreted by the duodenum which encourages the production of pancreatic juice

**secretion** /sɪˈkriːʃ(ə)n/ *noun* **1.** the process by which a substance is produced by a gland ○ *The pituitary gland stimulates the secretion of hormones by the adrenal gland.* **2.** a substance produced by a gland ○ *Sex hormones are bodily secretions.*

**secretor** /sɪˈkriːtə/ *noun* a person who secretes substances indicating ABO blood group into mucous fluids such as semen or saliva

**secretory** /sɪˈkriːtəri/ *adjective* referring to, accompanied by or producing a secretion

**secretory otitis media** /sɪˌkriːtəri əʊ ˌtaɪtɪs ˈmiːdiə/ *noun* same as **glue ear**

**section** /ˈsekʃən/ *noun* **1.** a part of something ○ *the middle section of the aorta* **2.** the action of cutting tissue **3.** a cut made in tissue **4.** a slice of tissue cut for examination under a microscope **5.** a part of a document such as an Act of Parliament ○ *She was admitted under section 5 of the Mental Health Act.*

**Section 47** /ˌsekʃən fɔːti ˈsev(ə)n/ *noun* a UK law under which a local authority has the power to seek an order from a magistrate's court authorising the removal of a person at severe risk from their home. The authority must have a doctor's certificate that the person is either suffering from a grave and chronic disease or is unable to look after himself or herself and is not receiving proper care and attention from other people.

**security blanket** /sɪˈkjʊərəti ˌblæŋkɪt/ *noun* a familiar blanket, toy or other object which a child carries around because it makes him or her feel safe

**sedate** /sɪˈdeɪt/ *verb* to calm a person by giving them a drug which acts on the nervous system and relieves stress or pain, and in larger doses makes the person sleep ○ *Elderly or confused patients may need to be sedated to prevent them wandering.* (NOTE: **sedating – sedated**)

**sedation** /sɪˈdeɪʃ(ə)n/ *noun* the act of calming someone using a sedative □ **under sedation** having been given a sedative ○ *He was* *still under sedation, and could not be seen by the police.*

**sedative** /ˈsedətɪv/ *noun* an anxiolytic or hypnotic drug such as benzodiazepine, which acts on the nervous system to help a person sleep or to relieve stress (*dated*) ○ *She was prescribed sedatives by the doctor.* ■ *adjective* acting to help a person sleep or to relieve stress

**sedentary** /ˈsed(ə)nt(ə)ri/ *adjective* involving a lot of sitting and little exercise

'...changes in lifestyle factors have been related to the decline in mortality from ischaemic heart disease. In many studies a sedentary lifestyle has been reported as a risk factor for ischaemic heart disease' [*Journal of the American Medical Association*]

**sedentary occupation** /ˌsed(ə)nt(ə)ri ˌɒkjʊˈpeɪʃ(ə)n/ *noun* a job where the workers sit down for most of the time

**sediment** /ˈsedɪmənt/ *noun* solid particles, usually insoluble, which fall to the bottom of a liquid

**sedimentation** /ˌsedɪmenˈteɪʃ(ə)n/ *noun* the action of solid particles falling to the bottom of a liquid

**sedimentation rate** /ˌsedɪmenˈteɪʃ(ə)n reɪt/ *noun* the rate at which solid particles are deposited from a solution, measured especially in a centrifuge

**segment** /ˈsegmənt/ *noun* a part of an organ or piece of tissue which is clearly separate from other parts

**segmental** /segˈment(ə)l/ *adjective* formed of segments

**segmental ablation** /segˌment(ə)l æˈbleɪʃ(ə)n/ *noun* a surgical operation to remove part of a nail, e.g. treatment for an ingrowing toenail

**segmental bronchi** /segˌment(ə)l ˈbrɒŋkiː/ *plural noun* air passages supplying a segment of a lung. Also called **tertiary bronchi**

**segmentation** /ˌsegmənˈteɪʃ(ə)n/ *noun* the movement of separate segments of the wall of the intestine to mix digestive juice with the food before it is passed along by the action of peristalsis

**segmented** /ˈsegməntɪd/ *adjective* formed of segments

**segregation** /ˌsegrɪˈgeɪʃ(ə)n/ *noun* **1.** the act of separating one person, group or thing from others, or of dividing people or things into separate groups which are kept apart from each other **2.** the separation of the alleles of each gene and their distribution to separate sex cells during the formation of these cells in organisms with paired chromosomes

**seizure** /ˈsiːʒə/ *noun* a fit, convulsion or sudden contraction of the muscles, especially in a heart attack, stroke or epileptic fit

**select** /sɪˈlekt/ *verb* to choose one person, thing or group, but not others ○ *She was selected to go on a midwifery course*

**selection** /sɪˈlekʃən/ *noun* an act of choosing one person, thing or group, but not others ○ *the selection of a suitable donor for a bone marrow transplant* ○ *The candidates for the post have to go through a selection process.*

**selective** /sɪˈlektɪv/ *adjective* choosing only one person, thing or group, and not others

**selective oestrogen receptor modulator** /sɪˌlektɪv ˈiːstrədʒ(ə)n rɪˌseptə ˌmɒdjʊleɪtə/, **selective estrogen receptor modulator** *noun* a drug which acts on specific oestrogen receptors to prevent bone loss without affecting other oestrogen receptors, e.g. raloxifene hydrochloride. Abbr **SERM**

**selective serotonin re-uptake inhibitor** /sɪˌlektɪv serəˌtəʊnɪn riːˈʌpteɪk ɪnˌhɪbɪtə/ *noun* a drug which causes a selective accumulation of serotonin in the central nervous system, and is used in the treatment of depression, e.g. fluoxetine. Abbr **SSRI**

COMMENT: The drug should not be started immediately after stopping an MAOI and should be withdrawn slowly.

**selenium** /səˈliːniəm/ *noun* a non-metallic trace element (NOTE: The chemical symbol is Se.)

**self-** /self/ *prefix* yourself

**self-abuse** /ˌself əˈbjuːs/ *noun* same as **self-harm**

**self-actualisation** /self ˌæktjuəlaɪˈzeɪʃ(ə)n/, **self-actualization** *noun* the successful development and use of personal talents and abilities

**self-admitted** /ˌself ədˈmɪtɪd/ *adjective* referring to a patient who has admitted himself or herself to hospital without being sent by a doctor

**self-care** /self ˈkeə/ *noun* the act of looking after yourself properly, so that you remain healthy

**self-catheterisation** /self ˌkæθɪtəraɪˈzeɪʃ(ə)n/, **self-catheterization** *noun* a procedure in which a person puts a catheter through the urethra into his or her own bladder to empty out the urine

**self-defence** /ˌself dɪˈfens/ *noun* the act of defending yourself when someone is attacking you

**self-examination** /ˌself ɪgˌzæmɪˈneɪʃ(ə)n/ *noun* the regular examination of parts of your own body for signs of disease

**self-governing hospital** /self ˌgʌvənɪŋ ˈhɒspɪt(ə)l/ *noun* in the UK, a hospital which earns its revenue from services provided to the District Health Authorities and family doctors. Also called **hospital trust**

**self-harm** /ˌself ˈhɑːm/ *noun* a deliberate act by which someone injures part of their body as the result of a personal trauma. Cutting and burning are two of the most common forms of self-harm. Also called **self-abuse, self-injury, self-mutilation, self-wounding**

**self-image** /self ˈɪmɪdʒ/ *noun* the opinion which a person has about how worthwhile, attractive, or intelligent he or she is

**self-injury** /ˌself ˈɪndʒəri/, **self-mutilation** /ˌself ˌmjuːtɪˈleɪʃ(ə)n/ *noun* same as **self-harm**

**self-retaining catheter** /self rɪˌteɪnɪŋ ˈkæθɪtə/ *noun* a catheter which remains in place until it is deliberately removed

**self-wounding** *noun* same as **self-harm**

**sella turcica** /ˌselə ˈtɜːsɪkə/ *noun* a hollow in the upper surface of the sphenoid bone in which the pituitary gland sits. Also called **pituitary fossa**

**semeiology** /ˌsiːmaɪˈɒlədʒi/ *noun* same as **symptomatology**

**semen** /ˈsiːmən/ *noun* a thick pale fluid containing spermatozoa, produced by the testes and seminal vesicles and ejaculated from the penis

**semi-** /semi/ *prefix* half

**semicircular** /ˌsemiˈsɜːkjʊlə/ *adjective* shaped like half a circle

**semicircular canal** /ˌsemisɜːkjʊlə kəˈnæl/ *noun* any one of three tubes in the inner ear which are partly filled with fluid and help to maintain balance. See illustration at EAR in Supplement
COMMENT: The three semicircular canals are on different planes. When a person's head moves, as when he or she bends down, the fluid in the canals moves and this movement is communicated to the brain through the vestibular section of the auditory nerve.

**semicircular duct** /ˌsemisɜːkjʊlə ˈdʌkt/ *noun* a duct in the semicircular canals in the ear

**semicomatose** /ˌsemiˈkəʊmətəʊs/ *adjective* almost unconscious or half asleep, but capable of being woken up

**semi-conscious** /ˌsemi ˈkɒnʃəs/ *adjective* half conscious, only partly aware of what is going on ○ *She was semi-conscious for most of the operation.*

**semi-liquid** /ˌsemi ˈlɪkwɪd/ *adjective* half liquid and half solid

**semilunar** /ˌsemiˈluːnə/ *adjective* shaped like half a moon

**semilunar cartilage** /ˌsemiˌluːnə ˈkɑːtəlɪdʒ/ *noun* same as **meniscus**

**semilunar valve** /ˌsemiˌluːnə ˈvælv/ *noun* either of two valves in the heart, the pulmonary valve and the aortic valve, through which blood flows out of the ventricles

**seminal** /ˈsemɪn(ə)l/ *adjective* referring to semen

**seminal fluid** /ˈsemɪn(ə)l ˌfluːɪd/ *noun* the fluid part of semen, formed in the epididymis and seminal vesicles

**seminal vesicle** /ˌsemɪn(ə)l ˈvesɪk(ə)l/ *noun* one of two glands at the end of the vas deferens which secrete the fluid part of semen.

See illustration at **urogenital system (male)** in Supplement

**seminiferous tubule** /ˌsemiˌnɪfərəs ˈtjuːbjuːl/ *noun* a tubule in the testis which carries semen

**seminoma** /ˌsemiˈnəʊmə/ *noun* a malignant tumour in the testis (NOTE: The plural is **seminomas** or **seminomata**)

**semipermeable** /ˌsemiˈpɜːmiəb(ə)l/ *adjective* allowing some types of particle to pass through but not others

**semipermeable membrane** /ˌsemi ˌpɜːmiəb(ə)l ˈmembreɪn/ *noun* a membrane which allows some substances in liquid solution to pass through but not others

**semiprone** /ˌsemiˈprəʊn/ *adjective* referring to a position in which someone lies face downwards, with one knee and one arm bent forwards and the face turned to one side

**semi-solid** /ˌsemi ˈsɒlɪd/ *adjective* half solid and half liquid

**SEN** *abbr* State Enrolled Nurse

**senescence** /sɪˈnesəns/ *noun* the ageing process

**senescent** /sɪˈnesənt/ *adjective* approaching the last stages of the natural life span

**Sengstaken tube** /ˈseŋzteɪkən tjuːb/ *noun* a tube with a balloon, which is passed through the mouth into the oesophagus to stop oesophageal bleeding [After Robert William Sengstaken (b. 1923), US surgeon]

**senile** /ˈsiːnaɪl/ *adjective* 1. referring to the last stages of the natural life span or the medical conditions associated with it 2. referring to someone whose mental faculties have become weak because of age

**senile cataract** /ˌsiːnaɪl ˈkætərækt/ *noun* a cataract which occurs in an elderly person

**senile dementia** /ˌsiːnaɪl dɪˈmenʃə/ *noun* mental degeneration affecting elderly people (*dated*)

**senile plaque** /ˈsiːnaɪl plæk/ *noun* a spherical deposit of beta amyloid in brain areas in Alzheimer's disease

**senilis** /səˈnaɪlɪs/ ♦ **arcus senilis**

**senility** /səˈnɪləti/ *noun* the deterioration of mental activity associated with the last stages of the natural life span

**senior** /ˈsiːniə/ *adjective* 1. older than another person or other people 2. holding a more important position than others ○ *He is the senior anaesthetist in the hospital.* ○ *Senior members of staff are allowed to consult the staff records.* ■ *noun* a senior person

**senna** /ˈsenə/ *noun* a laxative made from the dried fruit and leaves of a tropical tree

**sensation** /senˈseɪʃ(ə)n/ *noun* a feeling or information about something which has been sensed by a sensory nerve and is passed to the brain

**sense** /sens/ *noun* **1.** one of the five faculties by which a person notices things in the outside world: sight, hearing, smell, taste and touch ○ *When she had a cold, she lost her sense of smell.* **2.** the ability to discern or judge something ■ *verb* to notice something by means other than sight ○ *Teeth can sense changes in temperature.*

**sense of balance** /ˌsens əv ˈbæləns/ *noun* a feeling that keeps a person upright, governed by the fluid in the inner ear balance mechanism

**sense organ** /sens ˈɔːɡən/ *noun* an organ in which there are various sensory nerves which can detect environmental stimuli such as scent, heat or pain, and transmit information about them to the central nervous system, e.g. the nose or the skin

**sensibility** /ˌsensɪˈbɪlɪti/ *noun* the ability to detect and interpret sensations

**sensible** /ˈsensɪb(ə)l/ *adjective* **1.** showing common sense or good judgment **2.** able to be detected by the senses

**sensible perspiration** /ˌsensəb(ə)l ˌpɜːspəˈreɪʃ(ə)n/ *noun* drops of sweat which can be seen on the skin, secreted by the sweat glands

**sensitisation** /ˌsensɪtaɪˈzeɪʃ(ə)n/, **sensitization** *noun* **1.** the process of making a person sensitive to something **2.** an unexpected reaction to an allergen or to a drug, caused by the presence of antibodies which were created when the person was exposed to the drug or allergen in the past

**sensitise** /ˈsensɪtaɪz/, **sensitize** *verb* to make someone sensitive to a drug or allergen (NOTE: **sensitising – sensitised**)

**sensitised person** /ˌsensɪtaɪzd ˈpɜːs(ə)n/, **sensitized person** *noun* a person who is allergic to a drug

**sensitising agent** /ˈsensɪtaɪzɪŋ ˌeɪdʒənt/, **sensitizing agent** *noun* a substance which, by acting as an antigen, makes the body form antibodies

**sensitive** /ˈsensɪtɪv/ *adjective* **1.** able to detect and respond to an outside stimulus **2.** having an unexpected reaction to an allergen or to a drug, caused by the presence of antibodies which were created when the person was exposed to the drug or allergen in the past

**sensitivity** /ˌsensɪˈtɪvɪti/ *noun* **1.** the fact of being able to detect and respond to an outside stimulus **2.** the rate of positive responses in a test from persons with a specific disease. A high rate of sensitivity means a low rate of people being incorrectly classed as negative. Compare **specificity**

**sensorineural deafness** /ˌsensəriˌnjʊərəl ˈdefnəs/, **sensorineural hearing loss** /ˌsensəriˌnjʊərəl ˈhɪərɪŋ lɒs/ *noun* deafness caused by a disorder in the auditory nerves or the brain centres which receive impulses from the nerves. Also called **perceptive deafness**

**sensory** /ˈsensəri/ *adjective* referring to the detection of sensations by nerve cells

**sensory cortex** /ˌsensəri ˈkɔːteks/ *noun* the area of the cerebral cortex which receives information from nerves in all parts of the body (*dated*)

**sensory deprivation** /ˌsensəri ˌdeprɪˈveɪʃ(ə)n/ *noun* a condition in which a person becomes confused because they lack sensations

**sensory nerve** /ˈsensəri nɜːv/ *noun* a nerve which registers a sensation such as heat, taste or smell and carries impulses to the brain and spinal cord. Also called **afferent nerve**

**sensory neurone** /ˌsensəri ˈnjʊərəʊn/ *noun* a nerve cell which transmits impulses relating to sensations from the receptor to the central nervous system

**sensory receptor** /ˌsensəri rɪˈseptə/ *noun* a cell which senses a change in the surrounding environment, e.g. cold or pressure, and reacts to it by sending out an impulse through the nervous system. Also called **nerve ending**

**separate** *verb* /ˈsepəreɪt/ to move two or more people or things apart ○ *The surgeons believe it may be possible to separate the conjoined twins.* ○ *The retina has become separated from the back of the eye.* (NOTE: **separating – separated**) ■ *adjective* /ˈsep(ə)rət/ **1.** not touching, together or in the same place **2.** distinct and not related or the same

**separation** /ˌsepəˈreɪʃ(ə)n/ *noun* the act of separating or dividing two or more people or things, or the state of being separated

**separation anxiety** /ˌsepəˈreɪʃ(ə)n æŋ ˌzaɪəti/ *noun* a state of anxiety caused in someone, especially a young child, by the thought or fact of being separated from his or her mother or primary caregiver

**sepsis** /ˈsepsɪs/ *noun* the presence of bacteria and their toxins in the body, which kill tissue and produce pus, usually following the infection of a wound

**sept-** /sept/ *prefix* same as **septi-** (*used before vowels*)

**septa** /ˈseptə/ plural of **septum**

**septal** /ˈsept(ə)l/ *adjective* referring to a septum

**septal defect** /ˌsept(ə)l ˈdiːfekt/ *noun* a congenital condition in which a hole exists in the wall between the left and right sides of the heart allowing an excessive amount of blood to flow through the lungs, leading in severe cases to pulmonary hypertension and sometimes heart failure

**septate** /ˈsepteɪt/ *adjective* divided by a septum

**septi-** /septɪ/ *prefix* referring to sepsis

**septic** /'septɪk/ *adjective* referring to or produced by sepsis

**septicaemia** /ˌseptɪ'siːmiə/ *noun* a condition in which bacteria or their toxins are present in the blood, multiply rapidly and destroy tissue. ◊ **blood poisoning** (NOTE: The US spelling is **septicemia**.)

**septicaemic** /ˌseptɪ'siːmɪk/ *adjective* caused by septicaemia, associated with septicaemia (NOTE: The US spelling is **septicemic**.)

**septicaemic plague** /ˌseptɪsiːmɪk 'pleɪg/ *noun* a form of bubonic plague in which the symptoms are generalised throughout the body

**septic shock** /ˌseptɪk 'ʃɒk/ *noun* shock caused by bacterial toxins in the blood as a result of infection. There is a dramatic drop in blood pressure, preventing the delivery of blood to the organs. Toxic shock syndrome is one type of septic shock.

**septo-** /septəʊ/ *prefix* referring to a septum

**septoplasty** /'septəʊplæsti/ *noun* a surgical operation to straighten the cartilage in the septum (NOTE: The plural is **septoplasties**.)

**Septrin** /'septrɪn/ a trade name for co-trimoxazole

**septum** /'septəm/ *noun* a wall between two parts of an organ, e.g. between two parts of the heart or between the two nostrils in the nose. See illustration at HEART in Supplement (NOTE: The plural is **septa**.)

**septum defect** /'septəm ˌdiːfekt/ *noun* a condition in which a hole exists in a septum, usually the septum of the heart

**sequela** /sɪ'kwiːlə/ *noun* a disease or disorder that is caused by a disease or injury which the person had previously ○ *a case of osteomyelitis as a sequela of multiple fractures of the mandible* ○ *biochemical and hormonal sequelae of the eating disorders* ○ *Kaposi's sarcoma can be a sequela of Aids.* (NOTE: The plural is **sequelae**.)

**sequence** /'siːkwəns/ *noun* a series of things, numbers etc., which follow each other in order ■ *verb* **1.** to put things in order **2.** to show how amino acids are linked together in chains to form protein (NOTE: **sequences – sequencing – sequenced**)

**sequestra** /sɪ'kwestrə/ plural of **sequestrum**

**sequestration** /ˌsiːkwe'streɪʃ(ə)n/ *noun* **1.** the act of putting someone in an isolated place **2.** the loss of blood into spaces in the body, reducing the circulating volume. It can occur naturally or can be produced artificially by applying tourniquets. ○ *pulmonary sequestration* ○ *A dry hacking cough can cause sequestration of the peritoneum in the upper abdomen.* **3.** the formation of a sequestrum

**sequestrectomy** /ˌsiːkwɪ'strektəmi/ *noun* a surgical operation to remove a sequestrum (NOTE: The plural is **sequestrectomies**.)

**sequestrum** /sɪ'kwestrəm/ *noun* a piece of dead bone which is separated from whole bone (NOTE: The plural is **sequestra**.)

**ser-** /sɪər/ *prefix* same as **sero-** (used before vowels)

**sera** /'sɪərə/ *plural noun* plural of **serum**

**serine** /'serɪn/ *noun* an amino acid produced in the hydrolysis of protein

**serious** /'sɪəriəs/ *adjective* **1.** having very bad consequences ○ *He's had a serious illness.* ○ *There was a serious accident on the motorway.* ○ *There is a serious shortage of plasma.* **2.** thoughtful and not superficial or humorous ○ *a serious discussion on the appropriateness of the treatment* ○ *serious about becoming a GP*

**seriously** /'sɪəriəsli/ *adverb* in a serious way ○ *She is seriously ill.*

**SERM** *abbr* selective (o)estrogen receptor modulator

**sero-** /sɪərəʊ/ *prefix* **1.** referring to blood serum **2.** referring to the serous membrane

**seroconvert** /ˌsɪərəʊkən'vɜːt/ *verb* to produce specific antibodies in response to the presence of an antigen such as a bacterium or virus

**serological** /ˌsɪərə'lɒdʒɪk(ə)l/ *adjective* referring to serology

**serological diagnosis** /ˌsɪərəʊlɒdʒɪk(ə)l ˌdaɪəg'nəʊsɪs/ *noun* a diagnosis which comes from testing serum

**serological type** /ˌsɪərəlɒdʒɪk(ə)l 'taɪp/ *noun* same as **serotype**

**serology** /sɪə'rɒlədʒi/ *noun* the scientific study of serum and the antibodies contained in it

**seronegative** /ˌsɪərəʊ'negətɪv/ *adjective* referring to someone who gives a negative reaction to a serological test

**seropositive** /ˌsɪərəʊ'pɒzɪtɪv/ *adjective* referring to someone who gives a positive reaction to a serological test

**seropus** /'sɪərəʊˌpʌs/ *noun* a mixture of serum and pus

**serosa** /sɪ'rəʊsə/ *noun* same as **serous membrane** (NOTE: The plural is **serosas** or **serosae**.)

**serositis** /ˌsɪərəʊ'saɪtɪs/ *noun* inflammation of a serous membrane

**serotherapy** /ˌsɪərəʊ'θerəpi/ *noun* treatment of a disease using serum from immune people or immunised animals

**serotonin** /ˌsɪərə'təʊnɪn/ *noun* a compound which is a neurotransmitter and exists mainly in blood platelets. It is released after tissue is injured and is important in sleep, mood and vasoconstriction.

**serotype** /'sɪərəʊtaɪp/ *noun* **1.** a category of microorganisms or bacteria which have some antigens in common **2.** a series of common antigens which exists in microorganisms and bacteria ▶ also called **serological type** ■ *verb* to group microorganisms and bacteria according to their antigens (NOTE: **serotyping – sero-typed**)

**serous** /'sɪərəs/ *adjective* referring to, producing, or like serum

**serous membrane** /ˌsɪərəs 'membreɪn/ *noun* a membrane which both lines an internal cavity and covers the organs in the cavity, e.g. the peritoneum lining the abdominal cavity or pleura lining the chest cavity. Also called **serosa**

**serous pericardium** /ˌsɪərəs ˌperi'kɑːdiəm/ *noun* the inner part of the pericardium, forming a double sac which contains fluid to prevent the two parts of the pericardium from rubbing together

**serpens** /'sɜːpenz/ ♦ **erythema serpens**

**serpiginous** /səˈpɪdʒɪnəs/ *adjective* **1.** referring to an ulcer or eruption which creeps across the skin **2.** referring to a wound or ulcer with a wavy edge

**serrated** /səˈreɪtɪd/ *adjective* with a zigzag or saw-like edge

**serration** /səˈreɪʃ(ə)n/ *noun* one of the points in a zigzag or serrated edge

**Sertoli cells** /səˈtəuli selz/ *plural noun* cells which support the seminiferous tubules in the testis [Described 1865. After Enrico Sertoli (1842–1910), Italian histologist, Professor of Experimental Physiology at Milan, Italy.]

**sertraline** /'sɜːtrəliːn/ *noun* an antidepressant drug which extends the action of the neurotransmitter serotonin. It is also used in the treatment of obsessive-compulsive disorder and post-traumatic stress disorder.

**serum** /'sɪərəm/ *noun* **1.** a fluid which separates from clotted blood and is similar to plasma except that it has no clotting agents. Also called **blood serum 2.** blood serum taken from an animal which has developed antibodies to bacteria, used to give humans temporary immunity to a disease. Also called **antiserum 3.** any clear watery body fluid, especially a fluid that comes from a serous membrane (NOTE: The plural is **serums** or **sera**.)

COMMENT: Blood serum is plasma without the clotting agents. It contains salt and small quantities of albumin, globulin, amino acids, fats and sugars; its main component is water.

**serum albumin** /ˌsɪərəm 'ælbjumɪn/ *noun* a major protein in blood plasma

**serum bilirubin** /ˌsɪərəm bɪlɪ'ruːbɪn/ *noun* bilirubin in serum, converted from haemoglobin as red blood cells are destroyed

**serum globulin** /ˌsɪərəm 'glɒbjulɪn/ *noun* a major protein in blood serum that is an antibody

**serum glutamic–oxalacetic transaminase** /ˌsɪərəm gluːˌtæmɪk ˌɒksæləsiːtɪk trænsˈæmɪneɪz/ *noun* an enzyme excreted by damaged heart muscle, which appears in the blood of people who have had a heart attack. Abbr **SGOT**

**serum glutamic–pyruvic transaminase** /ˌsɪərəm gluːˌtæmɪk paɪˌruːvɪk trænsˈæmɪneɪz/ *noun* an enzyme secreted by the parenchymal cells of the liver, occurring in increased amounts in the blood of people with infectious hepatitis. Abbr **SGPT**

**serum hepatitis** /ˌsɪərəm ˌhepəˈtaɪtɪs/ *noun* a serious form of hepatitis transmitted by infected blood, unsterilised surgical instruments, shared needles or sexual intercourse. Also called **hepatitis B, viral hepatitis**

**serum sickness** /'sɪərəm ˌsɪknəs/ *noun* an allergic reaction to serum therapy which was formerly used as a way of boosting passive immunity

**serum therapy** *noun* the administration of treated serum, often from horses, formerly used as a way of boosting passive immunity

**serve** *verb* **1.** to give a person food or drink ○ *Lunch is served in the ward at 12:30.* **2.** to be useful or helpful to a person or group ○ *The clinic serves the local community well.* **3.** to have a particular effect or result ○ *The letter serves to remind you of your outpatients' appointment.* (NOTE: [all senses] **serves – serving – served**)

**service** /'sɜːvɪs/ *noun* **1.** the act or fact of serving a person or group **2.** a group of people working together

**sesamoid** /'sesəmɔɪd/, **sesamoid bone** /'sesəmɔɪd bəun/ *noun* any small bony nodule in a tendon, the largest being the kneecap

**sessile** /'sesaɪl/ *adjective* referring to something, especially a tumour, which has no stem. Opposite **pedunculate**

**session** /'seʃ(ə)n/ *noun* a visit to a therapist for treatment ○ *She has two sessions a week of physiotherapy.* ○ *The evening session had to be cancelled because the therapist was ill.*

**set** /set/ *verb* **1.** to put the parts of a broken bone back into their proper places and keep the bone fixed until it has mended ○ *The doctor set the man's broken arm.* **2.** (*of a broken bone*) to mend, to form a solid bone again ○ *His arm has set very quickly.* ○ *Her broken wrist is setting very well.* ◊ **reset** (NOTE: **setting – set**)

**settle** /'set(ə)l/ *verb* **1.** to begin to feel comfortable or at ease, or to make a person feel comfortable or at ease (NOTE: **settles – settling – settled**) **2.** (*of a sediment*) to fall to the bottom of a liquid **3.** (*of a parasite*) to attach itself, to stay in a part of the body ○ *The fluke settles in the liver.* (NOTE: **settles – settling – settled**)

**sever** /'sevə/ *verb* to cut something off ○ *His hand was severed at the wrist.* ○ *Surgeons tried to sew the severed finger back onto the patient's hand.*

**severe** /sɪ'vɪə/ *adjective* very bad or dangerous ○ *The patient experienced severe bleeding* ○ *A severe outbreak of whooping cough occurred during the winter.*

**severe acute respiratory disorder** /sɪ
ˌvɪə əˌkjuːt rɪˈspɪrət(ə)ri dɪsˌɔːdə/ *noun* full
form of **SARS**

**severely** /sɪˈvɪəli/ *adverb* very badly or dangerously ○ *Her breathing was severely affected.*

'…many severely confused patients, particularly
those in advanced stages of Alzheimer's disease, do
not respond to verbal communication' [*Nursing
Times*]

**severity** /sɪˈveriti/ *noun* the degree to which
something is bad or dangerous ○ *Treatment
depends on the severity of the attack.*

**sex** /seks/ *noun* **1.** one of two groups, male
and female, into which animals and plants can
be divided ○ *The sex of a baby can be identified before birth.* **2.** same as **sexual intercourse**

**sex act** /ˈseks ækt/ *noun* an act of sexual intercourse

**sexarche** /ˈseksɑːki/ *noun* the age when a
person first has sexual intercourse

**sex change** /ˈseks tʃeɪndʒ/ *noun* a surgical
operation accompanied by hormone treatment
to change someone's physical sex-linked characteristics from female to male or from male to
female

**sex chromosome** /ˈseks ˌkrəʊməsəʊm/
*noun* a chromosome which determines if a person is male or female

COMMENT: Out of the twenty-three pairs of
chromosomes in each human cell, two are
sex chromosomes, which are known as X and
Y. Females have a pair of X chromosomes
and males have a pair consisting of one X and
one Y chromosome. The sex of a baby is determined by the father's sperm. While the
mother's ovum only carries X chromosomes,
the father's sperm can carry either an X or a Y
chromosome. If the ovum is fertilised by a
sperm carrying an X chromosome, the embryo will contain the XX pair and so be female.
Disordered chromosomes affect sexual development: a person with an XO chromosome
pair (i.e. one X chromosome alone) has Turner's syndrome; a person with an extra X chromosome (making an XXY set) has Klinefelter's syndrome. Haemophilia is a disorder
linked to the X chromosome.

**sex      determination** /ˈseks   dɪtɜːmɪ
ˌneɪʃ(ə)n/ *noun* the way in which the sex of an
individual organism is fixed by the number of
chromosomes which make up its cell structure

**sex hormone** /seks ˈhɔːməʊn/ *noun* an oestrogen or androgen which promotes the growth
of secondary sexual characteristics

**sex-linkage** /ˈseks ˌlɪŋkɪdʒ/ *noun* the existence of characteristics which are transmitted
through the X chromosomes

**sex-linked** /ˈseks ˌlɪŋkt/ *adjective* **1.** referring to genes which are linked to X chromosomes **2.** referring to characteristics such as
colour-blindness    which    are    transmitted
through the X chromosomes

**sexology** /sekˈsɒlədʒi/ *noun* the study of sex
and sexual behaviour

**sex organ** /ˈseks ˌɔːgən/ *noun* an organ
which is associated with reproduction and sexual intercourse, e.g. the testes and penis in
men, and the ovaries, Fallopian tubes, vagina
and vulva in women

**sex selection** /ˈseks sɪˌlekʃ(ə)n/ *noun* the
determination of a baby's sex before conception by separating the spermatozoa carrying Y
chromosomes from those carrying X chromosomes

**sextuplet** /ˈsekstjʊplət/ *noun* one of six babies born to a mother at the same time

**sexual** /ˈsekʃuəl/ *adjective* referring to sex

**sexual act** /ˈsekʃuəl ækt/ *noun* an act of sexual intercourse

**sexual attraction** /ˌsekʃuəl əˈtrækʃ(ə)n/
*noun* a feeling of wanting to have sexual intercourse with someone

**sexual deviation** /ˌsekʃuəl diːviˈeɪʃ(ə)n/
*noun* any sexual behaviour which is not accepted as usual in the society in which you
live. Examples in Western society are sadism
and voyeurism.

**sexual intercourse** /ˌsekʃuəl ˈɪntəkɔːs/
*noun* physical contact between people which
involves stimulation of the genitals, especially
the insertion of a man's erect penis into a
woman's vagina with release of spermatozoa
from the penis by ejaculation, which may fertilise ova from the woman's ovaries. Also
called **sex, coitus, copulation**

**sexually transmitted disease** /ˌsekʃuəli
trænsˌmɪtɪd dɪˈziːz/, **sexually transmitted
infection**   /ˌsekʃuəli   trænsˌmɪtɪd   ɪn
ˈfekʃ(ə)n/ *noun* a disease or infection transmitted from an infected person to another person during sexual intercourse. Abbr **STD, STI**

COMMENT: Among the commonest STDs are
non-specific urethritis, genital herpes, hepatitis B and gonorrhoea; AIDS is also a sexually
transmitted disease. The spread of sexually
transmitted diseases can be limited by use of
condoms. Other forms of contraceptive offer
no protection against the spread of disease.

**sexual reproduction** /ˌsekʃuəl ˌriːprə
ˈdʌkʃən/ *noun* reproduction in which gametes
from two individuals fuse together

**SFD** *abbr* small for dates

**SGOT**   *abbr*   serum   glutamic-oxalacetic
transaminase

**SGPT** *abbr* serum glutamic-pyruvic transaminase

**shaft** /ʃɑːft/ *noun* **1.** the long central section
of a long bone **2.** main central section of the
erect penis

**shake** /ʃeɪk/ *verb* to move, or make something move, with short quick movements
(NOTE: **shaking – shook – shaken**)

**shaken baby syndrome** /ˌʃeɪkən ˈbeɪbi
ˌsɪndrəʊm/, **shaken infant syndrome** /

ˌʃeɪkən ˈɪnfənt ˌsɪndrəʊm/ *noun* a series of internal head injuries in a very young child, caused by being shaken violently. It can result in brain damage leading to speech and learning disabilities, paralysis, seizures and hearing loss, and may be life-threatening.

**shaky** /ˈʃeɪki/ *adjective* feeling weak and unsteady

**share** /ʃeə/ *verb* 1. to use or do something together with others 2. to divide something and give parts of it to different people or groups (NOTE: [all verb senses] **shares – sharing – shared**) ■ *noun* a single part of something divided among different people or groups

**shared care** /ˌʃeəd ˈkeə/ *noun* antenatal care given jointly by an obstetrician in a hospital together with a general practitioner or a midwife working in the community

**sharp** /ʃɑːp/ *adjective* 1. able to cut easily ○ *A surgeon's knife has to be kept sharp.* 2. hurting in a sudden and intense way ○ *She felt a sharp pain in her shoulder.*

**sharply** /ˈʃɑːpli/ *adverb* suddenly and to a significant extent ○ *His condition deteriorated sharply during the night.*

**sharps** /ʃɑːps/ *plural noun* objects with points, e.g. syringes (*informal*)

**shave** /ʃeɪv/ *noun* the removal of hair by cutting it off at skin level with a razor ■ *verb* to remove hair with a razor (NOTE: **shaving – shaved**)

**sheath** /ʃiːθ/ *noun* 1. a layer of tissue which surrounds a muscle or a bundle of nerve fibres 2. same as **condom**

**shed** /ʃed/ *verb* to lose blood or tissue ○ *The lining of the uterus is shed at each menstrual period.* ○ *He was given a transfusion because he had shed a lot of blood.* (NOTE: **shedding – shed**)

**sheet** /ʃiːt/ *noun* a large piece of cloth which is put on a bed ○ *The sheets must be changed each day.* ○ *The soiled sheets were sent to the hospital laundry.* ◊ **draw-sheet**

**shelf operation** /ˈʃelf ˌɒpəreɪʃ(ə)n/ *noun* a surgical operation to treat congenital dislocation of the hip in children, in which bone tissue is grafted onto the acetabulum

**sheltered accommodation** /ˌʃeltəd əˌkɒməˈdeɪʃ(ə)n/, **sheltered housing** /ˌʃeltəd ˈhaʊzɪŋ/ *noun* rooms or small flats provided for elderly people, with a resident supervisor or nurse

**shiatsu** /ʃiˈætsuː/ *noun* a form of healing massage in which the hands are used to apply pressure at acupuncture points on the body in order to stimulate and redistribute energy

**shift** /ʃɪft/ *noun* 1. a way of working in which one group of workers work for a period and are then replaced by another group ○ *She is working on the night shift.* ○ *The day shift comes on duty at 6.30 in the morning.* 2. the period of

time worked by a group of workers 3. a movement

**Shigella** /ʃɪˈgelə/ *noun* a genus of bacteria which causes dysentery

**shigellosis** /ˌʃɪgeˈləʊsɪs/ *noun* infestation of the digestive tract with *Shigella,* causing bacillary dysentery

**shin** /ʃɪn/ *noun* the front part of the lower leg

**shinbone** /ˈʃɪnbəʊn/ *noun* same as **tibia**

**shiner** /ˈʃaɪnə/ *noun* same as **black eye** (*informal*)

**shingles** /ˈʃɪŋgəlz/ *noun* same as **herpes zoster**

**shin splints** /ˈʃɪn splɪnts/ *plural noun* extremely sharp pains in the front of the lower leg, felt by athletes

**Shirodkar's operation** /ʃɪˈrɒdkɑːz ɒpəˌreɪʃ/, **Shirodkar pursestring** /ʃɪˌrɒdkɑː ˈpɜːsstrɪŋ/ *noun* a surgical operation to narrow the cervix of the uterus in a woman who experiences habitual abortion in order to prevent another miscarriage, the suture being removed before labour starts. Also called **pursestring operation** [After N. V. Shirodkar (1900–71), Indian obstetrician.]

**Shirodkar suture** /ʃɪˈrɒdkɑː ˌsuːtʃə/ *noun* a type of suture which is placed around a cervix to tighten it during pregnancy and prevent miscarriage. Also called **pursestring stitch**

**shiver** /ˈʃɪvə/ *verb* to tremble or shake all over the body because of cold or a fever, caused by the involuntary rapid contraction and relaxation of the muscles

**shivering** /ˈʃɪvərɪŋ/ *noun* the condition of trembling or shaking all over the body because of cold or a fever, caused by the involuntary rapid contraction and relaxation of the muscles

**shivery** /ˈʃɪvəri/ *adjective* trembling from cold, fear or a medical condition

**shock** /ʃɒk/ *noun* a state of weakness caused by illness or injury that suddenly reduces the blood pressure ○ *The patient went into shock.* ○ *Several of the passengers were treated for shock.* □ **traumatic shock** a state of shock caused by an injury which leads to loss of blood ■ *verb* to give someone an unpleasant surprise, and so put him or her in a state of shock ○ *She was still shocked several hours after the accident.* (NOTE: You say that someone is **in shock, in a state of shock** or that they **went into shock.**)

**shock lung** /ʃɒk ˈlʌŋ/ *noun* a serious condition in which a person's lungs fail to work following a trauma

**shock syndrome** /ˈʃɒk ˌsɪndrəʊm/ *noun* a group of symptoms, a pale face, cold skin, low blood pressure and rapid and irregular pulse, which show that someone is in a state of shock. ◊ **anaphylactic shock**

**shock therapy** /ˈʃɒk ˌθerəpi/, **shock treatment** /ˈʃɒk ˌtriːtmənt/ *noun* a method of treat-

# shoot

ing some mental disorders by giving an anaesthetised patient an electric shock to induce an epileptic convulsion

**shoot** /ʃuːt/ *verb* (*of pain*) to seem to move suddenly through the body with a piercing feeling ○ *The pain shot down his arm.*

**shooting** /'ʃuːtɪŋ/ *adjective* (*of pain*) sudden and intense

**short** /ʃɔːt/ *adjective* 1. not having enough of something 2. not very tall or long

**short-acting** /ˌʃɔːt 'æktɪŋ/ *adjective* effective only for a short period

**shortness of breath** /ˌʃɔːtnəs əv 'breθ/ *noun* the inability to breathe quickly enough to supply the oxygen needed

**short of breath** /ˌʃɔːt əv 'breθ/ *adjective* unable to breathe quickly enough to supply the oxygen needed ○ *After running up the stairs he was short of breath.*

**shortsighted** /ʃɔːt'saɪtɪd/ *adjective* same as **myopic**

**shortsightedness** /ˌʃɔːt'saɪtɪdnəs/ *noun* same as **myopia**

**shot** /ʃɒt/ *noun* same as **injection** (*informal*) ○ *The doctor gave her a tetanus shot.* ○ *He needed a shot of morphine to relieve the pain.*

**shoulder** /'ʃəʊldə/ *noun* a joint where the top of the arm joins the main part of the body ○ *He dislocated his shoulder.* ○ *She was complaining of pains in her shoulder or of shoulder pains.*

**shoulder blade** /'ʃəʊldə bleɪd/ *noun* same as **scapula**

**shoulder girdle** /'ʃəʊldə ˌgɜːd(ə)l/ *noun* same as **pectoral girdle**

**shoulder joint** /'ʃəʊldə dʒɔɪnt/ *noun* a ball and socket joint which allows the arm to rotate and move in any direction

**shoulder lift** /'ʃəʊldə lɪft/ *noun* a way of carrying a heavy person, in which the upper part of his or her body rests on the shoulders of two carriers

**shoulder presentation** /'ʃəʊldə ˌprez(ə)nˌteɪʃ(ə)n/ *noun* a position of a baby in the uterus, in which the shoulder will first appear

**show** /ʃəʊ/ *noun* the first discharge of blood at the beginning of childbirth ■ *verb* 1. to cause or allow something to be visible 2. to provide convincing evidence of something

**shrivel** /'ʃrɪv(ə)l/ *verb* to become dry and wrinkled (NOTE: **shrivelling – shrivelled**. The US spellings are **shriveling – shriveled**.)

**shuffling walk** /ˌʃʌf(ə)lɪŋ 'wɔːk/, **shuffling gait** /ˌʃʌf(ə)lɪŋ 'geɪt/ *noun* a way of walking in which the feet are not lifted off the ground, e.g. in Parkinson's disease

**shunt** /ʃʌnt/ *noun* 1. the passing of fluid through a channel which is not the usual one 2. a channel which links two different blood vessels and carries blood from one to the other ■ *verb* (*of blood*) to pass through a channel which

is not the usual one ○ *As much as 5% of venous blood can be shunted unoxygenated back to the arteries.*

**shunting** /'ʃʌntɪŋ/ *noun* a condition in which some of the deoxygenated blood in the lungs does not come into contact with air, and full gas exchange does not take place

**SI** *abbreviation* the international system of metric measurements. Full form **Système International**

**sial-** /saɪəl/ *prefix* same as **sialo-** (*used before vowels*)

**sialadenitis** /ˌsaɪəlˌædɪ'naɪtɪs/ *noun* inflammation of a salivary gland. Also called **sialoadenitis, sialitis**

**sialagogue** /saɪ'æləgɒg/ *noun* a substance which increases the production of saliva

**sialitis** /ˌsaɪəl'aɪtɪs/ *noun* same as **sialadenitis**

**sialo-** /saɪələʊ/ *prefix* 1. referring to saliva 2. referring to a salivary gland

**sialoadenitis** /ˌsaɪələʊˌædɪ'naɪtɪs/ *noun* same as **sialadenitis**

**sialogogue** /saɪ'æləgɒg/ *noun* same as **sialagogue**

**sialography** /ˌsaɪə'lɒgrəfi/ *noun* X-ray examination of a salivary gland. Also called **ptyalography**

**sialolith** /saɪ'æləʊlɪθ/ *noun* a stone in a salivary gland. Also called **ptyalith**

**sialorrhoea** /ˌsaɪələʊ'riːə/ *noun* the production of an excessive amount of saliva (NOTE: The US spelling is **sialorrhea**.)

**Siamese twins** /ˌsaɪəmiːz 'twɪnz/ *plural noun* same as **conjoined twins**

**sib** /sɪb/ *noun* same as **sibling** (*informal*)

**sibilant** /'sɪbɪlənt/ *adjective* referring to a sound which whistles

**sibling** /'sɪblɪŋ/ *noun* a brother or sister

**Sichuan flu** /ˌsɪtʃwaːn 'fluː/ *noun* a virulent type of flu which has the same symptoms as those of ordinary flu (e.g. fever, sore throat and aching muscles) but they are more pronounced (*informal*) (NOTE: The virus was first discovered in 1987 in Sichuan, a southwestern province of China.)

**sick** /sɪk/ *adjective* 1. having an illness ○ *He was sick for two weeks.* □ **to report** *or* **call in sick** to say officially that you are unwell and cannot work 2. about to vomit ○ *The patient got up this morning and felt sick.* □ **to be sick** to vomit ○ *The child was sick all over the floor.* □ **to make someone sick** to cause someone to vomit ○ *He was given something to make him sick.*

**sickbay** /'sɪkbeɪ/ *noun* a room in a factory or on a ship where people can visit a doctor for treatment

**sickbed** /'sɪkbed/ *noun* a bed where a person is lying sick ○ *She sat for hours beside her daughter's sickbed.*

**sick building syndrome** /ˌsɪk ˈbɪldɪŋ ˌsɪndrəum/ *noun* a condition in which many people working in a building feel ill or have headaches, caused by blocked air-conditioning ducts in which stale air is recycled round the building, often carrying allergenic substances or bacteria (*informal*)

**sicken for** /ˈsɪkən fɔː/ *verb* to feel the first symptoms of an illness (*informal*) ○ *She's looking pale – she must be sickening for something.*

**sickle cell** /ˈsɪk(ə)l sel/ *noun* a red blood cell shaped like a sickle, formed as a result of the presence of an unusual form of haemoglobin. Also called **drepanocyte**

**sickle-cell anaemia** /ˈsɪk(ə)l sel əˌniːmiə/ *noun* an inherited condition in which someone develops sickle cells which block the circulation, causing anaemia and pains in the joints and abdomen. Also called **drepanocytosis, sickle cell disease**

'...children with sickle-cell anaemia are susceptible to severe bacterial infection. Even children with the milder forms of sickle-cell disease have an increased frequency of pneumococcal infection' [*Lancet*]

COMMENT: Sickle-cell anaemia is a hereditary condition which is mainly found in people from Africa and the West Indies.

**sickle-cell chest syndrome** /ˌsɪk(ə)l sel ˈtʃest ˌsɪndrəum/ *noun* a common complication of sickle-cell disease, with chest pain, fever and leucocytosis

**sickle-cell disease** /ˈsɪk(ə)l sel dɪˌziːz/ *noun* same as **sickle-cell anaemia**. Abbr **SCD**

**sickle-cell trait** /ˈsɪk(ə)l sel ˌtreɪt/ *noun* a hereditary condition of the blood in which some red cells become sickle-shaped, but there are not enough affected cells to cause anaemia

**sicklist** /ˈsɪklɪst/ *noun* a list of people who are sick, e.g. children in a school or workers in a factory ○ *We have five members of staff on the sicklist.*

**sickly** /ˈsɪkli/ *adjective* (*usually of children*) subject to frequent sickness ○ *He was a sickly child, but now is a strong and healthy man.*

**sickness** /ˈsɪknəs/ *noun* **1.** a state of having an illness ○ *There is a lot of sickness in the winter months.* ○ *Many children are staying away from school because of sickness.* ◊ **seasickness, motion sickness 2.** a feeling of wanting to vomit

**sickroom** /ˈsɪkruːm/ *noun* a room where someone is ill ○ *Visitors are not allowed into the sickroom.*

**side** /saɪd/ *noun* **1.** the part of the body between the hips and the shoulder ○ *She was lying on her side.* **2.** the part of an object which is not the front, back, top or bottom ○ *The nurse wheeled the trolley to the side of the bed.*

**side-effect** /ˈsaɪd ɪˌfekt/ *noun* an effect produced by a drug or treatment which is not the main effect intended ○ *One of the side-effects of chemotherapy is that the patient's hair falls out.*

'...the treatment is not without possible side-effects, some of which can be particularly serious. The side-effects may include middle ear discomfort, claustrophobia, increased risk of epilepsy' [*New Zealand Medical Journal*]

**side rail** /ˈsaɪd ˌreɪl/ *noun* a rail at the side of a bed which can be lifted to prevent the person falling out

**sidero-** /saɪdərəu/ *prefix* referring to iron

**sideropenia** /ˌsaɪdərəˈpiːniə/ *noun* a lack of iron in the blood usually caused by insufficient iron in the diet

**siderophilin** /saɪdəˈrɒfəlɪn/ *noun* same as **transferrin**

**siderosis** /ˌsaɪdəˈrəusɪs/ *noun* **1.** a condition in which iron deposits form in tissue **2.** inflammation of the lungs caused by inhaling dust containing iron

**SIDS** *abbr* sudden infant death syndrome

**sight** /saɪt/ *noun* one of the five senses, the ability to see ○ *His sight is beginning to fail.* □ **to lose your sight** to become blind

**sighted** /ˈsaɪtɪd/ *adjective* able to see, as opposed to visually impaired

**sigmoid** /ˈsɪgmɔɪd/ *adjective* **1.** shaped like the letter S **2.** referring to the sigmoid colon ■ *noun* same as **sigmoid colon**

**sigmoid colon** /ˌsɪgmɔɪd ˈkəulɒn/ *noun* the fourth section of the colon which continues as the rectum. See illustration at DIGESTIVE SYSTEM in Supplement. Also called **pelvic colon, sigmoid, sigmoid flexure**

**sigmoidectomy** /ˌsɪgmɔɪˈdektəmi/ *noun* a surgical operation to remove the sigmoid colon (NOTE: The plural is **sigmoidectomies**.)

**sigmoid flexure** *noun* same as **sigmoid colon**

**sigmoidoscope** /sɪgˈmɔɪdəskəup/ *noun* a surgical instrument with a light at the end which can be passed into the rectum so that the sigmoid colon can be examined

**sigmoidoscopy** /ˌsɪgmɔɪˈdɒskəpi/ *noun* a procedure in which the rectum and sigmoid colon are examined with a sigmoidoscope

**sigmoidostomy** /ˌsɪgmɔɪˈdɒstəmi/ *noun* a surgical operation to bring the sigmoid colon out through a hole in the abdominal wall (NOTE: The plural is **sigmoidostomies**.)

**sign** /saɪn/ *noun* a movement, mark, colouring or change which has a meaning and can be recognised by a doctor as indicating a condition (NOTE: A change in function which is also noticed by the patient is a **symptom**.) ■ *verb* to write your name on a document such as a form or cheque, or at the end of a letter ○ *The doctor signed the death certificate.*

**significant** /sɪgˈnɪfɪkənt/ *adjective* important or worth noting ○ *No significant inflammatory responses were observed.*

**significantly** /sɪgˈnɪfɪkəntli/ *adverb* in an important or noteworthy manner ○ *He was not significantly better on the following day.*

**sign language** /'saɪn ˌlæŋgwɪdʒ/ *noun* a set of agreed signs made with the fingers and hands, used to indicate words by or for people who cannot hear or speak

**sildenafil citrate** /ˌsɪldənəfɪl 'saɪtreɪt/ *noun* an enzyme-inhibiting drug used in the treatment of male impotence

**silent** /'saɪlənt/ *adjective* **1.** not making any noise or talking **2.** not visible or showing no symptoms ○ *Genital herpes may be silent in women.* ○ *Graft occlusion is often silent with 80% of patients.*

**silica** /'sɪlɪkə/ *noun* a compound of silicon, the mineral which forms quartz and sand. Also called **silicon dioxide**

**silicon** /'sɪlɪkən/ *noun* a non-metallic chemical element (NOTE: The chemical symbol is **Si**.)

**silicon dioxide** /ˌsɪlɪkən daɪ'ɒksaɪd/ *noun* same as **silica**

**silicosis** /ˌsɪlɪ'kəʊsɪs/ *noun* a disease of the lungs caused by inhaling silica dust from mining or stone-crushing operations

COMMENT: This is a serious disease which makes breathing difficult and can lead to emphysema and bronchitis.

**silver** /'sɪlvə/ *noun* a white-coloured metallic element (NOTE: The chemical symbol is **Ag**.)

**silver nitrate** /ˌsɪlvə 'naɪtreɪt/ *noun* a salt of silver that is mixed with a cream or solution and used, e.g., to disinfect burns or to kill warts

**Silvester method** /sɪl'vestə ˌmeθəd/ *noun* a method of giving artificial respiration. The person lies on his or her back, then the first-aider brings the person's hands together on the chest and moves them above the person's head. ◊ **Holger-Nielsen method**

**Simmonds' disease** /'sɪməndz dɪˌziːz/ *noun* a condition of women due to postpartum haemorrhage, in which there is lack of activity in the pituitary gland, resulting in wasting of tissue, brittle bones and premature senility [Described 1914. After Morris Simmonds (1855–1925), German physician and pathologist.]

**simple** /'sɪmpəl/ *adjective* **1.** ordinary **2.** not very complicated

**simple epithelium** /ˌsɪmpəl ˌepɪ'θiːliəm/ *noun* an epithelium formed of a single layer of cells

**simple fracture** /ˌsɪmpəl 'fræktʃə/ *noun* a fracture where the skin surface around the damaged bone has not been broken and the broken ends of the bone are close together. Also called **closed fracture**

**simple tachycardia** /ˌsɪmpəl tæki'kɑːdiə/ *noun* same as **sinus tachycardia**

**simplex** /'sɪmpleks/ ♦ **herpes simplex**

**Sims' position** /'sɪmz pəˌzɪʃ(ə)n/ *noun* a position of the body in which the person lies on his or her left side with their left arm behind their back and their right knee and thigh flexed. It is used to allow the anal or vaginal area to be examined easily.

**simvastatin** /sɪm'væstɪn/ *noun* a drug which lowers lipid levels in the blood, used in the treatment of high cholesterol

**sinciput** /'sɪnsɪpʌt/ *noun* the part of the skull that includes the forehead and the area above it

**sinew** /'sɪnjuː/ *noun* same as **tendon**

**singer's nodule** /ˌsɪŋəz 'nɒdjuːl/ *noun* a small white polyp which can develop in the larynx of people who use their voice too much or too loudly

**single parent family** /ˌsɪŋg(ə)l ˌpeərənt 'fæm(ə)li/ *noun* a family which consists of a child or children and only one parent, e.g. because of death, divorce or separation

**single photon emission computed tomography** /ˌsɪŋg(ə)l ˌfəʊtɒn ɪˌmɪʃ(ə)n kəm ˌpjuːtɪd təˈmɒgrəfi/ *noun* a scan to study brain blood flow in conditions such as Alzheimer's disease

**singultus** /sɪŋ'gʌltəs/ *noun* same as **hiccup**

**sinistral** /'sɪnɪstrəl/ *adjective* relating to or located on the left side, especially the left side of the body

**sino-** /saɪnəʊ/ *prefix* referring to a sinus

**sinoatrial** /ˌsaɪnəʊ'eɪtriəl/ *adjective* relating to the sinus venosus and the right atrium of the heart

**sinoatrial node** /ˌsaɪnəʊ'eɪtriəl nəʊd/ *noun* a node in the heart at the junction of the superior vena cava and the right atrium, which regulates the heartbeat. Also called **SA node, sinus node**

**sinogram** /'saɪnəʊgræm/ *noun* an X-ray photograph of a sinus

**sinography** /saɪ'nɒgrəfi/ *noun* examination of a sinus by taking an X-ray photograph

**sinu-** /saɪnə/ *prefix* same as **sino-**

**sinuatrial** *adjective* same as **sinoatrial**

**sinus** /'saɪnəs/ *noun* **1.** a cavity inside the body, including the cavities inside the head behind the cheekbone, forehead and nose ○ *The doctor diagnosed a sinus infection.* **2.** a tract or passage which develops between an infected place where pus has gathered and the surface of the skin **3.** a wide venous blood space

**sinusitis** /ˌsaɪnə'saɪtɪs/ *noun* inflammation of the mucous membrane in the sinuses, especially the maxillary sinuses

**sinus nerve** /'saɪnəs nɜːv/ *noun* a nerve which branches from the glossopharyngeal nerve

**sinus node** /'saɪnəs nəʊd/ *noun* same as **sinoatrial node**

**sinusoid** /'saɪnəsɔɪd/ *noun* a specially shaped small blood vessel in the liver, adrenal glands and other organs

**sinus tachycardia** /ˌsaɪnəs tæki'kɑːdiə/ *noun* rapid beating of the heart caused by stimulation of the sinoatrial node. Also called **simple tachycardia**

**sinus venosus** /ˌsaɪnəs vəˈnəʊsɪs/ *noun* a cavity in the heart of an embryo, part of which develops into the coronary sinus and part of which is absorbed into the right atrium

**siphonage** /ˈsaɪfənɪdʒ/ *noun* the removal of liquid from one place to another with a tube, as used to empty the stomach of its contents

**Sippy diet** /ˈsɪpi ˌdaɪət/ *noun US* an alkaline diet of milk and dry biscuits as a treatment for peptic ulcers [After Bertram Welton Sippy (1866–1924), physician in Chicago, USA]

**sister** /ˈsɪstə/ *noun* 1. a female who has the same father and mother as someone ○ *He has three sisters.* ○ *Her sister works in a children's clinic.* 2. a senior nurse □ **sister in charge** a senior nurse in charge of a hospital ward

**sit** /sɪt/ *verb* 1. to rest with your weight largely supported by the buttocks 2. to cause a person to sit somewhere (NOTE: [all senses] **sitting – sat**)

**site** /saɪt/ *noun* 1. the position of something ○ *The X-ray showed the site of the infection.* 2. the place where something happened 3. the place where an incision is to be made in a surgical operation ■ *verb* to put something in a particular place, or be in a particular place ○ *The infection is sited in the right lung.* (NOTE: **siting – sited**)

'…arterial thrombi have a characteristic structure: platelets adhere at sites of endothelial damage and attract other platelets to form a dense aggregate' [*British Journal of Hospital Medicine*]

'…the sublingual site is probably the most acceptable and convenient for taking temperature' [*Nursing Times*]

'…with the anaesthetist's permission, the scrub nurse and surgeon began the process of cleaning up the skin round the operation site' [*NATNews*]

**situated** /ˈsɪtʃueɪtɪd/ *adjective* in a particular place ○ *The tumour is situated in the bowel.* ○ *The atlas bone is situated above the axis.*

**sit up** /ˌsɪt ˈʌp/ *verb* 1. to sit with your back straight ○ *The patient is sitting up in bed.* 2. to move from a lying to a sitting position (NOTE: **sitting up – sat up**)

**situs** /ˈsaɪtəs/ *noun* the position of an organ or part of the body, especially the usual position (NOTE: The plural is **situs**.)

**situs inversus** /ˌsaɪtəs ɪnˈvɜːsəs/, **situs inversus viscerum** /ˌsaɪtəs ɪnˌvɜːsəs ˈvɪsərəm/ *noun* a congenital condition, in which the organs are not on the usual side of the body, i.e. where the heart is on the right side and not the left

**sitz bath** /ˈsɪts bɑːθ/ *noun* a small low bath where someone can sit, but not lie down

**SI units** /ˌes ˈaɪ ˌjuːnɪts/ *plural noun* the units used in an international system of units for measuring physical properties such as weight, speed and light

**Sjögren's syndrome** /ˈʃɜːgrenz ˌsɪndrəʊm/ *noun* a chronic autoimmune disease in which the lacrimal and salivary glands become infiltrated with lymphocytes and plasma cells, and the mouth and eyes become dry

**skatole** /ˈskætəʊl/ *noun* another spelling of **scatole**

**skeletal** /ˈskelɪt(ə)l/ *adjective* referring to the skeleton

**skeletal muscle** /ˈskelɪt(ə)l ˌmʌs(ə)l/ *noun* a muscle attached to a bone, which makes a limb move

**skeleton** /ˈskelɪt(ə)n/ *noun* all the bones which make up a body

**Skene's glands** /ˈskiːnz glændz/ *noun* small mucous glands in the urethra in women [Described 1880. After Alexander Johnston Chalmers Skene (1838–1900), Scottish-born New York gynaecologist.]

**skia-** /skaɪə/ *prefix* referring to shadow

**skiagram** /ˈskaɪəgræm/ *noun* an old term for X-ray photograph

**skier's thumb** /ˌskiːəz ˈθʌm/ *noun* an injury to the thumb caused by falling directly onto it when it is outstretched, resulting in tearing or stretching of the ligaments of the main thumb joint

**skill** /skɪl/ *noun* an ability to do difficult work, which is acquired by training ○ *You need special skills to become a doctor.*

**skilled** /skɪld/ *adjective* having acquired a particular skill by training ○ *He's a skilled plastic surgeon.*

**skill mix** /ˈskɪl mɪks/ *noun* the range of different skills possessed by the members of a group or required for a particular job

**skin** /skɪn/ *noun* the tissue which forms the outside surface of the body ○ *His skin turned brown in the sun.* ○ *Skin problems in adolescents may be caused by diet.* (NOTE: For other terms referring to skin, see words beginning with **cut-, derm-, derma-, dermato-, dermo-.**)

COMMENT: The skin is the largest organ in the human body. It is formed of two layers: the epidermis is the outer layer, and includes the top layer of particles of dead skin which are continuously flaking off. Beneath the epidermis is the dermis, which is the main layer of living skin. Hairs and nails are produced by the skin, and pores in the skin secrete sweat from the sweat glands underneath the dermis. The skin is sensitive to touch and heat and cold, which are sensed by the nerve endings in the skin. The skin is a major source of vitamin D which it produces when exposed to sunlight.

**skin graft** /ˈskɪn grɑːft/ *noun* a layer of skin transplanted from one part of the body to cover an area where the skin has been destroyed ○ *After the operation she had to have a skin graft.*

**skinny** /ˈskɪni/ *adjective* very thin (*informal*)

**skin test** /ˈskɪn test/ *noun* a test for allergy, in which a substance is applied to the skin to see if a reaction occurs

**skull** /skʌl/ *noun* the eight bones which are fused or connected together to form the head, along with the fourteen bones which form the face. Also called **cranium** □ **skull fracture** a condition in which one of the bones in the skull has been fractured

**slash** /slæʃ/ *noun* a long cut with a knife ○ *He had bruises on his face and slashes on his hands.* ○ *The slash on her leg needs three stitches.* ■ *verb* **1.** to cut something with a knife or sharp edge □ **to slash your wrists** to try to kill yourself by cutting the blood vessels in the wrists **2.** to cut costs or spending sharply (*informal*)

**SLE** *abbr* systemic lupus erythematosus

**sleep** /sliːp/ *noun* the state or a period of resting, usually at night, when the eyes are closed and you are not conscious of what is happening ○ *You need to get a good night's sleep if you have a lot of work to do tomorrow.* ○ *He had a short sleep in the middle of the afternoon.* □ **to get to sleep** *or* **go to sleep** to start sleeping ■ *verb* to be in a state of sleep (NOTE: **sleeping – slept**)

COMMENT: Sleep is a period when the body rests and rebuilds tissue, especially protein. Most adults need eight hours' sleep each night. Children require more (ten to twelve hours) but older people need less, possibly only four to six hours. Sleep forms a regular pattern of stages: during the first stage the person is still conscious of his or her surroundings, and will wake on hearing a noise; afterwards the sleeper goes into very deep sleep (slow-wave sleep), where the eyes are tightly closed, the pulse is regular and the sleeper breathes deeply. During this stage the pituitary gland produces the growth hormone somatotrophin. It is difficult to wake someone from deep sleep. This stage is followed by rapid eye movement sleep (REM sleep), in which the sleeper's eyes are half open and move about, he or she makes facial movements, the blood pressure rises and he or she has dreams. After this stage the sleeper relapses into the first sleep stage again.

**sleep apnoea** /ˈsliːp æpˌniːə/ *noun* a condition related to heavy snoring, with prolonged respiratory pauses leading to cerebral hypoxia and subsequent daytime drowsiness

**sleeping pill** /ˈsliːpɪŋ pɪl/ *noun* a pill containing a drug, usually a barbiturate, which makes a person sleep ○ *She died of an overdose of sleeping pills.*

**sleeping sickness** /ˈsliːpɪŋ ˌsɪknəs/ *noun* an African disease, spread by the tsetse fly, where trypanosomes infest the blood. Also called **African trypanosomiasis**

COMMENT: Symptoms are headaches, lethargy and long periods of sleep. The disease is fatal if not treated.

**sleeping tablet** *noun* a tablet containing a drug, usually a barbiturate, which makes a person sleep

**sleeplessness** /ˈsliːpləsnəs/ *noun* ♦ **insomnia**

**sleep off** /ˌsliːp ˈɒf/ *verb* to recover from a mild illness or hangover by sleeping (NOTE: **sleeping off – slept off**)

**sleep terror disorder** /ˌsliːp ˈterə dɪsˌɔːdə/ *noun* a condition in which a person regularly wakes from sleep in a state of terror and confusion but remembers nothing about it in the morning

**sleepwalker** /ˈsliːpwɔːkə/ *noun* same as **somnambulist**

**sleepwalking** /ˈsliːpwɔːkɪŋ/ *noun* same as **somnambulism**

**sleepy** /ˈsliːpi/ *adjective* feeling ready to go to sleep (NOTE: **sleepier – sleepiest**)

**sleepy sickness** /ˈsliːpi ˌsɪknəs/ *noun* same as **lethargic encephalitis**

**slice** /slaɪs/ *noun* a thin flat piece of tissue which has been cut off ○ *He examined the slice of brain tissue under the microscope.*

**slide** /slaɪd/ *noun* a piece of glass, on which a tissue sample is placed, to be examined under a microscope ■ *verb* to move along smoothly ○ *The plunger slides up and down the syringe.* (NOTE: **sliding – slid**)

**sliding traction** /ˌslaɪdɪŋ ˈtrækʃ(ə)n/ *noun* traction for a fracture of a femur, in which weights are attached to pull the leg

**slight** /slaɪt/ *adjective* not very serious ○ *He has a slight fever.* ○ *She had a slight accident.*

**slim** /slɪm/ *adjective* pleasantly thin ○ *She has become slim again after being pregnant.* ■ *verb* to try to become thinner or weigh less ○ *She is trying to slim before she goes on holiday.* (NOTE: **slimming – slimmed**)

**slimming** /ˈslɪmɪŋ/ *noun* the use of a special diet or special food which is low in calories and which is supposed to stop a person getting fat

**sling** /slɪŋ/ *noun* a triangular bandage attached round the neck, used to support an injured arm and prevent it from moving ○ *She had her left arm in a sling.*

**slipped disc** /ˌslɪpt ˈdɪsk/ *noun* same as **displaced intervertebral disc, prolapsed intervertebral disc**

**slit lamp** /ˈslɪt læmp/ *noun* a piece of equipment which provides a narrow beam of light and is connected to a special microscope, used to examine the eye

**slough** /slaʊ/ *noun* dead tissue, especially dead skin, which has separated from healthy tissue ■ *verb* to lose dead skin which falls off

**slow-release vitamin tablet** /ˌsloʊ rɪˌliːs ˈvɪtəmɪn ˌtæblət/ *noun* a vitamin tablet which will dissolve slowly in the body and give a longer and more constant effect

**slow-wave sleep** /ˌsloʊ ˌweɪv ˈsliːp/ *noun* a period of sleep during which the sleeper sleeps deeply and the eyes do not move

COMMENT: During slow-wave sleep, the pituitary gland secretes the hormone somatotrophin.

**small** /smɔːl/ *adjective* **1.** not large ○ *His chest was covered with small red spots.* ○ *She has a small cyst in the colon.* **2.** young ○ *He had chickenpox when he was small.*

**small children** /ˌsmɔːl ˈtʃɪldrən/ *noun* young children, between about 1 and 10 years of age

**small for dates** /ˌsmɔːl fə ˈdeɪts/ *adjective* referring to an unborn baby which is small in comparison to the average size for that number of weeks. Abbr **SFD**

**small intestine** /ˌsmɔːl ɪnˈtestɪn/ *noun* a section of the intestine from the stomach to the caecum, consisting of the duodenum, the jejunum and the ileum

**small of the back** /ˌsmɔːl əv ðə ˈbæk/ *noun* the middle part of the back between and below the shoulder blades

**smallpox** /ˈsmɔːlpɒks/ *noun* a very serious, usually fatal, contagious disease caused by the pox virus, with a severe rash, leaving masses of small scars on the skin. Also called **variola**

COMMENT: It is more than 200 years since the first smallpox vaccine experiments and vaccination has proved effective in eradicating smallpox.

**small stomach** /ˌsmɔːl ˈstʌmək/ *noun* a stomach which is reduced in size after an operation, making the person unable to eat large meals

**smear** /smɪə/ *noun* a sample of soft tissue, e.g. blood or mucus, taken from a person and spread over a glass slide to be examined under a microscope

**smear test** /ˈsmɪə test/ *noun* same as **Papanicolaou test**

**smegma** /ˈsmegmə/ *noun* an oily secretion with an unpleasant smell which collects on and under the foreskin of the penis

**smell** /smel/ *noun* one of the five senses, the sense which is experienced through the nose ■ *verb* **1.** to notice the smell of something through the nose ○ *I can smell smoke.* ○ *He can't smell anything because he's got a cold.* **2.** to produce a smell ○ *The room smells of disinfectant.* (NOTE: **smelling – smelled** *or* **smelt**)

COMMENT: The senses of smell and taste are closely connected, and together give the real taste of food. Smells are sensed by receptors in the nasal cavity which transmit impulses to the brain. When food is eaten, the smell is sensed at the same time as the taste is sensed by the taste buds, and most of what we think of as taste is in fact smell, which explains why food loses its taste when someone has a cold and a blocked nose.

**smelling salts** /ˈsmelɪŋ ˌsɔːlts/ *noun* crystals of an ammonia compound which give off a strong smell and can revive someone who has fainted

**Smith-Petersen nail** /ˌsmɪθ ˈpiːtəs(ə)n neɪl/ *noun* a metal nail used to attach the fractured neck of a femur [Described 1931. After Marius Nygaard Smith-Petersen (1886–1953), Norwegian-born Boston orthopaedic surgeon.]

**Smith's fracture** /ˈsmɪθs ˌfræktʃə/ *noun* a fracture of the radius just above the wrist

**smog** /smɒg/ *noun* pollution of the atmosphere in towns, caused by warm damp air combining with smoke and exhaust fumes from cars

**smoke** /sməʊk/ *noun* a white, grey or black product made of small particles, given off by something which is burning ■ *verb* to breathe in smoke from a cigarette, cigar or pipe which is held in the lips ○ *Doctors are trying to persuade people to stop smoking.* (NOTE: **smoking – smoked**)

COMMENT: The connection between smoking tobacco, especially cigarettes, and lung cancer has been proved to the satisfaction of the British government, which prints a health warning on all packets of cigarettes. Smoke from burning tobacco contains nicotine and other substances which stick in the lungs, and can in the long run cause cancer and heart disease.

**smoke inhalation** /ˈsməʊk ɪnhəˌleɪʃ(ə)n/ *noun* the breathing in of smoke, as in a fire

**smoker** /ˈsməʊkə/ *noun* a person who smokes cigarettes

**smoker's cough** /ˌsməʊkəz ˈkɒf/ *noun* a dry asthmatic cough, often found in people who smoke large numbers of cigarettes

**smoking** /ˈsməʊkɪŋ/ *noun* the action of smoking a cigarette, pipe or cigar ○ *Smoking can injure your health.*

'…three quarters of patients aged 35–64 on GPs' lists have at least one major risk factor: high cholesterol, high blood pressure or addiction to tobacco. Of the three risk factors, smoking causes a quarter of heart disease deaths' [*Health Services Journal*]

**smooth** /smuːð/ *adjective* flat, not rough ■ *verb* to make something smooth ○ *She smoothed down the sheets on the bed.*

**smooth muscle** /smuːð ˈmʌs(ə)l/ *noun* a type of muscle found in involuntary muscles. Also called **unstriated muscle**

**SMR** *abbr* submucous resection

**snare** /sneə/ *noun* a surgical instrument made of a loop of wire, used to remove growths without the need of an incision

**sneeze** /sniːz/ *noun* a reflex action to blow air suddenly out of the nose and mouth because of irritation in the nasal passages ○ *She gave a loud sneeze.* ■ *verb* to blow air suddenly out of the nose and mouth because of irritation in the nasal passages ○ *The smell of flowers makes her sneeze.* ○ *He was coughing and sneezing and decided to stay in bed.* (NOTE: **sneezing – sneezed**)

COMMENT: A sneeze sends out a spray of droplets of liquid, which, if infectious, can then infect anyone who happens to inhale them.

**sneezing fit** /ˈsniːzɪŋ fɪt/ *noun* a sudden attack when someone sneezes many times

**Snellen chart** /ˈsnelən tʃɑːt/ *noun* a chart commonly used by opticians to test eyesight [Described 1862. After Hermann Snellen (1834–1908), Dutch ophthalmologist.]

COMMENT: The Snellen chart has rows of letters, the top row being very large, and the bottom very small, with the result that the more rows a person can read, the better his or her eyesight.

**Snellen type** /ˈsnelən taɪp/ *noun* different type sizes used on a Snellen chart

**sniff** /snɪf/ *noun* an act of breathing in air or smelling through the nose ○ *They gave her a sniff of smelling salts to revive her.* ■ *verb* to breathe in air or to smell through the nose ○ *He was sniffing because he had a cold.* ○ *She sniffed and said that she could smell smoke.*

**sniffle** /ˈsnɪf(ə)l/ *verb* to keep on sniffing because you have a cold or are crying (NOTE: **sniffling – sniffled**)

**sniffles** /ˈsnɪf(ə)lz/ *plural noun* a slight head cold, or an allergy that causes a running nose (*informal; used to children*) ○ *Don't go out into the cold when you have the sniffles.*

**snore** /snɔː/ *noun* a loud noise produced in the nose and throat when a person is asleep ■ *verb* to make a loud noise in the nose and throat when asleep (NOTE: **snoring – snored**)

COMMENT: A snore is produced by the vibration of the soft palate at the back of the mouth, and occurs when a sleeping person breathes through both mouth and nose.

**snoring** /ˈsnɔːrɪŋ/ *noun* noisy breathing while asleep

**snot** /snɒt/ *noun* mucus in the nose (*informal*)

**snow blindness** /ˈsnəʊ ˌblaɪndnəs/ *noun* temporary painful blindness caused by bright sunlight shining on snow

**snuffles** /ˈsnʌf(ə)lz/ *plural noun* the condition of breathing noisily through a nose which is blocked with mucus, which is usually a symptom of the common cold, but can sometimes be a sign of congenital syphilis (*informal; used to children*)

**soak** /səʊk/ *verb* to put something in liquid so that it absorbs some of it ○ *Use a compress made of cloth soaked in warm water.*

**social** /ˈsəʊʃ(ə)l/ *adjective* referring to society or to groups of people

**social disease** /ˌsəʊʃ(ə)l dɪˈziːz/ *noun US* sexually transmitted disease

**socialisation** /ˌsəʊʃ(ə)laɪˈzeɪʃ(ə)n/, **socialization** *noun* the process involved when young children are becoming aware of society and learning how they are expected to behave

**social medicine** /ˌsəʊʃ(ə)l ˈmed(ə)s(ə)n/ *noun* medicine as applied to treatment of diseases which occur in particular social groups

**social services** /ˌsəʊʃ(ə)l ˈsɜːvɪsɪz/ *plural noun* the special facilities which the government or local authorities provide to people in the community who need help, such as the eld-

erly, children whose parents have died or the unemployed

**social worker** /ˈsəʊʃ(ə)l ˌwɜːkə/ *noun* a government employee who works to provide social services to people in need and improve their living standards

**society** /səˈsaɪəti/ *noun* **1.** the community of people who live in a particular country and share its institutions and customs **2.** an organisation of people who have a shared interest

**sociopath** /ˈsəʊsiəpæθ/ *noun* same as **psychopath**

**socket** /ˈsɒkɪt/ *noun* a hollow part in a bone, into which another bone or organ fits ○ *The tip of the femur fits into a socket in the pelvis.*

**sodium** /ˈsəʊdiəm/ *noun* a chemical element which is the basic substance in salt (NOTE: The chemical symbol is **Na**.)

COMMENT: Sodium is an essential mineral and exists in the extracellular fluid of the body. Sweat and tears also contain a high proportion of sodium chloride.

**sodium balance** /ˈsəʊdiəm ˌbæləns/ *noun* the balance maintained in the body between salt lost in sweat and urine and salt taken in from food. The balance is regulated by aldosterone.

**sodium bicarbonate** /ˌsəʊdiəm baɪˈkɑːbənət/ *noun* sodium salt used in cooking, and also as a relief for indigestion and acidity. Also called **bicarbonate of soda**

**sodium chloride** /ˌsəʊdiəm ˈklɔːraɪd/ *noun* common salt

**sodium fusidate** /ˌsəʊdiəm ˈfjuːsɪdeɪt/ *noun* an antibiotic used mainly to treat penicillin-resistant staphylococcal infections

**sodium pump** /ˈsəʊdiəm pʌmp/ *noun* a cellular process in which sodium is immediately excreted from any cell which it enters and potassium is brought in

**sodium valproate** /ˌsəʊdiəm vælˈprəʊeɪt/ *noun* an anticonvulsant drug used especially to treat migraines, seizures and epilepsy

**sodokosis** /ˌsəʊdəʊˈkəʊsɪs/, **sodoku** /ˈsəʊdəʊkuː/ *noun* a form of rat-bite fever, in which swellings in the jaws do not occur

**sodomy** /ˈsɒdəmi/ *noun* anal sexual intercourse between men

**soft** /sɒft/ *adjective* not hard or not resistant to pressure

**soft chancre** /sɒft ˈʃæŋkə/ *noun* same as **soft sore**

**soften** /ˈsɒf(ə)n/ *verb* to make something soft, or become soft

**soft palate** /sɒft ˈpælət/ *noun* the back part of the palate leading to the uvula. ◊ **cleft palate**

**soft sore** /sɒft ˈsɔː/ *noun* a venereal sore with a soft base, situated in the groin or on the genitals and caused by the bacterium *Haemophilus ducreyi*. Also called **chancroid, soft chancre**

**soft tissue** /ˌsɒft ˈtɪʃuː/ *noun* skin, muscles, ligaments or tendons

**soil** /sɔɪl/ *noun* the earth in which plants grow ■ *verb* to make something dirty ○ *He soiled his sheets.* ○ *Soiled bedclothes are sent to the hospital laundry.*

**solar plexus** /ˌsəʊlə ˈpleksəs/ *noun* a nerve network situated at the back of the abdomen between the adrenal glands

**solar retinopathy** /ˌsəʊlə retɪˈnɒpəθi/ *noun* irreparable damage to the most sensitive part of the retina, the macula, caused by looking at the sun with no protection or inadequate protection, as when looking at an eclipse of the sun

**sole** /səʊl/ *noun* the part under the foot ○ *The soles of the feet are very sensitive.*

**soleus** /ˈsəʊliəs/ *noun* a flat muscle which goes down the calf of the leg (NOTE: The plural is **solei**.)

**solid** /ˈsɒlɪd/ *adjective* **1.** not soft or yielding **2.** hard and not liquid ○ *Water turns solid when it freezes.*

**solid food** /ˌsɒlɪd ˈfuːd/ *noun* food which is chewed and eaten, not drunk ○ *She is allowed some solid food.* or *She is allowed to eat solids.*
COMMENT: Solid foods are introduced gradually to babies and to patients who have had intestinal operations.

**solidify** /səˈlɪdɪfaɪ/ *verb* to become solid, or cause something to become solid ○ *Carbon dioxide solidifies at low temperatures.*

**solids** *noun* solid food

**soluble** /ˈsɒljʊb(ə)l/ *adjective* able to dissolve ○ *a tablet of soluble aspirin*

**soluble fibre** /ˌsɒljʊb(ə)l ˈfaɪbə/ *noun* a fibre in vegetables, fruit and pulses and porridge oats which is partly digested in the intestine and reduces the absorption of fats and sugar into the body, so lowering the level of cholesterol

**solute** /ˈsɒljuːt/ *noun* a solid substance which is dissolved in a solvent to make a solution

**solution** /səˈluːʃ(ə)n/ *noun* a mixture of a solid substance dissolved in a liquid

**solvent** /ˈsɒlv(ə)nt/ *noun* a liquid in which a solid substance can be dissolved

**solvent abuse** /ˈsɒlvənt əˌbjuːs/, **solvent inhalation** /ˌsɒlvənt ˌɪnhəˈleɪʃ(ə)n/ *noun* a type of drug abuse in which someone inhales the toxic fumes given off by particular types of volatile chemical. Also called **glue-sniffing**
'...deaths among teenagers caused by solvent abuse have reached record levels' [*Health Visitor*]

**soma** /ˈsəʊmə/ *noun* the body, as opposed to the mind (NOTE: The plural is **somata** or **somas**.)

**somat-** /ˈsəʊmət/ *prefix* same as **somato-** (used before vowels)

**somata** /ˈsəʊmətə/ plural of **soma**

**somatic** /səʊˈmætɪk/ *adjective* referring to the body, either as opposed to the mind, or as opposed to the intestines and inner organs. Compare **psychosomatic**

**somatic nerve** /səʊˈmætɪk nɜːv/ *noun* any of the sensory and motor nerves which control skeletal muscles

**somatic nervous system** /səʊˌmætɪk ˈnɜːvəs ˌsɪstəm/ *noun* the part of the nervous system that serves the sense organs and muscles of the body wall and limbs, and brings about activity in the voluntary muscles

**somato-** /ˈsəʊmətəʊ/ *prefix* **1.** referring to the body **2.** somatic

**somatology** /ˌsəʊməˈtɒlədʒi/ *noun* the study of both the physiology and anatomy of the body

**somatostatin** /ˌsəʊmətəʊˈstætɪn/ *noun* a hormone produced in the hypothalamus which helps to prevent the release of the growth hormone

**somatotrophic hormone** /ˌsəʊmətəˌtrɒfɪk ˈhɔːməʊn/, **somatotrophin** /ˌsəʊmətəˈtrəʊfɪn/ *noun* a growth hormone, secreted by the pituitary gland, which stimulates the growth of long bones (NOTE: The US term for somatotrophin is **somatotropin**.)

**somatropin** /ˌsəʊmətəʊˈtrəʊfɪn/ *noun* same as **growth hormone**

**-some** /səʊm/ *suffix* tiny cell bodies

**somnambulism** /sɒmˈnæmbjʊlɪz(ə)m/ *noun* a condition especially affecting children where the person gets up and walks about while still asleep. Also called **sleepwalking**

**somnambulist** /sɒmˈnæmbjʊlɪst/ *noun* a person who walks in his or her sleep. Also called **sleepwalker**

**somnambulistic** /sɒmnˌæmbjʊˈlɪstɪk/ *adjective* referring to somnambulism

**somnolent** /ˈsɒmnələnt/ *adjective* sleepy

**somnolism** /ˈsɒmnəlɪz(ə)m/ *noun* a trance which is induced by hypnotism

**Somogyi effect** /ˈʃɒmɒdʒi ɪˌfekt/, **Somogyi phenomenon** /ˈʃɒmɒdʒi fɪˌnɒmənən/ *noun* in diabetes mellitus, a swing to a high level of glucose in the blood from an extremely low level, usually occurring after an untreated insulin reaction during the night. It is caused by the release of stress hormones to counter low glucose levels.

**-somy** /ˈsəʊmi/ *suffix* the presence of chromosomes

**son** /sʌn/ *noun* a male child of a parent ○ *They have two sons and one daughter.*

**Sonne dysentery** /ˈsɒnə ˌdɪsəntri/ *noun* a common form of mild dysentery in the UK, caused by *Shigella sonnei* [Described 1915. After Carl Olaf Sonne (1882–1948), Danish bacteriologist and physician.]

**sonogram** /'səʊnəgræm/ noun a chart produced using ultrasound waves to find where something is situated in the body

**sonography** /sə'nɒgrəfi/ noun same as **ultrasonography**

**sonoplacentography** /ˌsəʊnəplæsən'tɒgrəfi/ noun the use of ultrasound waves to find how the placenta is placed in a pregnant woman

**sonotopography** /ˌsəʊnətə'pɒgrəfi/ noun the use of ultrasound waves to produce a sonogram

**soothe** /suːð/ verb to relieve pain or irritation or make a person less tense ○ The calamine lotion will soothe the rash. (NOTE: **soothing – soothed**)

**soothing** /'suːðɪŋ/ adjective relieving pain or irritation or making someone less tense ○ They played soothing music in the dentist's waiting room.

**sopor** /'səʊpə/ noun deep sleep or unconsciousness

**soporific** /ˌsɒpə'rɪfɪk/ noun a drug which makes a person go to sleep ■ adjective causing sleep

**sorbitol** /'sɔːbɪtɒl/ noun a white crystalline sweet alcohol which is used as a sweetener and a moisturiser, and in the manufacture of Vitamin C

**sordes** /'sɔːdiːz/ plural noun dry deposits round the lips of someone who has a fever

**sore** /sɔː/ noun a small wound on any part of the skin, usually with a discharge of pus ■ adjective **1.** rough and inflamed ○ a sore patch on the skin **2.** painful ○ My ankle still feels very sore.

**sore throat** /sɔː 'θrəʊt/ noun a condition in which the mucous membrane in the throat is inflamed, sometimes because the person has been talking too much, but usually because of an infection (informal)

**s.o.s.** adverb (on prescriptions) if necessary. Full form **si opus sit** (NOTE: It means that the dose should be taken once.)

**sotalol** /'sɒtəlɒl/ noun a drug used to treat an irregular heartbeat and high blood pressure

**souffle** /'suːf(ə)l/ noun a soft breathing sound, heard through a stethoscope

**sound** /saʊnd/ noun **1.** something which can be heard ○ The doctor listened to the sounds of the patient's lungs. ○ His breathing made a whistling sound. **2.** a long rod, used to examine or to dilate the inside of a cavity in the body ■ adjective strong and healthy ○ He has a sound constitution. ○ Her heart is sound, but her lungs are congested. ■ verb **1.** to make a particular noise ○ Her lungs sounded as if she had pneumonia. **2.** to examine the inside of a cavity using a rod

**sour** /'saʊə/ adjective not bitter, salt or sweet (NOTE: It is one of the basic tastes.)

**source** /sɔːs/ noun **1.** the substance which produces something ○ Sugar is a source of energy. ○ Vegetables are important sources of vitamins. **2.** the place where something comes from ○ The source of the allergy has been identified. ○ The medical team has isolated the source of the infection.

**space** /speɪs/ noun a place, empty area between things ○ An abscess formed in the space between the bone and the cartilage.

**spansule** /'spænsjuːl/ noun a drug in the form of a capsule which is specially designed to release its contents slowly in the stomach

**spare** /speə/ adjective extra or only used in emergencies ○ We have no spare beds in the hospital at the moment. ○ The doctor carries a spare set of instruments in her car. ■ verb to be able to give or spend something ○ Can you spare the time to see the next patient? ○ We have only one bed to spare at the moment. (NOTE: **sparing – spared**)

**spare part surgery** /ˌspeə 'pɑːt ˌsɜːdʒəri/ noun surgery in which parts of the body such as bones or joints are replaced by artificial pieces

**sparganosis** /ˌspɑːgə'nəʊsɪs/ noun a condition caused by the larvae of the worm Sparganum under the skin. It is widespread in East Asia.

**spasm** /'spæz(ə)m/ noun a sudden, usually painful, involuntary contraction of a muscle, as in cramp ○ The muscles in his leg went into spasm. ○ She had painful spasms in her stomach.

**spasmo-** /spæzməʊ/ prefix referring to a spasm

**spasmodic** /spæz'mɒdɪk/ adjective **1.** occurring in spasms **2.** happening from time to time

**spasmolytic** /ˌspæzmə'lɪtɪk/ noun a drug which relieves muscle spasms

**spasmus nutans** /ˌspæzməs 'njuːtənz/ noun a condition in which someone nods his or her head and at the same time has spasms in the neck muscles and rapid movements of the eyes

**spastic** /'spæstɪk/ adjective with spasms or sudden contractions of muscles ■ noun a person affected with cerebral palsy (NOTE: The noun sense is now considered to be offensive.)

**spastic colon** /ˌspæstɪk 'kəʊlɒn/ noun same as **mucous colitis**

**spastic diplegia** /ˌspæstɪk daɪ'pliːdʒə/ noun a congenital form of cerebral palsy which affects mainly the legs. Also called **Little's disease**

**spastic gait** /ˌspæstɪk 'geɪt/ noun a way of walking where the legs are stiff and the feet not lifted off the ground

**spasticity** /spæ'stɪstɪ/ *noun* a condition in which a limb resists passive movement. ◊ **rigidity**

**spastic paralysis** /ˌspæstɪk pə'ræləsɪs/ *noun* same as **cerebral palsy**

**spastic paraplegia** /ˌspæstɪk ˌpærə'pliːdʒə/ *noun* paralysis of one side of the body after a stroke

**spatula** /'spætjʊlə/ *noun* **1.** a flat flexible tool with a handle, used to scoop, lift, spread or mix things **2.** a flat wooden stick used to press the tongue down when the mouth or throat is being examined

**speak** /spiːk/ *verb* to say words or articulate sounds with the voice ○ *He is learning to speak again after a laryngectomy.* (NOTE: **speaking – spoke – spoken**)

**speak up** /ˌspiːk 'ʌp/ *verb* to speak more loudly ○ *Speak up, please – I can't hear you!*

**special** /'speʃ(ə)l/ *adjective* not ordinary, or for a specific purpose ○ *He has been given a special diet to cure his allergy.* ○ *She wore special shoes to correct a problem in her ankles.*

**special care baby unit** /ˌspeʃ(ə)l keə 'beɪbi ˌjuːnɪt/ *noun* a unit in a hospital which deals with premature babies or babies with serious disorders

**special health authority** /ˌspeʃ(ə)l 'helθ ɔːˌθɒrɪti/ *noun* a health authority which has unique national functions, or covers various regions. An example is UK Transplant, which manages the National Transplant Database and provides a 24-hour service for the matching and allocation of donor organs.

**special hospital** /ˌspeʃ(ə)l 'hɒspɪt(ə)l/ *noun* a hospital for people whose mental condition makes them a potential danger to themselves and/or others

**specialisation** /ˌspeʃəlaɪ'zeɪʃ(ə)n/, **specialization** *noun* **1.** the act of specialising in a particular branch of medicine **2.** a particular branch of medicine which a doctor specialises in

**specialise** /'speʃəlaɪz/, **specialize** *verb* **1.** to concentrate on a specific subject or activity **2.** to be an expert in a specific subject or area of knowledge (NOTE: **specialising – specialised**)

**specialised** /'speʃəlaɪzd/, **specialized** *adjective* **1.** designed for a particular purpose **2.** concentrating on a particular activity or subject ○ *specialised skills*

**specialise in** /'speʃəlaɪz ɪn/, **specialize in** *verb* to study or to treat one particular disease or one particular type of patient ○ *He specialises in children with breathing problems.* ○ *She decided to specialise in haematology.*

**specialism** /'speʃəlɪz(ə)m/ *noun* same as **speciality**

**specialist** /'speʃəlɪst/ *noun* a doctor who specialises in a particular branch of medicine

○ *He is a heart specialist.* ○ *She was referred to an ENT specialist.*

**specialist registrar** /ˌspeʃ(ə)lɪst 'redʒɪˌstrɑː/ *noun* a junior doctor in a hospital who is doing further specialist training

**speciality** /ˌspeʃi'æləti/ *noun* a particular activity or type of work which someone is specially trained for or very interested in. Also called **specialism, specialty**

**special school** /'speʃ(ə)l skuːl/ *noun* a school for children with disabilities

**specialty** /'speʃ(ə)lti/ *noun US* same as **speciality**

**species** /'spiːʃiːz/ *noun* a group of living things with the same characteristics and which can interbreed (NOTE: The plural is **species**.)

**specific** /spə'sɪfɪk/ *adjective* referring to a disease caused by one type of microorganism only. Opposite **non-specific** ■ *noun* a drug which is only used to treat one disease

**specific gravity** /spəˌsɪfɪk 'grævəti/ *noun* same as **relative density**

**specificity** /ˌspesɪ'fɪsəti/ *noun* the rate of negative responses in a test from persons free from a disease. A high specificity means a low rate of false positives. Compare **sensitivity**

**specific urethritis** /spəˌsɪfɪk jʊərɪ'θraɪtɪs/ *noun* inflammation of the urethra caused by gonorrhoea

**specimen** /'spesɪmɪn/ *noun* **1.** a small quantity of something given for testing ○ *He was asked to bring a urine specimen.* **2.** one item out of a group ○ *We keep specimens of diseased organs for students to examine.*

**spectacles** /'spektək(ə)lz/ *plural noun* glasses which are worn in front of the eyes to help correct problems in vision

COMMENT: Spectacles can correct problems in the focusing of the eye, such as shortsightedness, longsightedness and astigmatism. Where different lenses are required for reading, an optician may prescribe two pairs of spectacles, one for standard use and the other for reading. Otherwise, spectacles can be fitted with a divided lens (bifocals or varifocals).

**spectra** /'spektrə/ *plural of* **spectrum**

**spectrography** /spek'trɒgrəfi/ *noun* the recording of a spectrum on photographic film

**spectroscope** /'spektrəskəʊp/ *noun* an instrument used to analyse a spectrum

**spectrum** /'spektrəm/ *noun* **1.** the range of colours, from red to violet, into which white light can be split when it is passed through something (NOTE: Different substances in solution have different spectra.) **2.** the range of organisms that an antibiotic or chemical can kill (NOTE: The plural is **spectra** or **spectrums**.)

**specula** /'spekjʊlə/ *plural of* **speculum**

**specular** /'spekjʊlə/ *adjective* carried out using a speculum

**speculum** /'spekjʊləm/ *noun* a surgical instrument which is inserted into an opening in the body such as a nostril or the vagina to keep it open in order to allow a doctor to examine the inside (NOTE: The plural is **specula** or **speculums**.)

**speech** /spiːtʃ/ *noun* **1.** the ability to make intelligible sounds with the vocal cords **2.** a talk given to an audience

**speech block** /'spiːtʃ blɒk/ *noun* a temporary inability to speak, caused by the effect of nervous stress on the mental processes

**speech impediment** /'spiːtʃ ɪm,pedɪmənt/ *noun* an inability to speak easily or in the usual way because of the physical structure of the mouth or other disorders

**speech therapist** /'spiːtʃ ,θerəpɪst/ *noun* a qualified person who practises speech therapy

**speech therapy** /'spiːtʃ ,θerəpi/ *noun* treatment for a speech disorder such as stammering or one which results from a stroke or physical malformation

**spell** /spel/ *noun* a short period ○ *She has been having dizzy spells.* ○ *He had two spells in hospital during the winter.*

**sperm** /spɜːm/ *noun* same as **spermatozoon** (NOTE: The plural is **sperm**.)

**spermat-** /spɜːmət/ *prefix* same as **spermato-** (*used before vowels*)

**spermatic** /spɜː'mætɪk/ *adjective* referring to sperm

**spermatic artery** /spɜː,mætɪk 'ɑːtəri/ *noun* an artery which leads into the testes. Also called **testicular artery**

**spermatic cord** /spɜː,mætɪk 'kɔːd/ *noun* a cord running from the testis to the abdomen carrying the vas deferens, the blood vessels, nerves and lymphatics of the testis

**spermatid** /'spɜːmətɪd/ *noun* an immature male sex cell that develops into a spermatozoon

**spermato-** /spɜːmətəʊ/ *prefix* **1.** referring to sperm **2.** referring to the male reproductive system

**spermatocele** /'spɜːmətəsiːl/ *noun* a cyst which forms in the scrotum

**spermatocyte** /'spɜːmətəsaɪt/ *noun* an early stage in the development of a spermatozoon

**spermatogenesis** /,spɜːmətə'dʒenəsɪs/ *noun* the formation and development of spermatozoa in the testes

**spermatogonium** /,spɜːmətə'gəʊniəm/ *noun* a cell which forms a spermatocyte (NOTE: The plural is **spermatogonia**.)

**spermatorrhoea** /,spɜːmətə'rɪə/ *noun* the discharge of a large amount of semen frequently and without an orgasm (NOTE: The US spelling is **spermatorrhea**.)

**spermatozoon** /,spɜːmətə'zəʊɒn/ *noun* a mature male sex cell, which is ejaculated from the penis and is capable of fertilising an ovum.

Also called **sperm** (NOTE: The plural is **spermatozoa**.)

COMMENT: A human spermatozoon is very small and is formed of a head, neck and very long tail. A spermatozoon can swim by moving its tail from side to side. The sperm are formed in the testes and ejaculated through the penis. Each ejaculation may contain millions of sperm. Once a sperm has entered the female uterus, it remains viable for about three days.

**spermaturia** /,spɜːmə'tjʊəriə/ *noun* sperm in the urine

**sperm bank** /'spɜːm bæŋk/ *noun* a place where sperm can be stored for use in artificial insemination

**sperm count** /'spɜːm kaʊnt/ *noun* a calculation of the number of sperm in a quantity of semen

**sperm donor** /'spɜːm ,dəʊnə/ *noun* a male who gives sperm, for a fee, to allow a childless woman to bear a child

**spermi-** /spɜːmi/ *prefix* referring to sperm and semen

**spermicidal** /,spɜːmɪ'saɪd(ə)l/ *adjective* killing or able to kill sperm

**spermicidal jelly** /,spɜːmɪ,saɪd(ə)l 'dʒeli/ *noun* a jelly-like product which acts as a contraceptive

**spermicide** /'spɜːmɪsaɪd/ *noun* a substance which kills sperm

**spermio-** /spɜːmiəʊ/ *prefix* same as **spermi-**

**spermiogenesis** /,spɜːmiəʊ'dʒenəsɪs/ *noun* the stage of spermatogenesis during which a spermatid changes into a spermatozoon

**spheno-** /sfiːnəʊ/ *prefix* referring to the sphenoid bone

**sphenoid** /'sfiːnɔɪd/ *adjective* **1.** relating to the sphenoid bone **2.** shaped like a wedge ■ *noun* same as **sphenoid bone**

**sphenoid bone** /'sfiːnɔɪd bəʊn/ *noun* one of two bones in the skull which form the side of the socket of the eye. Also called **sphenoid**

**sphenoid sinus** /,sfiːnɔɪd 'saɪnəs/ *noun* one of the sinuses in the skull behind the nasal passage

**sphenopalatine ganglion** /,sfiːnəʊ ,pælətaɪn 'gæŋliɒn/ *noun* same as **pterygopalatine ganglion**

**spherocyte** /'sfɪərəʊsaɪt/ *noun* a red blood cell that is round rather than the usual disc shape

**spherocytosis** /,sfɪərəʊsaɪ'təʊsɪs/ *noun* a condition in which someone has spherocytes in the blood, causing anaemia, enlarged spleen and gallstones, as in acholuric jaundice

**sphincter** /'sfɪŋktə/, **sphincter muscle** /'sfɪŋktə ,mʌs(ə)l/ *noun* a circular band of muscle which surrounds an opening or passage in the body, especially the anus, and can narrow or close the opening or passage by contracting

**sphincterectomy** /ˌsfɪŋktə'rektəmi/ *noun* **1.** a surgical operation to remove a sphincter **2.** a surgical operation to remove part of the edge of the iris in the eye (NOTE: The plural is **sphincterectomies.**)

**sphincteroplasty** /'sfɪŋktərəˌplæsti/ *noun* a surgical operation to relieve a tightened sphincter (NOTE: The plural is **sphincteroplasties.**)

**sphincterotomy** /ˌsfɪŋktə'rɒtəmi/ *noun* a surgical operation to make an incision into a sphincter (NOTE: The plural is **sphincterotomies.**)

**sphincter pupillae muscle** /ˌsfɪŋktə 'pjuːpɪlaɪ ˌmʌs(ə)l/ *noun* an annular muscle in the iris which constricts the pupil

**sphyg** /sfɪg/ *noun* same as **sphygmomanometer** (*informal*)

**sphygmic** /'sfɪgmɪk/ *adjective* referring to the pulse of an artery

**sphygmo-** /sfɪgməʊ/ *prefix* referring to the pulse

**sphygmocardiograph** /ˌsfɪgməʊ 'kɑːdiəʊgrɑːf/ *noun* a device which records heartbeats and pulse rate

**sphygmograph** /'sfɪgməgrɑːf/ *noun* a device which records the pulse

**sphygmomanometer** /ˌsfɪgməʊmə 'nɒmɪtə/ *noun* an instrument which measures blood pressure in the arteries

COMMENT: The sphygmomanometer is a rubber sleeve connected to a scale with a column of mercury, allowing the nurse to take a reading. The rubber sleeve is usually wrapped round the arm and inflated until the blood flow is stopped. The blood pressure is determined by listening to the pulse with a stethoscope placed over an artery as the pressure in the rubber sleeve is slowly reduced, and by the reading on the scale.

**spica** /'spaɪkə/ *noun* a way of bandaging a joint where the bandage crosses over itself like the figure 8 on the inside of the bend of the joint (NOTE: The plural is **spicae** or **spicas.**)

**spicule** /'spɪkjuːl/ *noun* a small splinter of bone

**spigot** /'spɪgət/ *noun* the end of a pipe which is joined by insertion into the enlarged end of another pipe

**spina** /'spaɪnə/ *noun* **1.** a thin sharp piece of bone **2.** the vertebral column

**spina bifida** /ˌspaɪnə 'bɪfɪdə/ *noun* a serious condition in which part of the spinal cord protrudes through the spinal column. Also called **rachischisis**

COMMENT: Spina bifida takes two forms: a mild form, spina bifida occulta, where only the bone is affected, and there are no visible signs of the condition; and the serious spina bifida cystica where part of the meninges or spinal cord passes through the gap; it may result in paralysis of the legs, and mental impair-

ment is often present where the condition is associated with hydrocephalus.

**spinal** /'spaɪn(ə)l/ *adjective* referring to the spine ○ *She suffered spinal injuries in the crash.*

**spinal accessory nerve** /ˌspaɪn(ə)l ək 'sesəri nɜːv/ *noun* the eleventh cranial nerve which supplies the muscles in the neck and shoulders

**spinal anaesthesia** /ˌspaɪn(ə)l ˌænəs 'θiːziə/ *noun* local anaesthesia in which an anaesthetic is injected into the cerebrospinal fluid

**spinal anaesthetic** /ˌspaɪn(ə)l ˌænəs'θeɪ tɪk/ *noun* an anaesthetic given by injection into the spine, which results in large parts of the body losing the sense of feeling

**spinal block** /ˌspaɪn(ə)l 'blɒk/ *noun* analgesia produced by injecting the spinal cord with an anaesthetic

**spinal canal** /ˌspaɪn(ə)l kə'næl/ *noun* the hollow channel running down the back of the vertebrae, containing the spinal cord. Also called **vertebral canal**

**spinal column** /'spaɪn(ə)l ˌkɒləm/ *noun* same as **spine**

**spinal cord** /'spaɪn(ə)l kɔːd/ *noun* part of the central nervous system, running from the medulla oblongata to the filum terminale, in the vertebral canal of the spine (NOTE: For other terms referring to the spinal cord, see words beginning with **myel-, myelo-.**)

**spinal curvature** /ˌspaɪn(ə)l 'kɜːvətʃə/ *noun* unusual bending of the spinal column

**spinal fusion** /ˌspaɪn(ə)l 'fjuːʒ(ə)n/ *noun* a surgical operation to join two vertebrae together to make the spine more rigid. Also called **spondylosyndesis**

**spinal ganglion** /ˌspaɪn(ə)l 'gæŋgliən/ *noun* a cone-shaped mass of cells on the posterior root, the main axons of which form the posterior root of the spinal nerve

**spinal meningitis** /ˌspaɪn(ə)l ˌmenɪn'dʒaɪ ɪtɪs/ *noun* inflammation of the membranes around the spinal cord, which particularly affects young children

**spinal nerve** /'spaɪn(ə)l nɜːv/ *noun* one of the 31 pairs of nerves which lead from the spinal cord and govern mainly the trunk and limbs

**spinal puncture** /ˌspaɪn(ə)l 'pʌŋktʃə/ *noun* same as **lumbar puncture** (NOTE: The US term is **spinal tap.**)

**spinal shock** /'spaɪn(ə)l 'ʃɒk/ *noun* a loss of feeling in the lower part of the body below a point at which the spine has been injured

**spindle** /'spɪnd(ə)l/ *noun* **1.** a long thin structure **2.** a structure formed in cells during division to which the chromosomes are attached by their centromeres

**spine** /spaɪn/ *noun* **1.** the series of bones, the vertebrae, linked together to form a flexible supporting column running from the pelvis to the skull ○ *She injured her spine in the crash.* Also called **backbone, spinal column, vertebral column 2.** any sharp projecting part of a bone

COMMENT: The spine is made up of twenty-four ring-shaped vertebrae, with the sacrum and coccyx, separated by discs of cartilage. The hollow canal of the spine (the spinal canal) contains the spinal cord. See also note at vertebra.

**Spinhaler** /spɪnˈheɪlə/ a trade name for a device from which a person with breathing problems can inhale a preset dose of a drug

**spinnbarkeit** /ˈspɪnbɑːkaɪt/ *noun* a thread of mucus formed in the cervix which is used in determining the time of ovulation. At this time it can be drawn out on a glass slide to its maximum length.

**spino-** /spaɪnəʊ/ *prefix* **1.** referring to the spine **2.** referring to the spinal cord

**spinocerebellar tract** /ˌspaɪnəʊserəˌbelə ˈtrækt/ *noun* a nerve fibre in the spinal cord, taking impulses to the cerebellum

**spinous process** /ˌspaɪnəs ˈprəʊses/ *noun* a projection on a vertebra or a bone which looks like a spine

**spiral** /ˈspaɪrəl/ *adjective* running in a continuous circle upwards

**spiral bandage** /ˌspaɪrəl ˈbændɪdʒ/ *noun* a bandage which is wrapped round a limb, each turn overlapping the one before

**spiral ganglion** /ˌspaɪrəl ˈɡæŋɡliən/ *noun* a ganglion in the eighth cranial nerve which supplies the organ of Corti

**spiral organ** /ˌspaɪrəl ˈɔːɡən/ *noun* same as **organ of Corti**

**Spirillum** /spɪˈrɪləm/ *noun* one of the bacteria which cause rat-bite fever

**spiro-** /spaɪrəʊ/ *prefix* **1.** referring to a spiral **2.** referring to respiration

**spirochaetaemia** /ˌspaɪrəʊkɪˈtiːmiə/ *noun* the presence of spirochaetes in the blood (NOTE: The US spelling is **spirochetemia**.)

**spirochaete** /ˈspaɪrəʊkiːt/ *noun* a bacterium with a spiral shape, e.g. the one which causes syphilis (NOTE: The US spelling is **spirochete**.)

**spirogram** /ˈspaɪrəʊɡræm/ *noun* a record of someone's breathing made by a spirograph

**spirograph** /ˈspaɪrəʊɡrɑːf/ *noun* a device which records depth and rapidity of breathing

**spirography** /spaɪˈrɒɡrəfi/ *noun* the recording of a someone's breathing by use of a spirograph

**spirometer** /spaɪˈrɒmɪtə/ *noun* an instrument which measures the amount of air a person inhales or exhales

**spirometry** /spaɪˈrɒmətri/ *noun* a measurement of the vital capacity of the lungs by use of a spirometer

**spironolactone** /ˌspaɪrənəˈlæktəʊn/ *noun* a steroid which helps the body produce urine,

used in the treatment of oedema and hypertension

**spit** /spɪt/ *noun* saliva which is sent out of the mouth ■ *verb* to send liquid out of the mouth ○ *Rinse your mouth out and spit into the cup provided.* ○ *He spat out the medicine.* (NOTE: **spitting – spat**)

**Spitz-Holter valve** /ˌspɪts ˈhɒltə vælv/ *noun* a valve with a one-way system, surgically placed in the skull and used to drain excess fluid from the brain in hydrocephalus

**splanchnic** /ˈsplæŋknɪk/ *adjective* referring to viscera

**splanchnic nerve** /ˈsplæŋknɪk nɜːv/ *noun* any sympathetic nerve which supplies organs in the abdomen

**splanchnology** /splæŋkˈnɒlədʒi/ *noun* the study of the organs in the abdominal cavity

**spleen** /spliːn/ *noun* an organ in the top part of the abdominal cavity behind the stomach and below the diaphragm, which helps to destroy old red blood cells, form lymphocytes and store blood. See illustration at DIGESTIVE SYSTEM in Supplement

COMMENT: The spleen, which is the largest endocrine (ductless) gland, appears to act to remove dead blood cells and fight infection, but its functions are not fully understood and an adult can live healthily after his or her spleen has been removed.

**splen-** /splen/ *prefix* same as **spleno-** (*used before vowels*)

**splenectomy** /spleˈnektəmi/ *noun* a surgical operation to remove the spleen (NOTE: The plural is **splenectomies**.)

**splenic** /ˈsplenɪk/ *adjective* referring to the spleen

**splenic anaemia** /ˌsplenɪk əˈniːmiə/ *noun* a type of anaemia, caused by cirrhosis of the liver, in which the person has portal hypertension, an enlarged spleen and haemorrhages. Also called **Banti's syndrome**

**splenic flexure** /ˌsplenɪk ˈflekʃə/ *noun* a bend in the colon where the transverse colon joins the descending colon

**splenii** /ˈspliːnii/ *plural noun* plural of **splenius**

**splenitis** /spləˈnaɪtɪs/ *noun* inflammation of the spleen

**splenius** /ˈspliːniəs/ *noun* either of two muscles on each side of the neck that reach from the base of the skull to the upper back and rotate and extend the head and neck (NOTE: The plural is **splenii**.)

**spleno-** /spliːnəʊ/ *prefix* referring to the spleen

**splenomegaly** /ˌspliːnəʊˈmeɡəli/ *noun* a condition in which the spleen is unusually large, associated with several disorders including malaria and some cancers

**splenorenal** /ˌspliːnəʊˈriːn(ə)l/ *adjective* relating to both the spleen and the kidneys

**splenorenal anastomosis** /ˌspliːnəʊ ˌriːn(ə)l əˌnæstəˈməʊsɪs/ *noun* a surgical operation to join the splenic vein to a renal vein, as a treatment for portal hypertension

**splenovenography** /ˌspliːnəʊvəˈnɒɡrəfi/ *noun* X-ray examination of the spleen and the veins which are connected to it

**splint** /splɪnt/ *noun* a stiff support attached to a limb to prevent a broken bone from moving ○ *He had to keep his arm in a splint for several weeks.* ◊ **shin splints**

**splinter** /ˈsplɪntə/ *noun* a tiny thin piece of wood or metal which gets under the skin and can be irritating and cause infection

**splinter haemorrhage** /ˈsplɪntə ˌhem(ə)rɪdʒ/ *noun* a tiny line of haemorrhaging under the nails or in the eyeball

**split** /splɪt/ *verb* to divide something, or become divided (NOTE: **splitting – split**)

**split personality** /splɪt ˌpɜːsəˈnæləti/ *noun* same as **schizoid personality**

**split-skin graft** /ˌsplɪt ˌskɪn ˈɡrɑːft/ *noun* a type of skin graft in which thin layers of skin are grafted over a wound. Also called **Thiersch graft**

**spondyl** /ˈspɒndɪl/ *noun* same as **vertebra**

**spondyl-** /ˈspɒndɪl/ *prefix* same as **spondylo-** (*used before vowels*)

**spondylitis** /ˌspɒndɪˈlaɪtɪs/ *noun* inflammation of the vertebrae

**spondylo-** /ˈspɒndɪləʊ/ *prefix* referring to the vertebrae

**spondylolisthesis** /ˌspɒndɪləʊˈlɪsθəsɪs/ *noun* a condition in which one of the lumbar vertebrae moves forwards over the one beneath

**spondylosis** /ˌspɒndɪˈləʊsɪs/ *noun* stiffness in the spine and degenerative changes in the intervertebral discs, with osteoarthritis. This condition is common in older people.

**spondylosyndesis** /ˌspɒndɪləʊsɪnˈdiːsɪs/ *noun* same as **spinal fusion**

**sponge** /spʌndʒ/ *noun* a piece of light absorbent material, either natural or synthetic, used in bathing and cleaning

**sponge bath** /ˈspʌndʒ bɑːθ/ *noun* the act of washing someone in bed, using a sponge or damp cloth ○ *The nurse gave the elderly lady a sponge bath.*

**spongiform encephalopathy** /ˌspʌndʒi fɔːm enˌkefəˈlɒpəθi/ *noun* a brain disease in humans and animals in which areas of the brain slowly develop holes in their cells and begin to look like a sponge

**spongioblastoma** /ˌspʌndʒiəʊblæˈstəʊmə/ *noun* same as **glioblastoma** (NOTE: The plural is **spongioblastomas** or **spongioblastomata**.)

**spongiosum** /ˌspʌndʒiˈəʊsəm/ ♦ **corpus spongiosum**

**spongy** /ˈspʌndʒi/ *adjective* soft and full of holes like a sponge

**spongy bone** /ˈspʌndʒi bəʊn/ *noun* cancellous bone, light bone tissue which forms the inner core of a bone and also the ends of long bones. See illustration at **BONE STRUCTURE** in Supplement

**spontaneous** /spɒnˈteɪniəs/ *adjective* happening without any particular outside cause

**spontaneous abortion** /spɒnˌteɪniəs əˈbɔːʃ(ə)n/ *noun* same as **miscarriage**

**spontaneous delivery** /spɒnˌteɪniəs dɪˈlɪv(ə)ri/ *noun* a delivery of a baby which takes places naturally, without any medical or surgical help

**spontaneous pneumothorax** /spɒn ˌteɪniəs njuːməʊˈθɔːræks/ *noun* a condition occurring when an opening is created on the surface of the lung allowing air to leak into the pleural cavity

**spontaneous version** /spɒnˌteɪniəs ˈvɜːʃ(ə)n/ *noun* a movement of a fetus to take up another position in the uterus, caused by the contractions of the uterus during childbirth or by the movements of the baby itself before birth

**spoon** /spuːn/ *noun* an instrument with a long handle at one end and a small bowl at the other, used for taking liquid medicine ○ *a 5 ml spoon*

**spoonful** /ˈspuːnfʊl/ *noun* the quantity which a spoon can hold ○ *Take two 5 ml spoonfuls of the medicine twice a day.*

**sporadic** /spəˈrædɪk/ *adjective* referring to outbreaks of disease that occur as separate cases, not in epidemics

**spore** /spɔː/ *noun* a reproductive body of particular bacteria and fungi which can survive in extremely hot or cold conditions for a long time

**sporicidal** /ˌspɔːrɪˈsaɪd(ə)l/ *adjective* killing spores

**sporicide** /ˈspɔːrɪsaɪd/ *noun* a substance which kills bacterial spores

**sporotrichosis** /ˌspɔːrəʊtraɪˈkəʊsɪs/ *noun* a fungus infection of the skin which causes abscesses

**Sporozoa** /ˌspɔːrəˈzəʊə/ *noun* a type of parasitic Protozoa which includes Plasmodium, the cause of malaria

**sport** /spɔːt/ *noun* **1.** the playing of competitive physical games **2.** a competitive physical game

**sports injury** /ˈspɔːts ˌɪndʒəri/ *noun* an injury caused by playing a sport, e.g. a sprained ankle or tennis elbow

**sports medicine** /ˈspɔːts ˌmed(ə)sɪn/ *noun* the study of the treatment of sports injuries

**spot** /spɒt/ *noun* a small round mark or pimple ○ *The disease is marked by red spots on the chest.* □ **to break out in spots** *or* **to come out in spots** to have a sudden rash

**spotted fever** /ˌspɒtɪd ˈfiːvə/ *noun* same as **meningococcal meningitis**

**spotty** /'spɒti/ *adjective* covered with pimples

**sprain** /spreɪn/ *noun* a condition in which the ligaments in a joint are stretched or torn because of a sudden movement ■ *verb* to tear the ligaments in a joint with a sudden movement ○ *She sprained her wrist when she fell.*

**spray** /spreɪ/ *noun* **1.** a mass of tiny drops ○ *An aerosol sends out a liquid in a fine spray.* **2.** a special liquid for applying to an infection in a mass of tiny drops ○ *throat spray* or *nasal spray* ■ *verb* **1.** to send out a liquid in a mass of tiny drops ○ *They sprayed disinfectant everywhere.* **2.** to spray an area with liquid ○ *They sprayed the room with disinfectant.*

**spread** /spred/ *verb* to go out over a large area, or to cause something to do this ○ *The infection spread right through the adult population.* ○ *Sneezing in a crowded bus can spread infection.* (NOTE: **spreading – spread**)

'…spreading infection may give rise to cellulitis of the abdominal wall and abscess formation' [*Nursing Times*]

**Sprengel's deformity** /'spreŋgəlz dɪ,fɔːmɪti/, **Sprengel's shoulder** /,spreŋgəlz 'ʃəʊldə/ *noun* a congenitally malformed shoulder, in which one scapula is smaller and higher than the other [Described 1891. After Otto Gerhard Karl Sprengel (1852–1915), German surgeon.]

**sprue** /spruː/ *noun* same as **psilosis**

**spud** /spʌd/ *noun* a needle used to get a piece of dust or other foreign body out of the eye

**spur** /spɜː/ *noun* a sharp projecting part of a bone

**sputum** /'spjuːtəm/ *noun* mucus which is formed in the inflamed nose, throat or lungs and is coughed up ○ *She was coughing up bloodstained sputum.* Also called **phlegm**

**squama** /'skweɪmə/ *noun* a thin piece of hard tissue, e.g. a thin flake of bone or scale on the skin (NOTE: The plural is **squamae**.)

**squamo-** /skweɪməʊ/ *prefix* **1.** relating to the squamous part of the temporal bone **2.** scaly

**squamous** /'skweɪməs/ *adjective* thin and hard like a scale

**squamous bone** /'skweɪməs bəʊn/ *noun* a part of the temporal bone which forms the side of the skull

**squamous cell carcinoma** /,skweɪməs sel kɑːsɪ'nəʊmə/ *noun* a common type of cancer which usually develops in the outer layer of the skin, on the lips, or inside the mouth or oesophagus. Abbr **SCC**

**squamous epithelium** /,skweɪməs epɪ'θiːliəm/ *noun* epithelium with flat cells like scales, which forms the lining of the pericardium, the peritoneum and the pleura. Also called **pavement epithelium**

**squint** /skwɪnt/ *noun* a condition in which the eyes focus on different points. Also called **strabismus** ■ *verb* to have one eye or both eyes looking towards the nose ○ *Babies often*

*appear to squint, but it is corrected as they grow older.*

**SRN** *abbr* State Registered Nurse

**SSRI** *abbr* selective serotonin re-uptake inhibitor

**stab** /stæb/ *noun* a sudden burst of pain ○ *She had a stab of pain above her right eye.* ■ *verb* to cut by pushing the point of a knife into the flesh ○ *He was stabbed in the chest.* (NOTE: **stabbing – stabbed**)

**stabbing pain** /'stæbɪŋ peɪn/ *noun* pain which comes in a series of short sharp bursts ○ *He had stabbing pains in his chest.*

**stabilise** /'steɪbəlaɪz/, **stabilize** *verb* to make a condition stable ○ *We have succeeded in stabilising his blood sugar level.* (NOTE: **stabilising – stabilised**)

**stable** /'steɪb(ə)l/ *adjective* not changing ○ *Her condition is stable.*

**stable angina** /,steɪb(ə)l æn'dʒaɪnə/ *noun* angina which has not changed for a long time

**stab wound** /'stæb wuːnd/ *noun* a deep wound made by the point of a knife

**staccato speech** /stə,kɑːtəʊ 'spiːtʃ/ *noun* an unusual way of speaking with short pauses between each word

**Stacke's operation** /'stækiz ɒpə,reɪʃ(ə)n/ *noun* a surgical operation to remove the posterior and superior wall of the auditory meatus [After Ludwig Stacke (1859–1918), German otologist]

**stadium** /'steɪdiəm/ *noun* a particular stage of a disease (NOTE: The plural is **stadia**.)

**stadium invasioni** /,steɪdiəm ɪn,veɪʃi 'əʊni/ *noun* same as **incubation period**

**staff** /stɑːf/ *noun* people who work in an organisation such as a hospital, clinic or doctor's surgery ○ *We have 25 full-time medical staff.* ○ *The hospital is trying to recruit more nursing staff.* ○ *The clinic has a staff of 100.*

**staff midwife** /stɑːf 'mɪd,waɪf/ *noun* a midwife who is on the permanent staff of a hospital

**staff nurse** /'stɑːf nɜːs/ *noun* a nurse who is on the permanent staff of a hospital

**stage** /steɪdʒ/ *noun* a point in the development of a disease at which a decision can be taken about the treatment which should be given or at which distinctive developments take place ○ *The disease has reached a critical stage.* ○ *This is a symptom of the second stage of syphilis.*

'…memory changes are associated with early stages of the disease; in later stages, the patient is frequently incontinent, immobile and unable to communicate' [*Nursing Times*]

**stagger** /'stægə/ *verb* to move unsteadily from side to side while walking

**staging** /'steɪdʒɪŋ/ *noun* the process of performing tests to learn the extent of a disease within the body, in order to decide the best treatment for someone

**stagnant loop syndrome** /ˌstægnənt ˈluːp ˌsɪndrəʊm/ *noun* a condition which occurs in cases of diverticulosis or of Crohn's disease, with steatorrhoea, abdominal pain and megaloblastic anaemia

**stain** /steɪn/ *noun* a substance used to give colour to tissues which are going to be examined under the microscope ■ *verb* to treat a piece of tissue with a dye to increase contrast before it is examined under the microscope

> COMMENT: Some stains are designed to have an affinity only with those chemical, cellular or bacterial elements in a specimen that are of interest to a microbiologist; thus the concentration or uptake of a stain, as well as the overall picture, can be diagnostic.

**staining** /ˈsteɪnɪŋ/ *noun* the process of colouring tissue, bacterial samples or other materials to make it possible to examine them and to identify them under the microscope

**stalk** /stɔːk/ *noun* a piece of tissue which attaches a growth to the main tissue

**Stamey procedure** /ˈsteɪmi prəˌsiːdʒə/ *noun* a surgical operation to cure stress incontinence in women. A minor abdominal incision is made as well as a vaginal incision, and the neck of the bladder is stitched to the abdominal wall.

**stammer** /ˈstæmə/ *noun* a speech difficulty in which someone repeats parts of a word or the whole word several times or stops to try to pronounce a word ○ *He has a bad stammer.* ■ *verb* to speak with a stammer

**stammerer** /ˈstæmərə/ *noun* a person who stammers

**stammering** /ˈstæmərɪŋ/ *noun* difficulty in speaking, in which the person repeats parts of a word or the whole word several times or stops to try to pronounce a word. Also called **dysphemia**

**stamp out** /ˌstæmp ˈaʊt/ *verb* to remove something completely ○ *International organisations have succeeded in stamping out smallpox.* ○ *The government is trying to stamp out waste in the hospital service.*

**stand** /stænd/ *verb* **1.** to be in an upright position with your bodyweight resting on your feet, or to put a person in this position **2.** to get to your feet from a sitting position (NOTE: **stood**)

**standard** /ˈstændəd/ *adjective* usual, recommended or established ○ *It is standard practice to take the patient's temperature twice a day.* ■ *noun* **1.** something which has been agreed upon and is used to measure other things by **2.** a level of quality achieved by someone or something ○ *The standard of care in hospitals has increased over the last years.* ○ *The report criticised the standards of hygiene in the clinic.*

**standardise** /ˈstændədaɪz/, **standardize** *verb* to make all things of the same type follow the same standard

**Standard Precautions** /ˌstændəd prɪˈkɔːʃ(ə)nz/ *plural noun* the most recent set of guidelines for health care workers on dealing with blood, all body fluids, secretions and excretions (except sweat), non-intact skin and mucous membranes. They are designed to reduce the risk of transmission of microorganisms. The Standard Precautions are implemented automatically for everyone, as all patients are presumed to be potentially infectious.

**stand up** /ˌstænd ˈʌp/ *verb* **1.** to get up from being on a seat ○ *He tried to stand up, but did not have the strength.* **2.** to hold yourself upright ○ *She still stands up straight at the age of ninety-two.* (NOTE: **standing up – stood up**)

**stapedectomy** /ˌsteɪpɪˈdektəmi/ *noun* a surgical operation to remove the stapes (NOTE: The plural is **stapedectomies**.)

**stapedial mobilisation** /stəˌpiːdɪəl ˌməʊbɪlaɪˈzeɪʃ(ə)n/, **stapediolysis** /stəˌpiːdɪˈɒləsɪs/ *noun* a surgical operation to relieve deafness by detaching the stapes from the fenestra ovalis (NOTE: The plural of **stapediolysis** is **stapediolyses**.)

**stapes** /ˈsteɪpiːz/ *noun* one of the three ossicles in the middle ear, shaped like a stirrup. See illustration at EAR in Supplement

> COMMENT: The stapes fills the fenestra ovalis, and is articulated with the incus, which in turn articulates with the malleus.

**staph** /stæf/ *abbr* Staphylococcus

**staphylectomy** /ˌstæfɪˈlektəmi/ *noun* a surgical operation to remove the uvula (NOTE: The plural is **staphylectomies**.)

**staphylococcal** /ˌstæfɪləˈkɒk(ə)l/ *adjective* referring to Staphylococci

**staphylococcal poisoning** /ˌstæfɪləʊˌkɒkəl ˈpɔɪz(ə)nɪŋ/ *noun* poisoning by Staphylococci in food

**Staphylococcus** /ˌstæfɪləˈkɒkəs/ *noun* a bacterium which grows in a bunch like a bunch of grapes, and causes boils and food poisoning (NOTE: The plural is **Staphylococci**.)

**staphyloma** /ˌstæfɪˈləʊmə/ *noun* a swelling of the cornea or the white of the eye (NOTE: The plural is **staphylomas** or **staphylomata**.)

**staphylorrhaphy** /ˌstæfɪˈlɔːrəfi/ *noun* same as **palatorrhaphy** (NOTE: The plural is **staphylorrhaphies**.)

**staple** /ˈsteɪp(ə)l/ *noun* a small piece of bent metal, used to attach tissues together ■ *verb* to attach tissues with staples

**stapler** /ˈsteɪplə/ *noun* a device used in surgery to attach tissues with staples, instead of suturing

**starch** /stɑːtʃ/ *noun* the usual form in which carbohydrates exist in food, especially in bread, rice and potatoes. It is broken down by the digestive process into forms of sugar.

**starchy** /'stɑːtʃi/ *adjective* referring to food which contains a lot of starch ○ *He eats too much starchy food.*

**Starling's Law** /'stɑːlɪŋz lɔː/ *noun* a law that the contraction of the ventricles is in proportion to the length of the ventricular muscle fibres at the end of diastole

**startle reflex** /'stɑːt(ə)l ˌriːfleks/ *noun* the usual response of a young baby to a sudden loud noise or a sudden fall through the air, by contracting the limb and neck muscles

**starvation** /stɑːˈveɪʃ(ə)n/ *noun* the fact of having had very little or no food

**starvation diet** /stɑːˌveɪʃ(ə)n 'daɪət/ *noun* a diet which contains little nourishment, and is not enough to keep a person healthy

**starve** /stɑːv/ *verb* to have little or no food or nourishment ○ *The parents let the baby starve to death.*

**stasis** /'steɪsɪs/ *noun* a stoppage or slowing in the flow of a liquid, such as blood in veins, or food in the intestine

'A decreased blood flow in the extremities has been associated with venous stasis which may precipitate vascular complications' [*British Journal of Nursing*]

**-stasis** /steɪsɪs/ *suffix* referring to stoppage in the flow of a liquid

**stat.** /stæt/ *adverb* (*written on prescriptions*) immediately. Full form **statim**

**state** /steɪt/ *noun* the condition of something or of a person ○ *His state of health is getting worse.* ○ *The disease is in an advanced state.*

**State Enrolled Nurse** /ˌsteɪt ɪnˌrəʊld 'nɜːs/ *noun* Abbr **SEN**. Now called **second-level nurse**

**state of mind** /ˌsteɪt əv 'maɪnd/ *noun* a general feeling ○ *He's in a very miserable state of mind.*

**State Registered Nurse** /ˌsteɪt ˌredʒɪstəd 'nɜːs/ *noun* Abbr **SRN**. Now called **first-level nurse**

**statin** /'stætɪn/ *noun* a lipid-lowering drug which inhibits an enzyme in cholesterol synthesis, used to treat people with, or at high risk of developing, coronary heart disease

**-statin** /stætɪn/ *suffix* used in generic names of lipid-lowering drugs ○ *pravastatin*

**statistics** /stəˈtɪstɪks/ *plural noun* official figures which show facts ○ *Population statistics show that the birth rate is slowing down.*

**status** /'steɪtəs/ *noun* a state or condition

'…the main indications being inadequate fluid and volume status and need for evaluation of patients with a history of severe heart disease' [*Southern Medical Journal*]

'…the standard pulmonary artery catheters have four lumens from which to obtain information about the patient's haemodynamic status' [*RN Magazine*]

**status asthmaticus** /ˌsteɪtəs æsˈmætɪkəs/ *noun* an attack of bronchial asthma which lasts for a long time and results in exhaustion and collapse

**status epilepticus** /ˌsteɪtəs epɪˈleptɪkəs/ *noun* repeated and prolonged epileptic seizures without recovery of consciousness between them

**status lymphaticus** /ˌsteɪtəs lɪmˈfætɪkəs/ *noun* a condition in which the glands in the lymphatic system are enlarged

**statutory bodies** /ˌstætjʊt(ə)ri 'bɒdiz/ *plural noun* organisations set up by Acts of Parliament to carry out specific functions, e.g. the Nursing and Midwifery Council, set up to regulate the nursing and midwifery professions

**stay** /steɪ/ *noun* the time which someone spends in a place ○ *The patient is only in hospital for a short stay.* ■ *verb* to stop in a place for some time ○ *She stayed in hospital for two weeks.* ○ *He's ill with flu and has to stay in bed.*

**STD** *abbr* sexually transmitted disease

**steam inhalation** /ˌstiːm ɪnhəˈleɪʃ(ə)n/ *noun* a treatment for respiratory disease in which someone breathes in steam with medicinal substances in it

**steapsin** /stiˈæpsɪn/ *noun* an enzyme produced by the pancreas, which breaks down fats in the intestine

**stearic acid** /stiˌærɪk ˈæsɪd/ *noun* one of the fatty acids

**steat-** /'stiːət/, **steato-** /'stiːətəʊ/ *prefix* referring to fat

**steatoma** /ˌstiːəˈtəʊmə/ *noun* a cyst in a blocked sebaceous gland. ◊ **sebaceous cyst** (NOTE: The plural is **steatomata**.)

**steatopygia** /ˌstiːətəˈpɪdʒiə/ *noun* excessive fat on the buttocks

**steatorrhoea** /ˌstiːətəˈrɪə/ *noun* a condition in which fat is passed in the faeces

**Stein-Leventhal syndrome** /ˌstaɪn ˈlevəntɑːl ˌsɪndrəʊm/ *noun* ♦ **polycystic ovary syndrome** [Described 1935. After Irving F. Stein (b. 1887), US gynaecologist; Michael Leo Leventhal (1901–71), US obstetrician and gynaecologist.]

**Steinmann's pin** /ˌstaɪnmænz 'pɪn/ *noun* a pin for attaching traction wires to a fractured bone [Described 1907. After Fritz Steinmann (1872–1932), Swiss surgeon.]

**stellate** /'steleɪt/ *adjective* shaped like a star

**stellate fracture** /ˌsteleɪt 'fræktʃə/ *noun* a fracture of the kneecap shaped like a star

**stellate ganglion** /ˌsteleɪt 'gæŋɡliən/ *noun* a group of nerve cells in the neck, shaped like a star

**Stellwag's sign** /'stelvɑːɡz saɪn/ *noun* a symptom of exophthalmic goitre, where someone does not blink often, because the eyeball is protruding [After Carl Stellwag von Carion (1823–1904), ophthalmologist in Vienna, Austria]

**stem** /stem/ *noun* a thin piece of tissue which attaches an organ or growth to the main tissue

**steno-** /ˈstenəʊ/ *prefix* narrow or constricted

**stenose** /steˈnəʊs/ *verb* to make something narrow

**stenosed valve** /steˌnəʊst ˈvælv/ *noun* a valve which has become narrow or constricted

**stenosing condition** /steˌnəʊs kənˈdɪʃ(ə)n/ *noun* a condition which makes a passage narrow

**stenosis** /steˈnəʊsɪs/ *noun* a condition in which a passage becomes narrow

**stenostomia** /ˌstenəʊˈstəʊmiə/, **stenostomy** /steˈnɒstəmi/ *noun* the narrowing of an opening

**Stensen's duct** /ˌstensənz ˈdʌkt/ *noun* a duct which carries saliva from the parotid glands [Described 1661. After Niels Stensen (1638–86), Danish physician and priest, anatomist, physiologist and theologian.]

**stent** /stent/ *noun* a support of artificial material often inserted in a tube or vessel which has been sutured

**step** /step/ *noun* a movement of the foot and the leg as in walking ○ *He took two steps forward.* ○ *The baby is taking her first steps.*

**step up** /ˌstep ˈʌp/ *verb* to increase something (*informal*) ○ *The doctor has stepped up the dosage.*

**sterco-** /ˈstɜːkəʊ/ *prefix* referring to faeces

**stercobilin** /ˌstɜːkəˈbaɪlɪn/ *noun* a brown pigment which colours the faeces

**stercobilinogen** /ˌstɜːkəbərˈlɪnədʒen/ *noun* a substance which is broken down from bilirubin and produces stercobiline

**stercolith** /ˈstɜːkəlɪθ/ *noun* a hard ball of dried faeces in the bowel

**stercoraceous** /ˌstɜːkəˈreɪʃəs/ *adjective* **1.** made of or containing faeces **2.** similar to faeces

**stereognosis** /ˌsteriɒɡˈnəʊsɪs/ *noun* the ability to tell the shape of an object in three dimensions by means of touch

**stereoscopic vision** /ˌsteriəskɒpɪk ˈvɪʒ(ə)n/ *noun* the ability to judge the distance and depth of an object by binocular vision

**stereotactic** /ˌsteriəʊˈtæktɪk/ *adjective* referring to procedures which use coordinates put into a computer or scanner in order to locate and operate upon tumours precisely. Examples are biopsies, surgery or radiation therapy.

**stereotaxy** /ˌsteriəʊˈtæksi/, **stereotaxic surgery** /ˌsteriəʊˌtæksɪk ˈsɜːdʒəri/ *noun* a surgical procedure to identify a point in the interior of the brain, before an operation can begin, to locate exactly the area to be operated on

**stereotypy** /ˈsteriəʊtaɪpi/ *noun* the repetition of the same action or word again and again

**Sterets** /ˈsterəts/ a trademark for a type of swab used for cleaning the skin before an injection

**sterile** /ˈsteraɪl/ *adjective* **1.** with no harmful microorganisms present ○ *a sterile environment* **2.** not able to produce children

**sterile dressing** /ˌsteraɪl ˈdresɪŋ/ *noun* a dressing which is sold in a sterile pack, ready for use

**sterilisation** /ˌsterɪlaɪˈzeɪʃ(ə)n/, **sterilization** *noun* **1.** the action of making instruments or areas completely free from microorganisms which might cause infection **2.** a procedure that makes someone unable to have children

COMMENT: Sterilisation of a woman can be done by removing the ovaries or cutting the Fallopian tubes. Sterilisation of a man is carried out by cutting the vas deferens (vasectomy).

**sterilise** /ˈsterɪlaɪz/, **sterilize** *verb* **1.** to make something completely free from microorganisms which might cause infection **2.** to make someone unable to have children

**steriliser** /ˈsterəlaɪzə/, **sterilizer** *noun* a machine for sterilising surgical instruments by steam or boiling water

**sterilising** /ˈsterɪlaɪzɪŋ/ *adjective* able to kill microorganisms ○ *Wipe the surface with sterilising fluid.*

**sterility** /stəˈrɪlɪti/ *noun* **1.** the state of being free from microorganisms **2.** the state of being unable to have children

**Steri-Strips** /ˈsteri strɪps/ a trademark for thin paper strips which are placed over an incision in the skin. They help its edges to come together and form a scar.

**sternal** /ˈstɜːn(ə)l/ *adjective* referring to the breastbone

**sternal angle** /ˌstɜːn(ə)l ˈæŋɡ(ə)l/ *noun* the ridge of bone where the manubrium articulates with the body of the sternum

**sternal puncture** /ˌstɜːn(ə)l ˈpʌŋktʃə/ *noun* a surgical operation to remove a sample of bone marrow from the breastbone for testing

**sterno-** /ˈstɜːnəʊ/ *prefix* relating to the breastbone

**sternoclavicular** /ˌstɜːnəʊkləˈvɪkjʊlə/ *adjective* referring to the sternum and the clavicle

**sternoclavicular angle** /ˌstɜːnəʊkləˌvɪkjʊlə ˈæŋɡəl/ *noun* the angle between the sternum and the clavicle

**sternocleidomastoid muscle** /ˌstɜːnəʊˌklaɪdəʊˈmæstɔɪd ˌmʌs(ə)l/ *noun* a muscle in the neck, running from the breastbone to the mastoid process

**sternocostal** /ˌstɜːnəʊˈkɒst(ə)l/ *adjective* referring to the sternum and ribs

**sternocostal joint** /ˌstɜːnəʊˈkɒst(ə)l dʒɔɪnt/ *noun* a joint where the breastbone joins a rib

**sternohyoid** /ˌstɜːnəʊˈhaɪɔɪd/ *adjective* relating to the sternum and the hyoid bone

**sternohyoid muscle** /ˌstɜːnəʊˈhaɪɔɪd ˌmʌs(ə)l/ *noun* a muscle in the neck which runs from the breastbone into the hyoid bone

**sternomastoid** /ˌstɜːnəʊˈmæstɔɪd/ *adjective* referring to the breastbone and the mastoid

**sternomastoid tumour** /ˌstɜːnəʊ ˌmæstɔɪd ˈtjuːmə/ *noun* a benign tumour which appears in the sternomastoid muscle in newborn babies

**sternotomy** /stɜːˈnɒtəmi/ *noun* a surgical operation to cut through the breastbone, so as to be able to operate on the heart

**sternum** /ˈstɜːnəm/ *noun* same as **breastbone**

COMMENT: The sternum runs from the neck to the bottom of the diaphragm. It is formed of the manubrium (the top section), the body of the sternum and the xiphoid process. The upper seven pairs of ribs are attached to the sternum.

**sternutatory** /stɜːˈnjuːtətəri/ *noun* a substance which makes someone sneeze

**steroid** /ˈstɪərɔɪd/ *noun* any of several chemical compounds, including the sex hormones, which have characteristic ring systems and which affect the body and its functions

COMMENT: The word steroid is usually used to refer to corticosteroids. Synthetic steroids are used in steroid therapy, to treat arthritis, asthma and some blood disorders. They are also used by some athletes to improve their physical strength, but these are banned by athletic organisations and can have serious side-effects.

**steroidal** /stɪˈrɔɪdəl/ *adjective* containing steroids. Opposite **non-steroidal**

**sterol** /ˈstɪərɒl/ *noun* an insoluble substance which belongs to the steroid alcohols, e.g. cholesterol

**stertor** /ˈstɜːtə/ *noun* noisy breathing sounds in someone unconscious

**stertorous** /ˈstɜːt(ə)rəs/ *adjective* characterised by heavy snoring

**steth-** /steθ/, **stetho-** /ˈsteθə/ *prefix* referring to the chest

**stethograph** /ˈsteθəɡrɑːf/ *noun* an instrument which records breathing movements of the chest

**stethography** /steˈθɒɡrəfi/ *noun* the process of recording movements of the chest

**stethometer** /steˈθɒmɪtə/ *noun* an instrument which records how far the chest expands when a person breathes in

**stethoscope** /ˈsteθəskəʊp/ *noun* a surgical instrument with two earpieces connected to a tube and a metal disc, used by doctors to listen to sounds made inside the body, e.g. the sounds of the heart or lungs

**Stevens-Johnson syndrome** /ˌstiːvənz ˈdʒɒnsən ˌsɪndrəʊm/ *noun* a severe form of erythema multiforme affecting the face and genitals, caused by an allergic reaction to drugs [Described 1922. After Albert Mason Stevens (1884–1945); Frank Chambliss Johnson (1894–1934), physicians in New York, USA.]

**sthenia** /ˈsθiːniə/ *noun* a condition of great strength or vitality

**STI** *abbr* sexually transmitted infection

**stick** /stɪk/ *verb* to attach something, to fix things together, e.g. with glue ○ *In bad cases of conjunctivitis the eyelids can stick together.*

**sticking plaster** /ˈstɪkɪŋ ˌplɑːstə/ *noun* an adhesive plaster or tape used to cover a small wound or to attach a pad of dressing to the skin

**sticky** /ˈstɪki/ *adjective* able to become easily attached like glue

**sticky eye** /ˈstɪki aɪ/ *noun* a condition in babies in which the eyes remain closed because of conjunctivitis

**stiff** /stɪf/ *adjective* not able to be bent or moved easily ○ *My knee is stiff after playing football.*

**stiffly** /ˈstɪfli/ *adverb* in a stiff way ○ *He is walking stiffly because of the pain in his hip.*

**stiff neck** /stɪf ˈnek/ *noun* a condition in which moving the neck is painful, usually caused by a strained muscle or by sitting in a cold wind

**stiffness** /ˈstɪfnəs/ *noun* the fact of being stiff ○ *arthritis accompanied by stiffness in the joints*

**stigma** /ˈstɪɡmə/ *noun* a visible symptom which shows that someone has a particular disease (NOTE: The plural is **stigmas** or **stigmata**.)

**stilet** /staɪˈlet/ *noun* **1.** a fine wire used as a probe in surgery **2.** a wire inserted in a catheter to give it rigidity

**stillbirth** /ˈstɪlbɜːθ/ *noun* the birth of a dead fetus, more than 28 weeks after conception (*informal*)

**stillborn** /ˈstɪlbɔːn/ *adjective* referring to a baby born dead ○ *Her first child was stillborn.*

**Still's disease** /ˈstɪlz dɪˌziːz/ *noun* arthritis affecting children, similar to rheumatoid arthritis in adults [Described 1896. After Sir George Frederic Still (1868–1941), British paediatrician and physician to the king.]

**stimulant** /ˈstɪmjʊlənt/ *noun* a substance which makes part of the body function faster ○ *Caffeine is a stimulant.* ■ *adjective* increasing body function

COMMENT: Natural stimulants include some hormones, and drugs such as digitalis which encourage a weak heart. Drinks such as tea and coffee contain stimulants.

**stimulate** /ˈstɪmjʊleɪt/ *verb* to make a person or organ react, respond or function ○ *The therapy should stimulate the patient into attempting to walk unaided.* ○ *The drug stimulates the heart.*

**stimulation** /ˌstɪmjʊˈleɪʃ(ə)n/ *noun* the action of stimulating something

**stimulus** /ˈstɪmjʊləs/ *noun* something which has an effect on a person or a part of the body and makes them react (NOTE: The plural is **stimuli**.)

**sting** /stɪŋ/ *noun* the piercing of the skin by an insect which passes a toxic substance into the bloodstream ■ *verb* (*of an insect*) to make a hole in the skin and pass a toxic substance into the blood ○ *He was stung by a wasp.*

COMMENT: Stings by some insects such as tsetse flies can transmit a bacterial infection to a person. Other insects such as bees pass toxic substances into the bloodstream of the affected person, causing irritating swellings. Some people are strongly allergic to insect stings.

**stinging** /ˈstɪŋɪŋ/ *adjective* referring to a sharp unpleasant feeling of pricking or burning ○ *a sudden stinging sensation in the back of her leg*

**stirrup** /ˈstɪrəp/ *noun* same as **stapes**

**stirrup bone** /ˈstɪrəp bəʊn/ *noun* same as **stapes**

**stitch** /stɪtʃ/ *noun* **1.** same as **suture 2** ○ *He had three stitches in his head.* ○ *The doctor told her to come back in ten days' time to have the stitches taken out.* **2.** pain caused by cramp in the side of the body after running ○ *He had to stop running because he developed a stitch.* ■ *verb* same as **suture** ○ *They tried to stitch back the finger which had been cut off in an accident.*

**stitch abscess** /ˈstɪtʃ ˌæbses/ *noun* an abscess which forms at the site of a stitch or suture

**stock culture** /ˌstɒk ˈkʌltʃə/ *noun* the basic culture of bacteria, from which other cultures can be taken

**stocking** /ˈstɒkɪŋ/ *noun* a close-fitting piece of clothing to cover the leg

**Stokes–Adams syndrome** /ˌstəʊks ˈædəmz ˌsɪndrəʊm/ *noun* a loss of consciousness due to the stopping of the action of the heart because of asystole or fibrillation [After William Stokes (1804–78), Irish physician; Robert Adams (1791–1875), Irish surgeon]

**stoma** /ˈstəʊmə/ *noun* **1.** any opening into a cavity in the body **2.** the mouth **3.** a colostomy (*informal*) (NOTE: [all senses] The plural is **stomata**.)

**stomach** /ˈstʌmək/ *noun* **1.** the part of the body shaped like a bag, into which food passes after being swallowed and where the process of digestion continues ○ *She complained of pains in the stomach* or *of stomach pains.* ○ *He has had stomach trouble for some time.* See illustration at **DIGESTIVE SYSTEM** in Supplement **2.** the abdomen (*informal*) ○ *He had been kicked in the stomach.* (NOTE: For other terms referring to the stomach, see words beginning with **gastr-, gastro-**.)

COMMENT: The stomach is situated in the top of the abdomen, and on the left side of the body between the oesophagus and the duodenum. Food is partly broken down by hydro-

chloric acid and other gastric juices secreted by the walls of the stomach and is mixed and squeezed by the action of the muscles of the stomach, before being passed on into the duodenum. The stomach continues the digestive process started in the mouth, but few substances, except alcohol and honey, are actually absorbed into the bloodstream in the stomach.

**stomach ache** /ˈstʌmək eɪk/ *noun* pain in the abdomen or stomach, caused by eating too much food or by an infection

**stomach cramp** /ˈstʌmək kræmp/ *noun* a sharp spasm of the stomach muscles

**stomach hernia** *noun* same as **gastrocele**

**stomach pump** /ˈstʌmək pʌmp/ *noun* an instrument for sucking out the contents of the stomach, e.g. to extract a poison that has been swallowed

**stomach tube** /ˈstʌmək tjuːb/ *noun* a tube passed into the stomach to wash it out or to take samples of the contents

**stomach upset** /ˈstʌmək ˌʌpset/ *noun* a slight infection of the stomach ○ *She is in bed with a stomach upset.* Also called **upset stomach**

**stomach washout** /ˌstʌmək ˈwɒʃaʊt/ *noun* same as **gastric lavage**

**stomal** /ˈstəʊm(ə)l/ *adjective* referring to a stoma

**stomal ulcer** /ˌstəʊm(ə)l ˈʌlsə/ *noun* an ulcer in the region of the jejunum

**stomat-** /stəʊmət/ *prefix* same as **stomato-** (*used before vowels*)

**stomatitis** /ˌstəʊməˈtaɪtɪs/ *noun* inflammation of the inside of the mouth

**stomato-** /stəʊmətə/ *prefix* referring to the mouth

**stomatology** /ˌstəʊməˈtɒlədʒi/ *noun* a branch of medicine which studies diseases of the mouth

**-stomy** /stəmi/ *suffix* meaning an operation to make an opening

**stone** /stəʊn/ *noun* **1.** same as **calculus** (*informal*) (NOTE: For other terms referring to stones, see words beginning with **lith-, litho-**, or ending with **-lith**.) **2.** a measure of weight equal to 14 pounds or 6.35 kilograms ○ *He tried to lose weight and lost three stone.* ○ *She weighs eight stone ten* (i.e. 8 stone 10 pounds).

**stone-deaf** /ˌstəʊn ˈdef/ *adjective* totally deaf

**stool** /stuːl/ *noun* **1.** an act of emptying the bowels **2.** a piece of solid waste matter which is passed out of the bowels ○ *an abnormal stool* ○ *loose stools* ○ *a stool test* (NOTE: Often used in the plural.) ■ *verb* to pass a piece of solid matter out of the bowels

**stoop** /stuːp/ *noun* a position where especially the top of your back is bent forward ○ *He walks with a stoop.* ■ *verb* to have a stoop ○ *He is seventy-five and stoops.*

**stop needle** /'stɒp ˌniːd(ə)l/ *noun* a needle with a ring round it, so that it can only be pushed a specific distance into the body

**stoppage** /'stɒpɪdʒ/ *noun* an act of stopping the function of an organ

**storage disease** /'stɔːrɪdʒ dɪˌziːz/ *noun* a disease in which unusual amounts of a substance accumulate in a part of the body

**stove-in chest** /ˌstəʊv ɪn 'tʃest/ *noun* an injury resulting from an accident, where several ribs are broken and pushed towards the inside

**strabismal** /strə'bɪzm(ə)l/ *adjective* with the eyes focusing on different points

**strabismus** /strə'bɪzməs/ *noun* a condition in which the eyes focus on different points. Also called **squint, heterotropia**

**strabotomy** /strə'bɒtəmi/ *noun* a surgical operation to divide the muscles of the eye in order to correct a squint

**straight** /streɪt/ *adjective* with no irregularities such as bends, curves or angles

**straighten** /'streɪt(ə)n/ *verb* to make something straight, or become straight ○ *Her arthritis is so bad that she cannot straighten her knees.*

**strain** /streɪn/ *noun* **1.** a condition in which a muscle has been stretched or torn by a strong or sudden movement **2.** a group of microorganisms which are different from others of the same type ○ *a new strain of influenza virus* **3.** nervous tension and stress ○ *Her work is causing her a lot of strain.* ○ *He is suffering from nervous strain and needs to relax.* ■ *verb* to stretch a muscle too far ○ *He strained his back lifting the table.* ○ *She had to leave the game with a strained calf muscle.* ○ *The effort of running upstairs strained his heart.*

**strand** /strænd/ *noun* a thread

**strangle** /'stræŋɡəl/ *verb* to kill someone by squeezing the throat so that he or she cannot breathe or swallow

**strangulated** /'stræŋɡjʊleɪtɪd/ *adjective* referring to part of the body which is caught in an opening in such a way that the circulation of blood is stopped

**strangulated hernia** /ˌstræŋɡjʊleɪtɪd 'hɜːniə/ *noun* a condition in which part of the intestine is squeezed in a hernia and the supply of blood to it is cut off

**strangulation** /ˌstræŋɡjʊ'leɪʃ(ə)n/ *noun* the act of squeezing a passage in the body

**strangury** /'stræŋɡjʊri/ *noun* a condition in which very little urine is passed, although the person wants to urinate, caused by a bladder disorder or by a stone in the urethra

**strap** /stræp/ *verb* □ **to strap (up)** to wrap a bandage round a limb tightly, to attach tightly ○ *The nurses strapped up his stomach wound.* ○ *The patient was strapped to the stretcher.*

**strapping** /'stræpɪŋ/ *noun* wide strong bandages or adhesive plaster used to bandage a large part of the body

**Strategic Health Authority** /strəˌtiːdʒɪk 'helθ ɔːˌθɒrɪti/ *noun* in the UK, an organisation, accountable to government, that assesses the health needs of local people and ensures that local health services are commissioned and provided to meet those needs. Abbr **StHA**

**stratified** /'strætɪfaɪd/ *adjective* made of several layers

**stratified epithelium** /ˌstrætɪfaɪd epɪ'θiːliəm/ *noun* epithelium formed of several layers of cells

**stratum** /'strɑːtəm/ *noun* a layer of tissue forming the epidermis (NOTE: The plural is **strata**.)

COMMENT: The main layers of the epidermis are: the **stratum germinativum** or **stratum basale:** this layer produces the cells that are pushed up to form the other layers; the **stratum granulosum,** a layer with granular cells under the **stratum lucidum,** a thin clear layer of dead and dying cells, and the surface layer, or **stratum corneum,** a layer of dead keratinised cells which progressively fall off.

**strawberry mark** /'strɔːb(ə)ri mɑːk/ *noun* a red birthmark in children, which will often disappear in later life

**streak** /striːk/ *noun* a long thin line of a different colour

**strength** /streŋθ/ *noun* the fact of being strong ○ *After her illness she had no strength in her limbs.*

**strengthen** /'streŋθ(ə)n/ *verb* to make something strong

**strenuous** /'strenjuəs/ *adjective* referring to exercise which involves using a lot of force ○ *Avoid doing any strenuous exercise for some time while the wound heals.*

**strep throat** /ˌstrep 'θrəʊt/ *noun* an infection of the throat by a streptococcus (*informal*)

**strepto-** /streptə/ *prefix* referring to organisms which grow in chains

**streptobacillus** /ˌstreptəbə'sɪləs/ *noun* a type of bacterium which forms a chain

**streptococcal** /ˌstreptə'kɒk(ə)l/ *adjective* caused by a streptococcus

**streptococcus** /ˌstreptə'kɒkəs/ *noun* a genus of bacteria which grows in long chains, and causes fevers such as scarlet fever, tonsillitis and rheumatic fever (NOTE: The plural is **streptococci.**)

**streptodornase** /ˌstreptə'dɔːneɪs/ *noun* an enzyme formed by streptococci which can make pus liquid

**streptokinase** /ˌstreptə'kaɪneɪz/ *noun* an enzyme formed by streptococci which can break down blood clots and is therefore used in the treatment of myocardial infarction

**streptolysin** /strep'tɒləsɪn/ *noun* a toxin produced by streptococci in rheumatic fever, which acts to destroy red blood cells

**Streptomyces** /ˌstreptə'maɪsiːz/ *noun* a genus of bacteria used to produce antibiotics

**streptomycin** /ˌstreptə'maɪsɪn/ *noun* an antibacterial drug used mainly for the treatment of tuberculosis

**stress** /stres/ *noun* **1.** physical pressure on an object or part of the body **2.** a factor or combination of factors in a person's life which make him or her feel tired and anxious **3.** a condition in which an outside influence such as overwork or a mental or emotional state such as anxiety changes the working of the body and can affect the hormone balance

**stress disorder** /'stres dɪsˌɔːdə/ *noun* a disorder caused by stress

**stress fracture** /'stres ˌfræktʃə/ *noun* a fracture of a bone caused by excessive force, as in some types of sport. Also called **fatigue fracture**

**stress incontinence** /'stres ɪnˌkɒntɪnəns/ *noun* a condition in women in which the muscles in the floor of the pelvis become incapable of retaining urine when the intra-abdominal pressure is raised by coughing or laughing

**stress reaction** /'stres riˌækʃən/ *noun* a response to an outside stimulus which disturbs the usual physiological balance of the body

**stress-related illness** /ˌstres rɪˌleɪtɪd 'ɪlnəs/ *noun* an illness which is due in part or completely to stress

**stretch** /stretʃ/ *verb* to pull something out, or make something longer

**stretcher** /'stretʃə/ *noun* a folding bed, with handles, on which an injured person can be carried by two people ○ *She was carried out of the restaurant on a stretcher.* ○ *Some of the accident victims could walk to the ambulances, but there were several stretcher cases.*

**stretcher bearer** /'stretʃə ˌbeərə/ *noun* a person who helps to carry a stretcher

**stretcher case** /'stretʃə keɪs/ *noun* a person who is so ill that he or she has to be carried on a stretcher

**stretcher party** /'stretʃə ˌpɑːti/ *noun* a group of people who carry a stretcher and look after the person on it

**stretch mark** /'stretʃ mɑːk/ *noun* a mark on the skin of the abdomen of a pregnant woman or of a woman who has recently given birth. ◊ **striae gravidarum**

**stretch reflex** /'stretʃ ˌriːfleks/ *noun* a reflex reaction of a muscle which contracts after being stretched

**stria** /'straɪə/ *noun* a pale line on skin which is stretched, as in obese people (NOTE: The plural is **striae**.)

**striae gravidarum** /ˌstraɪiː ˌɡrævɪ 'deərəm/ *plural noun* the lines on the skin of

the abdomen of a pregnant woman or of a woman who has recently given birth

**striated** /straɪ'eɪtɪd/ *adjective* marked with pale lines

**striated muscle** /straɪˈeɪtɪd ˌmʌs(ə)l/ *noun* a type of muscle found in skeletal muscles whose movements are controlled by the central nervous system. Also called **striped muscle**

**strict** /strɪkt/ *adjective* severe, which must not be changed ○ *She has to follow a strict diet.* ○ *The doctor was strict with the patients who wanted to drink alcohol in the hospital.*

**stricture** /'strɪktʃə/ *noun* the narrowing of a passage in the body

**strictureplasty** /'strɪktʃərəʊˌplæsti/ *noun* a surgical operation in which a part of the intestine is widened

**stridor** /'straɪdɔː/, **stridulus** /'straɪdjʊləs/ *noun* a sharp high sound made when air passes an obstruction in the larynx. ◊ **laryngismus**

**strike-through** /'straɪk θruː/ *noun* blood absorbed right through a dressing so as to be visible on the outside

'If strike-through occurs, the wound dressing should be repadded, not removed' [*British Journal of Nursing*]

**string sign** /'strɪŋ saɪn/ *noun* a thin line which appears on the ileum, a sign of regional ileitis or Crohn's disease

**strip** /strɪp/ *noun* a long thin piece of material or tissue ○ *The nurse bandaged the wound with strips of gauze.* ○ *He grafted a strip of skin over the burn.* ■ *verb* to take off something, especially clothes ○ *The patients had to strip for the medical examination.* □ **to strip to the waist** to take off the clothes on the top part of the body

**striped muscle** /'straɪpt ˌmʌs(ə)l/ *noun* same as **striated muscle**

**stripper** /'strɪpə/ *noun* an instrument in the form of a flexible wire with an olive-shaped end used for stripping varicose veins

**stripping** /'strɪpɪŋ/ *noun* a surgical operation to remove varicose veins

**stroke** /strəʊk/ *noun* same as **cerebrovascular accident** ○ *He had a stroke and died.* ○ *She was paralysed after a stroke.* ■ *verb* to touch something or someone softly with the fingers

'…stroke is the third most frequent cause of death in developed countries after ischaemic heart disease and cancer' [*British Journal of Hospital Medicine*]

'…raised blood pressure may account for as many as 70% of all strokes. The risk of stroke rises with both systolic and diastolic blood pressure' [*British Journal of Hospital Medicine*]

COMMENT: There are two causes of stroke: cerebral haemorrhage (haemorrhagic stroke), when an artery bursts and blood leaks into the brain, and cerebral thrombosis (occlusive stroke), where a blood clot blocks an artery.

**stroke patient** /'strəʊk ˌpeɪʃ(ə)nt/ *noun* a person who has had a stroke

**stroke volume** /ˈstrəuk ˌvɒljuːm/ *noun* the amount of blood pumped out of the ventricle at each heartbeat

**stroma** /ˈstrəumə/ *noun* tissue which supports an organ, as opposed to the parenchyma or functioning tissues in the organ

**Strongyloides** /ˌstrɒndʒiˈlɔɪdiːz/ *noun* a parasitic worm which infests the intestines

**strongyloidiasis** /ˌstrɒndʒilɔɪˈdaɪəsɪs/ *noun* the fact of being infested with *Strongyloides* which enters the skin and then travels to the lungs and the intestines

**strontium** /ˈstrɒntiəm/ *noun* a metallic element (NOTE: The chemical symbol is **Sr**.)

**strontium-90** /ˌstrɒntiəm ˈnaɪnti/ *noun* an isotope of strontium which is formed in nuclear reactions and, because it is part of the fallout of nuclear explosions, can enter the food chain, attacking in particular the bones of humans and animals

**structure** /ˈstrʌktʃə/ *noun* the way in which an organ or muscle is formed

**struma** /ˈstruːmə/ *noun* a goitre

**strychnine** /ˈstrɪkniːn/ *noun* a poisonous alkaloid drug, made from the seeds of a tropical tree, and formerly used in small doses as a tonic

**Stryker frame** /ˈstraɪkə freɪm/ *noun* a special piece of equipment on which a patient can easily be rotated by a nurse, used for patients with spinal injuries

**ST segment** /ˌes ˈtiː ˌsegmənt/, **S-T segment** *noun* the part of an electrocardiogram, between the points labelled S and T, immediately before the last phase of the cardiac cycle. ◊ PQRST complex

**student** /ˈstjuːd(ə)nt/ *noun* a person who is studying at a college or university ○ *All the medical students have to spend some time in the hospital.*

**student nurse** /ˈstjuːd(ə)nt nɜːs/ *noun* a person who is studying to become a nurse

**study** /ˈstʌdi/ *noun* the act of examining something to learn about it ○ *She's making a study of diseases of small children.* ○ *They have finished their study of the effects of the drug on pregnant women.* ■ *verb* to examine something to learn about it ○ *He's studying pharmacy.* ○ *Doctors are studying the results of the screening programme.*

**stuffy** /ˈstʌfi/, **stuffed up** /ˌstʌft ˈʌp/ *adjective* referring to a nose which is blocked with inflamed mucous membrane and mucus (*informal*)

**stump** /stʌmp/ *noun* a short piece of a limb which is left after the rest has been amputated

**stun** /stʌn/ *verb* to knock someone out by a blow to the head

**stunt** /stʌnt/ *verb* to stop something growing ○ *The children's development was stunted by disease.*

**stupe** /stjuːp/ *noun* a wet medicated dressing used as a compress

**stupor** /ˈstjuːpə/ *noun* a state of being semiconscious ○ *After the party several people were found lying on the floor in a stupor.*

**Sturge-Weber syndrome** /ˌstɜːdʒ ˈwebə ˌsɪndrəum/ *noun* a dark red mark on the skin above the eye, together with similar marks inside the brain, possibly causing epileptic fits

**stutter** /ˈstʌtə/ *noun* a speech problem where someone repeats the sound at the beginning of a word several times ○ *He is taking therapy to try to cure his stutter.* ■ *verb* to speak with a stutter

**stuttering** /ˈstʌtərɪŋ/ *noun* same as **stammering**

**stye** /staɪ/ *noun* same as **hordeolum**

**stylet** /ˈstaɪlət/ *noun* **1.** a very thin piece of wire which is put into a catheter or hollow needle so that it will not become blocked when it is not being used **2.** any long thin pointed instrument

**stylo-** /staɪləu/ *prefix* referring to the styloid process

**styloglossus** /ˌstaɪləuˈglɒsəs/ *noun* a muscle which links the tongue to the styloid process

**styloid** /ˈstaɪlɔɪd/ *adjective* pointed

**styloid process** /ˈstaɪlɔɪd ˌprəusez/ *noun* a piece of bone which projects from the bottom of the temporal bone

**stylus** /ˈstaɪləs/ *noun* a long thin instrument used for applying antiseptics or ointments to the skin

**styptic** /ˈstɪptɪk/ *noun* a substance which stops bleeding ■ *adjective* used to stop bleeding

**styptic pencil** /ˌstɪptɪk ˈpens(ə)l/ *noun* a stick of alum, used to stop bleeding from small cuts

**sub-** /sʌb/ *prefix* underneath or below

**subabdominal** /ˌsʌbəbˈdɒmɪn(ə)l/ *adjective* beneath the abdomen

**subacute** /ˌsʌbəˈkjuːt/ *adjective* referring to a condition which is not acute but may become chronic

**subacute bacterial endocarditis** /ˌsʌbəkjuːt bækˌtɪəriəl ˌendəukɑːˈdaɪtɪs/, **subacute infective endocarditis** /ˌsʌbəkjuːt ɪnˌfektɪv ˌendəukɑːˈdaɪtɪs/ *noun* an infection of the membrane covering the inner surfaces of the heart caused by bacteria

**subacute combined degeneration of the spinal cord** /ˌsʌbəkjuːt kəmˌbaɪnd dɪ ˌdʒenəreɪʃ(ə)n əv ðə ˈspaɪn(ə)l kɔːd/ *noun* a condition, caused by Vitamin $B_{12}$ deficiency, in which the sensory and motor nerves in the spinal cord become damaged and the person has difficulty in moving

**subacute sclerosing panencephalitis** /ˌsʌbəkjuːt skləˌrəusɪŋ ˌpænenkefəˈlaɪtɪs/

*noun* a rare inflammatory disease of the brain, mostly affecting children. It is linked to having measles at a very young age, and is usually fatal.

**subarachnoid** /ˌsʌbəˈræknɔɪd/ *adjective* beneath the arachnoid membrane

**subarachnoid haemorrhage** /ˌsʌbəˌræknɔɪd ˈhem(ə)rɪdʒ/ *noun* bleeding into the cerebrospinal fluid of the subarachnoid space

**subarachnoid space** /ˌsʌbəˌræknɔɪd ˈspeɪs/ *noun* a space between the arachnoid membrane and the pia mater in the brain, containing cerebrospinal fluid

**subaxillary** /ˌsʌbækˈsɪləri/ *adjective* beneath the armpit

**subcartilaginous** /ˌsʌbkɑːtɪˈlædʒɪnəs/ *adjective* 1. beneath cartilage or a body part composed of cartilage 2. made partly of cartilage

**subclavian** /sʌbˈkleɪviən/ *adjective* underneath the clavicle

**subclavian artery** /sʌbˌkleɪviən ˈɑːtəri/ *noun* one of two arteries branching from the aorta on the left and from the innominate artery on the right, continuing into the brachial arteries and supplying blood to each arm

**subclavian vein** /sʌbˌkleɪviən ˈveɪn/ *noun* one of the veins which continue the axillary veins into the brachiocephalic vein

**subclinical** /sʌbˈklɪnɪk(ə)l/ *adjective* referring to a disease which is present in the body, but which has not yet developed any symptoms

**subconscious** /sʌbˈkɒnʃəs/ *noun* the part of a person's mental processes which he or she is not aware of most of the time, but which can affect his or her actions ∎ *adjective* present in the mind although a person is not aware of it

**subcortex** /sʌbˈkɔːteks/ *noun* the parts of the brain immediately beneath the cerebral cortex

**subcortical** /sʌbˈkɔːtɪk(ə)l/ *adjective* beneath a cortex

**subcostal** /sʌbˈkɒst(ə)l/ *adjective* below the ribs

**subcostal plane** /sʌbˌkɒst(ə)l ˈpleɪn/ *noun* an imaginary horizontal line drawn across the front of the abdomen below the ribs

**subcranial** /sʌbˈkreɪniəl/ *adjective* beneath the dome of the skull

**subculture** /ˈsʌbkʌltʃə/ *noun* a culture of bacteria which is taken from a stock culture

**subculturing** /sʌbˈkʌltʃərɪŋ/ *noun* the act of taking a culture of bacteria from a stock culture

**subcutaneous** /ˌsʌbkjuːˈteɪniəs/ *adjective* under the skin. Abbr **s.c.**

**subcutaneous injection** /ˌsʌbkjuːˌteɪniəs ɪnˈdʒekʃən/ *noun* same as **hypodermic injection**

**subcutaneous oedema** /ˌsʌbkjuːˌteɪniəs ɪˈdiːmə/ *noun* a fluid collecting under the skin, usually at the ankles

**subcutaneous tissue** /ˌsʌbkjuːˌteɪniəs ˈtɪʃuː/ *noun* fatty tissue under the skin

**subdural** /sʌbˈdjʊərəl/ *adjective* between the dura mater and the arachnoid

**subdural haematoma** /sʌbˌdjʊərəl hiːməˈtəʊmə/ *noun* a haematoma between the dura mater and the arachnoid which displaces the brain, caused by a blow on the head

**subglottis** /sʌbˈglɒtɪs/ *noun* the lowest part of the laryngeal cavity, below the vocal folds

**subinvolution** /ˌsʌbɪnvəˈluːʃ(ə)n/ *noun* a condition in which a part of the body does not go back to its former size and shape after having swollen or stretched, as in the case of the uterus after childbirth

**subject** /ˈsʌbdʒɪkt/ *noun* 1. a patient, a person who has a particular disease ○ *The hospital has developed a new treatment for arthritic subjects.* 2. something which is being studied or written about ○ *The subject of the article is 'Rh-negative babies'.*

**subjective** /səbˈdʒektɪv/ *adjective* representing the views or feelings of the person concerned and not impartial ○ *The psychiatrist gave a subjective opinion on the patient's problem.* Compare **objective**

**subject to** /ˈsʌbdʒekt tuː/ *adverb* likely to experience ○ *The patient is subject to fits.* ○ *After returning from the tropics she was subject to attacks of malaria.*

**sublimate** /ˈsʌblɪmeɪt/ *noun* a deposit left when a vapour condenses ∎ *verb* to convert violent emotion into action which is not antisocial

**sublimation** /ˌsʌblɪˈmeɪʃ(ə)n/ *noun* a psychological process in which violent emotions which would otherwise be expressed in antisocial behaviour are directed into actions which are socially acceptable

**subliminal** /sʌbˈlɪmɪn(ə)l/ *adjective* too slight to be noticed by the senses

**sublingual** /sʌbˈlɪŋgwəl/ *adjective* under the tongue

'...the sublingual region has a rich blood supply derived from the carotid artery and indicates changes in central body temperature more rapidly than the rectum' [*Nursing Times*]

**sublingual gland** /sʌbˈlɪŋgwəl glænd/ *noun* a salivary gland under the tongue

**subluxation** /ˌsʌblʌkˈseɪʃ(ə)n/ *noun* a condition in which a joint is partially dislocated

**submandibular** /ˌsʌbmænˈdɪbjʊlə/ *adjective* under the lower jaw

**submandibular ganglion** /sʌbmænˌdɪbjʊlə ˈgæŋgliən/ *noun* a ganglion associated with the lingual nerve, relaying impulses to the submandibular and sublingual salivary glands

**submandibular gland** /ˌsʌbmænˈdɪbjʊlə ˌglænd/, **submaxillary gland** /sʌbˈmæksɪləri

,glænd/ *noun* a salivary gland on each side of the lower jaw

**submental** /sʌb'ment(ə)l/ *adjective* under the chin

**submucosa** /ˌsʌbmjuː'kəʊsə/ *noun* tissue under a mucous membrane

**submucous** /sʌb'mjuːkəs/ *adjective* under a mucous membrane

**submucous resection** /sʌbˌmjuːkəs rɪ'sekʃən/ *noun* the removal of a bent cartilage from the septum in the nose. Abbr **SMR**

**subnormal** /sʌb'nɔːm(ə)l/ *adjective* with a mind which has not developed fully (NOTE: This term is regarded as offensive.)

**subnormality** /ˌsʌbnɔː'mælɪti/ *noun* a condition in which someone's mind has not developed fully (NOTE: This term is regarded as offensive.)

**suboccipital** /ˌsʌbɒk'sɪpɪt(ə)l/ *adjective* beneath the back of the head

**suborbital** /sʌb'ɔːbɪt(ə)l/ *adjective* beneath the eye socket

**subperiosteal** /ˌsʌbperi'ɒstiəl/ *adjective* immediately beneath the connective tissue around bones

**subphrenic** /sʌb'frenɪk/ *adjective* under the diaphragm

**subphrenic abscess** /sʌbˌfrenɪk 'æbses/ *noun* an abscess which forms between the diaphragm and the liver

**subside** /səb'saɪd/ *verb* to go down or become less violent ○ *After being given the antibiotics, her fever subsided.*

**substance** /'sʌbstəns/ *noun* a chemical material, e.g. a drug ○ *toxic substances released into the bloodstream* ○ *He became addicted to certain substances.*

**substance abuse** /'sʌbstəns əˌbjuːs/, **substance misuse** /'sʌbstəns mɪsˌjuːz/ *noun* the misuse or excessive use of drugs, alcohol or other substances for pleasure or to satisfy addiction, which often causes health, emotional or social problems for the user

**substance P** /ˌsʌbstəns 'piː/ *noun* a neurotransmitter involved in pain pathways

**substitution** /ˌsʌbstɪ'tjuːʃ(ə)n/ *noun* the act of replacing one thing with another

**substitution therapy** /ˌsʌbstɪ'tjuːʃ(ə)n ˌθerəpi/ *noun* a way of treating a condition by using a different drug from the one used before

**substrate** /'sʌbstreɪt/ *noun* a substance which is acted on by an enzyme

'...insulin is a protein hormone and the body's major anabolic hormone, regulating the metabolism of all body fuels and substrates' [*Nursing 87*]

**subsultus** /sʌb'sʌltəs/ *noun* a twitching of the muscles and tendons, caused by fever

**subtertian fever** /sʌbˌtɜːʃ(ə)n 'fiːvə/ *noun* a type of malaria, where the fever is present most of the time

**subthreshold** /'sʌbθreʃhəʊld/ *adjective* describing a stimulus that is not strong enough to have an effect

**subtotal** /sʌb'təʊt(ə)l/ *adjective* referring to an operation to remove most of an organ

**subtotal gastrectomy** /ˌsʌbtəʊt(ə)l gæ'strektəmi/ *noun* the surgical removal of all but the top part of the stomach in contact with the diaphragm

**subtotal hysterectomy** /ˌsʌbtəʊt(ə)l ˌhɪstə'rektəmi/ *noun* the surgical removal of the uterus, but not the cervix

**subtotal pancreatectomy** /ˌsʌbtəʊt(ə)l ˌpæŋkriə'tektəmi/ *noun* the surgical removal of most of the pancreas

**subtotal thyroidectomy** /ˌsʌbtəʊt(ə)l ˌθaɪrɔɪ'dektəmi/ *noun* the surgical removal of most of the thyroid gland

**subungual** /sʌb'ʌŋgwəl/ *adjective* under a nail

**succeed** /sək'siːd/ *verb* to do well at what one was trying to do ○ *Scientists have succeeded in identifying the new influenza virus.* ○ *They succeeded in stopping the flow of blood.*

**success** /sək'ses/ *noun* 1. the fact of doing something well, doing what one was trying to do ○ *They tried to isolate the virus but without success.* 2. something which goes well ○ *The operation was a complete success.*

**successful** /sək'sesf(ə)l/ *adjective* working well ○ *The operation was completely successful.*

**succession** /sək'seʃ(ə)n/ *noun* a line of happenings, one after the other ○ *She had a succession of miscarriages.*

**successive** /sək'sesɪv/ *adjective* following one after the other ○ *She had a miscarriage with each successive pregnancy.*

**succus** /'sʌkəs/ *noun* juice secreted by an organ

**succus entericus** /ˌsʌkəs en'terɪkəs/ *noun* juice formed of enzymes, produced in the intestine to help the digestive process

**succussion** /sə'kʌʃ(ə)n/ *noun* a splashing sound made when there is a large amount of liquid inside a cavity in the body, e.g. the stomach

**suck** /sʌk/ *verb* to pull liquid or air into the mouth or into a tube

**sucrase** /'suːkreɪz/ *noun* an enzyme in the intestine which breaks down sucrose into glucose and fructose

**sucrose** /'suːkrəʊs/ *noun* a sugar, formed of glucose and fructose, found in plants, especially in sugar cane, beet and maple syrup

**suction** /'sʌkʃən/ *noun* a force created by the action of sucking ○ *The dentist hooked a suction tube into the patient's mouth.*

**sudamen** /suˈdeɪmən/ *noun* a little blister caused by sweat (NOTE: The plural is **sudamina**.)

**sudden** /ˈsʌd(ə)n/ *adjective* happening quickly

**sudden death** /ˌsʌd(ə)n ˈdeθ/ *noun* death without any identifiable cause, not preceded by an illness

**sudden infant death syndrome** /ˌsʌd(ə)n ˌɪnfənt ˈdeθ ˌsɪndrəʊm/ *noun* the sudden death of a baby under the age of about twelve months in bed, without any identifiable cause. Abbr **SIDS**. Also called **cot death**

**Sudeck's atrophy** /ˈsuːdeks ˌætrəfi/ *noun* osteoporosis in the hand or foot [Described 1900. After Paul Hermann Martin Sudeck (1866–1938), German surgeon.]

**sudor** /ˈsuːdɔː/ *noun* sweat

**sudoriferous** /ˌsuːdəˈrɪfərəs/ *adjective* producing sweat

**sudorific** /ˌsuːdəˈrɪfɪk/ *noun* a drug which makes someone sweat

**suffer** /ˈsʌfə/ *verb* **1.** to have an illness for a long period of time ○ *I suffer from headaches.* **2.** to feel pain ○ *I didn't suffer much.* **3.** to receive an injury ○ *He suffered multiple injuries in the accident.*

**sufferer** /ˈsʌfərə/ *noun* a person who has a particular disease ○ *a drug to help asthma sufferers* or *sufferers from asthma*

**suffering** /ˈsʌf(ə)rɪŋ/ *noun* the experiencing of pain over a long period of time

**suffocate** /ˈsʌfəkeɪt/ *verb* to make someone stop breathing by cutting off the supply of air to his or her nose and mouth

**suffocation** /ˌsʌfəˈkeɪʃ(ə)n/ *noun* the act of making someone become unconscious by cutting off his or her supply of air

**suffuse** /səˈfjuːz/ *verb* to spread over or through something

**suffusion** /səˈfjuːʒ(ə)n/ *noun* the spreading of a red flush over the skin

**sugar** /ˈʃʊɡə/ *noun* any of several sweet carbohydrates (NOTE: For other terms referring to sugar, see words beginning with **glyc-, glyco-**.)

COMMENT: There are several natural forms of sugar: sucrose (in plants), lactose (in milk), fructose (in fruit), glucose and dextrose (in fruit and in body tissue). Edible sugar used in the home is a form of refined sucrose. All sugars are useful sources of energy, though excessive amounts of sugar can increase weight and cause tooth decay. Diabetes mellitus is a condition in which the body is incapable of absorbing sugar from food.

**sugar intolerance** /ˈʃʊɡər ɪnˌtɒlərəns/ *noun* diarrhoea caused by sugar which has not been absorbed

**suggest** /səˈdʒest/ *verb* to mention an idea ○ *The doctor suggested that she should stop smoking.*

**suggested daily intake** /səˌdʒestɪd ˌdeɪli ˈɪnteɪk/ *noun* the amount of a substance which

it is recommended a person should take in each day

**suggestibility** /səˌdʒestɪˈbɪlɪti/ *noun* a mental state in which somebody just accepts other people's ideas, attitudes or instructions, without questioning them. It is usually increased under hypnosis.

**suggestible** /səˈdʒestɪb(ə)l/ *adjective* easily influenced by other people

**suggestion** /səˈdʒestʃən/ *noun* **1.** an idea which has been mentioned ○ *The doctor didn't agree with the suggestion that the disease had been caught in the hospital.* **2.** (in psychiatry) the process of making a person's ideas change, by suggesting different ideas which the person can accept, such as that he or she is in fact cured

**suicidal** /ˌsuːɪˈsaɪd(ə)l/ *adjective* referring to someone who wants to kill himself ○ *He has suicidal tendencies.*

**suicide** /ˈsuːɪsaɪd/ *noun* the act of killing oneself □ **to commit suicide** to kill yourself ○ *After his wife died he committed suicide.*

**sulcus** /ˈsʌlkəs/ *noun* a groove or fold, especially between the gyri in the brain □ **lateral sulcus and central sulcus** two grooves which divide a cerebral hemisphere into lobes

**sulfa drug** /ˈsʌlfə drʌɡ/, **sulfa compound** /ˈsʌlfə ˌkɒmpaʊnd/ *noun* same as **sulfonamide**

**sulfasalazine** /ˌsʌlfəˈsæləziːn/ *noun* a drug belonging to the sulfonamide group of antibacterial drugs. It is used in the treatment of ulcerative colitis and Crohn's disease, and also of severe rheumatoid arthritis.

**sulfate** /ˈsʌlfeɪt/ *noun* same as **sulphate**

**sulfonamide** /sʌlˈfɒnəmaɪd/ *noun* a bacteriostatic drug, e.g. trimethoprim, used to treat bacterial infection, especially in the intestine and urinary system, but now less important due to increasing bacterial resistance

**sulfonylurea** /ˌsʌlfənaɪlˈjuːriːə/ *noun* any of a group of drugs which lower blood sugar, used in the treatment of diabetes

**sulfur** /ˈsʌlfə/ *noun* another spelling of **sulphur**

**sulphate** /ˈsʌlfeɪt/ *noun* a salt of sulphuric acid

**sulphur** /ˈsʌlfə/ *noun* a yellow non-metallic chemical element which is contained in some amino acids and is used in creams to treat some skin disorders (NOTE: The chemical symbol is **S**. Note also that words beginning **sulph-** are spelt **sulf-** in US English.)

**sulphuric acid** /sʌlˌfjʊərɪk ˈæsɪd/ *noun* a strong colourless oily corrosive acid which has many uses

**sumatriptan** /ˌsuːməˈtrɪptæn/ *noun* a drug which helps to narrow the blood vessels, used in the treatment of acute migraine

**sun** /sʌn/ *noun* the very hot and large star around which the earth travels and which gives light and heat

**sunbathing** /'sʌnbeɪðɪŋ/ *noun* the practice of lying in the sun to absorb sunlight

**sun blindness** /'sʌn ˌblaɪndnəs/ *noun* same as **photoretinitis**

**sunburn** /'sʌnbɜːn/ *noun* damage to the skin by excessive exposure to sunlight

**sunburnt** /'sʌnbɜːnt/ *adjective* referring to skin made brown or red by exposure to sunlight

**sunlight** /'sʌnlaɪt/ *noun* the light from the sun ○ *He is allergic to strong sunlight.*

COMMENT: Sunlight is essential to give the body Vitamin D, but excessive exposure to sunlight will not simply turn the skin brown, but also may burn the surface of the skin so badly that it dies and pus forms beneath. Constant exposure to the sun can cause cancer of the skin.

**sunscreen** /'sʌnskriːn/ *noun* a cream for rubbing into the skin that acts as a block against the harmful rays of the sun, used to reduce the risk of sunburn

**sunstroke** /'sʌnstrəʊk/ *noun* a serious condition caused by excessive exposure to the sun or to hot conditions, in which the person becomes dizzy and has a high body temperature but does not perspire

**super-** /suːpə/ *prefix* **1.** above **2.** extremely

**superciliary** /ˌsuːpə'sɪliəri/ *adjective* referring to the eyebrows

**superego** /ˌsuːpər'iːgəʊ/ *noun* (*in psychology*) the part of the mind which is a person's conscience, which is concerned with right and wrong

**superfecundation** /ˌsuːpəfiːkən'deɪʃ(ə)n/ *noun* a condition in which two or more ova produced at the same time are fertilised by different males

**superfetation** /ˌsuːpəfiː'teɪʃ(ə)n/ *noun* a condition in which an ovum is fertilised in a woman who is already pregnant

**superficial** /ˌsuːpə'fɪʃ(ə)l/ *adjective* on the surface, close to the surface or on the skin □ **superficial burn** burn on the skin surface

**superficial fascia** /ˌsuːpəfɪʃ(ə)l 'feɪʃə/ *plural noun* membranous layers of connective tissue found just under the skin

**superficial thickness burn** /ˌsuːpəfɪʃ(ə)l 'θɪknəs bɜːn/ *noun* same as **partial thickness burn**

**superficial vein** /ˌsuːpəfɪʃ(ə)l 'veɪn/ *noun* a vein which is near the surface of the skin

**superinfection** /'suːpərɪnˌfekʃən/ *noun* a second infection which affects the treatment of the first infection, because it is resistant to the drug used to treat the first

**superior** /suː'pɪəriə/ *adjective* (*of part of the body*) higher up than another part

**superior aspect** /suːˌpɪəriə 'æspekt/ *noun* a view of the body from above

**superior ganglion** /suːˌpɪəriə 'gæŋgliən/ *noun* a small collection of cells in the jugular foramen

**superiority** /suːˌpɪəri'ɒrɪti/ *noun* the fact of being better than something or someone else

**superiority complex** /suːˌpɪəri'ɒrɪti ˌkɒmˈpleks/ *noun* a condition in which a person feels he or she is better and more important than others and pays little attention to them

**superior mesenteric artery** /suːˌpɪəriə mes(e)nˌterɪk 'ɑːtəri/ *noun* one of the arteries which supply the small intestine

**superior vena cava** /suːˌpɪəriə ˌviːnə 'keɪvə/ *noun* a branch of the large vein into the heart, carrying blood from the head and the top part of the body. See illustration at **HEART** in Supplement

**supernumerary** /ˌsuːpə'njuːmərəri/ *adjective* extra, more than the usual number

'…allocation of supernumerary students to clinical areas is for their educational needs and not for service requirements' [*Nursing Times*]

**superovulation** /ˌsuːpərˌɒvjʊ'leɪʃ(ə)n/ *noun* an increased frequency of ovulation, or production of a large number of ova at one time. It is often caused by giving a woman with infertility problems gonadotrophin hormones to stimulate ovulation.

**supervise** /'suːpəvaɪz/ *verb* to manage or organise something ○ *The administration of drugs has to be supervised by a qualified person.* ○ *She has been appointed to supervise the transfer of patients to the new ward.*

**supervision** /ˌsuːpə'vɪʒ(ə)n/ *noun* management or organisation ○ *Elderly patients need constant supervision.* ○ *The sheltered housing is under the supervision of a full-time nurse.*

**supervisor** /'suːpəvaɪzə/ *noun* a person who supervises ○ *the supervisor of hospital catering services*

**supinate** /'suːpɪneɪt/ *verb* to turn the hand so that the palm faces upwards

**supination** /ˌsuːpɪ'neɪʃ(ə)n/ *noun* the act of turning the hand so that the palm faces upwards. Opposite **pronation**. See illustration at **ANATOMICAL TERMS** in Supplement

**supinator** /'suːpɪneɪtə/ *noun* a muscle which turns the hand so that the palm faces upwards

**supine** /'suːpaɪn/ *adjective* **1.** lying on the back. Opposite **prone 2.** with the palm of the hand facing upwards

'…the patient was to remain in the supine position, therefore a pad was placed under the Achilles tendon to raise the legs' [*NATNews*]

**supplement** /'sʌplɪmənt/ *noun* **1.** any extra nutrients that are taken to help a specific condition when someone is not getting all they need from their food ○ *vitamin and folic acid supplements* **2.** a pill or product regarded as helpful in improving health that can be bought without a prescription. Supplements are not tested in the same way as prescription drugs. ○ *dietary or food supplements* ■ *verb* to add on or increase above what is taken usually ○ *She supplemented her diet with folic acid when she was planning a pregnancy.*

**supply** /səˈplaɪ/ *noun* something which is provided ○ *The arteries provide a continuous supply of oxygenated blood to the tissues.* ○ *The hospital service needs a constant supply of blood for transfusion.* ○ *The government sent medical supplies to the disaster area.* ■ *verb* to provide or give something which is needed ○ *A balanced diet will supply the body with all the vitamins and trace elements it needs.* ○ *The brachial artery supplies the arm and hand.*

**support** /səˈpɔːt/ *noun* **1.** help to keep something in place ○ *The bandage provides some support for the knee.* ○ *He was so weak that he had to hold onto a chair for support.* **2.** a handle, a metal rail which a person can hold ○ *There are supports at the side of the bed.* ○ *The bath is provided with metal supports.* ■ *verb* **1.** to hold something ○ *He wore a truss to support a hernia.* **2.** to keep something in place

**support hose** /səˈpɔːt həʊz/ *plural noun* stockings that fit tightly to the legs, worn to help the flow of blood

**supportive** /səˈpɔːtɪv/ *adjective* helping or comforting someone in trouble ○ *Her family was very supportive when she was in hospital.* ○ *The local health authority has been very supportive of the hospital management.*

**support stocking** /səˈpɔːt ˌstɒkɪŋ/ *noun* a stocking worn to prevent postural hypotension and peripheral oedema

**support worker** /səˈpɔːt ˌwɜːkə/ *noun* someone who assists registered health service professionals as part of a team, e.g. as a nursing auxiliary or assistant, or in specialist areas such as mental health, speech therapy or physiotherapy

**suppository** /səˈpɒzɪt(ə)ri/ *noun* a piece of a soluble material such as glycerine jelly containing a drug, which is placed in the rectum to act as lubricant, or in the vagina, to treat disorders such as vaginitis, and is dissolved by the body's fluids

**suppress** /səˈpres/ *verb* to reduce the action of something completely, e.g. to remove a symptom or to stop the release of a hormone ○ *a course of treatment which suppresses the painful irritation* ○ *The drug suppresses the body's natural instinct to reject the transplanted tissue.* ○ *The release of adrenaline from the adrenal cortex is suppressed.*

**suppression** /səˈpreʃ(ə)n/ *noun* the act of suppressing something ○ *the suppression of allergic responses* ○ *the suppression of a hormone*

**suppressor T-cell** /səˌpresə ˈtiː sel/ *noun* a T-cell which stops or reduces the immune response to an antigen of B-cells and other T-cells

**suppurate** /ˈsʌpjʊreɪt/ *verb* to form and discharge pus

**suppurating** /ˈsʌpjʊreɪtɪŋ/ *adjective* purulent, containing or discharging pus

**suppuration** /ˌsʌpjʊˈreɪʃ(ə)n/ *noun* the formation and discharge of pus

**supra-** /suːprə/ *prefix* above or over

**supraglottis** /ˌsuːprəˈɡlɒtɪs/ *noun* the part of the larynx above the vocal folds, including the epiglottis

**supraoptic nucleus** /ˌsuːprəɒptɪk ˈnjuːkliəs/ *noun* a nucleus in the hypothalamus from which nerve fibres run to the posterior pituitary gland

**supraorbital** /ˌsuːprəˈɔːbɪt(ə)l/ *adjective* above the orbit of the eye

**supraorbital ridge** /ˌsuːprəɔːbɪt(ə)l ˈrɪdʒ/ *noun* the ridge of bone above the eye, covered by the eyebrow

**suprapubic** /ˌsuːprəˈpjuːbɪk/ *adjective* above the pubic bone or pubic area

**suprarenal** /ˌsuːprəˈriːn(ə)l/ *adjective* above the kidneys ■ *noun* same as **suprarenal gland**

**suprarenal area** /ˌsuːprəriːn(ə)l ˈeəriə/ *noun* the area of the body above the kidneys

**suprarenal cortical hormone** /ˌsuːprəriːn(ə)l ˌkɔːtɪk(ə)l ˈhɔːməʊn/ *noun* a hormone secreted by the cortex of the adrenal glands, e.g. cortisone

**suprarenal gland** /ˌsuːprəˈriːn(ə)l ɡlænd/, **suprarenal** /ˌsuːprəˈriːn(ə)l/ *noun* one of two endocrine glands at the top of the kidneys, which secrete adrenaline and other hormones

**suprarenal medulla** /ˌsuːprəriːn(ə)l meˈdʌlə/ *noun* same as **adrenal medulla**

**suprasternal** /ˌsuːprəˈstɜːn(ə)l/ *adjective* above the sternum

**supraventricular tachycardia** /ˌsʌbven ˌtrɪkjʊlə ˌtæki'kɑːdiə/ *noun* tachycardia coming from the upper chambers of the heart

**surface** /ˈsɜːfɪs/ *noun* the top layer of something ○ *The surfaces of the two membranes may rub together.*

**surfactant** /sɜːˈfæktənt/ *noun* a substance in the alveoli of the lungs which keeps the surfaces of the lungs wet and prevents lung collapse

**surgeon** /ˈsɜːdʒən/ *noun* a doctor who specialises in surgery (NOTE: Although surgeons are doctors, in the UK they are traditionally called 'Mr' and not 'Dr', so 'Dr Smith' may be a GP, but 'Mr Smith' is a surgeon.)

**surgeon general** /ˌsɜːdʒən ˈdʒen(ə)rəl/ *noun* US a government official responsible for all aspects of public health

**surgery** /ˈsɜːdʒəri/ *noun* **1.** the treatment of diseases or disorders by procedures which require an operation to cut into, to remove or to manipulate tissue, organs or parts ○ *The patient will need plastic surgery to remove the scars he received in the accident.* ○ *The surgical ward is for patients waiting for surgery.* ○ *Two of our patients had to have surgery.* ○ *She will have to undergo surgery.* **2.** a room where a doctor or dentist sees and examines patients ○ *There are ten patients waiting in the surgery.* ○ *Surgery hours are from 8.30 in the morning to 6.00 at night.*

**surgical** /ˈsɜːdʒɪk(ə)l/ *adjective* **1.** referring to surgery ○ *All surgical instruments must be sterilised.* **2.** referring to a disease which can be treated by surgery ○ *We manage to carry out six surgical operations in an hour.*

**surgical belt** /ˌsɜːdʒɪk(ə)l ˈbelt/ *noun* a fitted covering, worn to support part of the back, chest or abdomen

**surgical boot** /ˌsɜːdʒɪk(ə)l ˈbuːt/ *noun* a specially made boot for a person who has an unusually shaped foot, to support or correct it

**surgical care** /ˈsɜːdʒɪk(ə)l keə/ *noun* looking after patients who have had surgery

**surgical diathermy** /ˌsɜːdʒɪk(ə)l daɪəˈθɜːmi/ *noun* a procedure which uses a knife or electrode which is heated by a strong electric current until it coagulates tissue

**surgical emphysema** /ˌsɜːdʒɪk(ə)l ˌemfɪˈsiːmə/ *noun* air bubbles in tissue, not in the lungs

**surgical fixation** /ˌsɜːdʒɪk(ə)l fɪkˈseɪʃ(ə)n/ *noun* a method of immobilising something such as a bone either externally by the use of a splint or internally by a metal plate and screws

**surgical gloves** /ˈsɜːdʒɪk(ə)l ɡlʌvz/ *plural noun* thin plastic gloves worn by surgeons

**surgical hose** *noun* a strong elastic stocking worn to support a weak joint in a knee or to relieve varicose veins. Also called **elastic hose, surgical stocking**

**surgical intervention** /ˌsɜːdʒɪk(ə)l ˌɪntəˈvenʃən/ *noun* the treatment of disease or other condition by surgery

**surgically** /ˈsɜːdʒɪkli/ *adverb* using surgery ○ *The growth can be treated surgically.*

**surgical neck** /ˌsɜːdʒɪk(ə)l ˈnek/ *noun* the narrow part at the top of the humerus, where the arm can easily be broken

**surgical needle** /ˌsɜːdʒɪk(ə)l ˈniːd(ə)l/ *noun* a needle for sewing up surgical incisions

**surgical procedure** /ˌsɜːdʒɪk(ə)l prəˈsiːdʒə/ *noun* a surgical operation

**surgical shoe** /ˌsɜːdʒɪk(ə)l ˈʃuː/ *noun* a specially made boot for a person who has an unusually shaped foot, to support or correct it

**surgical spirit** /ˌsɜːdʒɪk(ə)l ˈspɪrɪt/ *noun* ethyl alcohol with an additive giving it an unpleasant taste, used as a disinfectant or for cleansing the skin. Also called **rubbing alcohol**

**surgical stocking** /ˌsɜːdʒɪk(ə)l ˈstɒkɪŋ/ *noun* same as **surgical hose**

**surgical ward** /ˈsɜːdʒɪk(ə)l wɔːd/ *noun* a ward for patients who have undergone surgery

**surgical wound** /ˈsɜːdʒɪk(ə)l wuːnd/ *noun* an incision made during a surgical operation

**surrogate** /ˈsʌrəɡət/ *adjective* taking the place of ■ *noun* someone or something that takes the place of another person or thing ◇ **surrogate mother 1.** a woman who has a child by artificial insemination for a woman who cannot become pregnant, with the intention of handing the child over to her when it is born **2.** a person who takes the place of a natural mother for someone

**surround** /səˈraʊnd/ *verb* to be all around something ○ *The wound is several millimetres deep and the surrounding flesh is inflamed.*

**survival** /səˈvaɪv(ə)l/ *noun* the act of continuing to live ○ *The survival rate of newborn babies has begun to fall.*

**survive** /səˈvaɪv/ *verb* to continue to live ○ *He survived two attacks of pneumonia.* ○ *The baby only survived for two hours.*

**survivor** /səˈvaɪvə/ *noun* a person who survives

**susceptibility** /səˌseptɪˈbɪlɪti/ *noun* lack of resistance to a disease

'...low birthweight has been associated with increased susceptibility to infection' [*East African Medical Journal*]

'...even children with the milder forms of sickle-cell disease have an increased frequency of pneumococcal infection. The reason for this susceptibility is a profound abnormality of the immune system' [*Lancet*]

**susceptible** /səˈseptɪb(ə)l/ *adjective* likely to catch a disease ○ *She is susceptible to colds* or *to throat infections.*

**suspect** *noun* /ˈsʌspekt/ a person who doctors believe may have a disease ○ *They are screening all typhoid suspects.* ■ *verb* /səˈspekt/ to think that someone may have a disease ○ *He is a suspected diphtheria carrier.* ○ *Several cases of suspected meningitis have been reported.*

'...those affected are being nursed in five isolation wards and about forty suspected sufferers are being barrier nursed in other wards' [*Nursing Times*]

**suspension** /səˈspenʃən/ *noun* a liquid with solid particles in it

**suspensory** /səˈspensəri/ *adjective* hanging down

**suspensory bandage** /səˌspensəri ˈbændɪdʒ/ *noun* a bandage to hold a part of the body which hangs

**suspensory ligament** /səˌspensəri ˈlɪɡəmənt/ *noun* a ligament which holds a part of the body in position. See illustration at **EYE** in Supplement

**sustain** /səˈsteɪn/ *verb* **1.** to keep, to support, to maintain something ○ *These bones can sustain quite heavy weights.* ○ *He is not eating* *enough to sustain life.* **2.** to experience an injury ○ *He sustained a severe head injury.*

**sustentacular** /ˌsʌstənˈtækjʊlə/ *adjective* referring to a sustentaculum

**sustentaculum** /ˌsʌstənˈtækjʊləm/ *noun* a part of the body which supports another part

**suture** /ˈsuːtʃə/ *noun* **1.** a fixed joint where two bones are fused together, especially the bones in the skull **2.** a procedure for attaching the sides of an incision or wound with thread, so that healing can take place. Also called **stitch 3.** a thread used for attaching the sides of a wound so that they can heal ■ *verb* to attach the sides of a wound or incision together with thread so that healing can take place. Also called **stitch**

COMMENT: Wounds are usually stitched using thread or catgut which is removed after a week or so. Sutures are either absorbable, made of a substance which is eventually absorbed into the body, or non-absorbable, in which case they need to be removed after a certain time.

**suxamethonium** /ˌsʌksəmɪˈθəʊniəm/ *noun* a drug similar to acetylcholine in structure, used as a muscle relaxant during surgery

**swab** /swɒb/ *noun* **1.** a cotton wool pad, often attached to a small stick, used, e.g., to clean a wound, to apply ointment or to take a specimen **2.** a specimen taken with a swab ○ *a cervical swab*

**swallow** /ˈswɒləʊ/ *verb* to make liquid, food and sometimes air go down from the mouth to the stomach ○ *Patients suffering from nosebleeds should try not to swallow the blood.*

**swallowing** /ˈswɒləʊɪŋ/ *noun* same as **deglutition**

**Swan-Ganz catheter** /ˌswɒn ˈgæntz ˌkæθɪtə/ *noun* a special catheter which can be floated through the right chamber of the heart into the pulmonary artery. The balloon at its tip is then inflated to measure arterial pressure.

**sweat** /swet/ *noun* a salty liquid produced by the sweat glands to cool the body as the liquid evaporates from the skin ○ *Sweat was running off the end of his nose.* ○ *Her hands were covered with sweat.* Also called **perspiration** ■ *verb* to produce moisture through the sweat glands and onto the skin ○ *After working in the fields she was sweating.*

**sweat duct** /ˈswet dʌkt/ *noun* a thin tube connecting the sweat gland with the surface of the skin

**sweat gland** /ˈswet glænd/ *noun* a gland which produces sweat, situated beneath the dermis and connected to the skin surface by a sweat duct

**sweat pore** /ˈswet pɔː/ *noun* a hole in the skin through which the sweat comes out

**sweet** /swiːt/ *adjective* one of the basic tastes, not bitter, sour or salt ○ *Sugar is sweet, lemons are sour.*

**swell** /swel/ *verb* to become larger, or cause something to become larger ○ *The disease affects the lymph glands, making them swell.* ○ *The doctor noticed that the patient had swollen glands in his neck.* ○ *She finds her swollen ankles painful.* (NOTE: **swelling – swelled – swollen**)

**swelling** /ˈswelɪŋ/ *noun* a condition in which fluid accumulates in tissue, making the tissue become large ○ *They applied a cold compress to try to reduce the swelling.*

**swimmer's cramp** /ˌswɪməz ˈkræmp/ *noun* spasms in arteries and muscles caused by cold water, or by swimming soon after a meal

**sycosis** /saɪˈkəʊsɪs/ *noun* a bacterial infection of hair follicles

**sycosis barbae** /saɪˌkəʊsɪs ˈbɑːbiː/ *noun* an infection of hair follicles on the sides of the face and chin. Also called **barber's itch, barber's rash**

**Sydenham's chorea** /ˌsɪdnəmz kɒˈriːə/ *noun* temporary chorea affecting children, frequently associated with endocarditis and rheumatism [Described 1686. After Thomas Sydenham (1624–89), English physician.]

**symbiosis** /ˌsɪmbaɪˈəʊsɪs/ *noun* a condition in which two organisms exist together and help each other to survive

**symblepharon** /sɪmˈblefərɒn/ *noun* a condition in which the eyelid sticks to the eyeball

**symbol** /ˈsɪmbəl/ *noun* a sign or letter which means something

**Syme's amputation** /ˌsaɪmz æmpjʊˈteɪʃ(ə)n/ *noun* a surgical operation to amputate the foot above the ankle [Described 1842. After James Syme (1799–1870), Edinburgh surgeon and teacher; one of the first to adopt antisepsis (Joseph Lister was his son-in-law), and also among the early users of anaesthesia.]

**symmetry** /ˈsɪmətri/ *noun* the regularity of structure and distribution of parts of the body, each side of the body being structurally similar to the other

**sympathectomy** /ˌsɪmpəˈθektəmi/ *noun* a surgical operation to cut part of the sympathetic nervous system, as a treatment of high blood pressure

**sympathetic** /ˌsɪmpəˈθetɪk/ *adjective* **1.** feeling or showing shared feelings, pity or compassion **2.** relating to or belonging to the sympathetic nervous system, or to one of its parts

**sympathetic nervous system** /ˌsɪmpəθetɪk ˈnɜːvəs ˌsɪstəm/, **sympathetic system** /ˌsɪmpəθetɪk ˈsɪstəm/ *noun* part of the autonomic nervous system, which leaves the spinal cord from the thoracic and lumbar regions to go to various important organs such as the heart, the lungs and the sweat glands, and which prepares the body for emergencies and vigorous muscular activity. ◊ **parasympathetic nervous system**

**sympatholytic** /ˌsɪmpəθəʊˈlɪtɪk/ *noun* a drug which stops the sympathetic nervous system working

**sympathomimetic** /ˌsɪmpəθəʊmɪˈmetɪk/ *adjective* referring to a drug such as dopamine hydrochloride which stimulates the activity of the sympathetic nervous system and is used in cardiac shock following myocardial infarction and in cardiac surgery

**sympathy** /ˈsɪmpəθi/ *noun* **1.** the feeling or expression of pity or sorrow for the pain or distress of somebody else **2.** the relationship between people which causes one of them to provoke a similar condition to their own in the other one. For example, when the first person yawns, the second feels an urge to yawn too. **3.** the influence produced on any part of the body by disease or change in another part

**symphysiectomy** /ˌsɪmfɪziˈektəmi/ *noun* a surgical operation to remove part of the pubic symphysis to make childbirth easier

**symphysiotomy** /ˌsɪmfɪziˈɒtəmi/ *noun* a surgical operation to make an incision in the pubic symphysis to make the passage for a fetus wider

**symphysis** /ˈsɪmfəsɪs/ *noun* the point where two bones are joined by cartilage which makes the joint rigid

**symphysis menti** /ˌsɪmfəsɪs ˈmenti/ *noun* a point in the front of the lower jaw where the two halves of the jaw are fused to form the chin

**symphysis pubis** /ˌsɪmfəsɪs ˈpjuːbɪs/ *noun* same as **pubic symphysis**

**symptom** /ˈsɪmptəm/ *noun* a change in the way the body works or a change in the body's appearance, which shows that a disease or disorder is present and which the person is aware of ○ *The symptoms of hay fever are a running nose and eyes.* ○ *A doctor must study the symptoms before making his diagnosis.* ○ *The patient presented all the symptoms of rheumatic fever.* (NOTE: If a symptom is noticed only by the doctor, it is a **sign**.)

**symptomatic** /ˌsɪmptəˈmætɪk/ *adjective* being a symptom of something ○ *The rash is symptomatic of measles.*

**symptomatology** /ˌsɪmptəməˈtɒlədʒi/ *noun* a branch of medicine concerned with the study of symptoms. Also called **semeiology**

**syn-** /sɪn/ *prefix* joint, or fused

**synalgia** /sɪˈnældʒə/ *noun* a pain which is felt in one part of the body, but is caused by a condition in another part, e.g. pain in the groin which can be a symptom of a kidney stone or pain in the right shoulder which can indicate gall bladder infection. Also called **referred pain**

**synapse** /ˈsaɪnæps/ *noun* a point in the nervous system where the axons of neurones are in contact with the dendrites of other neurones ■ *verb* to link something with a neurone

**synaptic** /sɪnˈæptɪk/ *adjective* referring to a synapse

**synaptic connection** /sɪnˌæptɪk kəˈnekʃ(ə)n/ *noun* a link between the dendrites of one neurone with another neurone

**synarthrosis** /ˌsɪnɑːˈθrəʊsɪs/ *noun* a joint, e.g. in the skull, where the bones have fused together

**synchondrosis** /ˌsɪnkɒnˈdrəʊsɪs/ *noun* a joint, as in children, where the bones are linked by cartilage, before the cartilage has changed to bone

**synchysis** /ˈsɪŋkɪsɪs/ *noun* a condition in which the vitreous humour in the eye becomes soft

**syncope** /ˈsɪŋkəpi/ *noun* a condition in which someone becomes unconscious for a short time because of reduced flow of blood to the brain. Also called **fainting fit**

**syncytium** /sɪnˈsɪʃiəm/ *noun* a continuous length of tissue in muscle fibres

**syndactyl** /sɪnˈdæktɪl/ *adjective* having two or more fingers or toes joined together when born

**syndactyly** /sɪnˈdæktɪli/, **syndactylism** /sɪnˈdæktɪlɪz(ə)m/ *noun* a condition in which two toes or fingers are joined together with tissue

**syndesm-** /sɪndesm/, **syndesmo-** /sɪndesməʊ/ *prefix* referring to ligaments

**syndesmology** /ˌsɪndesˈmɒlədʒi/ *noun* a branch of medicine which studies joints

**syndesmosis** /ˌsɪndesˈməʊsɪs/ *noun* a joint where the bones are tightly linked by ligaments

**syndrome** /ˈsɪndrəʊm/ *noun* a group of symptoms and other changes in the body's functions which, when taken together, show that a particular disease is present. ◊ **complex**

**synechia** /sɪˈnekiə/ *noun* a condition in which the iris sticks to another part of the eye

**syneresis** /sɪˈnɪərəsɪs/ *noun* the releasing of fluid as in a blood clot when it becomes harder

**synergism** /ˈsɪnədʒɪz(ə)m/ *noun* a situation where two or more things are acting together in such a way that both are more effective. Also called **synergy**

**synergist** /ˈsɪnədʒɪst/ *noun* a muscle or drug which acts with another and increases the effectiveness of both

**synergy** /ˈsɪnədʒi/ *noun* same as **synergism**

**syngeneic** /ˌsɪndʒəˈniːɪk/ *adjective* referring to individuals or tissues that have an identical or closely similar genetic make-up, especially one that will allow the transplanting of tissue without provoking an immune response

**syngraft** /ˈsɪngrɑːft/ *noun* same as **isograft**

**synoptophore** /sɪˈnɒptəfɔː/ *noun* an instrument used to correct a squint

**synostosed** /ˈsɪnɒˌstəʊzd/ *adjective* (of bones) fused together with new bone tissue

**synostosis** /ˌsɪnɒˈstəʊsɪs/ *noun* the fusing of two bones together by the formation of new bone tissue

**synovectomy** /ˌsɪnəʊˈvektəmi/ *noun* a surgical operation to remove the synovial membrane of a joint

**synovia** /saɪˈnəʊviə/ *noun* same as **synovial fluid**

**synovial** /saɪˈnəʊviəl/ *adjective* referring to the synovium

**synovial cavity** /saɪˌnəʊviəl ˈkæviti/ *noun* a space inside a synovial joint. See illustration at **SYNOVIAL JOINT** in Supplement

**synovial fluid** /saɪˌnəʊviəl ˈfluːɪd/ *noun* a fluid secreted by a synovial membrane to lubricate a joint. See illustration at **SYNOVIAL JOINT** in Supplement

**synovial joint** /saɪˌnəʊviəl ˈdʒɔɪnt/ *noun* a joint where the two bones are separated by a space filled with synovial fluid which nourishes and lubricates the surfaces of the bones. Also called **diarthrosis**

**synovial membrane** /saɪˌnəʊviəl ˈmembreɪn/, **synovium** *noun* a smooth membrane which forms the inner lining of the capsule covering a joint and secretes the fluid which lubricates the joint. See illustration at **SYNOVIAL JOINT** in Supplement

**synovioma** /ˌsɪnəʊviˈəʊmə/ *noun* a tumour in a synovial membrane

**synovitis** /ˌsaɪnəˈvaɪtɪs/ *noun* inflammation of the synovial membrane

**synovium** /sɪˈnəʊviəm/ same as **synovial membrane**

'70% of rheumatoid arthritis sufferers develop the condition in the metacarpophalangeal joints. The synovium produces an excess of synovial fluid which is abnormal and becomes thickened' [*Nursing Times*]

**synthesis** /ˈsɪnθəsɪs/ *noun* **1.** the process of combining different ideas or objects into a new whole **2.** a new unified whole resulting from the combination of different ideas or objects **3.** the formation of compounds through chemical reactions involving simpler compounds or elements **4.** in psychiatry, the fusing together of all the various elements of the personality (NOTE: The plural is **syntheses**.)

**synthesise** /ˈsɪnθəsaɪz/, **synthesize** *verb* to make a chemical compound from its separate components ○ *Essential amino acids cannot be synthesised.* ○ *The body cannot synthesise essential fatty acids and has to absorb them from food.*

**synthetic** /sɪnˈθetɪk/ *adjective* made by humans, made artificially

**synthetically** /sɪnˈθetɪkli/ *adverb* made artificially ○ *Synthetically produced hormones are used in hormone therapy.*

**syphilide** /ˈsɪfɪlaɪd/ *noun* a rash or open sore which is a symptom of the second stage of syphilis

**syphilis** /ˈsɪfəlɪs/ *noun* a sexually transmitted disease caused by a spirochaete *Treponema pallidum*

COMMENT: Syphilis is a serious sexually transmitted disease, but it is curable with penicillin injections if the treatment is started early. Syphilis has three stages: in the first, or primary, stage, a hard sore (chancre) appears on the genitals or sometimes on the mouth; in the second, or secondary, stage about two or three months later, a rash appears, with sores round the mouth and genitals. It is at this stage that the disease is particularly infectious. After this stage, symptoms disappear for a long time, sometimes many years. The disease reappears in the third, or tertiary, stage in many different forms: blindness, brain disorders, ruptured aorta or general paralysis leading to mental disorder and death. The tests for syphilis are the Wassermann test and the less reliable Kahn test.

**syring-** /sɪrɪndʒ/ *prefix* same as **syringo-** (used before vowels)

**syringe** /sɪˈrɪndʒ/ *noun* a medical instrument made of a tube with a plunger which either slides down inside the tube, forcing the contents out through a needle as in an injection, or slides up the tube, allowing a liquid to be sucked into it ■ *verb* to wash out the ears using a syringe

**syringo-** /sɪrɪŋgəʊ/ *prefix* referring to tubes, especially the central canal of the spinal cord

**syringobulbia** /sɪˌrɪŋgəʊˈbʌlbiə/ *noun* syringomyelia in the brain stem

**syringocystadenoma** /sɪˌrɪŋgəʊsɪstədɪˈnəʊmə/, **syringoma** /ˌsɪrɪŋˈgəʊmə/ *noun* a benign tumour in sweat glands and ducts

**syringomyelia** /sɪˌrɪŋgəʊmaɪˈiːliə/ *noun* a disease which forms cavities in the neck section of the spinal cord, affecting the nerves so that the person loses the sense of touch and pain

**syringomyelitis** /sɪˌrɪŋgəʊmaɪəˈlaɪtɪs/ *noun* a swelling of the spinal cord, which results in the formation of cavities in it

**syringomyelocele** /sɪˌrɪŋgəʊˈmaɪələʊsiːl/ *noun* a severe form of spina bifida where the spinal cord pushes through a hole in the spine

**systaltic** /sɪsˈtæltɪk/ *adjective* describing an organ such as the heart that contracts and relaxes alternately

**system** /ˈsɪstəm/ *noun* **1.** the body as a whole ○ *Amputation of a limb gives a serious shock to the system.* **2.** the arrangement of particular parts of the body so that they work together ○ *the lymphatic system*

**systematic desensitisation** /ˌsɪstəmætɪk diːˌsensɪtaɪˈzeɪʃ(ə)n/ *noun* a therapy for phobias and other anxiety disorders in which patients are gradually given longer and longer exposures to the object of their fears

**Système International d'Unités** /sɪˌstem ˌænteənæsjənuːl ˈduːnɪteɪ/ *noun* the International System of units. ◊ **SI**

**systemic** /sɪˈstiːmɪk/ *adjective* referring to or affecting the whole body ○ *Septicaemia is a systemic infection.*

**systemic circulation** /sɪˌstiːmɪk ˌsɜːkjʊˈleɪʃ(ə)n/ *noun* the circulation of blood around the whole body, except the lungs, starting with the aorta and returning through the venae cavae

**systemic lupus erythematosus** /sɪˌstiːmɪk ˌluːpəs ˌerɪθiːməˈtəʊsəs/ *noun* one of several collagen diseases which are forms of lupus, where red patches form on the skin and spread throughout the body. Abbr **SLE**

**systole** /ˈsɪstəli/ *noun* a phase in the beating of the heart when it contracts as it pumps blood out. Opposite **diastole** □ **the heart is in systole** the heart is contracting and pumping

**systolic** /sɪˈstɒlɪk/ *adjective* referring to the systole

**systolic murmur** /sɪˌstɒlɪk ˈmɜːmə/ *noun* a sound produced during systole which indicates an unusual condition of a heart valve

**systolic pressure** /sɪˌstɒlɪk ˈpreʃə/ *noun* the high point of blood pressure which occurs during the systole. Systolic pressure is always higher than diastolic pressure.

# T

**T** *symbol* tera-

**TAB** *abbr* typhoid-paratyphoid A and B ○ *He was given a TAB injection.* ○ *TAB injections give only temporary immunity against paratyphoid.* ◊ **TAB vaccine**

**tabes** /'teɪbiːz/ *noun* a condition in which someone is wasting away

**tabes dorsalis** /ˌteɪbiːz dɔːˈseɪlɪs/ *noun* a disease of the nervous system, caused by advanced syphilis, in which the person loses the sense of feeling, control of the bladder and the ability to coordinate movements of the legs, and has severe pains. Also called **locomotor ataxia**

**tabes mesenterica** /ˌteɪbiːz ˌmesen'terɪkə/ *noun* the wasting of glands in the abdomen

**tabetic** /tə'betɪk/ *adjective* wasting away or affected by tabes dorsalis

**tablet** /'tæblət/ *noun* **1.** a small flat round object containing medicine that is taken by swallowing ○ *a bottle of aspirin tablets* ○ *Take two tablets three times a day.* **2.** any tablet, pill or capsule taken by swallowing (*informal*)

**taboparesis** /ˌteɪbəʊpə'riːsɪs/ *noun* the final stage of syphilis in which the person has locomotor ataxia, general paralysis and mental deterioration

**TAB vaccine** /ˌtiː eɪ 'biː ˌvæksiːn/ *noun* a vaccine which immunises against typhoid fever and paratyphoid A and B

**tachy-** /tæki/ *prefix* fast

**tachyarrhythmia** /ˌtækiə'rɪðmiə/ *noun* a fast irregular heartbeat

**tachycardia** /ˌtæki'kɑːdiə/ *noun* a rapid beating of the heart

**tachyphrasia** /ˌtæki'freɪziə/, **tachyphasia** /ˌtæki'feɪziə/ *noun* a particularly rapid way of speaking, as occurs with some people with mental disorders

**tachyphyl(l)axis** /ˌtækifə'læksɪs/ *noun* an effect of a drug or neurotransmitter which becomes less with repeated doses

**tachypnoea** /ˌtækɪp'niːə/ *noun* very fast breathing

**tacrolimus** /ˌtækrə'liːməs/ *noun* a powerful immunosuppressant drug used to reduce the risk of organ transplant rejection

**tactile** /'tæktaɪl/ *adjective* able to be sensed by touch

**tactile anaesthesia** /ˌtæktaɪl ˌænəs'θiːziə/ *noun* the loss of the sensation of touch

**taenia** /'tiːniə/ *noun* **1.** a long ribbon-like part of the body **2.** a large tapeworm of the genus *Taenia*

COMMENT: The various species of *Taenia* which affect humans are taken into the body from eating meat which has not been properly cooked. The most obvious symptom of tapeworm infestation is a sharply increased appetite, together with a loss of weight. The most common infestations are with *Taenia solium*, found in pork, where the larvae develop in the body and can form hydatid cysts, and *Taenia saginata*, the adult form of which grows to between four and eight metres long in the human intestine.

**taeniacide** /'tiːniəsaɪd/ *noun* a substance which kills tapeworms

**taenia coli** /ˌtiːniə 'kəʊlaɪ/ *noun* the outer band of muscle running along the large intestine

**taeniafuge** /'tiːniəfjuːdʒ/ *noun* a substance which makes tapeworms leave the body

**taeniasis** /tiː'naɪəsɪs/ *noun* infestation of the intestines with tapeworms

**Tagamet** /'tægəmet/ a trade name for a preparation of cimetidine

**tai chi** /ˌtaɪ 'tʃiː/, **t'ai chi** *noun* an ancient Chinese system of exercises designed for health, self-defence and spiritual development

**take** /teɪk/ *verb* **1.** to swallow a medicine ○ *She has to take her tablets three times a day.* ○ *The medicine should be taken in a glass of water.* **2.** to do particular actions ○ *The dentist took an X-ray of his teeth.* ○ *The patient has been allowed to take a bath.* **3.** (*of graft*) to be accepted by the body ○ *The skin graft hasn't taken.* ○ *The kidney transplant took easily.* (NOTE: **taking – took – taken**)

**take after** /'teɪk ˌɑːftə/ *verb* to be like one or other parent ○ *He takes after his father.*

**take care of** /ˌteɪk ˈkeə əv/ *verb* to look after someone ○ *The nurses will take care of the accident victims.*

**take off** /ˌteɪk ˈɒf/ *verb* to remove something, especially clothes ○ *The doctor asked him to take his shirt off or to take off his shirt.*

**talc** /tælk/ *noun* a soft white powder used to dust on irritated skin

**talcum powder** /ˈtælkəm ˌpaʊdə/ *noun* scented talc

**tali** /ˈteɪli/ plural of **talus**

**talipes** /ˈtælɪpiːz/ *noun* a foot with a shape that does not allow usual walking, a congenital condition. Also called **cleft foot, club foot**

COMMENT: The most usual form of talipes (**talipes equinovarus**) is where the person walks on the toes because the foot is permanently bent forward. In other forms, the foot either turns towards the inside (**talipes varus**), towards the outside (**talipes valgus**) or upwards at the ankle (**talipes calcaneus**) so that the person cannot walk on the sole of the foot.

**tall** /tɔːl/ *adjective* high, usually higher than other people ○ *He's the tallest in the family – he's taller than all his brothers.* ○ *How tall is he?* ○ *He's 5 foot 7 inches (5'7") tall or 1.25 metres tall.*

**talo-** /teɪləʊ/ *prefix* referring to the ankle bone

**talus** /ˈteɪləs/ *noun* the top bone in the tarsus which articulates with the tibia and fibula in the leg, and with the calcaneus in the heel. Also called **anklebone**. See illustration at FOOT in Supplement (NOTE: The plural is **tali**.)

**tamoxifen** /təˈmɒksɪfen/ *noun* a drug which helps to prevent the actions of oestrogen, used especially in the treatment of breast cancer and some types of infertility

**tampon** /ˈtæmpɒn/ *noun* **1.** a wad of absorbent material put into a wound to soak up blood during an operation **2.** a cylindrical plug of soft material put into the vagina to absorb blood during menstruation

**tamponade** /ˌtæmpəˈneɪd/ *noun* **1.** the action of putting a tampon into a wound **2.** abnormal pressure on part of the body

**tan** /tæn/ *verb* (*of skin*) to become brown in sunlight ○ *He tans easily.* ○ *She is using a tanning lotion.*

**tannin** /ˈtænɪn/, **tannic acid** /ˈtænɪk ˈæsɪd/ *noun* a substance found in the bark of trees and in tea and other liquids, which stains brown

**tantalum** /ˈtæntələm/ *noun* a rare metal, used to repair damaged bones (NOTE: The chemical symbol is **Ta**.)

**tantalum mesh** /ˈtæntələm meʃ/ *noun* a type of net made of tantalum wire, used to repair cranial conditions

**tantrum** /ˈtæntrəm/ *noun* a sudden episode of bad behaviour, usually in a child, where the child throws things or lies on the floor and screams

**tap** /tæp/ *noun* **1.** a surgical procedure to drain off body fluid with a hollow needle or a tube **2.** a pipe with a closing valve and a handle which can be turned to make a liquid or gas come out of a container ■ *verb* **1.** to remove or drain liquid from part of the body. ◊ **spinal 2.** to hit someone or something lightly ○ *The doctor tapped his chest with his finger.*

**tape** /teɪp/ *noun* a long thin flat piece of material

**tapeworm** /ˈteɪpwɜːm/ *noun* a parasitic worm with a small head and long body like a ribbon. Tapeworms enter the intestine when a person eats raw meat or fish. The worms attach themselves with hooks to the side of the intestine and grow longer by adding sections to their bodies.

**tapotement** /təˈpəʊtmənt/ *noun* a type of massage where the therapist taps the person with his or her hands

**tapping** /ˈtæpɪŋ/ *noun* same as **paracentesis**

**target** /ˈtɑːɡɪt/ *noun* a place which is to be hit by something ◊ **target cell, target organ 1.** cell or organ which is affected by a drug, by a hormone or by a disease **2.** large red blood cell which shows a red spot in the middle when stained

'…the target cells for adult myeloid leukaemia are located in the bone marrow' [*British Medical Journal*]

**tarry stool** /ˌtɑːri ˈstuːl/ *noun* dark and sticky solid matter which is passed out of the bowels

**tars-** /tɑːs/ *prefix* same as **tarso-** (*used before vowels*)

**tarsal** /ˈtɑːs(ə)l/ *adjective* referring to the tarsus ■ *noun* same as **tarsal bone**

**tarsal bone** /ˈtɑːs(ə)l bəʊn/ *noun* one of seven small bones in the ankle, including the talus and calcaneus. Also called **tarsal**

**tarsalgia** /tɑːˈsældʒə/ *noun* a pain in the ankle

**tarsal gland** /ˈtɑːs(ə)l glænd/ *noun* same as **meibomian gland**

**tarsectomy** /tɑːˈsektəmi/ *noun* **1.** a surgical operation to remove one of the tarsal bones in the ankle **2.** a surgical operation to remove the tarsus of the eyelid

**tarsitis** /tɑːˈsaɪtɪs/ *noun* an inflammation of the edge of the eyelid

**tarso-** /tɑːsəʊ/ *prefix* **1.** relating to the ankle **2.** relating to the edge of the eyelid

**tarsorrhaphy** /tɑːˈsɒrəfi/ *noun* an operation to join the two eyelids together to protect the eye after an operation

**tarsotomy** /tɑːˈsɒtəmi/ *noun* an incision of the tarsus of the eyelid

**tarsus** /ˈtɑːsəs/ *noun* **1.** the seven small bones of the ankle. See illustration at FOOT in Supplement **2.** a connective tissue which supports an eyelid (NOTE: The plural is **tarsi**.)

COMMENT: The seven bones of the tarsus are: calcaneus, cuboid, the three cuneiforms, navicular and talus.

**tartar** /'tɑːtə/ *noun* a hard deposit of calcium which forms on teeth, and has to be removed by scaling. Also called **scale**

**tartrazine** /'tɑːtrəziːn/ *noun* a yellow substance (E102) added to food to give it an attractive colour. Although widely used, tartrazine provokes reactions in hypersensitive people and is banned in some countries.

**task allocation** /'tɑːsk ælə,keɪʃ(ə)n/ *noun* a system in which patient care is divided into tasks which are given to different nurses with specific skills

**taste** /teɪst/ *noun* one of the five senses, where food or substances in the mouth are noticed through the tongue ○ *She doesn't like the taste of onions.* ○ *He has a cold, so food seems to have lost all taste* or *seems to have no taste.* ■ *verb* 1. to notice the taste of something with the tongue ○ *I have a cold so I can't taste anything* ○ *You can taste the salt in this butter.* 2. to have a taste ○ *The tablets taste of peppermint.*

**taste bud** /'teɪst bʌd/ *noun* a tiny sensory receptor in the vallate and fungiform papillae of the tongue and in part of the back of the mouth
COMMENT: The taste buds can tell the difference between salt, sour, bitter and sweet tastes. The buds on the tip of the tongue identify salt and sweet tastes, those on the sides of the tongue identify sour, and those at the back of the mouth the bitter tastes. Note that most of what we think of as taste is in fact smell, and this is why when someone has a cold and a blocked nose, food seems to lose its taste. The impulses from the taste buds are received by the taste cortex in the temporal lobe of the cerebral hemisphere.

**taurine** /'tɔːriːn/ *noun* an amino acid which forms bile salts

**taxis** /'tæksɪs/ *noun* the procedure of pushing or massaging dislocated bones or hernias to make them return to their usual position

**-taxis** /tæksɪs/ *suffix* manipulation

**taxonomy** /tæk'sɒnəmi/ *noun* 1. the practice or principles of classification generally ○ *Any diagnostic task can be aided by a taxonomy of symptoms and a taxonomy of causes together with connections between them.* 2. the science of classifying plants, animals and microorganisms into increasingly broader categories based on shared features. Traditionally, organisms were grouped by physical resemblances, but recently other criteria such as genetic matching have also been used.

**Tay-Sachs disease** /,teɪ 'sæks dɪ,ziːz/ *noun* an inherited condition affecting the metabolism, characterised by progressive paralysis of the legs, blindness and learning disabilities [Described 1881. After Warren Tay (1843–1927), British ophthalmologist; Bernard Sachs (1858–1944), US neurologist.]

**TB** *abbr* tuberculosis ○ *He is suffering from TB.* ○ *She has been admitted to a TB sanatorium.*

**T bandage** /'tiː ,bændɪdʒ/ *noun* a bandage shaped like the letter T, used for bandaging the area between the legs

**TBI** *abbreviation* total body irradiation

**T-cell** /'tiː sel/ *noun* same as **T-lymphocyte**

**TCP** a trade name for various mild antiseptic liquids

**t.d.s., TDS** *adverb* (written on prescriptions) three times a day. Full form **ter in diem sumendus**

**tea** /tiː/ *noun* 1. the dried leaves of a plant used to make a hot drink 2. a hot drink made by pouring boiling water onto the dried leaves of a plant

**teach** /tiːtʃ/ *verb* 1. to give lessons in something ○ *Professor Smith teaches neurosurgery.* 2. to show someone how to do something ○ *She was taught first aid by her mother.* (NOTE: **teaching – taught**)

**teaching hospital** /'tiːtʃɪŋ ,hɒspɪt(ə)l/ *noun* a hospital attached to a medical school where student doctors work and study as part of their training

**team** /tiːm/ *noun* a group of people who work together ○ *The heart-lung transplant was carried out by a team of surgeons.*

**team nursing** /'tiːm ,nɜːsɪŋ/ *noun* a system in which the care of a group of patients is assigned to a team of four or five health workers, led by a professional nurse who assigns them various tasks. They meet at the beginning and end of each shift to exchange information.

**tear** /tɪə/ *noun* 1. a drop of the salty fluid which forms in the lacrimal gland. The fluid keeps the eyeball moist and clean and is produced in large quantities when a person cries. ○ *Tears ran down her face.* (NOTE: For other terms referring to tears, see words beginning with **dacryo-** or **lacrimal**.) □ **she burst into tears** she suddenly started to cry 2. /teə/ a hole or a split in a tissue often due to over-stretching ○ *An episiotomy was needed to avoid a tear in the perineal tissue.* ■ *verb* to make a hole or a split in a tissue by pulling or stretching it too much ○ *He tore a ligament in his ankle.* ○ *They carried out an operation to repair a torn ligament.* (NOTE: **tearing – tore – torn**)

**tear duct** /'tɪə dʌkt/ *noun* same as **lacrimal duct**

**tear gland** /'tɪə glænd/ *noun* same as **lacrimal gland**

**teat** /tiːt/ *noun* a rubber nipple on the end of a baby's feeding bottle

**technician** /tek'nɪʃ(ə)n/ *noun* a qualified person who does practical work in a laboratory or scientific institution ○ *He is a laboratory technician in a laboratory attached to a teaching hospital.*

**technique** /tek'niːk/ *noun* a way of doing scientific or medical work ○ *a new technique for treating osteoarthritis* ○ *She is trying out a new laboratory technique.*

'…few parts of the body are inaccessible to modern catheter techniques, which are all performed under local anaesthesia' [*British Medical Journal*]

'…the technique used to treat aortic stenosis is similar to that for any cardiac catheterization' [*Journal of the American Medical Association*]

'…cardiac resuscitation techniques used by over half the nurses in a recent study were described as 'completely ineffective'' [*Nursing Times*]

**tectorial membrane** /tek,tɔːriəl 'membreɪn/ *noun* a membrane in the inner ear which contains the hair cells which transmit impulses to the auditory nerve

**tectospinal tract** /,tektəʊ,spaɪn(ə)l 'trækt/ *noun* a tract which takes nerve impulses from the mesencephalon to the spinal cord

**TED** *abbr* thrombo-embolic deterrent stocking

**teeth** /tiːθ/ *plural of* **tooth**

**teething** /'tiːðɪŋ/ *noun* the period when a baby's milk teeth are starting to erupt, and the baby is irritable ○ *He is awake at night because he is teething.* ○ *She has teething trouble and won't eat.*

**Teflon** /'teflɒn/ *trademark* a synthetic polymer injected into the joints of the larynx to increase movement and help hoarseness of voice

**tegmen** /'tegmən/ *noun* the covering for an organ (NOTE: The plural is **tegmina**.)

**tegument** /'tegjʊmənt/ *noun* a covering, especially the protective outer covering of an organism

**tel-** /tel/ *prefix* same as **tele-** (*used before vowels*)

**tela** /'tiːlə/ *noun* a delicate part or tissue in the body with a fine or intricate pattern like a web

**telangiectasia** /te,lændʒiek'teɪsiə/ *noun* a condition in which the small blood vessels, especially in the face and thighs, are permanently dilated producing dark red blotches

**telangiectasis** /te,lændʒi'ektəsɪs/, **telangiectasia** /te,lændʒiek'teɪsiə/ *noun* small dark red spots on the skin, formed by swollen capillaries

**telangioma** /te,lændʒi'əʊmə/ *noun* a tumour or haematoma of the blood capillaries

**tele-** /teli/ *prefix* referring to distance

**teleceptor** /'telɪseptə/ *noun* a sensory receptor which receives sensations from a distance. These occur in the eyes, ears and nose. Also called **telereceptor**

**telemedicine** /'telimed(ə)sɪn/ *noun* the provision of diagnosis and health care from a distance using media such as interactive computer programs or off-site advisers

**telencephalon** /,telen'kefəlɒn/ *noun* same as **cerebrum**

**telepathy** /tə'lepəθi/ *noun* the apparent communication directly from one person's mind to

another person's, without the use of speech, writing or other signs or symbols

**teleradiography** /,telireɪdi'ɒgrəfi/ *noun* a type of radiography where the source of the X-rays is at a distance from the person being X-rayed

**teleradiology** /,telireɪdi'ɒlədʒi/ *noun* the process of transmitting scans and other images electronically so that they can be viewed by surgeons or other health care workers in different locations at the same time

**teleradiotherapy** /telireɪdiəʊ'θerəpi/ *noun* a type of radiotherapy, where the person being treated is some way away from the source of radiation

**telereceptor** /'telɪriseptə/ *noun* same as **teleceptor**

**telo-** /teləʊ/ *prefix* referring to an end

**telophase** /'teləʊfeɪz/ *noun* the final stage of mitosis, the stage in cell division after anaphase

**temazepam** /tə'mæzɪpæm/ *noun* a hypnotic drug used in the short-term treatment of insomnia

**temperature** /'temprɪtʃə/ *noun* **1.** the heat of the body or of the surrounding air, measured in degrees ○ *The doctor asked the nurse what the patient's temperature was.* ○ *His temperature was slightly above normal.* ○ *The thermometer showed a temperature of 99°F.* □ **to take a patient's temperature** to insert a thermometer in someone's body to see what his or her body temperature is ○ *They took his temperature every four hours.* ○ *When her temperature was taken this morning, it was normal.* **2.** illness when your body is hotter than normal ○ *He's in bed with a temperature.* ○ *Her mother says she's got a temperature, and can't come to work.*

COMMENT: The average body temperature is about 37° Celsius or 98° Fahrenheit. This temperature may vary during the day, and can rise if a person has taken a hot bath or had a hot drink. If the environmental temperature is high, the body has to sweat to reduce the heat gained from the air around it. If the outside temperature is low, the body shivers, because rapid movement of the muscles generates heat. A fever will cause the body temperature to rise sharply, to 40°C (103°F) or more. Hypothermia exists when the body temperature falls below about 35°C (95°F).

**temperature chart** /'temprɪtʃə tʃɑːt/ *noun* a chart showing changes in a person's temperature over a period of time

**temperature graph** /'temprɪtʃə grɑːf/ *noun* a graph showing how a person's temperature rises and falls over a period of time

**temper tantrum** /'tempə ,tæntrəm/ *noun* ➧ **tantrum**

**temple** /'tempəl/ *noun* the flat part of the side of the head between the top of the ear and the eye

**temporal** /'temp(ə)rəl/ *adjective* referring to the temple

**temporal arteritis** /,temp(ə)rəl ɑːtəˈraɪtɪs/ *noun* a headache caused by inflammation of the region over the temporal artery, usually occurring in older people

**temporal bone** /'tempərəl bəʊn/ *noun* one of the bones which form the sides and base of the cranium. See illustration at EAR in Supplement

COMMENT: The temporal bone is in two parts: the petrous part forms the base of the skull and the inner and middle ears, while the squamous part forms the side of the skull. The lower back part of the temporal bone is the mastoid process, while the part between the ear and the cheek is the zygomatic arch.

**temporal fossa** /,temp(ə)rəl 'fɒsə/ *noun* a depression in the side of the head, in the temporal bone above the zygomatic arch

**temporalis** /,tempə'reɪlɪs/, **temporalis muscle** /,tempə'reɪlɪs ,mʌs(ə)l/ *noun* a flat muscle running down the side of the head from the temporal bone to the coronoid process, which makes the jaw move up

**temporal lobe** /'temp(ə)rəl ləʊb/ *noun* the lobe above the ear in each cerebral hemisphere

**temporal lobe epilepsy** /,temp(ə)rəl ləʊb 'epɪlepsi/ *noun* epilepsy due to a disorder of the temporal lobe and causing impaired memory, hallucinations and automatism

**temporary** /'temp(ə)rəri/ *adjective* not permanent ○ *The dentist gave him a temporary filling.* ○ *The accident team put a temporary bandage on the wound.*

**temporo-** /tempərəʊ/ *prefix* **1.** referring to the temple **2.** referring to the temporal lobe

**temporomandibular** /,tempərəʊmæn'dɪbjʊlə/ *adjective* relating to the temporal bone and the mandible

**temporomandibular joint** /,tempərəʊ mæn'dɪbjʊlə ,dʒɔɪnt/ *noun* a joint between the jaw and the skull, in front of the ear

**temporomandibular syndrome** /,tempərəʊmæn'dɪbjʊlə ,sɪndrəʊm/ *noun* a painful condition affecting the temporomandibular joint and the muscles used for chewing, usually associated with a faulty meeting of the teeth in biting and sometimes causing clicking sounds

**tenacious** /tɪ'neɪʃəs/ *adjective* sticking or clinging to something else, especially a surface

**tenaculum** /tə'nækjʊləm/ *noun* a surgical instrument shaped like a hook, used to pick up small pieces of tissue during an operation

**tend** /tend/ *verb* **1.** □ **to tend to do something** to be inclined to do something as a normal process ○ *The prostate tends to enlarge as a man grows older.* **2.** to care for or attend to someone or something

**tendency** /'tendənsi/ *noun* the fact of being likely to do something □ **to have a tendency to something** to be likely to have something ○ *There is a tendency to obesity in her family.* ○ *The children of the area show a tendency to vitamin-deficiency diseases.*

'…premature babies have been shown to have a higher tendency to develop a squint during childhood' [*Nursing Times*]

**tender** /'tendə/ *adjective* referring to skin or a body part which is painful when touched ○ *The bruise is still tender.* ○ *Her shoulders are still tender where she got sunburnt.* ○ *A tender spot on the abdomen indicates that an organ is inflamed.*

**tenderness** /'tendənəs/ *noun* a feel of pain when touched ○ *Tenderness when pressure is applied is a sign of inflammation.*

**tendinitis** /,tendɪ'naɪtɪs/ *noun* an inflammation of a tendon, especially after playing sport, and often associated with tenosynovitis

**tendinous** /'tendɪnəs/ *adjective* referring to a tendon

**tendo calcaneus** /,tendəʊ kæl'keɪniəs/ *noun* the Achilles tendon, the tendon at the back of the ankle which connects the calf muscles to the heel and which acts to pull up the heel when the calf muscle is contracted

**tendon** /'tendən/ *noun* a strip of connective tissue which attaches a muscle to a bone. Also called **sinew** (NOTE: For other terms referring to a tendon, see words beginning with **teno-**.)

**tendonitis** /,tendə'naɪtɪs/ *noun* same as **tendinitis**

**tendon sheath** /'tendən ʃiːθ/ *noun* a tube of membrane which covers and protects a tendon

**tendovaginitis** /,tendəʊvædʒɪ'naɪtɪs/ *noun* an inflammation of a tendon sheath, especially in the thumb

**tenesmus** /tə'nezməs/ *noun* a condition in which someone feels the need to pass faeces, or sometimes urine, but is unable to do so and experiences pain

**tennis elbow** /,tenɪs 'elbəʊ/ *noun* an inflammation of the tendons of the extensor muscles in the hand which are attached to the bone near the elbow. Also called **lateral epicondylitis**

**teno-** /tenəʊ/ *prefix* referring to a tendon

**tenonitis** /,tenəʊ'naɪtɪs/ *noun* the inflammation of a tendon

**Tenon's capsule** /'tiːnɒns ,kæpsjuːl/ *noun* a tissue which lines the orbit of the eye [After Jacques René Tenon (1724–1816), French surgeon]

**tenoplasty** /'tenəplæsti/ *noun* a surgical operation to repair a torn tendon

**tenorrhaphy** /te'nɒrəfi/ *noun* a surgical operation to stitch pieces of a torn tendon together

**tenosynovitis** /,tenəʊ,saɪnə'vaɪtɪs/ *noun* a painful inflammation of the tendon sheath and the tendon inside. Also called **peritendinitis**

**tenotomy** /təˈnɒtəmi/ *noun* a surgical operation to cut through a tendon

**tenovaginitis** /ˌtenəʊˌvædʒɪˈnaɪtɪs/ *noun* inflammation of the tendon sheath, especially in the thumb

**TENS** /tens/ *abbreviation* a method of treating pain by applying electrodes to the skin. Small electric currents are passed through sensory nerves and the spinal cord. This suppresses the transmission of pain signals. ○ *a TENS unit or machine* Full form **transcutaneous electrical nerve stimulation**

**tense** /tens/ *adjective* **1.** (*of a muscle*) contracted **2.** nervous and worried ○ *The patient was very tense while she waited for the report from the laboratory.*

**tension** /ˈtenʃən/ *noun* **1.** the act of stretching or the state of being stretched **2.** an emotional strain or stress

**tension headache** /ˈtenʃən ˌhedeɪk/ *noun* a headache all over the head, caused by worry and stress

**tension pneumothorax** /ˈtenʃən njuːməʊˌθɔːræks/ *noun* a condition of the pneumothorax in which rupture of the pleura forms an opening like a valve, through which air is forced during coughing but cannot escape

**tensor** /ˈtensə/ *noun* a muscle which makes a joint stretch out

**tent** /tent/ *noun* a small shelter put over and around someone's bed so that gas or vapour can be passed inside

**tentorium cerebelli** /tenˌtɔːriəm ˌserəˈbeli/ *noun* a part of the dura mater which separates the cerebellum from the cerebral hemispheres

**tera-** /ˈterə/ *prefix* $10^{12}$. Symbol **T**

**terat-** /ˈterət/, **terato-** /ˈterətəʊ/ *prefix* congenitally unusual

**teratocarcinoma** /ˌterətəʊkɑːsɪˈnəʊmə/ *noun* a malignant teratoma, usually in the testes

**teratogen** /təˈrætədʒen/ *noun* a substance which causes the usual development of an embryo or fetus to be disrupted, e.g. the German measles virus

**teratogenesis** /ˌterətəˈdʒenəsɪs/ *noun* an unusual pattern of development in an embryo and fetus

**teratogenic** /ˌterətəˈdʒenɪk/ *adjective* **1.** having the tendency to produce physical disorders in an embryo or fetus **2.** relating to the production of physical disorders in an embryo or fetus

**teratology** /ˌterəˈtɒlədʒi/ *noun* the study of the unhealthy development of embryos and fetuses

**teratoma** /ˌterəˈtəʊmə/ *noun* a tumour, especially in an ovary or testis, which is formed of tissue not usually found in that part of the body

**terbutaline** /tɜːˈbjuːtəliːn/ *noun* a drug which relaxes muscles, used in the treatment

of respiratory disorders and to control premature labour

**teres** /ˈtɪəriːz/ *noun* one of two shoulder muscles running from the shoulder blade to the top of the humerus. The larger of the two muscles, the teres major, makes the arm turn towards the inside, and the smaller, the teres minor, makes it turn towards the outside.

**terfenadine** /tɜːˈfenədiːn/ *noun* an antihistamine used in the treatment of hay fever and urticaria

**term** /tɜːm/ *noun* **1.** a limited period of time, especially the period from conception to childbirth, or a point in time determined for an event □ **she was coming near to term** she was near the time when she would give birth **2.** part of a college or school year ○ *The anatomy exams are at the beginning of the third term.* **3.** a name or word for a particular thing

**terminal** /ˈtɜːmɪn(ə)l/ *adjective* **1.** referring to the last stage of a fatal illness ○ *The disease is in its terminal stages.* **2.** referring to the end, being at the end of something ○ *He is suffering from terminal cancer.* ■ *noun* an ending, a part at the end of an electrode or nerve

**terminal branch** /ˈtɜːmɪn(ə)l brɑːntʃ/ *noun* the end part of a neurone which is linked to a muscle. See illustration at **NEURONE** in Supplement

**terminale** /ˌtɜːmɪˈneɪli/ ♦ **filum terminale**

**terminal illness** /ˌtɜːmɪn(ə)l ˈɪlnəs/ *noun* an illness from which someone will soon die

**terminally ill** /ˌtɜːmɪnəli ˈɪl/ *adjective* very ill and about to die ○ *She was admitted to a hospice for terminally ill patients* or *for the terminally ill.*

**termination** /ˌtɜːmɪˈneɪʃ(ə)n/ *noun* the act of ending something □ **termination (of pregnancy)** abortion

**-terol** /terɒl/ *suffix* used in names of bronchodilators

**tertian** /ˈtɜːʃ(ə)n/ *adjective* referring to a fever with symptoms which appear every other day ■ *noun* a tertian fever or set of symptoms

**tertian fever** /ˈtɜːʃ(ə)n ˌfiːvə/ *noun* a type of malaria where the fever returns every two days. ◊ **quartan fever**

**tertiary** /ˈtɜːʃəri/ *adjective* third, coming after secondary and primary

**tertiary bronchi** /ˌtɜːʃəri ˈbrɒŋkiː/ *plural noun* ◊ **syphilis**. Same as **segmental bronchi**

**tertiary care** /ˌtɜːʃəri ˈkeə/, **tertiary health care** /ˌtɜːʃəri ˈhelθ keə/ *noun* highly specialised treatment given in a health care centre, often using very advanced technology. Compare **primary care**, **secondary care**

**test** /test/ *noun* a short examination to see if a sample is healthy or if part of the body is working well ○ *He had an eye test this morning.* ○ *Laboratory tests showed that she was a meningitis carrier.* ○ *Tests are being carried out on* *swabs taken from the operating theatre.* □ **the urine test was positive** the examination of the urine sample showed the presence of an infection or a diagnostic substance ■ *verb* to examine a sample of tissue to see if it is healthy or an organ to see if it is working well ○ *They sent the urine sample away for testing.* ○ *I must have my eyes tested.*

**testes** /'testiːz/ plural of **testis**

**testicle** /'testɪk(ə)l/ *noun* same as **testis**

**testicular** /te'stɪkjʊlə/ *adjective* referring to the testes ○ *Testicular cancer comprises only 1% of all malignant neoplasms in the male.*

**testicular artery** /te,stɪkjʊlə 'ɑːtəri/ *noun* same as **spermatic artery**

**testicular hormone** /te,stɪkjʊlə 'hɔːməʊn/ *noun* testosterone

**testis** /'testɪs/ *noun* one of two male sex glands in the scrotum. See illustration at **URO-GENITAL SYSTEM (MALE)** in Supplement. Also called **testicle** (NOTE: The plural is **testes**. For other terms referring to the testes, see words beginning with **orchi-**.)

COMMENT: The testes produce both spermatozoa and the sex hormone, testosterone. Spermatozoa are formed in the testes, and passed into the epididymis to be stored. From the epididymis they pass along the vas deferens through the prostate gland which secretes the seminal fluid, and are ejaculated through the penis.

**test meal** /'test miːl/ *noun* a test to check the secretion of gastric juices, no longer much used

**testosterone** /te'stɒstərəʊn/ *noun* a male sex hormone, secreted by the Leydig cells in the testes, which causes physical changes, e.g. the development of body hair and a deep voice, to take place in males as they become sexually mature

**test tube** /'test tjuːb/ *noun* a small glass tube with a rounded bottom, used in laboratories to hold samples of liquids

**test-tube baby** /'test tjuːb ,beɪbi/ *noun* a baby conceived through in vitro fertilisation in which the mother's ova are removed from the ovaries, fertilised with a man's spermatozoa in a laboratory, and returned to the mother's uterus to continue developing in the usual way

**tetanic** /te'tænɪk/ *adjective* referring to tetanus

**tetano-** /tetanəʊ/ *prefix* **1.** relating to tetanus **2.** relating to tetany

**tetanus** /'tet(ə)nəs/ *noun* **1.** the continuous contraction of a muscle, under repeated stimuli from a motor nerve **2.** an infection caused by *Clostridium tetani* in the soil, which affects the spinal cord and causes spasms in the muscles which occur first in the jaw. Also called **lock-jaw**

COMMENT: People who are liable to infection with tetanus, such as farm workers, should be immunised against it, and booster injections are needed from time to time.

**tetany** /'tetəni/ *noun* spasms of the muscles in the feet and hands, caused by a reduction in the level of calcium in the blood or by lack of carbon dioxide

**tetra-** /tetrə/ *prefix* four

**tetracycline** /,tetrə'saɪkliːn/ *noun* an antibiotic of a group used to treat a wide range of bacterial diseases such as chlamydia. However, they are deposited in bones and teeth and cause a permanent yellow stain in teeth if given to children.

COMMENT: Because of its side-effects tetracycline should not be given to children. Many bacteria are now resistant to tetracycline.

**tetradactyly** /,tetrə'dæktɪli/ *noun* a congenital condition in which a child has only four fingers or toes

**tetralogy of Fallot** /te,trælədʒi əv 'fæləʊ/ *noun* a disorder of the heart which makes a child's skin blue. Also called **Fallot's tetralogy**. ◊ **Blalock's operation, Waterston's operation**

COMMENT: The condition is formed of four conditions occurring together: the artery leading to the lungs is narrow, the right ventricle is enlarged, there is a disorder in the membrane between the ventricles and the aorta is not correctly placed.

**tetraplegia** /,tetrə'pliːdʒə/ same as **quadriplegia**

**textbook** /'tekstbʊk/ *noun* a book which is used by students ○ *a haematology textbook* or *a textbook on haematology*

**textbook case** /'tekstbʊk keɪs/ *noun* a case which shows symptoms which are exactly like those described in a textbook, a very typical case

**thalam-** /θæləm/ *prefix* same as **thalamo-** (used before vowels)

**thalamencephalon** /,θæləmen'kefəlɒn/ *noun* a group of structures in the brain linked to the brain stem, formed of the epithalamus, hypothalamus and thalamus

**thalamic syndrome** /θə'læmɪk ,sɪndrəʊm/ *noun* a condition in which someone is extremely sensitive to pain, caused by a disorder of the thalamus

**thalamo-** /θæləməʊ/ *prefix* referring to the thalamus

**thalamocortical tract** /,θæləməʊ ,kɔːtɪk(ə)l 'trækt/ *noun* a tract containing nerve fibres, running from the thalamus to the sensory cortex

**thalamotomy** /,θælə'mɒtəmi/ *noun* a surgical operation to make an incision into the thalamus to treat intractable pain

**thalamus** /'θæləməs/ *noun* one of two masses of grey matter situated beneath the cerebrum where impulses from the sensory neurones are transmitted to the cerebral cortex.

See illustration at BRAIN in Supplement (NOTE: The plural is **thalami**.)

**thalassaemia** /ˌθælæˈsiːmiə/ *noun* a hereditary disorder of which there are several forms caused by an anomalies in the protein component of the haemoglobin, leading to severe anaemia. It is found especially in people from Mediterranean countries, the Middle East and East Asia. Also called **Cooley's anaemia**

**thalidomide** /θəˈlɪdəmaɪd/ *noun* a synthetic drug given to pregnant women for morning sickness in the 1960s which caused babies to be born with stunted limbs. It is now used in the treatment of leprosy.

**thallium scan** /ˈθæliəm skæn/ *noun* a method of finding out about the blood supply to the heart muscle by scanning to see how the radioactive element thallium moves when injected into the bloodstream and where it attaches itself to the heart wall

**thanatology** /ˌθænəˈtɒlədʒi/ *noun* the study of the medical, psychological and sociological aspects of death and the ways in which people deal with it

**thaw** /θɔː/ *verb* to bring something which is frozen back to usual temperature

**theatre** /ˈθɪətə/ *noun* ♦ **operating theatre**

'While waiting to go to theatre, parents should be encouraged to participate in play with their children' [*British Journal of Nursing*]

**theatre gown** /ˈθɪətə ɡaʊn/ *noun* **1.** a loose piece of clothing worn by a person having an operation **2.** a long green robe worn over other clothes by a surgeon or nurse in an operating theatre

**theatre nurse** /ˈθɪətə nɜːs/ *noun* a nurse who is specially trained to assist a surgeon during an operation

**theca** /ˈθiːkə/ *noun* tissue shaped like a sheath

**thelarche** /ˈθelɑːki/ *noun* the beginning of the process of breast development in young women

**thenar** /ˈθiːnə/ *adjective* referring to the palm of the hand ■ *noun* the palm of the hand. Compare **hypothenar**

**thenar eminence** /ˌθiːnər ˈemɪnəns/ *noun* the ball of the thumb, the lump of flesh in the palm of the hand below the thumb

**theophylline** /θiˈɒfɪliːn/ *noun* a compound made synthetically or extracted from tea leaves which helps to widen blood vessels and airways, and to stimulate the central nervous system and heart. It is used in the treatment of breathing disorders.

**theory** /ˈθɪəri/ *noun* an argument which explains a scientific fact

**therapeutic** /ˌθerəˈpjuːtɪk/ *adjective* given in order to cure a disorder or disease

**therapeutic abortion** /ˌθerəpjuːtɪk əˈbɔːʃ(ə)n/ *noun* an abortion which is carried out because the health of the mother is in danger

**therapeutic index** /ˌθerəpjuːtɪk ˈɪndeks/ *noun* the ratio of the dose of a drug which causes cell damage to the dose of that drug which is typically needed to effect a cure, by which the safety of the drug is decided

**therapeutic radiographer** /ˌθerəpjuːtɪk ˌreɪdiˈɒɡrəfə/ *noun* someone specially trained to use X-rays or radioactive isotopes in the treatment of patients

**therapeutics** /ˌθerəˈpjuːtɪks/ *noun* the study of various types of treatment and their effect on patients

**therapist** /ˈθerəpɪst/ *noun* a person specially trained to give therapy ○ *an occupational therapist* ◊ **psychotherapist**

**therapy** /ˈθerəpi/ *noun* the treatment of a person to help cure a disease or disorder

**therm** /θɜːm/ *noun* a unit of heat equal to 100,000 British thermal units or $1.055 \times 10^8$ joules

**thermal** /ˈθɜːm(ə)l/ *adjective* referring to heat

**thermal anaesthesia** /ˌθɜːm(ə)l ˌænəsˈθiːziə/ *noun* the loss of the feeling of heat

**thermo-** /θɜːməʊ/ *prefix* referring to heat or temperature

**thermoanaesthesia** /ˌθɜːməʊˌænəsˈθiːziə/ *noun* a condition in which someone cannot tell the difference between hot and cold

**thermocautery** /ˌθɜːməʊˈkɔːtəri/ *noun* the procedure of removing dead tissue by heat

**thermocoagulation** /ˌθɜːməʊkəʊˌæɡjuˈleɪʃ(ə)n/ *noun* the procedure of removing tissue and coagulating blood by heat

**thermogram** /ˈθɜːməɡræm/ *noun* an infrared photograph of part of the body

**thermograph** /ˈθɜːməʊɡrɑːf/ *noun* a device that shows patterns of heat radiated from a body, used in diagnosis

**thermography** /θɜːˈmɒɡrəfi/ *noun* a technique, used especially in screening for breast cancer, where part of the body is photographed using infrared rays which record the heat given off by the skin and show variations in the blood circulating beneath the skin

**thermolysis** /θɜːˈmɒləsɪs/ *noun* a loss of body temperature, e.g. by sweating

**thermometer** /θəˈmɒmɪtə/ *noun* an instrument for measuring temperature

**thermophilic** /ˌθɜːməʊˈfɪlɪk/ *adjective* referring to an organism which needs a high temperature to grow

**thermoreceptor** /ˌθɜːməʊrɪˈseptə/ *noun* a sensory nerve which registers heat

**thermotaxis** /ˌθɜːməʊˈtæksɪs/ *noun* an automatic regulation of the body's temperature

**thermotherapy** /ˌθɜːməʊˈθerəpi/ *noun* treatment using heat, e.g. from hot water or infrared lamps, to treat conditions such as arthritis and bad circulation. Also called **heat therapy**

**thiamine** /ˈθaɪəmiːn/, **thiamin** /ˈθaɪəmɪn/ *noun* same as **Vitamin B₁**

**thicken** /'θɪkən/ *verb* **1.** to become wider or larger, or cause something to become wider or larger ○ *The walls of the arteries thicken under deposits of fat.* **2.** (*of liquid*) to become more dense and viscid and flow less easily ○ *The liquid thickens as its cools.*

**Thiersch graft** /'tɪəʃ grɑːft/, **Thiersch's graft** /'tɪəʃɪz grɑːft/ same as **split-skin graft**

**thigh** /θaɪ/ *noun* the top part of the leg from the knee to the groin

**thighbone** /'θaɪbəʊn/ *noun* the femur, the bone in the top part of the leg, which joins the acetabulum at the hip and the tibia at the knee (NOTE: For other terms referring to the thigh, see **femoral**.)

**thin** /θɪn/ *adjective* **1.** not fat ○ *His arms are very thin.* ○ *She's getting too thin – she should eat more.* ○ *He became quite thin after his illness.* **2.** not thick ○ *They cut a thin slice of tissue for examination under the microscope.* **3.** referring to blood which is watery (NOTE: **thinner – thinnest**)

**thiopental sodium** /ˌθaɪəʊpent(ə)l 'səʊdiəm/ *noun* a barbiturate drug used as a rapid-acting intravenous general anaesthetic. Also called **thiopentone**

**thiopentone** /ˌθaɪəʊ'pentəʊn/, **thiopentone sodium** /ˌθaɪəʊpentəʊn 'səʊdiəm/ *noun* same as **thiopental sodium** (NOTE: Its chemical formula is $C_{11}H_{17}N_2O2SNa$.)

**thioridazine** /ˌθaɪəʊ'rɪdəziːn/ *noun* a synthetic compound used as a tranquilliser for people who are suffering from a psychosis

**third-degree burn** /ˌθɜːd dɪˌgriː 'bɜːn/ *noun* a burn in which the skin and the tissues beneath it are severely damaged

**third-degree haemorrhoids** /θɜːd dɪ'griː/ *plural noun* haemorrhoids which protrude into the anus permanently

**third molar** /θɜːd 'məʊlə/ *noun* one of the four molars at the back of the jaw, which only appears at about the age of 20 and sometimes does not appear at all. Same as **wisdom tooth**

**thirst** /θɜːst/ *noun* a feeling of wanting to drink ○ *He had a fever and a violent thirst.*

**thirsty** /'θɜːsti/ *adjective* wanting to drink ○ *If the patient is thirsty, give her a glass of water.* (NOTE: **thirstier – thirstiest**)

**Thomas's splint** /'tɒməsɪz splɪnt/, **Thomas splint** /'tɒməs splɪnt/ *noun* a metal splint used to keep a fractured leg still. It has a padded ring at the hip attached to rods to which bandages are bound and a bar under the foot at the lower end. [Described 1875. After Hugh Owen Thomas (1834–91), British surgeon and bonesetter.]

**thorac-** /θɒːrəs/ *prefix* same as **thoraco-** (*used before vowels*)

**thoracectomy** /ˌθɒːrə'sektəmi/ *noun* a surgical operation to remove one or more ribs

**thoracentesis** /ˌθɒːrəsen'tiːsɪs/ *noun* same as **thoracocentesis**

**thoraces** /'θɒːrəsiːz/ plural of **thorax**

**thoracic** /θɒː'ræsɪk/ *adjective* referring to the chest or thorax

**thoracic aorta** /θɒːˌræsɪk eɪ'ɔːtə/ *noun* part of the aorta which crosses the thorax

**thoracic cavity** /θɒːˌræsɪk 'kævɪti/ *noun* the chest cavity, containing the diaphragm, heart and lungs

**thoracic duct** /θɒː'ræsɪk dʌkt/ *noun* one of the main terminal ducts carrying lymph, on the left side of the neck

**thoracic inlet** /θɒːˌræsɪk 'ɪnlət/ *noun* a small opening at the top of the thorax

**thoracic outlet** /θɒːˌræsɪk 'aʊtlet/ *noun* a large opening at the bottom of the thorax

**thoracic outlet syndrome** /θɒːˌræsɪk 'aʊtlet ˌsɪndrəʊm/ *noun* same as **scalenus syndrome**

**thoracic vertebrae** /θɒː'ræsɪk 'vɜːtɪbriː/ *plural noun* the twelve vertebrae in the spine behind the chest, to which the ribs are attached

**thoraco-** /θɒːrəkəʊ/ *prefix* relating to the thorax

**thoracocentesis** /ˌθɒːrəkəʊsen'tiːsɪs/ *noun* an operation in which a hollow needle is inserted into the pleura to drain fluid

**thoracolumbar** /ˌθɒːrəkəʊ'lʌmbə/ *adjective* referring to the thoracic and lumbar areas of the body

**thoracoplasty** /'θɒːrəkəʊplæsti/ *noun* a surgical operation to cut through the ribs to allow the lungs to collapse, formerly a treatment for pulmonary tuberculosis

**thoracoscope** /'θɒːrəkəskəʊp/ *noun* a surgical instrument, like a tube with a light at the end, used to examine the inside of the chest

**thoracoscopy** /ˌθɒːrə'kɒskəpi/ *noun* an examination of the inside of the chest, using a thoracoscope

**thoracotomy** /ˌθɒːrə'kɒtəmi/ *noun* a surgical operation to make a hole in the wall of the chest

**thorax** /'θɒːræks/ *noun* the cavity in the top part of the front of the body above the abdomen, containing the diaphragm, heart and lungs, and surrounded by the ribcage

**thread** /θred/ *noun* a thin piece of cotton, suture, etc. ○ *The surgeon used strong thread to make the suture.* ■ *verb* to insert a thin piece of cotton, suture, etc. through the eye of a needle

**thread vein** /'θred veɪn/ *noun* a fine vein that is visible through the skin

**threadworm** /'θredwɜːm/ *noun* a thin parasitic worm, *Enterobius vernicularis*, which infests the large intestine and causes itching round the anus. ♦ **Enterobius**. Also called **pinworm**

**thready** /'θredi/ *adjective* referring to a pulse which is very weak and can hardly be felt

**thready pulse** /ˌθredi ˈpʌls/ *noun* a very weak pulse which is hard to detect

**threatened abortion** /ˌθret(ə)nd ə ˈbɔːʃ(ə)n/ *noun* a possible abortion in the early stages of pregnancy, indicated by bleeding

**threonine** /ˈθriːəniːn/ *noun* an essential amino acid

**threshold** /ˈθreʃhəʊld/ *noun* **1.** the point at which something starts, e.g. where something can be perceived by the body or where a drug starts to have an effect ○ *She has a low hearing threshold.* **2.** the point at which a sensation is strong enough to be sensed by the sensory nerves

'…if intracranial pressure rises above the treatment threshold, it is imperative first to validate the reading and then to eliminate any factors exacerbating the rise in pressure' [*British Journal of Hospital Medicine*]

**thrill** /θrɪl/ *noun* a vibration which can be felt with the hands

**thrive** /θraɪv/ *verb* to do well, to live and grow strongly

**-thrix** /θrɪks/ *suffix* relating to a hair

**throat** /θrəʊt/ *noun* **1.** the top part of the tube which goes down from the mouth to the stomach **2.** the front part of the neck below the chin □ **to clear the throat** to give a little cough

COMMENT: The throat carries both food and air from the nose and mouth. It divides into the oesophagus, which takes food to the stomach, and the trachea, which takes air into the lungs.

**throb** /θrɒb/ *verb* **1.** (*of the heart*) to beat harder and faster than usual, especially from exertion or fear **2.** (*of a painful part of the body*) to experience pain which comes and goes regularly ○ *Once the local anaesthetic wore off his thumb began to throb.*

**throbbing** /ˈθrɒbɪŋ/ *adjective* referring to pain which comes again and again like a heart beat ○ *She has a throbbing pain in her finger.* ○ *He has a throbbing headache.*

**throbbing pain** /ˌθrɒbɪŋ ˈpeɪn/ *noun* pain which continues in repeated short attacks

**thrombectomy** /θrɒmˈbektəmi/ *noun* a surgical operation to remove a blood clot

**thrombin** /ˈθrɒmbɪn/ *noun* a substance which converts fibrinogen to fibrin and so coagulates blood

**thrombo-** /θrɒmbəʊ/ *prefix* **1.** referring to a blood clot **2.** referring to thrombosis

**thromboangiitis** /ˌθrɒmbəʊˌændʒiˈaɪtɪs/ *noun* a condition in which the blood vessels swell and develop blood clots along their walls

**thromboangiitis obliterans** /ˌθrɒmbəʊˌændʒiˌaɪtɪs əbˈlɪtərənz/ *noun* a disease of the arteries in which the blood vessels in a limb, usually the leg, become narrow, causing gangrene. Also called **Buerger's disease**

**thromboarteritis** /ˌθrɒmbəʊˌɑːtəˈraɪtɪs/ *noun* inflammation of an artery caused by thrombosis

**thrombocyte** /ˈθrɒmbəʊsaɪt/ *noun* same as **platelet**

**thrombocythaemia** /ˌθrɒmbəʊsaɪˈθiːmiə/ *noun* a disease in which someone has an unusually high number of platelets in the blood

**thrombocytopenia** /ˌθrɒmbəʊˌsaɪtəʊ ˈpiːniə/ *noun* a condition in which someone has an unusually low number of platelets in the blood

**thrombocytopenic** /ˌθrɒmbəʊˌsaɪtəʊ ˈpenɪk/ *adjective* referring to thrombocytopenia

**thrombocytosis** /ˌθrɒmbəʊsaɪˈtəʊsɪs/ *noun* an increase in the number of platelets in someone's blood

**thrombo-embolic deterrent stocking** /ˌθrɒmbəʊ emˌbɒlɪk dɪˈterənt ˌstɒkɪŋ/ *noun* a support stocking to prevent thrombus formation following surgery. Abbr **TED**

**thromboembolism** /ˌθrɒmbəʊ ˈembəlɪz(ə)m/ *noun* a condition in which a blood clot forms in one part of the body and moves through the blood vessels to block another, usually smaller, part

**thromboendarterectomy** /ˌθrɒmbəʊˌendɑːtəˈrektəmi/ *noun* a surgical operation to open an artery to remove a blood clot which is blocking it

**thromboendarteritis** /ˌθrɒmbəʊˌendɑːtə ˈraɪtɪs/ *noun* inflammation of the inside of an artery, caused by thrombosis

**thrombokinase** /ˌθrɒmbəʊˈkaɪneɪz/ *noun* an enzyme which converts prothrombin into thrombin, so starting the sequence for coagulation of blood. Also called **thromboplastin**

**thrombolysis** /θrɒmˈbɒləsɪs/ *noun* same as **fibrinolysis**

**thrombolytic** /θrɒmbəʊˈlɪtɪk/ *adjective* same as **fibrinolytic**

**thrombophlebitis** /ˌθrɒmbəʊflɪˈbaɪtɪs/ *noun* the blocking of a vein by a blood clot, sometimes causing inflammation

**thromboplastic** /ˌθrɒmbəʊˈplæstɪk/ *adjective* causing or increasing the formation of blood clots

**thromboplastin** /ˌθrɒmbəʊˈplæstɪn/ *noun* same as **thrombokinase**

**thrombopoiesis** /ˌθrɒmbəʊpɔɪˈiːsɪs/ *noun* the process by which blood platelets are formed

**thrombose** /θrɒmˈbəʊz/ *verb* to cause thrombosis in a blood vessel, or be affected by thrombosis

**thrombosis** /θrɒmˈbəʊsɪs/ *noun* the blocking of an artery or vein by a mass of coagulated blood

**thrombus** /ˈθrɒmbəs/ *noun* same as **blood clot**

**throw up** /ˌθrəʊ ˈʌp/ *verb* same as **vomit** (*informal*)

**thrush** /θrʌʃ/ *noun* an infection of the mouth or the vagina with the bacterium *Candida albicans*

**thumb** /θʌm/ *noun* the short thick finger, with only two bones, which is separated from the other four fingers on the hand

**thumb-sucking** /ˈθʌm ˌsʌkɪŋ/ *noun* the action of sucking a thumb ○ *Thumb-sucking tends to push the teeth forward.*

**thym-** /θaɪm/ *prefix* referring to the thymus gland

**thymectomy** /θaɪˈmektəmi/ *noun* a surgical operation to remove the thymus gland

**-thymia** /θaɪmiə/ *suffix* referring to a state of mind

**thymic** /ˈθaɪmɪk/ *adjective* referring to the thymus gland

**thymine** /ˈθaɪmiːn/ *noun* one of the four basic chemicals in DNA

**thymitis** /θaɪˈmaɪtɪs/ *noun* inflammation of the thymus gland

**thymocyte** /ˈθaɪməʊsaɪt/ *noun* a lymphocyte formed in the thymus gland

**thymol** /ˈθaɪmɒl/ *noun* a colourless compound which is made synthetically or extracted from thyme oil, used as an antiseptic

**thymoma** /θaɪˈməʊmə/ *noun* a tumour in the thymus gland

**thymus** /ˈθaɪməs/, **thymus gland** /ˈθaɪməs ɡlænd/ *noun* an endocrine gland in the front part of the top of the thorax, behind the breastbone

COMMENT: The thymus gland produces lymphocytes and is responsible for developing the system of natural immunity in children. It grows less active as the person becomes an adult. Lymphocytes produced by the thymus are known as T-lymphocytes or T-cells.

**thyro-** /θaɪrəʊ/ *prefix* referring to the thyroid gland

**thyrocalcitonin** /ˌθaɪrəʊkælsɪˈtəʊnɪn/ *noun* same as **calcitonin**

**thyrocele** /ˈθaɪrəʊsiːl/ *noun* swelling of the thyroid gland

**thyroglobulin** /ˌθaɪrəʊˈɡlɒbjʊlɪn/ *noun* protein stored in the thyroid gland which is broken down into thyroxine

**thyroglossal** /ˌθaɪrəʊˈɡlɒs(ə)l/ *adjective* referring to the thyroid gland and the throat

**thyroglossal cyst** /ˌθaɪrəʊɡlɒs(ə)l ˈsɪst/ *noun* a cyst in the front of the neck

**thyroid** /ˈθaɪrɔɪd/, **thyroid gland** *noun* /ˈθaɪrɔɪd ɡlænd/ an endocrine gland in the neck, which is activated by the pituitary gland and secretes a hormone which regulates the body's metabolism ■ *adjective* referring to the thyroid gland

COMMENT: The thyroid gland needs a supply of iodine in order to produce thyroxine. If the thyroid gland malfunctions, it can result in

hyperthyroidism (producing too much thyroxine) leading to goitre, or in hypothyroidism (producing too little thyroxine). Hyperthyroidism can be treated with carbimazole.

**thyroid cartilage** /ˌθaɪrɔɪd ˈkɑːtəlɪdʒ/ *noun* a large cartilage in the larynx, part of which forms the Adam's apple. See illustration at LUNGS in Supplement

**thyroid depressant** /ˈθaɪrɔɪd dɪˌpres(ə)nt/ *noun* a drug which reduces the activity of the thyroid gland

**thyroid dysfunction** /ˈθaɪrɔɪd dɪsˌfʌŋkʃ(ə)n/ *noun* malfunction of the thyroid gland

**thyroidectomy** /ˌθaɪrɔɪˈdektəmi/ *noun* a surgical operation to remove all or part of the thyroid gland

**thyroid extract** /ˈθaɪrɔɪd ˌekstrækt/ *noun* a substance extracted from thyroid glands of animals and used to treat hypothyroidism

**thyroid gland** /ˈθaɪrɔɪd ɡlænd/ *noun* same as **thyroid**

**thyroid hormone** /ˈθaɪrɔɪd ˌhɔːməʊn/ *noun* a hormone produced by the thyroid gland

**thyroiditis** /ˌθaɪrɔɪˈdaɪtɪs/ *noun* inflammation of the thyroid gland

**thyroid-stimulating hormone** /ˈθaɪrɔɪd ˌstɪmjʊleɪtɪŋ ˌhɔːməʊn/ *noun* a hormone secreted by the pituitary gland which stimulates the thyroid gland. Abbr **TSH**. Also called **thyrotrophin**

**thyroparathyroidectomy** /ˌθaɪrəʊˌpærə ˌθaɪrɔɪˈdektəmi/ *noun* a surgical operation to remove the thyroid and parathyroid glands

**thyroplasty** /ˈθaɪrəʊplæsti/ *noun* a surgical procedure performed on the cartilages of the larynx to improve the quality of the voice

**thyrotomy** /θaɪˈrɒtəmi/ *noun* a surgical opening made in the thyroid cartilage or the thyroid gland

**thyrotoxic** /ˌθaɪrəʊˈtɒksɪk/ *adjective* referring to severe hyperthyroidism

**thyrotoxic crisis** /ˌθaɪrəʊˌtɒksɪk ˈkraɪsɪs/ *noun* a sudden illness caused by hyperthyroidism

**thyrotoxic goitre** /ˌθaɪrəʊˌtɒksɪk ˈɡɔɪtə/ *noun* overactivity of the thyroid gland, as in hyperthyroidism

**thyrotoxicosis** /ˌθaɪrəʊtɒksɪˈkəʊsɪs/ *noun* same as **hyperthyroidism**

**thyrotrophin** /ˌθaɪrəʊˈtrəʊfɪn/ *noun* same as **thyroid-stimulating hormone** (NOTE: The US term is **thyrotropin**.)

**thyrotrophin-releasing hormone** /ˌθaɪrəʊˌtrəʊfɪn rɪˈliːsɪŋ ˌhɔːməʊn/ *noun* a hormone secreted by the hypothalamus, which makes the pituitary gland release thyrotrophin, which in turn stimulates the thyroid gland. Abbr **TRH**

**thyroxine** /θaɪˈrɒksiːn/ *noun* a hormone produced by the thyroid gland which regulates the body's metabolism and the conversion of food into heat, used in treatment of hypothyroidism

**TIA** *abbr* transient ischaemic attack

'…blood pressure control reduces the incidence of first stroke and aspirin appears to reduce the risk of stroke after TIAs by some 15%' [*British Journal of Hospital Medicine*]

**tibia** /'tɪbiə/ *noun* the larger of the two long bones in the lower leg between the knee and the ankle. Also called **shinbone**. Compare **fibula**

**tibial** /'tɪbiəl/ *adjective* referring to the tibia

**tibial artery** /'tɪbiəl ˌɑːtəri/ *noun* one of two arteries which run down the front and back of the lower leg

**tibialis** /ˌtɪbi'eɪlɪs/ *noun* one of two muscles in the lower leg running from the tibia to the foot

**tibial torsion** /ˌtɪbiəl 'tɔːʃ(ə)n/ *noun* a persistent slight twist in the tibia, caused by a cramped position in the uterus. It makes the feet of young children point inwards for up to a year after they begin to walk on their own, but it corrects itself as the leg grows.

**tibio-** /tɪbiəʊ/ *prefix* referring to the tibia

**tibiofibular** /ˌtɪbiəʊ'fɪbjʊlə/ *adjective* referring to both the tibia and the fibula

**tic** /tɪk/ *noun* an involuntary twitch of the muscles usually in the face (*informal*)

**tic douloureux** /tɪk duːlə'ruː/ *noun* same as **trigeminal neuralgia**

**tick** /tɪk/ *noun* a tiny parasite which sucks blood from the skin

**tick fever** /'tɪk ˌfiːvə/ *noun* an infectious disease transmitted by bites from ticks

**t.i.d., TID** *adverb* (*used on prescriptions*) three times a day. Full form **ter in die**

**tidal air** /'taɪd(ə)l ˌeə/, **tidal volume** /ˌtaɪd(ə)l 'vɒljuːm/ *noun* the amount of air that passes in and out of the body in breathing

**-tidine** /tɪdiːn/ *suffix* used for antihistamine drugs

**tie** /taɪ/ *verb* to attach a thread with a knot ○ *The surgeon quickly tied up the stitches.* ○ *The nurse had tied the bandage too tight.* (NOTE: **tying – tied**)

**timolol** /'tɪməlɒl/ *noun* a beta-blocker used in the treatment of migraine, high blood pressure and glaucoma

**tinct.** *abbr* tincture

**tincture** /'tɪŋktʃə/ *noun* a medicinal substance dissolved in alcohol

**tincture of iodine** /ˌtɪŋktʃər əv 'aɪədiːn/ *noun* a weak solution of iodine in alcohol, used as an antiseptic

**tinea** /'tɪniə/ *noun* ♦ ringworm

**tinea barbae** /ˌtɪniə 'bɑːbiː/ *noun* a fungal infection in the beard

**tinea capitis** /ˌtɪniə kə'paɪtɪs/ *noun* a fungal infection on the scalp

**tinea cruris** /ˌtɪniə 'kruːrɪs/ *noun* a fungal infection of the groin area, especially in hot climates

**tinea pedis** /ˌtɪniə 'pedɪs/ *noun* same as **athlete's foot**

**tingle** /'tɪŋgəl/ *verb* to have a pricking or stinging sensation in a body part

**tingling** /'tɪŋglɪŋ/ *noun* a feeling of pricking or stinging in a body part ○ *an unpleasant tingling down her arm* ■ *adjective* pricking or stinging ○ *a tingling sensation*

**tinnitus** /'tɪnɪtəs/ *noun* a condition in which someone hears a ringing sound in the ears

COMMENT: Tinnitus can sound like bells, or buzzing, or a loud roaring sound. In some cases it is caused by wax blocking the auditory canal, but it is also associated with Ménière's disease, infections of the middle ear and acoustic nerve conditions.

**tipped womb** /ˌtɪpt 'wuːm/ *noun US* same as **retroverted uterus**

**tired** /'taɪəd/ *adjective* feeling a need to rest

**tiredness** /'taɪədnəs/ *noun* the condition of being tired

**tired out** /ˌtaɪəd 'aʊt/ *adjective* feeling extremely tired ○ *She is tired out after the physiotherapy.*

**tissue** /'tɪʃuː/ *noun* a group of cells that carries out a specific function (NOTE: For other terms referring to tissue, see words beginning with **hist-, histo-**.)

COMMENT: Most of the body is made up of soft tissue, with the exception of the bones and cartilage. The main types of body tissue are connective, epithelial, muscular and nerve tissue.

**tissue culture** /'tɪʃuː ˌkʌltʃə/ *noun* tissue grown in a culture medium in a laboratory

**tissue plasminogen activator** /ˌtɪʃuː plæz'mɪnədʒən ˌæktɪveɪtə/ *noun* an agent given to cause fibrinolysis in blood clots. Abbr **TPA**

**tissue type** /'tɪʃuː taɪp/ *noun* the immunological characteristics of a tissue that determine whether or not it can be successfully transplanted into another person

**tissue typing** /'tɪʃuː ˌtaɪpɪŋ/ *noun* the process of identifying various elements in tissue from a donor and comparing them to those of the recipient to see if a transplant is likely to be rejected

**titanium** /taɪ'teɪniəm/ *noun* a light metallic element which does not corrode (NOTE: The chemical symbol is **Ti**.)

**titration** /taɪ'treɪʃ(ə)n/ *noun* the process of measuring the strength of a solution

**titre** /'tiːtə/ *noun* a measurement of the quantity of antibodies in a serum

**T-lymphocyte** /'tiː ˌlɪmfəsaɪt/ *noun* a lymphocyte formed in the thymus gland. Also called **T-cell**

**TNM classification** /ˌtiː en 'em ˌklæsɪfɪˌkeɪʃ(ə)n/ *noun* an internationally agreed standard which is the most widely used means for classifying the extent of cancer. T refers to the size of the tumour, N to the lymph node involvement and M to the presence or absence of metastasis.

**toco-** /ˈtəʊkəʊ/ *prefix* referring to childbirth

**tocography** /tɒˈkɒɡrəfi/ *noun* the process of recording the contractions of the uterus during childbirth

**tocopherol** /tɒˈkɒfərɒl/ *noun* one of a group of fat-soluble compounds which make up vitamin E, found in vegetable oils and leafy green vegetables

**toddler's diarrhoea** /ˌtɒdləz daɪəˈriːə/ *noun* a condition in which recurrent loose stools are produced, often containing partially digested food. It usually occurs in children between the ages of one and three years.

**Todd's paralysis** /ˈtɒdz pəˌræləsɪs/, **Todd's palsy** /ˈtɒdz ˌpɔːlzi/ *noun* a temporary paralysis of part of the body which has been the starting point of focal epilepsy

**toe** /təʊ/ *noun* one of the five separate parts at the end of the foot. Each toe is formed of three bones or phalanges, except the big toe, which only has two.

**toenail** /ˈtəʊneɪl/ *noun* a thin hard growth covering the end of a toe

**toileting** /ˈtɔɪlətɪŋ/ *noun* the act of helping someone to perform the actions of urinating or opening their bowels, including helping them to do so if they are unable to get out of bed or are incontinent

**toilet training** /ˈtɔɪlət ˌtreɪnɪŋ/ *noun* the process of teaching a small child to pass urine or faeces in a toilet, so that he or she no longer requires nappies

**tolbutamide** /tɒlˈbjuːtəmaɪd/ *noun* a drug which lowers blood-glucose levels by stimulating the pancreas to produce more insulin. It is used in the treatment of Type II diabetes.

**tolerance** /ˈtɒlərəns/ *noun* the ability of the body to tolerate a substance or an action ○ *He has been taking the drug for so long that he has developed a tolerance to it.*

'26 patients were selected from the outpatient department on grounds of disabling breathlessness, severely limiting exercise tolerance and the performance of activities of normal daily living' [*Lancet*]

**tolerate** /ˈtɒləreɪt/ *verb* **1.** not to be affected by the unpleasant effects of something, especially not to experience bad effects from being exposed to something harmful **2.** not to react to a drug through having developed a resistance to it

**-tome** /təʊm/ *suffix* **1.** a cutting instrument **2.** a segment ○ *a dermatome*

**tomo-** /ˈtəʊməʊ/ *prefix* referring to cutting or a section

**tomogram** /ˈtəʊməɡræm/ *noun* a picture of part of the body taken by tomography

**tomography** /təˈmɒɡrəfi/ *noun* the scanning of a particular part of the body using X-rays or ultrasound

**-tomy** /təmi/ *suffix* referring to a surgical operation

**tone** /təʊn/ *noun* the slightly tense state of a healthy muscle when it is not fully relaxed. Also called **tonicity**, **tonus**

**tongue** /tʌŋ/ *noun* the long muscular organ inside the mouth which can move and is used for tasting, swallowing and speaking. The top surface is covered with papillae, some of which contain taste buds. ○ *The doctor told him to stick out his tongue and say 'Ah'.* Also called **glossa** (NOTE: For other terms referring to the tongue, see **lingual** and words beginning with **gloss-**, **glosso-**.)

**tongue depressor** /ˈtʌŋ dɪˌpresə/ *noun* an instrument, usually a thin piece of wood, used by a doctor to hold someone's tongue down while the throat is being examined

**tongue-tie** /ˈtʌŋ taɪ/ *noun* the condition of being unable to move your tongue with the usual amount of freedom, because the small membrane which attaches the tongue to the floor of the mouth is unusually short

**tonic** /ˈtɒnɪk/ *adjective* referring to a muscle which is contracted ■ *noun* a substance which improves the someone's general health or which makes a tired person more energetic ○ *He is taking a course of iron tonic tablets.* ○ *She asked the doctor to prescribe a tonic for her anaemia.*

**tonicity** /təʊˈnɪsɪti/ *noun* same as tone

**tono-** /ˈtəʊnəʊ/ *prefix* referring to pressure

**tonography** /təʊˈnɒɡrəfi/ *noun* a measurement of the pressure inside an eyeball

**tonometer** /təʊˈnɒmɪtə/ *noun* an instrument which measures the pressure inside an organ, especially the eye

**tonometry** /təʊˈnɒmətri/ *noun* a measurement of pressure inside an organ, especially the eye

**tonsil** /ˈtɒns(ə)l/ *noun* an area of lymphoid tissue at the back of the throat in which lymph circulates and protects the body against germs entering through the mouth. Also called **palatine tonsil**

COMMENT: The tonsils are larger in children than in adults, and are more liable to infection. When infected, the tonsils become enlarged and can interfere with breathing.

**tonsillar** /ˈtɒnsɪlə/ *adjective* referring to the tonsils

**tonsillectomy** /ˌtɒnsɪˈlektəmi/ *noun* a surgical operation to remove the tonsils

**tonsillitis** /ˌtɒnsɪˈlaɪtɪs/ *noun* inflammation of the tonsils

**tonsillotome** /tɒnˈsɪlətəʊm/ *noun* a surgical instrument used in cutting into or removing the tonsils

**tonsillotomy** /ˌtɒnsɪˈlɒtəmi/ *noun* a surgical operation to make a cut into the tonsils

**tonus** /ˈtəʊnəs/ *noun* same as tone

**tooth** /tuːθ/ *noun* one of a set of bones in the mouth which are used to chew food (NOTE: The plural is **teeth**. For other terms relating to the teeth, see words beginning with **dent-**.)

COMMENT: A tooth is formed of a soft core of pulp, covered with a layer of hard dentine. The top part of the tooth, the crown, which can be seen above the gum, is covered with hard shiny enamel which is very hard-wearing. The lower part of the tooth, the root, which attaches the tooth to the jaw, is covered with cement, also a hard substance, but which is slightly rough and holds the periodontal membrane which links the tooth to the jaw. The milk teeth in a child appear over the first two years of childhood and consist of incisors, canines and molars. The permanent teeth which replace them are formed of eight incisors, four canines, eight premolars and twelve molars. The last four molars (the third molars or wisdom teeth), are not always present, and do not appear much before the age of twenty. Permanent teeth start to appear about the age of five to six. The order of eruption of the permanent teeth is: first molars, incisors, premolars, canines, second molars, wisdom teeth.

**toothache** /ˈtuːθeɪk/ *noun* a pain in a tooth. Also called **odontalgia**

**topagnosis** /ˌtəʊpəˈgnəʊsɪs/ *noun* an inability to tell which part of your body has been touched, caused by a disorder of the brain

**tophus** /ˈtəʊfəs/ *noun* a deposit of solid crystals in the skin or in the joints, especially in someone with gout (NOTE: The plural is **tophi**.)

**topical** /ˈtɒpɪk(ə)l/ *adjective* referring to a specific area of the external surface of the body ○ *suitable for topical application*

'…one of the most common routes of neonatal poisoning is percutaneous absorption following topical administration' [*Southern Medical Journal*]

**topical drug** /ˈtɒpɪk(ə)l drʌg/ *noun* a drug which is applied to a specific external part of the body only

**topically** /ˈtɒpɪkli/ *adverb* by putting on a specific external part of the body only ○ *The cream is applied topically.*

**topo-** /tɒpə/ *prefix* a place or region

**topographical** /ˌtɒpəˈgræfɪk(ə)l/ *adjective* referring to topography

**topography** /təˈpɒgrəfi/ *noun* the description of each particular part of the body

**tormina** /ˈtɔːmɪnə/ *noun* same as **colic**

**torpid** /ˈtɔːpɪd/ *adjective* describing a part of the body that has lost the ability to move or feel

**torpor** /ˈtɔːpə/ *noun* a condition in which someone seems sleepy or slow to react

**torsion** /ˈtɔːʃ(ə)n/ *noun* 1. the twisting of something, or a twisted state 2. the stress placed on an object which has been twisted

**torso** /ˈtɔːsəʊ/ *noun* the main part of the body, not including the arms, legs and head. Also called **trunk**

**torticollis** /ˌtɔːtɪˈkɒlɪs/ *noun* a condition of the neck, where the head is twisted to one side by contraction of the sternocleidomastoid muscle. Also called **wry neck**

**total** /ˈtəʊt(ə)l/ *adjective* 1. complete ○ *He has total paralysis of the lower part of the body.* 2. throughout the whole body

**total body irradiation** /ˌtəʊt(ə)l ˌbɒdi ɪˌreɪdiˈeɪʃ(ə)n/ *noun* treating the whole body with radiation

**total deafness** /ˌtəʊt(ə)l ˈdefnəs/ *noun* being unable to hear any sound at all. ◊ **hearing loss**

**total hip arthroplasty** /ˌtəʊt(ə)l ˈhɪp ˌɑːθrəʊplæsti/, **total hip replacement** /ˌtəʊt(ə)l ˈhɪp rɪˌpleɪsmənt/ *noun* the replacement of both the head of the femur and the acetabulum with an artificial joint

**total hysterectomy** /ˌtəʊt(ə)l ˌhɪstəˈrektəmi/ *noun* the surgical removal of the whole uterus

**total pancreatectomy** /ˌtəʊt(ə)l ˌpæŋkriəˈtektəmi/ *noun* the surgical removal of the whole pancreas together with part of the duodenum. Also called **Whipple's operation**

**total recall** /ˌtəʊt(ə)l rɪˈkɔːl/ *noun* the fact of being able to remember something in complete detail

**touch** /tʌtʃ/ *noun* one of the five senses, where sensations are felt by part of the skin, especially by the fingers and lips

COMMENT: Touch is sensed by receptors in the skin which send impulses back to the brain. The touch receptors can tell the difference between hot and cold, hard and soft, wet and dry, and rough and smooth.

**tough** /tʌf/ *adjective* unable to break or tear easily ○ *The meninges are covered by a layer of tough tissue, the dura mater.*

**Tourette's syndrome** /tuːˈrets ˌsɪndrəʊm/, **Tourette syndrome** /tuːˈret ˌsɪndrəʊm/ *noun* a condition which includes involuntary movements, tics, use of foul language and respiratory disorders. Also called **Gilles de la Tourette Syndrome**

**tourniquet** /ˈtɔːnɪkeɪ/ *noun* an instrument or tight bandage wrapped round a limb to constrict an artery, so reducing the flow of blood and stopping bleeding from a wound

**tox-** /tɒks/ *prefix* same as **toxo-** (used before vowels)

**toxaemia** /tɒkˈsiːmiə/ *noun* the presence of poisonous substances in the blood. ◊ **blood poisoning** (NOTE: The US spelling is **toxemia**.)

**toxaemia of pregnancy** /tɒkˌsiːmiə əv ˈpregnənsi/ *noun* a condition which can affect women towards the end of pregnancy, in which they develop high blood pressure and pass protein in the urine

**toxic** /ˈtɒksɪk/ *adjective* poisonous

**toxic goitre** /ˌtɒksɪk ˈɡɔɪtə/ *noun* a type of goitre due to hyperthyroidism in which the limbs tremble and the eyes protrude

**toxicity** /tɒkˈsɪsɪti/ *noun* **1.** the degree to which a substance is poisonous or harmful **2.** the amount of poisonous or harmful material in a substance

**toxico-** /tɒksɪkəʊ/ *prefix* referring to poison

**toxicogenic** /ˌtɒksɪkəʊˈdʒenɪk/ *adjective* same as **toxigenic**

**toxicologist** /ˌtɒksɪˈkɒlədʒɪst/ *noun* a scientist who specialises in the study of poisons

**toxicology** /ˌtɒksɪˈkɒlədʒi/ *noun* the scientific study of poisons and their effects on the human body

**toxicosis** /ˌtɒksɪˈkəʊsɪs/ *noun* poisoning

**toxic shock syndrome** /ˌtɒksɪk ˈʃɒk ˌsɪn↓drəʊm/ *noun* a serious condition caused by a staphylococcus infection of the skin or soft tissue. Its symptoms include vomiting, high fever, faintness, muscle aches, a rash and confusion. Abbr **TSS**

**toxigenic** /ˌtɒksɪˈdʒenɪk/ *adjective* caused or produced by a toxin. Also called **toxicogenic**

**toxin** /ˈtɒksɪn/ *noun* a poisonous substance produced in the body by microorganisms, and which, if injected into an animal, stimulates the production of antitoxins

**toxo-** /tɒksəʊ/ *prefix* referring to poison

**toxocariasis** /ˌtɒksəkəˈraɪəsɪs/ *noun* the infestation of the intestine with worms from a dog or cat. Also called **visceral larva migrans**

**toxoid** /ˈtɒksɔɪd/ *noun* a toxin which has been treated and is no longer poisonous, but which can still provoke the formation of antibodies. Toxoids are used as vaccines, and are injected into a patient to give immunity against specific diseases.

**toxoid-antitoxin** /ˌtɒksɔɪd ˌæntɪˈtɒksɪn/ *noun* a mixture of a toxoid and an antitoxin, used as a vaccine

**toxoplasmosis** /ˌtɒksəʊplæzˈməʊsɪs/ *noun* a disease caused by the parasite *Toxoplasma* which is carried by animals. Toxoplasmosis can cause encephalitis or hydrocephalus and can be fatal.

**TPA** *abbr* tissue plasminogen activator

**trabecula** /trəˈbekjʊlə/ *noun* a thin strip of stiff tissue which divides an organ or bone tissue into sections (NOTE: The plural is **trabeculae**.)

**trabeculectomy** /trəˌbekjʊˈlektəmi/ *noun* a surgical operation to treat glaucoma by cutting a channel through trabeculae to link with Schlemm's canal

**trace** /treɪs/ *noun* a very small amount ○ *There are traces of the drug in the blood sample.* ○ *The doctor found traces of alcohol in the patient's urine.* ■ *verb* to find someone or something that you are looking for

**trace element** /ˈtreɪs ˌelɪmənt/ *noun* a substance which is essential to the human body, but only in very small quantities

COMMENT: The trace elements are cobalt, chromium, copper, magnesium, manganese, molybdenum, selenium and zinc.

**tracer** /ˈtreɪsə/ *noun* a substance, often a radioactive one, injected into a substance in the body, so that doctors can follow its passage round the body

**trache-** /treɪki/ *prefix* same as **tracheo-** (NOTE: used before vowels)

**trachea** /trəˈkiːə/ *noun* the main air passage which runs from the larynx to the lungs, where it divides into the two main bronchi. It is about 10 cm long, and is formed of rings of cartilage and connective tissue. See illustration at LUNGS in Supplement. Also called **windpipe**

**tracheal** /trəˈkiːəl/ *adjective* referring to the trachea

**tracheal tugging** /trəˌkiːəl ˈtʌɡɪŋ/ *noun* the feeling that something is pulling on the windpipe when the person breathes in, a symptom of aneurysm

**tracheitis** /ˌtreɪkiˈaɪtɪs/ *noun* inflammation of the trachea due to an infection

**trachelorrhaphy** /ˌtreɪkiˈlɒrəfi/ *noun* a surgical operation to repair tears in the cervix of the uterus

**tracheo-** /treɪkiəʊ/ *prefix* relating to the trachea

**tracheobronchial** /ˌtreɪkiəʊˈbrɒŋkiəl/ *adjective* referring to both the trachea and the bronchi

**tracheobronchitis** /ˌtreɪkiəʊbrɒŋˈkaɪtɪs/ *noun* inflammation of both the trachea and the bronchi

**tracheo-oesophogeal** /ˌtreɪkiəʊ iːˌsɒfəˈdʒiːəl/ *adjective* referring to both the trachea and the oesophagus

**tracheostomy** /ˌtreɪkiˈɒstəmi/, **tracheotomy** /ˌtreɪkiˈɒtəmi/ *noun* a surgical operation to make a hole through the throat into the windpipe, so as to allow air to get to the lungs in cases where the trachea is blocked, as in pneumonia, poliomyelitis or diphtheria

COMMENT: After the operation, a tube is inserted into the hole to keep it open. The tube may be permanent if it is to bypass an obstruction, but can be removed if the condition improves.

**trachoma** /trəˈkəʊmə/ *noun* a contagious viral inflammation of the eyelids, common in tropical countries, which can cause blindness if the conjunctiva becomes scarred

**tract** /trækt/ *noun* **1.** a series of organs or tubes which allow something to pass from one part of the body to another **2.** a series or bundle of nerve fibres connecting two areas of the nervous system and transmitting nervous impulses in one or in both directions

'GI fistulae are frequently associated with infection because the effluent contains bowel organisms

which initially contaminate the fistula tract'
[*Nursing Times*]

**traction** /'trækʃən/ *noun* a procedure that consists of using a pulling force to straighten a broken or deformed limb ○ *The patient was in traction for two weeks.*

COMMENT: A system of weights and pulleys is fixed over the patient's bed so that the limb can be pulled hard enough to counteract the tendency of the muscles to contract and pull it back to its original position. Traction can also be used for slipped discs and other dislocations. Other forms of traction include frames attached to the body.

**tractotomy** /træk'tɒtəmi/ *noun* a surgical operation to cut the nerve pathway taking sensations of pain to the brain, as a treatment for severe pain that is hard to control

**tragus** /'treɪɡəs/ *noun* a piece of cartilage in the outer ear which projects forward over the entrance to the auditory canal

**training** /'treɪnɪŋ/ *noun* the process of educating by giving instruction and the opportunity to practise

**trait** /treɪt/ *noun* 1. a typical characteristic of someone 2. a genetically controlled characteristic

**trance** /trɑːns/ *noun* a condition in which a person is in a dream, but not asleep, and seems not to be aware of what is happening round him or her ○ *a hypnotic trance*

**tranexamic acid** /ˌtrænek,sæmɪk 'æsɪd/ *noun* a drug used to control severe bleeding

**tranquilliser** /'træŋkwɪlaɪzə/, **tranquillizer**, **tranquillising drug** /'træŋkwɪlaɪzɪŋ drʌɡ/ *noun* an antipsychotic, anxiolytic or hypnotic drug which relieves someone's anxiety and calms him or her down (*informal*) ○ *She's taking tranquillisers to calm her nerves.* ○ *He's been on tranquillisers ever since he started his new job.*

**trans-** /træns/ *prefix* through or across

**transaminase** /træn'sæmɪneɪz/ *noun* an enzyme involved in the transamination of amino acids

**transamination** /træns,æmɪ'neɪʃ(ə)n/ *noun* the process by which amino acids are metabolised in the liver

**transcendental meditation** /ˌtrænsen,dent(ə)l ,medɪ'teɪʃ(ə)n/ *noun* a type of meditation in which the same words or sounds are repeated silently

**transcription** /træn'skrɪpʃən/ *noun* 1. the act of copying something written, or of putting something spoken into written form 2. the first step in carrying out genetic instructions in living cells, in which the genetic code is transferred from DNA to molecules of messenger RNA, which then direct protein manufacture

**transcutaneous electrical nerve stimulation** /ˌtrænskjuː,teɪniəs ɪ,lektrɪk(ə)l 'nɜːv stɪmjʊ,leɪʃ(ə)n/ *noun* full form of **TENS**

**transdermal** /trænz'dɜːm(ə)l/ *adjective* referring to a drug which is released through the skin

**transdermal patch** /trænz,dɜːm(ə)l 'pætʃ/ *noun* a patch containing medication applied to the skin and releasing its contents into the body over a period of time

**transdiaphragmatic approach** /trænz ,daɪəfræɡ,mætɪk ə'prəʊtʃ/ *noun* an operation carried out through the diaphragm

**transection** /træn'sekʃ(ə)n/ *noun* 1. the act of cutting across part of the body 2. a sample of tissue which has been taken by cutting across a part of the body

**transfer** /træns'fɜː/ *verb* to pass from one place to another, or cause someone or something to pass from one place to another ○ *The hospital records have been transferred to the computer.* ○ *The patient was transferred to a special burns unit.*

**transference** /'trænsf(ə)rəns/ *noun* (*in psychiatry*) a condition in which someone transfers to the psychoanalyst the characteristics belonging to a strong character from his or her past such as a parent, and reacts as if the analyst were that person

**transferrin** /træns'ferɪn/ *noun* a substance found in the blood, which carries iron in the bloodstream. Also called **siderophilin**

**transfer RNA** /ˌtrænsfɜː ˌɑːr en 'eɪ/ *noun* RNA which attaches amino acids to protein chains being made at ribosomes

**transfix** /træns'fɪks/ *verb* to cut through a part of the body completely, e.g. when amputating a limb

**transfusion** /træns'fjuːʒ(ə)n/ *noun* the procedure of transferring blood or saline fluids from a container into a someone's bloodstream

**transient** /'trænziənt/ *adjective* not lasting long

**transient ischaemic attack** /ˌtrænziənt ɪ'skiːmɪk ə,tæk/ *noun* a mild stroke caused by a brief stoppage of blood supply to the brain. Abbr **TIA**

**transillumination** /ˌtrænsɪ,luːmɪ'neɪʃ(ə)n/ *noun* an examination of an organ by shining a bright light through it

**transitional** /træn'zɪʃ(ə)nəl/ *adjective* in the process of developing into something

**transitional epithelium** /træn,zɪʃ(ə)nəl epɪ'θiːliəm/ *noun* a type of epithelium found in the urethra

**translation** /træns'leɪʃ(ə)n/ *noun* 1. the act of putting something written or spoken in one language into words of a different language 2. the process by which information in messenger RNA controls the sequence of amino acids assembled by a ribosome during protein synthesis

**translocation** /ˌtrænsləʊ'keɪʃ(ə)n/ *noun* the movement of part of a chromosome to another part of the same chromosome or to a different chromosome pair, leading to genetic disorders

**translucent** /trænsˈluːs(ə)nt/ *adjective* allowing light to pass through, but not enough to allow objects on the other side to be clearly distinguished

**translumbar** /trænsˈlʌmbə/ *adjective* through the lumbar region

**transmigration** /ˌtrænzmaɪˈɡreɪʃ(ə)n/ *noun* the movement of a cell through a membrane

**transmission-based precautions** /træns mɪʃ(ə)n beɪst prɪˈkɔːʃ(ə)nz/ *plural noun* the most recent set of guidelines for health care workers on dealing with highly infectious diseases, to be used in addition to the Standard Precautions. There are three categories: Airborne Precautions, Droplet Precautions, and Contact Precautions, sometimes used in combination for diseases which can be transmitted in various ways.

**transmit** /trænzˈmɪt/ *verb* to pass something such as a message or a disease ○ *Impulses are transmitted along the neural pathways.* ○ *The disease is transmitted by lice.*

**transparent** /trænsˈpærənt/ *adjective* able to be seen through ○ *The cornea is a transparent tissue on the front of the eye.*

**transplacental** /ˌtrænspləˈsent(ə)l/ *adjective* through the placenta

**transplant** *noun* /ˈtrænsplɑːnt/ **1.** a procedure which involves taking an organ such as the heart or kidney, or tissue such as skin, and grafting it into someone to replace an organ or tissue which is diseased or not functioning properly ○ *She had a heart-lung transplant.* **2.** the organ or tissue which is grafted ○ *The kidney transplant was rejected.* ■ *verb* /trænsˈplɑːnt/ to graft an organ or tissue onto or into someone to replace an organ or tissue which is diseased or not functioning correctly

**transplantation** /ˌtrænsplɑːnˈteɪʃ(ə)n/ *noun* the act of transplanting something

'…bone marrow transplantation has the added complication of graft-versus-host disease' [*Hospital Update*]

**transport** /trænsˈpɔːt/ *verb* to carry someone or something to another place ○ *Arterial blood transports oxygen to the tissues.*

**transposition** /ˌtrænspəˈzɪʃ(ə)n/ *noun* a congenital condition where the aorta and pulmonary artery are placed on the opposite side of the body to their usual position

**transpyloric plane** /ˌtrænspaɪˌlɒrɪk ˈpleɪn/ *noun* a plane at right angles to the sagittal plane, passing midway between the suprasternal notch and the symphysis pubis. See illustration at ANATOMICAL TERMS in Supplement

**transrectal** /trænsˈrekt(ə)l/ *adjective* through the rectum

**transsexual** /trænzˈsekʃuəl/ *adjective* feeling uncomfortable with the birth gender ■ *noun* a person, especially a man, who feels uncomfortable with their birth gender

**transsexualism** /trænzˈsekʃuəlɪz(ə)m/ *noun* a condition in which a person, especially a man, feels uncomfortable with their birth gender

**transtubercular plane** /ˌtrænstjuː ˌbɜːkjʊlə ˈpleɪn/ *noun* an imaginary horizontal line drawn across the lower abdomen at the level of the projecting parts of the iliac bones. See illustration at ANATOMICAL TERMS in Supplement. Also called **intertubercular plane**

**transudate** /ˈtrænsjuːdeɪt/ *noun* a fluid which passes through the pores of a membrane. It contains less protein or solid material than an exudate.

**transudation** /ˌtrænsjuːˈdeɪʃ(ə)n/ *noun* the process of passing a fluid from the body's cells through the pores of a membrane

**transuretero-ureterostomy** /træns ˌjʊərɪtərəʊ ˌjʊərɪtəˈrɒstəmi/ *noun* a surgical operation in which both ureters are brought to the same side in the abdomen, because one is damaged or obstructed

**transurethral** /ˌtrænsjʊˈriːθrəl/ *adjective* through the urethra

**transurethral prostatectomy** /ˌtrænsjʊ ˌriːθrəl prɒstəˈtektəmi/, **transurethral resection** /ˌtrænsjʊˌriːθrəl rɪˈsekʃən/ *noun* a surgical operation to remove the prostate gland, where the operation is carried out through the urethra. Abbr **TUR**. Also called **resection of the prostate**

**transvaginal** /ˌtrænsvəˈdʒaɪn(ə)l/ *adjective* across or through the vagina

**transverse** /trænzˈvɜːs/ *adjective* across, at right angles to an organ

**transverse arch** /ˌtrænzˈvɜːs ɑːtʃ/ *noun* same as **metatarsal arch**

**transverse colon** /ˌtrænzvɜːs ˈkəʊlɒn/ *noun* the second section of the colon which crosses the body below the stomach. See illustration at DIGESTIVE SYSTEM in Supplement

**transverse fracture** /ˌtrænzvɜːs ˈfræktʃə/ *noun* a fracture where the bone is broken straight across

**transverse lie** /ˌtrænzvɜːs ˈlaɪ/ *noun* the position of a fetus across the body of the mother

**transverse plane** /ˌtrænzvɜːs ˈpleɪn/ *noun* a plane at right angles to the sagittal plane, running horizontally across the body. See illustration at ANATOMICAL TERMS in Supplement

**transverse presentation** /ˌtrænzvɜːs ˌprez(ə)nˈteɪʃ(ə)n/ *noun* a position of the baby in the uterus, where the baby's side will appear first, usually requiring urgent manipulation or caesarean section to prevent complications

**transverse process** /ˌtrænzvɜːs ˈprəʊses/ noun the part of a vertebra which protrudes at the side

**transvesical prostatectomy** /træns ˌvesɪk(ə)l prɒstəˈtektəmi/ noun an operation to remove the prostate gland, carried out through the bladder

**transvestism** /trænzˈvestɪz(ə)m/ noun the condition of liking to dress and behave as a member of the opposite sex

**transvestite** /trænzˈvestaɪt/ noun a person who dresses and behaves as a member of the opposite sex

**trapezium** /trəˈpiːziəm/ noun one of the eight small carpal bones in the wrist, below the thumb. See illustration at HAND in Supplement (NOTE: The plural is **trapeziums** or **trapezia**.)

**trapezius** /trəˈpiːziəs/ noun a triangular muscle in the upper part of the back and the neck, which moves the shoulder blade and pulls the head back

**trapezoid** /ˈtræpɪzɔɪd/, **trapezoid bone** / ˈtræpɪzɔɪd bəʊn/ noun one of the eight small carpal bones in the wrist, below the first finger. See illustration at HAND in Supplement

**trauma** /ˈtrɔːmə/ noun 1. a wound or injury 2. a very frightening or distressing experience which gives a person a severe emotional shock

**trauma centre** /ˈtrɔːmə ˌsentə/ noun a hospital or a department in a hospital that treats people who have complex, life-threatening injuries

**traumatic** /trɔːˈmætɪk/ adjective 1. caused by an injury 2. extremely frightening, distressing or shocking

**traumatic fever** /trɔːˌmætɪk ˈfiːvə/ noun a fever caused by an injury

**traumatic pneumothorax** /trɔːˌmætɪk njuːməʊˈθɔːræks/ noun pneumothorax which results from damage to the lung surface or to the wall of the chest, allowing air to leak into the space between the pleurae

**traumatology** /ˌtrɔːməˈtɒlədʒi/ noun a branch of surgery which deals with injuries received in accidents

**traveller's diarrhoea** /ˌtræv(ə)ləz daɪə ˈriːə/ noun diarrhoea that affects people who travel to foreign countries and which is due to contact with a different type of *E. coli* from the one they are used to. (*informal*)

**travel sickness** /ˈtræv(ə)l ˌsɪknəs/ noun same as **motion sickness**

**trazodone** /ˈtræzədəʊn/ noun an antidepressant drug which has a strong sedative effect, used in the treatment of depressive disorders accompanied by insomnia

**Treacher Collins syndrome** /ˌtriːtʃə ˈkɒlɪnz ˌsɪndrəʊm/ noun a hereditary disorder in which the lower jaw, the cheek bones, and the ear are not fully developed

**treat** /triːt/ verb to use medical methods to cure a disease or help a sick or injured person to recover ○ She has been treated with a new antibiotic. ○ She's being treated by a specialist for heart disease.

**treatment** /ˈtriːtmənt/ noun 1. actions taken to look after sick or injured people or to cure disease ○ He is receiving treatment for a slipped disc. 2. a particular way of looking after a sick or injured person or trying to cure a disease ○ cortisone treatment ○ This is a new treatment for heart disease.

**trematode** /ˈtremətəʊd/ noun a parasitic flatworm

**tremble** /ˈtrembəl/ verb to shake or shiver slightly

**trembling** /ˈtremblɪŋ/ noun rapid small movements of a limb or muscles ○ Trembling of the hands is a symptom of Parkinson's disease.

**tremens** /ˈtriːmenz/ ♦ delirium tremens

**tremor** /ˈtremə/ noun slight involuntary movements of a limb or muscle

**trench fever** /ˈtrenʃ ˌfiːvə/ noun a fever caused by Rickettsia bacteria, similar to typhus but recurring every five days

**trench foot** /ˌtrentʃ ˈfʊt/ noun a condition caused by exposure to cold and damp, in which the skin of the foot becomes red and blistered and in severe cases turns black when gangrene sets in. Also called **immersion foot** (NOTE: Trench foot was common among soldiers serving in the trenches during the First World War.)

**trench mouth** /ˌtrentʃ ˈmaʊθ/ noun ♦ gingivitis

**Trendelenburg's operation** /tren ˈdelənbɜːgz ɒpəˌreɪʃ(ə)n/ noun an operation to tie a saphenous vein in the groin before removing varicose veins [After Friedrich Trendelenburg (1844–1924), German surgeon]

**Trendelenburg's position** /tren ˈdelənbɜːgz pəˌzɪʃ(ə)n/, **Trendelenburg position** /trenˈdelənbɜːg pəˌzɪʃ(ə)n/ noun a position in which someone lies on a sloping bed with the head lower than the feet, and the knees bent. It is used in surgical operations to the pelvis and for people who have shock.

**Trendelenburg's sign** /trenˈdelənbɜːg saɪn/ noun a symptom of congenital dislocation of the hip, where the person's pelvis is lower on the opposite side to the dislocation

**trephination** /ˌtrɪfɪˈneɪʃ(ə)n/ noun a surgical operation which consists of removing a small part of the skull with a trephine in order to perform surgery on the brain

**trephine** /trɪˈfiːn/ noun a surgical instrument for making a round hole in the skull or for removing a round piece of tissue

**Treponema** /ˌtrepəˈniːmə/ *noun* a genus of bacteria which cause diseases such as syphilis or yaws

**treponematosis** /ˌtrepəniːməˈtəʊsɪs/ *noun* an infection by the bacterium *Treponema pertenue*. ◊ **yaws**

**TRH** *abbr* thyrotrophin-releasing hormone

**triad** /ˈtraɪæd/ *noun* three organs or three symptoms which are linked together in a group

**triage** /ˈtriːɑːʒ/ *noun* the system in which a doctor or nurse sees patients briefly in order to decide who should be treated first

**trial** /ˈtraɪəl/ *noun* a process of testing something such as a drug or treatment to see how effective it is, especially before allowing it to be used generally ○ *clinical trials* ○ *a six-month trial period* ○ *We're supplying it on a trial basis.* ■ *verb* to test something as part of a trial

**triamcinolone** /ˌtraɪæmˈsɪnələʊn/ *noun* a synthetic corticosteroid drug used in the treatment of skin, mouth and joint inflammations

**triangle** /ˈtraɪæŋɡəl/ *noun* **1.** a flat shape which has three sides **2.** part of the body with three sides

**triangular** /traɪˈæŋɡjʊlə/ *adjective* with three sides

**triangular bandage** /traɪˌæŋɡjʊlə ˈbændɪdʒ/ *noun* a bandage made of a triangle of cloth, used to make a sling for the arm

**triceps** /ˈtraɪseps/ *noun* a muscle formed of three parts, which are joined to form one tendon

**triceps brachii** /ˌtraɪseps ˈbreɪkiːiː/ *noun* a muscle in the back part of the upper arm which makes the forearm stretch out

**trich-** /trɪk/ *prefix* same as **tricho-** (*used before vowels*)

**trichiasis** /trɪˈkaɪəsɪs/ *noun* a painful condition in which the eyelashes grow in towards the eye and scratch the eyeball

**trichinosis** /ˌtrɪkɪˈnəʊsɪs/, **trichiniasis** /ˌtrɪkɪˈnaɪəsɪs/ *noun* a disease caused by infestation of the intestine by larvae of roundworms or nematodes, which pass round the body in the bloodstream and settle in muscles

COMMENT: The larvae enter the body in meat, especially pork, which has not been properly cooked.

**tricho-** /trɪkəʊ/ *prefix* **1.** referring to hair **2.** like hair

**Trichocephalus** /ˌtrɪkəˈsefələs/ *noun* same as **Trichuris**

**trichology** /trɪˈkɒlədʒi/ *noun* the study of hair and the diseases which affect it

**Trichomonas** /ˌtrɪkəˈməʊnəs/ *noun* a species of long thin parasite which infests the intestines

**Trichomonas vaginalis** /trɪkəˌməʊnəs vædʒɪˈneɪlɪs/ *noun* a parasite which infests the vagina and causes an irritating discharge

**trichomoniasis** /ˌtrɪkəʊməˈnaɪəsɪs/ *noun* infestation of the intestine or vagina with Trichomonas

**trichomycosis** /ˌtrɪkəʊmaɪˈkəʊsɪs/ *noun* a disease of the hair caused by a corynebacterium

**Trichophyton** /traɪˈkɒfɪtɒn/ *noun* a fungus which affects the skin, hair and nails

**trichophytosis** /ˌtrɪkəʊfaɪˈtəʊsɪs/ *noun* an infection caused by Trichophyton

**trichosis** /traɪˈkəʊsɪs/ *noun* any unusual condition of the hair

**trichotillomania** /ˌtrɪkəʊtɪləʊˈmeɪniə/ *noun* a condition in which a person pulls his or her hair out compulsively

**trichromatism** /traɪˈkrəʊmətɪz(ə)m/ *noun* vision which allows the difference between the three primary colours to be seen. Compare **dichromatism, monochromatism**

**trichrome stain** /ˈtraɪkrəʊm ˌsteɪn/ *noun* a stain in three colours used in histology

**trichuriasis** /ˌtrɪkjʊˈraɪəsɪs/ *noun* an infestation of the intestine with whipworms

**Trichuris** /trɪˈkjʊərɪs/ *noun* a thin round parasitic worm which infests the caecum. Also called **whipworm**

**tricuspid** /traɪˈkʌspɪd/ *noun* something which has three cusps, e.g. a tooth or leaf ■ *adjective* **1.** having three cusps or points **2.** referring to a tricuspid valve or tooth

**tricuspid valve** /traɪˈkʌspɪd vælv/ *noun* an inlet valve with three cusps between the right atrium and the right ventricle in the heart. See illustration at HEART in Supplement

**tricyclic antidepressant** /traɪˌsaɪklɪk ˌæntɪdɪˈpres(ə)nt/, **tricyclic antidepressant drug** /traɪˌsaɪklɪk ˌæntɪdɪˈpres(ə)nt drʌɡ/ *noun* a drug used to treat depression and panic disorder, e.g. amitriptyline and nortriptyline

COMMENT: Antimuscarinic and cardiac side-effects can occur; rapid withdrawal should be avoided.

**tridactyly** /traɪˈdæktɪli/ *noun* the condition of having only three fingers or toes

**trifocal lenses** /traɪˌfəʊk(ə)l ˈlenzɪz/, **trifocal glasses** /traɪˌfəʊk(ə)l ˈɡlɑːsɪz/, **trifocals** /traɪˈfəʊk(ə)lz/ *plural noun* spectacles which have three lenses combined in one piece of glass to give clear vision over different distances. ◊ **bifocal**

**trigeminal** /traɪˈdʒemɪn(ə)l/ *adjective* in three parts

**trigeminal ganglion** /traɪˌdʒemɪn(ə)l ˈɡæŋɡliən/ *noun* a sensory ganglion containing the cells of origin of the sensory fibres in the fifth cranial nerve. Also called **Gasserian ganglion**

**trigeminal nerve** /traɪˈdʒemɪn(ə)l nɜːv/ *noun* the fifth cranial nerve, formed of the ophthalmic nerve, the maxillary nerve and the mandibular nerve, which controls the sensory nerves in the forehead, face and chin, and the muscles in the jaw

**trigeminal neuralgia** /traɪˌdʒemɪn(ə)l njuˈrældʒə/ *noun* a disorder of the trigeminal nerve, which sends intense pains shooting across the face. Also called **tic douloureux**

**trigeminy** /traɪˈdʒemɪni/ *noun* an irregular heartbeat, where a regular beat is followed by two ectopic beats

**trigger** /ˈtrɪɡə/ *verb* to start something happening ○ *It is not known what triggers the development of shingles.*

**trigger finger** /ˈtrɪɡə ˌfɪŋɡə/ *noun* a condition in which a finger can bend but is difficult to straighten, probably because of a nodule on the flexor tendon

**triglyceride** /traɪˈɡlɪsəraɪd/ *noun* a substance such as fat which contains three fatty acids

**trigone** /ˈtraɪɡəʊn/ *noun* a triangular piece of the wall of the bladder, between the openings for the urethra and the two ureters

**trigonitis** /ˌtrɪɡəˈnaɪtɪs/ *noun* inflammation of the bottom part of the wall of the bladder

**trigonocephalic** /traɪˌɡɒnəkəˈfælɪk/ *adjective* referring to a skull which shows signs of trigonocephaly

**trigonocephaly** /traɪˌɡɒnəˈkef(ə)li/ *noun* a condition in which the skull is in the shape of a triangle, with points on either side of the face in front of the ears

**triiodothyronine** /traɪˌaɪədəʊˈθaɪrəniːn/ *noun* a hormone synthesised in the body from thyroxine secreted by the thyroid gland

**trimeprazine** /traɪˈmeprəziːn/ *noun* an antihistamine used to relieve the itching caused by eczema and various skin rashes, including allergic skin rashes caused by poison ivy

**trimester** /traɪˈmestə/ *noun* one of the three 3-month periods of a pregnancy

**trimethoprim** /traɪˈmiːθəprɪm/ *noun* a synthetic drug used in the treatment of malaria

**triphosphate** /traɪˈfɒsfeɪt/ ♦ **adenosine triphosphate**

**triple marker test** /ˌtrɪp(ə)l ˈmɑːkə test/ *noun* a blood test performed on pregnant women which can detect Down's syndrome in a fetus by analysing the relative levels of substances produced by the mother's placenta and the fetus itself

**triplet** /ˈtrɪplət/ *noun* one of three babies born to a mother at the same time

**triple vaccine** /ˌtrɪp(ə)l ˈvæksiːn/ *noun* a vaccine which induces protection against three diseases e.g. diphtheria, tetanus and whooping cough

**triploid** /ˈtrɪplɔɪd/ *adjective* referring to a cell where each chromosome, except the sex chromosome, occurs three times, which is not viable in humans

**triquetrum** /traɪˈkwetrəm/, **triquetral** /traɪˈkwetr(ə)l/, **triquetral bone** /traɪˈkwetr(ə)l bəʊn/ *noun* one of the eight small carpal bones in the wrist. See illustration at **HAND** in Supplement

**trismus** /ˈtrɪzməs/ *noun* a spasm in the lower jaw, which makes it difficult to open the mouth, a symptom of tetanus

**trisomic** /traɪˈsəʊmɪk/ *adjective* referring to Down's syndrome

**trisomy** /ˈtraɪsəʊmi/ *noun* a condition in which someone has three chromosomes instead of a pair

**trisomy 21** /ˌtraɪsəʊmi ˌtwenti ˈwʌn/ *noun* same as **Down's syndrome**

**tritanopia** /ˌtraɪtəˈnəʊpiə/ *noun* a rare form of colour blindness, in which someone cannot see blue. Compare **Daltonism, deuteranopia**

**trocar** /ˈtrəʊkɑː/ *noun* a surgical instrument or pointed rod which slides inside a cannula to make a hole in tissue to drain off fluid

**trochanter** /trəˈkæntə/ *noun* two bony lumps on either side of the top end of the femur where muscles are attached

COMMENT: The lump on the outer side is the greater trochanter, and that on the inner side is the lesser trochanter.

**trochlea** /ˈtrɒkliə/ *noun* any part of the body shaped like a pulley, especially part of the lower end of the humerus, which articulates with the ulna, or a curved bone in the frontal bone through which one of the eye muscles passes (NOTE: The plural is **trochleae**.)

**trochlear** /ˈtrɒkliə/ *adjective* referring to a ring in a bone

**trochlear nerve** /ˈtrɒkliə nɜːv/ *noun* the fourth cranial nerve which controls the muscles of the eyeball

**trochoid joint** /ˈtrəʊkɔɪd dʒɔɪnt/ *noun* a joint where a bone can rotate freely about a central axis as in the neck, where the atlas articulates with the axis. Also called **pivot joint**

**trolley** /ˈtrɒli/ *noun* a wheeled table for transporting patients ○ *The patient was placed on a trolley to be taken to the operating theatre.*

**troph-** /trɒf/ *prefix* same as **tropho-** (used before vowels)

**trophic** /ˈtrɒfɪk/ *adjective* relating to food and nutrition

**trophic ulcer** /ˌtrɒfɪk ˈʌlsə/ *noun* an ulcer caused by lack of blood, e.g. a bedsore

**tropho-** /trɒfəʊ/ *prefix* referring to food or nutrition

**trophoblast** /ˈtrɒfəʊblæst/ *noun* tissue which forms the wall of a blastocyst

**-trophy** /trəfi/ *suffix* **1.** nourishment **2.** referring to the development of an organ

**tropia** /ˈtrəʊpiə/ *noun* same as **squint**

**-tropic** /trɒpɪk/ *suffix* **1.** turning towards **2.** ferring to something which influences

**tropical** /'trɒpɪk(ə)l/ *adjective* located in or coming from areas around the equator where the climate is generally very hot and humid

**tropical disease** /,trɒpɪk(ə)l dɪ'ziːz/ *noun* a disease which is found in tropical countries, e.g. malaria, dengue or Lassa fever

**tropical medicine** /,trɒpɪk(ə)l 'med(ə)sɪn/ *noun* a branch of medicine which deals with tropical diseases

**tropical ulcer** /,trɒpɪk(ə)l 'ʌlsə/ *noun* a large area of infection which forms around a wound, found especially in tropical countries. Also called **Naga sore**

**trots** /trɒts/ □ **the trots** an attack of diarrhoea (*informal*)

**trouble** /'trʌb(ə)l/ *noun* a disorder or condition (*informal*) ○ *stomach trouble* ○ *treatment for back trouble*

**Trousseau's sign** /'truːsəʊz saɪn/ *noun* a spasm in the muscles in the forearm when a tourniquet is applied to the upper arm, which causes the index and middle fingers to extend. It is a sign of latent tetany, showing that the blood contains too little calcium. [After Armand Trousseau (1801–67), French physician]

**true rib** /,truː 'rɪb/ *noun* one of the top seven pairs of ribs which are attached to the breastbone. Compare **false rib**

**true vocal cords** /,truː 'vəʊk(ə)l ,kɔːdz/ *plural noun* the cords in the larynx which can be brought together to make sounds as air passes between them

**truncus** /'trʌŋkəs/ *noun* the main blood vessel in a fetus, which develops into the aorta and pulmonary artery

**trunk** /trʌŋk/ *noun* same as **torso**

**truss** /trʌs/ *noun* a belt worn round the waist, with pads, to hold a hernia in place

**trypanocide** /'trɪpənəʊsaɪd/ *noun* a drug which kills trypanosomes

**Trypanosoma** /,trɪpənəʊ'səʊmə/, **trypanosome** /'trɪpənəʊsəʊm/ *noun* a microscopic organism which lives as a parasite in human blood. It is transmitted by the bite of insects such as the tsetse fly and causes sleeping sickness and other serious illnesses.

**trypanosomiasis** /,trɪpənəʊsəʊ'maɪəsɪs/ *noun* a disease, spread by insect bites, where trypanosomes infest the blood. Symptoms are pains in the head, general lethargy and long periods of sleep.

COMMENT: In Africa, sleeping sickness, and in South America, Chagas' disease, are both caused by trypanosomes.

**trypsin** /'trɪpsɪn/ *noun* an enzyme converted from trypsinogen by the duodenum and secreted into the digestive system where it absorbs protein

**trypsinogen** /trɪp'sɪnədʒən/ *noun* an enzyme secreted by the pancreas into the duodenum

**tryptophan** /'trɪptəfæn/ *noun* an essential amino acid

**tsetse fly** /'tetsi flaɪ, 'setsi flaɪ/ *noun* an African insect which passes trypanosomes into the human bloodstream, causing sleeping sickness

**TSH** *abbr* thyroid-stimulating hormone

**TSS** *abbr* toxic shock syndrome

**tsutsugamushi disease** /,tsuːtsəgə 'muːʃi dɪ,ziːz/ *noun* a form of typhus caused by the Rickettsia bacteria, passed to humans by mites found in South East Asia. Also called **scrub typhus**

**tubal** /'tjuːb(ə)l/ *adjective* referring to a tube

**tubal ligation** /,tjuːb(ə)l laɪ'geɪʃ(ə)n/ *noun* a surgical operation to tie up the Fallopian tubes as a sterilisation procedure

**tubal occlusion** /,tjuːb(ə)l ə'kluːʒ(ə)n/ *noun* a condition in which the Fallopian tubes are blocked, either as a result of disease or surgery

**tubal pregnancy** /,tjuːb(ə)l 'pregnənsi/ *noun* the most common form of ectopic pregnancy, in which the fetus develops in a Fallopian tube instead of the uterus

**tube** /tjuːb/ *noun* **1.** a long hollow passage in the body **2.** a soft flexible pipe for carrying liquid or gas **3.** a soft plastic or metal pipe, sealed at one end and with a lid at the other, used to dispense a paste or gel

**tube feeding** /'tjuːb ,fiːdɪŋ/ *noun* the process of giving someone nutrients through a tube directly into their stomach or small intestine

**tuber** /'tjuːbə/ *noun* a swollen or raised area

**tuber cinereum** /,tjuːbə ,sɪnə'riəm/ *noun* the part of the brain to which the stalk of the pituitary gland is connected

**tubercle** /'tjuːbək(ə)l/ *noun* **1.** a small bony projection, e.g. on a rib **2.** a small infected lump characteristic of tuberculosis, where tissue is destroyed and pus forms

**tubercular** /tjʊ'bɜːkjʊlə/ *adjective* **1.** causing or referring to tuberculosis **2.** referring to someone who has tuberculosis **3.** with small lumps, though not always due to tuberculosis

**tuberculid** /tjʊ'bɜːkjʊlɪd/, **tuberculide** *noun* a skin wound caused by tuberculosis

**tuberculin** /tjʊ'bɜːkjʊlɪn/ *noun* a substance which is derived from the culture of the tuberculosis bacillus and is used to test people for the presence of tuberculosis

**tuberculin test** /tjʊ'bɜːkjʊlɪn test/ *noun* a test to see if someone has tuberculosis, in which someone is exposed to tuberculin and the reaction of the skin is noted

**tuberculosis** /tjʊ,bɜːkjʊ'ləʊsɪs/ *noun* an infectious disease caused by the tuberculosis bacillus, where infected lumps form in the tissue. Abbr **TB**

COMMENT: Tuberculosis can take many forms: the commonest form is infection of the lungs (pulmonary tuberculosis), but it can also attack the bones (Pott's disease), the skin (lupus), or the lymph nodes (scrofula). Tuberculosis is caught by breathing in bacillus or by eating contaminated food, especially unpasteurised milk. It can be passed from one person to another, and the carrier sometimes shows no signs of the disease. Tuberculosis can be cured by treatment with antibiotics, and can be prevented by inoculation with BCG vaccine. The tests for the presence of TB are the Mantoux test, the Heaf test and the patch test; it can also be detected by X-ray screening.

**tuberculous** /tjʊ'bɜːkjʊləs/ *adjective* referring to tuberculosis

**tuberose** /'tjuːbərəʊz/ *adjective* with lumps or nodules

**tuberose sclerosis** /ˌtjuːbərəʊs sklə'rəʊsɪs/ *noun* same as **epiloia**

**tuberosity** /ˌtjuːbə'rɒsɪti/ *noun* a large lump on a bone

**tuberous** /'tjuːbərəs/ *adjective* with lumps or nodules

**tubo-** /tjuːbəʊ/ *prefix* referring to a Fallopian tube or to the internal or external auditory meatus

**tuboabdominal** /ˌtjuːbəʊæb'dɒmɪn(ə)l/ *adjective* referring to a Fallopian tube and the abdomen

**tubocurarine** /ˌtjuːbəʊ'kjʊərəriːn/ *noun* a toxic alkaloid which is the active constituent of curare, used as a muscle relaxant

**tubo-ovarian** /ˌtjuːbəʊ əʊ'veəriən/ *adjective* referring to a Fallopian tube and an ovary

**tubotympanal** /ˌtjuːbəʊ'tɪmpən(ə)l/ *adjective* referring to the Eustachian tube and the tympanum

**tubular** /'tjuːbjʊlə/ *adjective* **1.** shaped like a tube **2.** referring to a tubule

**tubular bandage** /ˌtjuːbjʊlə 'bændɪdʒ/ *noun* a bandage made of a tube of elastic cloth

**tubular reabsorption** /ˌtjuːbjʊlə riːəb'sɔːpʃən/ *noun* the process by which some of the substances filtered into the kidney are absorbed back into the bloodstream by the tubules

**tubular secretion** /ˌtjuːbjʊlə sɪ'kriːʃ(ə)n/ *noun* the secretion of some substances into the urine by the tubules of the kidney

**tubule** /'tjuːbjuːl/ *noun* a small tube in the body. ◊ **renal tubule**

**tuft** /tʌft/ *noun* **1.** a small group of hairs **2.** a group of blood vessels. ◊ **glomerular tuft**

**tugging** /'tʌgɪŋ/ ♦ **tracheal tugging**

**tularaemia** /ˌtuːlə'riːmiə/ *noun* a disease of rabbits, caused by the bacterium *Pasteurella* or *Brucella tularensis,* which can be passed to humans. In humans, the symptoms are headaches, fever and swollen lymph nodes. Also called **rabbit fever** (NOTE: The US spelling is **tularemia**.)

**tulle gras** /'tjuːl grɑː/ *noun* a dressing made of open gauze covered with soft paraffin wax which prevents sticking

**tumefaction** /ˌtjuːmɪ'fækʃən/ *noun* swelling within body tissue, usually caused a build-up of blood or water

**tumescence** /tjuː'mes(ə)ns/ *noun* swollen tissue where liquid has accumulated underneath. ◊ **oedema**

**tumescent** /tjuː'mesənt/ *adjective* swollen or showing signs of swelling, usually as a result of a build-up of blood or water within body tissues

**tumid** /'tjuːmɪd/ *adjective* swollen

**tummy** /'tʌmi/ *noun* stomach or abdomen (*informal*)

**tummy ache** /'tʌmi eɪk/ *noun* stomach pain (*informal*)

**tumoral** /'tjuːmərəl/, **tumorous** /'tjuːmərəs/ *adjective* referring to a tumour

**tumour** /'tjuːmə/ *noun* an unusual swelling or growth of new cells ○ *The X-ray showed a tumour in the breast.* ○ *A brain tumour.* (NOTE: For other terms referring to tumours, see words beginning with **onco-**. The US spelling is **tumor**.)

**tunable dye laser** /ˌtjuːnəb(ə)l daɪ 'leɪzə/ *noun* a laser which coagulates fine blood vessels, used to blanch port wine stains

**tunica** /'tjuːnɪkə/ *noun* a layer of tissue which covers an organ

**tunica adventitia** /ˌtjuːnɪkə ˌædven'tɪʃə/ *noun* an outer layer of the wall of an artery or vein. Also called **adventitia**

**tunica albuginea testis** /ˌtjuːnɪkə ælbjuˌdʒɪniə 'testɪs/ *noun* a white fibrous membrane covering the testes and the ovaries

**tunica intima** /ˌtjuːnɪkə 'ɪntɪmə/ *noun* the inner layer of the wall of an artery or vein. Also called **intima**

**tunica media** /ˌtjuːnɪkə 'miːdiə/ *noun* the middle layer of the wall of an artery or vein. Also called **media**

**tunica vaginalis** /ˌtjuːnɪkə vædʒɪ'neɪlɪs/ *noun* a membrane covering the testes and epididymis

**tuning fork** /'tjuːnɪŋ fɔːk/ *noun* a metal fork which, if hit, gives out a perfect note, used in hearing tests such as Rinne's test

**tunnel vision** /ˌtʌn(ə)l 'vɪʒ(ə)n/ *noun* vision which is restricted to the area directly in front of the eye

**turbinate** /'tɜːbɪnət/ *adjective* **1.** having a shape like a spiral or an inverted cone **2.** referring to any of the three bones found on the walls of the nasal passages of mammals

**turbinate bone** /'tɜːbɪnət bəʊn/ *noun* ♦ **nasal conchae**

**turbinectomy** /ˌtɜːbɪ'nektəmi/ *noun* a surgical operation to remove a turbinate bone

**turbulent flow** /ˌtɜːbjʊlənt ˈfləʊ/ *noun* rushing or uneven flow of blood in a vessel, usually caused by a partial obstruction

**turcica** /ˈtɜːsɪkə/ ♦ **sella turcica**

**turgescence** /tɜːˈdʒes(ə)ns/ *noun* a swelling in body tissue caused by the accumulation of fluid

**turgid** /ˈtɜːdʒɪd/ *adjective* swollen with blood

**turgor** /ˈtɜːgə/ *noun* the condition of being swollen

**turn** /tɜːn/ *noun* a slight illness or attack of dizziness (*informal*) ■ *verb* **1.** to move the head or body to face in another direction **2.** to change into something different ○ *The solution is turned blue by the reagent.*

**Turner's syndrome** /ˈtɜːnəz ˌsɪndrəʊm/ *noun* a congenital condition in females, caused by the absence of one of the pair of X chromosomes, in which sexual development is retarded and no ovaries develop [Described 1938. After Henry Hubert Turner (b. 1892), US endocrinologist, Clinical professor of Medicine, Oklahoma University, USA.]

**turricephaly** /ˌtʌrɪˈsefəli/ same as **oxycephaly**

**tussis** /ˈtʌsɪs/ *noun* coughing

**tutor** /ˈtjuːtə/ *noun* a teacher, a person who teaches small groups of students

**tweezers** /ˈtwiːzəz/ *plural noun* an instrument shaped like small scissors, with ends which pinch and do not cut, used to pull out or pick up small objects

**twenty-four hour flu** /ˌtwenti ˌfɔː aʊə ˈfluː/ *noun* any minor illness similar to flu which lasts for a short period (*informal*)

**twenty-twenty vision** /ˌtwenti ˌtwenti ˈvɪʒ(ə)n/ *noun* perfect vision

**twice** /twaɪs/ *adverb* two times □ **twice daily** two times a day

**twilight myopia** /ˌtwaɪlaɪt maɪˈəʊpiə/ *noun* a condition of the eyes, in which someone has difficulty in seeing in dim light

**twilight sleep** /ˈtwaɪlaɪt ˌsliːp/ *noun* a type of anaesthetic sleep, in which the patient is semi-conscious but cannot feel any pain

**twilight state** /ˈtwaɪlaɪt steɪt/ *noun* a condition of epileptics and alcoholics in which the person can do some automatic actions, but is not conscious of what he or she is doing

COMMENT: Twilight state is induced at childbirth, by introducing anaesthetics into the rectum.

**twin** /twɪn/ *noun* one of two babies born to a mother at the same time

COMMENT: Twins occur at a rate of about one birth in 38. They are often found in the same family, where the tendency to have twins is passed through females.

**twinge** /twɪndʒ/ *noun* a sudden sharp pain ○ *He sometimes has a twinge in his right shoulder.*

**twist** /twɪst/ *verb* to hurt a joint by turning or bending it too much or the wrong way ○ *He twisted his ankle.*

**twitch** /twɪtʃ/ *noun* a small movement of a muscle in the face or hands ■ *verb* to make small movements of the muscles

**twitching** /ˈtwɪtʃɪŋ/ *noun* small movements of the muscles in the face or hands

**tylosis** /taɪˈləʊsɪs/ *noun* the development of a callus

**tympan-** /tɪmpən/ *prefix* same as **tympano-** (NOTE: used before vowels)

**tympanectomy** /ˌtɪmpəˈnektəmi/ *noun* a surgical operation to remove the tympanic membrane

**tympanic** /tɪmˈpænɪk/ *adjective* referring to the eardrum

**tympanic bone** /tɪmˈpænɪk bəʊn/ *noun* the part of the temporal bone that supports and partly surrounds the auditory canal

**tympanic cavity** /tɪmˌpænɪk ˈkævɪti/ *noun* the section of the ear between the eardrum and the inner ear, containing the three ossicles. Also called **middle ear, tympanum**

**tympanic membrane** /tɪmˌpænɪk ˈmembreɪn/ *noun* the membrane at the inner end of the external auditory meatus leading from the outer ear, which vibrates with sound and passes the vibrations on to the ossicles in the middle ear. Also called **tympanum, eardrum**. See illustration at EAR in Supplement

**tympanites** /ˌtɪmpəˈnaɪtiːz/ *noun* the expansion of the stomach with gas. Also called **meteorism**

**tympanitis** /ˌtɪmpəˈnaɪtɪs/ *noun* same as **otitis media**

**tympano-** /tɪmpənəʊ/ *prefix* referring to the eardrum

**tympanoplasty** /ˈtɪmpənəʊplæsti/ *noun* same as **myringoplasty**

**tympanosclerosis** /ˌtɪmpənəʊskləˈrəʊsɪs/ *noun* irreversible damage to the tympanic membrane and middle ear, starting with the replacement of tissues or fibrin by collagen and hyalin. Then calcification occurs, leading to deafness.

**tympanotomy** /ˌtɪmpəˈnɒtəmi/ *noun* same as **myringotomy**

**tympanum** /ˈtɪmpənəm/ *noun* **1.** same as **tympanic membrane 2.** same as **tympanic cavity**

**type A behaviour** /ˌtaɪp ˈeɪ bɪˌheɪvjə/ *noun* a behaviour pattern which may contribute to coronary heart disease, in which an individual is aggressive and over-competitive, and usually lives at a stressful pace. Compare **type B behaviour**

**type B behaviour** /ˌtaɪp ˈbiː bɪˌheɪvjə/ *noun* a behaviour pattern which is unlikely to contribute to coronary heart disease, in which an individual is patient, tolerant, not very competitive and lives at a more relaxed pace. Compare **type A behaviour**

**Type I diabetes mellitus** /taɪp ˌwʌn daɪə ˌbiːtiːz məˈlaɪtəs/ *noun* the type of diabetes mellitus in which the beta cells of the pancreas produce little or no insulin, and the person is completely dependent on injections of insulin for survival. It is more likely to develop in people under 30. Symptoms are usually severe and occur suddenly. Also called **insulin-dependent diabetes**

**Type II diabetes mellitus** /taɪp ˌtuː daɪə ˌbiːtiːz məˈlaɪtəs/ *noun* the type of diabetes mellitus in which cells throughout the body lose some or most of their ability to use insulin. It is more likely to develop in people who are over 40, who are overweight or obese, and who do not exercise regularly. It can be controlled in some cases with diet and exercise, but more severe cases may need oral medication which reduces glucose concentrations in the blood, or insulin injections, so that even cells with a poor uptake will capture enough insulin. Also called **non-insulin-dependent diabetes**

**typhlitis** /tɪˈflaɪtɪs/ *noun* inflammation of the caecum (large intestine)

**typho-** /taɪfəʊ/ *prefix* **1.** relating to typhoid fever **2.** relating to typhus

**typhoid** /ˈtaɪfɔɪd/, **typhoid fever** /ˌtaɪfɔɪd ˈfiːvə/ *noun* an infection of the intestine caused by *Salmonella typhi* in food and water

COMMENT: Typhoid fever gives a fever and diarrhoea and the person may pass blood in the faeces. It can be fatal if not treated. People who have had the disease may become carriers, and the Widal test is used to detect the presence of typhoid fever in the blood.

**typhus** /ˈtaɪfəs/ *noun* one of several fevers caused by the Rickettsia bacterium, transmitted by fleas and lice, producing a fever, extreme weakness and a dark rash on the skin. The test for typhus is the Weil-Felix reaction.

**typical** /ˈtɪpɪk(ə)l/ *adjective* showing the usual symptoms of a condition ○ *His gait was typical of a patient suffering from Parkinson's disease.*

**typically** /ˈtɪpɪkli/ *adverb* in a typical way

**tyramine** /ˈtaɪrəmiːn/ *noun* an enzyme found in cheese, beans, tinned fish, red wine and yeast extract, which can cause high blood pressure if found in excessive quantities in the brain. ◊ **monoamine oxidase**

**tyrosine** /ˈtaɪrəsiːn/ *noun* an amino acid in protein which is a component of thyroxine, and is a precursor to the catecholamines dopamine, noradrenaline and adrenaline

**tyrosinosis** /ˌtaɪrəʊsɪˈnəʊsɪs/ *noun* a condition in which there is irregular metabolism of tyrosine

# U

**UKCC** *abbr* United Kingdom Central Council for Nursing, Midwifery and Health Visiting

**ulcer** /ˈʌlsə/ *noun* an open sore in the skin or in a mucous membrane, which is inflamed and difficult to heal ○ *stomach ulcer*

**ulcerated** /ˈʌlsəreɪtɪd/ *adjective* covered with ulcers

**ulcerating** /ˈʌlsəreɪtɪŋ/ *adjective* developing into an ulcer

**ulceration** /ˌʌlsəˈreɪʃ(ə)n/ *noun* the development of an ulcer

**ulcerative** /ˈʌls(ə)rətɪv/ *adjective* referring to ulcers, or characterised by ulcers

**ulcerative colitis** /ˌʌls(ə)rətɪv kəˈlaɪtɪs/ *noun* severe pain in the colon, with diarrhoea and ulcers in the rectum, often with a psychosomatic cause

**ulceromembranous gingivitis** /ˌʌlsərəʊ ˌmembrənəs ˌdʒɪndʒɪˈvaɪtɪs/ *noun* inflammation of the gums, which can also affect the mucous membrane in the mouth

**ulcerous** /ˈʌlsərəs/ *adjective* **1.** referring to an ulcer **2.** like an ulcer

**ulitis** /juˈlaɪtɪs/ *noun* inflammation of the gums

**ulna** /ˈʌlnə/ *noun* the longer and inner of the two bones in the forearm between the elbow and the wrist. See illustration at HAND in Supplement. Compare **radius**

**ulnar** /ˈʌlnə/ *adjective* referring to the ulna

'…the whole joint becomes disorganised, causing ulnar deviation of the fingers resulting in the typical deformity of the rheumatoid arthritic hand' [*Nursing Times*]

**ulnar artery** /ˈʌlnər ˈɑːtəri/ *noun* an artery which branches from the brachial artery at the elbow and runs down the inside of the forearm to join the radial artery in the palm of the hand

**ulnar nerve** /ˈʌlnə nɜːv/ *noun* a nerve which runs from the neck to the elbow and controls the muscles in the forearm and some of the fingers

COMMENT: The ulnar nerve passes near the surface of the skin at the elbow, where it can easily be hit, giving the effect of the 'funny bone'.

**ulnar pulse** /ˈʌlnə pʌls/ *noun* a secondary pulse in the wrist, taken near the inner edge of the forearm

**ultra-** /ʌltrə/ *prefix* **1.** further than **2.** extremely

**ultrafiltration** /ˌʌltrəfɪlˈtreɪʃ(ə)n/ *noun* the process of filtering the blood to remove tiny particles, e.g. when the blood is filtered by the kidney

**ultramicroscopic** /ˌʌltrəˌmaɪkrəˈskɒpɪk/ *adjective* referring to something so small that it cannot be seen using a standard microscope

**ultrasonic** /ˌʌltrəˈsɒnɪk/ *adjective* referring to ultrasound

**ultrasonic probe** /ˌʌltrəsɒnɪk ˈprəʊb/ *noun* an instrument which locates organs or tissues inside the body using ultrasound

**ultrasonics** /ˌʌltrəˈsɒnɪks/ *noun* the study of ultrasound and its use in medical treatments

**ultrasonic waves** /ˌʌltrəsɒnɪk ˈweɪvz/ *plural noun* same as **ultrasound**

**ultrasonogram** /ˌʌltrəˈsɒnəgræm/ *noun* a picture made with ultrasound for the purpose of medical examination or diagnosis

**ultrasonograph** /ˌʌltrəˈsɒnəgrɑːf/ *noun* a machine which takes pictures of internal organs, using ultrasound

**ultrasonography** /ˌʌltrəsəˈnɒgrəfi/ *noun* the procedure of passing ultrasound waves through the body and recording echoes which show details of internal organs. Also called **echography**

**ultrasonotomography** /ˌʌltrəˌsɒnətəˈmɒ↓grəfi/ *noun* the procedure of making images using ultrasound of organs which are placed at different depths inside the body

**ultrasound** /ˈʌltrəsaʊnd/ *noun* very high frequency sound waves which can be reflected off internal body parts or off a fetus in the womb to create images for medical examination (NOTE: No plural for **ultrasound**.)

COMMENT: The very high frequency waves of ultrasound can be used to detect and record organs or growths inside the body, in a similar way to the use of X-rays, by recording the differences in echoes sent back from different tissues. Ultrasound is used routinely to monitor the development of a fetus in the womb, and to treat some conditions such as internal bruising. It can also destroy bacteria and calculi.

**ultrasound marker** /ˈʌltrəsaʊnd ˌmɑːkə/ noun an unusual physical characteristic seen in an ultrasound examination of a fetus which is an indication of the existence of a genetic or developmental disorder

**ultrasound probe** /ˈʌltrəsaʊnd prəʊb/ noun same as **ultrasonic probe**

**ultrasound scan** /ˈʌltrəsaʊnd skæn/ noun the examination of internal parts of the body, especially a fetus in the womb, using ultrasound technology

**ultrasound scanning** /ˈʌltrəsaʊnd ˌskænɪŋ/, **ultrasound screening** /ˈʌltrəsaʊnd ˌskriːnɪŋ/ noun a method of gathering information about the body by taking images using high-frequency sound waves

**ultrasound treatment** /ˈʌltrəsaʊnd ˌtriːtmənt/ noun the treatment of soft tissue inflammation using ultrasound waves

**ultraviolet** adjective referring to the short invisible rays beyond the violet end of the spectrum, which form the element in sunlight which tans the skin, helps the skin produce Vitamin D and kills bacteria. Abbr **UV**

**ultraviolet lamp** /ˌʌltrəˌvaɪələt ˈlæmp/ noun a lamp which gives off ultraviolet rays

**ultraviolet radiation** /ˌʌltrəˌvaɪələt reɪdi ˈeɪʃ(ə)n/, **ultraviolet rays** /ˌʌltrəˈvaɪələt reɪs/ noun short invisible rays of ultraviolet light. Abbr **UVR**

**umbilical** /ʌmˈbɪlɪk(ə)l/ adjective referring to the navel

**umbilical circulation** /ʌmˌbɪlɪk(ə)l ˌsɜːkjʊ ˈleɪʃ(ə)n/ noun the circulation of blood from the mother's bloodstream through the umbilical cord into the fetus

**umbilical cord** /ʌmˈbɪlɪk(ə)l kɔːd/ noun a cord containing two arteries and one vein which links the fetus inside the uterus to the placenta

COMMENT: The arteries carry the blood and nutrients from the placenta to the fetus and the vein carries the waste from the fetus back to the placenta. When the baby is born, the umbilical cord is cut and the end tied in a knot. After a few days, this drops off, leaving the navel marking the place where the cord was originally attached.

**umbilical hernia** /ʌmˌbɪlɪk(ə)l ˈhɜːniə/ noun a hernia which bulges at the navel, usually in young children. Also called **exomphalos**

**umbilical region** /ʌmˈbɪlɪk(ə)l ˌriːdʒ(ə)n/ noun the central part of the abdomen, below the epigastrium

**umbilicated** /ʌmˈbɪlɪkeɪtɪd/ adjective with a small depression, like a navel, in the centre

**umbilicus** /ʌmˈbɪlɪkəs/ noun same as **navel**

**umbo** /ˈʌmbəʊ/ noun a projecting part in the middle of the outer side of the eardrum

**un-** /ʌn/ prefix not

**unaided** /ʌnˈeɪdɪd/ adjective without any help ○ Two days after the operation, he was able to walk unaided.

**unblock** /ʌnˈblɒk/ verb to remove something which is blocking ○ An operation to unblock an artery.

**unciform bone** /ˈʌnsɪfɔːm bəʊn/ noun one of the eight small carpal bones in the wrist, shaped like a hook. Also called **hamate bone**

**uncinate** /ˈʌnsɪnət/ adjective shaped like a hook

**uncinate epilepsy** /ˌʌnsɪnət ˈepɪlepsi/ noun a type of temporal lobe epilepsy, in which the person has hallucinations of smell and taste

**unconditioned response** /ˌʌnkən ˌdɪʃ(ə)nd rɪˈspɒns/ noun a response to a stimulus which occurs automatically, by instinct, and has not been learned

**unconscious** /ʌnˈkɒnʃəs/ adjective not aware of what is happening ○ She was unconscious for two days after the accident. ■ noun □ **the unconscious** (in psychology) the part of the mind which stores feelings, memories or desires that someone cannot consciously call up. ◊ **subconscious**

**unconsciousness** /ʌnˈkɒnʃəsnəs/ noun the state of being unconscious, e.g. as a result of lack of oxygen or from some other external cause such as a blow on the head

**uncontrollable** /ˌʌnkənˈtrəʊləb(ə)l/ adjective not able to be controlled ○ The uncontrollable spread of the disease through the population.

**uncoordinated** /ˌʌnkəʊˈɔːdɪneɪtɪd/ adjective not working together ○ His finger movements are completely uncoordinated.

**uncus** /ˈʌŋkəs/ noun a projecting part of the cerebral hemisphere, shaped like a hook

**undecenoic acid** /ʌnˌdesɪnəʊɪk ˈæsɪd/, **undecylenic acid** /ʌnˌdɪsɪlenɪk ˈæsɪd/ noun a substance made from castor bean oil, used in the treatment of fungal infections such as thrush

**under-** /ʌndə/ prefix less than usual, too little

**undergo** /ˌʌndəˈɡəʊ/ verb to experience something such as a procedure or operation ○ He underwent an appendicectomy. ○ There are six patients undergoing physiotherapy.

**underhydration** /ˌʌndəhaɪˈdreɪʃ(ə)n/ noun the condition of having too little water in the body

**undernourished** /ˌʌndəˈnʌrɪʃt/ adjective having too little food

**underproduction** /ˌʌndəprəˈdʌkʃ(ə)n/ noun the act of producing less than normal

**undertake** /ˌʌndəˈteɪk/ verb to carry out a procedure such as a surgical operation ○ Replacement of the joint is mainly undertaken to relieve pain.

**underweight** /ˌʌndəˈweɪt/ *adjective* weighing less than is medically advisable ○ *He is several pounds underweight for his age.*

**undescended testis** /ˌʌndɪˌsendɪd ˈtestɪs/ *noun* a condition in which a testis has not descended into the scrotum

**undiagnosed** /ˌʌnˌdaɪəɡˈnəʊzd/ *adjective* not identified as a specific disease or disorder

**undigested** /ˌʌndaɪˈdʒestɪd/ *adjective* referring to food which is not digested in the body

**undine** /ˈʌndiːn/ *noun* a glass container for a solution to bathe the eyes

**undress** /ʌnˈdres/ *verb* to remove clothes

**undulant fever** /ˈʌndjʊlənt ˌfiːvə/ same as **brucellosis**

**unfit** /ʌnˈfɪt/ *adjective* not physically healthy

**ungual** /ˈʌŋɡwəl/ *adjective* referring to the fingernails or toenails

**unguent** /ˈʌŋɡwənt/ *noun* a smooth oily medicinal substance which can be spread on the skin to soothe irritations

**unguentum** /ʌŋˈɡwentəm/ *noun* (*in pharmacy*) an ointment

**unguis** /ˈʌŋɡwɪs/ same as **nail**

**unhealthy** /ʌnˈhelθi/ *adjective* **1.** not in good physical condition **2.** not helping someone to be healthy ○ *The children have a very unhealthy diet.*

**unhygienic** /ˌʌnhaɪˈdʒiːnɪk/ *adjective* not clean or good for health ○ *The conditions in the hospital laundry have been criticised as unhygienic.*

**uni-** /juːni/ *prefix* one

**unicellular** /ˌjuːnɪˈseljʊlə/ *adjective* referring to an organism formed of one cell

**uniform** /ˈjuːnɪfɔːm/ *noun* the set of official clothes worn by a group of people such as the nurses in a hospital to identify them ■ *adjective* the same or similar ○ *Healthy red blood cells are of a uniform shape and size.*

**unigravida** /ˌjuːnɪˈɡrævɪdə/ same as **primigravida**

**unilateral** /ˌjuːnɪˈlæt(ə)rəl/ *adjective* affecting one side of the body only

**unilateral oophorectomy** /ˌjuːnɪˌlæt(ə)rəl ˌəʊəfəˈrektəmi/ *noun* the surgical removal of one ovary

**union** /ˈjuːnjən/ *noun* the joining together of two parts of a fractured bone. Opposite **non-union.** ◊ **malunion**

**uniovular** /ˌjuːnɪˈɒvjʊlə/ *noun* consisting of, or coming from, one ovum

**uniovular twins** /ˌjuːnɪˌɒvjʊlə ˈtwɪnz/ *plural noun* same as **identical twins**

**unipara** /juːˈnɪpərə/ same as **primipara**

**unipolar** /ˌjuːnɪˈpəʊlə/ *adjective* referring to a neurone with a single process. Compare **bipolar.** See illustration at NEURONE in Supplement

**unipolar lead** /ˌjuːnɪpəʊlə ˈliːd/ *noun* an electric lead to a single electrode

**unipolar neurone** /juːnɪˌpəʊlə ˈnjʊərəʊn/ *noun* a neurone with a single process. Compare **multipolar neurone, bipolar neurone.** See illustration at NEURONE in Supplement

**unit** /ˈjuːnɪt/ *noun* **1.** a single part of a larger whole **2.** a part of a hospital that has a specialised function ○ *a burns unit* **3.** a named and agreed standard amount used for measuring something ○ *A gram is an SI unit of weight.* **4.** a quantity of a drug, enzyme, hormone or of blood, taken as a standard for measurement and producing a given effect ○ *three units of blood* ○ *a unit of insulin* **5.** a machine or device ○ *a waste-disposal unit*

'…the blood loss caused his haemoglobin to drop dangerously low, necessitating two units of RBCs and one unit of fresh frozen plasma' [*RN Magazine*]

**United Kingdom Central Council for Nursing, Midwifery, and Health Visiting** /juːˌnaɪtɪd ˌkɪŋdəm ˌsentrəl ˌkaʊnsəl fə ˌnɜːsɪŋ mɪdˌwɪfəri ənd ˈhelθ ˌvɪzɪtɪŋ/ *noun* in the UK from 1979 until April 2002, an organisation which regulated nurses, midwives, and health visitors. The UKCC and the four National Boards have now been replaced by the Nursing and Midwifery Council. Abbr **UKCC**

**univalent** /ˌjuːniˈveɪlənt/ *adjective* same as **monovalent**

**universal donor** /ˌjuːnɪvɜːs(ə)l ˈdəʊnə/ *noun* a person with blood group O, whose blood may be given to anyone

**Universal Precautions** /ˌjuːnɪvɜːs(ə)l prɪˈkɔːʃ(ə)nz/ *abbr* UP. ♦ **Standard Precautions**

**universal recipient** /ˌjuːnɪvɜːs(ə)l rɪˈsɪpiənt/ *noun* a person with blood group AB who can receive blood from all the other blood groups

**unmedicated dressing** /ʌnˌmedɪkeɪtɪd ˈdresɪŋ/ *noun* a sterile dressing with no antiseptic or other medication on it

**unprofessional conduct** /ʌnprəˌfeʃən(ə)l ˈkɒndʌkt/ *noun* action by a professional person such as a doctor or nurse which is considered wrong by the body which regulates the profession

'…refusing to care for someone with HIV-related disease may well result in disciplinary procedure for unprofessional conduct' [*Nursing Times*]

**unqualified** /ʌnˈkwɒlɪfaɪd/ *adjective* referring to someone who has no qualifications or no licence to practise

**unsaturated fat** /ʌnˌsætʃəreɪtɪd ˈfæt/ *noun* fat which does not have a large amount of hydrogen, and so can be broken down more easily

**unstable** /ʌnˈsteɪb(ə)l/ *adjective* referring to something which may change easily ○ *an unstable mental condition.*

**unstable angina** /ʌnˌsteɪb(ə)l ænˈdʒaɪnə/ *noun* angina which has suddenly become worse

**unsteady** /ʌnˈstedi/ *adjective* likely to fall down when walking ○ *She is still very unsteady on her legs.*

**unstriated muscle** /ˌʌnstraɪˌeɪtɪd ˈmʌs(ə)l/ *noun* same as **smooth muscle**

**unviable** /ʌnˈvaɪəb(ə)l/ *adjective* referring to a fetus that cannot live if born

**unwanted pregnancy** /ʌnˌwɒntɪd ˈpregnənsi/ *noun* a condition in which a woman becomes pregnant without wanting to have a child

**unwell** /ʌnˈwel/ *adjective* ill ○ *She felt unwell and had to go home.* (NOTE: Not used before a noun: **a sick woman** but **the woman was unwell**.)

**upper** /ˈʌpə/ *adjective* at the top, higher

**upper arm** /ˌʌpə ˈɑːm/ *noun* the part of the arm from the shoulder to the elbow

**upper limb** /ˌʌpə ˈlɪm/ *noun* an arm ○ *There was damage to the upper limbs only.*

**upper motor neurone** /ˌʌpə ˈməʊtə ˌnjʊərəʊn/ *noun* a neurone which takes impulses from the cerebral cortex

**upper respiratory infection** /ˌʌpə rɪ ˈspɪrət(ə)ri ɪnˌfekʃən/ *noun* an infection in the upper part of the respiratory system

**UPPP** *abbr* uvulopalatopharyngoplasty

**upset** *noun* /ˈʌpset/ a slight illness ■ *adjective* /ʌpˈset/ slightly ill

**upside down** /ˌʌpsaɪd ˈdaʊn/ *adverb* with the top turned to the bottom

**upside-down stomach** /ˌʌpsaɪd daʊn ˈstʌmək/ *adverb US* ♦ **diaphragmatic hernia**

**uracil** /ˈjʊərəsɪl/ *noun* a pyrimidine base, one of the four bases in RNA in which it pairs with thymine

**uraemia** /jʊˈriːmiə/ *noun* a disorder caused by kidney failure, where urea is retained in the blood, and the person develops nausea, convulsions and in severe cases goes into a coma (NOTE: The US spelling is **uremia**.)

**uraemic** /jʊˈriːmɪk/ *adjective* referring to uraemia, or having uraemia (NOTE: The US spelling is **uremic**.)

**uran-** /jʊərən/ *prefix* referring to the palate

**uraniscorrhaphy** /ˌjʊərənɪˈskɒrəfi/ *noun* same as **palatorrhaphy**

**urataemia** /ˌjʊərəˈtiːmiə/ *noun* a condition in which urates are present in the blood, e.g. in gout

**urate** /ˈjʊəreɪt/ *noun* a salt of uric acid found in urine

**uraturia** /ˌjʊərəˈtjʊəriə/ *noun* the presence of excessive amounts of urates in the urine, e.g. in gout

**urea** /jʊˈriːə/ *noun* a substance produced in the liver from excess amino acids, and excreted by the kidneys into the urine

**urease** /ˈjʊərieɪz/ *noun* an enzyme which converts urea into ammonia and carbon dioxide

**urecchysis** /jʊˈrekɪsɪs/ *noun* a condition in which uric acid leaves the blood and enters connective tissue

**uresis** /jʊˈriːsɪs/ *noun* the act of passing urine

**ureter** /jʊˈriːtə, ˈjʊərɪtə/ *noun* one of the two tubes which take urine from the kidneys to the urinary bladder. See illustration at **KIDNEY** in Supplement. Also called **urinary duct**

**ureter-** /jʊriːtə/ *prefix* same as **uretero-** (*used before vowels*)

**ureteral** /jʊˈriːtərəl/ *adjective* referring to the ureters

**ureterectomy** /ˌjʊərɪtəˈrektəmi/ *noun* the surgical removal of a ureter

**ureteric** /ˌjʊərɪˈterɪk/ *adjective* same as **ureteral**

**ureteric calculus** /ˌjʊərɪterɪk ˈkælkjʊləs/ *noun* a kidney stone in the ureter

**ureteric catheter** /ˌjʊərɪterɪk ˈkæθɪtə/ *noun* a catheter passed through the ureter to the kidney, to inject an opaque solution into the kidney before taking an X-ray

**ureteritis** /ˌjʊərɪtəˈraɪtɪs/ *noun* inflammation of a ureter

**uretero-** /jʊriːtərəʊ/ *prefix* referring to the ureter

**ureterocele** /jʊˈriːtərəʊsiːl/ *noun* swelling in a ureter caused by narrowing of the opening where the ureter enters the bladder

**ureterocolostomy** /jʊˌriːtərəʊkɒˈlɒstəmi/ *noun* a surgical operation to implant the ureter into the sigmoid colon, so as to bypass the bladder

**ureteroenterostomy** /jʊˌriːtərəʊˌentə ˈrɒstəmi/ *noun* an artificially formed passage between the ureter and the intestine

**ureterolith** /jʊˈriːtərəʊlɪθ/ *noun* a stone in a ureter

**ureterolithotomy** /jʊˌriːtərəʊlɪˈθɒtəmi/ *noun* the surgical removal of a stone from the ureter

**ureterolysis** /ˌjʊərɪtəˈrɒləsɪs/ *noun* a surgical operation to free one or both ureters from adhesions or surrounding tissue

**ureteroneocystostomy** /jʊˌriːtərəʊ ˌniːəʊsaɪˈstɒstəmi/ *noun* a surgical operation to transplant a ureter to a different location in the bladder

**ureteronephrectomy** /jʊˌriːtərəʊnɪ ˈfrektəmi/ *noun* same as **nephroureterectomy**

**ureteroplasty** /jʊˈriːtərəʊplæsti/ *noun* a surgical operation to repair a ureter

**ureteropyelonephritis** /jʊˌriːtərəʊ ˌpaɪələʊnɪˈfraɪtɪs/ *noun* inflammation of the ureter and the pelvis of the kidney to which it is attached

**ureteroscope** /jʊˈriːtərəʊskəʊp/ *noun* an instrument which is passed into the ureter and up into the kidneys, usually used to locate or remove a stone

**ureteroscopy** /ˌjuərɪtəˈrɒskəpi/ *noun* an examination of the ureter with a ureteroscope

**ureterosigmoidostomy** /juˌriːtərəʊsɪgˌmɔɪˈdɒstəmi/ same as **ureterocolostomy**

**ureterostomy** /ˌjuərɪtəˈrɒstəmi/ *noun* a surgical operation to make an artificial opening for the ureter into the abdominal wall, so that urine can be passed directly out of the body

**ureterotomy** /ˌjuərɪtəˈrɒtəmi/ *noun* a surgical operation to make an incision into the ureter, mainly to remove a stone

**ureterovaginal** /juˌriːtərəʊvəˈdʒaɪn(ə)l/ *adjective* referring to the ureter and the vagina

**urethr-** /juəriːθr/ *prefix* same as **urethro-** (used before vowels)

**urethra** /juˈriːθrə/ *noun* a tube which takes urine from the bladder to be passed out of the body. See illustration at **UROGENITAL SYSTEM** in Supplement

COMMENT: In males, the urethra serves two purposes: the discharge of both urine and semen. The male urethra is about 20cm long; in women it is shorter, about 3cm and this relative shortness is one of the reasons for the predominance of bladder infection and inflammation (cystitis) in women. The urethra has sphincter muscles at either end which help control the flow of urine.

**urethral** /juˈriːθr(ə)l/ *adjective* referring to the urethra

**urethral catheter** /juˌriːθr(ə)l ˈkæθɪtə/ *noun* a catheter passed up the urethra to allow urine to flow out of the bladder, used to empty the bladder before an abdominal operation. Also called **urinary catheter**

**urethral stricture** /juˌriːθrəl ˈstrɪktʃə/ *noun* a condition in which the urethra is narrowed or blocked by a growth. Also called **urethrostenosis**

**urethritis** /ˌjuərəˈθraɪtɪs/ *noun* inflammation of the urethra

**urethro-** /juriːθrəʊ/ *prefix* referring to the urethra

**urethrocele** /juˈriːθrəsiːl/ *noun* **1.** a swelling formed in a weak part of the wall of the urethra **2.** prolapse of the urethra in a woman

**urethrogram** /juˈriːθrəgræm/ *noun* an X-ray photograph of the urethra

**urethrography** /juərɪˈθrɒgrəfi/ *noun* X-ray examination of the urethra

**urethroplasty** /juˈriːθrəplæsti/ *noun* a surgical operation to repair a urethra

**urethrorrhaphy** /juərɪˈθrɒrəfi/ *noun* a surgical operation to repair a torn urethra

**urethrorrhoea** /juˌriːθrəˈriːə/ *noun* the discharge of fluid from the urethra, usually associated with urethritis

**urethroscope** /juˈriːθrəskəʊp/ *noun* a surgical instrument, used to examine the interior of a man's urethra

**urethroscopy** /juərɪˈθrɒskəpi/ *noun* an examination of the inside of a man's urethra with a urethroscope

**urethrostenosis** /juˌriːθrəʊstəˈnəʊsɪs/ *noun* same as **urethral stricture**

**urethrostomy** /juərɪˈθrɒstəmi/ *noun* a surgical operation to make an opening for a man's urethra between the scrotum and the anus

**urethrotomy** /juərɪˈθrɒtəmi/ *noun* a surgical operation to open a blocked or narrowed urethra. Also called **Wheelhouse's operation**

**uretic** /juˈriːtɪk/ *adjective* referring to the passing of urine

**urge** /ɜːdʒ/ *noun* a strong need to do something

**urge incontinence** /ˈɜːdʒ ɪnˌkɒntɪnəns/ *noun* a condition in which someone feels a very strong need to urinate and cannot retain their urine

**urgent** /ˈɜːdʒənt/ *adjective* needing to be done quickly ○ *She had an urgent operation for strangulated hernia.*

**urgently** /ˈɜːdʒəntli/ *adverb* immediately ○ *The relief team urgently requires more medical supplies.*

**-uria** /juəriə/ *suffix* **1.** a condition of the urine **2.** a disease characterised by a condition of urine

**uric acid** /ˌjuərɪk ˈæsɪd/ *noun* a chemical compound which is formed from nitrogen in waste products from the body and which also forms crystals in the joints of people who have gout

**uricacidaemia** /ˌjuərɪkæsɪdˈiːmiə/ *noun* same as **lithaemia**

**uricosuric** /ˌjuərɪkəˈsjuərɪk/ *noun* a drug which increases the amount of uric acid excreted in the urine

**uridrosis** /ˌjuərɪˈdrəʊsɪs/ *noun* a condition in which excessive urea forms in the sweat

**urin-** /juərɪn/ *prefix* same as **urino-** (used before vowels)

**urinalysis** /ˌjuərɪˈnæləsɪs/ *noun* the analysis of urine, to detect diseases such as diabetes mellitus

**urinary** /ˈjuərɪn(ə)ri/ *adjective* referring to urine

**urinary bladder** /ˌjuərɪn(ə)ri ˈblædə/ *noun* a sac where the urine collects after passing from the kidneys through the ureters, before being passed out of the body through the urethra. See illustration at **KIDNEY**, **UROGENITAL SYSTEM (MALE)** in Supplement

**urinary catheter** /ˌjuərɪn(ə)ri ˈkæθɪtə/ *noun* same as **urethral catheter**

**urinary duct** /ˈjuərɪn(ə)ri dʌkt/ *noun* same as **ureter**

**urinary incontinence** /ˌjuərɪn(ə)ri ɪnˈkɒntɪnəns/ *noun* the involuntary emission of urine

**urinary obstruction** /ˌjʊərɪn(ə)ri əbˈstrʌkʃən/ *noun* a blockage of the urethra, which prevents urine being passed

**urinary retention** /ˌjʊərɪn(ə)ri rɪˈtenʃən/ *noun* the inability to pass urine, usually because the urethra is blocked or because the prostate gland is enlarged. Also called **urine retention**

**urinary system** /ˌjʊərɪn(ə)ri ˈsɪstəm/ *noun* a system of organs and ducts which separate waste liquids from the blood and excrete them as urine, including the kidneys, bladder, ureters and urethra

**urinary tract** /ˈjʊərɪn(ə)ri trækt/ *noun* the set of tubes down which the urine passes from the kidneys to the bladder and from the bladder out of the body

**urinary tract infection** /ˈjʊərɪn(ə)ri trækt ɪnˌfekʃən/ *noun* a bacterial infection of any part of the urinary system. Symptoms are usually a need to urinate frequently and pain on urination. Abbr **UTI**

**urinate** /ˈjʊərɪneɪt/ *verb* to pass urine from the body

**urination** /ˌjʊərɪˈneɪʃ(ə)n/ *noun* the passing of urine out of the body. Also called **micturition**

**urine** /ˈjʊərɪn/ *noun* a yellowish liquid, containing water and waste products, mainly salt and urea, which is excreted by the kidneys and passed out of the body through the ureters, bladder and urethra

**urine retention** /ˈjʊərɪn rɪˌtenʃ(ə)n/ *noun* same as **urinary retention**

**uriniferous** /ˌjʊərɪˈnɪfərəs/ *adjective* carrying urine

**uriniferous tubule** /ˌjʊərɪˌnɪf(ə)rəs ˈtjuːbjuːl/ *noun* same as **renal tubule**

**urino-** /ˈjʊərɪnəʊ/ *prefix* referring to urine

**urinogenital** /ˌjʊərɪnəʊˈdʒenɪt(ə)l/ *adjective* same as **urogenital**

**urinometer** /ˌjʊərɪˈnɒmɪtə/ *noun* an instrument which measures the specific gravity of urine

**urobilin** /ˌjʊərəʊˈbaɪlɪn/ *noun* a yellow pigment formed when urobilinogen comes into contact with air

**urobilinogen** /ˌjʊərəʊbaɪˈlɪnədʒən/ *noun* a colourless pigment formed when bilirubin is reduced to stercobilinogen in the intestines

**urocele** /ˈjʊərəsiːl/ *noun* a swelling in the scrotum which contains urine

**urochesia** /ˌjʊərəˈkiːziə/ *noun* the passing of urine through the rectum, due to injury of the urinary system (NOTE: The US spelling is **urochezia**.)

**urochrome** /ˈjʊərəkrəʊm/ *noun* the pigment which colours the urine yellow

**urodynamics** /ˌjʊərəʊdaɪˈnæmɪks/ *plural noun* the active changes which occur during the function of the bladder, urethral sphincter and pelvic floor muscles

**urogenital** /ˌjʊərəʊˈdʒenɪt(ə)l/ *adjective* referring to the urinary and genital systems. Also called **urinogenital**

**urogenital diaphragm** /jʊərəˌdʒenɪt(ə)l ˌdaɪəˈfræm/ *noun* a fibrous layer beneath the prostate gland through which the urethra passes

**urogenital system** /ˌjʊərəʊˈdʒenɪt(ə)l ˌsɪstəm/ *noun* the whole of the urinary tract and reproductive system

**urogram** /ˈjʊərəgræm/ *noun* an X-ray picture of the urinary tract, or of a part of it

**urography** /jʊˈrɒgrəfi/ *noun* an X-ray examination of part of the urinary system after injection of radio-opaque dye

**urokinase** /ˌjʊərəʊˈkaɪneɪz/ *noun* an enzyme formed in the kidneys, which begins the process of breaking down blood clots

**urolith** /ˈjʊərəlɪθ/ *noun* a stone in the urinary system

**urological** /ˌjʊərəˈlɒdʒɪk(ə)l/ *adjective* referring to urology

**urologist** /jʊˈrɒlədʒɪst/ *noun* a doctor who specialises in urology

**urology** /jʊˈrɒlədʒi/ *noun* the scientific study of the urinary system and its diseases

**urostomy** /jʊˈrɒstəmi/ *noun* the surgical creation of an artificial urethra

**urticaria** /ˌɜːtɪˈkeəriə/ *noun* an allergic reaction to injections, particular foods or plants where the skin forms irritating reddish patches. Also called **hives, nettle rash**

**USP** *abbr* United States Pharmacopeia. ♦ **pharmacopoeia**

**usual** /ˈjuːʒʊəl/ *adjective* expected or typical

**uter-** /ˈjuːtə/ *prefix* same as **utero-** (used before vowels)

**uteri** /ˈjuːt(ə)ri/ plural of **uterus**

**uterine** /ˈjuːtəraɪn/ *adjective* referring to the uterus

**uterine cavity** /ˌjuːtəraɪn ˈkævɪti/ *noun* the inside of the uterus

**uterine fibroid** /ˌjuːtəraɪn ˈfaɪbrɔɪd/, **uterine fibroma** /ˌjuːtəraɪn faɪˈbrəʊmə/ *noun* same as **fibroid tumour**

**uterine procidentia** /ˌjuːtəraɪn prəʊsɪˈdenʃə/, **uterine prolapse** /ˌjuːtəˌraɪn ˈprəʊlæps/ *noun* a condition in which part of the uterus has passed through the vagina, usually after childbirth

COMMENT: Uterine procidentia has three stages of severity: in the first the cervix descends into the vagina, in the second the cervix is outside the vagina, but part of the uterus is still inside, and in the third stage, the whole uterus passes outside the vagina.

**uterine retroflexion** /ˌjuːtəraɪn ˌretrəʊˈflekʃ(ə)n/ *noun* a condition in which the uterus bends backwards away from its usual position

**uterine retroversion** /ˌjuːtəraɪn retrəʊ
ˈvɜːʃ(ə)n/ *noun* a condition in which the uterus slopes backwards away from its usual position

**uterine subinvolution** /ˌjuːtəraɪn ˌsʌb
ɪnvəˈluːʃ(ə)n/ *noun* a condition in which the
uterus does not go back to its previous size after childbirth

**uterine tube** /ˈjuːtəraɪn tjuːb/ *noun* same as
**Fallopian tube**

**utero-** /juːtərəʊ/ *prefix* referring to the uterus

**uterocele** /ˈjuːtərəsiːl/ *noun* a hernia of the
uterus. Also called **hysterocele**

**uterogestation**        /ˌjuːtərədʒeˈsteɪʃ(ə)n/
*noun* a standard pregnancy, where the fetus develops in the uterus

**uterography** /ˌjuːtəˈrɒɡrəfi/ *noun* an X-ray
examination of the uterus

**utero-ovarian** /ˌjuːtərəʊ əʊˈveəriən/ *adjective* referring to the uterus and the ovaries

**uterosalpingography**        /ˌjuːtərəʊsælpɪŋ
ˈɡɒɡrəfi/ same as **hysterosalpingography**

**uterovesical** /ˌjuːtərəʊˈvesɪk(ə)l/ *adjective*
referring to the uterus and the bladder

**uterus** /ˈjuːt(ə)rəs/ *noun* the hollow organ in
a woman's pelvic cavity, behind the bladder
and in front of the rectum in which the embryo
develops before birth. Also called **womb**. See
illustration at **UROGENITAL SYSTEM (FEMALE)** in
Supplement (NOTE: For other terms referring to
the uterus, see words beginning with **hyster-,
hystero-, metr-, metro-.**)

COMMENT: The top of the uterus is joined to the
Fallopian tubes which link it to the ovaries,
and the lower end (cervix uteri) opens into the
vagina. When an ovum is fertilised it becomes
implanted in the wall of the uterus and develops into an embryo inside it. If fertilisation and
pregnancy do not take place, the lining of the
uterus (endometrium) is shed during menstruation. At childbirth, strong contractions of the
wall of the uterus (myometrium) help push the
baby out through the vagina.

**uterus didelphys** /ˌjuːt(ə)rəs daɪˈdelfɪs/
*noun* same as **double uterus**

**UTI** *abbr* urinary tract infection

**utricle** /ˈjuːtrɪk(ə)l/, **utriculus** /jʊˈtrɪkjʊləs/
*noun* a large sac inside the vestibule of the ear,
which relates information about the upright
position of the head to the brain

**UV** *abbreviation* ultraviolet

**UV-absorbing lens** /juː ˌviː əbˌzɔːbɪŋ
ˈlenz/ *noun* a lens devised to absorb UVR in
order to protect the eyes against the sun

**uvea** /ˈjuːviə/ *noun* a layer of organs in the
eye beneath the sclera, formed of the iris, the
ciliary body and the choroid. Also called **uveal
tract**

**uveal** /ˈjuːviəl/ *adjective* referring to the uvea

**uveal tract** /ˈjuːviəl trækt/ *noun* same as
**uvea**

**uveitis** /ˌjuːviˈaɪtɪs/ *noun* inflammation of
any part of the uvea

**uveoparotid fever** /ˌjuːviəˈpærətɪd ˌfiːvə/,
**uveoparotid syndrome** /ˌjuːviəˈpærətɪd
ˌsɪndrəʊm/ *noun* inflammation of the uvea
and of the parotid gland

**UVR** *abbr* ultraviolet radiation

**uvula** /ˈjuːvjʊlə/ *noun* a piece of soft tissue
which hangs down from the back of the soft
palate

**uvular** /ˈjuːvjʊlə/ *adjective* referring to the
uvula

**uvulectomy** /ˌjuːvjʊˈlektəmi/ *noun* the surgical removal of the uvula

**uvulitis** /ˌjuːvjʊˈlaɪtɪs/ *noun* inflammation
of the uvula

**uvulopalatopharyngoplasty** /ˌjuːvjʊləʊ
ˌpælətəʊfəˈrɪŋɡəʊplæsti/ *noun* a surgical operation to remove the uvula and other soft tissue in the palate, in order to widen the airways
and treat the problem of snoring. Abbr **UPPP**

# V

**vaccinate** /ˈvæksɪneɪt/ *verb* to introduce vaccine into a person's body in order to make the body create its own antibodies, so making the person immune to the disease (NOTE: You vaccinate someone **against** a disease.)

**vaccination** /ˌvæksɪˈneɪʃ(ə)n/ *noun* the action of vaccinating someone

> COMMENT: Originally the words **vaccination** and **vaccine** applied only to smallpox immunisation, but they are now used for immunisation against any disease. Vaccination is mainly given against cholera, diphtheria, rabies, smallpox, tuberculosis, and typhoid.

**vaccine** /ˈvæksiːn/ *noun* a substance which contains antigens to a disease or a weak form of a disease, used to protect people against it

**vaccinotherapy** /ˌvæksɪnəʊˈθerəpi/ *noun* the treatment of a disease with a vaccine

**vacuole** /ˈvækjuəʊl/ *noun* a space in a fold of a cell membrane

**vacuum** /ˈvækjuəm/ *noun* a space which is completely empty of all matter, including air

**vacuum extraction** /ˈvækjuəm ɪkˌstrækʃən/ *noun* the procedure of pulling on the head of the baby with a suction instrument to aid birth

**vacuum extractor** /ˈvækjuəm ɪkˌstræktə/ *noun* a surgical instrument formed of a rubber suction cup which is used in vacuum extraction during childbirth

**vacuum suction** /ˈvækjuəm ˌsʌkʃən/ *noun* a method used to achieve an abortion, after dilatation of the cervix. Also called **aspiration**

**vagal** /ˈveɪɡ(ə)l/ *adjective* referring to the vagus nerve

**vagal tone** /ˌveɪɡ(ə)l ˈtəʊn/ *noun* the action of the vagus nerve to slow the beat of the sinoatrial node

**vagin-** /vədʒaɪn/ *prefix* referring to the vagina

**vagina** /vəˈdʒaɪnə/ *noun* a passage in a woman's reproductive tract between the entrance to the uterus, the cervix, and the vulva, able to stretch enough to allow a baby to pass through during childbirth. See illustration at UROGENITAL SYSTEM (FEMALE) in Supplement (NOTE: For other terms referring to the vagina, see words beginning with **colp-, colpo-**.)

**vaginal** /vəˈdʒaɪn(ə)l/ *adjective* referring to the vagina

**vaginal bleeding** /vəˌdʒaɪn(ə)l ˈbliːdɪŋ/ *noun* bleeding from the vagina

**vaginal delivery** /vəˌdʒaɪn(ə)l dɪˈlɪv(ə)ri/ *noun* the birth of a baby through the mother's vagina, without surgical intervention

**vaginal diaphragm** /vəˌdʒaɪn(ə)l ˈdaɪəfræm/ *noun* a circular contraceptive device for women, which is inserted into the vagina and placed over the neck of the uterus before sexual intercourse

**vaginal discharge** /vəˌdʒaɪn(ə)l ˈdɪstʃɑːdʒ/ *noun* the flow of liquid from the vagina

**vaginal douche** /vəˌdʒaɪn(ə)l ˈduːʃ/ *noun* **1.** the process of washing out the vagina **2.** a device or liquid for washing out the vagina

**vaginal examination** /vəˌdʒaɪn(ə)l ɪɡˌzæmɪˈneɪʃ(ə)n/ *noun* the act of checking the vagina for signs of disease or growth

**vaginalis** /ˌvædʒɪˈneɪlɪs/ *noun* **1.** same as **Trichomonas vaginalis 2.** same as **tunica vaginalis**

**vaginal orifice** /vəˌdʒaɪn(ə)l ˈɒrɪfɪs/ *noun* an opening leading from the vulva to the uterus

**vaginal proctocele** /vəˌdʒaɪn(ə)l ˈprɒktəsiːl/ *noun* a condition associated with prolapse of the uterus, where the rectum protrudes into the vagina

**vaginal suppository** *noun* same as **pessary 1**

**vaginectomy** /ˌvædʒɪˈnektəmi/ *noun* a surgical operation to remove the vagina or part of it

**vaginismus** /ˌvædʒɪˈnɪzməs/ *noun* a painful contraction of the vagina which prevents sexual intercourse

**vaginitis** /ˌvædʒɪˈnaɪtɪs/ *noun* inflammation of the vagina which is mainly caused by the bacterium *Trichomonas vaginalis* or by a fungus *Candida albicans*

**vaginography** /ˌvædʒɪˈnɒɡrəfi/ *noun* an X-ray examination of the vagina

**vaginoplasty** /vəˈdʒaɪnəplæsti/ *noun* a surgical operation to graft tissue on to the vagina

**vaginoscope** /'vædʒɪnəʊskəʊp/ *noun* same as **colposcope**

**vago-** /veɪgəʊ/ *prefix* referring to the vagus nerve

**vagotomy** /veɪ'gɒtəmi/ *noun* a surgical operation to cut through the vagus nerve which controls the nerves in the stomach, as a treatment for peptic ulcers

**vagus** /'veɪgəs/, **vagus nerve** /'veɪgəs nɜːv/ *noun* either of the tenth pair of cranial nerves which carry sensory and motor neurons serving the heart, lungs, stomach, and various other organs and control swallowing. Also called **pneumogastric nerve**

**valgus** /'vælgəs/, **valgum** /'vælgəm/, **valga** /'vælgə/ *adjective* turning outwards. ◊ **hallux valgus**. Compare **varus**

**validity** /və'lɪdɪti/ *noun* (*of a study*) the fact of being based on sound research and methods which exclude alternative explanations of a result

**valine** /'veɪliːn/ *noun* an essential amino acid

**Valium** /'væliəm/ a trade name for diazepam

**vallate papillae** /,væleɪt pə'pɪliː/ *plural noun* large papillae which form a line towards the back of the tongue and contain taste buds

**vallecula** /və'lekjʊlə/ *noun* a natural depression or fissure in an organ as between the hemispheres of the brain (NOTE: The plural is **valleculae**.)

**Valsalva's manoeuvre** /væl'sælvəz mə,nuːvə/ *noun* the process of breathing out while holding the nostrils closed and keeping the mouth shut, used in order to test the functioning of the Eustachian tubes or to adjust the pressure in the middle ear

**value** /'væljuː/ *noun* **1.** the degree to which something is useful or necessary ○ *food with low nutritional value* **2.** a number or amount that is unknown and is shown as a symbol ■ *plural noun* **values** the views someone has about the appropriate way to behave ○ *respect for different cultural values*

**valve** /vælv/ *noun* a flap which opens and closes to allow liquid to pass in one direction only, e.g. in the heart, blood vessels or lymphatic vessels

**valvotomy** /væl'vɒtəmi/ *noun* a surgical operation to cut into a valve to make it open wider

**valvula** /'vælvjʊlə/ *noun* a small valve (NOTE: The plural is **valvulae**.)

**valvular** /'vælvjʊlə/ *adjective* referring to a valve

**valvular disease of the heart** /,vælvjʊlə dɪ,ziːz əv ðiː 'hɑːt/ *noun* an inflammation of the membrane which lines the valves of the heart. Abbr **VDH**

**valvulitis** /,vælvjʊ'laɪtɪs/ *noun* inflammation of a valve in the heart

**valvuloplasty** /'vælvjʊləʊplæsti/ *noun* surgery to repair valves in the heart without opening the heart

'…in percutaneous balloon valvuloplasty a catheter introduced through the femoral vein is placed across the aortic valve and into the left ventricle; the catheter is removed and a valve-dilating catheter bearing a 15mm balloon is placed across the valve' [*Journal of the American Medical Association*]

**valvulotomy** /,vælvjʊ'lɒtəmi/ *noun* same as **valvotomy**

**vancomycin** /,væŋkəʊ'maɪsɪn/ *noun* an antibiotic which is effective against some bacteria which are resistant to other antibiotics. Strains of bacteria resistant to vancomycin have now developed.

**van den Bergh test** /,væn den 'bɜːg ,test/ *noun* a test of blood serum to see if a case of jaundice is caused by an obstruction in the liver or by haemolysis of red blood cells [After A.A. Hijmans van den Bergh (1869–1943), Dutch physician]

**vaporise** /'veɪpəraɪz/, **vaporize** *verb* to turn a liquid into a vapour

**vaporiser** /'veɪpəraɪzə/, **vaporizer** *noun* a device which warms a liquid to which medicinal oil has been added, so that it provides a vapour which someone can inhale

**vapour** /'veɪpə/ *noun* **1.** a substance in the form of a gas **2.** steam from a mixture of a liquid and a medicinal oil (NOTE: The US spelling is **vapor**.)

**Vaquez-Osler disease** /væ,keɪz 'ɒslə dɪ,ziːz/ *noun* same as **polycythaemia vera** [After Henri Vaquez (1860–1936), French physician, Sir William Osler (1849–1919), Professor of Medicine in Montreal, Philadelphia, Baltimore and then Oxford]

**vara** /'veərə/ *adjective* same as **varus**

**variant CJD** /,veəriənt ,siːdʒeɪ 'diː/ *noun* a form of Creutzfeldt-Jakob disease which was observed first in the 1980s, especially affecting younger people. Abbr **vCJD**

**variation** /,veəri'eɪʃ(ə)n/ *noun* a change from one level to another ○ *There is a noticeable variation in his pulse rate.* ○ *The chart shows the variations in the patient's temperature over a twenty-four hour period.*

**varicectomy** /,væri'sektəmi/ *noun* a surgical operation to remove a vein or part of a vein

**varicella** /,væri'selə/ *noun* same as **chickenpox**

**varicella-zoster virus** /,væriselə 'zɒstə ,vaɪrəs/ *noun* a herpes virus that causes chickenpox and shingles

**varices** /'værisiːz/ plural of **varix**

**varicocele** /'værikəʊsiːl/ *noun* swelling of a vein in the spermatic cord which can be corrected by surgery

**varicose** /'værikəʊs/ *adjective* **1.** affected with or having varicose veins **2.** designed for the treatment of varicose veins **3.** relating to or producing swelling

**varicose eczema** /ˌværɪkəʊs ˈeksɪmə/ *noun* eczema which develops on the legs, caused by bad circulation. Also called **hypostatic eczema**

**varicose ulcer** /ˌværɪkəʊs ˈʌlsə/ *noun* an ulcer in the leg as a result of bad circulation and varicose veins

**varicose vein** /ˌværɪkəʊs ˈveɪn/ *noun* a vein, usually in the legs, which becomes twisted and swollen

**varicosity** /ˌværɪˈkɒsɪti/ *noun* (*of veins*) the condition of being swollen and twisted

**varicotomy** /ˌværɪˈkɒtəmi/ *noun* a surgical operation to make a cut into a varicose vein

**varifocals** /ˈveəriˌfəʊk(ə)lz/ *plural noun* spectacles with lenses which have varying focal lengths from top to bottom, for looking at things at different distances from the wearer

**variola** /vəˈraɪələ/ *noun* same as **smallpox**

**varioloid** /ˈveəriəlɔɪd/ *noun* a type of mild smallpox which affects people who have already had smallpox or have been vaccinated against it

**varix** /ˈveəriks/ *noun* a swollen blood vessel, especially a swollen vein in the leg (NOTE: The plural is **varices**.)

**Varolii** /vəˈrəʊliː/ ♦ **pons Varolii**

**varus** /ˈveərəs/, **varum** /ˈveərəm/, **vara** /ˈveərə/ *adjective* turning inwards. ◊ **coxa vara**. Compare **valgus**

**vary** /ˈveəri/ *verb* **1.** to change ○ *The dosage varies according to the age of the patient.* **2.** to try different actions ○ *The patient was recommended to vary her diet.*

**vas** /væs/ *noun* a tube in the body (NOTE: The plural is **vasa**.)

**vas-** /væs/ *prefix* same as **vaso-**

**vasa efferentia** /ˌveɪsə efəˈrentiə/ *plural noun* the group of small tubes which sperm travel down from the testis to the epididymis

**vasa vasorum** /ˌveɪsə veɪˈsɔːrəm/ *plural noun* tiny blood vessels in the walls of larger blood vessels

**vascular** /ˈvæskjʊlə/ *adjective* referring to blood vessels

**vascular dementia** /ˌvæskjʊlə dɪˈmenʃə/ *noun* a form of mental degeneration due to disease of the blood vessels in the brain

**vascularisation** /ˌvæskjʊləraɪˈzeɪʃ(ə)n/, **vascularization** *noun* the development of new blood vessels

**vascular lesion** /ˌvæskjʊlə ˈliːʒ(ə)n/ *noun* damage to a blood vessel

**vascular system** /ˈvæskjʊlə ˌsɪstəm/ *noun* the series of vessels such as veins, arteries and capillaries, carrying blood around the body

**vasculitis** /ˌvæskjʊˈlaɪtɪs/ *noun* inflammation of a blood vessel

**vas deferens** /ˌvæs ˈdefərenz/ *noun* see illustration at UROGENITAL SYSTEM (MALE) in Supplement. also called **ductus deferens**, **sperm duct** (NOTE: The plural is **vasa deferentia**.)

**vasectomy** /vəˈsektəmi/ *noun* a surgical operation to cut a vas deferens, in order to prevent sperm travelling from the epididymis up the duct. ◊ **bilateral vasectomy**

**vas efferens** /ˌvæs ˈefərenz/ *noun* one of many tiny tubes which take the spermatozoa from the testis to the epididymis (NOTE: The plural is **vasa efferentia**.)

**vaso-** /veɪzəʊ/ *prefix* **1.** referring to a blood vessel **2.** referring to the vas deferens

**vasoactive** /ˌveɪzəʊˈæktɪv/ *adjective* having an effect on the blood vessels, especially constricting the arteries

**vasoconstriction** /ˌveɪzəʊkənˈstrɪkʃən/ *noun* a contraction of blood vessels which makes them narrower

**vasoconstrictor** /ˌveɪzəʊkənˈstrɪktə/ *noun* a chemical substance which makes blood vessels become narrower, so that blood pressure rises, e.g. ephedrine hydrochloride

**vasodilatation** /ˌveɪzəʊˌdaɪləˈteɪʃ(ə)n/, **vasodilation** /ˌveɪzəʊdaɪˈleɪʃ(ə)n/ *noun* the relaxation of blood vessels, especially the arteries, making them wider and leading to increased blood flow or reduced blood pressure

**vasodilator** /ˌveɪzəʊdaɪˈleɪtə/ *noun* a chemical substance which makes blood vessels become wider, so that blood flows more easily and blood pressure falls, e.g. hydralazine hydrochloride

'Volatile anaesthetic agents are potent vasodilators and facilitate blood flow to the skin.' [*British Journal of Nursing*]

**vaso-epididymostomy** /ˌveɪzəʊ ˌepɪdɪdɪˈmɒstəmi/ *noun* a surgical operation to reverse a vasectomy in which the cut end of the vas deferens is joined to a tubule within the epididymis above a blockage in it

**vasoinhibitor** /ˌveɪzəʊɪnˈhɪbɪtə/ *noun* a chemical substance that reduces or stops the activity of the nerves that control the widening or narrowing of the blood vessels

**vasoligation** /ˌveɪzəlaɪˈgeɪʃ(ə)n/ *noun* a surgical operation to tie the vasa deferentia to prevent infection entering the epididymis from the urinary system

**vasomotion** /ˌveɪzəˈməʊʃ(ə)n/ *noun* the control of the diameter of blood vessels and thus of blood flow. ◊ **vasoconstriction**, **vasodilatation**

**vasomotor** /ˌveɪzəʊˈməʊtə/ *adjective* referring to the control of the diameter of blood vessels

**vasomotor centre** /ˌveɪzəʊˈməʊtə ˌsentə/ *noun* a nerve centre in the brain which changes the rate of heartbeat and the diameter of blood vessels and so regulates blood pressure

**vasomotor nerve** /ˌveɪzəʊˈməʊtə nɜːv/ noun a nerve in the wall of a blood vessel which affects the diameter of the vessel

**vasopressin** /ˌveɪzəʊˈpresɪn/ noun same as **antidiuretic hormone**

**vasopressor** /ˌveɪzəʊˈpresə/ noun a substance which increases blood pressure by narrowing the blood vessels

**vasospasm** /ˈveɪzəʊspæzm/ noun a muscle spasm causing the fingers to become cold, white and numb. ◊ **Raynaud's disease**

**vasovagal** /ˌveɪzəʊˈveɪg(ə)l/ adjective referring to the vagus nerve and its effect on the heartbeat and blood circulation

**vasovagal attack** /ˌveɪzəʊˈveɪg(ə)l əˌtæk/ noun a fainting fit as a result of a slowing down of the heartbeats caused by excessive activity of the vagus nerve

**vasovasostomy** /ˌveɪzəʊvəˈsɒstəmi/ noun a surgical operation to reverse a vasectomy

**vasovesiculitis** /ˌveɪzəʊvesɪkjuˈlaɪtɪs/ noun inflammation of the seminal vesicles and a vas deferens

**vastus intermedius** /ˌvæstəs ˌɪntəˈmiːdiəs/, **vastus medialis** /ˌvæstəs ˌmiːdiˈeɪlɪs/, **vastus lateralis** /ˌvæstəs ˌlætəˈreɪlɪs/ noun three of the four parts of the quadriceps femoris, the muscle of the thigh (NOTE: The fourth is the rectus femoris.)

**vault** /vɔːlt/ noun □ **vault of the skull** part of the skull which includes the frontal bone, the temporal bones and the occipital bone

**VBAC** abbr vaginal birth after Caesarean section

**vCJD** abbr variant CJD

**VD** abbr venereal disease

**VD clinic** /ˌviː ˈdiː ˌklɪnɪk/ noun a clinic specialising in the diagnosis and treatment of venereal diseases

**VDH** abbr valvular disease of the heart

**vectis** /ˈvektɪs/ noun a curved surgical instrument used in childbirth

**vector** /ˈvektə/ noun an insect or animal which carries a disease and can pass it to humans ○ The tsetse fly is a vector of sleeping sickness.

**vegan** /ˈviːgən/ noun someone who does not eat meat, dairy produce, eggs or fish and eats only vegetables and fruit ■ adjective involving a diet of only vegetables and fruit

**vegetarian** /ˌvedʒɪˈteəriən/ noun someone who does not eat meat, but eats mainly vegetables and fruit and sometimes dairy produce, eggs or fish ■ adjective involving a diet without meat

**vegetation** /ˌvedʒɪˈteɪʃ(ə)n/ noun a growth on a membrane, e.g. on the cusps of valves in the heart

**vegetative** /ˈvedʒɪtətɪv/ adjective 1. referring to growth of tissue or organs 2. referring

to a state after brain damage, where a person is alive and breathing but shows no responses

**vehicle** /ˈviːɪk(ə)l/ noun a liquid in which a dose of a drug is put

**vein** /veɪn/ noun a blood vessel which takes deoxygenated blood containing waste carbon dioxide from the tissues back to the heart (NOTE: For other terms referring to veins see words beginning **phleb-, phlebo-** or **vene-, veno-**.)

**vena cava** /ˌviːnə ˈkeɪvə/ noun one of two large veins which take deoxygenated blood from all the other veins into the right atrium of the heart. See illustration at HEART in Supplement, KIDNEY in Supplement (NOTE: The plural is **venae cavae**.)

COMMENT: The superior vena cava brings blood from the head and the top part of the body, while the inferior vena cava brings blood from the abdomen and legs.

**vene-** /veni/ prefix referring to veins

**venene** /vəˈniːn/ noun a mixture of different venoms, used to produce antivenene

**venepuncture** /ˈvenɪpʌŋktʃə/ noun the act of puncturing a vein either to inject a drug or to take a blood sample

**venereal** /vəˈnɪəriəl/ adjective 1. relating to sex acts or sexual desire 2. relating to the genitals 3. referring to an infection or disease which is transmitted through sexual intercourse ○ venereal warts

**venereal disease** /vɪˈnɪəriəl dɪˌziːz/ noun a disease which is passed from one person to another during sexual intercourse. Abbr **VD** (NOTE: Now usually called a **sexually transmitted disease (STD)**.)

**venereal wart** /vəˌnɪəriəl ˈwɔːt/ noun a wart on the genitals or in the urogenital area

**venereologist** /vəˌnɪəriˈɒlədʒɪst/ noun a doctor who specialises in the study of venereal diseases

**venereology** /vəˌnɪəriˈɒlədʒi/ noun the scientific study of venereal diseases

**venereum** /vəˈnɪəriəm/ ◆ **lymphogranuloma venereum**

**veneris** /ˈvenərɪs/ ◆ **mons**

**venesection** /ˌvenɪˈsekʃən/ noun an operation where a vein is cut so that blood can be removed, e.g. when taking blood from a donor

**venipuncture** /ˈvenɪpʌŋktʃə/ noun same as **venepuncture**

**veno-** /viːnəʊ/ prefix referring to veins

**venoclysis** /vəˈnɒkləsɪs/ noun the procedure of slowly introducing a saline or other solution into a vein

**venogram** /ˈviːnəgræm/ noun same as **phlebogram**

**venography** /vɪˈnɒgrəfi/ noun same as **phlebography**

**venom** /ˈvenəm/ noun a poison in the bite of a snake or insect

COMMENT: Depending on the source of the bite, venom can have a wide range of effects, from a sore spot after a bee sting, to death from a scorpion. Antivenene will counteract the effects of venom, but is only effective if the animal which gave the bite can be correctly identified.

**venomous** /ˈvenəməs/ *adjective* referring to an animal which has poison in its bite ○ *The cobra is a venomous snake.* ○ *He was bitten by a venomous spider.*

**venosus** /vɪˈnəʊsəs/ ♦ **ductus venosus**

**venous** /ˈviːnəs/ *adjective* referring to the veins

'…venous air embolism is a potentially fatal complication of percutaneous venous catheterization' [*Southern Medical Journal*]

'…a pad was placed under the Achilles tendon to raise the legs, thus aiding venous return and preventing deep vein thrombosis' [*NATNews*]

**venous bleeding** /ˌviːnəs ˈbliːdɪŋ/ *noun* bleeding from a vein

**venous blood** /ˈviːnəs blʌd/ *noun* same as **deoxygenated blood**

**venous haemorrhage** /ˌviːnəs ˈhem(ə)rɪdʒ/ *noun* the escape of blood from a vein

**venous system** /ˈviːnəs ˌsɪstəm/ *noun* a system of veins which brings blood back to the heart from the tissues

**venous thrombosis** /ˌviːnəs θrɒmˈbəʊsɪs/ *noun* the blocking of a vein by a blood clot

**venous ulcer** /ˌviːnəs ˈʌlsə/ *noun* an ulcer in the leg, caused by varicose veins or by a blood clot

**ventilation** /ˌventɪˈleɪʃ(ə)n/ *noun* the act of breathing air in or out of the lungs, so removing waste products from the blood in exchange for oxygen. ◊ **dead space**

**ventilator** /ˈventɪleɪtə/ *noun* a machine which pumps air into and out of the lungs of someone who has difficulty in breathing ○ *The newborn baby was put on a ventilator.* Also called **respirator**

**ventilatory failure** /ˈventɪleɪtri ˌfeɪljə/ *noun* a failure of the lungs to oxygenate the blood correctly

**Ventimask** /ˈventɪmɑːsk/ a trademark for a type of oxygen mask

**Ventolin** /ˈventəlɪn/ a trade name for salbutamol

**ventouse** /ˈventuːs/ *noun* a cup-like vacuum device attached to the top of an unborn baby's head in the process of delivery, used to enable a distressed baby to be born quickly

**ventral** /ˈventr(ə)l/ *adjective* **1.** referring to the abdomen **2.** referring to the front of the body. Opposite **dorsal**

**ventricle** /ˈventrɪk(ə)l/ *noun* a cavity in an organ, especially in the heart or brain. See illustration at **HEART** in Supplement

COMMENT: There are two ventricles in the heart: the left ventricle takes oxygenated blood from the pulmonary vein through the left atrium, and pumps it into the aorta to circulate round the body; the right ventricle takes blood from the veins through the right atrium, and pumps it into the pulmonary artery to be passed to the lungs to be oxygenated. There are four ventricles in the brain, each containing cerebrospinal fluid. The two lateral ventricles in the cerebral hemispheres contain the choroid processes which produce cerebrospinal fluid. The third ventricle lies in the midline between the two thalami. The fourth ventricle is part of the central canal of the hindbrain.

**ventricul-** /ventrɪkjʊl/ *prefix* referring to a ventricle in the brain or heart

**ventricular** /venˈtrɪkjʊlə/ *adjective* referring to the ventricles

**ventricular fibrillation** /venˌtrɪkjʊlə ˌfaɪbrɪˈleɪʃ(ə)n/ *noun* a serious heart condition where the ventricular muscles flutter and the heart no longer beats. Abbr **VF**

**ventricular folds** /venˈtrɪkjʊlə fəʊldz/ *plural noun* same as **vocal cords**

**ventricular septal defect** /venˌtrɪkjʊlə ˈsept(ə)l dɪˌfekt/ *noun* a condition in which blood can flow between the two ventricles of the heart, because the intraventricular septum has not developed properly. Abbr **VSD**. Compare **atrial septal defect**

**ventriculitis** /ˌventrɪkjʊˈlaɪtɪs/ *noun* inflammation of the brain ventricles

**ventriculoatriostomy** /venˌtrɪkjʊləʊˌeɪtrɪˈɒstəmi/ *noun* an operation to relieve pressure caused by excessive quantities of cerebrospinal fluid in the brain ventricles

**ventriculogram** /venˈtrɪkjʊləgræm/ *noun* an X-ray picture of the ventricles of the brain

**ventriculography** /ˌventrɪkjʊˈlɒgrəfi/ *noun* a method of taking X-ray pictures of the ventricles of the brain after air has been introduced to replace the cerebrospinal fluid

**ventriculo-peritoneal shunt** /venˌtrɪkjʊləʊ ˌperɪtəˌniːəl ˈʃʌnt/ *noun* an artificial drain used in hydrocephalus to drain cerebrospinal fluid from the ventricles

**ventriculoscopy** /venˌtrɪkjʊˈlɒskəpi/ *noun* an examination of the brain using an endoscope

**ventriculostomy** /venˌtrɪkjʊˈlɒstəmi/ *noun* a surgical operation to pass a hollow needle into a ventricle of the brain so as to reduce pressure, take a sample of fluid or enlarge the ventricular opening to prevent the need for a shunt

**ventro-** /ventrəʊ/ *prefix* **1.** ventral **2.** referring to the abdomen

**ventrofixation** /ˌventrəʊfɪkˈseɪʃ(ə)n/ *noun* a surgical operation to treat retroversion of the uterus by attaching the uterus to the wall of the abdomen

**ventrosuspension** /ˌventrəʊsəˈspenʃən/ *noun* a surgical operation to treat retroversion of the uterus

**Venturi mask** /venˈtjʊəri mɑːsk/ *noun* a type of disposable mask which gives the person a controlled mixture of oxygen and air

**Venturi nebuliser** /venˈtjʊəri ˌnebjʊlaɪzə/ *noun* a type of nebuliser which is used in aerosol therapy

**venule** /ˈvenjuːl/ *noun* a small vein or vessel leading from tissue to a larger vein

**verapamil** /vəˈræpəmɪl/ *noun* a synthetic compound which helps to prevent the movement of calcium ions across membranes. It is used in the treatment of angina pectoris, hypertension and irregular heartbeat.

**verbigeration** /ˌvɜːbɪdʒəˈreɪʃ(ə)n/ *noun* a condition seen in people with mental disorders, in which they keep saying the same words over and over again

**vermicide** /ˈvɜːmɪsaɪd/ *noun* a substance which kills worms in the intestine

**vermiform** /ˈvɜːmɪfɔːm/ *adjective* shaped like a worm

**vermiform appendix** /ˌvɜːmɪfɔːm əˈpendɪks/ *noun* same as **appendix 1**

**vermifuge** /ˈvɜːmɪfjuːdʒ/ *noun* a substance which removes worms from the intestine

**vermillion border** /vəˌmɪliən ˈbɔːdə/ *noun* the external red parts of the lips

**vermis** /ˈvɜːmɪs/ *noun* the central part of the cerebellum, which forms the top of the fourth ventricle

**vermix** /ˈvɜːmɪks/ *noun* a vermiform appendix

**vernix caseosa** /ˌvɜːnɪks keɪsiˈəʊsə/ *noun* an oily substance which covers a baby's skin at birth

**verruca** /vəˈruːkə/ *noun* a small hard harmless growth on the sole of the foot, caused by a virus (NOTE: Verrucas are a type of wart. The plural is **verrucas** or **verrucae**.)

**version** /ˈvɜːʃ(ə)n/ *noun* the procedure of turning a fetus in a uterus so as to put it in a better position for birth

**vertebra** /ˈvɜːtɪbrə/ *noun* one of twenty-four ring-shaped bones which link together to form the backbone. See illustration at CARTILAGINOUS JOINT in Supplement (NOTE: The plural is **vertebrae**.)

COMMENT: The top vertebra (the atlas) supports the skull; the first seven vertebrae in the neck are the cervical vertebrae; then follow the twelve thoracic or dorsal vertebrae which are behind the chest and five lumbar vertebrae in the lower part of the back. The sacrum and coccyx are formed of five sacral vertebrae and four coccygeal vertebrae which have fused together.

**vertebral** /ˈvɜːtɪbrəl/ *adjective* referring to the vertebrae

**vertebral artery** /ˌvɜːtɪbrəl ˈɑːtəri/ *noun* one of two arteries which go up the back of the neck into the brain

**vertebral canal** /ˌvɜːtɪbrəl kəˈnæl/ *noun* same as **spinal canal**

**vertebral column** /ˈvɜːtɪbrəl ˌkɒləm/ *noun* the series of bones and discs linked together to form a flexible column running from the base of the skull to the pelvis. Also called **backbone, spinal column**. See illustration at PELVIS in Supplement

**vertebral disc** /ˌvɜːtɪbrəl ˈdɪsk/ *noun* same as **intervertebral disc**

**vertebral foramen** /ˌvɜːtɪbrəl fəˈreɪmən/ *noun* a hole in the centre of a vertebra which links with others to form the vertebral canal through which the spinal cord passes

**vertebral ganglion** /ˌvɜːtəbrəl ˈɡæŋɡliən/ *noun* a ganglion in front of the origin of the vertebral artery

**vertebro-basilar insufficiency** /ˌvɜːtɪbrəʊ ˌbæzɪlə ˌɪnsəˈfɪʃənsi/ *noun* a brainstem ischaemia due to temporary occlusion of the arteries

**vertex** /ˈvɜːteks/ *noun* the top of the skull

**vertex delivery** /ˈvɜːteks dɪˌlɪv(ə)ri/ *noun* a normal birth, where the baby's head appears first

**vertigo** /ˈvɜːtɪɡəʊ/ *noun* **1.** feelings of dizziness or giddiness caused by a malfunction of the sense of balance **2.** a fear of heights, as a result of a sensation of dizziness which is felt when high up, especially on a tall building ○ *She won't sit near the window – she suffers from vertigo.*

**very low density lipoprotein** /ˌveri ləʊ ˌdensəti ˌlɪpəʊˈprəʊtiːn/ *noun* a fat produced by the liver after food has been absorbed and before it becomes low density lipoprotein. Abbr **VLDL**

**vesical** /ˈvesɪk(ə)l/ *adjective* referring to the bladder

**vesicant** /ˈvesɪkənt/ *noun* a substance which makes the skin blister. Also called **epispastic**

**vesicle** /ˈvesɪk(ə)l/ *noun* **1.** a small blister on the skin, e.g. caused by eczema **2.** a sac which contains liquid

**vesico-** /ˈvesɪkəʊ/ *prefix* referring to the urinary bladder

**vesicofixation** /ˌvesɪkəʊfɪkˈseɪʃ(ə)n/ *noun* same as **cystopexy**

**vesicostomy** /ˌvesɪˈkɒstəmi/, **vesicotomy** /ˌvesɪˈkɒtəmi/ *noun* same as **cystostomy**

**vesicoureteric reflux** /ˌvesɪkəʊjʊəri ˌterɪk ˈriːflʌks/ *noun* the flowing of urine back from the bladder up the ureters during urination, which may carry infection from the bladder to the kidneys. Also called **vesicoureteric reflux**

**vesicouretic** /ˌvesɪkəʊjʊˈretɪk/ *adjective* relating to the urinary bladder and the ureters

**vesicouretic reflux** /ˌvesɪkəʊjʊˌretɪk ˈriːflʌks/ *noun* same as **vesicoureteric reflux**

**vesicovaginal** /ˌvesɪkəʊvəˈdʒaɪn(ə)l/ *adjective* referring to the bladder and the vagina

**vesicovaginal fistula** /ˌvesɪkəʊvəˌdʒaɪn(ə)l ˈfɪstjʊlə/ *noun* an unusual opening between the bladder and the vagina

**vesicular** /vəˈsɪkjʊlə/ *adjective* referring to a vesicle

**vesicular breathing** /vəˌsɪkjʊlə ˈbriːðɪŋ/, **vesicular breath sound** /vəˌsɪkjʊlə ˈbreθ saʊnd/ *plural noun* the sound made during the normal breathing process

**vesiculation** /vəˌsɪkjʊˈleɪʃ(ə)n/ *noun* the formation of blisters on the skin

**vesiculectomy** /ˌvesɪkjʊˈlektəmi/ *noun* a surgical operation to remove a seminal vesicle

**vesiculitis** /vəˌsɪkjʊˈlaɪtɪs/ *noun* inflammation of the seminal vesicles

**vesiculography** /vəˌsɪkjʊˈlɒɡrəfi/ *noun* an X-ray examination of the seminal vesicles

**vesiculopapular** /vəˌsɪkjʊləʊˈpæpjʊlə/ *adjective* referring to a skin disorder which has both blisters and papules

**vesiculopustular** /vəˌsɪkjʊləʊˈpʌstjʊlə/ *adjective* referring to a skin disorder which has both blisters and pustules

**vessel** /ˈves(ə)l/ *noun* **1.** a tube in the body along which liquid flows, especially a blood vessel **2.** a container for fluids

**vestibular** /veˈstɪbjʊlə/ *adjective* referring to a vestibule, especially the vestibule of the inner ear

**vestibular folds** /veˈstɪbjʊlə fəʊldz/ *plural noun* folds in the larynx above the vocal folds, which are not used for speech. Also called **false vocal cords**

**vestibular glands** /veˈstɪbjʊlə ɡlændz/ *plural noun* the glands at the point where the vagina and vulva join, which secrete a lubricating substance

**vestibular nerve** /veˈstɪbjʊlə nɜːv/ *noun* the part of the auditory nerve which carries information about balance to the brain

**vestibule** /ˈvestɪbjuːl/ *noun* a cavity in the body at the entrance to an organ, especially the first cavity in the inner ear or the space in the larynx above the vocal cords or a nostril. See illustration at EAR in Supplement

**vestibulocochlear nerve** /ˌvesˌtɪbjʊləʊ ˈkɒkliə ˌnɜːv/ *noun* the eighth cranial nerve which governs hearing and balance. Also called **acoustic nerve, auditory nerve**

**vestigial** /vesˈtɪdʒiəl/ *adjective* existing in a rudimentary form ○ *The coccyx is a vestigial tail.*

**VF** *abbr* ventricular fibrillation □ **in VF** referring to someone whose heart is no longer able to beat

**viability** /ˌvaɪəˈbɪlɪti/ *noun* the fact of being viable ○ *The viability of the fetus before the 22nd week is doubtful.*

**viable** /ˈvaɪəb(ə)l/ *adjective* referring to a fetus which can survive if born ○ *A fetus is viable by about the 28th week of pregnancy.*

**Viagra** /vaɪˈæɡrə/ a trade name for sildenafil citrate

**vial** /ˈvaɪəl/ *noun* same as **phial**

**Vibramycin** /ˌvaɪbrəˈmaɪsɪn/ a trade name for doxycycline

**vibrate** /vaɪˈbreɪt/ *verb* to move rapidly and continuously

**vibration** /vaɪˈbreɪʃ(ə)n/ *noun* rapid and continuous movement ○ *Speech is formed by the vibrations of the vocal cords.*

**vibration white finger** /vaɪˌbreɪʃ(ə)n ˈwaɪt ˌfɪŋɡə/ *noun* a condition caused by long-term use of a chain saw or pneumatic drill, which affects the circulation in the fingers

**vibrator** /vaɪˈbreɪtə/ *noun* a device to produce vibrations, which may be used for massages

**Vibrio** /ˈvɪbriəʊ/ *noun* a genus of Gram-negative bacteria which are found in water and cause cholera

**vibrissae** /vaɪˈbrɪsiː/ *plural noun* hairs in the nostrils or ears

**vicarious** /vɪˈkeəriəs/ *adjective* done by one organ or agent in place of another

**vicarious menstruation** /vɪˌkeəriəs ˌmenstruˈeɪʃ(ə)n/ *noun* the discharge of blood other than by the vagina during menstrual periods

**victim** /ˈvɪktɪm/ *noun* a person who is injured in an accident or who has caught a disease ○ *The victims of the rail crash were taken to the local hospital.* □ **to fall victim to something** to become a victim of or to experience bad effects from something ○ *Half the people eating at the restaurant fell victim to salmonella poisoning.*

**vigour** /ˈvɪɡə/ *noun* a combination of positive attributes expressed in rapid growth, large size, high fertility and long life in an organism (NOTE: The US spelling is **vigor**.)

**villous** /ˈvɪləs/ *adjective* shaped like a villus, or formed of villi

**villus** /ˈvɪləs/ *noun* a tiny projection like a finger on the surface of a mucous membrane (NOTE: The plural is **villi**.)

**vinblastine** /vɪnˈblæstiːn/ *noun* an alkaloid drug used in the treatment of cancer

**vincristine** /vɪnˈkrɪstiːn/ *noun* an alkaloid drug similar to vinblastine, also used in the treatment of cancer. It works by blocking cell division and is highly toxic.

**vinculum** /ˈvɪŋkjʊləm/ *noun* a thin connecting band of tissue (NOTE: The plural is **vincula**.)

**violent** /ˈvaɪələnt/ *adjective* very strong, very severe ○ *He had a violent headache.* ○ *Her reaction to the injection was violent.*

**violently** /ˈvaɪələntli/ *adverb* in a strong way ○ *He reacted violently to the antihistamine.*

**violet** /ˈvaɪələt/ *noun* a dark, purplish blue colour at the end of the visible spectrum

**viraemia** /vaɪˈriːmiə/ *noun* a virus in the blood (NOTE: The US spelling is **viremia**.)

**viral** /ˈvaɪrəl/ *adjective* caused by a virus, or referring to a virus

**viral hepatitis** *noun* same as **serum hepatitis**

**viral infection** /ˈvaɪrəl ɪnˌfekʃən/ *noun* an infection caused by a virus

**viral pneumonia** /ˌvaɪrəl njuːˈməʊniə/ *noun* a type of inflammation of the lungs caused by a virus. Also called **virus pneumonia**

**virgin** /ˈvɜːdʒɪn/ *noun* a female who has not experienced sexual intercourse

**virginity** /vəˈdʒɪnɪti/ *noun* the condition of a female who has not experienced sexual intercourse

**virile** /ˈvɪraɪl/ *adjective* like a man, with strong male characteristics

**virilisation** /ˌvɪrɪlaɪˈzeɪʃ(ə)n/, **virilization** *noun* the development of male characteristics in a woman, caused by a hormone imbalance or therapy

**virilism** /ˈvɪrɪlɪz(ə)m/ *noun* male characteristics such as body hair and a deep voice in a woman

**virology** /vaɪˈrɒlədʒi/ *noun* the scientific study of viruses

**virulence** /ˈvɪrʊləns/ *noun* **1.** the ability of a microorganism to cause a disease **2.** the degree of effect of a disease

**virulent** /ˈvɪrʊlənt/ *adjective* **1.** referring to the ability of a microorganism to cause a disease ○ *an unusually virulent strain of the virus* **2.** referring to a disease which develops rapidly and has strong effects

**virus** /ˈvaɪrəs/ *noun* a parasite consisting of a nucleic acid surrounded by a protein coat that can only develop in other cells. Viruses cause many diseases including the common cold, AIDS, herpes and polio. (NOTE: Antibiotics have no effect on viruses, but effective vaccines have been developed for some viral diseases.)

**virus pneumonia** *noun* same as **viral pneumonia**

**viscera** /ˈvɪsərə/ *plural noun* the internal organs, e.g. the heart, lungs, stomach and intestines

**visceral** /ˈvɪsərəl/ *adjective* referring to the internal organs

**visceral larva migrans** /ˌvɪsərəl ˌlɑːvə ˈmaɪɡrænz/ *noun* same as **toxocariasis**

**visceral muscle** /ˈvɪsərəl ˌmʌs(ə)l/ *noun* a smooth muscle in the wall of the intestine which makes the intestine contract

**visceral pericardium** /ˌvɪsərəl ˌperiˈkɑːdiəm/ *noun* the inner layer of serous pericardium, attached to the wall of the heart

**visceral peritoneum** /ˌvɪsərəl ˌperitəʊˈniːəm/ *noun* part of the peritoneum which covers the organs in the abdominal cavity

**visceral pleura** /ˌvɪsərəl ˈplʊərə/ *noun* a membrane attached to the surface of a lung. See illustration at LUNGS in Supplement

**visceral pouch** /ˈvɪsərəl paʊtʃ/ *noun* same as **pharyngeal pouch**

**viscero-** /vɪsərəʊ/ *prefix* relating to the viscera

**visceromotor** /ˌvɪsərəˈməʊtə/ *adjective* controlling the movement of viscera

**visceroptosis** /ˌvɪsərəˈtəʊsɪs/ *noun* a movement of an internal organ downwards from its usual position

**visceroreceptor** /ˌvɪsərəʊriˈseptə/ *noun* a receptor cell which reacts to stimuli from organs such as the stomach, heart and lungs

**viscid** /ˈvɪsɪd/ *adjective* referring to a liquid which is sticky and slow-moving

**viscosity** /vɪˈskɒsɪti/ *noun* the state of a liquid which moves slowly

**viscous** /ˈvɪskəs/ *adjective* referring to a liquid which is thick and slow-moving

**viscus** /ˈvɪskəs/ ♦ **viscera**

**visible** /ˈvɪzɪb(ə)l/ *adjective* able to be seen ○ *There were no visible symptoms of the disease.*

**vision** /ˈvɪʒ(ə)n/ *noun* the ability to see, eyesight ○ *After the age of 50, many people's vision begins to fail.*

**vision centre** /ˈvɪʒ(ə)n ˌsentə/ *noun* the point in the brain where the nerves relating to the eye come together

**visit** /ˈvɪzɪt/ *noun* **1.** a short stay with someone, especially to comfort a patient ○ *The patient is too weak to have any visits.* ○ *He is allowed visits of ten minutes only.* **2.** a short stay with a professional person ○ *They had a visit from the district nurse.* ○ *She paid a visit to the chiropodist.* ○ *On the patient's last visit to the physiotherapy unit, nurses noticed a great improvement in her walking.* ■ *verb* to stay a short time with someone ○ *I am going to visit my brother in hospital.* ○ *She was visited by the health visitor.*

**visiting times** /ˈvɪzɪtɪŋ taɪmz/ *plural noun* the times of day when friends are allowed into a hospital to visit patients

**visitor** /ˈvɪzɪtə/ *noun* a person who visits ○ *Visitors are allowed into the hospital on Sunday afternoons.* ○ *How many visitors did you have this week?*

**visual** /ˈvɪʒʊəl/ *adjective* referring to sight or vision

**visual acuity** /ˌvɪʒʊəl əˈkjuːɪti/ *noun* the ability to see objects clearly

**visual area** /ˌvɪʒʊəl ˈeəriə/ *noun* the part of the cerebral cortex which is concerned with sight

**visual axis** /ˌvɪʒʊəl ˈæksɪs/ *noun* the line between the object on which the eye focuses, and the fovea

**visual cortex** /ˌvɪʒʊəl ˈkɔːteks/ *noun* the part of the cerebral cortex which receives information about sight

**visual field** /ˈvɪʒʊəl fiːlᵈd/ *noun* the area which can be seen without moving the eye. Also called **field of vision**

**visualisation** /ˌvɪʒʊəlaɪˈzeɪʃ(ə)n/, **visualization** *noun* **1.** a technique in which an image of an internal organ or other part of the body is produced by using X-rays or other means such as magnetic resonance imaging **2.** a technique in which someone creates a strongly positive mental picture of something such as the way in which they would like to solve a problem, in order to help them cope with it

**visually impaired** /ˌvɪʒʊəli ɪmˈpeəd/ *adjective* having difficulty in seeing because of an eye condition

**visually impaired person** /ˌvɪʒʊəli ɪmˌpeəd ˈpɜːs(ə)n/ *noun* a person whose eyesight is not clear

**visual purple** /ˌvɪʒʊəl ˈpɜːp(ə)l/ *noun* same as **rhodopsin**

**vitae** /ˈvaɪtiː/ ◆ **arbor vitae**

**vital** /ˈvaɪt(ə)l/ *adjective* very important or necessary for life ○ *If circulation is stopped, vital nerve cells begin to die in a few minutes.* ○ *Oxygen is vital to the human system.*

**vital capacity** /ˌvaɪt(ə)l kəˈpæsɪti/ *noun* the largest amount of air which a person can exhale at one time

**vital centre** /ˌvaɪt(ə)l ˈsentə/ *noun* a group of nerve cells in the brain which govern a particular function of the body such as the five senses

**vital organs** /ˌvaɪt(ə)l ˈɔːɡənz/ *plural noun* the most important organs in the body, without which a human being cannot live, e.g. the heart, lungs and brain

**vital signs** /ˌvaɪt(ə)l ˈsaɪnz/ *plural noun* measurements of pulse, breathing and temperature

**vital statistics** /ˌvaɪt(ə)l stəˈtɪstɪks/ *plural noun* a set of official statistics relating to the population of a place, such as the percentage of live births per thousand, the incidence of particular diseases and the numbers of births and deaths

**vitamin** /ˈvɪtəmɪn/ *noun* an essential substance not synthesised in the body, but found in most foods, and needed for good health

**Vitamin A** /ˌvɪtəmɪn ˈeɪ/ *noun* a vitamin which is soluble in fat and can be formed in the body from precursors but is mainly found in food such as liver, vegetables, eggs and cod liver oil. Also called **retinol**

COMMENT: Lack of Vitamin A affects the body's growth and resistance to disease and can cause night blindness or xerophthalmia. Carotene (the yellow substance in carrots) is a precursor of Vitamin A, which accounts for the saying that eating carrots helps you to see in the dark.

**Vitamin B₁** /ˌvɪtəmɪn biː ˈwʌn/ *noun* a vitamin found in yeast, liver, cereals and pork. Also called **thiamine**

**Vitamin B₂** /ˌvɪtəmɪn biː ˈtuː/ *noun* a vitamin found in eggs, liver, green vegetables, milk and yeast. Also called **riboflavine**

**Vitamin B₆** /ˌvɪtəmɪn biː ˈsɪks/ *noun* a vitamin found in meat, cereals and molasses. Also called **pyridoxine**

**Vitamin B₁₂** /ˌvɪtəmɪn biː ˈtwelv/ *noun* a vitamin found in liver and kidney, but not present in vegetables. Also called **cyanocobalamin**

**Vitamin B complex** /ˌvɪtəmɪn biː ˈkɒmpleks/ *noun* a group of vitamins such as folic acid, riboflavine and thiamine

**Vitamin C** /ˌvɪtəmɪn ˈsiː/ *noun* a vitamin which is soluble in water and is found in fresh fruit, especially oranges and lemons, raw vegetables and liver. Also called **ascorbic acid**

**Vitamin D** /ˌvɪtəmɪn ˈdiː/ *noun* a vitamin which is soluble in fat and is found in butter, eggs and fish. It is also produced by the skin when exposed to sunlight. It helps in the formation of bones, and lack of it causes rickets in children.

**vitamin deficiency** /ˈvɪtəmɪn dɪˌfɪʃ(ə)nsi/ *noun* a lack of necessary vitamins ○ *He is suffering from Vitamin A deficiency.* ○ *Vitamin C deficiency causes scurvy.*

**Vitamin E** /ˌvɪtəmɪn ˈiː/ *noun* a vitamin found in vegetables, vegetable oils, eggs and wholemeal bread

**Vitamin K** /ˌvɪtəmɪn ˈkeɪ/ *noun* a vitamin found in green vegetables such as spinach and cabbage, and which helps the clotting of blood and is needed to activate prothrombin

**vitelline sac** /vɪˈtelaɪn sæk/ *noun* a sac attached to an embryo, where the blood cells first form

**vitellus** /vɪˈteləs/ *noun* the yolk of an egg (ovum)

**vitiligo** /ˌvɪtiˈlaɪɡəʊ/ *noun* a condition in which white patches appear on the skin. Also called **leucoderma**

**vitrectomy** /vɪˈtrektəmi/ *noun* a surgical operation to remove some or all of the vitreous humour of the eye

**vitreous** /ˈvɪtriəs/ *adjective* **1.** having the characteristics of glass **2.** relating to the vitreous humour of the eye

**vitreous body** /ˈvɪtriəs ˌbɒdi/ *noun* same as **vitreous humour**

**vitreous detachment** /ˌvɪtriəs dɪˈtætʃmənt/ *noun* the separation of the vitreous humour from the retina, often due to natural ageing when the vitreous humour thins, but also occurring in other conditions such as diabetes

**vitreous humour** /ˌvɪtriəs ˈhjuːmə/ *noun* a transparent jelly which fills the main cavity behind the lens in the eye. See illustration at EYE in Supplement

**vitritis** /vɪˈtraɪtɪs/ *noun* same as **hyalitis**

**vitro** /ˈviːtriəʊ/ **♦ in vitro**

**Vitus** /ˈvaɪtəs/ **♦ St Vitus's dance**

**viviparous** /vɪˈvɪpərəs/ *adjective* referring to animals which bear live young, such as humans, as opposed to birds and reptiles which lay eggs

**vivisection** /ˌvɪvɪˈsekʃən/ *noun* the act of dissecting a living animal as an experiment

**vocal** /ˈvəʊk(ə)l/ *adjective* referring to the voice

**vocal cords** /ˈvəʊk(ə)l kɔːdz/ *plural noun* a pair of fibrous sheets of tissue which span the cavity of the voice box (**larynx**) and produce sounds by vibrating. Also called **ventricular folds**

**vocal folds** /ˈvəʊk(ə)l fəʊldz/ *plural noun* same as **vocal cords**

**vocal folds abducted** /ˌvəʊk(ə)l fəʊldz əb ˈdʌktɪd/ *noun* the usual condition of the vocal cords in quiet breathing

**vocal folds adducted** /ˌvəʊk(ə)l fəʊldz ə ˈdʌktɪd/ *noun* the position of the vocal cords for speaking

**vocal fremitus** /ˌvəʊk(ə)l ˈfremɪtəs/ *noun* a vibration of the chest when a person speaks or coughs

**vocal ligament** /ˈvəʊk(ə)l ˌlɪgəmənt/ *noun* a ligament in the centre of the vocal cords

**vocal resonance** /ˌvəʊk(ə)l ˈrezənəns/ *noun* a sound heard by a doctor when he or she listens through a stethoscope to the chest while a person is speaking

**voice** /vɔɪs/ *noun* the sound made when a person speaks or sings □ **to lose one's voice** not to be able to speak because of a throat infection □ **his voice has broken** his voice has become deeper and adult, with the onset of puberty

**voice box** /ˈvɔɪs bɒks/ *noun* the larynx, a hollow organ containing the vocal cords at the back of the throat, which produces sounds

**volar** /ˈvəʊlə/ *adjective* referring to the palm of the hand or sole of the foot

**volatile** /ˈvɒlətaɪl/ *adjective* referring to a liquid which turns into gas at room temperature

**volatile oils** /ˌvɒlətaɪl ˈɔɪlz/ *plural noun* concentrated oils from plants used in cosmetics and as antiseptics

**volitantes** /ˌvɒlɪˈtæntiːz/ **♦ muscae volitantes**

**volition** /vəˈlɪʃ(ə)n/ *noun* the ability to use the will

**Volkmann's canal** /ˈfɒlkmɑːnz kəˌnæl/ *noun* a canal running horizontally through compact bone, carrying blood to the Haversian systems [After Richard von Volkmann (1830–89), German surgeon]

**Volkmann's contracture** /ˈfɒlkmɑːnz kən ˌtræktʃə/ *noun* a fibrosis and tightening of the muscles of the forearm because blood supply has been restricted, leading to contraction of the fingers

**volsella** /vɒlˈselə/ *noun* a type of surgical forceps with claw-like hooks at the end of each arm. Also called **vulsella**

**volume** /ˈvɒljuːm/ *noun* an amount of a substance

**voluntary** /ˈvɒlənt(ə)ri/ *adjective* done because one wishes to do it

**voluntary admission** /ˌvɒlənt(ə)ri əd ˈmɪʃ(ə)n/ *noun* the process of taking someone into a psychiatric hospital with the person's consent

**voluntary movement** /ˌvɒlənt(ə)ri ˈmuːvmənt/ *noun* a movement directed by the person's willpower, using voluntary muscles, e.g. walking or speaking

**voluntary muscle** /ˈvɒlənt(ə)ri ˌmʌs(ə)l/ *noun* a muscle which is consciously controlled. It is usually made up of striated fibres.

COMMENT: Voluntary muscles work in pairs where one contracts and pulls, while the other relaxes to allow the bone to move.

**volunteer** /ˌvɒlənˈtɪə/ *noun* a person who offers to do something for free, without being paid ○ *The hospital relies on voluntary help with sports for disabled children* ○ *They are asking for volunteers to test the new cold cure.* ■ *verb* to offer to do something for free ○ *The research team volunteered to test the new drug on themselves.*

**volvulus** /ˈvɒlvjʊləs/ *noun* a condition in which a loop of intestine is twisted and blocked, so cutting off its blood supply

**vomer** /ˈvəʊmə/ *noun* a thin flat vertical bone in the septum of the nose

**vomica** /ˈvɒmɪkə/ *noun* **1.** a cavity in the lungs containing pus **2.** the act of vomiting pus from the throat or lungs

**vomit** /ˈvɒmɪt/ *noun* partly digested food which has been brought up from the stomach into the mouth ○ *His bed was covered with vomit.* ○ *She died after choking on her own vomit.* Also called **vomitus** ■ *verb* to bring up partly digested food from the stomach into the mouth ○ *He had a fever, and then started to vomit.* ○ *She vomited her breakfast.*

**vomiting** /ˈvɒmɪtɪŋ/ *noun* the act of bringing up vomit into the mouth. Also called **emesis**

**vomitus** /ˈvɒmɪtəs/ *noun* same as **vomit**

**von Hippel-Lindau syndrome** /vɒn ˌhɪp(ə)l ˈlɪndaʊ ˌsɪndrəʊm/ *noun* a disease in which angiomas of the brain are related to angiomas and cysts in other parts of the body

**von Recklinghausen's disease** /ˌvɒn ˈreklɪŋhaʊz(ə)nz dɪˌziːz/ *noun* **1.** same as **neurofibromatosis 2.** same as **osteitis fibrosis cystica** [Described 1882. After Friedrich Daniel von Recklinghausen (1833–1910), Professor of Pathology at Strasbourg, France.]

**von Willebrand's disease** /ˌvɒn ˈvɪlɪ
brændz dɪˌziːz/ *noun* a hereditary blood disease, occurring in both sexes, in which the mucous membrane starts to bleed without any apparent reason. It is caused by a deficiency of a
clotting factor in the blood, called von Willebrand's factor. [Described 1926. After E. A. von
Willebrand (1870–1949), Finnish physician.]
**von Willebrand's factor** /ˌvɒn ˈvɪlɪ
brændz ˌfæktə/ *noun* a protein substance in
plasma involved in platelet aggregation
**voyeurism** /ˈvwaɪɜːrɪz(ə)m/ *noun* a condition in which a person experiences sexual
pleasure by watching others having intercourse
**VSD** *abbr* ventricular septal defect
**vu** /vuː/ ♦ déjà vu
**vulgaris** /vʌlˈgeərɪs/ ♦ lupus vulgaris
**vulnerable** /ˈvʌln(ə)rəb(ə)l/ *adjective* likely
to catch a disease because of being in a weakened state ○ *Premature babies are especially
vulnerable to infection.*
**vulsella** /vʌlˈselə/, **vulsellum** /vʌlˈseləm/
*noun* same as **volsella**
**vulv-** /vʌlv/ *prefix* referring to the vulva (*used
before vowels*)
**vulva** /ˈvʌlvə/ *noun* a woman's external sexual organs, at the opening leading to the vagina.
◊ **kraurosis vulvae** (NOTE: For other terms referring to the vulva, see words beginning with **epi-
si-**.)
  COMMENT: The vulva is formed of folds (the labia), surrounding the clitoris and the entrance
  to the vagina.
**vulvectomy** /vʌlˈvektəmi/ *noun* a surgical
operation to remove the vulva
**vulvitis** /vʌlˈvaɪtɪs/ *noun* inflammation of
the vulva, causing intense irritation
**vulvovaginitis** /ˌvʌlvəʊvædʒɪˈnaɪtɪs/ *noun*
inflammation of the vulva and vagina

# W

**wad** /wɒd/ *noun* a pad of material used to put on a wound ○ *The nurse put a wad of absorbent cotton over the sore.*

**wadding** /'wɒdɪŋ/ *noun* material used to make a wad ○ *Put a layer of cotton wadding over the eye.*

**waist** /weɪst/ *noun* the narrow part of the body below the chest and above the buttocks

**wait** /weɪt/ *verb* to stay somewhere until something happens or someone arrives ○ *He has been waiting for his operation for six months.* ○ *There are ten patients waiting to see Dr Smith.*

**waiting list** /'weɪtɪŋ lɪst/ *noun* a list of people waiting for admission to hospital usually for treatment of non-urgent disorders ○ *The length of waiting lists for non-emergency surgery varies enormously from one region to another.* ○ *It is hoped that hospital waiting lists will get shorter.*

**waiting room** /'weɪtɪŋ ruːm/ *noun* a room at a doctor's or dentist's surgery where people wait ○ *Please sit in the waiting room – the doctor will see you in ten minutes.*

**waiting time** /'weɪtɪŋ taɪm/ *noun* the period between the time when someone's name has been put on the waiting list and his or her admission into hospital

**wake** /weɪk/ *verb* **1.** to interrupt someone's sleep ○ *The nurse woke the patient.* or *The patient was woken by the nurse.* **2.** to stop sleeping ○ *The patient had to be woken to have his injection.* (NOTE: **waking – woke – woken**)

**wakeful** /'weɪkf(ə)l/ *adjective* wide awake, not wanting to sleep

**wakefulness** /'weɪkfʊlnəs/ *noun* the condition of being wide awake

**wake up** /ˌweɪk 'ʌp/ *verb* to stop sleeping, or stop someone sleeping ○ *The old man woke up in the middle of the night and started calling for the nurse.*

**Waldeyer's ring** /ˌvɑːldaɪəz 'rɪŋ/ *noun* a ring of lymphoid tissue made by the tonsils and adenoid [Described 1884. After Heinrich Wilhelm Gottfried Waldeyer-Hartz (1836–1921), German anatomist.]

**walk** /wɔːk/ *verb* to go on foot ○ *The baby is learning to walk.* ○ *He walked when he was only eleven months old.* ○ *She can walk a few steps with a Zimmer frame.*

**walking distance** /'wɔːkɪŋ ˌdɪstəns/ *noun* the distance which someone can walk before they experience pain in their muscles, which shows the effectiveness of the blood supply to their legs

**walking frame** /'wɔːkɪŋ freɪm/ *noun* a metal frame used by people who have difficulty in walking. ◊ **Zimmer frame**

**wall** /wɔːl/ *noun* the side part of an organ or a passage in the body ○ *An ulcer formed in the wall of the duodenum.* ○ *The doctor made an incision in the abdominal wall.* ○ *They removed a fibroma from the wall of the uterus* or *from the uterine wall.*

**wall eye** /'wɔːl aɪ/, **walleye** *noun* an eye which is very pale or which is squinting so strongly that only the white sclera is visible

**Wangensteen tube** /'wæŋɡənstiːn tjuːb/ *noun* a tube which is passed into the stomach to remove the stomach's contents by suction [Described 1832. After Owen Harding Wangensteen (1898–1980), US surgeon.]

**ward** /wɔːd/ *noun* a room or set of rooms in a hospital, with beds for the patients ○ *He is in Ward 8B.* ○ *The children's ward is at the end of the corridor.*

**ward manager** /'wɔːd ˌmænɪdʒə/ *noun* a nurse in charge of a ward

**ward nurse** /'wɔːd nɜːs/ *noun* a nurse who works in a hospital ward

**ward sister** /'wɔːd ˌsɪstə/ *noun* a senior nurse in charge of a ward

**warfarin** /'wɔːf(ə)rɪn/ *noun* a colourless crystalline compound used to help prevent the blood clotting

**warm** /wɔːm/ *adjective* quite hot, pleasantly hot ○ *The patients need to be kept warm in cold weather.*

**warn** /wɔːn/ *verb* to tell someone that a danger is possible ○ *The children were warned about the dangers of solvent abuse.* ○ *The doctors warned her that her husband would not live more than a few weeks.*

**warning** /'wɔːnɪŋ/ *noun* written or spoken information about a danger ○ *There's a warning on the bottle of medicine, saying that it should be kept away from children.* ○ *Each packet of cigarettes has a government health warning printed on it.* ○ *The health department has given out warnings about the danger of hypothermia.*

**wart** /wɔːt/ *noun* a small hard harmless growth on the skin, usually on the hands, feet or face, caused by a virus (NOTE: Warts on the feet are called **verrucas**.)

**washbasin** /'wɒʃbeɪs(ə)n/ *noun* a bowl in a kitchen or bathroom where you can wash your hands

**washout** /'wɒʃaʊt/ *noun* a thorough cleaning with a liquid, especially water

**Wassermann reaction** /'wɒsəmæn rɪ ˌækʃ(ə)n/, **Wassermann test** /'wɒsəmæn test/ *noun* a blood serum test to see if someone has syphilis. Abbr **WR** [Described 1906. After August Paul von Wassermann (1866–1925), German bacteriologist.]

**waste** /weɪst/ *adjective* referring to material or matter which is useless ○ *The veins take blood containing waste carbon dioxide back into the lungs.* ○ *Waste matter is excreted in the faeces or urine.* ■ *verb* to use more of something than is needed ○ *The hospital kitchens try not to waste a lot of food.*

**waste away** /ˌweɪst ə'weɪ/ *verb* to become thinner ○ *When he caught the disease he simply wasted away.*

**waste product** /ˌweɪst 'prɒdʌkt/ *noun* a substance which is not needed in the body and is excreted in urine or faeces

**wasting** /'weɪstɪŋ/ *noun* a condition in which a person or a limb loses weight and becomes thin

**wasting disease** /'weɪstɪŋ dɪˌziːz/ *noun* a disease which causes severe loss of weight or reduction in size of an organ

**water** /'wɔːtə/ *noun* **1.** the liquid essential to life which makes up a large part of the body ○ *Can I have a glass of water please?* ○ *They suffered dehydration from lack of water.* □ **water on the knee** fluid in the knee joint under the kneecap, caused by a blow on the knee **2.** urine (*informal*) ○ *He passed a lot of water during the night.* ○ *She noticed blood streaks in her water.* ○ *The nurse asked him to give a sample of his water.* ■ *plural noun* **waters** the fluid in the amnion in which a fetus floats (*informal*) Also called **amniotic fluid** ■ *verb* (of the eyes) to fill with tears or saliva (NOTE: For other terms referring to water, see words beginning with **hydr-, hydro-**.)

COMMENT: Since the body is formed of about 50% water, the average adult needs to drink about 2.5 litres (5 pints) of fluid each day. Water taken into the body is passed out again as urine or sweat.

**water balance** /'wɔːtə ˌbæləns/ *noun* a state where the water lost by the body, e.g. in urine or sweat, is made up by water absorbed from food and drink

**water bed** /'wɔːtə bed/ *noun* a mattress made of a large heavy plastic bag filled with water, used to prevent bedsores

**waterbrash** /'wɔːtəbræʃ/ *noun* a condition caused by dyspepsia, in which there is a burning feeling in the stomach and the mouth suddenly fills with acid saliva

**water-hammer pulse** /'wɔːtə ˌhæmə pʌls/ *noun* same as **Corrigan's pulse**

**Waterhouse-Friderichsen syndrome** /ˌwɔːtəhaʊs 'friːdərɪksən ˌsɪndrəʊm/ *noun* a condition caused by blood poisoning with meningococci, in which the tissues of the adrenal glands die and haemorrhage [Described 1911 by Rupert Waterhouse (1873–1958), physician at Bath, UK; described 1918 by Carl Friderichsen (b. 1886), Danish physician]

**watering eye** /ˌwɔːtərɪŋ 'aɪ/ *noun* an eye which fills with tears because of an irritation

**waterproof** /'wɔːtəpruːf/ *adjective* not allowing water through ○ *Put a waterproof sheet on the baby's bed.*

**water sac** /'wɔːtə sæk/ *noun* ♦ **amnion**

**Waterston's operation** /'wɔːtəstənz ˌɒpəreɪʃ(ə)n/ *noun* a surgical operation to treat Fallot's tetralogy, in which the right pulmonary artery is joined to the ascending aorta [After David James Waterston (1910–85), paediatric surgeon in London, UK]

**waterworks** /'wɔːtəwɜːks/ *plural noun* same as **urinary system** (*informal*)

**watery** /'wɔːt(ə)ri/ *adjective* liquid, like water ○ *He passed some watery stools.*

**Watson-Crick helix** /ˌwɒts(ə)n 'krɪk ˌhiːlɪks/ *noun* a molecular model for DNA in which the organic base pairs are linked by hydrogen bonds which form the rungs of a ladder spiralling in the form of a helix

**Watson knife** /ˌwɒtsən 'naɪf/ *noun* a type of very sharp surgical knife for skin transplants

**wax** /wæks/ *noun* a soft yellow substance produced by bees or made from petroleum

**WBC** *abbr* white blood cell

**weak** /wiːk/ *adjective* not strong ○ *After his illness he was very weak.* ○ *She is too weak to dress herself.* ○ *He is allowed to drink weak tea or coffee.*

**weaken** /'wiːkən/ *verb* to make something or someone weak, or become weak ○ *He was weakened by the disease and could not resist further infection.* ○ *The swelling is caused by a weakening of the wall of the artery.*

**weakness** /'wiːknəs/ *noun* the fact of lacking strength ○ *The doctor noticed the weakness of the patient's pulse.*

**weak pulse** /ˌwiːk 'pʌls/ *noun* a pulse which is not strong, which is not easy to feel

**weal** /wiːl/ *noun* a small area of skin which swells because of a sharp blow or an insect bite

**wean** /wiːn/ *verb* to make a baby stop breast-feeding and take other liquid or solid food, or to make a baby start to eat solid food after having only had liquids to drink ○ *The baby was breastfed for two months and then was gradually weaned onto the bottle.*

**wear** /weə/ *verb* to become damaged through being used ○ *The cartilage of the knee was worn from too much exercise.* (NOTE: **wearing – wore – worn**)

**wear and tear** /ˌweər ən ˈteə/ *noun* the normal use which affects an organ ○ *A heart has to stand a lot of wear and tear.* ○ *The wear and tear of a strenuous job has begun to affect his heart.*

**wear off** /ˌweər ˈɒf/ *verb* to disappear gradually ○ *The effect of the painkiller will wear off after a few hours.* ○ *He started to open his eyes, as the anaesthetic wore off.*

**webbing** /ˈwebɪŋ/ *noun* the condition of having an extra membrane of skin joining two structures in the body together

**Weber-Christian disease** /ˌweɪbə ˈkrɪstʃən dɪˌziːz/ *noun* a type of panniculitis where the liver and spleen become enlarged [After Frederick Parkes Weber (1863–1962), British physician; Henry Asbury Christian (1876–1951), US physician]

**Weber's test** /ˈweɪbəz test/ *noun* a test to see if both ears hear correctly, where a tuning fork is struck and the end placed on the head [After Friedrich Eugen Weber-Liel (1832–91), German otologist]

**web space** /ˈweb speɪs/ *noun* the soft tissue between the bases of the fingers and toes

**Wechsler scales** /ˈvekslə skeɪlz/ *plural noun* a set of standardised scales for measuring someone's IQ. There are three separate versions developed for different age groups.

**wee** /wiː/ *verb* same as **urinate** (*informal*)

**weep** /wiːp/ *verb* 1. to cry 2. (*of a wound*) to ooze fluid

**Wegener's granulomatosis** /ˌvegənəz ˌɡrænjʊləʊməˈtəʊsɪs/ *noun* a disease of connective tissue, where the nasal passages, lungs and kidneys are inflamed and ulcerated, with formation of granulomas. It is usually fatal.

**weigh** /weɪ/ *verb* 1. to measure how heavy something is ○ *The nurse weighed the baby on the scales.* 2. to have a particular weight ○ *She weighed seven pounds (3.5 kilos) at birth.* ○ *A woman weighs less than a man of similar height.* ○ *The doctor asked him how much he weighed.* ○ *I weigh 120 pounds* or *I weigh 54 kilos.*

**weight** /weɪt/ *noun* 1. how heavy someone or something is ○ *What's the patient's weight?* □ **her weight is only 105 pounds** she weighs only 105 pounds □ **to lose weight** to get thinner ○ *She's trying to lose weight before she*

goes on holiday. □ **to put on weight** to become fatter ○ *He's put on a lot of weight in the last few months.* □ **to gain in weight** to become fatter or heavier 2. something which is heavy ○ *Don't lift heavy weights, you may hurt your back.*

**weight gain** /ˈweɪt ˌɡeɪn/ *noun* the fact of becoming fatter or heavier

**weight loss** /ˈweɪt ˌlɒs/ *noun* the fact of losing weight or of becoming thinner ○ *Weight loss can be a symptom of certain types of cancer.*

**Weil-Felix reaction** /ˌvaɪl ˈfeɪlɪks rɪˌækʃən/, **Weil-Felix test** /ˌvaɪl ˈfeɪlɪks test/ *noun* a test to see if someone has typhus, in which the person's serum is tested for antibodies against *Proteus vulgaris* [Described 1916. After Edmund Weil (1880–1922) Austrian physician and bacteriologist; Arthur Felix (1887–1956), British bacteriologist.]

**Weil's disease** /ˈvaɪlz dɪˌziːz/ *noun* same as **leptospirosis** [Described 1886. After Adolf Weil (1848–1916), physician in Estonia who also practised in Wiesbaden, Germany.]

**welder's flash** /ˌweldəz ˈflæʃ/ *noun* a condition in which the eye is badly damaged by very bright light

**welfare** /ˈwelfeə/ *noun* 1. good health, good living conditions ○ *They look after the welfare of the old people in the town.* 2. money paid by the government to people who need it ○ *He exists on welfare payments.*

**well** /wel/ *adjective* healthy ○ *He's not a well man.* ○ *You're looking very well after your holiday.* ○ *He's quite well again after his flu.* ○ *She's not very well, and has had to stay in bed.*

**well-baby clinic** /ˌwel ˈbeɪbi ˌklɪnɪk/ *noun* a clinic where parents can ask a doctor or nurse any questions they have about their child's growth and development. Their babies can be weighed and measured and their development monitored.

**wellbeing** /ˈwel ˌbiːɪŋ/ *noun* the state of being in good health and having good living conditions ○ *She is responsible for the wellbeing of the patients under her care.*

**well-man clinic** /ˌwel ˈmæn ˌklɪnɪk/ *noun* a clinic just for men where they can get checkups, advice and health information

**well-woman clinic** /ˌwel ˈwʊmən ˌklɪnɪk/ *noun* a clinic which specialises in preventive medicine for women, e.g. breast screening and cervical smear tests, and gives advice on pregnancy, contraception and the menopause

**wen** /wen/ *noun* a cyst which forms in a sebaceous gland

**Werdnig-Hoffmann disease** /ˌvɜːdnɪɡ ˈhɒfmən dɪˌziːz/ *noun* a disease in which the spinal muscles atrophy, making the muscles of the shoulders, arms and legs weak. In its most severe form, infants are born floppy, have feeding and breathing problems and rarely live more than two or three years.

**Werner's syndrome** /'wɜːnəz ˌsɪndrəʊm/ noun an inherited disorder involving premature ageing, persistent hardening of the skin, underdevelopment of the sex organs and cataracts

**Wernicke-Korsakoff syndrome** /ˌvɜːnɪkə 'kɔːsəkɒf ˌsɪndrəʊm/ noun a form of brain damage caused by severe nutritional deficiencies in people with long-term alcoholism

**Wernicke's encephalopathy** /ˌvɜːnɪkəz enˌkefə'lɒpəθi/ noun a condition caused by lack of Vitamin B, which often affects alcoholics and in which the person is delirious, moves the eyes about rapidly, walks unsteadily and is subject to constant vomiting [Described 1875. After Karl Wernicke (1848–1905), Breslau psychiatrist and neurologist.]

**Wertheim's operation** /'vɜːthaɪmz ɒpəˌreɪʃ(ə)n/ noun a surgical operation to remove the uterus, the lymph nodes which are next to it and most of the vagina, the ovaries and the Fallopian tubes, as treatment for cancer of the uterus [Described 1900. After Ernst Wertheim (1864–1920), Austrian gynaecologist.]

**West Nile fever** /ˌwest 'naɪl ˌfiːvə/ noun a mosquito-borne viral infection which causes fever, pains, enlarged lymph nodes and sometimes inflammation of the brain

**wet** /wet/ adjective not dry, covered in liquid ○ He got wet waiting for the bus in the rain and caught a cold. ○ The baby has nappy rash from wearing a wet nappy. ■ verb to make the bed wet by urinating while asleep ○ He is eight years old and he still wets his bed every night.

**wet beriberi** /ˌwet ˌberi'beri/ noun beriberi in which the body swells with oedema

**wet burn** /wet 'bɜːn/ noun same as **scald**

**wet dream** /wet driːm/ noun same as **nocturnal emission**

**wet dressing** /ˌwet 'dresɪŋ/ noun ♦ **compress**

**Wharton's duct** /ˌwɔːt(ə)nz 'dʌkt/ noun a duct which takes saliva into the mouth from the salivary glands under the lower jaw [After Thomas Wharton (1614–73), English physician and anatomist at St Thomas's Hospital, London, UK]

**Wharton's jelly** /ˌwɔːt(ə)nz 'dʒeli/ noun a jelly-like tissue in the umbilical cord

**wheal** /wiːl/ same as **weal**

**Wheelhouse's operation** /'wiːlhaʊsɪz ˌɒpəreɪʃ(ə)n/ noun same as **urethrotomy** [After Claudius Galen Wheelhouse (1826–1909), British surgeon]

**wheeze** /wiːz/ noun a whistling noise in the bronchi ○ The doctor listened to his wheezes. ■ verb to make a whistling sound when breathing ○ When she has an attack of asthma, she wheezes and has difficulty in breathing.

**wheezing** /'wiːzɪŋ/ noun whistling noises in the bronchi when breathing. Wheezing is often found in people with asthma and is also associated with bronchitis and heart disease.

**wheezy** /'wiːzi/ adjective making a whistling sound when breathing ○ She was quite wheezy when she stopped running.

**whiplash injury** /'wɪplæʃ ˌɪndʒəri/ noun an injury to the vertebrae in the neck, caused when the head jerks backwards, often occurring in a car that is struck from behind

**whiplash shake syndrome** /ˌwɪplæʃ 'ʃeɪk ˌsɪndrəʊm/ noun in young babies, a series of internal head injuries caused by being shaken violently. They can result in brain damage leading to speech and learning disabilities, paralysis, seizures, blindness and hearing loss. They are often life-threatening.

**Whipple's disease** /'wɪp(ə)lz dɪˌziːz/ noun a disease in which someone has difficulty in absorbing nutrients and passes fat in the faeces, the joints are inflamed and the lymph glands enlarged [Described 1907. After George Hoyt Whipple (1878–1976), US pathologist. Nobel prize for Pathology and Medicine 1934.]

**Whipple's operation** /'wɪp(ə)lz ɒpəˌreɪʃ(ə)n/ noun same as **pancreatectomy**

**whipworm** /'wɪpwɜːm/ noun same as **Trichuris**

**white** /waɪt/ adjective of a colour like snow or milk ○ White patches developed on his skin. ○ Her hair has turned quite white. (NOTE: **whiter – whitest**) ■ noun the main part of the eye which is white ○ The whites of his eyes turned yellow when he developed jaundice.

**white blood cell** /ˌwaɪt 'blʌd ˌsel/ noun a colourless blood cell which contains a nucleus but has no haemoglobin, is formed in bone marrow and creates antibodies. Abbr **WBC**. Also called **leucocyte**

**white commissure** /ˌwaɪt 'kɒmɪsjʊə/ noun part of the white matter in the spinal cord near the central canal

**white corpuscle** /ˌwaɪt 'kɔːpʌs(ə)l/ noun same as **white blood cell**

**white finger** /ˌwaɪt 'fɪŋɡə/ noun a condition in which a finger has a mottled discoloured appearance because its blood vessels are damaged. The thumb is usually not affected. Very severe cases can result in finger loss. It occurs most commonly in Raynaud's disease.

**whitehead** /'waɪthed/ noun a small white swelling formed when a sebaceous gland becomes blocked

**white leg** /ˌwaɪt 'leg/ noun a condition which affects women after childbirth, in which a leg becomes pale and inflamed as a result of lymphatic obstruction. Also called **milk leg**, **phlegmasia alba dolens**

**white matter** /'waɪt ˌmætə/ noun nerve tissue in the central nervous system which contains more myelin than grey matter

**white noise instrument** /ˌwaɪt ˈnɔɪz ˌɪn strʊmənt/ *noun* a small electronic device worn in the ear. It combines sounds of many different frequencies. It is used to mask internal noise in the ear due to tinnitus.

**whites** /waɪts/ *plural noun* same as **leucorrhoea** (*informal*)

**whitlow** /ˈwɪtləʊ/ *noun* an inflammation caused by infection near the nail in the fleshy part of the tip of a finger. Also called **felon**

**WHO** *abbr* World Health Organization

**whoop** /wuːp, huːp/ *noun* a loud noise made when inhaling by a person who has whooping cough

**whooping cough** /ˈhuːpɪŋ kɒf/ *noun* an infectious disease caused by *Bordetella pertussis* affecting the bronchial tubes, common in children, and sometimes very serious. Also called **pertussis**

COMMENT: A person with whooping cough coughs very badly and makes a characteristic 'whoop' when he or she breathes in after a coughing fit. Whooping cough can lead to pneumonia, and is treated with antibiotics. Vaccination against whooping cough is given to infants.

**Widal reaction** /viːˈdɑːl rɪˌækʃən/, **Widal test** /viːˈdɑːl test/ *noun* a test to detect typhoid fever. A sample of the person's blood is put into a solution containing typhoid bacilli, or anti-typhoid serum is added to a sample of bacilli from the person's faeces. If the bacilli agglutinate, i.e. form into groups, this indicates that the person has typhoid fever. [Described 1896. After Georges Fernand Isidore Widal (1862–1929), French physician and teacher.]

**Willis** /ˈwɪlɪs/ ♦ **circle of Willis**

**willpower** /ˈwɪlˌpaʊə/ *noun* the fact of having a strong will ○ *The patient showed the willpower to start walking again unaided.*

**Wilms' tumour** /ˈvɪlmz ˌtjuːmə/ *noun* same as **nephroblastoma** [Described 1899. After Max Wilms (1867–1918), Professor of Surgery at Leipzig, Basle and Heidelberg.]

**Wilson's disease** /ˈwɪlsənz dɪˌziːz/ *noun* a hereditary disease where copper deposits accumulate in the liver and the brain, causing cirrhosis. Also called **hepatolenticular degeneration** [Described 1912. After Samuel Alexander Kinnier Wilson (1878–1937), British neurologist.]

**wind** /wɪnd/ *noun* 1. gas which forms in the digestive system and escapes through the anus ○ *The baby is suffering from wind.* Also called **flatus** 2. an uncomfortable feeling caused by the accumulation of gas in the upper digestive system ○ *He has pains in the stomach caused by wind.* Also called **flatulence** □ **to break wind** to bring up gas from the stomach, or to let gas escape from the anus

**windburn** /ˈwɪndbɜːn/ *noun* redness and inflammation of the skin caused by exposure to harsh wind

**window** /ˈwɪndəʊ/ *noun* a small opening in the ear

**windpipe** /ˈwɪndpaɪp/ *noun* same as **trachea**

**wiring** /ˈwaɪərɪŋ/ *noun* 1. a network of wires 2. a neurological or physiological structure or process which controls a function in the body 3. the act of fixing a piece of bone in place using wires

**wisdom tooth** /ˈwɪzdəm tuːθ/ *noun* one of the four teeth in the back of the jaw which only appear at about the age of 20 and sometimes do not appear at all. Also called **third molar**

**witch hazel** /ˈwɪtʃ ˌheɪz(ə)l/ *noun* a lotion made from the bark of a tree, used to check bleeding and harden inflamed tissue and bruises. Also called **hamamelis**

**withdrawal** /wɪðˈdrɔːəl/ *noun* 1. a loss of interest in having contact with other people, which leads to a person becoming isolated 2. a period during which a person who has been addicted to a drug stops taking it and experiences unpleasant symptoms

'…she was in the early stages of physical withdrawal from heroin and showed classic symptoms: sweating, fever, sleeplessness and anxiety' [*Nursing Times*]

**withdrawal symptom** /wɪðˈdrɔːəl ˌsɪmptəm/ *noun* an unpleasant physical condition, e.g. vomiting, headaches or fever, which occurs when someone stops taking an addictive drug

**Wolff-Parkinson-White syndrome** /wʊlf ˌpɑːkɪns(ə)n ˈwaɪt ˌsɪndrəʊm/ *noun* a condition within the heart's conducting tissue which makes the heart beat dangerously fast. It can be fatal.

**womb** /wuːm/ *noun* same as **uterus** (NOTE: For other terms referring to the womb, see words beginning with **hyster-**, **hystero-**, **metr-**, **metro-**, **uter-**, **utero-**.)

**women's ward** /ˈwɪmɪnz wɔːd/, **women's hospital** /ˈwɪmɪnz ˌhɒspɪt(ə)l/ *noun* a ward or hospital for female patients. ◊ **well-woman clinic**

**Wood's lamp** /ˈwʊdz læmp/ *noun* an ultraviolet lamp which allows a doctor to see fluorescence , e.g. in the hair of someone who has a fungal infection [After Robert Williams Wood (1868–1955), US physicist]

**woolsorter's disease** /ˈwʊlsɔːtəz dɪˌziːz/ *noun* a form of anthrax which affects the lungs

**word blindness** /ˈwɜːd ˌblaɪndnəs/ *noun* same as **alexia**

**work-related upper limb disorder** /ˌwɜːk rɪˌleɪtɪd ˌʌpə ˈlɪm dɪsˌɔːdə/ same as **repetitive strain injury**. Abbr **WRULD**.

**World Health Organization** /ˌwɜːld ˈhelθ ɔːgənaɪˌzeɪʃ(ə)n/ *noun* an organisation, part of the United Nations, which aims to improve health in the world. Abbr **WHO**

**worm** /wɜːm/ *noun* a long thin animal with no legs or backbone, which can infest the human body, especially the intestines

**wound** /wuːnd/ *noun* damage to external tissue which allows blood to escape ○ *He had a knife wound in his leg.* ○ *The doctors sutured the wound in his chest.* □ **gunshot wound** wound caused by a pellet or bullet from a gun ■ *verb* to harm someone by making a hole in the tissue of the body ○ *She was wounded three times in the head.*

**wound dehiscence** /wuːnd dɪˈhɪs(ə)ns/ *noun* the splitting open of a surgical incision

**wound healing** /ˈwuːnd ˌhiːlɪŋ/ *noun* the replacement of dead tissue with new tissue

**WR** *abbr* Wassermann reaction

**wrench** /rentʃ/ *verb* to injure part of the body by twisting it suddenly and forcibly

**wrinkle** /ˈrɪŋkəl/ *noun* a fold in the skin

**wrinkled** /ˈrɪŋkəld/ *adjective* covered with wrinkles

**wrist** /rɪst/ *noun* a joint between the hand and forearm ○ *He sprained his wrist and can't play tennis tomorrow.* See illustration at **HAND** in Supplement (NOTE: For other terms referring to the wrist, see words beginning with **carp-, carpo-.**)

COMMENT: The wrist is formed of eight small bones in the hand which articulate with the bones in the forearm. The joint allows the hand to rotate and move downwards and sideways. The joint is easily fractured or sprained.

**wrist drop** /ˈrɪst drɒp/ *noun* paralysis of the wrist muscles, caused by damage to the radial nerve in the upper arm, which causes the hand to hang limp

**wrist joint** /ˈrɪst dʒɔɪnt/ *noun* a place where the wrist joins the arm

**writer's cramp** /ˌraɪtəz ˈkræmp/ *noun* a painful spasm of the muscles in the forearm and hand which comes from writing too much

**writhe** /raɪð/ *verb* □ **to writhe in pain** to twist and turn because the pain is very severe

**WRULD** *abbr* work-related upper limb disorder

**wry neck** /ˈraɪ nek/, **wryneck** *noun* same as **torticollis**

**Wuchereria** /ˌvʊkəˈrɪəriə/ *noun* a type of tiny nematode worm which infests the lymph system, causing elephantiasis

# X

**xanth-** /zænθ/ *prefix* same as **xantho-** (used before vowels)

**xanthaemia** /zæn'θi:miə/ *noun* same as **carotenaemia** (NOTE: The US spelling is **xanthemia**.)

**xanthelasma** /ˌzænθə'læzmə/ *noun* the formation of little yellow fatty tumours on the eyelids

**xanthine** /'zænθi:n/ *noun* **1.** an intermediate product in the breakdown of nucleic acids to uric acid, found in blood, body tissue and urine **2.** a derivative of xanthine, e.g. caffeine or theophylline

**xantho-** /zænθəʊ/ *prefix* yellow

**xanthochromia** /ˌzænθə'krəʊmiə/ *noun* yellow colour of the skin as in jaundice

**xanthoma** /zæn'θəʊmə/ *noun* a yellow fatty mass, often on the eyelids and hands, found in people with a high level of cholesterol in the blood (NOTE: The plural is **xanthomata**.)

**xanthomatosis** /ˌzænθəmə'təʊsɪs/ *noun* a condition in which several small masses of yellow fatty substance appear in the skin or some internal organs, caused by an excess of fat in the body

**xanthopsia** /zæn'θɒpsiə/ *noun* a disorder of the eyes, making everything appear yellow

**xanthosis** /zæn'θəʊsɪs/ *noun* yellow colouring of the skin, caused by eating too much food containing carotene

**X chromosome** /'eks ˌkrəʊməsəʊm/ *noun* a chromosome that determines sex. Compare **Y chromosome**. ◊ **sex chromosome**

**xeno-** /zenəʊ/ *prefix* different

**xenograft** /'zenəɡrɑːft/ *noun* tissue taken from an individual of one species and grafted on an individual of another species. Also called **heterograft**. Opposite **homograft**

**xenotransplantation** /ˌzenəʊtrænsplɑːn teɪʃ(ə)n/ *noun* the process of transplanting organs from one species to another, especially from animals to humans

**xero-** /zɪərəʊ/ *prefix* dry

**xeroderma** /ˌzɪərə'dɜːmə/ *noun* a skin disorder where dry scales form on the skin

**xerophthalmia** /ˌzɪərɒf'θælmiə/ *noun* a condition of the eye, in which the cornea and conjunctiva become dry because of a lack of Vitamin A

**xeroradiography** /ˌzɪərəʊˌreɪdi'ɒɡrəfi/ *noun* an X-ray technique used in producing mammograms on selenium plates

**xerosis** /zɪ'rəʊsɪs/ *noun* extreme dryness of skin or mucous membrane

**xerostomia** /ˌzɪərə'stəʊmiə/ *noun* dryness of the mouth, caused by lack of a saliva

**xiphi-** /zɪfɪ/ *prefix* relating to the xiphoid process

**xiphisternal plane** /ˌzɪfɪˌstɜːn(ə)l 'pleɪn/ *noun* an imaginary horizontal line across the middle of the chest at the point where the xiphoid process starts

**xiphisternum** /ˌzɪfɪ'stɜːnəm/ *noun* same as **xiphoid process**

**xiphoid process** /'zɪfɔɪd ˌprəʊses/, **xiphoid cartilage** /'zɪfɔɪd ˌkɑːtɪlɪdʒ/ *noun* the bottom part of the breastbone which is cartilage in young people but becomes bone by middle age. Also called **ensiform cartilage**, **xiphisternum**

**X-linked** /'eks ˌlɪŋkt/ *adjective* relating to the genes situated on the X chromosome

**X-linked disease** /'eks ˌlɪŋkt dɪˌziːz/ *noun* a genetic disorder caused by a mutation on the X chromosome which only appears in males, e.g. one form of haemophilia

**X-ray** /'eks reɪ/, **x-ray** *noun* **1.** a ray with a very short wavelength, which is invisible, but can go through soft tissue and register as a photograph on a film. X-rays are used in diagnosis in radiography, and in treating disease by radiotherapy. ○ *The X-ray examination showed the presence of a tumour in the colon.* **2.** a photograph taken using X-rays ○ *The dentist took some X-rays of the patient's teeth.* ○ *He pinned the X-rays to the light screen.* **3.** an examination in which X-ray photographs are taken ○ *All the staff had to have chest X-rays.* ■ *verb* to take an X-ray photograph of a patient ○ *There are six patients waiting to be X-rayed.*

COMMENT: Because X-rays go through soft tissue, it is sometimes necessary to make internal organs opaque so that they will show up on the film. In the case of stomach X-rays, people take a barium meal before being photographed (contrast radiography); in other cases, such as kidney X-rays, radioactive substances are injected into the bloodstream or into the organ itself. X-rays are used not only in radiography for diagnosis but as a treatment in radiotherapy as rapidly dividing cells such as cancer cells are most affected. Excessive exposure to X-rays, either as a person being treated, or as a radiographer, can cause radiation sickness.

**X-ray imaging** /'eks reɪ ˌɪmɪdʒɪŋ/ *noun* the process of showing X-ray pictures of the inside of part of the body on a screen

**X-ray photograph** /ˌeks reɪ 'fəʊtəgrɑːf/ *noun* a picture produced by exposing sensitive film to X-rays ○ *He was examining the X-ray photographs of the patient's chest.*

**X-ray screening** /'eks reɪ ˌskriːnɪŋ/ *noun* a method of gathering information about the body by taking images using X-rays. It is carried out by a radiographer or radiologist.

**Xylocaine** /'zaɪləkeɪn/ a trade name for a preparation of lignocaine

**xylometazoline hydrochloride** /ˌzaɪləʊ mə,tæzəliːn ˌhaɪdrə'klɔːraɪd/, **xylometazoline** /ˌzaɪləʊmə'tæzəliːn/ *noun* a drug which helps to narrow blood vessels, used in the treatment of colds and sinusitis

**xylose** /'zaɪləʊz/ *noun* pentose which has not been metabolised

**XYY syndrome** /ˌeks waɪ 'waɪ ˌsɪndrəʊm/ *noun* an extremely rare condition in males in which they have two Y chromosomes instead of one. They grow faster than normal, and their final height is approximately 7cm above average. Many experience severe acne during adolescence.

# Y

**yawn** /jɔːn/ *noun* a reflex action when tired or sleepy, in which the mouth is opened wide and after a deep intake of air, the breath exhaled slowly ○ *His yawns made everyone feel sleepy.* ■ *verb* to open the mouth wide and breathe in deeply and then breathe out slowly

**yawning** /'jɔːnɪŋ/ *noun* the act of opening the mouth without conscious control and slowly releasing a deep breath, usually a sign of tiredness or boredom

**yaws** /jɔːz/ *noun* a tropical disease caused by the spirochaete *Treponema pertenue*. Symptoms include fever with raspberry-like swellings on the skin, followed in later stages by bone malformation. Also called **framboesia, pian**. ◊ **treponematosis**

**Y chromosome** /'waɪ ˌkrəʊməsəʊm/ *noun* a chromosome that determines sex, it is carried by males and is shorter than an X chromosome. Compare **X chromosome**. ◊ **sex chromosome**

**yeast** /jiːst/ *noun* a fungus which is used in the fermentation of alcohol and in making bread. It is a good source of Vitamin B.

**yellow** /'jeləʊ/ *adjective* of a colour like that of the sun or of gold ○ *His skin turned yellow when he had hepatitis.* ○ *The whites of the eyes become yellow as a symptom of jaundice.* ■ *noun* a colour like that of the sun or of gold

**yellow atrophy** /ˌjeləʊ 'ætrəfi/ *noun* an old name for severe damage to the liver

**yellow elastic fibrocartilage** /ˌjeləʊ ɪˌlæstɪk ˌfaɪbrəʊ'kɑːtɪlɪdʒ/ *noun* flexible cartilage, e.g. in the ear and epiglottis

**yellow fever** /'jeləʊ ˌfiːvə/ *noun* an infectious disease, occurring especially in Africa and South America, caused by an arbovirus carried by the mosquito *Aedes aegypti*. It affects the liver and causes jaundice. There is no known cure and it can be fatal, but vaccination can prevent it.

**yellow fibre** /ˌjeləʊ 'faɪbə/ *noun* same as **elastic fibre**

**yellow marrow** *noun* ♦ **marrow**

**yellow spot** /'jeləʊ spɒt/ *noun* same as **macula lutea**

**Yersinia pestis** /jɜːˌsɪniə 'pestɪs/ *noun* a bacterium which causes plague

**yin and yang** /ˌjɪn ənd 'jæŋ/ *noun* the two opposite and complementary principles of Chinese philosophy which are thought to exist in varying proportions in all things. They are sometimes thought of as femininity and masculinity.

**yoga** /'jəʊgə/ *noun* **1.** a Hindu discipline which promotes spiritual unity with a Supreme Being through a system of postures and rituals **2.** any one of dozens of systems and methods derived from or based on Hindu yoga. Many include breathing exercises and postures which are thought to aid health.

**yolk sac** /'jəʊk sæk/ *noun* same as **vitelline sac**

**yuppie flu** /ˌjʌpi 'fluː/ *noun* ♦ **myalgic encephalomyelitis** (*informal*)

# Z

**Zadik's operation** /'zeɪdɪks ɒpəˌreɪʃ(ə)n/ *noun* a surgical operation to remove the whole of an ingrowing toenail

**Zantac** /'zæntæk/ a trade name for ranitidine

**zidovudine** /zɪ'dəʊvjʊdiːn/ *noun* azidothymidine or AZT, a drug used in the treatment of AIDS, which helps to slow the progress of the disease

**Zimmer frame** /'zɪmə freɪm/ a trademark for a metal frame used by people who have difficulty in walking ○ *She managed to walk some steps with a Zimmer frame.* ◊ **walking frame**

**zinc** /zɪŋk/ *noun* a white metallic trace element (NOTE: The chemical symbol is **Zn**.)

**zinc ointment** /zɪŋk 'ɔɪntmənt/ *noun* a soothing ointment made of zinc oxide and oil

**zinc oxide** /zɪŋk 'ɒksaɪd/ *noun* a compound of zinc and oxygen, which forms a soft white soothing powder used in creams and lotions (NOTE: Its chemical formula is $ZnO$.)

**Zollinger-Ellison syndrome** /ˌzɒlɪndʒər 'elɪs(ə)n ˌsɪndrəʊm/ *noun* a condition in which tumours are formed in the islet cells of the pancreas together with peptic ulcers [Described 1955. After Robert Milton Zollinger (b. 1903), Professor of Surgery at Ohio State University, USA; Edwin H. Ellison (1918–70), Associate Professor of Surgery at Ohio State University, USA.]

**zona** /'zəʊnə/ *noun* **1.** same as **herpes zoster** **2.** a zone or area

**zona pellucida** /ˌzəʊnə pɪ'luːsɪdə/ *noun* a membrane which forms around an ovum

**zone** /zəʊn/ *noun* an area of the body

**zonula** /'zɒnjʊlə/, **zonule** /'zɒnjuːl/ *noun* a small area of the body

**zonule of Zinn** /ˌzɒnjuːl əv 'zɪn/ *noun* a suspensory ligament of the lens of the eye

**zonulolysis** /ˌzɒnjuː'lɒləsɪs/ *noun* the removal of a zonule by dissolving it

**zoo-** /zəʊ/ *prefix* relating to animals

**zoonosis** /ˌzəʊɒ'nəʊsɪs/ *noun* a disease which a human can catch from an animal (NOTE: The plural is **zoonoses**.)

**zoster** /'zɒstə/ ♦ **herpes zoster**

**Z-plasty** /'zed ˌplæsti/ *noun* a technique used in plastic surgery. A deep Z-shaped incision is made to relieve tension in the area of a scar, or to change the direction of a scar.

**zygoma** /zaɪ'gəʊmə/ *noun* same as **zygomatic arch** (NOTE: The plural is **zygomata**.)

**zygomatic** /ˌzaɪgə'mætɪk/ *adjective* referring to the zygomatic arch

**zygomatic arch** /ˌzaɪgəmætɪk 'aːtʃ/ *noun* the ridge of bone across the temporal bone, running between the ear and the bottom of the eye socket. Also called **zygoma**

**zygomatic bone** /ˌzaɪgəmætɪk 'bəʊn/ *noun* a bone which forms the prominent part of the cheek and the lower part of the eye socket. Also called **cheekbone, malar bone**

**zygomatic process** /ˌzaɪgəmætɪk 'prəʊses/ *noun* one of the bony projections which form the zygomatic arch

**zygomycosis** /ˌzaɪgəmaɪ'kəʊsɪs/ *noun* a disease caused by a fungus which infests the blood vessels in the lungs

**zygote** /'zaɪgəʊt/ *noun* a fertilised ovum, the first stage of development of an embryo

**zym-** /zaɪm/ *prefix* (*used before vowels*) **1.** enzymes **2.** fermentation

**zymogen** /'zaɪmədʒen/ *noun* same as **proenzyme**

**zymosis** /zaɪ'məʊsɪs/ *noun* same as **fermentation**

**zymotic** /zaɪ'mɒtɪk/ *adjective* referring to zymosis

# SUPPLEMENT

# Anatomical Terms

The body is always described as if standing upright with the palms of the hands facing forward. There is only one central vertical plane, termed the *median* or *sagittal* plane, and this passes through the body from front to back. Planes parallel to this on either side are *parasagittal* or *paramedian* planes. Vertical planes at right angles to the median are called *coronal* planes. The term *horizontal* (or *transverse*) plane speaks for itself. Two specific horizontal planes are (a) the *transpyloric,* midway between the suprasternal notch and the symphysis pubis, and (b) the *transtubercular* or *intertubercular* plane, which passes through the tubercles of the iliac crests. Many other planes are named from the structures they pass through.

Views of the body from some different points are shown on the diagram; a view of the body from above is called the *superior aspect,* and that from below is the *inferior aspect.*

*Cephalic* means toward the head; *caudal* refers to positions (or in a direction) towards the tail. *Proximal* and *distal* refer to positions respectively closer to and further from the centre of the body in any direction, while *lateral* and *medial* relate more specifically to relative sideways positions, and also refer to movements. *Ventral* refers to the abdomen, front or anterior, while *dorsal* relates to the back of a part or organ. The hand has a *dorsal* and a *palmar* surface, and the foot a *dorsal* and a *plantar* surface.

Note that *flexion of the thigh* moves it forward while *flexion of the leg* moves it backwards; the movements of *extension* are similarly reversed. Movement and rotation of limbs can be *medial,* which is with the front moving towards the centre line, or *lateral,* which is in the opposite direction. Specific terms for limb movements are *adduction,* towards the centre line, and *abduction,* which is away from the centre line. Other specific terms are *supination* and *pronation* for the hand, and *inversion* and *eversion* for the foot.

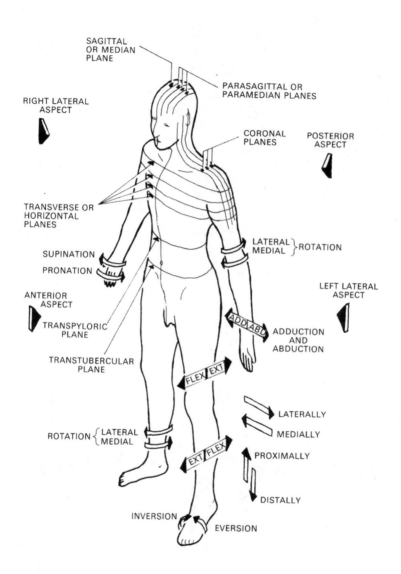

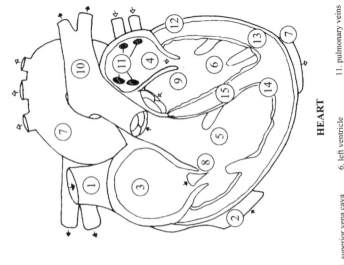

## LUNGS

1. thyroid cartilage
2. cricoid cartilage
3. trachea
4. main bronchus
5. superior lobe bronchus
6. middle lobe bronchus
7. inferior lobe bronchus
8. superior lobe
9. middle lobe
10. inferior lobe
11. oblique fissure
12. horizontal fissure
13. cardiac notch
14. visceral pleura
15. parietal pleura
16. pleural cavity
17. alveolus
18. alveolar duct
19. bronchiole

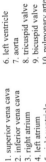

## HEART

1. superior vena cava
2. inferior vena cava
3. right atrium
4. left atrium
5. right ventricle
6. left ventricle
7. aorta
8. tricuspid valve
9. bicuspid valve
10. pulmonary artery
11. pulmonary veins
12. epicardium
13. myocardium
14. endocardium
15. septum

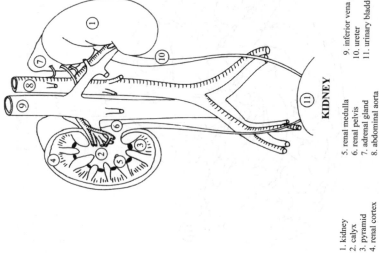

**DIGESTIVE SYSTEM**

1. liver
2. pancreas
3. spleen
4. gall bladder
5. stomach
6. duodenum

7. jejunum
8. ileum
9. ascending colon
10. transverse colon
11. descending colon

12. sigmoid colon
13. caecum
14. appendix
15. rectum
16. anus

**KIDNEY**

1. kidney
2. calyx
3. pyramid
4. renal cortex

5. renal medulla
6. renal pelvis
7. adrenal gland
8. abdominal aorta

9. inferior vena cava
10. ureter
11. urinary bladder

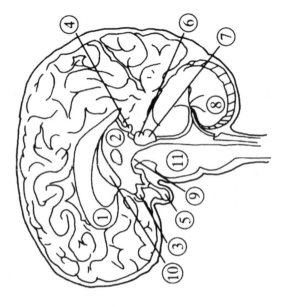

## NEURON

(a) multipolar     (b) bipolar     (c) unipolar

1. nucleus
2. Nissl granules
3. neurofibrilla
4. dendrite
5. axon
6. myelin sheath
7. Schwann cell nucleus
8. node of Ranvier
9. neurilemma
10. terminal branch

## BRAIN

1. corpus callosum
2. thalamus
3. hypothalamus
4. pineal body
5. pituitary gland
6. superior colliculi
7. inferior colliculi
8. cerebellum
9. cerebral peduncle
10. fornix cerebri
11. pons

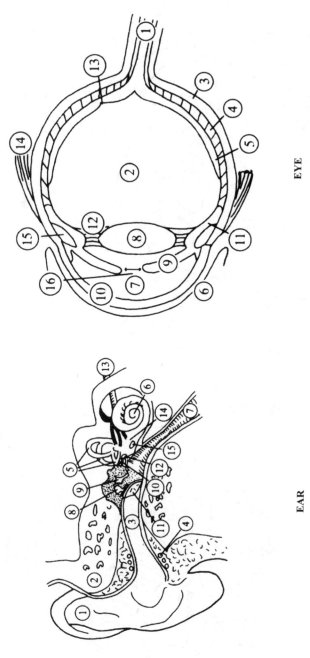

**EAR**

1. pinna
2. temporal bone
3. external auditory meatus
4. ceruminous glands
5. semicircular canals
6. cochlea
7. Eustachian tube
8. malleus
9. incus
10. stapes
11. tympanic membrane (eardrum)
12. round window
13. auditory nerve
14. vestibule
15. oval window

**EYE**

1. optic nerve
2. vitreous humour
3. sclera
4. choroid
5. retina
6. conjunctiva
7. aqueous humour
8. lens
9. iris
10. cornea
11. ciliary body
12. suspensory ligament
13. fovea
14. muscle
15. ciliary muscle
16. pupil

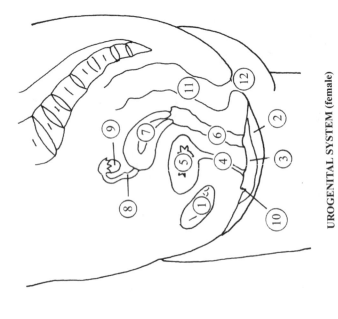

## UROGENITAL SYSTEM (male)

1. penis
2. scrotum
3. testis
4. epididymis
5. ductus deferens
6. seminal vesicle
7. ejaculatory duct
8. prostate gland
9. glans
10. urinary bladder
11. urethra
12. rectum
13. anus
14. corpus cavernosum
15. corpus songiosum
16. pubic bone

## UROGENITAL SYSTEM (female)

1. pubic bone
2. labia majora
3. labia minora
4. urethra
5. urinary bladder
6. vagina
7. uterus
8. Fallopian tube
9. ovary
10. clitoris
11. rectum
12. anus

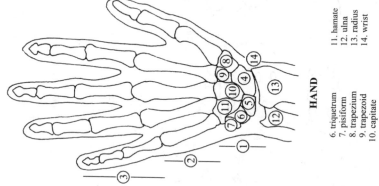

**FOOT**

1. tarsus
2. metatarsus
3. phalanges
4. cuneiforms
5. navicular
6. cuboid
7. calcaneus
8. talus

**HAND**

1. carpus
2. metacarpus
3. phalanges
4. scaphoid
5. lunate
6. triquetrum
7. pisiform
8. trapezium
9. trapezoid
10. capitate
11. hamate
12. ulna
13. radius
14. wrist

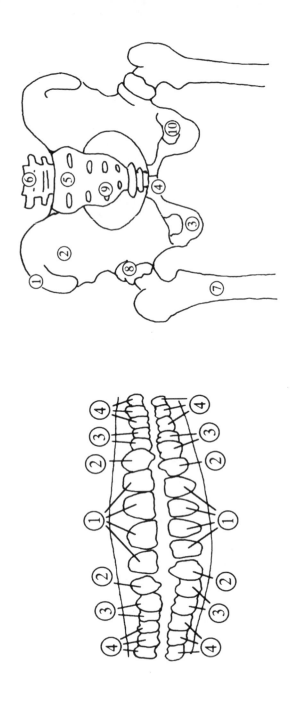

**PELVIS**

1. iliac crest
2. ilium
3. ischium
4. pubis
5. sacrum
6. vertebral column
7. femur
8. hip joint
9. sacral foramen
10. obturator foramen

**TEETH**

1. incisors
2. canines
3. premolars
4. molars

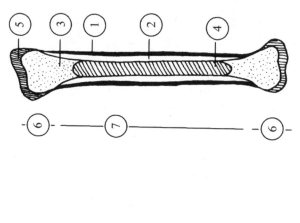

## BONE STRUCTURE

1. periosteum
2. compact bone
3. cancellous (spongy) bone (red marrow)
4. medullary cavity (yellow marrow)
5. articular cartilage
6. epiphysis
7. diaphysis

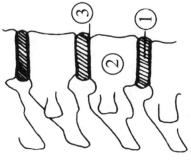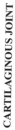

## CARTILAGINOUS JOINT

1. intervertebral disc
2. vertebra
3. hyaline cartilage

## SYNOVIAL JOINT

1. bone
2. articular cartilage
3. synovial membrane
4. synovial cavity and fluid
5. joint capsule (ligament)